OPERATIVE
OTOLARYNGOLOGY

HEAD AND NECK SURGERY

Volume 2

OPERATIVE OTOLARYNGOLOGY

HEAD AND NECK SURGERY

Second Edition

Editor

Eugene N. Myers, MD

Distinguished Professor and Emeritus Chair
Department of Otolaryngology
University of Pittsburgh School of Medicine
Professor
Department of Oral and Maxillofacial Surgery
University of Pittsburgh School of Dental Medicine
Pittsburgh, Pennsylvania

Associate Editors

Ricardo L. Carrau, MD
David E. Eibling, MD
Berrylin J. Ferguson, MD
Robert L. Ferris, MD, PhD
Grant S. Gillman, MD
Suman Golla, MD
Jennifer R. Grandis, MD
Barry E. Hirsch, MD
Jonas T. Johnson, MD
Yael Raz, MD
Clark A. Rosen, MD
Barry M. Schaitkin, MD
Carl H. Snyderman, MD
Elizabeth H. Toh, MD

Department of Otolaryngology
University of Pittsburgh School of Medicine
Pittsburgh, Pennsylvania

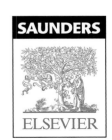

SAUNDERS

ELSEVIER

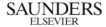

SAUNDERS
ELSEVIER

1600 John F. Kennedy Blvd.
Suite 1800
Philadelphia, PA 19103-2899

OPERATIVE OTOLARYNGOLOGY: HEAD AND NECK SURGERY   ISBN: 978-1-4160-2445-3
Second Edition

Library of Congress Cataloging-in-Publication Data
Operative otolaryngology : head and neck surgery / editor, Eugene N. Myers ; associate editors, Ricardo L. Carrau . . . [et al.].—2nd ed.
     p. ; cm.
  Includes bibliographical references and index.
  ISBN 978-1-4160-2445-3 (alk. paper)
  1. Otolaryngology, Operative.   I. Myers, Eugene N., 1933-   II. Carrau, Ricardo L.
  [DNLM: 1. Otorhinolaryngologic Surgical Procedures.   2. Otorhinolaryngologic Diseases—surgery. WV 168 O612 2008]
RF51.O6145 2008
617.5′1059—dc22   2007040207

Inset cover image courtesy of Dr. Francis Marchal.

ISBN: 978-1-4160-2445-3

Acquisitions Editor: Scott Scheidt
Developmental Editor: Rachel Yard
Publishing Services Manager: Frank Polizzano
Senior Project Manager: Robin E. Hayward
Cover Designer: Ellen Zanolle
Design Direction: Ellen Zanolle

Printed in China.

Last digit is the print number: 9   8   7   6   5   4   3

The Second Edition of *Operative Otolaryngology: Head and Neck Surgery* is dedicated to the faculty of the Department of Otolaryngology at the University of Pittsburgh School of Medicine and our wonderful colleagues in the Departments of Dermatology, Neurological Surgery, Ophthalmology, Oral and Maxillofacial Surgery, and Plastic Surgery. This book is also dedicated to our patients, who have taught us well over the years.

CONTRIBUTORS

Stephanie Moody Antonio, MD
Assistant Professor, Department of Otolaryngology, Eastern Virginia Medical School, Norfolk, Virginia
Chapter 123

Jeffrey Balzer, PhD
Associate Professor, Department of Neurological Surgery, University of Pittsburgh School of Medicine; University of Pittsburgh Medical Center, Pittsburgh, Pennsylvania
Chapter 130

Thomas W. Braun, DMD, PhD
Professor and Dean, Department of Oral and Maxillofacial Surgery, University of Pittsburgh School of Dental Medicine; Chair, Department of Dental Medicine, UPMC Presbyterian-Shadyside, Pittsburgh, Pennsylvania
Chapter 21

John F. Caccamese, Jr., DMD, MD, FACS
Assistant Professor and Residency Program Director, Department of Oral and Maxillofacial Surgery, University of Maryland Medical Center, R. Adams Cowley Shock Trauma Center, Baltimore, Maryland
Chapter 91

Ricardo L. Carrau, MD, FACS
Professor, Department of Otolaryngology, University of Pittsburgh School of Medicine; University of Pittsburgh Medical Center, Pittsburgh, Pennsylvania
Chapters 2, 6, 15, 18, 20, 30, 42, 45, 52, 53, 54, 70, 96, 100, 101, 103, 104, 105, 106

C. Y. Joseph Chang, MD
Clinical Professor, Department of Otolaryngology–Head and Neck Surgery, University of Texas-Houston Medical School; University of Texas-Houston Medical Center, Houston, Texas
Chapter 123

Bernard J. Costello, DMD, MD, FACS
Assistant Professor and Program Director, Department of Oral and Maxillofacial Surgery, University of Pittsburgh School of Dental Medicine; Chief, Pediatric Oral and Maxillofacial Surgery, Children's Hospital of Pittsburgh, Pittsburgh, Pennsylvania
Chapters 83, 91

Frederic W.-B. Deleyiannis, MD, MPhil, MPH
Associate Professor of Plastic and Reconstructive Surgery, Departments of Surgery and Otolaryngology, University of Pittsburgh School of Medicine, Pittsburgh, Pennsylvania
Chapters 81, 87

David E. Eibling, MD, FACS
Professor, Department of Otolaryngology, University of Pittsburgh School of Medicine, Pittsburgh, Pennsylvania
Chapters 8, 33, 35, 48, 49, 50, 57, 67, 78

Johnathan A. Engh, MD
Assistant Professor, Department of Neurological Surgery, University of Pittsburgh School of Medicine, Pittsburgh, Pennsylvania
Chapter 130

Berrylin J. Ferguson, MD, FACS
Associate Professor, Department of Otolaryngology, University of Pittsburgh School of Medicine; Director, Division of Sino-Nasal Disorders and Allergy, University of Pittsburgh Medical Center, Pittsburgh, Pennsylvania
Chapters 1, 3, 12, 19

Robert L. Ferris, MD, PhD, FACS
Associate Professor, Vice Chair for Clinical Operations, and Chief, Division of Head and Neck Surgery, Departments of Otolaryngology and Immunology; Co-Leader, Cancer Immunology Program, University of Pittsburgh Cancer Institute, Pittsburgh, Pennsylvania
Chapters 24, 28, 46, 66, 73

Peter F. Ferson, MD
Professor, Department of Surgery, Heart, Lung, and Esophageal Surgery Institute, University of Pittsburgh School of Medicine; Chief, Thoracic Surgery, Pittsburgh Health Care System
Chapter 67

Andrew S. Florea, MD
Assistant Professor, Department of Otolaryngology–Head and Neck Surgery, Loma Linda University School of Medicine; Chief, Division of Laryngology, Loma Linda University Medical Center, Loma Linda, California
Chapters 39, 40

Rebecca E. Fraioli, MD

Resident, Department of Otolaryngology, University of Pittsburgh Medical Center, Pittsburgh, Pennsylvania
Chapters 58, 61

Paul A. Gardner, MD

Assistant Professor, Department of Neurosurgery, University of Pittsburgh School of Medicine; University of Pittsburgh Medical Center, Pittsburgh, Pennsylvania
Chapter 106

Brian R. Gastman, MD

Assistant Professor, Department of Otolaryngology and Surgery, Divisions of Otolaryngology and Plastic Surgery, University of Maryland School of Medicine, Baltimore, Maryland
Chapter 81

Grant S. Gillman, MD, FRCS(C)

Assistant Professor, Department of Otolaryngology, University of Pittsburgh School of Medicine; Director, Division of Facial Plastic Surgery, UPMC Shadyside, Pittsburgh, Pennsylvania
Chapters 24, 84, 86, 89, 90

Suman Golla, MD, FACS

Associate Professor, Department of Otolaryngology, University of Pittsburgh School of Medicine, Pittsburgh, Pennsylvania
Chapters 5, 23

Jennifer R. Grandis, MD, FACS

Professor, Department of Otolaryngology and Pharmacology, University of Pittsburgh School of Medicine; Vice Chair for Research, UPMC Endowed Chair in Head and Neck Cancer Surgical Research, Program Leader, Head and Neck Cancer Program, University of Pittsburgh Cancer Institute, Pittsburgh, Pennsylvania
Chapters 58, 61

Anil Gungor, MD

Director, Department of Otolaryngology–Head and Neck Surgery, Anadolu Foundation Healthcare/Johns Hopkins, Istanbul, Turkey
Chapter 83

Alyssa Hackett, MD

Visiting Research Instructor, Department of Otolaryngology, University of Pittsburgh School of Medicine; University of Pittsburgh Medical Center, Pittsburgh, Pennsylvania
Chapter 107

Trevor Hackman, MD

Resident, Department of Otolaryngology, University of Pittsburgh Medical Center, Pittsburgh, Pennsylvania
Chapter 102

Bridget Hathaway, MD

Assistant Professor, Department of Otolaryngology, University of Pittsburgh School of Medicine, Pittsburgh, Pennsylvania
Chapter 54

Barry E. Hirsch, MD, FACS

Professor, Departments of Otolaryngology, Neurological Surgery, and Communication Science and Disorders, University of Pittsburgh School of Medicine; Director, Division of Otology/Neurotology, University of Pittsburgh Medical Center, Pittsburgh, Pennsylvania
Chapters 108, 109, 111, 112, 113, 114, 117, 119, 121, 123, 124, 125, 126

Michael Horowitz, MD

Professor, Department of Neurological Surgery and Radiology, University of Pittsburgh School of Medicine; Chief, Department of Neurosurgery, UPMC Presbyterian, Pittsburgh, Pennsylvania
Chapter 130

Jonas T. Johnson, MD

Professor and Eugene N. Myers, MD Chair, Department of Otolaryngology, University of Pittsburgh School of Medicine, Pittsburgh, Pennsylvania
Chapters 9, 11, 13, 21, 26, 34, 44, 47, 55, 62, 63, 76, 77

Amin B. Kassam, MD

Professor and Chair, Department of Neurological Surgery, University of Pittsburgh School of Medicine; Director, Minimally Invasive endoNeurosurgery Center, University of Pittsburgh Medical Center, Pittsburgh, Pennsylvania
Chapters 6, 18, 79, 96, 100, 101, 103, 104, 105, 106, 124, 130

Karen M. Kost, MD, FRCSC

Associate Professor, Department of Otolaryngology, and Director of the Voice Laboratory, McGill University; Site Director, Department of Otolaryngology, Montreal General Hospital, Montreal, Quebec, Canada
Chapter 68

Priya Krishna, MD
Assistant Professor, Department of Otolaryngology, University of Pittsburgh School of Medicine; Laryngologist, University of Pittsburgh Voice Center, University of Pittsburgh Medical Center, Pittsburgh, Pennsylvania
Chapter 36

Stephen Y. Lai, MD, PhD, FACS
Assistant Professor, Department of Otolaryngology and Pharmacology, University of Pittsburgh School of Medicine, Pittsburgh, Pennsylvania
Chapter 55

John Y. K. Lee, MD
Assistant Professor, Department of Neurological Surgery, University of Pennsylvania School of Medicine; Pennsylvania Hospital, Philadelphia, Pennsylvania
Chapter 130

Li-Xing Man, MD
Resident, Department of Otolaryngology, University of Pittsburgh School of Medicine, Pittsburgh, Pennsylvania
Chapter 1

Ernest K. Manders, MD
Professor, Department of Surgery, Division of Plastic and Reconstructive Surgery, University of Pittsburgh School of Medicine, Pittsburgh, Pennsylvania
Chapter 82

Arpita I. Mehta, MD
Resident, Department of Otolaryngology, University of Pittsburgh Medical Center, Pittsburgh, Pennsylvania
Chapter 116

Eugene N. Myers, MD, FACS, FRCS Edin (Hon)
Distinguished Professor and Emeritus Chair, Department of Otolaryngology, University of Pittsburgh School of Medicine; University of Pittsburgh Medical Center, Pittsburgh, Pennsylvania
Chapters 4, 8, 10, 22, 25, 27, 29, 31, 32, 35, 43, 51, 56, 60, 64, 65, 68, 69, 71, 72, 74, 75, 76

Jayakar V. Nayak, MD, PhD
Chief Resident, Department of Otolaryngology, University of Pittsburgh Medical Center, Pittsburgh, Pennsylvania
Chapter 87

Mark W. Ochs, DMD, MD
Professor and Chair, Department of Oral and Maxillofacial Surgery, University of Pittsburgh School of Dental Medicine; Head, Hospital Dentistry, University of Pittsburgh Medical Center, Pittsburgh, Pennsylvania
Chapters 92, 93

Yael Raz, MD
Assistant Professor, Department of Otolaryngology, University of Pittsburgh School of Medicine; University of Pittsburgh Medical Center, Pittsburgh, Pennsylvania
Chapters 107, 110, 115, 116, 118, 120

Clark A. Rosen, MD, FACS
Associate Professor, Department of Otolaryngology, University of Pittsburgh School of Medicine; Director, University of Pittsburgh Voice Center, University of Pittsburgh Medical Center, Pittsburgh, Pennsylvania
Chapters 36, 37, 38, 39, 40, 41, 59

Ramon Ruiz, DMD, MD
Clinical Assistant Professor, Department of Oral and Maxillofacial Surgery, University of North Carolina at Chapel Hill, Chapel Hill, North Carolina; Director, Pediatric Craniomaxillofacial Surgery, Arnold Palmer Hospital for Children and Winnie Palmer Hospital for Women and Babies, Orlando, Florida
Chapter 83

James M. Russavage, MD, DMD
Assistant Professor, Department of Surgery, Division of Plastic and Reconstructive Surgery, University of Pittsburgh School of Medicine, Pittsburgh, Pennsylvania
Chapter 81

Barry M. Schaitkin, MD, FACS
Professor, Department of Otolaryngology, University of Pittsburgh School of Medicine; UPMC Shadyside, Pittsburgh, Pennsylvania
Chapters 7, 14, 15, 16, 17, 88, 99

Jacob Sedgh, MD
Resident, Department of Otolaryngology, University of Pittsburgh Medical Center, Pittsburgh, Pennsylvania
Chapter 1

Libby J. Smith, DO
Assistant Professor, Department of Otolaryngology, University of Pittsburgh School of Medicine; Laryngologist, University of Pittsburgh Voice Center, University of Pittsburgh Medical Center, Pittsburgh, Pennsylvania
Chapters 37, 38

Carl H. Snyderman, MD, FACS
Professor, Department of Otolaryngology, University of Pittsburgh School of Medicine; Co-Director, Center for Cranial Base Surgery, University of Pittsburgh Medical Center, Pittsburgh, Pennsylvania
Chapters 2, 6, 18, 20, 79, 95, 96, 98, 100, 101, 103, 104, 105, 106

John C. Sok, MD, PhD
Resident, Department of Otolaryngology, University of Pittsburgh Medical Center, Pittsburgh, Pennsylvania
Chapter 59

Ryan J. Soose, MD
Assistant Professor, Department of Otolaryngology, University of Pittsburgh School of Medicine; University of Pittsburgh Medical Center, Pittsburgh, Pennsylvania
Chapters 30, 42, 45, 52, 53, 70

S. Tonya Stefko, MD
Assistant Professor, Departments of Ophthalmology, Otolaryngology, and Neurosurgery, University of Pittsburgh School of Medicine; Director, Orbital, Oculoplastics and Aesthetic Surgery, University of Pittsburgh Medical Center, Pittsburgh, Pennsylvania
Chapters 94, 95, 97, 98

Michele St. Martin, MD, MBA
Assistant Professor, Department of Otolaryngology, University of Florida College of Medicine, Gainesville, Florida
Chapters 115, 121, 124

Elizabeth H. Toh, MD, FACS
Assistant Professor, Department of Otolaryngology, University of Pittsburgh School of Medicine; Attending/Faculty, University of Pittsburgh Medical Center, Pittsburgh, Pennsylvania
Chapters 102, 111, 122, 127, 128, 129, 131

Alec Vaezi, MD, PhD
Resident, Department of Otolaryngology, University of Pittsburgh Medical Center, Pittsburgh, Pennsylvania
Chapter 126

Allan D. Vescan, MD, FRCS(C)
Lecturer in the Department of Otolaryngology–Head and Neck Surgery, University of Toronto Faculty of Medicine; Staff Surgeon, Otolaryngology–Head and Neck Surgery, Mount Sinai Hospital/University Health Network, Toronto, Ontario, Canada
Chapters 96, 100, 101, 104, 105

William A. Wood, MD
Resident, Department of Otolaryngology, University of Pittsburgh Medical Center, Pittsburgh, Pennsylvania
Chapters 120, 131

Robert F. Yellon, MD
Associate Professor, Department of Otolaryngology, University of Pittsburgh School of Medicine; Director of Clinical Services and Co-Director, Department of Pediatric Otolaryngology, Children's Hospital of Pittsburgh, Pittsburgh, Pennsylvania
Chapter 85

Yu-Lan Mary Ying, MD
Resident, Department of Otolaryngology, University of Pittsburgh Medical Center, Pittsburgh, Pennsylvania
Chapters 122, 129

John A. Zitelli, MD
Clinical Associate Professor, Departments of Dermatology and Otolaryngology, University of Pittsburgh School of Medicine, Pittsburgh, Pennsylvania
Chapter 80

PREFACE

We are very pleased and proud to present the Second Edition of *Operative Otolaryngology: Head and Neck Surgery*. This book was written by members of our Department of Otolaryngology together with our colleagues in the Departments of Dermatology, Neurological Surgery, Ophthalmology, Oral and Maxillofacial Surgery, and Plastic Surgery, all from the University of Pittsburgh Medical Center. We have a long record of excellent relationships with our colleagues and without them we would not have been able to become leaders in subspecialty areas requiring intense multidisciplinary collaboration such as head and neck surgery, surgery of the cranial base, and neuro-otology.

In reviewing the table of contents from the First Edition, I was astonished to see how many of the procedures we described are now either completely obsolete or rarely used. The specialty of otolaryngology has evolved dramatically over the decade since the publication of the First Edition. We are now in an era in which very exciting new developments in technology have set the stage not only for new and improved surgical techniques but also for maintaining an excellent quality of life for our patients.

The Second Edition has 131 chapters compared with 125 in the First Edition. However, many of the original chapters were eliminated or consolidated under other headings so that we have been able to add 30 new chapters while only having to add an overall total of 6 chapters. Forty-six new authors have played a major role in producing this book. These new authors are all on the faculty of the University of Pittsburgh School of Medicine and bring great vigor and talent to those chapters that reflect their special areas of interest. Exciting new work in the field of otology includes the new techniques for BAHA surgery and updates the fast-moving field of cochlear implantation. Functional endoscopic sinus surgery was too new to be included in the previous edition. Here, these techniques are described in detail, as is the management of many of the vexing complications encountered with this type of surgery. The improvement in the quality of life of these patients is remarkable.

Great emphasis has been placed on the endonasal endoscopic management of tumors at the base of the skull and the unique complications encountered. In our institution, we have pioneered the two-team approach, which includes an otolaryngologist/head and neck surgeon and a neurosurgeon working simultaneously to allow two-hand dissection. Almost all tumors, both benign and malignant, in this anatomical area can be removed endoscopically. Transnasal endoscopic surgery also allows for decompression of the optic nerve in patients with Graves' disease, traumatic injury, or orbital/skull base tumors. This technique can be done quickly with no side effects and the immediate return of vision is quite dramatic. Transnasal dacryocystorhinostomy is a helpful technique in the management of tearing. Cerebrospinal fluid leaks of all sizes are now managed successfully endoscopically.

The endoscope now plays an increasingly important role in removal of tumors of the thyroid and parathyroid glands. These techniques, in select patients, provide a bloodless surgical field with the possibilities for great exposure and complete removal of small- to medium-size tumors. The scarring is minimal and this technique has been well received.

The innovative use of the endoscope coupled with the CO_2 laser allows for the excision of both benign and malignant tumors of the larynx. This technique was not included in the previous edition but is well described herein. The selective neck dissection, which wasn't widely used at the time of the First Edition, is also described here.

In the last ten years, we have developed one of the leading centers for the care of the voice. The University of Pittsburgh Voice Center has three fellowship-trained laryngologists in conjunction with a cadre of well-trained speech-language pathologists who provide care for the professional voice. They have contributed the entire section on laryngology, which is all new to this edition. Since many patients require Botox injection for various spasmodic conditions in the larynx, our laryngologists have also become quite expert in the technique of injection of Botox in the management of Frey's syndrome, another addition to the book.

The operative techniques described in this book are augmented with detailed information regarding preoperative evaluation and postoperative care since the philosophy of our department is that preoperative evaluation and postoperative care play important roles in the outcome of the procedure.

We've dedicated this book to our department, our colleagues, and our patients, who are the beneficiaries of these advances in surgery in our field. We hope our readers will benefit from the innovative advances that have taken place in this field and are described in this book.

Eugene N. Myers, MD

ACKNOWLEDGMENTS

We gratefully acknowledge the enormous contributions of our editorial coordinator, Mary Jo Tutchko. Mary Jo was also the editorial coordinator for the First Edition and brings the same wisdom, maturity, incredible work ethic, and stamina to the Second Edition. Without her single-handed efforts, producing this book would not have been possible.

We also acknowledge the efficient and good natured help from Rebecca S. Gaertner, Helen Sofio, and Maria Lorusso from Elsevier, for all their help in making this Second Edition possible.

CONTENTS

VIDEOS

resected with a back-biting rongeur. The sphenoidotomy is enlarged.

Video 103-7. Sphenoid septations are carefully removed with a drill or rongeurs while avoiding injury to the internal carotid artery.

Video 103-8. The bone of the sella is thinned with a drill and then removed with a 1-mm Kerrison rongeur while being careful to direct the tip tangential to the carotid artery.

Video 103-9. A left middle meatal antrostomy is performed and the sphenopalatine artery is identified at the foramen at the posterosuperior corner of the sinus.

Video 103-10. The bone of the sphenopalatine foramen and pterygopalatine space is removed with a 1-mm Kerrison rongeur and the sphenopalatine artery is ligated.

Video 103-11. Bone surrounding the vidian artery and nerve (pterygoid canal) is carefully drilled to determine the plane of the petrous carotid artery.

Chapter 106

Video 106-1. Overview of the surgical field after sphenoidotomy and resection of the posterior nasal septum. The surgical field extends from the floor of the sphenoid sinus superiorly to the level of the soft palate inferiorly and to the eustachian tubes laterally.

Video 106-2. The mucosa, underlying paraspinal muscles, and dense pharyngobasilar fascia of the nasopharynx are resected to expose the underlying bone of the clivus and C1.

Video 106-3. The outer cortical bone of the clivus is removed from the floor of the sphenoid sinus to the foramen magnum with a 3-mm hybrid bit. This facilitates resection of the dense pharyngobasilar fascia.

Video 106-4. The central ring of C1 is removed with the drill and the defect is widened laterally with a Kerrison rongeur. Note the excessive mobility of C1 in this patient with rheumatoid degeneration.

Video 106-5. The odontoid is hollowed out with a drill until a thin shell of cortical bone remains.

Video 106-6. The base of the dens is detached from the body of C2 and the shell of remaining bone is dissected free from the surrounding ligamentous attachments.

Video 106-7. The rheumatoid pannus is thinned with an ultrasonic aspirator until transmitted pulsations are evident.

Video 106-8. In the absence of a cerebrospinal fluid leak, the surgical defect is covered with fibrin glue.

Chapter 113

Video 113-1. Canal injection.

Video 113-2. Twelve- and 6-o'clock incisions.

Video 113-3. Back elevation of the posterior canal conchal flap.

Video 113-4. Postauricular elevation of the posterior canal flap.

Video 113-5. Connection of the canal incisions and retraction with a tracheostomy tape.

Video 113-6. Anterior canal wall incision.

Video 113-7. Dissection of the medial canal skin.

Video 113-8. Canal skin elevated medially at the annulus.

Video 113-9. Removal of the superior and anterior canal/tympanic membrane epithelium.

Video 113-10. Retrograde elevation of the anterior canal wall skin.

Video 113-11. Anterior canalplasty.

Video 113-12. Access to the anterior annulus.

Video 113-13. Curettage of the annulus sulcus.

Video 113-14. Inspection of the middle ear and ossicular chain.

Video 113-15. Removal of the incus.

Video 113-16. Preparation of the fascial graft.

Video 113-17. Placement of the fascial graft medial to and around the malleus handle.

Video 113-18. Preparation of the canal wall skin.

Video 113-19. Trimming of the canal wall skin.

Video 113-20. Replacement of the canal wall skin.

Video 113-21. Placement of the medial rosebud packing.

Video 113-22. Placement of Merocel balls in the packing.

Video 113-23. Placement of Merocel balls in the lateral rosebud packing.

Chapter 114

Video 114-1. Left ear. Reinforced Silastic sheeting is placed under the handle of the malleus.

Video 114-2. Left ear. Reinforced Silastic sheeting has been placed in the middle ear. A fascial graft is positioned lateral to the Silastic sheeting and rests on the bony annulus.

Video 114-3. Left ear. The incus is removed from the attic along with a focus of tympanosclerosis.

Video 114-4. The incus is held with toothed forceps. A battery-powered drill is used to sculpt the incus for placement between the stapes and malleus.

Video 114-5. Right ear. An Applebaum prosthesis is positioned between the stapes and the eroded long process of the incus.

Video 114-6. Partial ossicular replacement prosthesis with a trimmable shaft. It is cut on a measuring block and then placed on the stapes.

Video 114-7. Type IV tympanoplasty. The incus is sculpted with a drill for placement of the long process on the footplate and creation of a notch underneath the malleus.

Video 114-8. A 5-mm titanium sizing total ossicular replacement prosthesis is placed between the stapes footplate and tympanic membrane. A thin piece of cartilage will be necessary.

Video 114-9. The prosthesis is positioned on the stapes footplate and supported with pledgets of wet Gelfoam.

Video 114-10. The lateral chain is palpated and found to be fixed. The incudostapedial joint is separated.

Video 114-11. Fracture of the malleus handle at the proximal handle is demonstrated.

Chapter 115

Video 115-1. Removal of squamous epithelium from the scutum.

Chapter 117

Video 117-1. Stapes down-fracture. The stapes superstructure is down-fractured with a curved pick and removed.

Video 117-2. Right ear. The vein graft is positioned over the stapedotomy.

Video 117-3. Right ear. A Robinson prosthesis is placed next to and rested against the incus.

Video 117-4. Right ear. The well of the Robinson prosthesis is easily positioned under the lenticular process of the incus.

Video 117-5. Right ear. A few attempts may be needed to properly position the well of the prosthesis.

Video 117-6. A small piece of vein is placed over the incus to further secure the bucket handle into position. This is termed a "band-aid."

Video 117-7. Right ear. The stapedial tendon and posteriori crus are vaporized with a CO_2 laser. The footplate is fenestrated.

Video 117-8. Right ear. The footplate is being vaporized in a rosette pattern with a CO_2 laser.

Video 117-9. Right ear. The edges of the stapedotomy are thinned with the laser and the opening enlarged with a footplate pick.

Video 117-10. A wire-Teflon prosthesis is positioned in the fenestration and hooked onto the incus.

Video 117-11. A hand-held laser is used to heat the Nitinol prosthesis to tighten it on the incus.

Video 117-12. Right ear with obliterative otosclerosis. The stapes footplate is initially thinned with a small diamond burr mounted on a micro ear drill.

Video 117-13. A graft of perichondrium is placed medial to the tympanic membrane and lateral to the stapes prosthesis to avoid extrusion.

Chapter 121

Video 121-1. Left ear treated via a transcanal approach for separation of the incudostapedial joint and removal of the incus. Note the facial nerve tumor located superior to the stapes.

Video 121-2. A facial nerve neuroma of the horizontal and vertical segments of the left ear is being dissected at the second genu.

Video 121-3. The facial nerve tumor in the left ear is being carefully dissected from the fallopian canal and arch of the stapes.

Video 121-4. The areolar and adventitial layers are dissected from the end of the nerve to be grafted. The epineurium is left around the nerve fascicle.

Chapter 124

Video 124-1. Right translabyrinthine approach. The internal auditory canal is outlined and the superior trough is being developed.

Video 124-2. A high jugular bulb must be decompressed to provide access to the internal auditory canal and inferior trough.

Video 124-3. The dura of the posterior fossa is opened with a Beaver blade. A microscissors completes this opening at the porus of the internal auditory canal.

Video 124-4. The dural covering the internal auditory canal is opened, providing access to the lateral aspect of the tumor in the fundus.

Video 124-5. Following removal of most of the cerebellopontine angle portion of the tumor, the proximal eighth nerve is divided. The facial nerve is identified more medially.

Video 124-6. A suture of 4-0 silk is used to reapproximate the dura of the posterior fossa.

Video 124-7. Strips of abdominal fat are placed through the dura and fill the mastoid cavity. Fibrin glue is used to further secure the dural closure.

Video 124-8. Right retrosigmoid approach. Opening the cisterna magna and exposing the lower cranial nerves.

Video 124-9. The origin of the facial nerve can typically be identified before starting dissection of the tumor. The facial nerve originates from the brain stem in close proximity to the ninth cranial nerve. Using a Kartush facial nerve stimulator, the location of the facial nerve can be verified. Once its position is confirmed visually and with electrical stimulation, a pledget of Teflon felt is placed over the nerve for protection and as a marker for subsequent tumor dissection.

Video 124-10. After confirming that the facial nerve is not on the posterior surface of the tumor, surface vessels are bipolared, the tumor is then biopsied, debulked with an ultrasonic aspirator, and excised following the same sequence of operative techniques.

Video 124-11. The petrosal vein (Dandy's vein) is located superiorly and laterally in the posterior fossa, just inferior to the tentorium. The video clip demonstrates bipolar cautery and division of the vessel before tumor removal.

Video 124-12. The inferior pole of the tumor is dissected from the proximal eighth and seventh cranial nerves. Once the dissection plane is defined, pledgets of Teflon are placed to maintain separation of tumor from the surrounding normal structures.

Video 124-13. The dura over the posterior surface of the porus is cauterized with a bipolar forceps. This region is incised with a no. 15 blade. A flap of dura pedicled on the posterior lip of the porus is developed.

Video 124-14. The posterior wall of the internal auditory canal is being drilled. The flap of dura based on the lip of the porus remains intact but will be subsequently excised.

Video 124-15. Using a diamond burr, troughs are created above superior and inferior to the interior auditory canal as the dissection is taken laterally toward the fundus.

Video 124-16. A narrow dissector is used to palpate the limits of dissection in an extradural plane superior and inferior to the tumor to determine whether adequate bone removal has been achieved.

Video 124-17. The dura of the internal auditory canal is opened. The tumor is dissected from the superior fold of dura seeking the location of the facial nerve.

Video 124-18. Using a nerve stimulator, the tumor is dissected and the facial nerve is identified in the anterior superior quadrant of the internal auditory canal.

Video 124-19. The tumor is dissected from the facial nerve using an excavator.

Video 124-20. The inferior and lateral aspects of the tumor are rolled from the fundus of the internal auditory canal. The lateral fibers of the vestibular nerve are sharply divided.

Video 124-21. The facial nerve often gets compressed at the proximal internal auditory canal (IAC) near the porus. The tumor is being dissected off the facial nerve at the mid and proximal portions of the IAC.

Video 124-22. The tumor is removed from the proximal internal auditory canal and cerebellopontine angle with ultrasonic aspiration and dissection.

Video 124-23. Excision of the remaining tumor is now undertaken from a medial to lateral direction keeping the facial nerve in view.

Video 124-24. If the tumor is adherent to the facial nerve, meticulous dissection in a piecemeal fashion is necessary for final removal.

Chapter 125

Video 125-1. Using microbipolar forceps facilitates hemostasis during removal of the tumor.

Video 125-2. Tumor resection is performed through the facial recess approach with cup forceps.

Video 125-3. Cotton soaked with adrenalin is used to control bleeding during tumor dissection.

Chapter 131

Video 131-1. The posterior semicircular canal is skeletonized and blue-lined midway between its ampulla and the common crus. A central bony island is left over the membranous labyrinth. This remaining bone is removed using a sharp pick, taking care to leave the membranous labyrinth intact. The membranous canal is then plugged with bone wax.

Plastic and Reconstructive Surgery

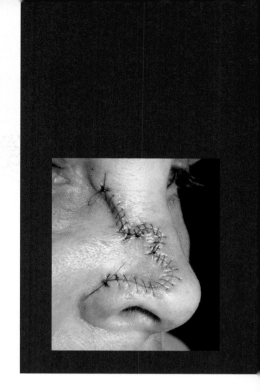

Chapter **80**

Management of Skin Cancer of the Head and Neck

John A. Zitelli

Cancer of the skin is the most common form of cancer in humans. The incidence of skin cancer is greater than that of all other forms of cancer combined and is increasing faster than any other cancer, largely because of an aging population and the popularity of sun exposure during the last half-century. Skin cancer is most common in the 60- to 80-year-old age group, and as our life expectancy and this segment of the population have increased, the incidence of skin cancer has risen dramatically. In addition, since discovery of the health benefits of vitamins in the early 20th century, particularly the role of sunlight and production of vitamin D, sun exposure was advocated for its health benefits. As leisure time increased and convenient transportation offered sunny vacations to those living in colder climates, the lifetime exposure to ultraviolet light increased as well, thereby expanding the age range and incidence of skin cancer in each age group. Skin cancer contributes in part to the practice of most specialties in medicine, and because the majority of skin cancers arise on sun-exposed areas of the head and neck, it is an important part of operative otolaryngology. Together, these and other epidemiologic factors have resulted in a virtual epidemic of skin cancer that requires the expertise of multiple specialties of medicine.

Malignant neoplasms may arise from any cell type in the skin, and thus there are numerous forms of skin cancer to consider. Cancer may arise from the epidermis (epidermal precursor cells [basal cell carcinoma], differentiated epidermal cells [squamous cell carcinoma], and melanocytes [melanoma]), neuroendocrine cells (Merkel cell carcinoma), adnexal skin cells (sebaceous glands [sebaceous carcinoma], eccrine glands [eccrine carcinoma, microcystic adnexal carcinoma], and apocrine glands [extramammary Paget's disease]), fibroblasts (dermatofibrosarcoma protuberans [DFSP], atypical fibroxanthoma, and malignant fibrous histiocytoma), endothelial cells (angiosarcoma), and smooth muscle (leiomyosarcoma). Each type of skin cancer has a unique appearance, biologic behavior, prognosis, and response to treatment, so knowledge of each type is important before treatment is begun. This chapter discusses the biology and operative management of the most common forms of skin cancer of the head and neck.

PATIENT SELECTION

Selection of patients for surgical management of skin cancer is not difficult. Most patients are surgical candidates. Most skin cancers are small (<2 cm) and can be treated under local anesthesia in the office, ambulatory surgery center, or hospital outpatient setting with or without sedation. Many common contraindications to surgery do not apply to these smaller operative procedures. For example, patients taking anticoagulants such as aspirin or warfarin (Coumadin) may safely continue their medications for most skin cancer surgery. The risk of complications from thrombosis caused by discontinuing their medications (i.e., stroke or heart attack) is more serious than the uncommon and less serious complication of bleeding or hematoma (<1%). Age is also rarely a contraindication to surgery. Most skin cancers are treated by simple operative procedures that have very few risks or complications and are not disruptive, even to fragile elderly patients. A short operative procedure in 1 day is often less disruptive than managing chronic nonhealing skin ulcers from untreated skin cancer.

Contraindications to Surgery

Although contraindications to surgery for skin cancer are rare, a few situations should be considered. The first issue is life expectancy rather than age. One must consider, all together, the type of skin cancer, its biologic behavior, and the patient's health and life expectancy. For example, basal cell carcinoma is a slowly growing tumor that may be asymptomatic for years. Therefore, treatment is no emergency, and there may be no need to treat a small nonulcerated basal cell carcinoma in a patient with other metastatic disease and a life expectancy of less than 1 year. On the other hand, treatment of nodular melanoma in an independent 95-year-old patient may be curative and allow the family to celebrate the potential 100-year mark. Each patient and each tumor must be considered individually, but health and life expectancy are more important than age when considering the need to treat skin cancer.

Another important consideration in patient selection and the decision for surgery is the extent of disease and the impact of surgery. Although surgery for skin cancer is rarely serious or life-threatening, there are occasions when extensive or invasive tumors may require surgery that has a significant mortality rate and impact on quality of life after surgery or is unlikely to achieve cure. In these rare cases the balance of risks and benefits must be weighed carefully. Is it worthwhile to remove one eye because of a slowly growing basal cell carcinoma in an elderly patient who has little or no vision in the other eye? Is temporal bone resection for management of a "close positive margin" after excision of squamous cell carcinoma worth the mortality risk? In difficult management cases, discussions and informed consent must include a realistic probability of results from treatment versus no treatment, as well as the possibility of alternative forms of therapy or palliative treatment.

When selecting patients for surgery it is also important to discuss nonoperative alternatives. Although surgery usually offers a simple treatment with little pain, delivers specimens for a pathologist to evaluate the success of removal, and is usually accompanied by an aesthetic reconstruction, there are significant reasons to consider alternative methods. The single most common treatment of skin cancer today is the use of destructive techniques such as curettage and electrodesiccation, laser destruction, cryosurgery, radiation therapy, or topical treatment with chemotherapy and immunomodulating creams. Altogether, they offer cure rates similar to those of surgical excision in properly selected patients after considering variables such as tumor type, size, location, and patient expectations of cosmetic results.

Curettage with electrodesiccation is the technique commonly used for small noninvasive basal cell carcinomas less than 2 cm in diameter and very small squamous cell carcinomas. Under local anesthesia, a circular knife 2 to 6 mm in diameter is used in a scraping motion to remove the tumor, which is soft in comparison to the normal surrounding dermis. Scraping removes the majority of the tumor, and this portion of the procedure is followed by electrodessication of the wound, which destroys an additional 3 to 4 mm of skin and soft tissue. This procedure is not useful if the tumor involves fat, cartilage, or tissue, for which one cannot feel the contrast between tumor and normal skin with the curette. Similarly, it is not useful in scar tissue, recurrent skin cancers in scar tissue, or hard infiltrating tumors that cannot be separated from normal dermis. After removal of the tumor and wider destruction with electrodesiccation, the wound heals by secondary intention, and a pale but acceptable scar is often left in carefully chosen locations.

Laser destruction is often successful for superficial skin cancers confined largely to the epidermis and superficial dermis, such as superficial basal cell carcinoma and Bowen's disease or microinvasive squamous cell carcinoma. Like electrodesiccation and curettage, the wounds are left to heal by secondary intention, and pale white scars often result. Two advantages of laser destruction are its ability to destroy very superficial layers of skin with less destruction than occurs with curettage and electrodesiccation and its ability to detect focal invasive areas of tumor during vaporization by their unique "bubbling" reaction as opposed to the simple shrinkage of underlying normal dermis.

Cryosurgical treatment of skin cancer uses liquid nitrogen as a coolant to freeze tumor and adjacent skin and kill cells by dehydration or the formation of intracellular ice crystals, which will burst the cell. It is often claimed as a method to kill cancer cells and preserve a viable framework of collagen that heals with less scarring than with other techniques. However, in practice, the cosmetic result is similar to that achieved with other destructive techniques, and the results are quite operator dependent because there is no way to accurately judge the depth of destruction without significant experience.

Radiation therapy for skin cancer was once a popular alternative to surgery that was used by dermatologists and radiation oncologists alike. It too is quite operator dependent because experience is needed to estimate not only the width of the surgical margin but, with more difficulty, the depth of tumor invasion as well. In practice it is inconvenient for most patients because 10 to

30 visits are required, and it is also the most expensive treatment option. The advantage of radiation therapy is that it provides a cure rate similar to that of surgery without most of the risks and complications of surgery. Nowadays it is most useful as an adjunct to surgery, especially for tumors whose surgical margins are positive but inoperable or whose margins are questionable but at high risk for recurrence, as well as for adjunctive treatment around the surgical site to provide local control if there is a high risk for satellite metastases. It is commonly used, for example, after excision of high-risk squamous cell carcinoma and Merkel cell carcinoma. It is also used as a nonoperative adjunct to elective management of high-risk lymph node metastases.

Another nonoperative option for head and neck skin cancer is *topical therapy*. The use of topical chemotherapy, specifically, 5-fluorouracil cream and topical immunomodulators such as imiquimod, has been tried with some success. However, it must be emphasized that fluorouracil and imiquimod have been approved by the Food and Drug Administration only for superficial skin cancer and imiquimod is not approved for use on the head and neck. The results of current studies show short-term success rates of 80%, and long-term cure rates will probably be significantly lower. The cost is high, the results are interim, and their use is limited. Some may consider topical therapy for widespread superficial disease that would otherwise be inoperable or for very superficial tumors that with excision might result in significant cosmetic deformity.

Besides nonoperative alternatives to routine surgical excision of skin cancer, there is one operative alternative to consider when selecting patients for surgery—*Mohs surgery*. Mohs surgery is a method of complete histologic control of the surgical margin.[1] Like routine excisional surgery, Mohs surgery is an excisional method performed under local anesthesia but differs from routine excision by the method of evaluating the surgical margin. In contrast to routine excision and pathologic evaluation (with or without frozen section control), in which less than 0.1% of the margin is sampled, Mohs surgery literally examines 100% of the margin. By examining the entire surgical margin of the excision and accurately mapping any positive areas within the wound, the excision can be continued until a negative margin is ensured with almost certainty. The result is a low recurrence rate, the ability to remove tumor with very narrow margins, and a method to preserve valuable normal skin for reconstruction. Mohs surgery as an alternative to routine excision is most useful for skin cancers that might be at higher risk for recurrence, such as those in the midface and ears because the depth or lateral margins are difficult to estimate, for previously treated skin cancers that have recurred or those excised with positive margins, or for cancer in areas where the smallest possible wound is important to achieve the best cosmetic or functional result. This surgery is not time consuming, but like routine excision it usually requires a half- or full-day time commitment for patients. Its costs compare favor-

Table 80-1	AVERAGE COST OF TREATING SKIN CANCER BY DIFFERENT METHODS*
Method	**Cost ($)**
Destruction	652
Office excision/permanent section	1167
Mohs surgery	1243
Office excision/frozen sections	1400
Ambulatory surgery/frozen section	1973
Radiation therapy	4558

*Based on a 1.5-cm facial skin cancer.
From Cook J, Zitelli JA: Mohs micrographic surgery: A cost analysis. J Am Acad Dermatol 39:698-703, 1998.

ably with other office procedures, but it does require special fellowship training.

In times of limited health care dollars, the cost of treatment must also be considered in patient selection. A comparison of costs for the most common treatment options is presented in Table 80-1, including the cost from the time of initial evaluation up to and including 5 years of follow-up screening.[2]

Syndromes and Predisposing Factors

It is important to recognize a few common syndromes and predisposing factors that often influence the surgical decision and management of skin cancer.

Basal cell nevus syndrome has cutaneous findings of multiple basal cell carcinomas, including tiny pits in the stratum corneum of the palms and plantar surfaces of the fingers, toes, hands, and feet; the characteristic facial appearance of frontal bossing and wide-set eyes; and internal findings of jaw cysts, skeletal abnormalities, and calcification of the falx cerebri. The difficulty in treating patients with basal cell nevus syndrome is that tumors begin to appear at an early age (often before puberty) and they number in the hundreds over a lifetime. Patients usually become discouraged because of the need for frequent treatment and are often lost to follow-up, only to reappear with multiple difficult-to-treat lesions. Effective lifetime care should include counseling to prevent discouragement and lack of regular follow-up routine care, treatment planning to minimize loss of work/school and quality time, and selection of treatment with a high cure rate to prevent multiple repeat treatments and minimize deformity. Thus far, chemoprophylactic treatment either topically or with systemic retinoids has not proved useful in the long term. Effective management often requires the resources of multiple forms of treatment and multiple specialists over a lifetime. These patients are often very difficult to manage.

Muir-Torres syndrome is a form of familial polyposis characterized by multiple sebaceous tumors of the skin, particularly sebaceous carcinoma and adenoma, and adenocarcinoma of the colon and small intestine. Sebaceous carcinoma behaves like squamous cell carcinoma in its risk of metastasis, and treatment is similar. Any patient with even a single sebaceous carcinoma of the skin should be counseled about the possibility of Muir-Torres syndrome and be referred for colonoscopy and genetic counseling. Most patients have only a few skin cancers, and they are curable if treated early. Important in the long-term management of these patients is patient education about the risk of colon cancer, affected family members, and the need for self-examination of the skin; routine gastrointestinal follow-up; and regular lifetime skin cancer screening.

The *syndrome of multiple trichoepitheliomas* is important to recognize when selecting patients for treatment. A trichoepithelioma is a benign neoplasm of the hair follicle that often simulates basal cell carcinoma both clinically and histologically. Patients with this syndrome have increasing numbers of small papules on the medial aspect of the cheeks, nose, and upper lip, as well as on the ear and elsewhere on the face. Management difficulties arise because (1) the tumors resemble basal cell carcinoma clinically and histologically; lesions may be misdiagnosed as basal cell carcinoma if an accurate clinical description is not given to the pathologist or if an expert pathologist is not available to examine the lesion; (2) these patients often have true basal cell carcinomas developing within benign trichoepitheliomas that require adequate treatment; and (3) excision of basal cell carcinomas in these patients is complicated by difficulty assessing the pathology margin because of confusion between benign trichoepithelioma and malignant basal cell carcinoma at the margin. In general, a single lesion that looks different from the other dozens of lesions or any lesion that is enlarging or ulcerated should undergo biopsy and be interpreted by an experienced dermatopathologist.

Dysplastic nevus syndrome, or *atypical mole syndrome,* is another syndrome important to recognize in the management of skin cancer, especially melanoma. Dysplastic nevus syndrome is inherited as an autosomal dominant trait with incomplete penetrance and is characterized by frequent spontaneous mutations. Recognized only in the last 2 decades, there is still considerable confusion and controversy surrounding both diagnosis and management. A dysplastic nevus is clinically recognized as a pigmented mole and is usually larger than a normal nevus or greater than 6 mm in diameter. It is nonuniform in pigmentation with slight variations of brown. The pigment at the border appears to diffuse into the surrounding skin, in contrast to the clear distinction at the border of normal nevi. The importance of dysplastic nevus syndrome is its association with an increased lifetime risk for melanoma. Patients with dysplastic nevus syndrome usually have multiple dysplastic nevi on the trunk, as well as on the head, neck, and scalp. Although the normal population has a 1% lifetime risk of melanoma, patients with common dysplastic nevus syndrome have an approximately 5% risk. Patients with even a single dysplastic nevus may have an increased risk for melanoma, but those with multiple nevi and a family history of melanoma together have the highest risk for melanoma, approaching 100%.

Management problems in a patient with dysplastic nevus syndrome arise around the controversy regarding diagnosis and treatment. Dysplastic nevi resemble melanoma in some ways, both clinically and histologically. Biopsies are common because of the irregular clinical appearance similar to melanoma, and pathologists may have difficulty distinguishing the pattern of atypical cells from melanoma or describe the common but benign finding of cellular atypia and dysplasia and comment that margins are still positive. Ambiguous pathology reports often leave management decisions to be made by the clinician, who may be confused about the unresolved controversy. Important facts are that dysplastic nevi are benign and do not to be excised. Melanomas that arise in these patients, although they may appear in preexisting nevi, often develop in normal skin. Elective removal of all or most dysplastic nevi is not recommended for decreasing the risk of melanoma. Because dysplastic nevi are benign and commonly show atypia and dysplasia, they do not need to be either excised or re-excised if a biopsy specimen shows a positive margin. Some pathologists write this recommendation to absolve themselves from the responsibility of not having looked at an entire lesion (if the margin is positive, some of the dysplastic nevus remains in a patient who has not been examined histologically). They also point out the later difficulty in making a histopathologic diagnosis from a biopsy specimen of a recurrent nevus that even more closely falsely resembles melanoma.

In general, it is important to recognize and diagnose this syndrome to counsel patients to minimize lifetime exposure to ultraviolet light, to perform regular self-examination of skin, to have yearly checkups by dermatologists, and to understand the genetics for children and close family members.

Associated Diseases

Along with syndromes, some cutaneous conditions have important associations with skin cancer. *Oral lichen planus* is a chronic inflammatory condition involving both skin and mucous membranes. On the lips, whitening of the vermilion, ulceration, thickening of the epidermis, and induration caused by the inflammatory response together can simulate squamous cell carcinoma both clinically and histologically. Despite the possibility of lichen planus simulating squamous cell carcinoma, it also predisposes one to the development of true invasive squamous cell carcinoma. As with many other conditions, it is important to match the findings on a biopsy report to the clinical picture.

Skin cancer is also a serious and almost universal long-term complication in *solid organ transplant* patients or other patients who are chronically immunosuppressed and represents an experiment in nature, thus emphasizing the important role of immune surveillance in preventing skin cancer. Skin cancer in transplant patients is similar to skin cancer in patients with basal cell nevus syndrome in that transplant patients often become discouraged with the overwhelming number of skin cancers, the need for frequent treatment, and the time and effort required to keep up with treatment. Worse yet is that the majority of skin cancers are squamous cell carcinoma and squamous cell carcinoma in situ. Neglected or recurrent disease may be life-threatening and is often the cause of death in transplant patients. This emphasizes the need for early effective treatment and constant surveillance, follow-up, and patient education. Coordinating medical management with the transplant team to keep immunosuppressive drugs at their lowest possible dose is often advisable.

Other forms of *immunosuppression* are also associated with an increased risk for skin cancer. Human immunodeficiency virus–positive patients with low CD4+ lymphocyte counts have a higher risk for squamous cell carcinoma and often other forms of skin cancer as well. Chronic infection with human papillomavirus plays an important role in the development of squamous cell carcinoma in these immunosuppressed patients. Immunosuppression not only predisposes patients to skin cancer but also complicates and compromises the prognosis of patients at high risk for metastatic disease or those with known metastatic disease. Again, coordination of their care to balance the risks and benefits of immunosuppression is an important part of patient selection for surgery.

PREOPERATIVE EVALUATION

The *patient's history* plays a small but important role in the preoperative evaluation. In general, lesions that have not undergone change for many years tend to be benign, whereas a history of increasing size or growth is a signal to consider malignancy and therefore biopsy. A history of previous treatment of skin cancer is a signal that the original treatment failed because of inadequate treatment, usually secondary to unrecognized positive margins. It is important to remember that routine pathology can only sample surgical margins and a report of clear margins is only an estimate of clear margins. In the face of recurrence, retreatment with routine surgery is associated with a much higher recurrence rate than treatment of the primary lesions is, and therefore Mohs surgery may be indicated.

Physical examination, however, plays a very important role in the preoperative evaluation. It is important to incorporate tumor location, size, and depth into the decision-making process. To assess size and therefore tumor margins it is extremely important to tightly stretch the skin under very bright light such as that of an examination or operating room light. Clues to tumor extension of basal cell carcinoma and squamous cell carcinoma may include subtle pink from the vascular response induced by inflammation, scar-like white or yellow from fibrosis and tumor infiltration, a more shiny pearly appearance from underlying tumor lobules, and lack of normal fine skin wrinkling. Extension of superficial basal cell carcinoma or squamous cell carcinoma in situ beyond invasive disease may stimulate dermatitis and have a totally difference appearance than the primary tumor. Tumor depth may be more difficult to estimate beyond simple palpation and movement over underlying structures such as attachment to bone.

Estimating melanoma margins is more difficult on the head and neck than on the trunk and extremities. Normal skin lesions such as lentigines, freckles, seborrheic keratoses, and actinic keratoses may all camouflage the margin. Furthermore, in situ extensions at the edge of a melanoma on the skin of the head and neck are often amelanotic and simulate dermatitis or may be totally invisible.

Palpation for signs of local, regional, or metastatic disease in the form of satellite metastases, in transit metastases, and lymph node metastases is necessary for skin cancers with a risk of metastatic disease, especially squamous cell carcinoma, melanoma, Merkel cell carcinoma, malignant fibrous histiocytoma, and sebaceous carcinoma.

Adjunctive testing to evaluate the lymph nodes for metastatic disease has limited value. Computed tomography (CT), magnetic resonance imaging (MRI), and ultrasound may be useful in obese patients, in whom palpation of early clinical disease is difficult. Sentinel lymph node biopsy is a technique that has not been proved to improve survival, and research results on its benefit are limited to improvements in staging. Similarly, preoperative testing with CT or MRI to determine the extent of invasion is rarely helpful except in the largest cases, and even then they are helpful only to get an estimate of the likelihood of bone invasion, orbit invasion, or involvement of vital structures of the neck. The resolution of these tests can estimate the extent of gross tumor involvement but cannot detect microscopic extensions of skin cancer in soft tissue, which are often located just millimeters from the main tumor mass.

Histopathology laboratory results are an essential part of the preoperative evaluation, and a histologic diagnosis is important before definitive surgery is planned. The tumor type determines the need for evaluation of metastases, as well as the width of the surgical margin. Because many types of skin cancer and other benign diseases have a similar appearance, the proper diagnosis is important before planning excision. Furthermore, one should always be sure that the pathology results correlate with the clinical picture. Biopsies are often small samples of a larger lesion and may not represent the entire tumor. Sometimes the microscopic appearance of one skin cancer simulates another tumor. A melanoma can be confused with a superficial basal cell carcinoma, and a Merkel cell carcinoma can be confused with cutaneous lymphoma. The clinician must be sure that the patient's history, the appearance, and the histopathology results all correlate; otherwise, another biopsy may be indicated.

SURGICAL APPROACH

Tumor Type

The goal of surgery is complete removal of skin cancer with clear margins as determined by histopathology.

This goal is achieved by careful selection of patients, careful surgical planning, and extensive examination of the margins by the pathologist. The surgical approach differs according to tumor type.

Basal Cell Carcinoma

Careful selection and planning should achieve a 5-year cure rate of 90% to 95% for basal cell carcinoma (Fig. 80-1). For primary basal cell carcinoma 2 cm or less in diameter that has clearly visible margins, a surgical margin 4 mm wide should be adequate.[3] The depth of the surgical margin is more difficult to estimate and depends a great deal on tumor location and clinical judgment. Histopathologic variants such as morphea-form or sclerosing basal cell carcinoma and micronodular and even superficial basal cell carcinoma require wider margins than 4 mm, as well as the aid of careful intraoperative frozen section control during excision. Similarly, tumors larger than 2 cm in diameter and recurrent tumors require a wider margin to achieve acceptable cure rates. The best chance for cure is the first operation, and although 1- to 2-mm margins often cure some basal cell carcinomas, 5-year cure rates are only 50% to 60% and are considered inadequate for such narrow margins.

Squamous Cell Carcinoma

Even though squamous cell carcinoma is associated with a significant risk for metastases, the goal of surgery is still complete removal with negative surgical margins (Fig. 80-2). Extra wide margins, excised in the hope of including microscopic satellite metastases, do not improve survival or local control. However, squamous cell carcinoma usually requires wider surgical margins than basal cell carcinoma does to achieve clear margins of the primary tumor. For low-risk squamous cell carcinomas 2 cm or less in diameter in areas such as the cheek and neck and not invading fat, a surgical margin of 4 mm is acceptable. For moderate-risk squamous cell carcinomas up to 2 cm in diameter, a 6-mm margin is necessary to approach a 95% chance of achieving clear surgical margins. For high-risk squamous cell carcino-

mas greater than 2 cm in diameter, those on the temple, scalp, or lip, or those invading fat, a 9-mm surgical margin is necessary to achieve an acceptable chance of negative margins.[4] If histopathologic sampling confirms negative margins with these clinical margin widths, the risk for local persistence of tumor is minimized to an acceptable level.

Keratoacanthoma is a variant of squamous cell carcinoma that often shows extremely rapid growth of a dome-shaped nodule. Although keratoacanthomas have been reported to spontaneously involute without treatment, these tumors can be aggressive, destructive, and otherwise indistinguishable from true squamous cell carcinoma, including the ability to metastasize. Complete surgical excision is the treatment of choice.

Squamous cell carcinoma in situ appears as a superficial scaly lesion that may be small or large. Although the malignant atypical cells are limited to the epidermis, the difficulty in treatment occurs when the atypical cells extend down hair follicles into the dermis. In this case, either deep destruction or full-thickness skin excision is required to achieve effective cure rates. When there is little or no follicular extension, superficial destruction with curettage, cryosurgery, or laser surgery is quite effective. Left untreated or inadequately treated, squamous cell carcinoma in situ often progresses to true invasive squamous cell carcinoma with metastatic potential.

Melanoma

Successful excision of melanoma on the head and neck (Fig. 80-3) is more difficult than excision on the trunk

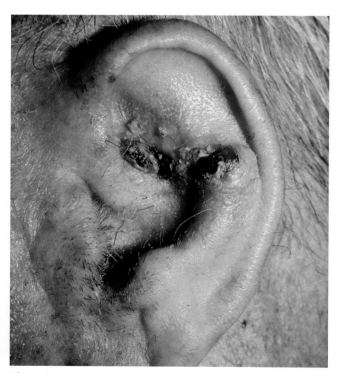

Figure 80-2. Squamous cell carcinoma of the ear.

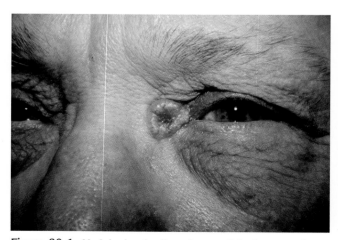

Figure 80-1. Nodular basal cell carcinoma of the inner canthus.

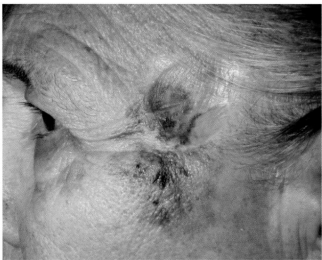

Figure 80-3. Locally recurrent melanoma on the temple.

and extremities because melanoma margins are more difficult to visualize, amelanotic melanomas are more common, and surgical margins are often reduced because of cosmetic and functional concerns. Therefore, these melanomas recur at the surgical margin in 9% to 18% of cases because of inadequate excision. The previously published recommendation of a 5-mm margin for melanoma in situ has no scientific basis and often results in inadequate excision and recurrence of both melanoma in situ and invasive melanoma. When possible, 1.2-cm margins are likely to clear melanoma on the head and neck in 97% of cases.[5] When this margin cannot be excised, very careful histopathologic examination of the more narrow margins is necessary to confirm clear margins. Melanomas that recur at previously treated surgical margins may be due to previous inadequate excision rather than metastatic disease. In the former case the histopathology of the biopsy specimen generally shows an intraepidermal component. Metastases are usually located in the dermis or subcutaneous tissue. Melanoma recurrences as a result of previous inadequate excision have a much better prognosis than metastatic recurrences do, and their prognosis is still accurately related to tumor thickness.

The value of elective lymph node dissection for melanoma of the head and neck is still unproven. The interim results of the Multicenter Selective Lymphadenectomy Trial I (MSLT I) have shown no survival benefit for sentinel lymph node biopsy and complete lymph node dissection in patients with microscopically positive disease.[6] Possible benefits of sentinel lymph node biopsy include a slight improvement in estimating a patient's prognosis in comparison with Breslow's thickness alone, although this may be true only for melanomas 2 to 4 mm thick. For other thicknesses, the benefit of sentinel lymph node biopsy in estimating prognosis is no better than Breslow's thickness. Early detection of microscopically positive disease with complete lymph node dissection may also aid in improved regional control, which can be an important benefit in the head and neck, especially in patients who may otherwise neglect regular follow-up or self-palpation of lymph nodes and be seen instead with advanced regional nodal disease. The final results of the MSLT II trial will hopefully provide further evidence to guide clinical decisions about sentinel lymph node biopsy.

The benefits of radiation treatment in the management of high-risk, but clinically negative nodes is currently unproven and is being investigated. For now, management of melanoma is still a surgical issue. There is no adjuvant treatment that significantly prolongs survival. Early treatment with complete removal of primary disease is the most important factor. Surgical removal of local, in transit, and regional disease can still salvage a significant number of patients with metastases. Teaching patients to palpate nodes and soft tissue is an important part of surgical management.

Adnexal Neoplasms

Cancer may arise within any skin structure, such as sebaceous glands and eccrine sweat glands, or differentiate toward the structures. Sebaceous carcinoma is a malignant tumor of sebaceous glands that often arises on the eyelids or skin of the head and neck. Its malignant potential is similar to that of squamous cell carcinoma and it should be treated as such. Microcystic adnexal carcinoma and eccrine carcinoma appear clinically similar to basal cell carcinoma but often show more extensive subclinical invasion. To minimize local recurrence, wider margins are necessary than for basal cell carcinoma to prevent recurrence. In addition, complete margin examination or Mohs surgery will minimize the high rate of recurrence.

Trichoepitheliomas are benign tumors of hair follicles. Clinically and histologically they may resemble basal cell carcinoma. Therefore, single or isolated trichoepitheliomas are often treated as basal cell carcinoma, especially if they are large, ulcerated, or growing. Patients with multiple trichoepithelioma lesions do not require treatment; however, these patients often have associated basal cell carcinomas that develop from their benign tumors and will require treatment consisting of complete excision of the basal cell carcinoma portion but not the trichoepithelioma portion often seen at the margin.

Merkel Cell Carcinoma

Merkel cell carcinoma arises from neuroendocrine cells populating the skin and is characterized by a pink or red papule or nodule. It is rarely diagnosed clinically but instead undergoes biopsy when a red papule persists or enlarges. This tumor has biologic behavior similar to that of melanoma, with a very high risk of metastatic disease. The microscopic extensions of Merkel cell carcinoma are much wider and deeper than clinical estimates, and therefore wide and deep margins (i.e., 2 cm) are recommended to provide the best chance of complete removal and minimize the risk of local recurrence. Careful histologic examination of the surgical margins is important to validate complete excision. Mohs surgery can be helpful to ensure total excision. If negative margins are not possible or are in question, radiation treatment may improve local control because this tumor is very radiosensitive. The role of sentinel lymph node biopsy and elective node dissection may be similar to that in melanoma, although there is no proven benefit.

Dermatofibrosarcoma Protuberans

DFSP is a tumor of fibroblast origin that is manifested as a dermal subcutaneous mass and often as a nodular tumor greater than 2 cm in diameter. Although these tumors rarely metastasize, local recurrence rates are high because of difficulty clinically estimating the microscopic extent of the tumor. DFSP invades the dermis and fibrous septa between the fat lobules, so its microscopic extent is much wider and deeper than is visible or palpable. Imaging studies are of limited value because they cannot detect the microscopic involvement of fat lobules accurately. Wide lateral margins of 2 to 2.5 cm of normal-appearing skin may be adequate to clear the lateral margins, but the deep margins are often the most difficult to estimate. Careful histologic margin control is important to achieve negative surgical margins. Mohs surgery is very effective and results in both the lowest recurrence rate and the narrowest margins possible.

Angiosarcoma

Angiosarcoma is a malignant tumor of blood vessels. In its early stage it is a purple papule or nodule, but most often it is seen as a large flat plaque resembling a bruise or ecchymosis that covers wide areas of the scalp and forehead. Clipping or shaving the hair is necessary to see the full extent of these lesions in hair-bearing areas. Surgical management is difficult. Small lesions may be surgically excised with success, but local recurrence rates and regional metastatic rates are high. Surgical margins are difficult to evaluate histologically because growth of the malignant vessel is subtle. Large lesions may not be amenable to surgery because of their extreme size. Angiosarcoma is a radiosensitive tumor, and therefore radiation therapy plays a role in the adjuvant treatment of small lesions to provide local control; radiotherapy also plays a role in the primary treatment of large lesions that are not amenable to surgery. Adjuvant chemotherapy has no proven value for local disease.

Atypical Fibroxanthoma/ Malignant Fibrous Histiocytoma

Atypical fibroxanthoma is a skin cancer often seen in sun-exposed areas. It resembles squamous cell carcinoma or basal cell carcinoma because of the presence of a pink papule or erosion. It is usually diagnosed only after biopsy. Tumors involving the dermis and superficial fat are termed *atypical fibroxanthoma* and rarely metastasize. Deeper tumors involving subcutaneous tissue or muscle are labeled *malignant fibrous histiocytoma* and have a high risk of metastatic disease. Surgical treatment of atypical fibroxanthoma is excision with margins similar to those for squamous cell carcinoma, and treatment of malignant fibrous histiocytoma is wide and deep excision, similar to treatment of Merkel cell carcinoma or melanoma. Elective regional node management is unnecessary for atypical fibroxanthoma and has no proven value for malignant fibrous histiocytoma.

Tumors of Uncertain Behavior

Surgeons are often faced with tumors on the head and neck with uncertain biologic behavior. Spitz nevi are benign nevi manifested as enlarging red papules, usually in children or young adults. The difficulty with this lesion is that it resembles a nodular form of amelanotic melanoma both clinically and histologically. A classic lesion in a young person who also has a histologic diagnosis of benign Spitz nevus from a dermatopathologist may not require excision; however, lesions arising in adults or those showing cellular atypia or nonclassic features histologically may be more difficult to distinguish accurately from melanoma. These uncertain lesions should be excised and treated as though they were melanoma, that is, with negative surgical margins documented histologically by careful examination of margins.

Dysplastic nevi are also benign lesions that are seen on the head and neck and can clinically resemble melanoma because of their large diameter, irregular borders, and irregular pigment. Lesions for which biopsy reports describe the cellular atypia or dysplasia common in benign lesions do not require excision. However, a description of severe atypia may be an indication that the pathologist cannot distinguish the lesion from melanoma with certainty. With these lesions, a discussion with the pathologist may be helpful to understand whether the diagnosis is benign, malignant, or uncertain. Pigmented lesions of uncertain diagnosis should be excised with margins as though they were melanoma and negative surgical margins determined histologically. Benign dysplastic nevi do not require excision even if the biopsy margins are positive.

Many other cutaneous lesions have overlapping features with their benign and malignant counterparts. Desmoplastic trichoepithelioma can resemble morphea or sclerosing basal cell carcinoma both clinically and histologically. Other tumors of follicular origin may be difficult to distinguish from basal cell carcinoma with follicular differentiation. Ultimately, the clinician must process the information described by the pathologist along with the clinical picture to decide whether to manage it as a benign or malignant lesion.

Evaluating Surgical Margins

The goal of treating skin cancer is to excise or destroy the tumor completely with no visible tumor behind. One advantage of surgical excision is the ability to evaluate the margins of the tissue removed at the time of surgery and assess the completeness of removal. In contrast, destructive techniques and radiation therapy rely on a certain amount of guesswork in estimating the margin without the benefit of a tissue specimen to accurately evaluate the success of removal.

Routine processing of tissue specimens by pathologists involves only a sampling of the margin. Most pathologists "bread loaf" specimens and sample both lateral and deep margins for tumor involvement; however, it is important to understand that these sampling techniques examine less than 0.1% of the margin, thus giving the surgeon at best only an estimate of the status of the surgical margin.[7] It is important for the surgeon to keep this in mind when interpreting the pathology report. For example, a biopsy of a malignant lesion that was not removed with the intent to include standard surgical margins may be reported by the pathologist to have negative margins even when there is visible tumor remaining. For this reason it is always important to excise skin cancer with adequate margins of normal skin and only then use the pathologist's report to validate the results of excision.

If the goal of surgery is complete excision and if the surgeon relies on the pathologist to measure the success of excision, the surgeon must understand the process of margin examination. Intraoperative frozen sections give a quick estimate of margins. Frozen sections of the skin and subcutaneous tissue are technically difficult to cut, and intraoperative examination usually samples only a very small portion, far less than the 0.1% of permanent section. Frozen section results are followed by more accurate results from permanent section, but these results are available only days afterward. Permanent sections are of better quality for visualization but still often provide examination of only a small sample of the margins.

Some pathologists are willing to examine a greater portion of the margin by processing strips of tissue from lateral and deep margins obtained with tangential cuts. This more complete examination can be useful in evaluating a high-risk infiltrating skin cancer or those whose margins are difficult to visualize clinically. Such sections have been termed peripheral in continuity tissue examination or en face tissue sectioning.

Mohs surgery provides the most complete margin examination and literally examines 100% of the surgical margin. With Mohs surgery, the tissue is excised in a way that allows the entire margin to be flattened into a two-dimensional, one-plane tissue "patty." This patty is cut into pieces for processing like a puzzle, and then the edges are dyed and numbered for individual identification. Each specimen is processed so that the entire outer surface is examined microscopically, and the results of the examination are marked on the puzzle-like map of specimens. In this way any remaining tumor at the margin can be located within the wound by using the wound map. Remaining tumor is re-excised in the positive area, reprocessed in the same fashion, and repeated if necessary until its true tumor-free plane is reached. Mohs surgery requires special fellowship training because the surgeon also acts as the pathologist to better understand correlation of the pathology results with the clinical tumor margin. With this method of excision and complete margin examination, the rate of complete excision and skin cancer cure is the highest of any method. In addition, the initial surgical margin is narrower than traditional margins and relies on the complete examination to detect any positive remaining areas. This initial margin is often negative and results in smaller wounds than those after traditional excision. Mohs surgery is useful when conservation of tissue is important around cosmetic and functional structures of the head and neck. It is also useful for infiltrative tumors or tumors with poorly defined margins, especially recurrent tumors or tumors excised with positive margins. Mohs surgeons are an important part of the multispecialty team for the treatment of skin cancer. They often contribute by completely excising the cancer and working with colleagues for reconstruction after Mohs surgery. They can also be helpful to clear soft tissue margins and identify any remaining tumor near vital structures of the head and neck, such as invasion of bone; perineural invasion extending into the infraorbital, supraorbital, or other important foramen; and invasion of the parotid gland close to the facial nerve.

A pathology report with a final diagnosis of a positive margin should be taken seriously. Approximately 10% to 12% of excision specimens of head and neck cancer are positive for tumor at the margin. Without further treatment, at least a third will recur and may be difficult to cure after recurrence. Therefore, it is recommended that the first attempt at excision try to achieve clear surgical margins. For high-risk tumors or excisions requiring complex reconstruction, complete margin examination or Mohs surgery should be undertaken to ensure clear margins. Otherwise, routine surgery should be followed by delayed reconstruction until negative margins are confirmed by permanent paraffin pathology sections. When margins are positive, re-excision should be attempted. Mohs surgery can also be helpful to identify any positive margin and remove remaining tumor. When surgery is not an option for treatment of the positive margin, radiation therapy may be considered, but the chance for cure is lower than with surgically or pathologically documented negative margins.

Tumor Location

The surgical approach to skin cancer considers not only the type of skin cancer but also the location of the tumor. The incidence of skin cancer by tumor type varies according to location. For example, sebaceous carcinoma is most common in the eyelids, squamous cell carcinoma is more common on the lower lip, and basal cell carcinoma is more common on the upper lip. The biologic behavior of skin cancer also varies considerably in different locations, and the surgical approach must consider the unique anatomic difference of each location.

Eyelids

Basal cell carcinoma, squamous cell carcinoma, melanoma, and sebaceous carcinoma are the most common cancers of the periocular region. In this location, tumor clinical margins are often indistinct, especially with superficial basal cell carcinoma on the thin skin of the eyelid and those infiltrating into the lid margin and tarsal plate, thus making it very difficult to achieve negative histologic margins with narrow surgical margins. In the inner canthus region, basal cell carcinoma tends to invade deeply, and when the tumor appears to be fixed to bone, it often involves the lacrimal drainage system or extends into the orbit. The reason for deep extension of small tumors is not the often quoted "embryonic fusion plane" theory. Instead, it is well documented that basal cell carcinomas are stromal dependent for continued growth. That is, they will invade tissue only with the appropriate stromal components. Basal cell carcinoma grows slowly and poorly in fatty tissue, but it grows more quickly in fascia and muscle. With little protective fat in the periocular region, basal cell carcinoma quickly invades through the dermis and into the deeper tissues of the medial and lateral canthus and orbital septum. These extensions are invisible and hard to predict, and the small microscopic extensions do not appear on current imaging systems such as MRI or CT. Mohs surgery or careful complete margin examination is important for successful management of skin cancer in this location.

Ears

Basal cell carcinoma, squamous cell carcinoma, atypical fibroxanthoma, and melanoma are most common on the ears. Chondrodermatitis nodularis helicis or focal pressure dermatitis of the ear can simulate skin cancer, thus emphasizing the value of biopsy before initiating surgical excision. On the ear, skin cancer margins are difficult to outline with certainty, and recurrence rates are high. Tumors tend to invade through the thin skin quickly down to perichondrium and spread laterally with little visual surface change. This is particularly true on the antihelix and conchal bowl, as well as extensions down into the external canal. Tumors rarely invade cartilage, but sacrificing cartilage may be necessary to achieve negative surgical margins during excision. In the preauricular and postauricular sulcus, the lack of fat allows tumor to invade quickly, and deep negative surgical margins are often difficult to achieve.

Lips

Basal cell carcinoma is the most common tumor on the upper lip, whereas squamous cell carcinoma is the most frequently seen tumor on the lower lip. Squamous cell carcinoma on the lower lip is often associated with a dense inflammatory infiltrate, which makes the true depth of invasion difficult to assess. The tumor frequently feels deeper than is seen microscopically. However, the in situ component of squamous cell carcinoma on the lip often extends laterally much wider than appears clinically. One option in the treatment of lip lesions is to excise the invasive portion surgically and treat the in situ component with a more conservative approach such as laser destruction of the vermilion.

Nose

Basal cell carcinoma, squamous cell carcinoma, melanoma, and Merkel cell carcinoma are often seen on the nose. In this location, depth of tumor invasion is most difficult to estimate, especially on the lower third of the nose. The lack of fat allows early invasive tumors easy access to muscle and fibrous tissue. Underlying cartilage also makes it difficult to palpate tumors adequately to determine tumor depth with confidence. Squamous cell carcinoma arising from the nasal septum frequently invades deeply to the bone of the nasal spine. Recurrence rates for all skin cancers are high for these reasons, and therefore very careful examination of margins or Mohs surgery is helpful to ensure clear pathology margins.

Cheeks

All forms of skin cancer are seen on the cheeks, including DFSP and angiosarcoma. The fat is often a barrier to invasion of deeper structures until the cancer becomes very large. Involvement of the medial portion of the cheek adjacent to the nose or the lateral preauricular aspect of the cheeks is associated with the most difficulty during excision because of enhancement of tumor invasiveness by the superficially located muscle or aponeurotic layers.

Forehead, Temple, and Scalp

All forms of skin cancer are seen in these locations. Squamous cell carcinoma tends to be aggressive in these locations, with satellite metastases being a common complication of large tumors. Management of multiple satellite and in transit metastases includes surgical excision when possible and the use of adjuvant wide-field radiation for local and regional control when multiple widespread metastasis has occurred. The bone of the skull acts as a strong barrier to invasion, but when the periosteum is removed during excision and the bone is pitted, the surgeon can safely assume that early bone invasion has occurred. In this case the outer cortex should be removed with an osteotome or burr or by excision, followed by split-thickness skin grafting. Early bone invasion is not easily seen with imaging studies and must be part of the intraoperative assessment of these tumors.

Neck

Skin cancers of the neck are the least difficult. Estimating depth and lateral margins is rarely complex, and the excess loose skin makes reconstruction straightforward. Care must be taken to avoid the greater auricular nerve on the lateral infra-auricular aspect of the neck and the spinal accessory nerve on the posterior lateral portion of the neck.

Reconstruction

The surgical approach to skin cancer must also include plans for surgical reconstruction. Before reconstructing any wound after excision of skin cancer, it is important to have reasonable certainty that the excision margins are clear of tumor. Re-excision for positive margins is very difficult, especially after local flaps, complicated repairs, or repair with extensive undermining of tissue has occurred. Reasonable certainty of negative margins includes evidence-based width of surgical margins around well-defined primary lesions with convincing clinical judgment that the margins are clear. However, for large, deep, recurrent, or poorly defined tumors, reasonable certainty should include negative histopathologic margins by extensive examination of the margin or by Mohs surgery. Otherwise, reasonable certainty occurs only with delayed reconstruction after margins have been determined to be negative by permanent paraffin sections.

In most locations, reconstructive choices are predictable and results are reproducible. The following discussion of reconstruction choices covers the majority of defects after excision of skin cancer; however, each defect is unique and each has its own challenges. Selection of the method of repair depends mainly on (1) the likelihood of negative margins, (2) the laxity and availability of adjacent skin for closure, and (3) the desire of the patient for a good cosmetic outcome.

Periorbital Repair

One of the first considerations of periorbital reconstruction is protection of the eyes, especially the cornea. Poorly planned repairs may result in ectropion with exposure-induced desiccation of the conjunctiva or keratitis from drying of the cornea. Suture must be placed in a manner that prevents irritation of the globe as well. Eyelid margin repair is often best done by an oculoplastic surgeon. In the skin around the eye within the orbital rim, primary closure is easily performed if special care is taken to move tissue horizontally, even if the orientation of the ellipse is somewhat oblique. It is important to have the patient open the eye and for the surgeon to check for lid apposition or displacement after placing the first key suture. Larger defects of the lower lid can be repaired with rotation flaps based inferiorly and laterally. Care should be taken to design the flap by extending the lateral incision superiorly so that during rotation when the superior portion of the flap moves medially and inferiorly, the eyelid is not pulled down. A full-thickness skin graft also provides a good cosmetic result, especially in the medial and lateral canthus areas. On the lower lid, the inevitable shrinkage of the graft increases the risk of ectropion, and therefore it is a secondary choice. For treatment of defects of the brow, the surgeon must plan to move hair-bearing skin and maintain brow continuity even if brow length is shortened. Vertically oriented primary closure for small defects and island pedicle flaps for larger defects work well. Rarely, hair-bearing full-thickness composite grafts can be harvested from the temples with special care to maintain proper orientation of the hair follicles, even to the point of a double graft in which the top graft of hair faces inferior and lateral and the bottom half of the graft faces superior and lateral.

Ears

Helical wound defects are the most common challenging reconstruction of the ear. When the defect preserves cartilage and provides a good vascular base, a full-thickness skin graft from the postauricular donor site provides a very good cosmetic result. For defects that extend to cartilage or include cartilage but are less than 1 to 1.5 cm, helical rim advancement flaps work well (Fig. 80-4). During design it is important to cut anteriorly through the skin and cartilage but not through the posterior skin. Instead, undermining with separation of the posterior skin from the cartilage leaves a large vascular base for the helical rim flap. If the cut extends through anterior skin, cartilage, and posterior skin, only a small base of the helix is left to provide vascular supply to the flap, and the tip is often compromised. For large defects on the helical rim, an advancement flap from the postauricular surface through the postauricular sulcus can be performed as either a one- or two-stage procedure. This provides a reproducible repair and may require cartilage replacement from the ipsilateral conchal bowl if cartilage is missing in the helical rim. For superficial defects on the scapha, split-thickness skin grafts from the postauricular mastoid work well. Defects inside the rim of the scapha heal nicely by secondary intention without the need for repair. Defects of the external canal should be grafted if they involve more than half the circumference to prevent stenosis of the canal. Very large defects consisting of more than half the ear may do best with a prosthesis rather than surgical reconstruction. When planning to use a prosthesis, salvage of the tragus is important to help hide the prosthetic border. Wedge resection of the ear often results in an inferior cosmetic result when compared with other reconstruction choices and should be avoided if possible.

Upper Lip

Most wounds up to 1 to 1.5 cm can be repaired as a vertically oriented primary closure.[8] There is no value in attempting to avoid cutting through the vermilion border and the inferior triangle and using laterally based incisions above it such as an A-to-T closure. Vertical incisions around the vermilion should extend around the lip and superiorly onto the labial mucosa. The caveat is to avoid ending Burow's triangle on the vermilion or lip margin because this often results in inferior displacement of the lip.

Defects of the philtrum can be closed primarily only if they are very small. Larger superficial defects down to muscle can be grafted with donor skin from the preauricular, postauricular, or conchal bowl skin or from Burow's triangle harvested from above the defect and extending to the inferior columella. Large and deep defects of the medial aspect of the lip into muscle near the philtral crest that are too large for primary closure can be closed with horizontally moving advancement flaps using a perialar crescent and, if necessary, another Burow's triangle lateral to the commissure of the mouth. Defects of the lateral portion of the lip are

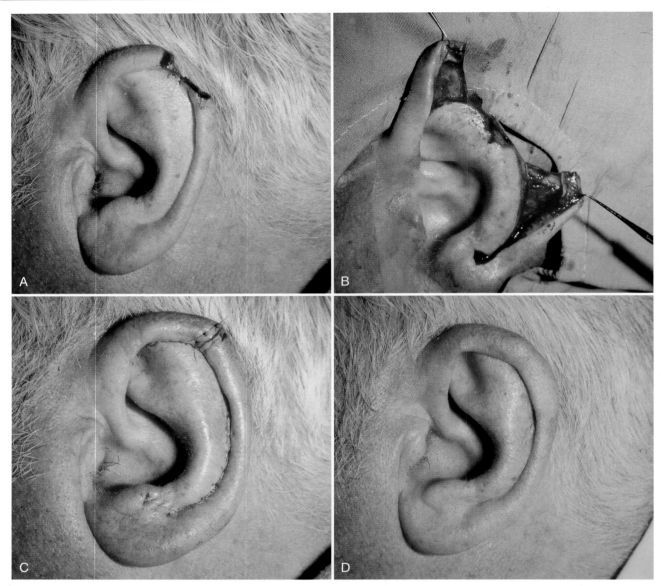

Figure 80-4. Helical rim advancement flap. **A,** Defect after excision of basal cell carcinoma. **B,** Bilateral helical rim advancement flaps elevated with a broad posterior base. **C,** Immediate postoperative result. **D,** Cosmetic result after 6 months.

more easily repaired. Superior lateral defects respond nicely to island pedicle flap repair (Fig. 80-5). Preferably, these flaps are designed within the cosmetic unit of the lip and nasolabial fold. If necessary, the flap may be designed to include the medial cheek skin as well. It is important for the apex of the triangular island pedicle flap to be oriented vertically at the most inferior portion to prevent distortion of the commissure or upward pull of the lip. For large inferior lateral defects of the upper lip, inferior or laterally based transposition flaps may be helpful. Rarely are Karapanzic or Abbé flaps necessary.

Lower Lip

Primary closure of defects of the lower lip is usually possible even if the defects extend up to half of the width of the lip. For the best cosmetic result, primary closure is not a simple wedge resection. A fusiform or elliptical excision of skin is performed so that the superior triangle, if it involves the vermilion, extends around the lip and then inferiorly onto the labial mucosa. For larger defects, some muscle may be excised to minimize bulk on closure, but less muscle than skin should always be excised. Next, both the skin and mucosa are undermined above the muscle and laterally to elevate flaps of skin and mucosa. The muscle is closed first, and then the skin and mucosa are advanced over the muscle and closed in layered fashion. Squamous cell carcinoma arising from the vermilion of the lower lip often presents a problem of dealing with extensive in situ disease along large portions of the vermilion. To minimize the deformity of excision, one option is to excise the inva-

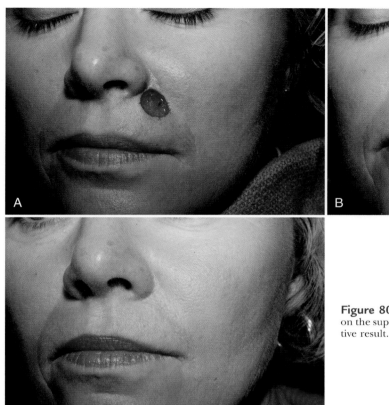

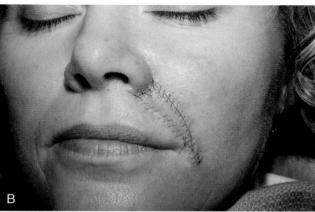

Figure 80-5. Island pedicle flap reconstruction of the lip. **A,** Defect on the superior lateral aspect of the upper lip. **B,** Immediate postoperative result. **C,** Cosmetic result after 6 months.

sive portion of squamous cell carcinoma, make plans for primary closure, and then treat the in situ portion with carbon dioxide laser destruction or alternatively with superficial vermilionectomy and mucosal advancement. Very large defects on the lip are fortunately very rare but may require full-thickness cheek advancement with a turnover of labial or buccal mucosa to re-create the mucosa and vermilion of the lip.

Nose

Reconstruction of the nose requires a mastery of local flaps and grafts.[9] For purposes of discussion, the nose can be divided into reconstruction of the upper two thirds and reconstruction of the lower third of the nose. For defects of the upper two thirds of the nose, the skin is less sebaceous than the lower third. Very large defects in the nasal sidewall and dorsum can be repaired with full-thickness skin grafts and good cosmetic results achieved if the wound depth is not significantly greater than the thickness of the grafted skin from postauricular or supraclavicular donor sites. For very deep defects, especially in thick sebaceous skin on the nose, a forehead flap provides a good result. Small midline defects up to 1 cm on the nose can be closed primarily with long vertical incisions extending from the nasal root to the inferior nasal tip and including extensive undermining at the level of perichondrium and nasal bone, essentially skeletonizing the nasal tip and dorsum. This

technique may narrow the nose slightly but usually provides an excellent cosmetic result. Small defects on the nasal sidewall can also be closed primarily or may be closed with small inferior and laterally based transposition flaps.

The lower third of the nose is more difficult to repair because of the unique thick sebaceous skin, limited opportunity to recruit nearby skin, and the need to prevent distortion of the tip or alar rim. For defects of the tip, long primary closure as noted earlier usually works well with wounds less than 1 cm in diameter. Defects on the lateral tip or sidewall up to 1.5 cm can be repaired with a bilobed flap (Fig. 80-6).[10] For defects of the lower sidewall and ala, a single-stage nasolabial flap using cheek skin can provide a very good result if care is taken in the design to excise Burow's triangle superiorly and advance the cheek skin while closing the donor site by tacking the suture line to the immobile tissue above periosteum in the area of the lateral ala and the triangular portion of the upper lip. This preserves the alar crease, prevents tenting across the nasolabial fold, and minimizes the risk of trapdooring. The flap should be trimmed of excess fat before suturing into the defect (Fig. 80-7). Defects of the ala alone may be repaired with a two-stage nasolabial interpolation flap, especially if cartilage is necessary to support the alar rim.[11] Large defects on the tip and ala can be repaired nicely with a two-stage forehead flap

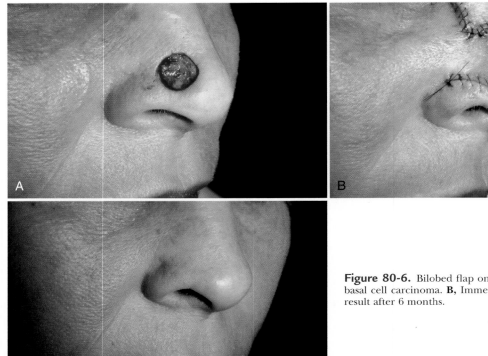

Figure 80-6. Bilobed flap on the nose. **A,** Defect after excision of a basal cell carcinoma. **B,** Immediate postoperative result. **C,** Cosmetic result after 6 months.

(Fig. 80-8). Grafts on the lower third of the nose are useful when the defect is small and no deeper than the thickness of grafted skin. The conchal bowl of the ear is a very good donor site for this area because the skin of the ear matches the skin of the nose better than any other donor skin. In addition, the donor site can heal by secondary intention by simply removing a small plug of cartilage in the center of the wound to allow granulation tissue to cover the remainder of cartilage and promote re-epithelialization of the wound.

Forehead, Temple, and Scalp

The majority of wounds on the forehead can be closed primarily, often even wounds up to 2 cm in diameter. However, contrary to popular practice, vertically oriented closures provide better results than horizontal closures do. Very small defects less than 1 cm may be closed horizontally. Anything 1 cm or larger may lift the brow and create asymmetry or an irregular pattern in the horizontal wrinkle lines of the forehead, and horizontal closures often result in a persistent numb area above the wound that is disturbing to patients. Skin grafts on the forehead are noticeable and are rarely a good choice for repair. In fact, when no good options for closure exist, allowing the wound to heal by secondary intention is usually better than a skin graft.

On the temple and lateral aspect of the forehead, primary closures are most useful, but with orientation along radial lines so that the closure is vertical on the lateral part of the forehead but horizontal when located lateral to the canthus. Transposition flaps may also be useful on the temple and lateral aspect of the forehead, especially near the hairline. In this area, special care to avoid the temporal branch of the facial nerve during excision and undermining is important.

Scalp

Most scalp wounds less than 2 cm in diameter can be closed primarily after wide undermining below the galea. For larger defects in hair-bearing skin, a very large rotation flap may cover the wound. Scalp skin stretches very little, and large wounds require a very large rotation flap. Healing by secondary intention is often a good choice, even in hair-bearing areas, because the defect contracts significantly and may result in a wound smaller than any secondary defect created during rotation of large flaps. Skin grafts on a balding scalp are a good choice for repair if the wound cannot be closed primarily. When periosteum is removed and bone is exposed, large flaps may be necessary to cover exposed bone. Burring of the bone to cause bleeding, followed by the application of a split-thickness skin graft, is a possible option, but burring of the outer cortex destroys its barrier function to invasion by tumor. Tumor recurrence in this area can then easily invade the bone, thus making treatment of recurrences a high-risk operation. Burring of bone as management of exposed bone should be a last resort.

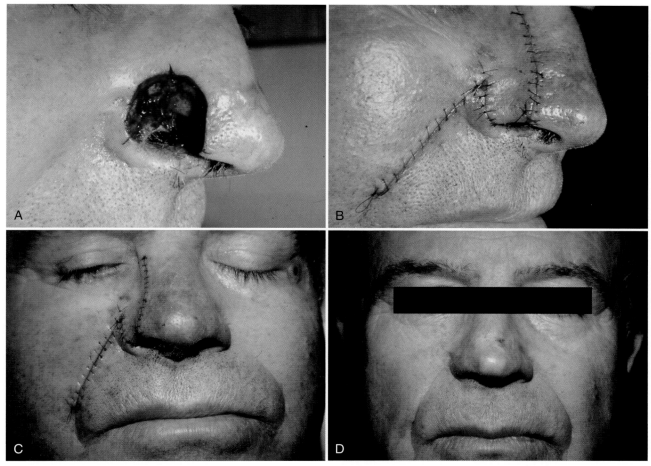

Figure 80-7. Single-stage nasolabial flap reconstruction of the nose. **A,** Defect of the ala with loss of the alar rim. **B,** Immediate postoperative result with the flap turned under the alar rim. **C,** Immediate result with preservation of all creases and sulci. **D,** Cosmetic result after 6 months.

Cheeks

The loose skin of the cheeks makes primary closure possible even for very large defects. Closures are usually oriented vertically in the lateral and preauricular parts of the cheek, are crescent shaped in the midcheek area, and are obliquely oriented parallel to the nasolabial fold for medial cheek defects. For large superior medial cheek defects unable to be closed primarily, full cheek rotation flaps provide good results (Fig. 80-9). Large wounds on the midportion of the cheek may be repaired with island pedicle flaps. Large lateral and inferior wounds can be repaired with transposition flaps consisting of loose skin from the neck area as well.

Neck

The neck, like the cheek, has the advantage of large amounts of loose skin, and therefore almost all wounds can be closed primarily or with transposition flaps.

POSTOPERATIVE MANAGEMENT

The immediate concerns during the postoperative period are pain and bleeding. Most patients claim that the aching or pain after skin cancer surgery is handled well by acetaminophen for minor procedures and minor narcotic pain relievers for larger procedures, especially for wounds under tension or those involving muscle. Bleeding is a risk, particularly in the first 6 to 8 hours postoperatively, and is minimized by careful intraoperative hemostasis, a well-placed dressing that applies pressure over the wound and undermined areas, and instructions to the patient to minimize physical activity. Patients should be instructed that if bleeding occurs, steady pressure for 20 minutes should stop most bleeding episodes.

After 4 weeks, when the wound has developed tensile strength, patients may massage their wounds to minimize swelling and firmness of the scar. Rarely is any scar revision worthwhile before 3 months. At 3 months dermabrasion of wounds on the nose may be helpful, and at 6 months re-evaluation of wounds for any other revision surgery can be considered.

Managing Open Wounds

Some wounds are best managed without reconstruction. Small biopsy wounds; wounds after excision of

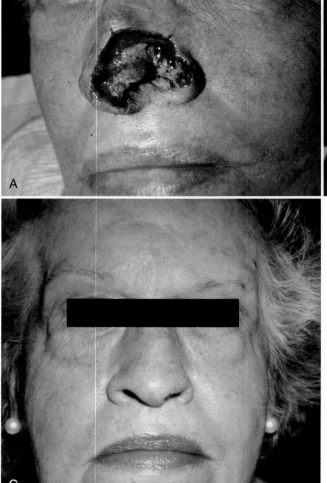

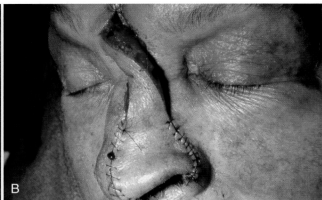

Figure 80-8. Paramedian forehead flap for large nasal reconstruction. **A,** Full-thickness defect of the nasal tip, ala, sidewall, and vestibular dome. **B,** Reconstruction with mucosal advancement for nasal lining, cartilage graft for support, and a paramedian forehead flap for skin coverage. **C,** Cosmetic result after 6 months.

small cancers at the medial canthus, alar crease, ear, forehead, and scalp; and even large graft donor sites may heal better by secondary intention than by reconstruction. Wounds in concave areas heal with better cosmetic results than do wounds on convex surfaces. Scars from wounds on pigmented skin or a red, ruddy complexion will be more noticeable than the same scar in pale, white skin. A scar is better camouflaged in skin with other lesions such as lentigines or keratoses than in flawless, smooth skin. All wounds contract and can therefore create distortion of nearby structures during healing, such as eclabion and ectropion. With these predictable events in mind, one can make a better informed decision about which wounds can heal and which wounds should be repaired.

COMPLICATIONS

Aside from pain and bleeding, most postoperative complications appear in the first few weeks. Surgical site infections are noted as early as 48 hours but most commonly 5 to 7 days after surgery. An infection is almost always *red* and *painful*. Purulent discharge may not be present. Redness may also be due to normal wound healing or be exaggerated by a tight closure, excess intraoperative electrocoagulation to control brisk bleeding, or poor tissue handling or suturing technique. The diagnosis of a surgical site infection is a clinical diagnosis by the surgeon alone. There is no absolute set of criteria for infection. Even culture results do not define infection; they serve as only a guide for appropriate antibiotic therapy once a diagnosis is made.

Hematoma at the surgical site should be drained if possible and can usually be achieved through a 1- to 2-cm opening in the incision line. Local anesthesia may be necessary if the blood is coagulated, and pressure is necessary to evacuate the hematoma. Interstitial hematomas occur when blood and fluid infiltrate the tissue without a pooled collection. They cannot be drained. Fortunately, interstitial hematomas resolve quickly and completely.

Necrosis of flaps and grafts may begin to occur at 1 week and develop over the subsequent few weeks. Because it is difficult to estimate the true extent of

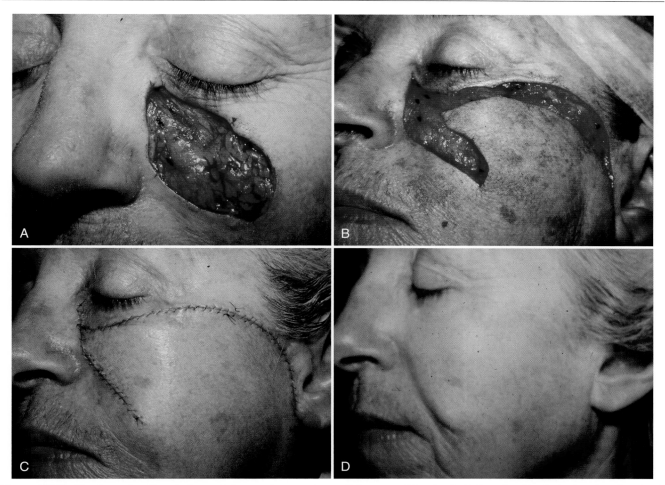

Figure 80-9. Cheek rotation flap. **A,** Large defect on the superior medial aspect of the cheek. **B,** Rotation flap incised and undermined. **C,** Immediate postoperative result. **D,** Cosmetic result at 6 months.

tissue loss in the first week or two, it is better to delay any decision to débride tissue until the full extent of necrosis is evident by the appearance of a black eschar or autolysis and separation of fully necrotic skin. Many times dark or violaceous tissue will heal nicely without the need for débridement. Early débridement is discouraged.

One frustrating event in the postoperative course is an open wound that fails to heal. Nonhealing wounds are often caused by one of three conditions. The most common is overgrowth of *Candida albicans* caused by the topical application of antibiotics and the use of occlusive dressings continuously for 3 weeks or longer. There may be no clinical evidence of infection by yeast. By simply adding or switching to a topical antiyeast medication, healing can be promoted. If the wound does not respond to antiyeast medications, the failure to heal may be related to a skin condition called erosive pustular dermatosis. This commonly occurs on the scalp and forehead, although it can be seen elsewhere as superficial erosions with thick yellow and greasy crusts. This condition responds

quickly to the topical application of potent corticosteroid creams.

When exuberant granulation tissue appears elevated over the wound edges, scraping it with a curette or scalpel may promote wound healing. Local anesthesia with epinephrine plus a pressure dressing is helpful to control oozing and bleeding. If the granulation tissue is only minimally elevated, it does not interfere with healing and no manipulation is necessary. Topical treatment of granulation tissue with silver nitrate or other caustic agents delays wound healing and is not recommended.

PATIENT EDUCATION

An important part of the postoperative management of patients after skin cancer surgery is education of the patient. Patients should be advised of their prognosis and risk for recurrence locally, regionally, and systemically, all of which differ according to tumor type, size, location, and treatment. Patients should be advised about their family risk as well. Patients with a history of melanoma and dysplastic nevus syndrome may have family members at increased risk who should be evaluated. Patients with sebaceous carcinoma are at increased risk for gastrointestinal malignancies because of its association with familial polyposis, and their families should also be screened.

Patients with a tumor at risk for regional recurrence in lymph nodes should be instructed in self-palpation of lymph nodes. Instruction should emphasize the method of palpation and that most regional disease is discovered first by the patient. Instruction may result in earlier detection by the patient before regularly scheduled follow-up appointments. One should emphasize the method of palpation and advise that involved nodes are not usually painful. They should also be instructed to palpate for satellite and in transit disease.

Most skin cancers are associated with ultraviolet light exposure. Patients should be instructed to minimize exposure to ultraviolet light through the liberal use of sunscreens and protective clothing. Sunscreens should absorb ultraviolet light in both the UVA and UVB range. Most people do not apply sunscreens liberally enough to get the absorption indicated on the label by the sun protective factor (SPF) value, so UVB protection ratings of SPF 30 or higher are better than a rating of 15. Sources of artificial light in tanning booths are just as harmful as sunlight and should be avoided as well.

FOLLOW-UP

Patients with a history of skin cancer have at least a 40% risk of a second skin cancer within the first 5 years after surgery and a higher risk if they have squamous cell carcinoma or a history of multiple skin cancers. For this reason they should be instructed in self-examination of their skin at least monthly with a description of the appearance of skin cancer. They should also be advised to undergo full-body skin examination by a dermatologist at least yearly to detect new skin cancers early. Follow-up schedules to observe for signs of local, regional, or distant disease depend on the tumor type and stage. For example, patients with high-risk tumors such as Merkel cell carcinoma, thick melanomas, or deep squamous cell carcinomas may be monitored every 2 months, whereas those with uncomplicated low-risk basal cell carcinoma should be scheduled for yearly follow-up.

Follow-up for evaluation of the cosmetic result of reconstruction varies with the procedure. Repairs at risk of contraction and distortion may benefit from the injection of high-dose intralesional steroids (triamcinolone, 40 mg/mL) 1 month after surgery in areas such as the lower eyelid or upper lip. Dermabrasion of suture lines on the thick sebaceous skin of the nose occasionally helps and is valuable at 3 months. Most other surgical revisions are best delayed until 6 months because of spontaneous improvement in the early stages of wound healing.

PEARLS

- Always have a pathology report from a biopsy of the lesion and understand its significance before planning surgery.
- Know the literature about skin cancer. There are standards for treatment that include surgical margins, laboratory and imaging evaluations, and the value of adjuvant therapy, including surgery, radiation therapy, immunotherapy, and chemotherapy.
- Learn how to visualize tumor margins with bright lights and stretching the skin.
- Respect the need for clear surgical margins and learn the meaning of the pathologist's interpretation of clear surgical margins.
- Practice quality assurance to improve the quality of patient care and the results of surgery.

PITFALLS

- Failure to respect local recurrence of disease results in a high risk for persistent disease when retreating recurrent cancer.
- The use of surgical excision as the only option for treating skin cancer overlooks important alternative choices, including destruction, Mohs surgery, radiation therapy, and topical therapy.
- Immediate reconstruction after excision of complex cancer before clear margins are documented may result in buried and fragmented persistent tumor and more difficult re-excision and repair options.
- Failure to seek the help of other specialists for difficult cancers may adversely affect patient care.
- Failure to arrange and ensure continued patient care may result in missed or delayed treatment of recurrent disease, as well as discovery of new primary skin cancers.

References

1. Zitelli JA: Mohs surgery—concepts and misconceptions. Int J Dermatol 24:541-548, 1985.
2. Cook J, Zitelli JA: Mohs micrographic surgery: A cost analysis. J Am Acad Dermatol 39:698-703, 1998.
3. Wolf DJ, Zitelli JA: Surgical margins for basal cell carcinoma. Arch Dermatol 123:213-215, 1987.
4. Brodland DG, Zitelli JA: Surgical margins for excision of primary cutaneous squamous cell carcinoma. J Am Acad Dermatol 27:241-248, 1992.
5. Bricca GM, Brodland DG, Ren D, et al: Cutaneous head and neck melanoma treated with Mohs micrographic surgery. J Am Acad Dermatol 52:92-100, 2005.
6. Morton DL, Cochran AJ, Thompson JF, et al: Sentinel node biopsy for early-stage melanoma: Accuracy and morbidity in MSLT-I, an international multicenter trial. Ann Surg 242:302-313, 2005.

7. Abide JM, Nahai F, Bennett RG: The meaning of surgical margins. Plast Reconstr Surg 73:492-497, 1984.

8. Zitelli JA, Brodland DG: A regional approach to reconstruction of the upper lip. J Dermatol Surg Oncol 17:143-148, 1991.

9. Burget GC, Menick FJ: Aesthetic Reconstruction of the Nose. Chicago, CV Mosby, 1994.

10. Zitelli JA: The bilobed flap in nasal reconstruction. Arch Dermatol 125:957-959, 1989.

11. Zitelli JA: The nasolabial flap as a single-stage procedure. Arch Dermatol 126:1445-1448, 1990.

Chapter **81**

Microvascular Reconstruction of the Head and Neck

Frederic W.-B. Deleyiannis, Brian R. Gastman, and James M. Russavage

The goals of reconstruction are to restore premorbid function and quality of life. Successful reconstruction requires careful consideration of both the surgical defect and patient-specific variables, such as general health, radiation status, and dental rehabilitation. Cardiac, vascular, and pulmonary disease, as well as alcoholism, are common in patients with cancer of the head and neck and may independently have an impact on survival and limit reconstructive options. For example, the fibula would be a poor donor site in an individual with severe lower extremity peripheral vascular disease. Radiation induces soft tissue fibrosis, in particular, perivascular fibrosis. Therefore, a history of previous radiation therapy with its anticipated decreased vascularity may guide reconstructive options toward using a pedicled or free flap instead of a skin graft.

The anticipated defect should be classified according to the extent of rigid, soft tissue, and neurologic components. When possible, resected tissue should be reconstructed with tissue that duplicates both the appearance and the function of the resected tissue. Epithelium can be used to resurface mucosal or skin defects, muscle can be used to restore bulk and motion, and palatal and mandibular skeletal defects can be reconstructed with bone. Skin grafts, local or regional flaps, prosthetic devices, and free tissue transfer are among the range of options that the reconstructive surgeon must possess to customize the reconstruction to an individual patient.

Free tissue transfer offers a well-accepted, superior ability to restore form and function with certain major head and neck defects. Microvascular surgery provides distinct advantages for reconstruction of osseous defects of the mandible, large glossectomy defects, total or near-total pharyngeal defects, and complex defects of the midface and skull base.

PATIENT SELECTION AND PREOPERATIVE EVALUATION

Early experience with free flaps was primarily concerned with free skin flaps (i.e., the free groin flap and free dorsalis pedis artery flap). As experience with microsurgery grew and knowledge about vascular anatomy expanded, transfer of musculocutaneous and osteocutaneous flaps became as commonplace as transfer of free cutaneous flaps. Theoretically, any tissue with a defined vascular circuit can be transferred as a free flap, but for head and neck reconstruction, eight free flaps are particularly useful: the radial forearm, parascapular and scapular, lateral arm, rectus abdominis, fibula, iliac crest, and anterolateral thigh flaps.

Radial Forearm Free Flap

The radial forearm free flap (RFFF) is a fasciocutaneous free flap that derives it blood supply from branches of the radial artery running in the intermuscular septum between the brachioradialis and flexor carpi radialis muscles.[1] The major advantage of the RFFF is the large amount of thin forearm skin that can be harvested for reconstruction of any associated intraoral or external skin defect. A segment of radius vascularized by vessels passing from the radial artery through the lateral intermuscular septum and perforating vessels through the muscle belly of the flexor pollicis longus may be transferred with the RFFF (Fig. 81-1). Approximately 10 cm of bone can be harvested between the insertion of the pronator teres and the insertion of the brachioradialis. A "boat-shaped" osteotomy as opposed to right-angle bone cuts may help avoid the complication of fracture.[2] Only 30% of the cross-sectional area of the radius should be removed to preserve the structural integrity

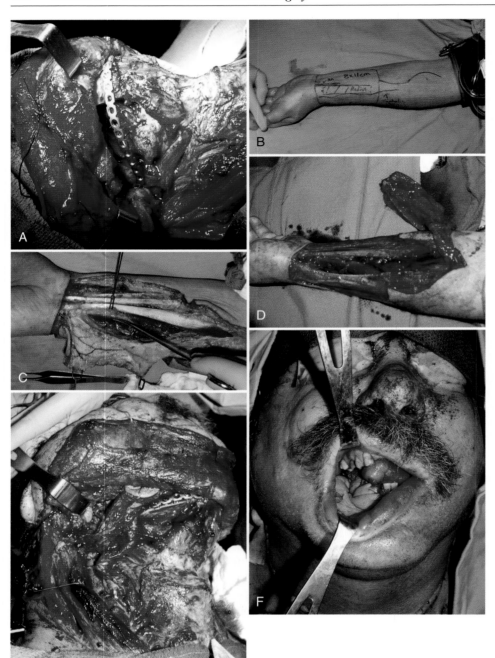

Figure 81-1. Osteocutaneous radial forearm free flap for a lateral mandibular defect. **A,** Lateral mandibular and floor of the mouth defect after resection of T4 carcinoma. **B,** Flap design with the radius, skin paddle, cephalic vein, and radial artery marked. **C,** Perforators to the radius from the radial artery traversing through the flexor pollicis longus and pronator quadratus identified. **D,** Keel-shaped osteotomies from the insertion point of the brachioradialis to the origin of the pronator teres. **E,** Inset of the radius with the skin paddle used for reconstruction of the floor of the mouth. **F,** Final closure.

of the radius. Provided that the periosteum is carefully preserved on the volar and radial aspects of the segment of the radius, one or two osteotomies may be performed from the medullary aspect to allow reconstruction of anterior symphyseal and parasymphyseal defects. Whereas the anterior projection of the anterior mandible can be re-created with an osteotomized radial forearm osteocutaneous flap, the vertical height of the anterior mandible cannot be created. The bony segment of the radius is usually too thin to allow placement of osseointegrated implants. The antebrachial cutaneous

nerves of the forearm can be incorporated into the flap to make the RFFF a sensate flap. However, spontaneous return of flap sensation has been documented in patients who underwent reconstruction of the oral cavity with noninnervated flaps.[3]

An Allen's test should be performed before harvesting or RFFF to assess the adequacy of ulnar collateral circulation to the hand. If a positive Allen's test is detected, one should use a different flap for reconstruction or be prepared to replace the radial artery with a vein graft.

Scapular and Parascapular Fasciocutaneous and Osteocutaneous Flaps

The branching pattern of the circumflex scapular artery and vein permits the harvest of a number of fasciocutaneous and osteocutaneous flaps for reconstruction of the oral cavity. The scapular flap is based on the horizontal cutaneous branch of the circumflex scapular artery (Fig. 81-2). The parascapular flap is based on the descending cutaneous branch of the circumflex scapular artery. Up to 14 cm of the lateral border of the scapula vascularized by periosteal branches from the circumflex scapular artery and vein can be isolated. Unlike other osteocutaneous flaps, the scapular bone and the two skin paddles can be orientated independently of one another for reconstruction of complex three-dimensional defects.[4] In addition, the latissimus dorsi and serratus anterior muscles vascularized by the thoracodorsal artery and vein can be harvested with the scapular flaps based on the common vascular pedicle of the subscapular artery and vein.

The disadvantages of these flaps are that they require harvesting in the lateral position, the lateral border of the scapula is quite thin and may preclude secondary osseointegration, and the segmental periosteal blood supply may be compromised if multiple osteotomies are required to shape the scapula for anterior defects. The skin on the back can also be the thickest in the body, and with obesity these flaps can be quite thick.

Lateral Arm Flap

The lateral arm flap is a reliable fasciocutaneous flap that has the distinct advantages that its vascular supply, the profunda brachii artery, is a nonessential artery whose harvest does not jeopardize the vascular supply to the upper extremity and the donor site can be closed

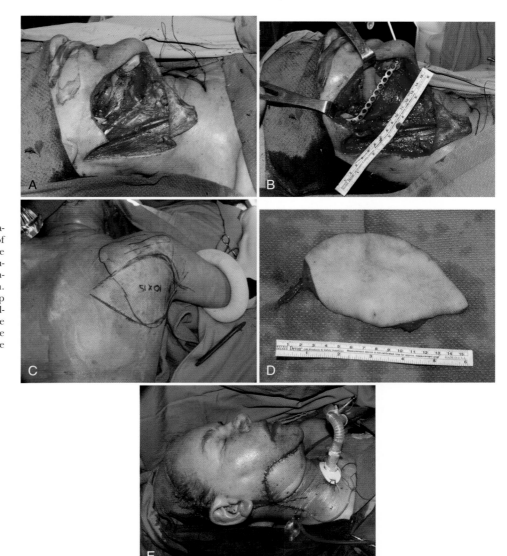

Figure 81-2. Scapular fasciocutaneous flap. **A,** Composite resection of the lateral mandible, floor of the mouth, and cheek skin. **B,** Mandibular continuity restored with a reconstruction plate. **C,** Flap design. **D,** Scapular flap harvested. **E,** Flap inset with a strip of skin de-epithelialized to allow two skin paddles—one for the cheek and neck skin and one for reconstruction of the floor of the mouth.

with a linear scar.[5] The axis of the flap is centered on the lateral intermuscular septum, which is located between the triceps posteriorly and the brachialis and the brachioradialis anteriorly (Fig. 81-3). After the profunda brachii branches from the brachial artery, it travels in the spiral groove with the radial nerve. As the profunda brachii enters the septum, it divides into anterior and posterior radial collateral arteries. The posterior radial collateral artery supplies the lateral arm flap. The vascular pedicle is usually ligated in the spiral groove, but additional length can be obtained by dissecting deep to the lateral and long head of the triceps. The posterior cutaneous nerve of the arm, which is closely associated with the posterior radial collateral artery, can be incorporated into the flap to make the lateral arm flap a sensate flap. Donor site complications, including radial nerve palsy and hyperesthesia of the proximal lateral forearm skin caused by damage to the posterior cutaneous nerve of the forearm, have been reported but are seldom seen.

Rectus Abdominis Free Musculocutaneous Flap

The rectus abdominis free musculocutaneous flap is based on periumbilical perforators from the deep inferior epigastric arteries.[6] Incorporation of the periumbilical perforators permits the skin paddle to be oriented in virtually any direction from the midline (Fig. 81-4). After the perforators are identified, the anterior rectus sheath is incised medial to the linea semilunaris and lateral to the linea alba. To preserve the strength of the abdominal wall, the anterior rectus sheath should not be harvested below the arcuate line. Inferiorly, the anterior rectus sheath is incised vertically to completely expose the rectus muscle. The deep inferior epigastric pedicle is identified after the rectus muscle is bluntly dissected free from the posterior rectus sheath. The vascular pedicle, up to 15 cm in length, is exposed all the way to the origin of the vessels from the external iliac artery and vein. The intercostal nerves that supply the rectus muscle and overlying skin are mixed sensory and motor nerves, but microanastomosis to a sensory nerve in the head and neck has not yet resulted in a report of restoration of sensation. Closure of the abdominal wall can be accomplished by direct approximation of the residual anterior fascial margins. Few reports have quantified the functional effect of harvesting a single rectus muscle on lifestyle. Most surgeons would agree that unless patients are engaged in vigorous physical activity, harvest of a unilateral rectus muscle has little impact.

Fibular Free Flap

The fibula is our first line choice for mandibular reconstruction (Fig. 81-5). It can be transferred as a free osseous, free osteocutaneous, or free osteomuscular flap.[7] The skin of the lateral aspect of the calf is supplied by septocutaneous perforators that traverse the posterior crural septum between the posterior compartment muscles (the gastrocnemius and soleus) and the

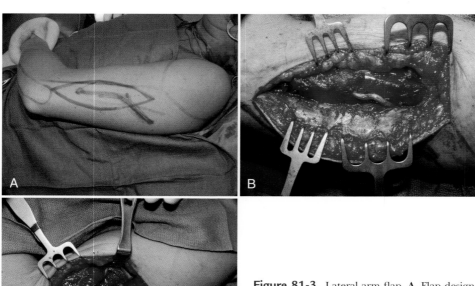

Figure 81-3. Lateral arm flap. **A,** Flap design with the position of the posterior radial collateral artery marked in red. **B,** Radial nerve identified. **C,** Flap harvested.

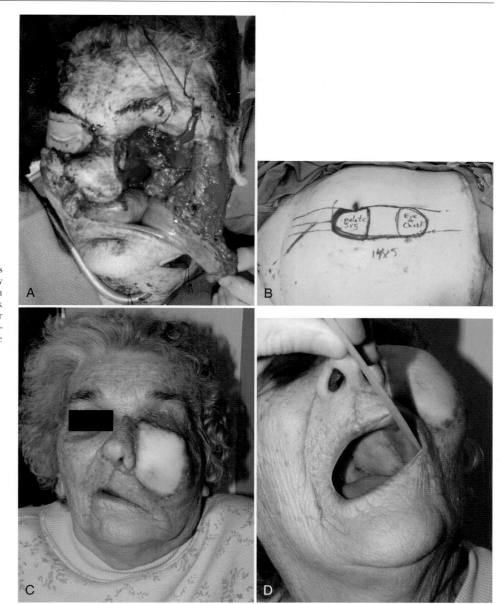

Figure 81-4. Rectus myocutaneous free flap. **A,** Total orbitomaxillectomy defect. **B,** Flap design with two skin paddles—one for orbit and cheek skin reconstruction and the other for palate reconstruction. **C,** Postoperative frontal view. **D,** Postoperative view of the palatal reconstruction.

lateral anterior compartment muscles (the peroneus longus and brevis). Musculocutaneous perforators that run through the flexor hallucis and soleus may also supply the skin. Consequently, when harvesting an osteocutaneous fibular flap, one should include a cuff of flexor hallucis and soleus muscle to protect these perforators. Even with care taken to protect the septocutaneous and musculocutaneous perforators, loss of the skin paddle has been reported in 5% to 10% of cases. The fibula may be harvested with a lateral cuff of soleus muscle without a skin paddle and be used to replace oral lining by allowing the exposed muscle to mucosalize. The fibula will provide up to 26 cm of bone vascularized by the peroneal artery and its two venae comitantes. The peroneal artery provides both endosteal and periosteal blood supply to the fibula, and con-

sequently blood supply to multiple bony segments of the fibula can be maintained through these segmental periosteal perforators after multiple osteotomies of the fibula. The cross-sectional area of the fibula approximates the cross-sectional area of the midbody of the mandible and is ideally suited for placement of osseointegrated implants for dental rehabilitation.

The need for preoperative vascular assessment before fibular transfer is controversial. Large series performed without preoperative imaging have reported no adverse sequelae, yet given the prevalence of risk factors for peripheral vascular disease in the head and neck cancer population, others have stressed the need for vascular evaluation. According to Futran and colleagues, ankle-arm index screening and color flow Doppler imaging may be more economical and efficient ways to

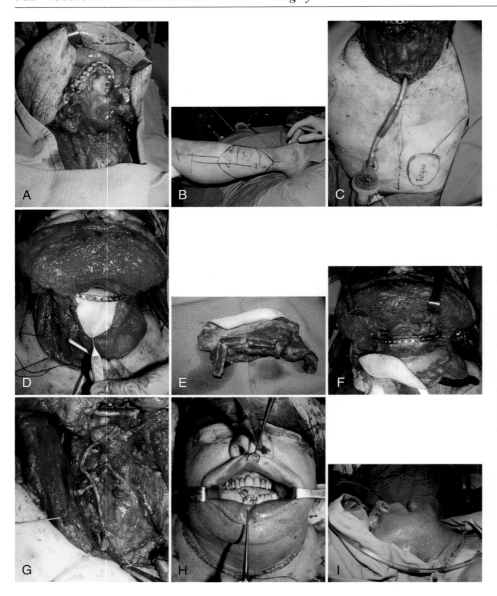

Figure 81-5. Fibular osteocutaneous free flap and pectoralis major myocutaneous flap for near-total mandibulectomy and total glossectomy. **A,** Near-total mandibulectomy and total glossectomy defect. **B,** Osteocutaneous fibular free flap design with the skin perforators (P) marked. The skin paddle is to be used for floor of the mouth and anterior tongue reconstruction. **C,** Pectoralis flap for posterior tongue reconstruction. **D,** Inset of the pectoralis flap. **E,** Closing wedge osteotomies of the fibula. **F,** Inset of the fibular free flap with the skin paddle to be rotated over the plate and sewn to the pectoralis flap. **G,** Inset of the greater saphenous vein graft into the proximal internal jugular vein stump. Both internal jugular veins had been ligated during the resection. **H,** Final inset—oral cavity. **I,** Final inset—lateral view.

evaluate the vasculature of the lower extremity than angiography or magnetic resonance angiography.[8]

Two criticisms of use of the fibular free flap have been the height discrepancy between the fibular bone and the native mandible and the inability to reconstruct associated large soft tissue defects (e.g., large glossectomy defects or through-and-through defects). Recent innovations have addressed these criticisms. Jones and associates described a "double-barrel" technique in which the fibula is folded on itself to effectively double the height of the neomandible.[9] In conjunction with a fibula free flap, large soft tissue defects can be repaired with a second flap, either an RFFF or a pectoralis myocutaneous flap. After free fibula harvest, most patients will have some decrease in their range of motion of ankle plantar flexion and dorsiflexion and loss of knee and ankle strength. However, as demonstrated by Anthony and coworkers, these decreases are not severe

enough to have an impact on patients' daily activities.[10]

Iliac Crest

As the popularity of the fibula flap has grown, the indications for use of an iliac crest free flap have decreased. The iliac crest will provide a large segment of corticocancellous bone, up to 14 cm in length, vascularized by the deep circumflex iliac artery and its two venae comitantes.[11] The deep circumflex iliac vessels can be dissected to their origin from the external iliac vessels to provide a pedicle length between 8 and 10 cm. The height of the native mandible can be matched by harvesting an appropriate amount of bone from the iliac crest (Fig. 81-6). Depending on the location of the mandibular defect, preoperative planning with models of the mandible and iliac crest will help the surgeon pattern the segment of

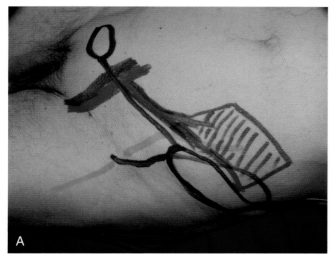

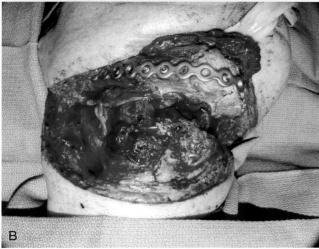

Figure 81-6. Iliac crest—internal oblique free flap. **A,** Flap design with the expected internal oblique muscle harvest indicated in purple. **B,** Iliac crest inset for restoration of an anterior mandibular defect.

the iliac crest bone on the ipsilateral or contralateral iliac crest to use the normal curve of the superior iliac crest. Cutaneous perforators along the medial aspect of the iliac crest supply an area of overlying skin that can be harvested with the bone as an osteocutaneous flap. To preserve these cutaneous perforators, a cuff of external oblique muscle, internal oblique muscle, and transversus abdominis muscle through which the perforators traverse should be harvested. The thickness of the overlying subcutaneous tissue can make an osteocutaneous iliac crest flap too bulky for intraoral use. To decrease the bulkiness, one can harvest the iliac crest bone with a paddle of internal oblique muscle (supplied by the ascending branch of the deep circumflex artery), which is then skin-grafted.

Femoral nerve injury, hernia, gait disturbance, and pain are potential donor site morbidities. Harvest of the internal oblique muscle can also cause denervation of the rectus abdominis through interruption of its motor nerve supply, which runs between the internal oblique and transversus abdominis. Forrest and coauthors reported on donor site complications in 82 patients who underwent transfer of a free iliac crest flap.[12] Sensory disturbances (27%), contour irregularity (20%), poor scar (12%), hernia (10%), gait disturbance (11%), and pain lasting longer than 1 year (8%) were documented.

Jejunal Free Flap

The jejunal free flap was the first free tissue transfer reported in the literature in 1959. Its continued use for circumferential pharyngeal defects is a testimony to its time-tested importance in head and neck reconstruction. This flap can be used as a mucosal tube or as a patch. Its advantages for pharyngeal reconstruction include a diameter that matches that of the cervical esophagus, the potential for peristalsis, and innate secretory ability. Large series report success rates higher than 90% with fistula rates between 15% and 20%.[13] The jejunum can now be harvested laparoscopically, thereby reducing much of the postoperative convalescence.[14]

Some of the relative disadvantages of this flap include abdominal complication rates as high as 5.8%.[15] Tracheoesophageal puncture (TEP) speech may be less discernible than that with other flaps because of the intrinsic moistness of the jejunum. The serosa of the flap may also impede neovascularization, which may place the flap in jeopardy if the pedicle is divided during subsequent head and neck surgery. In addition, the plicae circularis of the jejunum may trap food and cause significant halitosis.

Flap harvest is usually performed by qualified general surgeons and may be done simultaneously with the extirpative procedure. Preoperative bowel preparation is not essential. The jejunal arteries arise from the superior mesenteric artery and form a series of vascular arcades that run in the mesentery. Large segments of jejunum can be harvested by proximally dividing a single jejunal vessel that feeds multiple arcades.

To limit ischemia to the jejunum, one should divide the pedicle only after the pharyngeal defect and recipient vessels have been prepared. During inset, if there is a size mismatch at the level of the base of tongue, the antimesenteric border may be divided to "open" up the proximal end. Any redundancy in the jejunum after inset may cause the jejunum to fold on itself and become a barrier to food transport. To prevent such redundancy, we perform the base of the tongue inset first and then the vascular microanastomosis. With perfusion re-established the jejunum expands, and after this expansion we resect any redundant jejunum before completing the mucosal anastomosis to the cervical esophagus. A jejunal feeding tube is usually placed because long-term supplementation may be required even after oral intake of food has begun.

Anterolateral Thigh Flap

The anterolateral thigh free flap has recently gained popularity in soft tissue reconstruction of the head and neck.[16] It is a perforator flap derived from the descending branch of the lateral circumflex femoral artery. Its advantages include a long pedicle with a suitable vessel diameter and the possibility of harvesting the flap with thigh musculature (the vastus lateralis, rectus femoris, tensor fasciae lata, or any combination of these muscles) or as a sensate flap (by incorporating the anterior branch of the lateral cutaneous nerve of the thigh). Because of its distance from the head and neck, harvest can be performed simultaneously with tumor extirpation.

Flap elevation begins by mapping the cutaneous perforators with a pencil Doppler probe. These perforators are located by first marking the midpoint between the anterior superior iliac spine and the superolateral corner of the patella (Fig. 81-7A and B). A circle centered at this midpoint is then drawn with a radius of 3 cm. The majority of the cutaneous perforators are located in the inferolateral quadrant of this circle. The flap is then harvested with its center over these perforators and its long axis parallel to that of the thigh. The flap can be elevated with or without the fascia lata (suprafascial dissection). The skin and subcutaneous tissue of the flap are raised until the perforator or perforators to the skin are defined. Once the skin vessel or vessels are seen, they are dissected until the main pedicle is reached (Fig. 81-7C). If the skin vessel is a musculocutaneous perforator (the majority of patients), harvest includes intramuscular dissection through the vastus lateralis muscle. If the skin vessel is a septocutaneous perforator, the dissection is simpler and proceeds between the vastus lateralis and rectus femoris muscles.[16] The length of the pedicle is 8 to 16 cm, with a vessel diameter larger than 2 mm.

A skin defect of less than 9 cm in width can be closed primarily without any reported evidence of compartment syndrome. Larger defects require skin grafting. A distinct disadvantage is the thickness of the flap in overweight individuals. However, the flap can be trimmed to the subdermal fat level for use as a thinner flap (4 mm). In subfascial dissections, loss of the fascia lata may leave a bulge in the lateral aspect of the thigh. The vastus lateralis muscle is a major constituent of the quadriceps femoris. However, in cases in which the vastus lateralis has been taken for reconstructive purposes, nearly normal quadriceps function has been reported.[17]

SURGICAL APPROACHES

Mandibular Defects

The indications for mandibular reconstruction remain a subject of legitimate controversy. The fact that major mandibular resection carries with it significant functional and cosmetic sequelae is undisputed, but the effect of mandibular resection on function is highly variable. The level of postoperative disability depends on (1) the preoperative condition of the oral cavity (including the presence or absence of viable teeth), (2) the extent of mandible to be included in the resection, (3) the site of the tumor (anterior versus lateral), and (4) the soft tissues to be resected. When the mandible is resected with an accompanying large soft tissue defect, the mandibular defect is sometimes "incidental" to the

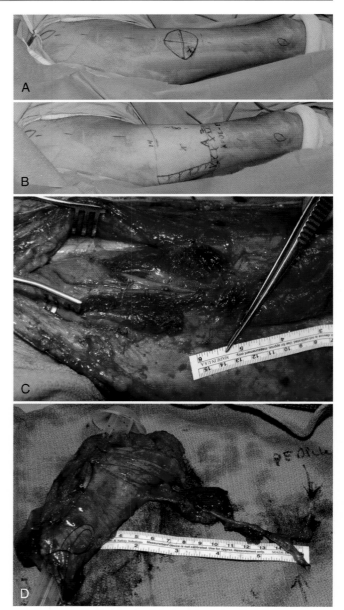

Figure 81-7. Anterior lateral thigh flap (ALTF). **A,** *Circle* marking the location of the cutaneous perforator. **B,** Flap design based on the location of the perforator. **C,** A single musculocutaneous perforator supplies the entire flap. **D,** Total pharyngeal reconstruction using the ALTF. The fascia lata has been wrapped around the reconstruction for an additional layer of closure.

rest of the wound. Closure of the soft tissue defect with restoration of function and coverage of the planned mandibular reconstruction becomes the primary goal.

The extent of mandibular resection is critical in predicting the disability secondary to surgery. Some patients function well after segmental lateral mandibulectomy without restoration of mandibular continuity. However, a contour deformity of the lower third of the face will develop in patients whose defects have not been reconstructed, and the pull of the contralateral muscles of mastication displaces the remaining mandible toward the side of the defect. In patients with dentition this results in malocclusion. For these reasons, most surgeons offer patients primary reconstruction of lateral mandibular defects.

Numerous reports have supported the use of a reconstruction plate with soft tissue coverage to reconstruct pure lateral mandibular defects (see Fig. 81-2). Soft tissue coverage has generally been provided by a pectoralis myocutaneous flap or an RFFF. Delayed reconstructive failure secondary to external plate exposure or plate fracture has generally been reported to occur in 5% to 7% of cases. For lateral mandibular defects, Shpitzer and colleagues advocate the use of an osteocutaneous free flap.[18] In their report comparing three different reconstruction techniques for lateral mandibular defects (plate and pectoralis major myocutaneous flap [PMMF], plate and RFFF, and osteocutaneous flap), plates had to be removed in 7 of the 27 patients in the PMMF group and 2 of the 16 patients in the RFFF group. None of the 14 osteocutaneous free flaps failed. Speech was also best in the osteocutaneous free flap group.

Anterior mandibular resection can leave a patient an oral cripple. When reconstruction is not attempted, the retained segments of the mandible tend to collapse toward the midline. This lack of support results in an Andy Gump deformity with associated oral incontinence and cosmetic deformity. Schusterman and associates, in a study of the use of AO plates for immediate mandibular reconstruction, noted an unacceptably high rate of plate failure in patients with anterior defects.[19] Plate extrusion developed in four of the six patients (66%) who underwent reconstruction of anterior defects with a plate and soft tissue flap. Free tissue transfer of a composite osteocutaneous flap was thus advocated as the reconstructive method of choice. However, all centers do not report such a high rate of anterior plate failure. In an evaluation of 51 cases of primary mandibular reconstruction with the titanium hollow-screw reconstruction plate, Irish and coauthors reported a 19% incidence of plate failure in patients with anterior defects and a 13% incidence of failure with lateral defects.[20] In their experience with 102 stainless steel and titanium bridging plates, the success rate was 83% for lateral defects and 65% for anterior defects at 2-year follow-up.[21]

Given the long-term problems of plate fracture and exposure, we prefer to perform free vascularized bony reconstruction for both lateral defects and anterior defects (see Figs. 81-1 and 81-5). In patients who are unwilling or unable to undergo free vascularized bone transfer becomes of significant comorbidity, poor prognosis, or lack of recipient vessels, we perform a plate and soft tissue flap reconstruction. If the goal of reconstruction with a pectoralis flap is simply to close the wound and allow a patient to avoid complications, one should consider using a pectoralis flap only for soft tissue reconstruction without restoration of mandibular continuity with a reconstruction plate.[22]

Glossectomy Defects

Restoration of tongue function after ablative surgery remains a major challenge for the reconstructive surgeon. The ultimate goal is to restore form and function, but the complex set of intrinsic and extrinsic muscles that provide coordinated motor activity cannot be duplicated by reinnervated muscle flaps. It is unrealistic to expect a unidirectional, reinnervated muscle, such as the rectus abdominis, to mimic the complex pattern of muscle contraction in the native tongue. The attainable goals of tongue reconstruction are preservation of the mobility of the remaining tongue, restoration of bulk so that the neotongue can contact the palate to assist in articulation and swallowing, and restoration of sensation.

The extent of the glossectomy and the presence or absence of an associated mandibulectomy defect determine one's approach to reconstruction.[23] Because of the different functions of the two regions, the tongue is divided into the mobile anterior part and the tongue base. The mobility of the anterior tongue is critical for articulation, mastication, and the oral phase of swallowing. The tongue base is critical in completing the pharyngeal phase of swallowing. The approach to reconstructing the mobile tongue should involve the use of thin, sensate, pliable tissues that maintain maximum mobility and potentially restore sensation. Defects of the tongue base present a separate problem. The volume of the tongue base must be restored so that it can contact the pharyngeal walls and generate force to drive the food bolus through the pharynx.

The combination of a segmental mandibulectomy defect and a partial glossectomy defect involving the mobile tongue or both the mobile tongue and base of tongue is a more challenging reconstruction. The reconstructive options begin with first choosing the optimal flap for tongue reconstruction and then considering the options for the mandible. Two free flaps, in particular, a forearm flap with a fibular flap, may be necessary for complex composite defects. For segmental defects less than 8 cm and with significant tongue defects, an osteocutaneous RFFF is often our first choice. Lateral composite mandibular defects may be reconstructed with a fasciocutaneous free flap or a pedicled flap and a mandibular reconstruction plate. Soft tissue reconstruction without restoration of lateral mandibular continuity can also yield satisfactory outcomes.

Total tongue reconstruction involves creating bulk for the neotongue and positioning the neotongue so that its vertical height is sufficient to achieve contact with the palate. Free musculocutaneous flaps, in particular, the rectus abdominis free flap, have the advantage that the muscle of the flap can be used as a platform for positioning the overlying fat and skin components. Drill holes placed in the mandible can be used to secure the muscle. The tendinous inscriptions in the rectus abdominis flap offer better purchase for sutures than do those directly placed in muscle. Fasciocutaneous free flaps, such as forearm, scapular, parascapular, or anterolateral thigh, can also be de-epithelialized and folded on themselves to create additional bulk and help maintain the position of the neotongue. Total tongue defects can also be reconstructed with a pectoralis major myocutaneous flap (see Fig. 81-5C and D).

Because of its bulk, an iliac crest osteocutaneous flap should be considered for reconstruction of total glossectomy defects with anterior mandibular defects.

Pharyngectomy Defect

The major goal of pharyngeal reconstruction is restoration of swallowing. Laryngeal preservation in the setting of a major pharyngeal defect is especially challenging because aspiration is inevitable. In addition to the patient's preoperative function, designing a reconstruction that can minimize aspiration may be the critical issue that determines whether patients will be able to keep their larynx. It is important to choose a flap that can be inset at the level of the hypopharynx both to prevent stenosis and to not be too bulky and cause obstruction. Although the pectoralis major flap has been used with success, the radial forearm flap offers many advantages.[24] Its pliability allows exact replacement of the hypopharyngeal mucosa. In addition, with a radial forearm flap a nonvascularized rib graft can be used to reconstruct the infrastructure of the larynx.[25] Anastomosis of an antebrachial cutaneous nerve of the forearm flap with the superior laryngeal nerve may assist the neopharynx in regaining sensation.

In most cases of advanced laryngopharyngeal or pharyngeal carcinoma the larynx is resected. When a strip of hypopharyngeal mucosa remains after total laryngopharyngectomy, controversy exists concerning the relative benefits of resecting the remaining mucosa and converting the defect to a circumferential defect. Preservation of the remaining mucosa and incorporation of this mucosa into the reconstruction may reduce the risk of stenosis. However, the additional suture lines may place the reconstruction at greater risk for a fistula than is the case with a tubed free flap.

For circumferential defects the jejunal free flap has been the "gold standard."[26] It requires no tubing and thus one less suture line. Most studies report that the jejunal free flap has stenosis and fistula rates that are lower than or equal to those of tubed fasciocutaneous flaps.[27] The major alternative to the jejunum is a tubed RFFF (Fig. 81-8). Its advantages over the jejunum include the lack of abdominal harvest, better TEP speech, and the ability to create separate skin paddles for cervical skin reconstruction.[27] The use of a Montgomery stent may lower fistula and stenosis rates.[28] The anterolateral thigh free flap may also be used for pharyngeal reconstruction and has the additional advantage that the fascia lata may be included to provide an extra layer of closure for the neopharynx (see Fig. 81-7D). Studies are ongoing to determine the effectiveness of this reconstruction.[29]

If the cervical esophageal resection extends below the thoracic inlet, most reconstructive surgeons would not place a reconstructive suture line within the chest because of the increased morbidity of a salivary leak. Gastric pull-up continues to be the gold standard for defects that extend below the thoracic inlet.

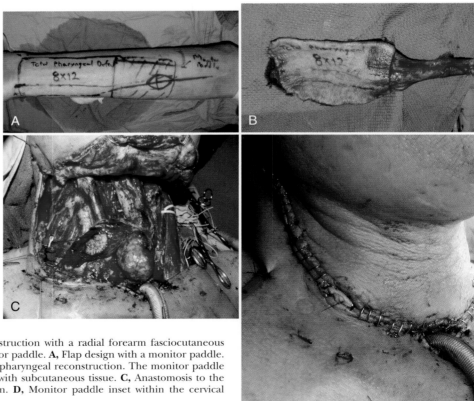

Figure 81-8. Total pharyngeal reconstruction with a radial forearm fasciocutaneous free flap (RFFF) harvested with a monitor paddle. **A,** Flap design with a monitor paddle. **B,** The RFFF tubed for circumferential pharyngeal reconstruction. The monitor paddle is connected to the tubed skin paddle with subcutaneous tissue. **C,** Anastomosis to the right transverse cervical artery and vein. **D,** Monitor paddle inset within the cervical incision.

Midface and Maxillectomy Defects

Defects in the midface occur after resection of tumors that arise from the paranasal sinuses, palate, overlying skin, nasal cavity, skull base, orbital contents, or oral mucosa. As a result, extensive midface reconstructions may require independently reconstructing the palate, orbit, cheek, and bony midface (maxilla and zygoma).

Recently, Cordeiro and Santamaria proposed a classification system and algorithm for reconstruction of maxillectomy and midfacial structures.[30] The temporalis muscle, soft tissue free flaps (rectus abdominis and radial forearm), nonvascularized bone (rib or calvaria), and vascularized bone flaps (osteocutaneous RFFF) were used to construct a variety of maxillectomy defects. Palatal defects were closed only with soft tissue (see Fig. 81-4). The nonvascularized and vascularized bone was used for osseous reconstruction of the zygoma, maxilla, and orbital floor.

Other algorithms containing many other free flaps and designs have been adopted.[31] Many have focused on various osteocutaneous flaps such as the fibula and the iliac crest. These latter flaps allow osteointegration of implants for dental rehabilitation.[32] In cases of combined midface and lip resection, oral competency can be restored by using local flaps, such as the Abbé lip switch flap, in combination with free tissue transfer.

Skull Base Defects

Although small defects can and should be reconstructed with local flaps, such as pericranial or temporoparietal fascial flaps, many defects in the expanding spectrum of extirpative endeavors will require free tissue transfer.[33] The main reconstructive needs of skull base defects include separating the intracranial and extracranial spaces to avoid intracranial infections, obliterating the dead space with coverage of vital structures, preventing brain herniation, diminishing the risk of cerebrospinal fluid leakage, and restoring cosmesis.

The rectus and latissimus myocutaneous (or myofascial) free flaps (Fig. 81-9) are two of the flaps commonly chosen.[34] The rich vascular supply of the flaps' muscle component can allow neovascularization of dural reconstructions and free bone grafts, and their large subcutaneous fat and skin islands can obliterate dead space and be used to reconstruct any skin deficit. In some instances of massive resection, multiple flaps may be needed. In such cases the subscapular artery system allows a combination of flaps based on one pedicle. For example, a latissimus dorsi myocutaneous flap may be harvested with a scapular osteocutaneous or fasciocutaneous flap.[35]

POSTOPERATIVE MANAGEMENT: FREE FLAP MONITORING

The gold standard for assessing the viability of a free tissue transfer remains clinical examination. We prefer nursing assessment of all flaps (with Doppler examination of the pedicle) every hour for the first 72 hours and physician assessment every 6 hours. Color, turgor, temperature, evidence of edema, quantity and quality of blood extravasation after pinprick, and quality of the Doppler sound are all basic methods of assessment. The arterial signal should increase in strength during subsequent postoperative days. The venous signal should be augmentable.

Signs of venous congestion include bluish discoloration, increased warmth and swelling, and quick and bluish blood return after pinprick (Fig. 81-10). The arterial Doppler sound may be "hammer-like," indicative of outflow obstruction, and there may be loss of the venous signal. With arterial compromise the flap appears pale, feels cool, and has a loss or delay of bright red blood with pinprick of the flap. The Doppler sound may be present but can be faint, and areas thought to represent skin perforators may be lost totally, an indication of early loss of vascular inflow. If there is any

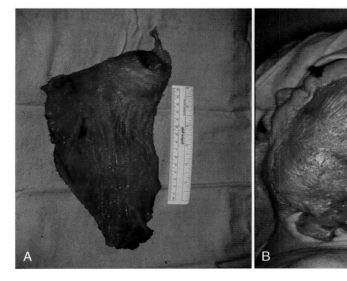

Figure 81-9. Latissimus dorsi free flap. **A,** Muscle harvested. **B,** Reconstruction of the lateral temporal bone resection.

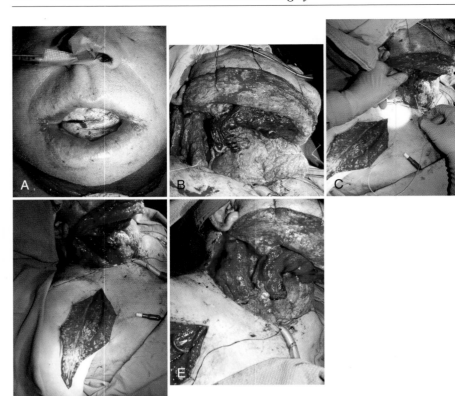

Figure 81-10. Venous outflow obstruction and restoration (postoperative day 1, same patient as in Fig. 81-5). **A,** Venous congestion of a fibular free flap: bluish blood with pinprick of a flap skin paddle. **B,** Saphenous vein graft and internal jugular vein clotted. **C,** Clots in the venae comitantes of the fibular flap cleared with a no. 3 Fogarty catheter. **D,** Cephalic vein rotated from the right upper extremity to the neck. **E,** Restoration of venous outflow with anastomosis of the cephalic vein to the peroneal vena comitans.

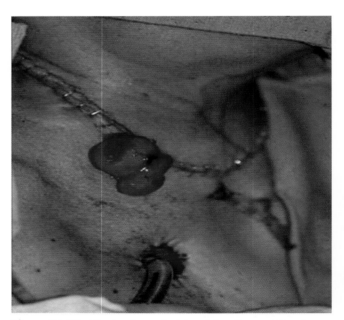

Figure 81-11. Monitor loop of a jejunal free flap used for pharyngeal reconstruction.

concern about vascular inflow or outflow obstruction, the patient should be returned to the operating room immediately for surgical exploration.

Most fasciocutaneous flaps that are buried, such as for pharyngeal defects, can allow a small skin paddle to be separately incorporated into the cervical skin closure. This permits clinical assessment and pinprick examination. Later, as an outpatient under local anesthesia, this skin island can be removed, and the cervical skin suture line can be reapproximated. Because of its vasculature arcade, a small portion of the jejunum can be separated from the rest of the flap and externalized for monitoring (Fig. 81-11). Afterward (approximately 3 to 5 days after surgery), this segment can be removed by ligating the base with a suture. When assessing buried flaps without an externalized portion, one can rely on a Doppler signal that is transmitted through the cervical apron flap. However, such assessment can be inaccurate if one mistakes the carotid artery and internal jugular vein as the vascular supply to the flap. Although we do not routinely use them, implantable Doppler systems are also available for monitoring flaps.[36]

PEARLS

- Any redundancy in the jejunum after inset may cause the jejunum to fold on itself and become a barrier to food transport. To prevent such redundancy, the base of the tongue inset should be performed first and then the vascular microanastomosis. With perfusion re-established, the jejunum expands. After this expansion, any redundant jejunum should be resected before completing the mucosal anastomosis to the cervical esophagus.

- For flaps that are buried, such as the radial forearm fasciocutaneous free flap for pharyngeal defects, a small skin paddle can be separately incorporated in the cervical skin closure to allow clinical assessment and pinprick examination.
- For maxillectomy and midface defects, volume and surface area requirements will dictate whether a rectus free flap or a radial forearm free flap should be selected. Relatively large-volume defects (e.g., total maxillectomy) are commonly reconstructed with a rectus free flap with separate skin paddles designed for reconstruction of the palate and skin.
- Through-and-through composite segmental defects of the mandible can often be reconstructed with a single osteocutaneous radial forearm free flap or fibular free flap. A large skin paddle should be harvested with the flap so that an area of skin can be de-epithelialized to create two skin paddles—one for oral cavity reconstruction and the other for cutaneous reconstruction.
- If there are no recipient veins in the neck for microanastomosis, the cephalic vein can be transected distally in the arm and rotated to the head and neck for microanastomosis.

PITFALLS

- The pedicle length of a rectus abdominis flap may be insufficient to reach the neck, especially when the mandible is intact. Careful planning of the skin paddle and intramuscular dissection of the pedicle from the rectus muscle may be necessary to ensure adequate length.
- Aggressive harvest (>40%) of the radial bone may lead to pathologic fracture of the radius. Prophylactic plating of the radius should be considered to prevent fracture.
- Irreversible ischemic changes in the jejunum can occur within 2 hours. The jejunal vessels should be divided and transferred from the abdomen only after the recipient vessels have been isolated for microanastomosis.
- Failure to recognize venous congestion will lead to total loss of the flap. Leeches should be used only as treatment of venous congestion after problems with the microanastomosis and pedicle have been excluded by surgical exploration.
- Harvest of a fibular free flap in patients with peripheral vascular disease (an ankle-arm index <1.0) but with three-vessel runoff may still lead to delayed wound healing at the harvest site and failure of complete take of a skin graft on the lower extremity cutaneous defect.

References

1. Jacobson MC, Franssen E, Fliss DM, et al: Free forearm flap in oral reconstruction. Functional outcome. Arch Otolaryngol Head Neck Surg 121:959-964, 1995.
2. Bardsley AF, Soutar DS, Elliot D, Batchelor AG: Reducing morbidity in the radial forearm flap donor site. Plast Reconstr Surg 86:287-292, discussion 293-294, 1990.
3. Close LG, Truelson JM, Milledge RA, Schweitzer C: Sensory recovery in noninnervated flaps used for oral cavity and oropharyngeal reconstruction. Arch Otolaryngol Head Neck Surg 121:967-972, 1995.
4. Swartz WM, Banis JC, Newton ED, et al: The osteocutaneous scapular flap for mandibular and maxillary reconstruction. Plast Reconstr Surg 77:530-545, 1986.
5. Ninkovic M, Harpf C, Schwabegger AH, Rumer-Moser A: The lateral arm flap. Clin Plast Surg 28:367-374, 2001.
6. Urken ML, Turk JB, Weinberg H, et al: The rectus abdominis free flap in head and neck reconstruction. Arch Otolaryngol Head Neck Surg 117:857-866, 1991.
7. Hidalgo DA, Rekow A: A review of 60 consecutive fibula free flap mandible reconstructions. Plast Reconstr Surg 96:585-596, discussion 597-602, 1995.
8. Futran ND, Stack BC Jr, Zaccardi MJ: Preoperative color flow Doppler imaging for fibula free tissue transfers. Ann Vasc Surg 12:445-450, 1998.
9. Jones NF, Swartz WM, Mears DC, et al: The "double barrel" free vascularized fibular bone graft. Plast Reconstr Surg 81:378-385, 1988.
10. Anthony JP, Rawnsley JD, Benhaim P, et al: Donor leg morbidity and function after fibula free flap mandible reconstruction. Plast Reconstr Surg 96:146-152, 1995.
11. Urken ML, Vickery C, Weinberg H, et al: The internal oblique–iliac crest osseomyocutaneous free flap in oromandibular reconstruction. Report of 20 cases. Arch Otolaryngol Head Neck Surg 115:339-349, 1989.
12. Forrest C, Boyd B, Manktelow R, et al: The free vascularized iliac crest tissue transfer: Donor site complications associated with eighty-two cases. Br J Plast Surg 45:89-93, 1992.
13. Theile DR, Robinson DW, Theile DE, Coman WB: Free jejunal interposition reconstruction after pharyngolaryngectomy: 201 consecutive cases. Head Neck 17:83-88, 1995.
14. Wadsworth JT, Futran N, Eubanks TR: Laparoscopic harvest of the jejunal free flap for reconstruction of hypopharyngeal and cervical esophageal defects. Arch Otolaryngol Head Neck Surg 128:1384-1387, 2002.
15. Shangold LM, Urken ML, Lawson W: Jejunal transplantation for pharyngoesophageal reconstruction. Otolaryngol Clin North Am 24:1321-1342, 1991.
16. Wei FC, Jain V, Celik N, et al: Have we found an ideal soft-tissue flap? An experience with 672 anterolateral thigh flaps. Plast Reconstr Surg 109:2219-2226, discussion 2227-2230, 2002.
17. Huang LY, Lin H, Liu YT, et al: Anterolateral thigh vastus lateralis myocutaneous flap for vulvar reconstruction after radical vulvectomy: A preliminary experience. Gynecol Oncol 78:391-393, 2000.
18. Shpitzer T, Neligan PC, Gullane PJ, et al: The free iliac crest and fibula flaps in vascularized oromandibular reconstruction: Comparison and long-term evaluation. Head Neck 21:639-647, 1999.
19. Schusterman MA, Reece GP, Kroll SS, Weldon ME: Use of the AO plate for immediate mandibular reconstruction in cancer patients. Plast Reconstr Surg 88:588-593, 1991.
20. Irish JC, Gullane PJ, Gilbert RW, et al: Primary mandibular reconstruction with the titanium hollow screw reconstruction plate: Evaluation of 51 cases. Plast Reconstr Surg 96:93-99, 1995.
21. Gullane P, Boyd B, Brown D: Primary mandibular reconstruction: Using plate and flap. Proceedings of the Third International Conference on Head and Neck Cancer. Head Neck Cancer 3:807-823, 1993.
22. Deleyiannis FWB, Carolyn C, Lee E, et al: Reconstruction of the lateral mandibulectony defect: Management based on prognosis and the location and volume of the soft tissue resection. Laryngoscope 116:2071-2080, 2006.

23. Urken ML, Moscoso JF, Lawson W, Biller HF: A systematic approach to functional reconstruction of the oral cavity following partial and total glossectomy. Arch Otolaryngol Head Neck Surg 120:589-601, 1994.

24. Schuller DE, Mountain RE, Nicholson RE, et al: One-stage reconstruction of partial laryngopharyngeal defects. Laryngoscope 107:247-253, 1997.

25. Urken ML, Blackwell K, Biller HF: Reconstruction of the laryngopharynx after hemicricoid/hemithyroid cartilage resection. Preliminary functional results. Arch Otolaryngol Head Neck Surg 123:1213-1222, 1997.

26. Disa JJ, Pusic AL, Hidalgo DA, Cordeiro PG: Microvascular reconstruction of the hypopharynx: Defect classification, treatment algorithm, and functional outcome based on 165 consecutive cases. Plast Reconstr Surg 111:652-660, discussion 661-663, 2003.

27. Azizzadeh B, Yafai S, Rawnsley JD, et al: Radial forearm free flap pharyngoesophageal reconstruction. Laryngoscope 111:807-810, 2001.

28. Varvares MA, Cheney ML, Gliklich RE, et al: Use of the radial forearm fasciocutaneous free flap and Montgomery salivary bypass tube for pharyngoesophageal reconstruction. Head Neck 22:463-468, 2000.

29. Chana JS, Wei FC: A review of the advantages of the anterolateral thigh flap in head and neck reconstruction. Br J Plast Surg 57:603-609, 2004.

30. Cordeiro PG, Santamaria E: A classification system and algorithm for reconstruction of maxillectomy and midfacial defects. Plast Reconstr Surg 105:2331-2346, discussion 2347-2348, 2000.

31. Kelley P, Klebuc M, Hollier L: Complex midface reconstruction: Maximizing contour and bone graft survival utilizing periosteal free flaps. J Craniofac Surg 14:413-416, 2003.

32. Anthony JP, Foster RD, Sharma AB, et al: Reconstruction of a complex midfacial defect with the folded fibular free flap and osseointegrated implants. Ann Plast Surg 37:204-210, 1996.

33. Chang DW, Robb GL: Microvascular reconstruction of the skull base. Semin Surg Oncol 19:211-217, 2000.

34. Besteiro JM, Aki FE, Ferreira MC, et al: Free flap reconstruction of tumors involving the cranial base. Microsurgery 15:9-13, 1994.

35. Evans GR, Luethke RW: A latissimus/scapula combined myoosseous free flap based on the subscapular artery used for elbow reconstruction. Ann Plast Surg 30:175-179, 1993.

36. Swartz WM, Jones NF, Cherup L, Klein A: Direct monitoring of microvascular anastomoses with the 20-MHz ultrasonic Doppler probe: An experimental and clinical study. Plast Reconstr Surg 81:149-161, 1988.

Chapter 82

Regional Pedicle Flaps

Ernest K. Manders

The use of pedicle flaps has significantly improved the safety and functional outcomes of head and neck surgery. The reliability and ready availability of pedicle flaps make them the most commonly used means of reconstructing defects created in the course of extirpative surgery. Because of the aggressiveness of today's chemotherapy and radiation therapy protocols, the ability to bring oxygenated tissue with a nourishing blood supply to the surgical defect has been critical. Moreover, many of these flaps can be created and transferred without needing to reposition the patient intraoperatively. They do not require microvascular expertise, along with the painstaking time spent under the microscope, nor do they tend to significantly increase the duration of the operative procedure. This chapter presents an overview of the relevant anatomy, steps for technical execution, and common complications of pedicled flaps for the head and neck.

Several excellent general references and atlases have been prepared to assist surgeons contemplating head and neck reconstruction with regional flaps. Three excellent sources are listed at the beginning of the reference section.[1-3]

PECTORALIS MAJOR FLAP

The pectoralis major flap is the most commonly used muscle or myocutaneous flap worldwide in head and neck surgery and certainly one of the most reliable of all the pedicle flaps.[4-7] It has a long tradition of use in reconstruction of the oral cavity and oropharynx and can be used with a cutaneous island or as a myofascial flap alone (Fig. 82-1). Its ability to protect the great vessels of the neck is literally a lifesaving attribute.

The pectoralis major muscle provides the bulk of the flap and is nourished by the pectoral branches of the thoracoacromial artery. The thoracoacromial artery branches from the subclavian artery deep to the clavicle and enters the underside of the pectoralis major muscle at about the midpoint of the clavicle. One can draw the course of the thoracoacromial artery on the skin of the chest by marking the clavicle at its midpoint. If one draws a line from the xyphoid to the acromion and constructs a perpendicular to this line that meets the midpoint of the clavicle, the artery's course corresponds to the vertical perpendicular and the medial portion of the line from xyphoid to acromion. When elevating the pectoralis major, the artery can be seen running in fat on the underside of the muscle.

Additionally, the lateral thoracic artery enters the lateral portion of the sternal head of the pectoralis major muscle but is routinely sacrificed during harvest to maximize the arc of rotation of the flap. Usually, this will not compromise flap viability, but a wary surgeon is advised to inspect the course of the thoracoacromial first. Some authors have reported that perhaps one in seven patients has a sternal portion of the muscle served predominantly by a branch of the lateral thoracic artery.

The skin overlying the medial aspect of the pectoralis major muscle is nourished by perforators from the internal mammary artery, especially those arising from rib interspaces 2, 3, and 4, with perforators from interspaces 3 and 4 playing particularly prominent roles. These perforators are the arterial input for the classic deltopectoral flap.

The origin of the pectoralis major is divided into three segments: clavicular, sternocostal, and the aponeurosis of the external oblique. The clavicular origin arises from the medial third of the clavicle. The sternocostal origin arises from the sternum and the first six ribs. The third origin arises from the attachment of the inferior edge of the pectoralis muscle to the aponeurosis and the fascia of the external oblique muscle. The insertion of the pectoralis major runs deep to the deltoid and inserts on the greater tubercle of the humerus. The medial edge of the deltoid and the tendinous insertion of the pectoralis major are almost

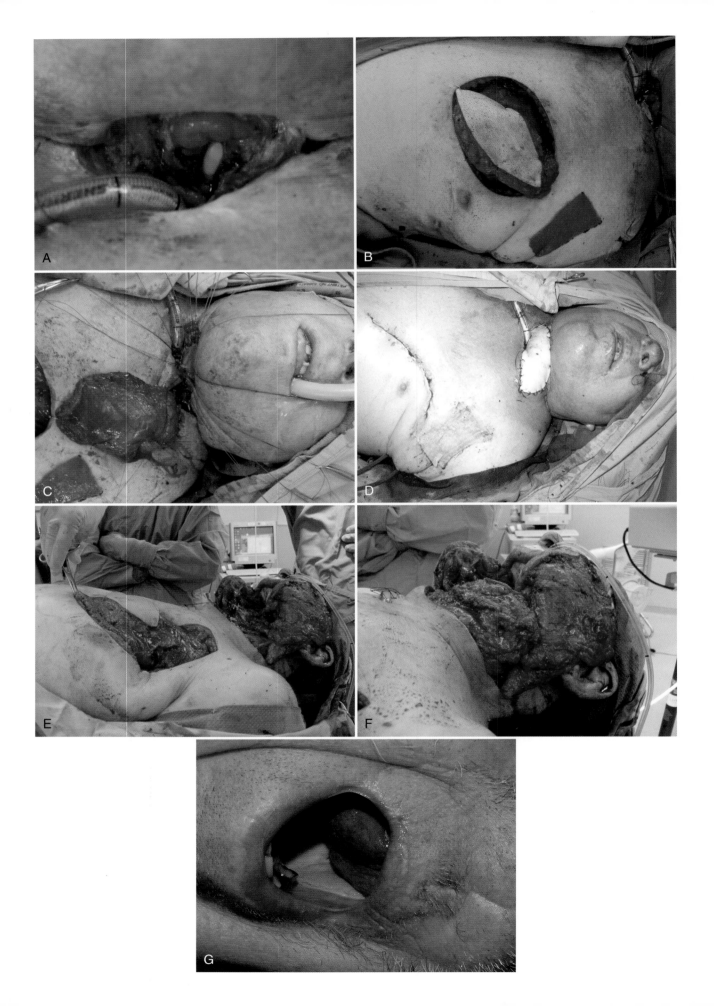

indistinguishable from one another. The cephalic vein can be used as a guide to differentiate between them. The thoracoacromial artery will run the length of the muscle on its deep surface as described earlier.

The pectoralis muscle mass stretches across the superior anterior aspect of the chest, where it acts to abduct and medially rotate the humerus. Use of the muscle in construction of a flap does not cause significant functional disability. Because of the length available in this flap, the pectoralis major muscle can be used for defects ranging from the lower part of the neck such as a stoma after laryngectomy, the upper part of the neck, the tongue and floor of the mouth, and the lateral head/auricular area.

A skin island is often used to replace mucosa when a pectoralis major myocutaneous flap is positioned in the site of the defect. The skin island is fed by perforators of the thoracoacromial system emerging from the anterior surface of the muscle. If the skin island is extended off the boundaries of the muscle in any direction, the portion of skin extending beyond the muscle will have a random blood supply and can be less reliable. However, the skin island can be placed anywhere on the anterior surface of the muscle that would be usable in filling the defect. This is often approximated during surgery by positioning a towel at the origin of the thoracoacromial artery below the clavicle and extending inferiorly to the inferior edge of the skin island. In this way the arc of rotation and the length of the muscle on its pedicle can be evaluated to ensure adequate advancement.

The incision for liberating the pectoralis major muscle from the overlying skin and the underlying chest wall can be varied, depending on the concerns of the patient and the needs of the reconstructive procedure. Typically, the skin island is positioned near the end of the flap, close to the caudal portion of the muscle origin. It is often possible to dissect out the muscle through an incision in the inframammary fold. If a skin flap is needed, the skin and subcutaneous tissue can be incised to expose the pectoralis muscle, which can then be raised through these incisions around the skin island. The skin island is fed by perforators from the thoracoacromial artery running through the muscle, and thus care must be taken to not undercut or shear the skin island from the muscle. Several stay sutures tacking the skin island to the muscle are helpful toward this end, and the inferior sutures may be left long to help bring the flap up into its final position. The use of long stay sutures wrapped around the surgeon's finger provides traction and flexibility as the surgeon pulls the flap below the neck skin overlying the

clavicle. The crucial technical detail to be observed in flap advancement is making the tunnel under the clavicular skin large enough to easily accommodate the bulk of the muscle. Sometimes it will be necessary to incise this skin and place a skin graft over the muscle.

Any area of the skin island directly over the muscle should have a good blood supply. Portions of the skin that extend beyond the pectoralis will be random, and their survivability is less reliable. Flaps may be harvested with one skin island, two as in the case of a bilobed flap, or no skin island at all. Inclusion of rib has been used when osseous reconstruction is needed, although this is much less commonly done today now that experience with osteocutaneous free flaps is so extensive. If the fifth rib is harvested along with the flap, care must be taken to not separate the muscle from the fifth rib because the rib derives its blood supply from perforators running through the muscle to the periosteum over the surface of the rib.

In a female patient, a curvilinear incision inferior to the breast, in the breast crease, can avoid the more obvious scarring that can still be seen with low neck lines when the incision runs on the anterior chest wall. In addition, the fibrofatty breast tissue can easily be elevated away off the muscle as a complete unit when making an incision in the inframammary fold.

As the pectoralis muscle is lifted off the chest wall, it must be divided at its medial origin and lateral insertion. The connection of the muscle to the proximal end of the humerus will ultimately need to be released to allow enough mobility for the flap to fill a defect in the head and neck region. These muscle divisions are best accomplished with electrocautery. Care must be taken to avoid disruption of the feeder vessels on the undersurface of the pectoralis major. The nerve supply to the pectoralis major muscle arises from the lateral (C5 to C7) and medial (C8, T1) pectoral nerves. These nerves are often cut when raising this flap to provide an adequate arc of rotation. This causes some long-term atrophy of the muscle, which is often advantageous in head and neck reconstruction.

The muscle may be released medially from the sternum and laterally at the anterior axillary line near its insertion. It may then be brought over the clavicle, under the supraclavicular skin, and into the defect. Alternatively, the muscle may be divided on either side of the thoracoacromial vascular bundle down to the distal end of the flap, which may be larger and even include a cutaneous portion. This flap is like a lollipop and creates less of a deformity in the neck. However, it does not have the expanse of tissue to cover deep neck structures, including the great vessels, that the wider pectoralis major flap does.

When positioning this flap the operator must be careful to not overly twist, kink, or crimp the vascular pedicle. If the operator's hand can be comfortably placed below the skin of the inferior portion of the neck and supraclavicular area from the neck incision into the chest incision, there is little danger the vascular pedicle will be compromised. Similarly, experimenting with the most natural pattern for the flap to fill the defect can

Figure 82-1. Pectoralis myocutaneous flap. **A,** Defect for a pectoralis myocutaneous flap. **B,** Incision for flap elevation. **C,** Pectoralis flap ready for coverage of the defect. **D,** Pectoralis myocutaneous flap in place. **E,** Pectoralis flap for closure of the oral cavity. **F,** Flap in place. **G,** Pectoralis myocutaneous flap lining the oral cavity in another patient.

avoid excessive rotation and reduction of the blood supply.

Complications are fortunately relatively infrequent with this flap, and hence it is used frequently in head and neck reconstruction. Full necrosis of the flap is uncommon. Partial necrosis is not uncommon, however, although local wound care is typically sufficient to resolve problems encountered with healing. On occasion, a split-thickness skin graft will need to be used for coverage of a donor site defect. This is preferable to having the chest wound break down later because of a closure that is too tight. The operator must be wary of tension on the donor site closure when a large skin island has been harvested. A skin graft whose appearance bothers the patient can probably be removed later with the technique of serial excision.

Using at least two suction drains helps avoid but cannot absolutely prevent a postoperative hematoma. Particularly if the patient's blood pressure is elevated or if an episode of excessive coughing occurs, a sudden bulge in the donor area may herald a subcutaneous hematoma. Of course, careful hemostasis must be obtained as the flap is harvested to help avoid this complication.

When advanced, the flap can be wrapped around bone or reconstruction plates (or both). A cutaneous paddle can be intraoral, extraoral, or both if a bridge of skin between the paddles is de-epithelialized and buried. The surgeon soon learns that myocutaneous flaps to the head and neck must be suspended adequately to obtain the best results. External cutaneous paddles in particular will invariably settle and appear to hang with time, and patients should be advised of this possibility. Later corrective surgery is frequently possible to achieve a significant measure of improvement.

LATISSIMUS DORSI FLAP

The latissimus dorsi flap remains the most generally dependable and versatile flap in the reconstructive surgery armamentarium.[8-10] It is a broad flat muscle of considerable length. It originates from an aponeurosis that joins the posterior layer of the thoracolumbar fascia from about the sixth thoracic vertebra to the posterior iliac crest. The muscle inserts into the intertubercular groove of the humerus. Its considerable length allows it to easily reach the head and neck area as a pedicled flap (Fig. 82-2). For this purpose it may be tunneled subcutaneously over the pectoralis major, under the pectoralis major insertion fibers and over the lateral aspect of the clavicle, or under the clavicle itself. In the head and neck area the latissimus dorsi flap may be used for surface reconstruction, and it may also be advanced into the oral cavity and even used for esophageal reconstructions. If a skin paddle is required, it is best to base it on the middle of the muscle because the most distal portion at the origin is not reliably well perfused.

The muscle is approached with the patient bumped up to expose the back or in a decubitus position. A transverse incision high in the axilla is extended along the posterior axillary fold to expose the lateral border of the muscle. The dissection separates the overlying back skin and subcutaneous tissue from the posterior aspect of the muscle, except where a cutaneous portion may be required. Electrocautery is used to release the muscle from its origin. The anterior dissection should respect the long thoracic artery to the serratus muscle, where it lies just a centimeter or so behind and under the anterior border of the latissimus muscle. The thoracodorsal artery serves the latissimus muscle. The thoracodorsal neurovascular bundle is relatively large and may easily be traced to its origin from the subscapular artery. For transposition to the region of the head and neck, painstaking vascular dissection is required so that the muscle can be mobilized on its vascular leash and advanced to above the ear, the maxilla, or across the base of the neck as needed.

As for reconstructions with the pectoralis major muscle, it is essential that the latissimus be supported with multiple sutures so that it does not descend and thereby dehisce the wound or create a sagging flap that

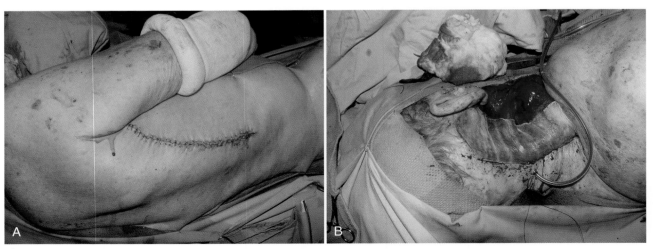

Figure 82-2. Latissimus dorsi flap. **A,** Latissimus dorsi donor site incision. **B,** Latissimus flap in place with a skin graft.

is less functional and attractive than when inset in the operating room. Some sagging late is almost always a problem, but early dehiscence must be avoided.

STERNOCLEIDOMASTOID MUSCLE FLAP

The sternocleidomastoid (SCM) flap can be based either from its inferior origin on the sternum and clavicle or from its superior insertion on the mastoid process[11,12] because of the multiple arterial blood supply to the muscle along its course. The principal blood supply to the SCM is via the occipital artery at the superior aspect of the muscle. Further inferiorly along its course the muscle receives blood from the postauricular artery, branches from the superior thyroid artery, and branches from the thyrocervical trunk. A skin island can be incorporated with this flap and derives its blood supply from perforators running through the SCM. Motor neural input to the SCM comes from branches of the spinal accessory nerve. In addition, C2 and C3 supply innervation, with disagreement whether this innervation is motor or sensory in nature.

There is some controversy about using the SCM flap when cervical metastases from an upper aerodigestive tract malignancy are present. Spread down the internal jugular chain lymph nodes can bring the cervical metastases into contact with the SCM, and in this situation a different reconstructive option should be considered. If the SCM must be excised to complete the neck dissection, another flap must obviously be considered.

Evaluation of the arc of rotation that will best allow the flap to fill the defect will determine how the flap will be pedicled. Basing the flap superiorly or inferiorly will allow sufficient length to place the skin island in the oral cavity. Occasionally, periosteum from the clavicle or full- or split-thickness clavicle can be incorporated as part of an SCM flap. This necessitates a superiorly based flap, which carries with it the advantage of preserving the most robust arterial feeders, namely, the occipital and the superior thyroid. Its disadvantage is that the platysma muscle overlies the SCM in the caudal neck. This extra layer of tissue between the SCM and the skin island reduces the perforators that supply the skin in this region, and authors have noted a substantial rate of partial or complete skin island necrosis. This is even more common in an irradiated neck. The inferiorly based SCM flap carries with it the advantage of a more robust supply of skin perforators because the platysma does not cross between the SCM and the skin in this region of the neck. The disadvantage of a inferiorly based flap is that it relies on caudal arterial supply to the SCM muscle, branches off the thyrocervical trunk, which places the blood supply to the muscle as a whole in more jeopardy.

To incorporate periosteum for repair of the anterior tracheal wall or part of the larynx, care must be taken to elevate the periosteum in continuity with the SCM muscle to preserve the blood supply. This also holds true for partial-thickness or full-thickness clavicle. Clavicular bone can then be used to repair anterior

tracheal/laryngeal defects. Meyer has popularized this technique, which has been ascribed to Lindholm.[13] It is recommended that if periosteum is being used as a patch to repair the anterior tracheal wall, a tracheostomy tube be placed inferior to the defect and either a T tube (with the tracheostomy tube inserted into it) or a Montgomery laryngeal stent (with through-and-through stay sutures brought out through the skin and traversing from one side of the neck to the other while passing through the stent) be placed within the airway. In this manner, the flaccid periosteum will be stented to prevent collapse into the airway lumen. The Montgomery stent or T tube would need to be removed later in the operating room.

Raising the SCM flap generally does not present unique challenges to the head and neck surgeon. All the vital structures of the carotid sheath, as well as the hypoglossal nerve, lie deep to the SCM muscle. In addition, the carotid sheath lies deep to the omohyoid muscle in the inferior aspect of the neck. The hypoglossal nerve lies deep to the digastric muscle more superiorly. Therefore, the SCM muscle may be raised relatively quickly if the omohyoid and digastric muscles are identified deep to it. Superiorly, one must be cognizant of cranial nerve XI as it courses superiorly. It will split the SCM muscle as it descends in the neck.

The arc of rotation must be carefully considered when planning this flap. In the case of a superiorly based flap, preservation of the superior thyroid artery will improve the blood supply but often restricts the arc of rotation. Generally, two of the three arterial supplies to the SCM muscle are sacrificed for the sake of attaining adequate rotation.

When the periosteum or clavicle is incorporated as part of the flap, the sternal head of the muscle can often be sacrificed for ease of placement of the clavicular head and periosteum or bone into the defect. Occasionally, looping the clavicular head deep to the sternal head will accomplish the same task without sacrifice of the sternal head.

TRAPEZIUS MUSCLE FLAP

Use of a cutaneous trapezius muscle flap extends back to 1842, when Mutter used it for the release of burn contractures in the neck. The three varieties of trapezius flap (superior, lateral island, and lower island) have been well described by many surgeons. These concepts are defined in the following text as they relate to specific flaps.[14-17]

The trapezius is a triangular muscle that extends along the midline of the spine from the skull base to the about the 10th thoracic vertebra. It inserts on the lateral third of the clavicle, the scapular spine, and the acromion. It defines the posterior border of the posterior triangle of the neck. The trapezius functions to elevate and retract the shoulder and rotate the scapula.

Motor innervation of the trapezius is supplied by the spinal accessory nerve, cranial nerve XI. Contributions from C2 to C4 are also present, but it is unclear to what degree they play a role in functioning of the muscle. The blood supply to the trapezius is from the occipital artery, paraspinous perforators, the transverse cervical artery, and the dorsal scapular artery.

There are three distinct ways that the trapezius muscle can be used as a flap for head and neck reconstruction, as described in the following sections.

Superior Trapezius Flap

This flap is based on the occipital artery and the paraspinous perforators. It extends from the occiput, along the anterior border of the trapezius toward the shoulder, and then back again medially up to the midline of the spine. It creates a long tongue of tissue, both muscle and skin, for use in the head and neck. Elevation of this flap relies on elevation of the trapezius muscle with the skin overlying it remaining attached. This flap has been described as being divided into three angiosomes. The first is the most medial; it extends from the midline of the spine toward the shoulder and receives its blood supply from the occipital artery and the paraspinous perforators. The second angiosome extends laterally from this one and receives its blood supply from the transverse cervical artery as it courses over the clavicle. The last angiosome extends laterally from the second and ends over the deltoid muscle. This last angiosome receives its blood supply from a branch of the thoracoacromial artery. Choke arteries that run through the skin allow the paraspinous perforators to supply the third angiosome if the transverse cervical artery is interrupted, such as during the course of neck dissection. This flap can then be swung medially onto the neck to repair loss of cutaneous tissue on the neck. A skin graft is required for closure of the donor site defect. Either intervening skin from the neck that is covered by the flap is removed so that the entire length of the flap can be inset, or the underlying neck skin can be left in place and the base of the flap taken down and replaced in its original location as a delayed secondary procedure.

Lateral Island Flap

In this flap the transverse cervical artery (TCA) and vein (TCV) must be meticulously dissected in the inferior portion of the posterior triangle of the neck and traced to their entry into the trapezius muscle. The skin island is situated along the anterior edge of the trapezius and extends inferiorly along the back of the patient. Care must be taken to preserve the pedicle artery and vein, especially if neck dissection has previously been performed. Additionally, the TCA and TCV may pass through portions of the brachial plexus and not allow harvest of the flap because of an inability to rotate the flap into position. Once the TCA and TCV have been dissected in the root of the neck and followed to their insertion in the trapezius muscle, the skin island can be adjusted so that the vascular pedicle is centered in the skin island. After the pedicle has been secured, a skin incision is made around the skin island and through the trapezius muscle. The skin and muscle island is then elevated off the underlying muscles while paying atten-

tion to not disrupt the vascular pedicle. The pedicle and attached skin/muscle island are then swung into position in the neck. Greater arc of rotation can be obtained when medial dissection along the pedicle frees the pedicle from surrounding tissue. Closure of the donor site defect can then be accomplished, frequently without a skin graft, as long as wide undermining is done.

Lower Trapezius Island Flap

This flap has the longest arc of rotation of any of the three; however, it does require exposure of the patient's back and therefore positioning the patient in the decubitus position is required (Fig. 82-3). The arm is adducted and medially rotated. The lower trapezius flap is based on the TCA and possibly the dorsal scapular artery (DSA). The skin island is positioned between the spine and the medial edge of the scapula. Dissection starts by incising the skin from the distal tip of the skin island superiorly toward the clavicle. Wide undermining of the medial and lateral skin is then accomplished. The inferior lateral edge of the trapezius muscle is identified and then dissected from the underlying muscles by proceeding in a superior direction. The skin island remains attached to the trapezius muscle as it is elevated. The DSA and dorsal scapular vein (DSV) will be encountered as they penetrate from the underlying rhomboids into the inferior portion of the trapezius muscle. With digital pressure the artery can be compressed lightly and bleeding from the edge of the skin island assessed. If deemed adequate, the DSA and DSV can be ligated and the dissection continued superiorly. The trapezius muscle must be freed from its attachments along the spine. In doing this the paraspinous perforators must be cauterized or ligated. Additionally, the attachments to the scapular spine must be incised. The TCA and TCV will be identified as the superior edge of the levator scapulae and the rhomboid minor are encountered. The DSA enters the trapezius from the deep musculature, between the rhomboid major and minor, inferior to the entry of the TCA. This flap will often yield a lengthy pedicle sufficient to reach to the auricle or side of the face.

TEMPOROPARIETAL FASCIAL FLAP

The temporoparietal fascial flap is useful for reconstruction of the ear, the orbit, the anterior cranial base, the superior and middle thirds of the face, and even the oral cavity (Fig. 82-4).[18-20] The anatomy is quite straightforward in that the flap is based on the parietal branch or the superficial temporal artery and vein. These vessels ascend just anterior to the auricle and branch approximately 2 to 4 cm above the zygomatic arch. They must be preserved when raising the flap, especially as one approaches the base of the flap. A Doppler monitor may be helpful in guiding dissection.

The flap is approached with a scalp incision from the root of the helix of the ear to the top of the temporal fossa. The scalp is raised off the deeper soft tissues

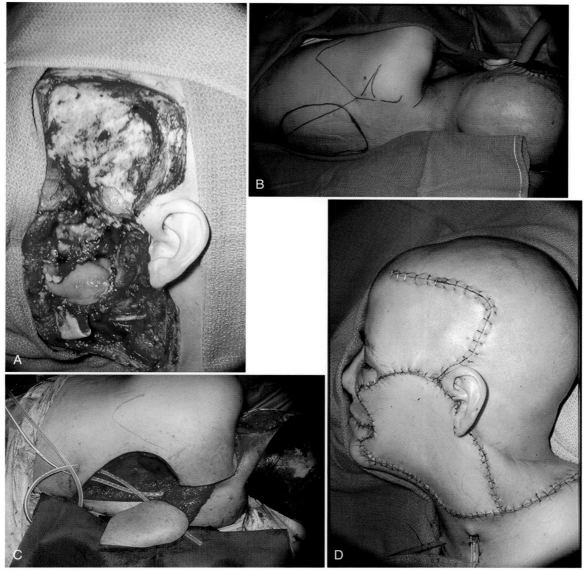

Figure 82-3. Trapezius flap. **A,** Defect of the face and scalp. **B,** Planning of the trapezius flap. **C,** Elevation of the trapezius flap. **D,** Reconstruction with the trapezius flap. *(Courtesy of Dr. B. Chandrasekhar.)*

in an adipose plane below the hair follicles. Care must be exerted here so that no areas of alopecia are created by dissection that is too superficial. The soft tissues are incised in an arc paralleling the line of origin of the temporalis muscle, and the flap is raised off the deep temporalis fascia itself. Anteriorly, care must be taken to avoid injury to the temporal branch of the facial nerve. The flap includes the galea and may be extended somewhat by including periosteum above the line of origin of the temporalis. The flap is narrowed as the base of the pedicle is approached at the point where the parietal branch of the superficial temporal artery enters the flap.

Closure of the donor defect is direct, and there should be no observable donor defect. The flap can be buried or covered with a split-thickness skin graft with

great success. It will reach the orbit and the oral cavity with ease. This flap is without peer in covering the cartilage framework of the external ear.

TEMPORALIS MUSCLE FLAP

The temporalis muscle flap is particularly useful for reconstruction of defects in the region of the auricle, the orbit and infratemporal fossa, and the hard palate and even intraoral defects (Fig. 82-5).[21-23] It is not used with a cutaneous component because a scalp defect and an area of alopecia would be created.

The temporalis muscle is fan shaped and passes under the zygomatic arch to insert on the coronoid process of the mandible. There are two major vascular inputs, the anterior and the posterior deep temporal

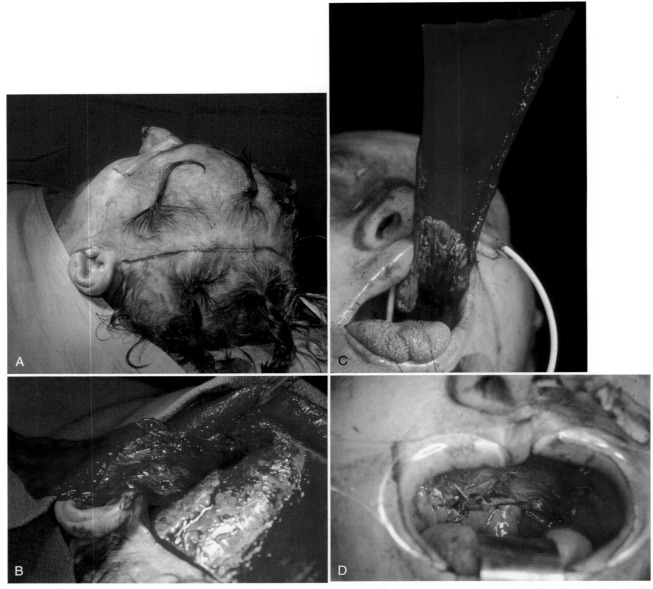

Figure 82-4. Temporoparietal fascia (TPF) flap. **A,** Planning the TPF flap incision. **B,** Elevation of the TPF flap. **C,** Delivery of the TPF flap into the oral cavity. **D,** TPF flap in place to close an intraoral defect. *(Courtesy of Dr. Michael Carstens.)*

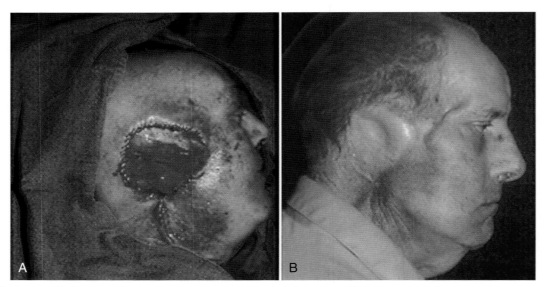

Figure 82-5. Temporalis flap. **A,** Defect in the auricular area covered with a temporalis flap. **B,** Late follow-up of the temporalis flap.

arteries. After freeing its origin, the muscle can be turned posteriorly over a defect in the auricular area or moved anteriorly to fill the orbit. If a portion of the zygomatic arch is removed, the muscle may be advanced caudally to the lower border of the mandible.

Flap elevation is quite easy, and the challenge to the surgeon is usually moving the muscle where it is needed once the origin is released. Most commonly it is directed toward the orbit, the infratemporal fossa, or the hard palate.

DELTOPECTORAL FLAP

The deltopectoral flap was once the most commonly used flap in head and neck surgery, but it has largely been superseded by the pectoralis major flap, which is more robust and can be raised and inset with confidence without a delay procedure.[24-26] The deltopectoral flap can be used with great success for reconstruction of defects of the middle and lower thirds of the face, the oral cavity, the neck, and the esophagus (Fig. 82-6).

It is raised over the upper part of the chest, based in the peristernal area, and extended laterally and cephalad to the deltoid region. It may even be extended to the posterior aspect of the shoulder if delayed. It is perfused by the first through third peristernal perforators of the internal mammary artery. A flap 10 cm in width and 20 cm in length can be reliably raised and used with a high likelihood of success. Longer flaps should be delayed. The fascia of the pectoralis major muscle may be raised with the flap.

When the end of the flap is inset for its intended purpose, the proximal portion of the flap that is not inset as part of the reconstruction may be tubed. Later, 2 or 3 weeks after elevation, the flap may be divided with inset of the base of the flap into the donor area, or the redundant flap may simply be excised. Skin grafting is usually required to close the donor site wound, and the resulting defect is noticeable.

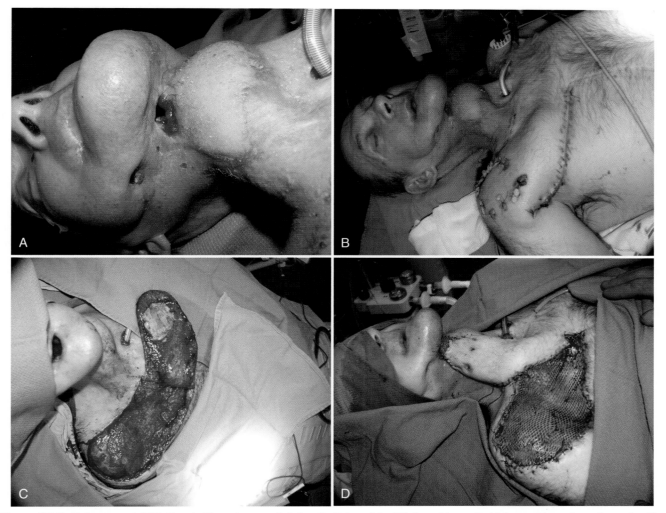

Figure 82-6. Deltopectoral (DP) flap. **A,** Hypopharyngeal defect. **B,** Delay of the DP flap with a split-thickness skin graft on the underside. **C,** Elevation of the DP flap with a skin graft for lining at the site of the defect. **D,** DP flap in place with a skin graft placed over the donor defect. *(Courtesy of Dr. Frederic W.-B. Deleyiannis.)*

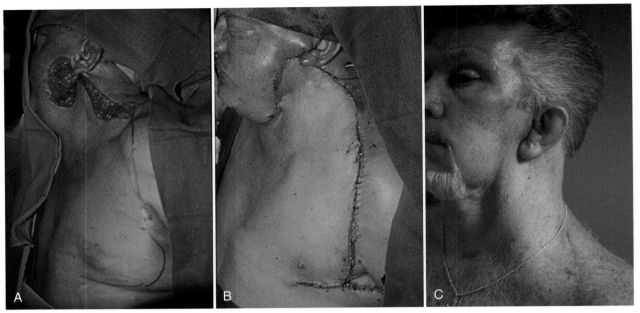

Figure 82-7. Cervicopectoral flap. **A**, Defect requiring closure. **B**, Elevation and advancement of the cervicopectoral flap with elimination of the defect. **C**, The flap has healed completely and the patient has undergone postoperative radiation therapy. *(Courtesy of Dr. James Russavage.)*

CERVICOPECTORAL FLAP

The cervicopectoral flap is a skin flap of large proportions that affords coverage of lateral neck and cheek defects.[27] The blood supply is essentially that of the deltopectoral flap. The skin flap is raised from the inferior border of the neck or cheek defect across the trapezius muscle 2 cm behind its anterior border and down across the acromioclavicular point of the shoulder and the top of the anterior axillary fold (Fig. 82-7). A backcut may be needed to facilitate full rotation, and dog-ears at the anterior jaw line and in the axilla should be excised at the time of closure. The flap is raised in a plane just deep to the platysma muscle and the anterior pectoral fascia, and care must be exercised to avoid disruption of the internal thoracic perforators medially at the very base of the flap.

The cervicopectoral flap has skin color and texture like that of the resected skin, although depending on the cephalad border it may not carry bearded skin. It can be assessed via fluorescein perfusion before full inset to ensure reconstruction with fully viable tissue. Extensive mobilization will allow closure of defects measuring 10 cm in diameter with a very satisfactory appearance at the site of reconstruction and a minimal donor site defect. The scar is quite acceptable and the flap is robust. To achieve the advancement possible with this flap, the surgeon must undermine extensively. The plane is easily entered and traversed, and there is very low morbidity. In view of the ready availability of this flap and the excellent tissue match, this flap is probably underused for head and neck reconstruction.

CONCLUSION

This listing will provide the head and neck surgeon with a number of options for restoring cover and continence at places where defects are created. As pointed out, these flaps do not require much time and can bring a long extirpative operation to a fairly rapid conclusion. Familiarity with these techniques will prove lifesaving for some patients. Local pedicled flaps have been one of the factors that have transformed head and neck surgery to the safer and predictable endeavor that it is today. These flaps are a welcome alternative at crucial moments in the treatment of patients stricken with neoplasms of the head and neck.

PEARLS

- A good working knowledge of the anatomy of the muscles of the head and neck and upper thorax is essential for the successful use of pedicle flaps.
- The pectoralis major flap is almost always a good alternative for reconstruction of head and neck defects.
- The latissimus dorsi and the cervicopectoral flaps are often excellent choices for head and neck reconstruction.
- Planning can afford both lining at the mucosal level and skin cover when both are needed.
- When flaps are passed subcutaneously, the passageway must be large to avoid constriction of the pedicle.

PITFALLS

- A lack of respect for the vascular anatomy of a pedicle flap will often result in compromise of the flap and even its loss.
- Be on the lookout for a lateral thoracic contribution that is the dominant artery serving the sternal portion of the pectoralis major muscle.
- Do not forget that fluorescein testing of flaps can help one ensure a successful reconstruction. Failure to test when in doubt may result in a necrotic flap.
- Support for the flaps with multiple suture suspensions and no tension along the line of the flap is essential for aesthetically pleasing reconstructions.
- Do not forget that flaps can be revised with benefit when the primary mission of closure and recovery is accomplished, and do not forget to assure the patient of this.

References

1. Baker SR, Swanson NA: Local Flaps in Facial Reconstruction. St Louis, CV Mosby, 1995.
2. Strauch B, Vasconez LO, Hall-Findlay EJ: Grabb's Encyclopedia of Flaps. Boston, Little, Brown, 1990.
3. Mathes SJ, Nahai F: Reconstructive Surgery: Principles, Anatomy, and Techniques. New York, Churchill Livingstone, 1997.
4. Ariyan S: The pectoralis major myocutaneous flap: A versatile flap for reconstruction in the head and neck. Plast Reconstr Surg 63:73-81, 1979.
5. Freeman JL, Walker EP, Wilson JSP, Shaw HJ: The vascular anatomy of the pectoralis major flap. Br J Plast Surg 34:3-10, 1981.
6. Tobin GR: Pectoralis major segmental anatomy and segmentally split pectoralis major flaps. Plast Reconstr Surg 75:814-824, 1985.
7. Baek SM, Lawson W, Biller HF: An analysis of 133 pectoralis major myocutaneous flaps. Plast Reconstr Surg 69:460-467, 1982.
8. Barton FE, Spicer TE, Byrd HS: Head and neck reconstruction with the latissimus dorsi myocutaneous flap: Anatomic observations and report of 60 cases. Plast Reconstr Surg 71:199-204, 1983.
9. Watson JS, Robertson GA, Lendrum J, et al: Pharyngeal reconstruction using the latissimus dorsi myocutaneous flap. Br J Plast Surg 35:401-407, 1982.
10. Yamamoto K, Takagi N, Miyashita Y, et al: Facial reconstruction with latissimus dorsi myocutaneous island flap following total maxillectomy. J Craniomaxillofac Surg 15:288-294, 1987.
11. Zhao YF, Zhang WF, Zhao JH: Reconstruction of intraoral defects after cancer surgery using cervical pedicle flaps. J Oral Maxillofacial Surg 59:1142-1146, 2001.
12. Charles GA, Hamaker RC, Singer MI: Sternocleidomastoid myocutaneous flap. Laryngoscope 97:970-974, 1987.
13. Meyer R: Current treatment of stenoses. In Reconstructive Surgery of the Trachea. New York, Thieme, 1982, pp 80-82.
14. Mathes SJ, Vasconez LO: The cervicohumeral flap. Plast Reconstr Surg 61:7-12, 1978.
15. Baek SM, Biller HF, Krespi YP, Lawson W: The lower trapezius island myocutaneous flap. Ann Plast Surg 5:108-114, 1980.
16. Chandrasekhar B, Terez JJ, Kokal WA, et al: The inferior trapezius musculocutaneous flap in head and neck surgery. Ann Plast Surg 21:201-209, 1988.
17. Panje W: Myocutaneous trapezius flap. Head Neck Surg 2:206-212, 1980.
18. Abul-Hassan HS, Asher GVD, Acland RD: Surgical anatomy and blood supply of the fascial layers of the temporal region. Plast Reconstr Surg 77:17-24, 1986.
19. Antonyshyn O, Gruss JS, Bart BD: Versatility of temporal muscle and fascial flaps. Br J Plast Surg 41:118-131, 1988.
20. Carstens MH, Greco RJ, Hurwitz DJ, Tolhurst DE: Clinical applications of the subgaleal fascia. Plast Reconstr Surg 87:615-626, 1991.
21. Bakamjian VY, Souther SG: Use of temporal muscle flap for reconstruction after orbitomaxillary resections for cancer. Plast Reconstr Surg 56:171-177, 1975.
22. Koranda FC, McMahon MF, Jernstorm VR: The temporalis muscle flap for intraoral reconstruction. Arch Otorhinolaryngol 113:740-743, 1987.
23. Reese AB, Jones IS: Exenteration of the orbit and repair by transplantation of the temporalis muscle. Am J Ophthalmol 51:217-222, 1961.
24. Bakamjian VY: A two-stage method of pharyngoesophageal reconstruction with a primary pectoral skin flap. Plast Reconstr Surg 36:173-184, 1965.
25. Mendelson BC, Woods JE, Masson JK: Experience with the deltopectoral flap. Plast Reconstr Surg 59:360-365, 1977.
26. Krizek TJ, Robson MC: Potential pitfalls in the use of the deltopectoral flap. Plast Reconstr Surg 50:326-332, 1972.
27. Becker DW: A cervicopectoral rotation flap for cheek coverage. Plast Reconstr Surg 61:868-870, 1978.

Chapter **83**

Cleft Lip and Palate: Comprehensive Treatment and Technique

Anil Gungor, Ramon Ruiz, and Bernard J. Costello

Comprehensive treatment of cleft lip and palate deformities requires thoughtful consideration of the anatomic complexities of the deformity and the delicate balance between intervention and growth. Comprehensive and coordinated care from infancy through adolescence is essential to achieve an ideal outcome. Surgeons with formal training and experience in all phases of care must be actively involved in planning and treatment.[1,2] Specific goals of surgical care for children born with a cleft lip and palate include:

- Normalized aesthetic appearance of the lip and nose
- Intact primary and secondary palates
- Normalized speech, language, and hearing
- Nasal airway patency
- Class I occlusion with normal masticatory function
- Good dental and periodontal health
- Normal psychosocial development

What makes these goals challenging in some children is the wide spectrum of cleft lip, palate, and nasal deformities. The range of manifestations from one affected child to another is highly variable. An asymptomatic bifid uvula is an example of a clinically inconsequential cleft. A relatively simple deformity may include a submucous cleft palate that causes speech abnormality after an uneventful adenoidectomy. An occult cleft lip with an intact philtral ridge and symmetrical Cupid's bow and an otherwise normal-looking child with a small notch in the alveolar ridge are other such examples of minimal deformities. Unfortunately, the other end of the spectrum includes wide bilateral clefts of the lip and palate or facial dysplasia with several associated anomalies (Fig. 83-1).

A cleft surgeon has the tasks of addressing anatomic and functional deficiencies at the initial evaluation and planning for future functional and aesthetic needs. Success in these endeavors is dependent on many factors, including the severity of disruption of bone, cartilage, and soft tissue. Surgical skill and technique matched to the nature and severity of the deformity are the fundamental factors in obtaining superior results. Attention to all aspects of care, such as anatomic variants, the biology of scar formation, parent education, and cooperation, is very important in determining success. A healthy and collaborative team environment is essential in achieving these goals.

This chapter presents a technical overview of the reconstruction of cleft lip and palate deformities. Surgical reconstruction of clefts requires that surgeons undertaking this important work maintain a cognitive understanding of the complex malformation itself, the varied operative techniques used, facial growth considerations, and the psychosocial health of the patient and family. The objectives of this chapter are to present the overall staged reconstructive approach for repair of cleft lip and palate from infancy through the time of skeletal maturity, as well as a focused discussion of the specific surgical procedures involved in primary repair of clefts of the lip and palate.

CLASSIFICATION OF CLEFTS

Classification of clefts is necessary to describe the deformities, to study causative factors, and to compare results of treatment undertaken. Several classification systems have been described.[2-5] Simple classification systems are valuable for everyday use and are easy to understand; they provide broad groups with large numbers of patients in each group for research and analysis. However, simple classification systems fail to detail the variations in severity of cleft manifestations. As a consequence, there has been a tendency to use more

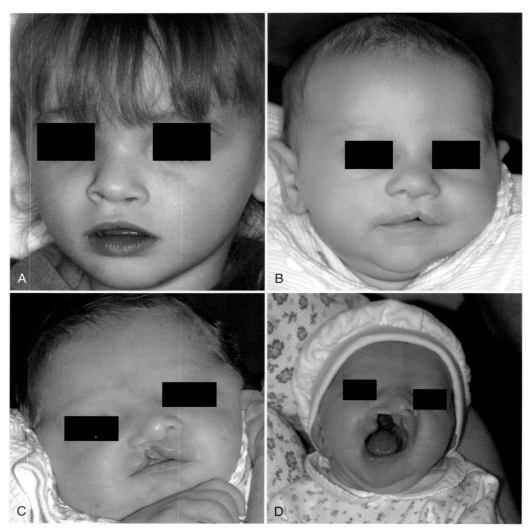

Figure 83-1. Because cleft lips come in a variety of configurations, each repair must be individually customized to establish the most normal morphology. **A,** Microform left unilateral cleft lip only, not requiring repair. **B,** Minor left incomplete unilateral cleft lip only. **C,** Right incomplete unilateral cleft lip and palate with a Simonart band. **D,** Wide right complete unilateral cleft lip and palate.

complex classification systems, which are more difficult to use clinically but provide better information for research and outcomes analysis.

There is infinite variation in the configuration of clefts, and a compromise between simple and complex classification systems has to be reached. Regardless of complexity, all classification systems use basic nasal (ala, dome, columella, nostril sill, septum, vomer), labial (vermilion, philtrum, Cupid's bow, Lister's tubercle, red and white lines, prolabium), and palatal (incisive foramen, primary and secondary palate, hard and soft palate, alveolar process, attachment to septum) landmarks for reporting.

The LAHSHAL system is a basic and useful classification that allows easy compilation of data. Starting from the patient's right side, the cleft status is recorded as C(omplete), I(ncomplete), or X (absent) for the L(ip), A(lveolus), H(ard palate), S(oft palate), H(ard palate), A(lveolus), and L(ip) (Table 83-1). Craniofa-

Table 83-1	CLASSIFICATION OF CLEFTS					
Right						**Left**
L	A	H	S	H	A	L
I	C	C	C	X	X	X

This example is for a unilateral right incomplete cleft lip (I) with a complete cleft alveolus (A) and hard (H) and soft (S) palates. The vomer is attached to the left side of the hard palate. The alveolus and lip on the left side are intact.

C, complete; I, incomplete; X, no cleft.

cial clefting may be described with Tessier's orbitocentric system of numbering (Fig. 83-2).

INTERDISCIPLINARY CARE

Successful management of the child born with a cleft lip and palate requires coordinated care provided by

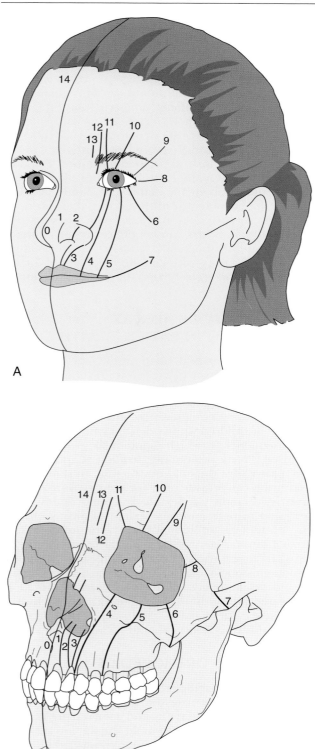

Figure 83-2. A and **B,** Complex facial clefts can be classified according to Tessier's orbitocentric system of numbering. Clefts may involve all tissue planes, including the skin, mucosa, bone, teeth, muscle, brain, peripheral nerve, and other specialized structures.

individuals from a number of different specialties, including otolaryngology, oral and maxillofacial surgery, plastic surgery, genetics/dysmorphology, speech/language pathology, orthodontics, prosthodontics, and others.[1,2,6] Because care is provided over the entire course of the child's development, long-term follow-up is critical to ensure complete and comprehensive care.

Rehabilitation of a patient with a cleft is best performed as an interdisciplinary effort. Most children with clefts have multiple interrelated issues, and several team models are available to address these issues in an interdisciplinary fashion. Key members of the team are the cleft surgeon or surgeons, orthodontist, and speech-language pathologist. Cleft surgeons may be trained plastic surgeons, oral and maxillofacial surgeons, or otolaryngologists. Other key persons may include the pediatric dentist, geneticist/dysmorphologist, pediatrician, psychologist, and social worker. The team director may or may not be a cleft surgeon but should be a nonbiased participant in care. The formation of interdisciplinary cleft teams serves two key objectives of successful cleft care: (1) coordinated care provided by all the necessary disciplines and (2) continuity of care with close interval follow-up of the patient throughout periods of active growth and ongoing stages of reconstruction.

In a carousel team, patients are seen on the same day by all specialists. Comprehensive evaluation is not performed, at the time of decision making information may be incomplete, and one practitioner's treatment decision may not reflect the complete status of the patient until all the information can be reviewed by everyone involved. In a triage team, one gatekeeper organizes outpatient referrals to specialists through multiple visits. This approach is often costly and requires a team meeting of all the practitioners to provide comprehensive care.

Multidisciplinary teams have many specialists, but they may not necessarily be cooperative or interactive. The best organization of care occurs when multidisciplinary teams are also interdisciplinary. Interdisciplinary teams work together to come up with the best treatment plan for a given patient. In this treatment model, decisions are based on a collaborative process, and each member is cognizant of other members' treatment priorities.

PRENATAL DIAGNOSIS

Team involvement ideally starts in the prenatal period.[1,2,7,8] Prenatal diagnosis by ultrasound presents an opportunity to introduce team members and their roles early in the process and provides reassurance, familiarity, and a structured approach for the various issues, including counseling, treatment, and feeding approaches. Prenatal sonographic detection of clefts is often dependent on cleft type and severity. When a cleft is present, the overall detection rate is approximately 65% (isolated cleft palate, 22%; isolated cleft lip, 67%; cleft lip and palate, 93%).[1]

Additional testing may be warranted to evaluate the possibility of associated deformities, syndromes, and sequences that could affect the birthing process. Exceptionally skilled ultrasonographers can visualize airway development and other abnormalities that may require early intervention with fetal surgery, ex utero intrapartum procedures, extracorporeal membrane oxygenation, or surgical airway management (tracheotomy) at the time of delivery. Evaluations of any associated malformations are completed via three-dimensional ultrasound, magnetic resonance imaging, and other genetic evaluations. These detailed evaluations can be very helpful in understanding the nature of various deformities, the likelihood of an uneventful birth, and the need for additional evaluation and treatment.

SEQUENCING OF PROCEDURES

Because of many different treatment philosophies, the timing of treatment interventions varies from one cleft center to another. Therefore, it is difficult to produce a timing regimen that everyone agrees on.[1,2,9-11] A sample timeline of staged reconstruction of cleft lip and palate deformities is presented in Table 83-2. This is a general timeline and requires an individualized approach based on aesthetic and functional priorities.

Table 83-2	TIMELINE FOR STAGED RECONSTRUCTION OF CLEFT LIP AND PALATE DEFORMITIES
Procedure	**Timing**
Airway evaluation and intervention	After initial assessment when necessary
Presurgical orthopedics, nasoalveolar molding, lip adhesion	Before lip repair in select cases
Cleft lip/nasal repair	After 10 wk
Cleft palate repair	9-18 mo
Myringotomy and tubes	At the time of lip or palate repair, depending on the presence of middle ear effusion and hearing status
Pharyngeal flap or pharyngoplasty	3-5 yr or later, depending on speech development
Maxillary/alveolar reconstruction with bone grafting	6-9 yr, depending on dental development
Cleft orthognathic surgery	14-16 yr in girls, 16-18 yr in boys
Cleft septorhinoplasty	After 5 yr of age but preferably at skeletal maturity after orthognathic surgery when possible
Cleft lip revision	Anytime after initial remodeling and scar maturation, but best after 5 yr of age

The timing of cleft lip and palate repair is controversial. Despite a number of meaningful advancements in the care of patients with cleft lip and palate, there is a lack of consensus regarding the timing and specific techniques used during each stage of cleft reconstruction. Surgeons must continue to carefully balance the functional needs, aesthetic concerns, and the issue of ongoing growth when deciding how and when to intervene. In no other type of deformity is the effect of early surgery on growth more apparent than in the treatment of cleft lip and palate deformities. The decision to surgically manipulate the tissues of a growing child should not be made lightly and should take into account the possible growth restriction that can occur with early surgery. Nevertheless, many patients with congenital deformities will benefit from early surgical intervention for functional or psychosocial reasons. Understanding the growth and development of the craniofacial skeleton is essential to the treatment planning process.[1,2]

MANAGEMENT OF AIRWAY OBSTRUCTION IN PATIENTS WITH CLEFTS

Features of the airway depend on the type of cleft and its severity. An intact palate provides tongue support and prevents glossoptosis. Lacking this support, a child with a wide cleft palate will have obstruction of the upper airway of varying severity. This obstruction is pronounced in children with associated syndromes and the Robin sequence in which mandibular growth is compromised. Prone positioning, feeding adaptation, and time may resolve the mild obstruction. In some cases a nasal airway can provide relief for a few weeks to months. Airway evaluation via flexible and rigid endoscopy is warranted to determine the extent of airway obstruction, as well as additional airway compromise (i.e., choanal atresia, laryngotracheomalacia, subglottic stenosis). In severe cases of obstruction, surgical options include glossopexy, mandibular distraction osteogenesis, and tracheotomy. Difficult intubation should be anticipated, and additional equipment such as a Bullard laryngoscope, laryngeal mask airway, or flexible endoscopic intubation devices should be available.

PRESURGICAL ORTHOPEDICS

Presurgical orthopedic (PSO) devices are used to mechanically manipulate the position of the alveolar segments before definitive lip and nasal repair. A custom acrylic prosthesis is used to mold the lip and maxillary dental arch. As the greater segment is pushed into position, space is cut away within the palatal plate to allow the lesser segment to drift into the proper arch form. When the lip has an incomplete cleft, the alveolar segments are usually molded into a reasonable arch form, and maxillary arch orthopedic devices are not necessary.

Nasoalveolar molding is a technique that combines maxillary arch orthopedics with a PSO device and lip and nasal contour shaping via nasal-vestibular projec-

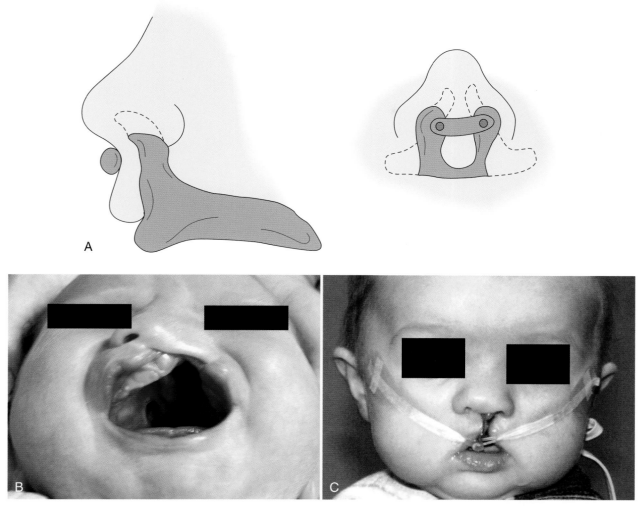

Figure 83-3. A, Frontal and lateral views of the Grayson nasoalveolar molding (NAM) appliance showing the nasal projections that help mold the nasal cartilage and maxillary segments into a more appropriate configuration before repair. **B,** Segments before the use of NAM. **C,** Segments after NAM but before closure.

tion (Fig. 83-3).[12-17] The importance of this technique is emphasized by surgeons who advocate primary nasal repair at the time of lip repair for children with wide clefts and severe nasal deformities, especially those with a very short columella. Successful use of PSO devices requires a dedicated pediatric dentist or orthodontist, a good laboratory, and diligent parents. Noncompliance can be a problem, so for this and other reasons, some centers rely on pin-retained prostheses. However, these appliances have been associated with significant midface growth restriction.[17]

Some surgeons perform a surgical lip adhesion procedure at about 3 months to mold the alveolar segments into better position before definitive repair. Effective PSO devices may obviate the need for a lip adhesion procedure and the additional anesthetic required for it.[18] Although initial results are reportedly good, use of these devices and their efficacy are still controversial because long-term outcome studies showing improved aesthetics, higher retention of dentition, and better dental arch form are still not available.[1,2,14-16,19]

LIP ADHESION

In exceptionally wide unilateral or bilateral clefts or in extremely asymmetrical bilateral clefts, it may be helpful to approximate the segments of the cleft lip before definitive lip repair to achieve a better relationship of both the lip structures and the dental arches. In this technique, which is used by some surgeons, small flaps of tissue are advanced across the cleft site (Fig. 83-4). Care is taken to not disturb natural landmarks, and a through-and-through horizontal tension suture is placed. When used, lip adhesion is usually completed at 3 months of age. The definitive lip repair is then completed 3 to 6 months later by excising the scar and reapproximating the remaining lip structures.

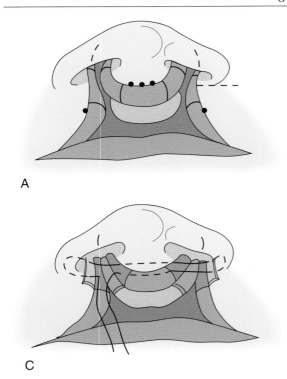

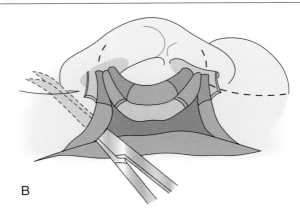

Figure 83-4. Example of the lip adhesion technique used by some surgeons as a first stage in closing wide clefts. **A,** Flaps are designed to bridge the defect. **B,** Undermining allows approximation. **C,** A retention suture may be used before closure for additional support. *(From Senders CW: Presurgical orthopedics. Facial Plast Surg Clinics North Am 4:333-342, 1996.)*

PRIMARY UNILATERAL CLEFT LIP REPAIR

Unilateral clefts of the lip and nose have a high degree of variability, and thus each repair design is unique (see Fig. 83-1). One repair technique preferred by the authors for cleft lip and nasal deformities is shown in Figures 83-5 and 83-6 and is usually performed after 10 weeks of age. The goal of the repair is to create a three-layered closure of skin, muscle, and mucosa in which hypoplastic tissue at the cleft margins is excised and normal tissues are approximated. Critical in the process is reconstruction of the orbicularis oris musculature into a continuous, functional sphincter. The Millard rotation-advancement technique has the advantage of allowing each of the incision lines to fall within the natural contours of the lip and nose.[1,2,20,21] This is an advantage because it is difficult to achieve "mirror image" symmetry in a unilateral cleft lip and nose with the normal side immediately adjacent to the surgical site. A Z-plasty technique such as the Randall-Tennison repair may not achieve this level of symmetry because the Z-shaped scar is directly adjacent to the linear non-clefted philtrum. Achieving symmetry is more difficult when the rotation portion of the cleft is quite short in comparison with the advancement segment. There is a great degree of variability in repair techniques from surgeon to surgeon. Several techniques are discussed as examples of unilateral and bilateral lip repair.

All landmarks are carefully marked with the use of operating loupes and surgical calipers (Fig. 83-5A). Marking starts with identification of the low point (midline) (1) and the peak (2) of Cupid's bow on the

noncleft side (NCS). The distance between these two points is used to determine the position of the peak of Cupid's bow on the cleft side (CS) (3). The alar base on the NCS (4), the columellar base (5), and the commissures (6 and 7) are marked. The lateral peak of Cupid's bow (8) is marked by taking the distance from the CS commissure and the width of the vermilion into account. The combined vertical height of the wet and dry vermilion at point 8 should match the vertical height of the vermilion at point 3. Therefore, 8 can be placed within 1 to 2 mm of the measured distance (matching the distance between 2 and 6) from the commissure to match the vermilion in height.

The tip of the advancement flap (9) is marked so that the distance between points 8 and 9 matches the distance between 2 and 5 (see Fig. 83-5A). The surgeon must avoid discolored, hypoplastic skin with increased vascular patterns when designing the flap. The slightest difference in color here will be highly visible against the contrast provided by the NCS lip and columella skin.

The rotation incision is followed by a very small (<1 mm) releasing cut (y) made high in the lip in a near-perpendicular angle to the rotation incision (see Fig. 83-5B). This should allow the NCS to drop down without tension and create a symmetrical prolabium with minimal transgression of the upper philtral column.

The orbicularis oris is dissected from the skin along the rotation and advancement flaps (see Fig. 83-5C). The dissection is performed to facilitate layered closure. If feasible, the muscle may be interdigitated. The mucosal closure is started in the sulcus and extended

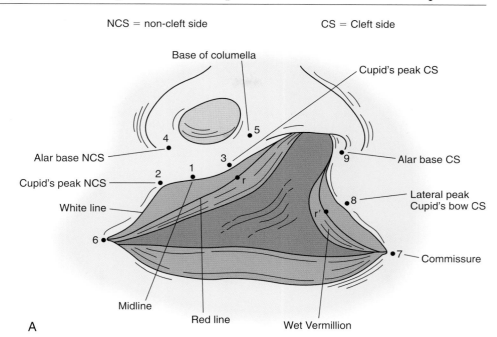

NCS = non-cleft side   CS = Cleft side

Base of columella

Cupid's peak CS

Alar base NCS

Cupid's peak NCS

White line

Midline

Red line

Alar base CS

Lateral peak
Cupid's bow CS

Commissure

Wet Vermillion

3-r = 8-r′ (to align red line)

Figure 83-5. A, Key landmarks of a unilateral cleft lip repair are marked with a fine marking instrument. **B,** Hypoplastic tissue is excised by following the key landmarks, and a variety of backcuts can be made to address symmetry.

A

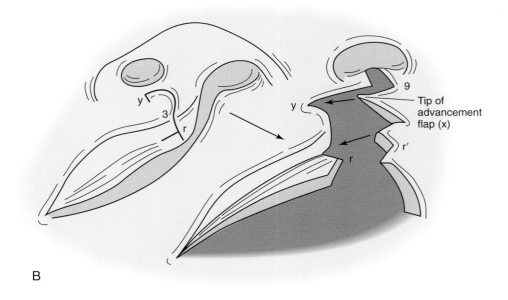

Tip of
advancement
flap (x)

B

toward the wet vermilion with 4-0 chromic or polyglycolic acid suture. The skin is closed with 5-0 or 6-0 nylon or with absorbable suture (see Fig. 83-5D).

Primary nasal reconstruction may be considered at the time of lip repair to reposition the displaced lower lateral cartilage and alar tissue. Several techniques have been advocated, and considerable variation exists with respect to the exact nasal reconstruction performed by each surgeon.[1,2,12,22] Primary nasal repair may be achieved by releasing and reshaping the lower lateral cartilage and alar base and augmenting the area with

allogeneic subdermal grafts or even formal open rhinoplasty. Because lip repair is done at such an early point in growth and development, the authors prefer minimal surgical dissection because of the effects of scarring on subsequent growth of these tissues. McComb described a technique that has become popular in which the lower lateral cartilage is dissected free from the alar base and the surrounding attachments through the incision at the alar crease.[22]

The lower lateral cartilage is dissected free of skin (including that between the medial crura and dome)

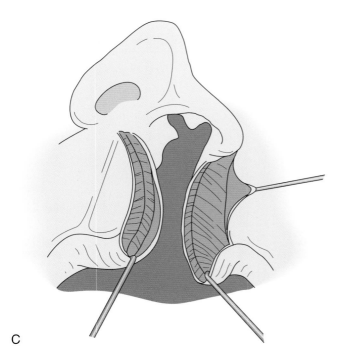

C

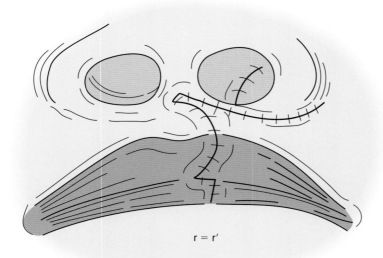

$$r = r'$$

D

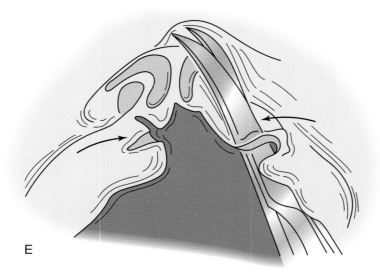

E

Figure 83-5, cont'd C, A three-layered closure is achieved by first reconstructing the oral mucosa and nasal floor and then the orbicularis oris musculature. The skin flaps should be passively closed without tension. **D,** The rotation and advancement flaps are inset for optimized symmetry in all three dimensions. **E,** Limited nasal dissection can be used to reposition the lower lateral cartilage, as well as the lateral alar tissue. These tissues must be released from their abnormal insertions and repositioned for better symmetry. A nasal bolster or silicone nasal formers may be placed at the end of the procedure.

(see Fig. 83-5E) and suspended to the ipsilateral upper lateral cartilage with a looping suture (see Fig. 83-1D). If necessary, interdomal and suspension sutures (see Fig. 83-1E) may be used to reposition and reorient the nasal tip. This modification requires extended dissection. The dislocated nasal septum is released, transposed, and secured through the membranous septal incision. The nasal ala is then repositioned to address symmetry in all three dimensions. In most complete unilateral clefts, the alar base has to be dissociated from the lateral aspect of the lip and piriform aperture by extending the circumalar incision to allow these elements to move independently. The advancement flap will be advanced more than the ala. The tip of the advancement flap may then be anchored to the membranous septum. The nostril may be stented for several weeks or longer with silicone nostril retainers or bolsters to prevent distortion in nostril shape.

Parents may feed their child immediately by the same methods that were used preoperatively. Arm restraints are routinely used to protect the lip from trauma for approximately 2 weeks. Antibiotic ointment may be applied in the first few days, followed by gentle massage several times per day starting 2 weeks after repair to encourage remodeling of the scar.

PRIMARY BILATERAL LIP REPAIR

Bilateral cleft lip repair can be one of the most challenging technical procedures performed. The lack of quality tissue and the widely displaced segments are major challenges to achieving exceptional results, but superior technique and adequate mobilization of the tissue flaps generally yield excellent aesthetic results (Figs. 83-7 to 83-9). Additionally, the columella may be quite short in length, and the premaxillary segment may be significantly rotated. Adequate mobilization of the segments and attention to the details of using only appropriately developed tissue will yield excellent results, even in individuals with significant asymmetry.

Although often more challenging than most unilateral repairs, the technique for bilateral cleft lip and nose reconstruction is similar in concept to that for unilateral repair. Markings are made with a fine marking instrument at key landmarks while being sure to not include any hypoplastic tissue from within the cleft (Fig. 83-7). Points 12 and 13 should be made at the beginning of the good white roll and vermilion, with a small backcut extending laterally to allow advancement under the prolabial tissue. Points 8 to 12 and 7 to 13 should be equal in length, and the measurement at 2 to 4 should be no longer than 3 mm. This tissue will stretch significantly later as remodeling of the lip occurs. Incisions within the nares should be made carefully so that one does not excise too much tissue and make the nares quite small. Backcuts around the alar base should be long enough to allow nasal dissection, release of alar tissue from the piriform rim, and advancement medially to reconstruct the nares.

Some surgeons have used operative techniques involving banked fork flaps to surgically lengthen the

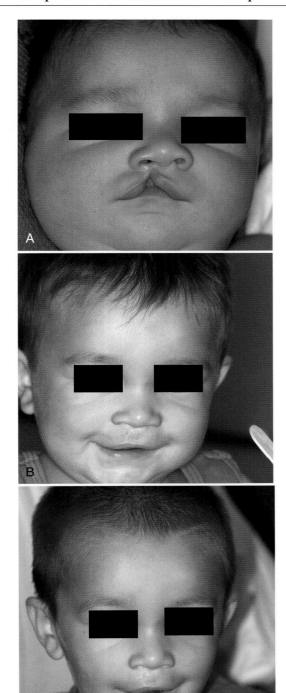

Figure 83-6. A, Three-month-old child with a right-sided incomplete unilateral cleft lip. Note the short philtrum near the midline, which must be rotated downward to avoid notching and to improve symmetry. **B,** Nine-month-old boy after rotation-advancement repair of his cleft lip and nasal deformities. **C,** The same child in **B** 2½ years after his cleft lip and nasal repairs.

columella and preserve hypoplastic tissue. Early and aggressive tissue flaps in the nostril and columella areas do not look natural after significant growth has occurred and result in abnormal tissue contours. Although surgical attempts at lengthening the columella may look

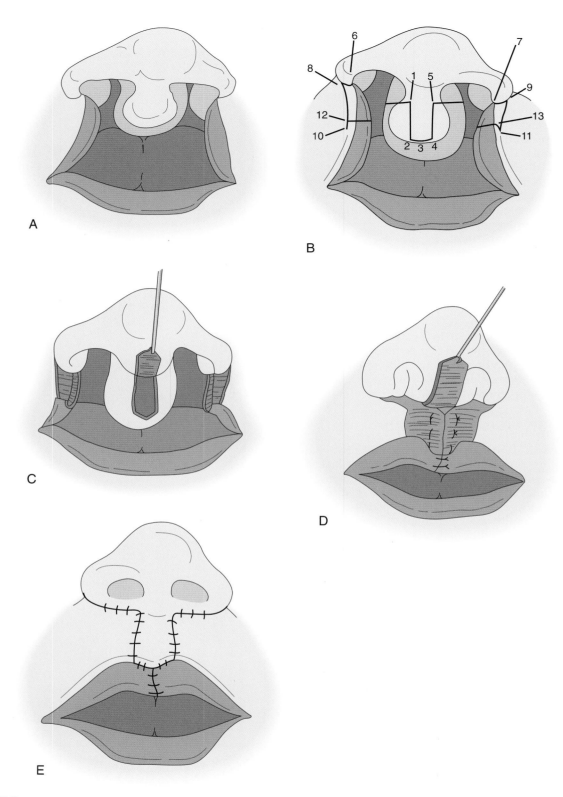

Figure 83-7. A, The bilateral cleft of the lip and maxilla shown here is complete and highlights the nature of hypoplastic tissue along the cleft edges. The importance of the nasal deformity is evident in the shorter columella and disrupted nasal complexes. **B,** Markings of the authors' preferred repair are shown with an emphasis on excision of hypoplastic tissue and approximating more normal tissue with the advancement flaps. Measurements should be roughly equal in the following fashion: 1 to 2 = 6 to 10; 5 to 4 = 7 to 11; 1 to 2 = 5 to 4; and 6 to 10 = 7 to 11. **C,** A new philtrum is created by excising the lateral hypoplastic tissue and elevating the philtrum superiorly. Additionally, the lateral advancement flaps are dissected into three distinct layers (skin, muscle, and mucosa). Nasal floor reconstruction also occurs in conjunction with these advancement flaps. **D,** The orbicularis oris musculature is approximated in the midline with multiple interrupted or mattress sutures, or both. This is a critical step in total reconstruction of a functional lip. There is no musculature present in the premaxillary segment, and it must be brought to the midline from each lateral advancement flap. The nasal floor flaps are sutured at this time as well. The new vermilion border is reconstructed in the midline with good white roll tissue advanced from the lateral flaps. **E,** Final approximation of the skin and mucosal tissues is performed in a manner that leaves the healing incision lines in the natural contours of the lip and nose.

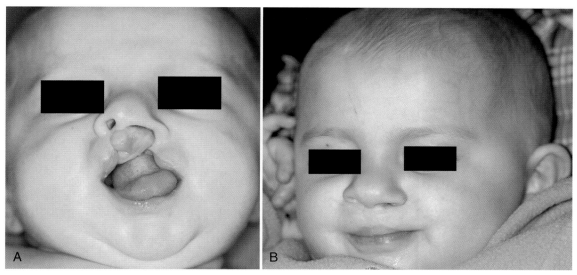

Figure 83-8. A, Presurgical appearance of a bilateral cleft lip and palate with impressive asymmetry and rotation of the premaxillary segment. Note the significant nasal asymmetry and bunching of the orbicularis oris laterally. **B,** The same child at 14 months of age. No presurgical orthopedic appliances were used.

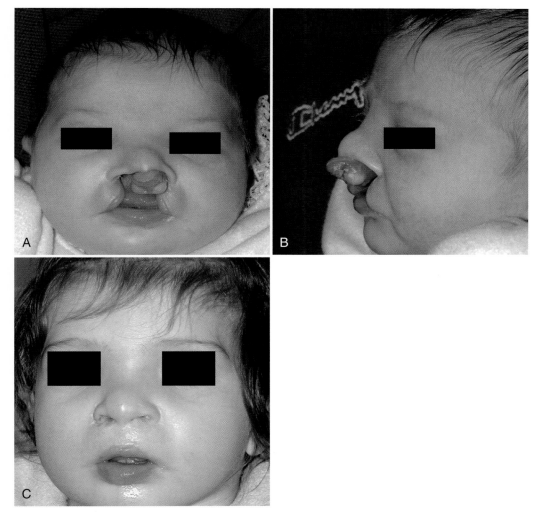

Figure 83-9. A, Presurgical frontal view of a wide bilateral cleft lip and palate with significant asymmetry and lack of columella length. **B,** Presurgical left lateral view of a wide bilateral cleft lip and palate with a protrusive premaxillary segment. Note the short length of the columella. **C,** The same child after repair of her bilateral cleft lip and palate. No presurgical taping or orthopedic appliances were used.

good initially, they frequently appear abnormally long and excessively angular later in life. Revision of these iatrogenic deformities is difficult, and some of the contour irregularities will not be able to be revised adequately. Usually, if the hypoplastic tissue is excised and incisions within the medial nasal base and columella are avoided, the long-term aesthetic results are excellent.

The authors prefer a primary nasal reconstruction that can be performed in a fashion similar to the unilateral technique described by McComb.[1,2,22] Other open rhinoplasty techniques involving either a direct incision on the nasal tip or prolabial unwind-ing techniques have been suggested.[12] As with most early maneuvers, aggressive rhinoplasty at this time may result in early scarring that affects the growth potential of the surrounding tissues and makes revision more difficult and long-term aesthetics less than ideal.

CLEFT LIP REVISION

Despite even the most superb techniques, many patients who undergo cleft lip repair will benefit from at least a minor revision at some point in life. Although revision procedures are often viewed as optional phases of cleft lip reconstruction, surgeons must advise families of this likelihood. The hard and soft tissues of the maxillofacial complex grow and change as a child grows, and the repaired lip is affected. Bilateral clefts will benefit from lip revision more often than unilateral clefts will. The majority of lip growth is complete after the age of 5 years, and this may be the best time to consider revision of the lip because the psychosocial benefits before entering school may be considerable. Alternatively, revision of the lip can be delayed until the teenage years, when most maxillofacial growth is complete. It is preferable to wait until orthognathic surgery is completed (if this becomes necessary) because these procedures will considerably change the contour and shape of the nose and lips.

The surgical objectives of cleft lip revision include excision of residual scar, reapproximation of key anatomic landmarks such as the vermilion-cutaneous junction and vermilion-mucosal junction, and leveling of vertical lip lengths (philtral columns). Repair of the orbicularis oris muscle as a distinct layer is critical to an acceptable outcome. Although small scar revisions may be considered in some patients, many patients will benefit from a revision that completely reconstructs the area by excision of the scar, dissection of the tissues into three layers (skin, muscle, and mucosa), and a reconstruction that achieves improved symmetry and form. As with the primary repair, 6-0 or smaller sutures may be used to minimize stitch marks. Postoperative care includes careful early wound care and avoidance of extended sun exposure, similar to the instructions for primary repairs.

PALATOPLASTY

There are two main goals of cleft palate repair during infancy: (1) closure of the oral-nasal communication involving the embryologic secondary palate and (2) anatomic repair of the musculature within the soft palate, which is important for normal production of speech. The soft palate, or velum, is part of the complex coupling and decoupling of the oral and nasal cavities involved in the production of speech. When a cleft of the soft palate is present, abnormal muscle insertions are located at the posterior edge of the hard palate. Surgery must not simply be aimed at closing the palatal defect, but rather at release of abnormal muscle insertions to create muscle continuity with improved orientation so that the velum may serve as a dynamic structure. Despite successful repair of the palate, a significant number of children who undergo cleft palate repair will still require speech therapy and have difficulty closing the velum for a variety of reasons.

Several techniques of palatoplasty with a substantial number of modifications may be found in the literature. Three popular techniques are discussed, including:

- Two-flap palatoplasty with intravelar veloplasty
- V-Y pushback with intravelar veloplasty
- Furlow palatoplasty

Before each procedure, the type and severity of the cleft, position of the segments, degree of septum deviation, width of the cleft, length and symmetry of the soft palate, and mobility of the soft palate and pharyngeal walls have to be considered. It is helpful to measure and record palatal width, length, and other cleft dimensions with calipers.

The patient is placed supine with the neck slightly extended, and a shoulder roll is used. A cleft mouth retractor is used to maximally open the mouth and at the same time secure the endotracheal tube in a midline position against the tongue. A small throat pack may be fitted in the hypopharynx around the tube. Incisions are marked with a marking pen, gentian violet, or methylene blue. Lidocaine with epinephrine solution is injected into the submucosal tissue and subperiosteal plane and around the palatine foramen. Subperiosteal injections can facilitate undermining of the mucoperiosteal flaps and improve hemostasis. The surgeon should avoid injecting into the neurovascular bundle. If vomer flaps are planned, the vomer is injected.

A variety of blades, including nos. 11, 15, and Beaver 6300 blades, are used to dissect the flaps. A small half-circle cutter is helpful when the cleft space is narrow. The PS 5 is a fine all-purpose $^3/_8$-inch cutter. The PS 4 cutter takes larger bites when required. In careful hands, a cutting needle may be less traumatic than a taper needle. However, if there is any tension on the wound, tapered needles may be used to avoid mucosal damage.

Two-Flap Palatoplasty with Intravelar Veloplasty

In the authors' practice this repair is the most appropriate technique for a complete unilateral cleft palate repair (Fig. 83-10).[1,2,23,24] The nasal flaps may be designed so that a strip of mucoperiosteum is left on the medial

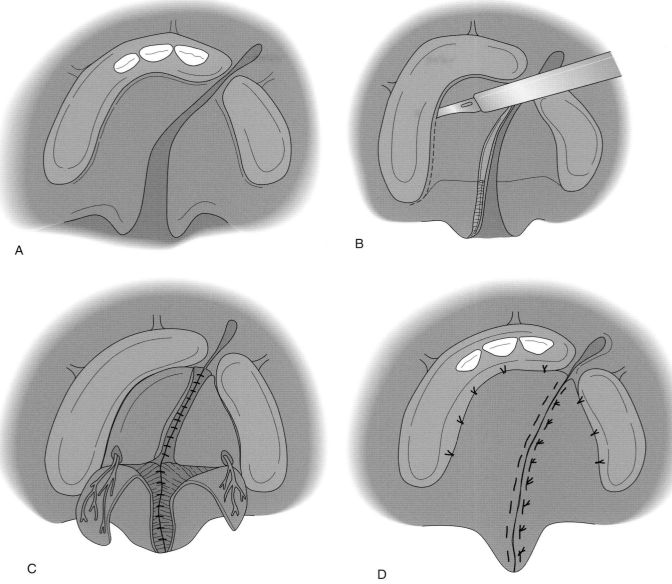

Figure 83-10. **A,** A unilateral cleft of the primary and secondary palates is shown with typical involvement from the anterior vestibule to the uvula. **B,** The Bardach palatoplasty technique requires two large full-thickness mucoperiosteal flaps to be elevated from each palatal shelf. The anterior portion (anterior to the incisive foramen) of the cleft is not reconstructed until the mixed-dentition stage. **C,** A layered closure is performed in the Bardach palatoplasty by reapproximating the nasal mucosa. The muscle bellies of the levator palatini are elevated off their abnormal insertions on the posterior palate. They are then reapproximated in the midline to create a dynamic functional sling for speech purposes. **D,** Once the nasal mucosa and musculature of the soft palate are approximated, the oral mucosa is closed in the midline. The lateral releasing incisions are quite easily closed primarily because of the length gained from the depth of the palate. In rare cases, with very wide clefts, a portion of the lateral incisions may remain open and granulate by secondary intention.

edge of the hard palate. The wider the cleft, the wider the strip of mucoperiosteum left on the medial edge of flap. The width and angle of the palatal shelves are also considered when designing the incisions. When these flaps are elevated and mobilized to reconstruct the nasal mucosal layer, they should meet each other without tension. On the soft palate, the incisions should follow the subtle transition line between the nasal and oral mucosa into the tip of the uvula. In a wide cleft

(gaps larger than 15 mm), vomer flaps may be designed to aid in closure centrally.

Laterally, the flaps are designed to include oral mucoperiosteum only (see Fig. 83-10B). Gingiva should be avoided. The incision line moves laterally at the junction of the alveolus, and the palatal shelf recovers its posterior direction quickly once the lateral aspect of the alveolus is reached and may continue 0.5 to 1 cm into the soft palate.

The oral mucosa is separated from the nasal mucosa toward the tip of the uvula with a superficial incision. Mucoperiosteal incisions on the hard palate have to be firm, perpendicular to the palatal plane, and should reach the palatal shelf with a continuous clean cut. Hemostasis with a fine needle tip electrocautery or bipolar electrocautery at low setting may be performed.

Elevation of mucoperiosteum is started anterolaterally with a Woodson or other small elevator. Gentle subperiosteal elevation of the tip of the flap is performed. After elevation of the tip, a Freer elevator is used to continue subperiosteal elevation posteriorly to visualize and elevate tissue around the neurovascular bundle. All muscular and tendinous attachments to the hard palate shelf are detached with a combination of sharp and blunt dissection while leaving the flap attached to the hard palate by the neurovascular bundle and lateral pedicle.

The soft palate is transposed medially by entering the space of Ernst with a blunt instrument (Metzenbaum scissors). To obtain more medial mobilization, infracture of the hamulus may be performed but is rarely necessary. Veau's muscle inserts into the periosteum on the posterior edge of the hard palate in concert with the tensor aponeurosis after it rounds the hamulus. (Veau's muscle is a clefted muscle consisting of the levator and the palatopharyngeus.) Some surgeons divide the tendon to mobilize muscles toward the medial aspect.

Gentle traction is used to pull the neurovascular bundle out of the greater palatine foramen (see Fig. 83-10C); the palatine foramen is surrounded by a periosteal cone that can be incised superficially on either side and posteriorly to allow maximal mobilization of the flap. Additional dissection is necessary to provide maximal mobility of the flap.

Complete dissection of Veau's muscle from the hard palate and nasal mucoperiosteum follows. Attachments are stripped from the nasal mucoperiosteum with sharp scissors and scalpel. Precise dissection allows lengthening of the palate and posterior/medial transfer of muscles to create a functional muscle sling. This reconstruction is termed an intravelar velarplasty. Dissection of muscle from the nasal and oral mucosa is more extensive than described in traditional two-flap palatoplasty techniques. Complete dissection with repositioning and tightening of the palatopharyngeus and levator in a posterior position is, for some, theoretically more physiologic.

Once the flaps are mobilized, closure of the nasal layer begins anteriorly and should be tension free (see Fig. 83-10C). Sutures are tied in knots on the nasal surface. The difference in length between the two flaps is considered and spacing of the sutures adjusted at this stage. There should be no tension at the hard palate–soft palate junction. The soft palate muscles are repositioned (overlapped if necessary) and sutured together with two or three mattress sutures (3-0 to 4-0 resorbable suture). The oral layer is then closed with single resorbable 4-0 or 5-0 interrupted or mattress

sutures and knots tied in the oral surface (see Fig. 83-10D).

The combined flaps are anchored (tagged) to the nasal mucoperiosteal closure with a 4-0 resorbable suture at about the midpoint, and the tip is secured to the alveolus with two to four sutures. These steps prevent dead space between the oral and nasal layers and stabilize the flaps. The same objective can be achieved by using three to four vertical mattress sutures through both the oral and nasal layers. Exposed bone laterally may be filled with microfibrillar collagen. A tongue suture (3-0 silk/nylon) is applied to aid in tongue advancement acutely in the rare instance of postoperative obstruction. Surgeons should minimize the time that the mouth gag retractor is activated during the procedure to avoid more severe swelling.

V-Y Pushback with Intravelar Veloplasty

For many surgeons, the V-Y pushback operation is the most appropriate technique for repair of a posterior (soft palate) cleft with limited extension into the hard palate (e.g., Robin-type cleft with unilateral or bilateral incomplete hard palate involvement). Design principles are similar to those for two-flap palatoplasty but include a V to Y incision design on the hard palate for theoretical retropositioning of the soft palate. Mucoperiosteum over the primary palate in front of the incisive foramen is left intact, and flaps are designed to leave this area in a V form. For closure, the flaps slide posteriorly to close the gap, and transposition of this junction into a Y form occurs. (This posterior displacement is limited to the tip of the mucoperiosteal flaps, is minimal, and should not be confused with what is frequently called a pushback palatoplasty in which posterior displacement aims to reposition the velar muscles.) Intravelar veloplasty and the remaining repair are identical to those used for the two-flap technique. Generally, a vomer flap is not necessary. The flaps are secured to the anterior mucoperiosteum with several sutures. This technique is not a good choice for a wide bilateral cleft that involves the incisive foramen area because a residual fistula will remain that is often difficult to close and may affect speech.

Furlow Palatoplasty

The Furlow technique closes the palate by mirror image Z-plasties of the oral and nasal sides of the soft palate (Fig. 83-11A to D).[1,2,25] Palatal muscles are carried in the posteriorly based flaps of each Z-plasty to construct an overlapping retropositioned palatal muscle sling. In some studies, this technique is associated with a lower frequency of velopharyngeal insufficiency (VPI) than noted with other palatoplasty techniques and at times is recommended for the treatment of VPI after another type of repair as a secondary procedure.[1,2,25,26]

The landmarks that determine the flap angles and flap design include the hamuli, the posterior edge of the hard palate, the base of the uvular halves, and the eustachian tube orifice (torus tubarius) (see Fig. 83-11E). The hamulus is palpable as a small bony eleva-

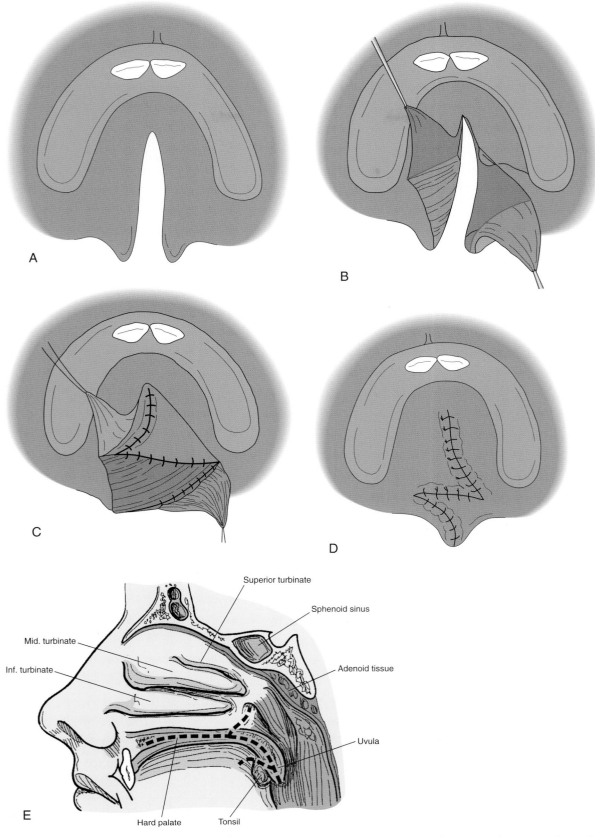

E

| Label positions in figure E: |
| Superior turbinate |
| Sphenoid sinus |
| Mid. turbinate |
| Inf. turbinate |
| Adenoid tissue |
| Uvula |
| Hard palate |
| Tonsil |

Figure 83-11. A, A complete cleft of the secondary palate (both hard and soft) is shown from the incisive foramen to the uvula. **B,** The Furlow double-opposing Z-plasty technique requires that separate Z-plasty flaps be developed on the oral and then the nasal side. Note the cutbacks creating the nasal side flaps, highlighted in blue. **C,** The flaps are then transposed to theoretically lengthen the soft palate. A nasal side closure is completed in standard fashion anterior to the junction of the hard and soft palate. Generally, this junction is the highest area of tension and can be difficult to close. This contributes to the higher fistula rate in this type of repair at this location. **D,** The oral side flaps are then transposed and closed in similar fashion to complete closure of the palate. **E,** Lateral view of nasal and palatal anatomy. The lateral extension of incisions in the Furlow palatoplasty sometimes requires that the incision be extended to the torus tubarius region. Care is taken to reposition the palatal musculature that is abnormally inserted on the posterior palate in conjunction with the double-opposing Z-plasty flaps.

tion of the pterygoid plate just medial and posterior to the maxillary tuberosity. Thus, when marking the flaps, the surgeon should remember that the Z-plasties are not two dimensional and that the angles do not need to be at 60 degrees each because flap design is based on the anatomy of the palate, not the geometry of the Z-plasty.

The lateral limbs of the incisions on the oral side and at the level of hamulus are extended to allow advancement of the flaps (see Fig. 83-11B). This incision can be extended around the maxillary tuberosity as a short backcut when necessary. For limited soft palate clefts, only the soft palate incisions and flaps are elevated without the need for hard palate releasing incisions.

The left myomucosal flap (oral) is posteriorly based. The muscle is dissected from the nasal mucosa with scissors, and the levator muscle is carefully preserved. The palatal muscles are separated from the aponeurosis and from the medial side of the superior constrictor to mobilize the flap for rotation. Once the oral flaps are raised, the nasal Z flaps are incised. On the left, the anteriorly based flap (nasal) is elevated as a mucosal flap. On the right, the posteriorly based (nasal) flap is elevated with the muscle. Each lateral limb incision ends just medial to the eustachian tube orifice (torus).

The left anteriorly based (nasal) mucosal flap is incised from the uvula along the dissected edge of the cleft muscle to the left torus. The right posteriorly based (nasal) mucosal-muscle flap is created by an incision from the posterior hard palate to near the torus while taking care to include velar cleft muscle in the flap. However, the mucosal incision on this flap is not extended completely up to the torus to facilitate subsequent closure.

The nasal side is closed by first transposing the left nasal mucosal (anteriorly based) flap transversely to the distal portion of the right nasal incision stepwise from the distal to the proximal aspects to the posterior hard palate nasal mucoperiosteum until the end of the flap reaches near the right torus. When tension is present, avoidance of the natural inclination to sew the distal tip of the flap to its ultimate location first helps protect the fragile tip of the flap. Next, the right myomucosal flap is transposed until the tip of the flap reaches the opposite superior constrictor muscle at the torus (see Fig. 83-11C). This flap is sutured to the nasal mucosal flap anteriorly. The muscle of the posteriorly based oral myomucosal flap on the left side is then secured to the right tonsillar pillar. The right anteriorly based mucosal flap is sutured in stepwise manner across to the oral mucosa on the opposite side.

Retention sutures through the muscle of the posteriorly based right-sided nasal flap may be placed through the base of the oral flap on the opposite side to relieve tension. Mucoperiosteal flaps (when present) are brought into the horizontal plane and sutured. Usually, no bone is exposed and no raw nasal area on the soft palate is left to contract and shorten the palate.

Postoperative care includes a liquid diet and placement of arm restraints for approximately 2 weeks to allow adequate mucosal healing. Careful follow-up and regular visits with a speech pathologist are important.

CLEFT PALATE, MIDDLE EAR, AND SPEECH

Speech characteristics associated with a cleft palate include abnormal nasal resonance, abnormal nasal airflow and altered laryngeal voice quality, nasal or facial grimace, and atypical consonant production (Table 83-3). In patients with clefts, abnormal nasal resonance is typically manifested as hypernasality secondary to VPI. Inadequate nasal resonance (hyponasality) may also occur as result of obstruction. Hypernasality and hyponasality can occur together (mixed nasality). Altered laryngeal voice quality commonly includes hoarseness and reduced volume. Nasal or facial grimace is an unconscious compensation mechanism to inhibit airflow through the nose. As a result of these issues and other factors, there is a risk of articulation disorders and other speech abnormalities.

Chronic Otitis Media

The cleft palate population has a high incidence of mild to moderate hearing loss. Early onset of otitis media with effusion (OME) is a universal finding in infants with unrepaired cleft palates, and the pathology is causally related to an inherent defect in the opening

Table 83-3	COMMON SPEECH ABNORMALITIES SEEN IN PATIENTS WITH CLEFT PALATE

Hypernasality: Failure of the palate to separate the oral and nasal cavities during non-nasal consonant production. Oral phonemes substituted by nasal sounds (m, n, ng)

Hyponasality: Reduction of the nasal airflow that occurs with the nasal consonants /m/, /n/, and /ng/. Usually not present with velopharyngeal insufficiency but may be noted when large adenoid or posterior nasal airway obstruction is present with an incompetent velopharyngeal valve

Cul-de-sac resonance: Air enters the nasal cavity but cannot escape because of anterior nasal blockage. Muffled sound quality

Nasal emission: Airflow normal with nasal consonants; abnormal with plosives, fricatives, and affricates. Determined with mirror testing. May be audible or inaudible

Nasal snort, /s/ phoneme, and other fricatives: In a patient with an initially closed velopharyngeal valve, as intraoral pressure increases, air escapes from the nose

Stops glottal: Plosive consonant produced by vocal fold valving

Chronic hoarseness: Vocal hyperfunction secondary to compensation at the laryngeal level

mechanism of the eustachian tube that results in persistent collapse of the tubal lumen.[27,28] Treatment of this condition requires evacuation of the effusion and insertion of ventilation tubes. In children with a cleft lip and palate, present and persistent OME should be addressed at the time of lip repair, which usually takes place at around 3 months of age. In children with a cleft palate only, persistent OME should be addressed when diagnosed, in a separate procedure, and should not wait for palate repair. In the author's opinion (A.G.), long-term tubes (T tubes) should be used when possible. This option may not be available in a very small ear. In both groups, ears need to be reevaluated shortly before palate repair and regular tubes replaced with long-term ventilation tubes at the time of palate repair. After successful palate repair, most children with a cleft lip and palate will not be scheduled for another surgical procedure for several years. The shorter retaining period and high extrusion rate of regular tubes make them less than ideal in many instances. Even after palate repair, eustachian tube function remains deficient in a large percentage of these children, and ear problems (infections, hearing loss, or both) are most prevalent in the 4- to 6-year-old age group. Ear problems persist at a substantial level until the age of 12 years, and children with a cleft lip and palate have a prolonged recovery and a substantial incidence of late sequelae.[28] T tubes are retained longer and will therefore obviate the need for repeated tube insertion, which presents additional unnecessary anesthesia risk for the child, as well as increases the cost of care substantially in the first 5 years of the child's life. Evaluation of the ear and hearing should be undertaken every 6 months.

Submucous Cleft Palate

A submucous cleft palate is a microform or incomplete version of a complete cleft of the embryologic secondary palate. It is characterized by the presence of a bifid uvula, a translucent midline known as the zona pellucida (caused by diastasis of the soft palate muscles),

and lack of a posterior nasal spine causing palpable notching of the posterior hard palate. A submucous cleft palate may be asymptomatic throughout life or become symptomatic after adenoidectomy, as well as after natural involution of the adenoid tissue. It is important to inspect the uvula carefully and palpate the posterior hard palate before an adenoidectomy. When considering adenoidectomy in any patient, if the posterior palatal spine cannot be palpated and a midline notch is present, partial (anterior) adenoidectomy should be considered. In general, submucous cleft palates are repaired only when they cause symptomatic speech abnormalities.

VELOPHARYNGEAL INCOMPETENCE

The secondary palate is composed of a hard (bone) palate anteriorly and a soft palate or "velum" posteriorly. Within the soft palate, the levator veli palatini muscle forms a dynamic sling that elevates the velum toward the posterior pharyngeal wall during the production of certain sounds. Other muscle groups within the velum, the tonsillar pillar region, and the pharyngeal walls also affect the quality of resonance during speech formation. The combination of the soft palate and pharyngeal wall musculature jointly forms what is described as the velopharyngeal valve mechanism (Fig. 83-12). This mechanism functions as a sphincter valve for regulating airflow between the oral and nasal cavities to create a combination of orally based and nasally based sounds.

Children born with a cleft palate have, by definition, a malformation that has a dramatic impact on the anatomic components of the velopharyngeal valve mechanism. Specifically, clefting of the secondary palate causes division of the musculature of the velum into separate muscle bellies with abnormal insertions along the posterior edge of the hard palate (see Fig. 83-12). VPI is a major functional concern for patients with a cleft. Regardless of the repair type, the incidence of VPI

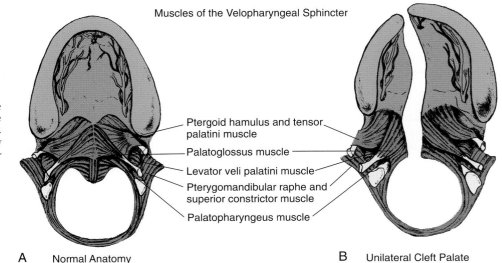

Muscles of the Velopharyngeal Sphincter

Figure 83-12. Anatomy of the palate and velopharyngeal valve mechanism. **A,** Normal anatomy. **B,** Unilateral cleft of the primary and secondary palate with associated anatomic abnormalities.

Ptergoid hamulus and tensor palatini muscle
Palatoglossus muscle
Levator veli palatini muscle
Pterygomandibular raphe and superior constrictor muscle
Palatopharyngeus muscle

A   Normal Anatomy

B   Unilateral Cleft Palate

after primary palate repair varies in studies from 5% to higher than 50%.[1,2,29,30]

VPI is defined as inadequate closure of the nasopharyngeal airway port during speech production. The exact cause of VPI after successful cleft palate repair is a complex problem that remains difficult to define completely. Incomplete surgical repair of the musculature is one cause of VPI, but even muscles that have been appropriately realigned and reconstituted may fail to heal normally or function properly. In addition, it must be considered that the repaired cleft palate is only one factor contributing to velopharyngeal valve function and that other abnormalities related to oropharyngeal morphology, nerve innervation, lateral and posterior pharyngeal wall motion, and nasal airway dynamics may all contribute to velopharyngeal valve dysfunction. For example, a short, scarred soft palate that does not elevate well may be compensated by recruitment and hypertrophy of muscular tissue within the posterior pharyngeal wall (Passavant's ridge).

Approximately 20% of children with VPI after palatoplasty will eventually require management involving additional palatal surgery. Left untreated, nasal air escape–related resonance problems will lead to other speech abnormalities, namely, abnormal compensatory articulation. These abnormal, compensatory misarticulations further complicate problems with speech formation and decrease speech intelligibility in patients with cleft palate–related VPI.

After the initial cleft palate repair, periodic evaluations are important to assess the speech and language development of each child. Typically, this involves a standardized screening examination performed by a speech and language pathologist as part of an annual visit to the cleft palate team. Detailed studies that include the use of videofluoroscopy and nasopharyngoscopy may be indicated. Videofluoroscopy is used to radiographically examine the upper airway with the aid of an oral contrast agent. This technique allows dynamic testing of the velopharyngeal valve mechanism with views of the musculature in action. In addition, details of upper airway anatomy, including residual palatal fistulas, can be visualized and their contribution to speech dysfunction evaluated during the study. For a videofluoroscopy study to be of diagnostic value it must include multiple views of the velopharyngeal valve mechanism, and a speech pathologist must be present to administer verbal testing in the radiology suite.

Nasopharyngoscopy allows direct visualization of the upper airway and specifically the velopharyngeal valve mechanism from the nasopharynx. This technique avoids the radiation exposure associated with videofluoroscopy but requires preparation of the nose with a topical anesthetic, skillful maneuvering of the scope, and a compliant patient. Once the endoscope is inserted, observations of palatal function, airway morphology, and pharyngeal wall motion are made while the patient is verbally tested by the speech pathologist. The opportunity for direct visualization of the velopharyngeal valve mechanism in action during speech formation provides information that is critical to clinical decision making related to secondary palatal surgery in cases of confirmed or suspected VPI.

With videofluoroscopy and nasoendoscopy, the closure pattern of the palate is documented and should be differentiated. The closure pattern may help determine the success of various secondary palatal procedures designed to augment anatomic deficiencies.

- The most common pattern of closure (55% of the normal population) is coronal closure. It consists of posterior movement of the soft palate to the posterior pharyngeal wall with little movement from the lateral walls. Approximately 45% of patients with VPI have this pattern of closure.
- The sagittal closure pattern is seen in 10% to 15% of the population. Primary closure is by lateral wall movement without significant anterior-to-posterior closure. This pattern is seen in approximately 10% of children with VPI.
- Circular closure includes lateral wall movement and posterior movement of the soft palate. It occurs in approximately 10% of the population and 20% of children with VPI. Circular closure with Passavant's ridge includes lateral wall and soft palate movement, as well as anterior movement of the posterior pharyngeal wall. This pattern is seen in 20% of the normal population and in 25% of children with VPI.

Secondary palatal surgery in young children is indicated when VPI is causing hypernasal speech on a consistent basis and is related to the anatomic problem. The exact timing of surgery for VPI remains controversial, however, with recommendations ranging from 2.5 to older than 5 years. In such a young age group, variables such as the child's language and articulation development and lack of compliance during speech evaluation compromise the diagnostic accuracy of preoperative assessment. The decision to proceed with additional surgery for VPI is not an isolated surgical judgment. The authors believe that lack of palatal movement in the anterior-posterior direction benefits most often from a pharyngeal flap, and frequently the lack of lateral wall motion is best treated by sphincter pharyngoplasty. There is considerable variation in surgical technique for each of these procedures, and each can be customized to fit the particular closure pattern of each patient.

TONSILLECTOMY AND ADENOIDECTOMY IN CHILDREN WITH CLEFTS

The age group of children evaluated for VPI certainly coincides with the period when enlargement of the tonsils and adenoids is most common. This issue is not well addressed in the literature and, if ignored, has a tendency to disrupt the positive outcome of cleft palate repair.

Severely enlarged tonsils can interfere with elevation and closure of the palate. Careful observation of the tonsil–soft palate relationship during oropharyngeal examination, as well as nasoendoscopy, will disclose the impact of tonsil enlargement. A repeat speech evaluation should be performed 6 to 8 weeks after tonsillectomy and the presence and severity of VPI reassessed.

Enlarged adenoids aid velopharyngeal closure. After adenoidectomy, occult VPI suddenly becomes overt and decompensated speech patterns can be dramatic. VPI after adenoidectomy in the general population occurs in less than 1% of cases. Of these, approximately one third can be observed to have findings of mild VPI before adenoidectomy. The risk for VPI after adenoidectomy is increased in children with developmental delay, generalized hypotonia, mental retardation, submucous cleft palate, family history of VPI, and history of feeding problems in early childhood.

If a subsequent pharyngeal flap is not planned, adenoidectomy in a child with a repaired or submucous cleft palate or in a child with other risk factors as mentioned earlier should be limited to the anterior one half of the adenoid tissue (closest to the choanae and torus) while leaving the height and posterior one half of the adenoid tissue intact for adequate velar closure. Adenoidectomy in this age group is frequently indicated for recurrent or chronic sinonasal infections and for recurrent or chronic otitis media. One of the rare causes of VPI is closure of the palate against asymmetrical adenoid tissue, which can be adequately identified only with nasoendoscopy.

A major cause of obstructive sleep apnea in children is adenotonsillar hypertrophy. Failure to recognize the impact of adenotonsillar hypertrophy in a child with sleep-disordered breathing, snoring, or mild apnea can lead to severe obstructive sleep apnea after creation of a pharyngeal flap to treat VPI. Performing an adenoidectomy after a pharyngeal flap is in place is difficult and may carry a higher risk of bleeding. A moderately enlarged mass of adenoid tissue can become severely obstructive after a few months and interfere with the function of a pharyngeal flap. When adenoidectomy is required before treatment of VPI, appropriate surgical planning may include removal of the obstructive adenoid tissue at least 4 to 6 weeks before creation of a pharyngeal flap.

Enlarged tonsils obstructing the view of the posterior pillars may interfere with the elongation of flaps for pharyngoplasty. When necessary, conservative tonsillectomy (preservation of both the anterior and posterior tonsil pillars) is planned before pharyngoplasty. The lateral pharyngeal ports can become obstructed by enlarged tonsils several months after a successful pharyngeal flap procedure and cause speech disturbance, obstructive sleep apnea, or both. Nasoendoscopy will show this problem and tonsillectomy can alleviate it. It should be noted that adenoidectomy and tonsillectomy in patients with clefting is a controversial area and that treatment plans must be individualized.

OPERATIVE TECHNIQUES FOR VELOPHARYNGEAL INSUFFICIENCY

Contemporary surgical management of VPI generally involves the use of two types of procedures: a pharyngeal flap and sphincter pharyngoplasty.[1,2,29] The use of autogenous or alloplastic implants for augmentation of the posterior pharyngeal wall has been described but is not a commonly used procedure. More recently, some surgeons have advocated performance of a second palatoplasty operation in an attempt at palatal lengthening in a patient with VPI. This may become an alternative in some patients with short gaps posteriorly.

A superiorly based pharyngeal flap remains the standard approach for surgical management of VPI. Using 14F catheters for guidance, the technique advocated by the authors limits the combined size of the lateral ports to less than 20 mm^2, the maximal velopharyngeal port opening during clinically normal speech. Surgical maneuvers are directed at recruiting tissue by developing a superiorly based soft tissue flap from the posterior pharyngeal wall (Fig. 83-13). The soft palate is then divided along the midsagittal plane from the junction of the hard and soft palate to the uvula, and the flap from the posterior pharyngeal wall is inset within the nasal layer of the soft palate. A superiorly based flap may be covered with mucosal flaps on both the dorsal and ventral surfaces, thus increasing the viability of the flap, reducing flap contracture, and expediting mucosal healing. As a result, a large nasopharyngeal opening that cannot be completely closed by the patient's velopharyngeal valve mechanism is converted into two (right and left) lateral pharyngeal ports. Closure of these ports is easier for the patient to accomplish as long as adequate lateral pharyngeal wall motion is present.

The high overall success rate and the flexibility to design the dimensions and position of the flap itself are advantages of the superiorly based pharyngeal flap procedure. Disadvantages of the pharyngeal flap procedure are primarily related to the possibility of nasal obstruction, resulting in trapping of mucus and the potential for exacerbation of obstructive sleep apnea.

Inferiorly based pharyngeal flaps for the management of VPI are rarely used and tend to cause downward pull on the soft palate after healing and contracture of the flap. The result may be a tethered palate with decreased ability to elevate during the formation of speech sounds. Moreover, should postoperative hemorrhage occur, an inferiorly based flap obscures the donor site for access to the bleeding site, and to control the bleeding, the flap may need to be sacrificed in some instances. A superiorly based flap leaves the donor site fully accessible.

Dynamic sphincter pharyngoplasty is another option for the surgical management of VPI. The operative procedure involves the creation of two superiorly based myomucosal flaps that include each posterior tonsil pillar (Fig. 83-14). Each flap is elevated with care taken to include as much of the palatopharyngeal muscle as possible. It may be difficult to raise flaps in patients with velocardiofacial syndrome, because the internal carotid arteries may take a median course in the posterior pharynx. The flaps are then attached and inset within a horizontal incision made high on the posterior pharyngeal wall. These flaps are designed to

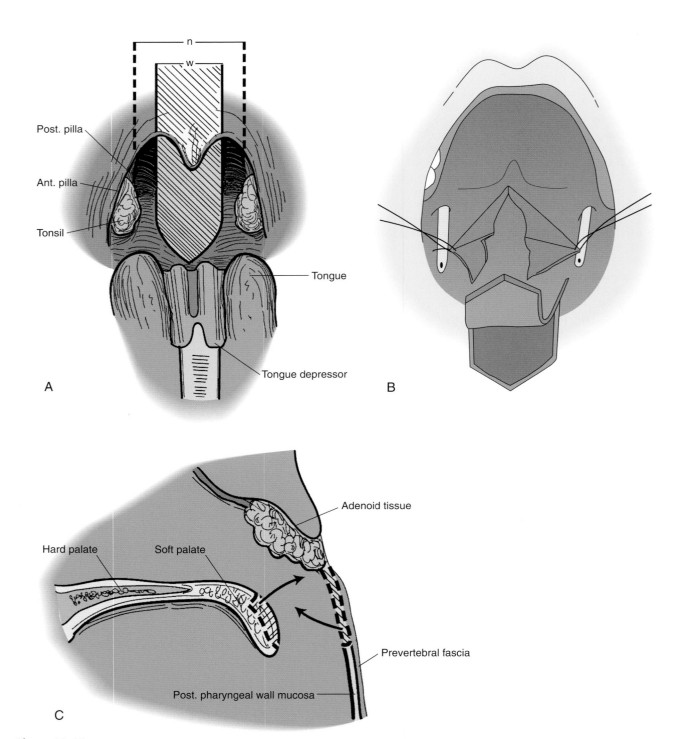

Figure 83-13. Superiorly based pharyngeal flap. **A,** Elevation of a myomucosal flap from the prevertebral fascia and division of the soft palate tissues. **B,** Dissection of the oral, nasal, and muscular layers for insetting the flap. **C,** Sagittal view of soft palatal anatomy in preparation for insetting the pharyngeal flap at the appropriate vertical height.

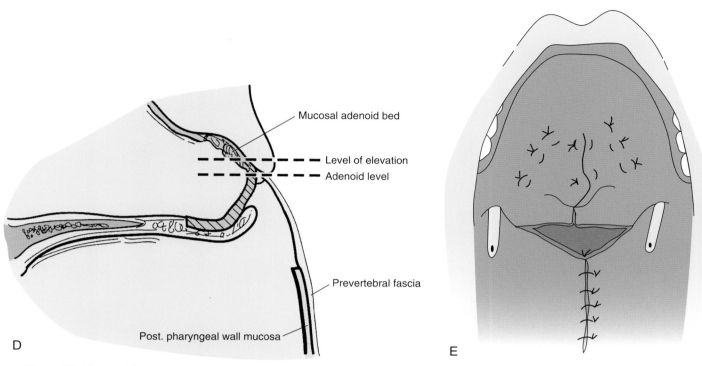

Figure 83-13, cont'd D, Sagittal close-up view indicating the relationship between adenoid tissue and the pharyngeal flap. **E,** Insertion of the flap with closure of the oral mucosa over the raw defect to decrease scarring.

be anastomosed either end to end (if short) or side to side (overlap) (if long) (see Fig. 83-14).

The goal of this procedure is creation of a single nasopharyngeal port (instead of the two ports of the pharyngeal flap) that has a contractile ridge posteriorly to improve velopharyngeal valve function. Transposed flaps should be high in the nasopharynx, at the level of the velopharyngeal closure. VPI may persist if positioning is incorrect or narrowing is inadequate. Ideally, at the completion of the procedure, the flaps should not be visible during oropharyngeal examination.

The main advantage of sphincter pharyngoplasty over a superiorly based flap is a lower rate of complications related to nasal airway obstruction, as described earlier. Despite this theoretical advantage, there is no convincing evidence that pharyngoplasty procedures achieve superior outcomes in the resolution of VPI. In addition, the use of a sphincter pharyngoplasty technique may be associated with increased scarring along the tonsillar pillar region.

Some surgeons advocate the use of revision palatoplasty instead of a pharyngeal flap or pharyngoplasty procedure for the management of patients with VPI. Specifically, either aggressive repositioning of the musculature with a two-flap palatoplasty and intravelar velarplasty or a Furlow double-opposing Z-plasty is carried out to facilitate velopharyngeal valve closure. The ideal patient for a revision Furlow procedure is a child younger than 12 years with poor levator reconstruction, a short palate with a gap of less than 10 mm,

and 50% to 75% lateral pharyngeal wall movement. An older patient with a 5-mm or smaller gap and good lateral wall movement may also be a good candidate. Long-term speech results of revision Furlow procedures are unavailable at present, but some surgeons strongly advocate this technique. Thus, the exact choice for each patient still remains controversial and is best tailored according to each surgeon's individual experience.

PALATAL FISTULA REPAIR

Fistulas can occur in patients who undergo repair of cleft palates. The recommended timing of closure may vary significantly and remains a controversial topic.[1,2,30-33] Some surgeons or speech pathologists may advocate aggressive management with early closure of any fistula present after the initial palate repair. The authors prefer to take a more long-range view of fistulas and delay surgery for several years whenever possible. Fistulas that have a negative impact on speech may be closed earlier.

In infants, closure of a small, nonfunctional fistula can generally be deferred until later in childhood. In such cases, fistula repair may be incorporated into any future procedures such as pharyngeal surgery for VPI or bone graft reconstruction of the cleft maxilla and alveolus, as long as there is no functional speech or feeding-related concerns. When a large (>5 mm) fistula is present, there is a greater likelihood that functional impairment will be encountered, such as nasal air

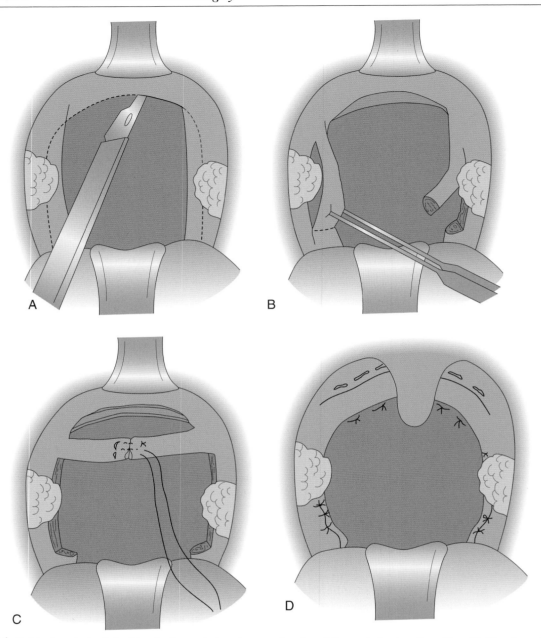

Figure 83-14. Sphincteroplasty. **A,** Incision in the posterior pharyngeal wall and the posterior tonsillar pillars. **B,** Elevation of the tonsillar pillar–myomucosal flaps. **C,** Approximation in the central pharyngeal area to customize the size of the central port. **D,** Sutured flaps placed in the posterior pharyngeal walls and posterior-lateral pharyngeal walls.

escape affecting speech, nasal reflux of food and liquids, and hygiene-related difficulties. In clinical situations in which significant functional problems exist, earlier closure of a persistent fistula is indicated. As part of the decision-making process, surgeons must weigh the benefits of repair against the negative effects on subsequent maxillary growth of a second palatal surgery involving stripping of mucoperiosteum.

Another consideration in planning the exact timing of closing a fistula is the type of technique being used for the repair. Closure of a fistula with local flaps or repeat palatoplasty may be undertaken during infancy

and early childhood. On the other hand, in cases in which the use of a tongue flap is considered, the child must be old enough to cooperate with the perioperative regimen.

Operations currently used for fistula repair include local palatal flaps, modifications of the von Langenbeck and two-flap palatoplasty techniques, palatoplasty with incorporation of a pharyngeal flap, and the use of a tongue flap. Other regional flaps, including tongue, buccal mucosa, buccinator myomucosal, temporalis muscle, and vascularized tissue transfer, are used less frequently.

When less than 4 mm in diameter, the fistula may be closed with an edge-based turnover flap for nasal lining, followed by a large oral mucoperiosteal rotation flap. In this manner, the nasal and oral suture lines are staggered. In some hard palate fistulas or large fistulas, dissection resembling palate repair with palatal mucoperiosteal flap elevation and separate nasal and oral closure is necessary. Depending on the location, closure of larger fistulas is aided by flaps from the buccal sulcus or pharynx.

When a large fistula is located within the anterior two thirds of the hard palate, another excellent choice for repair is an anteriorly based dorsal tongue flap. First, turnover flaps are developed to close the nasal side of the palatal defect with multiple interrupted sutures. Next, this technique calls for the development of an anteriorly based tongue flap that is approximately 5 cm in length by one third to two thirds the width of the tongue. The tongue flap is elevated along the underlying musculature and then inset with multiple mattress sutures for closure of the oral side. The recipient bed within the tongue is closed primarily. After the initial surgery, the tongue flap is allowed to heal for approximately 2 weeks. At that time the patient is returned to the operating room. The flap is sectioned and the stump at the donor site is freshened and inset into the tongue. The use of laterally and posteriorly based tongue flaps has also been advocated. In our opinion, an anteriorly based flap is better tolerated by most patients and allows the greatest degree of tongue mobility with less risk of tearing the flap from its palatal insertion. Some surgeons use maxillomandibular fixation for 2 weeks while the flap becomes vascularized.

MAXILLARY AND ALVEOLAR CLEFT BONE GRAFTING

Approximately 75% of patients with clefts will have clefts that involve the alveolus, maxilla, nasal floor, and piriform rim. The vast majority of surgeons advocate reconstruction of this portion of the cleft during mixed dentition before eruption of the permanent canine or lateral incisor.[1,2,34] This approach allows continuity of the maxillary arch, support for the erupting teeth, reconstruction of the congenital defect, support of the nasal base, and closure of the residual cleft/fistula. Frequently, orthodontic maxillary expansion is required to match the arch compatibility of the mandible before performing the grafting procedure. Such expansion is performed by a skilled orthodontist over a period of several months before surgery in a coordinated fashion.

The technique used by most surgeons involves layered closure of the defect with a multiple-flap technique that mobilizes attached gingiva into the cleft defect where the tooth/teeth will ideally erupt (Fig. 83-15). Both anterior vestibular and palatal flaps are necessary, because the defect courses from the piriform rim to alveolus and back to the incisive foramen region. Some patients may have a residual hard palatal fistula that can be repaired at the same time.

The iliac crest is the most common donor site for bone graft reconstruction at the cleft site. Other sites have also been recommended, but the best results continue to be achieved with cancellous bone procured from the anterior iliac crest via a minimal 3- to 5-cm incision posterior and lateral to the anterior iliac spine. The cartilaginous cap of the iliac crest is directly incised with a blade, and a small trapdoor is elevated medially. Curettes are used to procure enough bone to fill the defect. Although attempts have been made to use allogeneic bone products or synthetic material, outcomes have been poor in comparison with autogenous iliac crest.[1,2,34]

Watertight closure is desirable for the nasal side of the closure, and resorbable sutures with tapered needles are used throughout. This can be tested by using a bulb syringe with irrigation in the naris. Defects are repaired with horizontal mattress or interrupted suture techniques. The bone graft taken from the iliac crest is then placed in the site while remembering to fill the entire defect up to the piriform rim rather than just at the alveolus. The oral mucosa is then mobilized to close the remaining oral cavity layer in a tension-free manner.

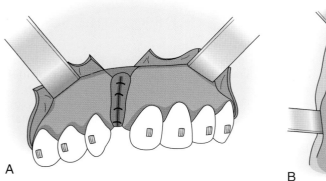
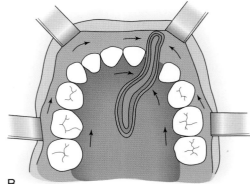

A

B

Figure 83-15. A and **B,** Four-flap technique of advancing much-needed attached mucosa into the residual cleft of the primary palate with simultaneous closure of the oral-nasal fistula and placement a of cancellous iliac crest bone graft. *(From Fonseca RJ: Davis Reconstructive Preprosthetic OMS. Philadelphia, WB Saunders, 1995, p 996.)*

Patients with bilateral clefts of the anterior palate benefit from placement of a postoperative acrylic splint made before surgery for stabilization of the premaxillary segment. The splint can be wired to orthodontic mechanics or bonded with a dental bonding agent to the teeth for several weeks during healing of the mucosal tissue.

Patients are placed on a liquid diet for 2 weeks and told to avoid using straws. Once the initial mucosal healing is complete, the diet can be advanced slowly over the next several weeks. The splint is removed when the mucosal tissues are more completely healed. Patients should brush their teeth, but not directly over the repair sites. Gentle mouth rinses of saline or chlorhexidine may be used to keep the dentition and oral cavity clean as well.

CLEFT RHINOPLASTY

Congenital clefts that involve the lip, nose, and underlying skeletal structure will cause a complex three-dimensional deformity of the nasal complex that affects both form and function. In the case of a complete unilateral cleft, the typical nasal deformity is characterized by splaying of the alar base, inferior displacement of the alar rim, deviation of the nasal tip, and irregularity of the caudal nasal septum.[1,2,30] Abnormal fibrous insertions exist between the lateral crus of the lower lateral cartilage and the lateral piriform rim on the cleft side. At the time of the initial lip repair procedure, maneuvers for primary nasal reconstruction include dissection along the lower lateral cartilage to separate the overlying skin from the cartilage and sharp release of the fibrous insertions along the piriform rim so that the nostril can be repositioned appropriately. Despite effective primary cleft lip and nasal repair during infancy, most patients will demonstrate enough residual nasal dysmorphology that secondary nasal surgery for correction of the cleft-associated malformation or improvement in nasal airflow will be beneficial later in life.

The timing of cleft nasal revision surgery also remains controversial. Some surgeons take a more aggressive approach and undertake extensive nasal reconstruction during early childhood. Our philosophy is to delay the definitive cleft rhinoplasty until the nasal complex is close to mature size. When possible, early nasal surgery should be performed after bone graft reconstruction of the maxilla so that a stable bony foundation along the piriform rim and nasal base exists first. If the patient's reconstructive treatment plan also requires maxillary advancement, nasal surgery should be delayed until approximately 6 months after the orthognathic procedure. This allows a more predictable outcome and long-lasting improvement in nasal function and facial aesthetics. Early surgery is reserved for individuals with severe airway or nasal airflow problems or children who endure psychosocial consequences such as teasing at school.

Secondary cleft-nasal reconstruction will often require dorsal reduction, lower lateral cartilage sculpting, cartilage grafting, and nasal osteotomies. Cartilage grafting is a critical component of the final nasal reconstruction and is used for augmentation of the dysmorphic lower lateral cartilage and improvement of nasal tip projection. Several different donor sites may be used, including auricular cartilage, nasal septum, and rib cartilage. Ear cartilage is most useful in situations in which augmentation of hypoplastic cleft-side lower lateral cartilage is required. Septal cartilage is most easily accessible and provides an excellent scaffold for repositioning of the lower lateral cartilage and improvement of nasal tip symmetry and projection. Unfortunately, patients may be scheduled for definitive nasal reconstruction after having previously undergone septal cartilage harvest and not have sufficient quantity for a second septal cartilage graft. In such cases, the use of costochondral cartilage is another excellent option. Rib cartilage provides adequate amounts of graft material but requires a distant donor surgical site. We have found this type of cartilage graft to provide excellent strength for support of the nasal tip and alar complex. These techniques are best carried out through an open approach. A transcolumellar splitting incision is combined with marginal incisions to provide wide access and direct visualization of the nasal dorsum, upper and lower lateral cartilage, and nasal septum.

A similar rationale is applied when considering the timing of secondary nasal reconstruction in a patient with a bilateral cleft lip, but the specific dysmorphology addressed is somewhat different. Generally, nasal asymmetry is less problematic, and the dysmorphology is characterized by deficient columellar length. Many surgeons have focused on secondary lengthening of the columella through the use of banked forked flaps or columellar lengthening with soft tissue flaps from the floor of the nose and alar flaps. Unfortunately, these types of surgical procedures often result in a distorted columellar-labial angle, excessive scars that extend onto the nasal tip, and additional distortion of the broad nasal tip. We find that using septal cartilage strut grafts attached to the caudal nasal septum and lower lateral cartilage yields the most natural-looking results. The objective is correction of the underlying cartilaginous anatomy with stretching of the overlying soft tissue envelope instead of direct surgical manipulation of the columellar skin.

CLEFT ORTHOGNATHIC SURGERY

The technical details and integrated orthodontic-surgical treatment planning for orthognathic correction are beyond the scope of this chapter, but the treatment concepts warrant comment inasmuch as more than 35% of patients who undergo cleft repairs will benefit from orthognathic surgery to treat malocclusion.[35,36] Most commonly, midface hypoplasia results in an underbite that causes functional and aesthetic problems. Additionally, facial asymmetry is common in patients who have previously undergone cleft repairs in infancy. These procedures are performed at the end of growth in the craniomaxillofacial skeleton, usually 14 to 16 years of age in girls and 16 to 18 years in boys. In

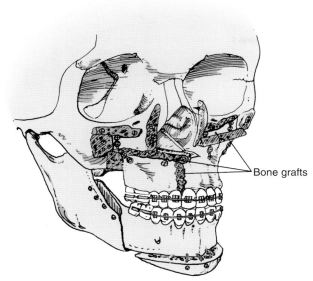

Bone grafts

Figure 83-16. A Le Fort I osteotomy, bilateral sagittal splits, and genioplasty osteotomies are shown for a patient with maxillary hypoplasia associated with early surgery required for a unilateral cleft lip and palate. Onlay bone grafts may be helpful for improving facial contour. *(From Ruiz RL, Costello BJ, Turvey T: Orthognathic surgery in the cleft patient. In Oral and Maxillofacial Surgery Clinics of North America: Secondary Cleft Surgery. Philadelphia, WB Saunders, 2002, pp 491-507.)*

rare instances, midface advancement may be indicated earlier. Coordinated care with a skilled orthodontist is very important to achieve the optimal result and consists of planning and several phases of orthodontic therapy both before and after orthognathic surgery.

Usually, a Le Fort I osteotomy is indicated for patients with maxillary hypoplasia and malocclusion. In many cases, bilateral sagittal split osteotomies and genioplasty are helpful in treating the malocclusion and improving facial balance (Fig. 83-16). Traditional orthognathic surgery is dependent on precise placement of fixation to ensure the optimal occlusion and facial balance to avoid relapse. Recently, distraction osteogenesis has been used in patients who require exceptionally large advancement of the midface.[37] Although the technique shows little or no improvement over traditional osteotomy techniques in most patients, it may be helpful in some patients who require larger advancement.

CONCLUSIONS

Comprehensive care of patients with clefts requires an interdisciplinary approach that demands precise surgical execution of the various procedures necessary to correct cleft deformities, as well as frequent long-term follow-up. Clinicians experienced in the comprehensive interdisciplinary care of patients with clefts are best equipped to deal with these concerns. Treatment of patients with cleft and craniofacial deformities should be free of bias and should include team care that is patient, family, and community oriented. Only in this fashion can the overall treatment be optimally successful. This type of care maximizes patients' ability to grow into adulthood and succeed in life without focusing on their deformity.

PEARLS

- Marking the key landmarks is important to obtain the best result, and the temptation to keep hypoplastic tissue should be discouraged.
- Nasoalveolar molding appliances may be helpful in reapproximating the segments to allow easier surgical repair, and they may improve the aesthetic result of the lip and nose.
- A three-layered closure is the key to both functional and aesthetic repair of the lip.
- Some nasal asymmetry is expected in wide unilateral clefts, but this can be minimized by conservative primary nasal reconstruction.
- Nasal bolsters or silicone nasal stents can be used to help mold the nose in the postoperative period.
- Arm restraints may be used for the first 2 weeks to help avoid injury to the lip repair, but they should be removed occasionally to allow range of motion of the arms.
- Palate repair requires adequate mobilization of tissues to allow the most tension-free closure possible.
- Releasing the nasal and palatal periosteum, as well as the tensor veli palatine muscle or Veau's muscle, is helpful in gaining additional mobilization.

PITFALLS

- Patients with syndromes, dysmorphology, and wide palates are more prone to fistulas.
- A common pitfall is to incompletely reconstruct the musculature of the lip or palate.
- Another common pitfall occurs when the surgeon leaves considerable dead space within the layers of the repair. Placement of at least several sutures through each of the layers is important in preventing dead space.
- Careful wound care is necessary because some bolsters used to help mold the nose may cause pressure necrosis of the columella or nasal base if placed too tightly or kept in place for too long.
- A common pitfall occurs when the surgeon fails to mobilize enough muscle to create an active levator sling that is posteriorly displaced.
- Failure to preserve the vascular pedicle may result in necrosis of the tissues.

References

1. Posnick JC: The staging of cleft lip and palate reconstruction: Infancy through adolescence. In Posnick JC (ed): Craniofacial and Maxillofacial Surgery in Children and Young Adults. Philadelphia, WB Saunders, 2000, pp 785-826.

2. Costello BJ, Ruiz RL: Cleft lip and palate: Comprehensive treatment and primary repair. In Milaro M, Larsen PE, Waite PD, Ghali G (eds): Peterson's Oral and Maxillofacial Surgery. Hamilton, Ontario, BC Decker, 2004, pp 839-858.

3. Tolarova MM, Cervenka J: Classification and birth prevalence of orofacial clefts. Am J Med Genet 75:126-137, 1998.

4. Cohen MM: Etiology and pathogenesis of orofacial clefting. Cleft lip and palate: A physiological approach. Oral Maxillofac Clin North Am 12:379-397, 2000.

5. Tessier P: Anatomical classification of facial, cranio-facial, and latero-facial clefts. J Maxillofac Surg 4:69-92, 1976.

6. Parameters for the evaluation and treatment of patients with cleft lip/palate or other craniofacial anomalies. American Cleft Palate–Craniofacial Association. March, 1993 Cleft Palate Craniofac J 30(Suppl):S1-S16, 1993.

7. Cash C, Set P, Coleman N: The accuracy of antenatal ultrasound in the detection of facial clefts in a low-risk screening population. Ultrasound Obstet Gynecol 18:432-436, 2001.

8. Pretorius DH, House M, Nelson TR, Hollenbach KA: Evaluation of normal and abnormal lips in fetuses: Comparison between three- and two-dimensional sonography. AJR Am J Roentgenol 165:1233-1237, 1995.

9. Dorf DS, Curtin JW: Early cleft palate repair and speech outcome. Plast Reconstr Surg 70:74-81, 1982.

10. Dorf DS, Curtin JW: Early cleft palate repair and speech outcome: A ten year experience. In Bardach J, Morris HL (eds): Multidisciplinary Management of Cleft Lip and Palate. Philadelphia, WB Saunders, 1990, pp 341-348.

11. Copeland M: The effect of very early palatal repair on speech. Br J Plast Surg 43:676-682, 1990.

12. Grayson BH, Cutting CB, Wood R: Preoperative columella lengthening in bilateral cleft lip and palate. Plast Reconstr Surg 92:1422-1423, 1993.

13. Grayson BH, Santiago PE, Brecht LE, et al: Presurgical nasoalveolar molding in infants with cleft lip and palate. Cleft Palate Craniofac J 36:486-498, 1999.

14. Ross RB, MacNamera MC: Effect of presurgical infant orthopedics on facial esthetics in complete bilateral cleft lip and palate. Cleft Palate Craniofac J 31:410-411, 1994.

15. Grayson BH, Cutting CB, Wood R: Preoperative columella lengthening in bilateral cleft lip and palate. Plast Reconstr Surg 92:1422-1423, 1993.

16. Grayson BH, Santiago PE, Brecht LE, et al: Presurgical nasoalveolar molding in infants with cleft lip and palate. Cleft Palate Craniofac J 36:486-498, 1999.

17. Berkowitz S: The comparison of treatment results in complete cleft lip/palate using conservative approach vs. Millard-Latham PSOT procedure. Semin Orthod 1996;2:169-184.

18. Randall P, Graham WP: Lip adhesion in the repair of bilateral cleft lip. In Grabb WC, Rosenstein SW, Bzoch KR (eds): Cleft Lip and Palate. Boston, Little, Brown, 1971.

19. Pruzansky S: Pre-surgical orthopedics and bone grafting for infants with cleft lip and palate: A dissent. Cleft Palate J 1:164-187, 1964.

20. Millard DR: Cleft Craft, vol 1. Boston, Little, Brown, 1976, pp 165-173.

21. Millard DR: A primary camouflage of the unilateral harelip. In Transactions of the International Congress of Plastic Surgeons. Baltimore, Williams & Wilkins, 1957, pp 160-166.

22. McComb H: Primary correction of unilateral cleft lip nasal deformity: A 10 year review. Plast Reconstr Surg 75:791-799, 1985.

23. Shaw WC, Asher-McDade C, Brattstrom V, et al: A six-center international study of treatment outcome in patients with clefts of the lip and palate. Part 5. General discussion and conclusions. Cleft Palate Craniofac J 29:413-418, 1992.

24. Bardach J, Nosal P: Geometry of the two-flap palatoplasty. In Bardach J, Salyer K (eds): Surgical Techniques in Cleft Lip and Palate, 2nd ed. St Louis, Mosby–Year Book, 1991.

25. Furlow LT Jr: Cleft palate repair by double opposing Z-plasty. Plast Reconstr Surg 78:724-738, 1986.

26. Randall P, LaRossa D, Solomon M, Cohen M: Experience with the Furlow double-reversing Z-plasty for cleft palate repair. Plast Reconstr Surg 77:569-576, 1986.

27. Doyle WJ, Cantekin EI, Bluestone CD: Eustachian tube function in cleft palate children. Ann Otol Rhinol Laryngol 89(Suppl 68):34-40, 1980.

28. Sheahan P, Miller I, Sheahan JN, et al: Incidence and outcome of middle ear disease in cleft lip and/or cleft palate. Int J Pediatr Otorhinolaryngol 67:785-793, 2003.

29. Costello BJ, Ruiz RL, Turvey T: Surgical management of velopharyngeal insufficiency in the cleft patient. In Oral and Maxillofacial Surgery Clinics of North America: Secondary Cleft Surgery. Philadelphia, WB Saunders, 2002, pp 539-51.

30. Ruiz RL, Costello BJ: Secondary cleft surgery. In Milaro M, Larsen PE, Waite PD, Ghali G (eds): Peterson's Oral and Maxillofacial Surgery. Hamilton, Ontario, BC Decker, 2004, pp 871-886.

31. Reid DAC: Fistulae in the hard palate following cleft palate surgery. Br J Plast Surg 78:739-747, 1986.

32. Abyholm FE, Borchgrevink HH, Eskeland G: Palatal fistulae following cleft palate surgery. Scand J Plast Reconstr Surg 13:295-300, 1979.

33. Cohen SR, Kalinowski J, La Rossa D, et al: Cleft palate fistulas: A multivariate statistical analysis of prevalence, etiology, and surgical management. Plast Reconstr Surg 87:1041-1047, 1991.

34. Boyne PJ, Sands NR: Secondary bone grafting of residual alveolar and palatal clefts. J Oral Surg 30:87-92, 1972.

35. Posnick JC, Tompson B: Cleft-orthognathic surgery. Complications and long-term results. Plast Reconstr Surg 96:255-266, 1995.

36. Ruiz RL, Costello BJ, Turvey T: Orthognathic surgery in the cleft patient. In Oral and Maxillofacial Surgery Clinics of North America: Secondary Cleft Surgery. Philadelphia, WB Saunders, 2002, pp 491-507.

37. Costello BJ, Ruiz RL: The role of distraction osteogenesis in orthognathic surgery of the cleft patient. Selected Readings Oral Maxillofac Surg 10:1-27, 2002.

Otoplasty

Grant S. Gillman

Auricular characteristics are inherited as an autosomal dominant trait with variable penetrance. Many of those who are born with an auricular deformity are subject to teasing and ridicule in childhood and become very self-conscious of the appearance of their ears in adolescence and adulthood. Surgical correction of prominent or protuberant ears (Fig. 84-1) may yield very gratifying results with relatively simple surgery. Nonetheless, correct analysis of the deformity preoperatively and a well-designed and well-executed surgical plan are fundamental requirements for optimal patient satisfaction and stable long-term results. With a good result, patients will derive both psychological and cosmetic benefit.

The purpose of corrective surgery is to re-establish what are considered "normal contour lines" (Fig. 84-2) of the external ear, as well as the relationship of the external ear to the scalp.

PATIENT SELECTION

Patients will generally be in one of three categories:

- Absence of the antihelical fold (thereby unfurling the upper half of the ear and increasing the auriculomastoid angle)
- A deep overly projected conchal bowl (increasing lateral projection of the ear and the conchomastoid angle)
- Both of the above (Fig. 84-3)

Any of these patients are considered appropriate for otoplasty. As with all cosmetic procedures, the patient must be psychologically stable, be well motivated, and have realistic expectations about the surgical outcome. It is important that the patient recognize that although the goal is perfection, "improvement" with a natural appearance and without complications is an acceptable result.

The timing of the procedure is guided by the patient's own awareness of the deformity. By 5 years of age, the auricle has achieved about 80% to 85% of adult size, so it is preferable to wait until at least this age before considering surgery. If the deformity is exceptionally emotionally disturbing to the child, the procedure may be performed just before the child begins school. There is no end point beyond which the surgery could not be performed; however, as the ear cartilage ages, it loses its flexibility, thereby restricting the response to surgical manipulation.

PREOPERATIVE PLANNING

Preoperative planning begins with an evaluation of the deformity.[1] First, one has to decide whether the problem is due to absence of the antihelical fold, a deep conchal bowl, or both. Simple observation will reveal whether there is a weak or absent antihelical fold. In such cases, gentle finger pressure on the helical rim to create an antihelical fold and set the ear back should indicate whether this corrects the problem sufficiently or whether there is still some protrusion contributed by the depth of the conchal bowl. It is also important to note right-left symmetry preoperatively. Frequently, the two sides are asymmetric, and it is useful to point this out to the patient and the patient's family.

The surgical goals[1-3] are

- A natural looking, pleasing appearance of the auricular correction
- Creation of an antihelical fold with smooth edges and contour and without sharp edges, ridges, or unsightly scarring
- Reasonable symmetry between the two ears
- An enduring, stable long-term result
- Minimal or no complications, with preservation of a postauricular sulcus

Preoperative photodocumentation is mandatory and should include an anterior full face view, a posterior full head view, full right and left lateral views, and close-up lateral views.

Reasonable surgical outcomes, as well as possible complications, are discussed preoperatively (see later). Ultimately, ears that do not attract attention to themselves will be the measure of success to the patient.

SURGICAL TECHNIQUES[3-5]

Otoplasty for protuberant ears in children is usually performed under general anesthesia. In older children and adults, local anesthesia with or without intravenous sedation can be used.

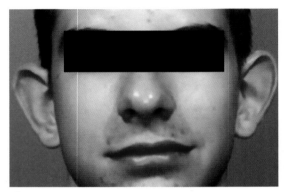

Figure 84-1. Typical patient with protuberant ears.

The position and site of the planned antihelical fold is determined by gently furling the ear with fingers on the helical rim until a pleasing natural antihelical fold is apparent. Markings are made symmetrically on either side of the fold to guide the site of later placement of horizontal mattress sutures.

To gauge the amount of postauricular skin to be removed, the ear is manually set back against the scalp and the amount of redundant skin determined. An ellipse is then marked on the posterior auricle to outline the skin excision. The width of the ellipse is thus individualized but generally measures 15 mm (±5 mm) at its maximal width. Conservatism is warranted because more skin can be excised incrementally at any time if need be. The ellipse incorporates the postauricular sulcus but is not centered on the sulcus—it is biased toward the posterior auricular surface so that more skin is removed from the ear than from the scalp. In addition, within about 5 to 7 mm of the lobular attachment inferiorly or the helical root superiorly, the ellipse curves onto the auricle so the scars will not extend beyond the sulcus and risk being visible on a lateral view.

The face, both ears, and the surrounding occipital areas are prepared with an antiseptic solution and draped into the sterile field. The postauricular skin is injected with 1% lidocaine with 1 : 100,000 epinephrine. A broad-spectrum antibiotic is administered intravenously before commencing surgery. If the ears are asymmetric, the ear with the more significant deformity is usually done first.

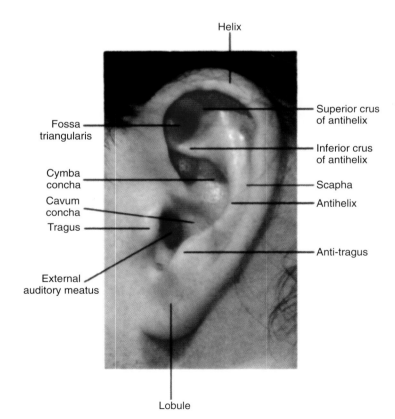

Figure 84-2. Normal auricular anatomy.

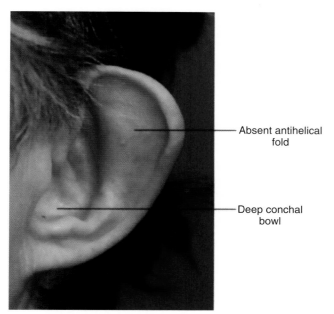

Figure 84-3. Auricular deformity commonly seen in an otoplasty patient: an ill-defined antihelical fold and a deep conchal bowl.

Absent antihelical fold

Deep conchal bowl

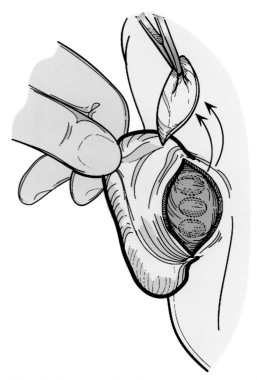

Figure 84-4. Excision of a skin ellipse, as well as partial-thickness "discs" of conchal cartilage to facilitate retrodisplacement of the auricle.

The ear is retracted forward and the ellipse of post-auricular skin is excised with a no. 15 blade as outlined (Fig. 84-4). A strip of premastoid soft tissue is excised with electrocautery to ultimately help create space for the auricular setback. With wide two-pronged hooks or

Senn retractors placed in the lateral aspect of the incision, the remaining postauricular skin is undermined out to the helical rim in a supraperichondrial plane.

At this point, aligning the wound incision margins (folding the ear back) demonstrates the extent to which the conchal bowl cartilage is interfering with the auricular setback. This maneuver also demonstrates how the conchal cartilage pivots forward at the posterior margin of the external auditory meatus as the ear is set back. To prevent iatrogenic meatal stenosis, a vertically oriented ellipse of conchal bowl cartilage is excised medially just behind the ear canal. The ellipse is about 1 to 1.5 cm in height and approximately 1 cm in maximal width. Incremental excision allows additional removal if need be. There is often some contact between the posterior aspect of the conchal cartilage and the premastoid region as well that can impede satisfactory setback of the ear. In this case one tangentially shaves partial-thickness discs of cartilage from the posterior aspect of the conchal cartilage behind the external auditory canal to further facilitate retrodisplacement of the ear. In addition to preventing inadvertent canal stenosis, this addresses the overly deep protruding conchal bowl as well.

Creation of an antihelical fold is the next step. Markings on either side of the future antihelical fold were made earlier. A no. 15 blade can be used to score the cartilage posteriorly along the line of the fold so that the "spring" of the cartilage is weakened. Incisional approaches to creating an antihelical fold will tend to create a sharp, unnatural-looking antihelical fold. Scoring the cartilage to weaken the spring works better together with the Mustardé sutures.

To ease placement of the cartilage-contouring horizontal (Mustardé) sutures posteriorly, it is useful to initially place two temporary percutaneous contouring sutures[6] from the anterior (lateral) aspect of the auricle to create and maintain an antihelical fold while the Mustardé sutures are placed posteriorly. This allows the surgeon to move the ear forward and back while placing the Mustardé sutures without concern that these sutures may loosen or become released. The anterior temporary contouring sutures (4-0 Prolene or silk on Keith needles) are placed in horizontal mattress fashion around the proposed antihelical fold, with both needles passed from the side of the conchal bowl, through into the wound posteriorly, and then back through the auricular skin anteriorly close to the helical rim (Fig. 84-5). Two such temporary sutures are placed and then tightened until a pleasing antihelical fold is created.

Attention is then turned posteriorly to placement of the Mustardé sutures.[7] Two to four 4-0 Mersilene (or similar) sutures are placed through the full thickness of the auricular cartilage in horizontal mattress fashion (as described by Mustardé) (Fig. 84-6) around the neofold and tightened as the anterior temporary sutures hold the position of the fold. Care is taken to ensure that as the Mustardé sutures are placed they do not penetrate the skin anteriorly (Fig. 84-7) and that they are not overtightened, which would create a fold with an unnatural sharp edge. Slight overcorrection will help account

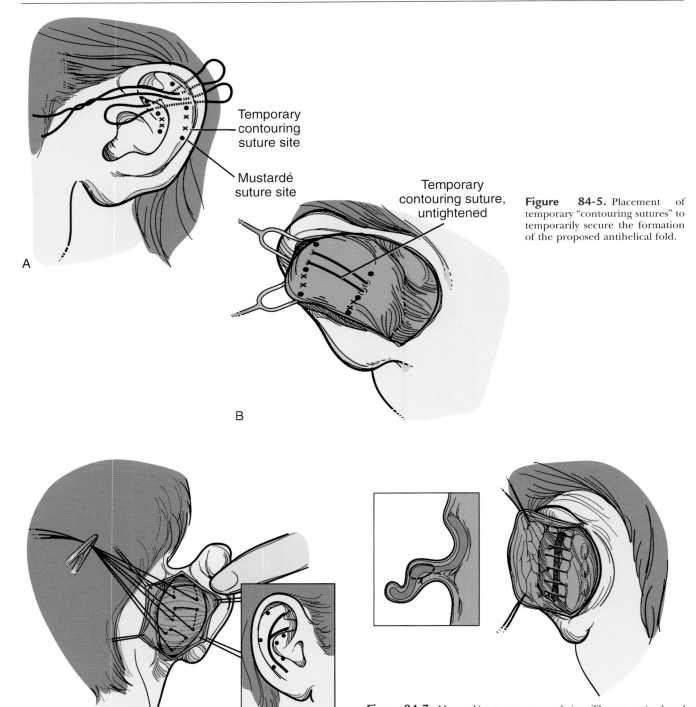

Temporary contouring suture site

Mustardé suture site

Temporary contouring suture, untightened

Figure 84-5. Placement of temporary "contouring sutures" to temporarily secure the formation of the proposed antihelical fold.

A

B

Figure 84-6. Mustardé horizontal mattress sutures as seen from behind the ear.

Figure 84-7. Mustardé sutures—coronal view. The suture is placed through the full thickness of the cartilage without penetrating the anterior skin.

for some reprotrusion that often occurs with time. Once the Mustardé sutures are secured, the temporary contouring sutures can be removed.

At this point the position of the ear is further secured with setback sutures. Conchomastoid 4-0 Mersilene suture is placed from the posterior aspect of the

conchal bowl cartilage to the premastoid fascia or periosteum. One or two such sutures may be required. If this suture is placed too far back on the cartilage or too far forward on the mastoid, anterior rotation of the conchal cartilage may be exaggerated and result in some stenosis or compromise of the external auditory canal. Care is thus taken to ensure that the suture passes on the cartilage and the mastoid fascia are either at the same anterior/posterior point or that the pass on the mastoid side is slightly behind the point of purchase on the cartilage.

If some protrusion of the superior pole of the ear still remains, a similar type of setback suture may be placed at a point on the cartilage superiorly in the region of the triangular fossa back to the premastoid soft tissue.

Once one is satisfied with the position of the ear, the skin is closed with 5-0 plain or fast-absorbing gut suture.

Finally, Xeroform gauze or cotton soaked in mineral oil is contoured to the lateral surface of the ear and placed in the postauricular sulcus as well. Fluffs are then applied and a lightly compressive mastoid-type dressing is secured. The dressing should not be so tight that epidermolysis of the skin ensues.

POSTOPERATIVE MANAGEMENT

The dressing is removed on the fifth to seventh postoperative day. Thereafter, the patient is asked to wear a supportive headband at night for 2 to 3 weeks. Incisions can be cleaned with a cotton swab soaked in fresh hydrogen peroxide, and antibiotic ointment can be gently applied to the postauricular incision. Pain medication is usually required only for the first several days. When instructing the parents or the patient, one must advise them of the signs of possible complications at the surgical site, which would probably be manifested as increasing pain, discomfort, or erythema. Patients who experience such signs should contact the surgeon as soon as possible.

A typical patient, preoperatively and postoperatively, is presented in Figures 84-8 and 84-9.

COMPLICATIONS[3]

Early

Hematoma is signaled by an inordinate amount of pain, especially unilateral. Treatment includes exploration of the wound, hemostatic control, irrigation with an antibiotic solution, and closure. Untreated hematoma risks secondary cartilage necrosis and a deformed ear.

Infection usually takes 3 to 4 days to become evident. Unilateral severe pain disproportionate to the physical findings should raise suspicion. If cellulitis is present, treatment with systemic broad-spectrum antibiotics (covering gram-positive cocci and *Pseudomonas*) is warranted in an effort to prevent progression to perichondritis or chondritis, which can result in cartilage loss and an auricular deformity. Treatment of the latter, which fortunately is rare, requires surgical drainage and débridement.

Constriction/stenosis of the external auditory canal results from failure to excise the anterior portion of the conchal cartilage or from over-rotation of the conchal bowl with the setback sutures. Treatment requires excision of that portion of the cartilage.

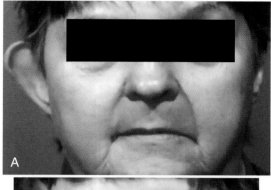
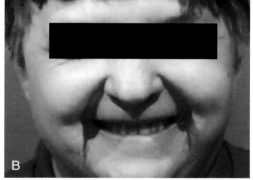

Figure 84-8. Preoperative (**A**) and postoperative (**B**) photos of a patient with a unilateral protuberant ear.

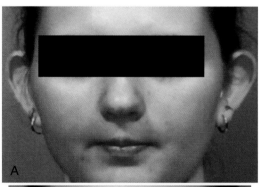
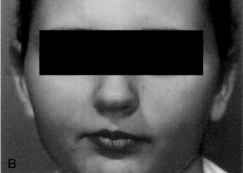

Figure 84-9. Preoperative (**A**) and postoperative (**B**) photos of a patient with bilateral protuberant ears.

Loss of the postauricular sulcus can result from over-resection of skin. Proper preoperative planning and incremental skin excision intraoperatively when needed will avoid this problem.

An overly compressive dressing can lead to epidermolysis/pressure necrosis of the auricular skin. Treatment involves conservative wound care.

Late

Cosmetically unacceptable results include overcorrection, undercorrection, asymmetries, sharp unnatural contours or ridges, and gross asymmetry. All these complications are largely avoidable with proper preoperative planning and intraoperative attention to detail. Cartilage-cutting techniques (as opposed to the cartilage-contouring technique described herein) have a higher overall rate of cosmetic irregularities.

Minor asymmetry is not uncommon and should be discussed with the patient preoperatively as realistically being possible and not indicative of an unacceptable result. Gross asymmetry, on the other hand, is not acceptable. Undercorrection of the middle third of the ear as a result of untreated conchal protrusion creates a convex appearance on frontal view and requires correction with excision of the anterior portion of the conchal bowl and setback sutures. Undercorrection of the superior or inferior pole of the ear will result in a concave appearance on frontal view (the "telephone deformity") and may require secondary revision.

Some degree of reprotrusion or suture release at the superior pole is not uncommon. Braided sutures such as Mersilene for the Mustardé mattress sutures are less likely to release than a monofilament suture material. Patients should be forewarned of this possibility. If minor, the patient is still frequently sufficiently pleased with the overall result that no treatment is necessary. If significant deformity develops, revision may be necessary.

Hypertrophic scarring/keloids can occur, but well-planned incisions and tension-free closure may help prevent this complication from developing. If hypertrophic scarring or keloids are noted early, intralesional triamcinolone (Kenalog) injections every 3 to 4 weeks may control the problem. Otherwise, excision and serial steroid injections may be required.

PEARLS

- Preoperative evaluation of the patient should establish the cause of the deformity (absence of an antihelical fold, a deep conchal bowl, or both), which guides the operative plan.
- It is important to establish proper expectations preoperatively, particularly with respect to the potential for minor persisting asymmetry postoperatively. Document and photodocument.
- The amount of skin excised should facilitate the auricular setback but not obliterate the postauricular sulcus.
- Mustardé sutures should be tightened to create a smooth, natural-appearing antihelical fold.
- Setback sutures (conchomastoid and scaphoid) can further assist in retrodisplacing the ear without having to excise more skin or cartilage.

PITFALLS

- Failure to plan appropriately or establishing inappropriate expectations is the precursor of most complications.
- Overexcision of postauricular skin can lead to overcorrection (and obliteration of the postauricular sulcus), which can be more difficult to address than undercorrection.
- Overtightening of the Mustardé sutures can create a ridge-like appearance that is unnatural and displeasing to the patient.
- Incomplete hemostasis at the time of closure can predispose to hematoma, infection, and subsequent cartilage necrosis.
- Unilateral severe or disproportionate pain may be indicative of skin necrosis, hematoma, or infection and requires prompt visual examination of the patient.

References

1. Becker DG, Lai SS, Wise JB, Steiger JD: Analysis in otoplasty. Facial Plast Surg Clin N Am 14:63-71, 2006.
2. Nuara MJ, Mobley SR: Nuances of otoplasty: A comprehensive review of the past 20 years. Facial Plast Surg Clin N Am 14:89-102, 2006.
3. Adamson PA, Litner JA: Otoplasty technique. Facial Plast Surg Clin N Am 14:79-87, 2006.
4. Ducic Y, Hilger PA: Effective step-by-step technique for the surgical treatment of protruding ears. J Otolaryngol 28(2):59-64, 1999.
5. Cheney ML, Rounds M: Otoplasty. Facial Plast Surg Clin N Am 5:319-328, 1997.
6. Hilger P, Khosh MM, Nishioka G, Larrabee WF: Modification of the Mustardé otoplasty technique using temporary contouring sutures. Plast Reconstr Surg 100:1585-1586, 1997.
7. Mustardé JC: Correction of prominent ears using simple mattress sutures. Br J Plast Surg 16:170-178, 1963.

Chapter 85

Reconstruction of Microtia

Robert F. Yellon

Auricular reconstruction for microtia is challenging, yet rewarding. Many lessons about the limitations of surgery may be learned as a surgeon acquires the skills and judgment required for successful auricular reconstruction. For example, the competing goals of a well-projected, detailed auricular graft and a thin, intact, vascularized skin flap to show that detail must be accommodated through compromise. The limitations of blood supply and tension on the skin flap must not be exceeded to avoid the complications of flap loss and infection, which may necessitate the creation of an auricle with a thicker skin flap than would be ideal for aesthetic purposes. Meticulous attention to detail and atraumatic tissue handling are critical for achieving excellent results, with the caveat that an auricle constructed by a surgeon may fail to rival that of normal embryonic development.

Most cases of microtia are unilateral, with an 8 : 1 ratio of unilateral to bilateral cases. The majority of patients are male. Microtia usually, but not always, occurs in conjunction with aural atresia. In general, reconstruction of the microtia is completed before reconstruction of the aural atresia.

PATIENT SELECTION

The best chance for successful auricular cartilage grafting is when the blood supply to the recipient site has not been impaired by previous surgery and scarring. Although some surgeons have advocated starting microtia reconstruction as early as 2 years of age, most surgeons prefer to wait until the child is older. Reconstruction may be started as early as 4 years of age in a large boy with bilateral microtia. In contrast, for a petite child with unilateral microtia, one may wait to begin reconstruction at 7 years of age. The longer the surgeon waits to begin, the more rib cartilage is available and the more cooperative children are because they understand the surgical process. However, the longer the surgeon waits to begin reconstruction, the more psychological trauma may occur because of ridicule from the other children and the longer the child has to wait for possible reconstruction of aural atresia with the associated limitations of maximal conductive hearing loss. Nonetheless, the recent availability of the bone-anchored hearing aid gives the surgeon a new option for improving hearing at an age as early as 3 years with minimal impairment of the potential for auricular cartilage grafting.[1]

Most patients with microtia are candidates for reconstruction. Exceptions are those with previous extensive surgery in the area of the auricle, burns, tumors, or radiation in the area. Relative contraindications to reconstruction include highly uncooperative children and those with very severe hemifacial microsomia. In the setting of severe hemifacial microsomia, formal angiography may be required to ensure that the blood supply from the superficial temporal and occipital arteries is adequate. No major surgery should be performed if the blood supply is inadequate because of congenital absence of the vessels. A small, minimally projecting graft may be placed in the case of severe hemifacial microsomia with slightly diminished blood supply if one takes into consideration the limited capacity of the recipient area to support a large graft.

PREOPERATIVE EVALUATION

At the initial consultation for an infant with microtia, the focus should be on hearing function. Audiologic testing of the normal ear should be undertaken with determination of sound-field response and otoacoustic emissions. If testing is inconclusive and for bilateral cases, auditory brain stem response testing may be required. Bone-anchored hearing aids are available and worn as an external headband device for infants and children who are too young for definitive reconstructive surgery. Computed tomography of the temporal bones is performed late in the first year of life to determine whether the child has adequate anatomy for consideration of aural atresia reconstruction in the future. Computed tomography is also important to detect the occasional case of congenital cholesteatoma that requires surgical removal at an early age. The child is evaluated at 6- to 12-month intervals until it is determined that that child is ready for definitive reconstruction.

The parents must be made aware that the reconstructed auricle will be a great improvement over the microtic vestige but it will not be completely normal. Realistic expectations are important. Photographs depicting the various stages of surgery are valuable for educating families. The timing of reconstructive surgery is discussed, with most children beginning between the ages of 4 and 7 years, as discussed earlier. The surgical process of staged procedures is explained, with most children requiring four stages of reconstruction as described later. Two to 3 months is allowed for healing between stages. Thus, the overall process may be completed in about 1 year. Additional surgery for scar revision or refinement of cosmetic results may be necessary. The possibility of bleeding, infection, pneumothorax, flap loss, cartilage graft loss, scarring, and poor cosmetic results must be discussed with the parents.

The parents and child should be informed that after each stage of reconstruction a mastoid dressing will be worn for approximately 2 weeks. Tape will be used to fix the dressing to the child's hair to make it less likely that an uncooperative child will pull the dressing off, which can lead to complications. The family needs to know that the child will not like the frequent dressing changes with pulling of the hair during tape removal, but it will be worth the struggle in the long run. A very short haircut is recommended.

A template of the normal ear (if present) is made from x-ray film and will be used to determine the dimensions of the reconstructed auricle. The optimal position of the reconstructed auricle is determined by the distance from the lateral canthus, the brow, and the position of the normal ear. The axis of a normal auricle is about 30 degrees from the vertical position, with the superior aspect of the auricle being in a more posterior position. With hemifacial microsomia, considerable judgment is required to select the best position for the new auricle because the two sides of the head and face are not symmetrical.

SURGICAL APPROACHES

Most surgeons prefer grafting of costal cartilage for auricular reconstruction and use the method of Brent as described later.[2] Alternatives include prefabricated implants instead of cartilage and osseointegrated implants for a clip-on prosthetic auricle.

Stage 1

Sculpting an auricle out of costal cartilage takes skill and practice. Preoperative practice carving a block of soap or soft wood is recommended. Prophylactic perioperative antimicrobials are administered before all stages of microtia reconstruction. Figure 85-1 shows grade 2 microtia with a well-formed lower auricle and deficiency of the upper two thirds of the auricle. For harvest of costal cartilage, a curvilinear incision is made along the lower medial border of the *contralateral* rib cage because it has a more favorable curve for reconstruction of the auricle. The upper portion of the rectus abdominis muscle is dissected, preserved, and retracted laterally to allow exposure of the intercostal muscles and ribs. Preservation of the rectus abdominis muscle, rather than transecting it, decreases the chance of future chest wall deformity caused by a depression at the rib harvest site.[3] The two lowest floating ribs are harvested along with the synchondrosis of the sixth and seventh ribs (Fig. 85-2). With the floating ribs, cartilage is harvested all the way laterally until the bony-cartilaginous junction is reached. A suction drain is placed through a separate incision.

Young children have a relative deficiency of cartilage, and therefore pieces of cartilage are often stacked up to provide adequate bulk and lateral projection for details of the reconstructed auricle. In the occasional teen or adult with a generous amount of rib cartilage, the cartilage may be carved as a solid block, with adequate thickness and projection and little or no stacking required. This is called a closed or solid framework. In younger children, the various pieces of cartilage are

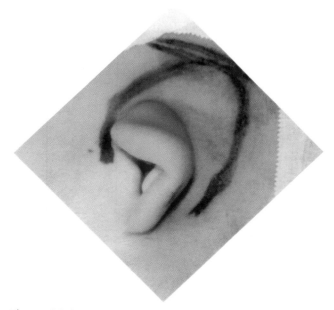

Figure 85-1. Grade 2 microtia with deficiency of the upper two thirds of the auricle. The planned site of placement of an auricular graft is marked.

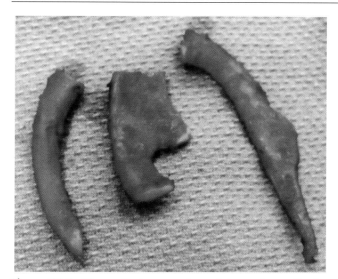

Figure 85-2. The cartilaginous portions of the two lowest floating ribs have been harvested along with all but the superior 4 mm of the synchondrosis of the sixth and seventh ribs.

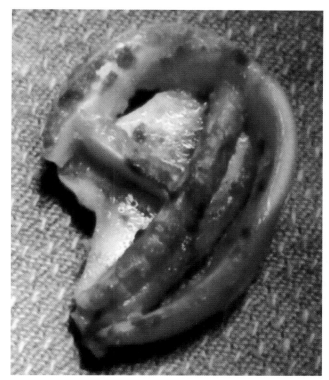

Figure 85-3. An open-type framework has been created from rib cartilage segments. Note how the cartilage fragments have been stacked to increase detail and lateral projection. Also note how the surface details are separated to allow the skin flap to drape in between the details or they will not be seen as separate entities.

carved and stacked with open spaces between the portions. This is called an open framework. The perichondrium is harvested along with the ribs, with great care taken to not enter the pleural space. The portion of rib cartilage containing the synchondrosis is used as the body or central portion of the framework. The helix is created by attaching a long floating rib segment around the perimeter of the body. This floating rib may be trimmed to achieve the proper projection and contour. The perichondrium and cartilage around the outer rim of the helix can be scored with partial-thickness incisions to "break the spring" so that the helical cartilage can wrap around the body with less tension. The various pieces of cartilage are attached via 4-0 clear nylon mattress sutures with the knots tied on the deep side of the graft, or superficially placed knots may later extrude through the skin flap. Additional pieces of cartilage may be stacked for creation of the antihelix and crura (Fig. 85-3). Occasionally, if adequate cartilage is available, the tragus may be attached to the main auricular cartilage graft with sutures during the first stage of reconstruction. The overall cartilage graft for the auricle is fashioned to be 2 to 3 mm smaller than the template from the opposite auricle. The additional 2 to 3 mm will be provided by the overlying skin flap.

To create the recipient bed for the cartilage graft, an incision is made anterior to the microtic vestige, and a thin flap is created just deep to the subdermal plexus. The flap is elevated for approximately 2 to 3 cm past the position marked for the auricle to allow a loose pocket without tension. This decreases the chance of flap loss and improves the details seen in the graft as the loose skin of the flap drapes into the depressions between the prominent areas of the cartilage graft. Two tiny suction drains are placed through separate incisions. The wounds are closed and the suction drains are activated. One drain is placed around the helix and the second is placed in the space between the anterior and posterior crura (Fig. 85-4). The microtic vestige is not resected at this time because if there is partial loss of the skin flap, the skin of the vestige may be used as a graft to cover the defect. A sterile mastoid dressing is placed. The drains are removed when the drainage has tapered off.

Stage 2

After 8 to 12 weeks, if healing has been complete, the second stage of microtia reconstruction may be undertaken. If there have been areas of skin breakdown or tenuous blood supply after any stage of microtia reconstruction, it is wise to defer the next stage until healing is complete.

Figure 85-5 shows the auricle of a child with initial grade 3 microtia who has healed after the first stage of reconstruction with implantation of an auricular cartilage graft. The microtic lobule is too anterior and superior and needs to be transposed to a more posterior and inferior position. The second stage of microtia reconstruction is essentially a Z-plasty. The skin at the recipient site is elevated and transposed to the site where the lobule had been. The cartilaginous reconstructed auricle has developed a fibrous capsule around it, and flap elevation should be performed in a plane outside this capsule. The lobular and skin flaps are elevated sufficiently to allow transposition and closure of the wounds without tension. The microtic vestige is resected

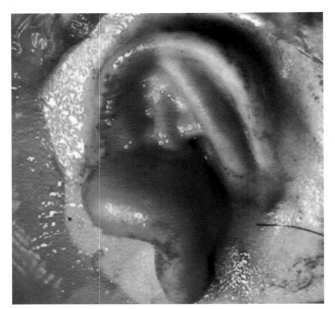

Figure 85-4. An auricular cartilage graft has been implanted and the two suction drains have been activated. Note how one drain is placed between the crura to drain that space.

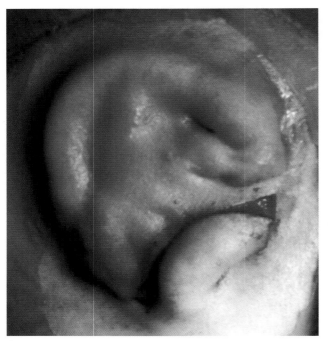

Figure 85-5. Second stage of reconstruction for a child with grade 3 microtia. Incisions have been made and flaps have been elevated for Z-plasty.

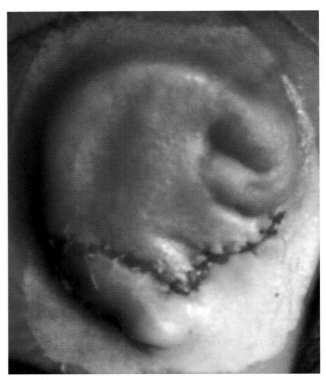

Figure 85-6. Completed reconstruction of second stage microtia with transposition of the lobule. Note how the lobule flap has been tapered and beveled to provide a smooth transition from the lobule to the rest of the auricle.

Stage 3

After the second stage, an additional 2 to 3 months is required for healing. The third stage of microtia reconstruction involves elevation of the auricle, which is in a pocket under the scalp. Elevation increases the lateral projection of the auricle and defines the helix and postauricular sulcus. Figure 85-7 shows the auricle of a child who has completed the first two stages of reconstruction and is ready for elevation of the auricle. An incision is made approximately 4 mm superior and posterior to the reconstructed helix (Fig. 85-8). The incision is carried down to the plane of the temporalis fascia. The auricle is elevated in this plane with a generous, undisturbed anterior pedicle left for the blood supply. The excess skin attached to the auricular graft is gently tacked down to the helical rim with 4-0 chromic suture. Excessive tension on the helical skin is avoided to prevent skin flap loss. The scalp is undermined via the postauricular incision in posterior and superior directions in the plane of the temporalis fascia (Fig. 85-9). Heavy sutures are used in a horizontal mattress fashion to advance the elevated scalp in anterior and inferior directions. Lighter sutures are used to further advance the skin edges. The goal is to hide the free edge of the scalp incision under the auricular cartilage graft for cosmetic purposes and, at the same time, decrease the size of the area requiring skin grafting on the scalp medial to the auricle. A split-thickness skin graft is harvested from the hip area or upper, inner

during the second stage of reconstruction. The lobular flap is carefully thinned and beveled to allow a smooth and natural transition from the helix of the cartilage graft to the lobule. Resection of tissue and beveling the lobule medially decrease the natural lateral rotation of the lobule (Fig. 85-6). Insufficient thinning and beveling will result in a "stuck-on" appearance of the lobule. No drains are required. The mastoid dressing and activity limitations are the same as described earlier.

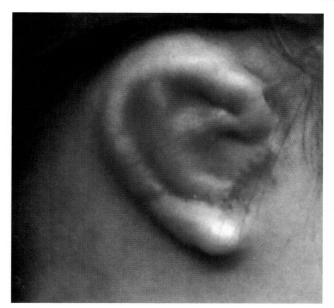

Figure 85-7. Auricle of a child who has completed the first two stages of reconstruction and is ready for elevation of the auricle.

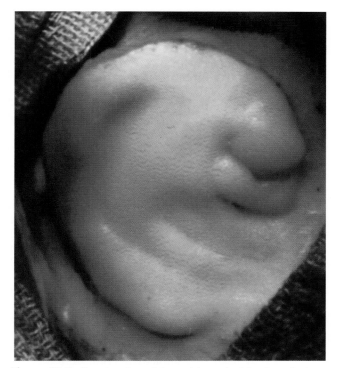

Figure 85-8. For elevation of the auricle, an incision is made 4 mm superior and posterior to the helical rim.

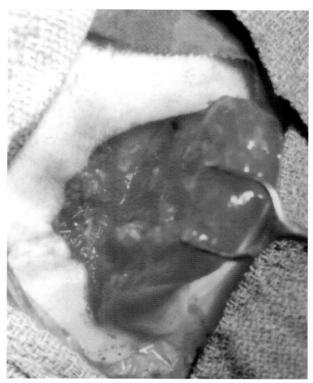

Figure 85-9. The scalp has been undermined in superior and posterior directions and heavy mattress sutures have been placed to advance the scalp flap in inferior and anterior directions. Such advancement hides the scalp incision medial to the auricle and decreases the size of the area requiring skin grafting.

aspect of the arm. The skin graft is cut to the appropriate size and shape. A few perforations are made in the skin graft to allow drainage of blood and serous fluid. The skin graft is then sewn in place in the postauricular area with 4-0 chromic suture. One end of all these sutures is left long for later use in tying down the bolster over the postauricular skin graft. An iodine-impregnated bolster is fashioned in the shape of an orange

wedge and packed into the postauricular area. The ends of the sutures are tied over the bolster securing the skin graft (Fig. 85-10). The mastoid dressing is placed as described earlier. The bolster is removed in the office after 8 to 12 days.

Stage 4

The tragus may be attached to the main auricular cartilage graft during the first stage of reconstruction if adequate cartilage is available, as described previously. If this was not possible, the final stage of microtia reconstruction is creation of the tragus and conchal bowl. This stage is performed after 2 to 3 months have elapsed for healing after the third stage. Two methods have been described for creation of the tragus during the final stage. One method, originally described by Tanzer,[4] involves creation of an anteriorly based flap in the area of the future tragus (Fig. 85-11). This method may be used for bilateral microtia reconstruction or when the family does not want the normal ear to be operated on in cases of unilateral microtia. A rectangular-shaped piece of cartilage is harvested from the conchal area of the auricular cartilage graft. The conchal area is carefully excavated and deepened while taking care to watch out for the occasional superficial aberrant facial nerve. The rectangular cartilage graft is placed at the base of the anteriorly based flap (Fig. 85-12). The skin flap is folded over the rectangular cartilage graft, and a 3-0

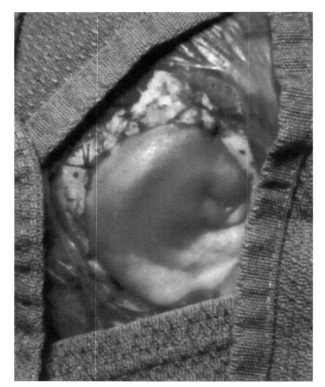

Figure 85-10. A wedge-shaped bolster has been tied in over the postauricular skin graft to secure it.

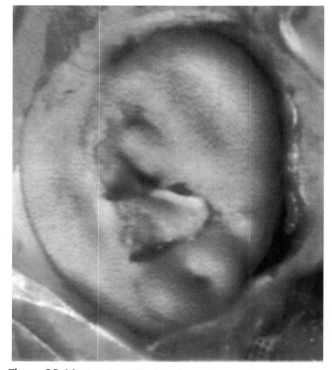

Figure 85-11. A U-shaped incision is used for creation of the tragus by the anteriorly based flap method.

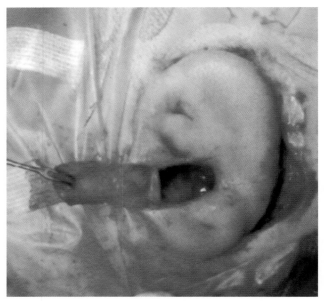

Figure 85-12. A rectangular cartilage graft for the tragus has been harvested from the conchal area of the reconstructed auricle and placed at base of the anteriorly pedicled skin flap.

nylon mattress stitch is placed through all layers to create the tragus (Fig. 85-13). A full-thickness skin graft is placed in the conchal bowl. An iodine-impregnated bolster is tied in place with sutures. The mastoid dressing is placed and the bolster is removed in the office after 8 to 12 days. Figure 85-14 shows the final result.

Another method of tragal reconstruction was described by Brent[2] and is used for unilateral cases of microtia. The reconstructed auricle is usually flatter than the normal auricle. A chondrocutaneous graft is harvested from the lateral posterior aspect of the concha of the normal ear (Fig. 85-15). Harvesting of this graft decreases the projection of the normal ear, which serves to improve bilateral frontal symmetry of the auricles (Fig. 85-16). A J-shaped incision is made at the site of the planned tragus (Fig. 85-17). The skin in the conchal area is elevated and some of the soft tissues are resected by careful blunt and sharp dissection as described earlier to deepen the conchal bowl. The surgeon must be alert to the possibility of the occasional aberrant facial nerve (Fig. 85-18). A full-thickness skin graft is placed. The previously harvested chondrocutaneous graft is placed into the J-shaped incision and fixed in place with a 3-0 nylon mattress suture. The graft is placed in a manner that allows the composite graft to be angled from a more anterior position medially and a more posterior position laterally. This serves to create a shadow in the conchal bowl that mimics an ear canal (Fig. 85-19). A bolster is placed for 8 to 10 days, and the mastoid dressing is placed as described previously. The bolster is removed in the office after 8 to 12 days (Fig. 85-20).

Staging of Surgery for Bilateral Microtia

Auricular cartilage grafts for first-stage microtia reconstruction are performed as unilateral procedures

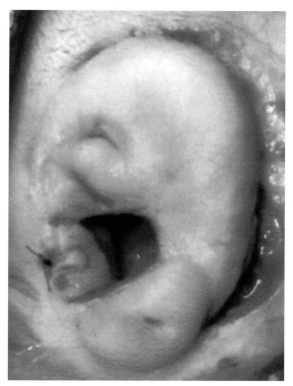

Figure 85-13. The anteriorly based flap has been folded over the rectangular cartilage graft and secured with a nylon mattress suture to create the tragus.

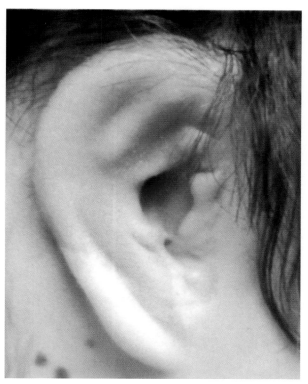

Figure 85-14. Final result after completion of stage 4 of reconstruction with the anteriorly based flap method of tragal reconstruction.

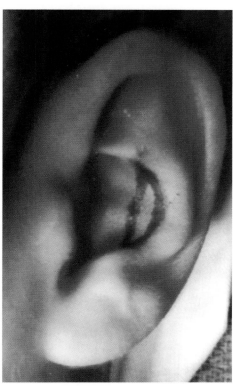

Figure 85-15. Planned incisions for otoplasty and the chondrocutaneous graft that is harvested from the lateral posterior aspect of the concha of the normal ear.

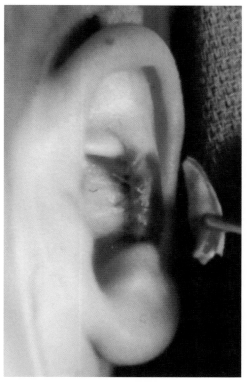

Figure 85-16. Otoplasty and harvest of the chondrocutaneous composite graft are performed to decrease lateral projection of normal auricle. This serves to improve frontal symmetry of the two auricles. The composite graft will be used for tragal reconstruction.

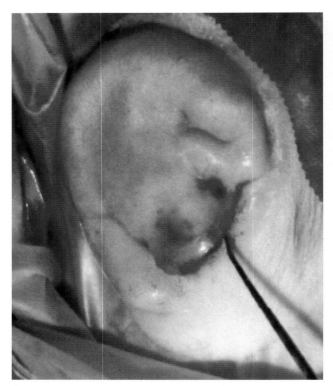

Figure 85-17. A second method of tragal reconstruction requires a J-shaped incision at the site of the planned tragus.

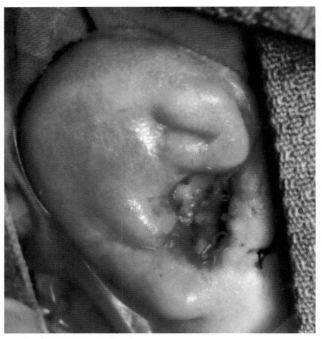

Figure 85-19. The chondrocutaneous composite graft has been positioned to create the posterior border of the tragus. The skin flap has been draped into the conchal bowl. A full-thickness skin graft has been sewn into the conchal bowl between the pedicled skin flap and the composite graft. Note how the reconstructed tragus casts a shadow that gives the appearance of an external auditory canal.

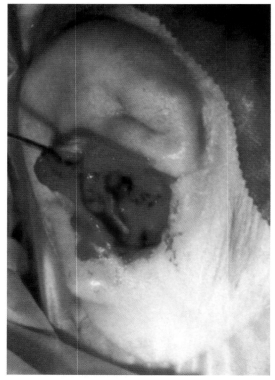

Figure 85-18. The conchal bowl has been excavated after the skin flap was elevated. Care is taken to avoid a possible aberrant facial nerve during excavation.

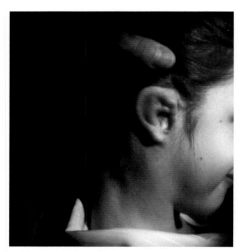

Figure 85-20. Final result after completion of four stages of microtia reconstruction with a J-shaped incision and a chondrocutaneous composite graft for tragal reconstruction.

because of the extensive nature of these surgeries. Third-stage microtia reconstruction with auricular elevation is also performed as a unilateral procedure because the posterior scalp tissue can be advanced only to one side at a time. Second-stage microtia reconstruction with lobule transposition and fourth-stage reconstruction with creation of the tragus by the anteriorly pedicled flap method may be performed bilaterally during the same anesthetic because of the more limited areas involved in these stages.

Revision Surgery

Revision surgery may be performed to enlarge the size of the postauricular sulcus with a full-thickness skin graft. A scar band with partial obliteration of the sulcus often occurs at the junction of the superior two thirds and inferior third of the sulcus because of skin graft loss secondary to limited blood supply in this area. A second area that may require revision is the transition of the lobule to the auricle. If the transition of the lobule to the auricular graft is not smooth and the lobule has a notched or "stuck-on" appearance, revision may be needed.

POSTOPERATIVE MANAGEMENT

Most surgeons prefer to continue prophylactic perioperative antimicrobial agents for 10 days. It is critical to fix the mastoid dressing to a young child's hair with tape to avoid having the child remove the dressing. Without taping to hair, young children will nearly always remove their dressing, which can lead to complications of infection, bleeding, and flap loss. The discomfort of hair pulling during dressing changes is well worth the avoidance of complications and preservation of good results. The dressing is changed on postoperative days 1, 3, and 7, and it is removed after 14 days. Contact sports are avoided for a total of 6 weeks.

PEARLS

- The surgeon should invariably choose to preserve the blood supply to avoid complications when balancing aesthetics versus blood supply.
- To minimize bleeding and to save time, bipolar scissors are excellent for removing intercostal muscles from the ribs. Retraction of the ribs with a two-pronged skin hook improves exposure during rib harvest.
- Small areas of flap loss usually respond to antimicrobials and gentle local wound care.
- Reducing the lateral projection of the cartilage graft to permit closure without tension allows healing of moderately sized areas of flap loss.

PITFALLS

- Unless a bridge of approximately 4 mm of cartilage is left in situ at the superior aspect of the synchondrosis, the undesirable late chest wall deformity of splaying out of the ribs may occur.[2]
- If the pleural space was entered but the visceral pleura of the lung has not been violated, a red rubber suction tube is placed while the anesthesiologist provides positive pressure to evacuate the pleural air. The catheter is withdrawn and the wound is closed. No chest tube is required unless the visceral pleura was violated.
- If the cut edges of the ribs remaining in the chest are not beveled so that the edges are smooth, painful irritation of the pleura and intercostal muscles may result.
- If adequate space between the surface details of the auricular graft is not provided, the skin will not drape in between the details and the details will not be seen as separate entities.
- Large areas of flap loss require a temporoparietal pedicled flap with a full-thickness skin graft to provide adequate blood supply and coverage.
- Unless Doppler or angiographic evaluation of the superficial temporal and occipital arteries is used to identify and preserve the vascular pedicle of the temporoparietal flap,[5] flap loss is more likely to occur.

References

1. Priwin C, Stenfelt S, Granstrom G, et al: Bilateral bone-anchored hearing aids (BAHAs): An audiometric evaluation. Laryngoscope 114:77-84, 2004.
2. Brent B: Technical advances in ear reconstruction with autogenous rib cartilage grafts: Personal experience with 1200 cases. Plast Reconstr Surg 104:319-334, discussion 335-338, 1999.
3. Eavey RD, Ryan DP: Refinements in pediatric microtia reconstruction. Arch Otolaryngol Head Neck Surg 122:617-620, 1996.
4. Tanzer RC: Total reconstruction of the external ear. Plast Reconstr Surg Transplant Bull 23:1-15, 1959.
5. Park C, Lew DH, Yoo WM: An analysis of 123 temporoparietal fascial flaps: Anatomic and clinical considerations in total auricular reconstruction. Plast Reconstr Surg 104:1295-1306, 1999.

Basic Rhinoplasty

Grant S. Gillman

Perhaps no other procedure combines the degree of artistic and technical detail affecting both form and function to the same extent as cosmetic rhinoplasty, which is what makes it the most challenging, humbling, and variable of all cosmetic procedures in facial plastic surgery. No single procedure is suitable to all patients, no single procedure is embraced by all surgeons, and the goals or desired changes will vary from one individual to the next.

Given the number of variables that come into play with each patient, no two operations are ever exactly the same. Each case is unique, and only through thoughtful preoperative analysis,[1-3] commitment to technical detail, critical and honest evaluation of one's postoperative results, ongoing education, and years of experience can the surgeon deliver consistent and predictable results. Finally, rhinoplasty surgery requires not only an appreciation of the artistic but also an awareness of the potential impact that changes may impart on nasal function so that nasal airflow is preserved or improved but not compromised.

The goal of this chapter is to outline some of the principles behind basic rhinoplasty maneuvers and the most commonly requested changes—dorsal reduction, tip refinement, and changes (increase or decrease) in nasal tip projection. In most cases, combinations of procedures are carried out, and it is incumbent on the rhinoplasty surgeon to understand the dynamic interplay[4,5] between techniques to properly anticipate what is necessary to help achieve the desired result.

PREOPERATIVE PLANNING

Preoperative evaluation begins by establishing the issues that are of greatest concern to the patient to clarify what the patient hopes to achieve through rhinoplasty surgery. A complete medical history is obtained. In particular, a history of any previous nasal surgery is elicited and medications reviewed. Any anticoagulant medications (including products containing warfarin [Coumadin], aspirin, or ibuprofen and any herbal products) should be discontinued 7 to 10 days before surgery to minimize the likelihood of excessive or unnecessary bleeding intraoperatively or postoperatively.

A thorough assessment[1-3] of the nose follows, which should include an evaluation of the nasal airway, skin thickness, dorsal height, tip definition, rotation and projection, alignment of the nose (straight versus crooked), and identification of any preoperative asymmetry.

Based on the patient's desires and findings on physical examination, a surgical plan is developed. The operation should be individualized according to the deformity, characteristics of the patient's tissues, and the patient's objectives. In this way a "game plan" unique to the individual patient is formulated.

The operative plan is then discussed with the patient and realistic expectations are set. The typical postoperative course, as well as potential complications and their relative frequency, are reviewed.

It is equally important to consider the limitations imposed by the patient's tissues and what may *not* be achievable and to clearly convey this information to the patient. The goal of surgery is to create a natural-looking nose without the tell-tale signs of surgery—one that harmonizes well with the other facial features. A conservative change is always preferable to overcorrection.

Preoperative photography must be done routinely and should include full facial frontal, right and left lateral, right and left oblique, and nasal base views. Close-up views are optional in general but preferable in cases in which there is obvious asymmetry preoperatively or a crooked nose.

ANESTHESIA

Rhinoplasty can be carried out under deep intravenous sedation or general anesthesia according to the preference of the patient and surgeon. Because intraoperative bleeding is inevitable, a general anesthetic provides maximal airway protection against aspiration and is thus preferred in most circumstances. In either case, the nose is also injected with 10 to 15 mL of 1% lidocaine with 1:100,000 adrenaline and the mucosa is decongested with oxymetazoline pledgets. The minimal amount of infiltrative anesthesia required to facilitate hemostasis without overly distorting the nose is recommended.

SURGICAL APPROACHES

Surgical approaches to rhinoplasty can be broadly classified as endonasal or external. Endonasal approaches to rhinoplasty are more difficult to learn and master because of somewhat more limited visual access, and for that reason most surgeons and certainly the less experienced are best served by the external approach for maximal exposure of the surgical anatomy. Consequently, only the external rhinoplasty approach will be outlined herein.

The basic principles underlying design of the columellar incision in external rhinoplasty are intended to minimize the chance of an unsightly conspicuous scar across the columella.[6] For this reason the incision is irregularized rather than linear and placed across the narrowest portion of the columella. A variety of incisions are used (gull-wing, stair-step, inverted-V incisions), but the basic rationale that underlies each of them is the same. We prefer a five-cornered, inverted V transcolumellar incision because the angles of the incision facilitate meticulous alignment at the end of surgery, which helps better camouflage the resulting scar.

A five-cornered inverted-V incision (Fig. 86-1) is marked across the narrowest portion of the columella. The transcolumellar incision is joined at a precise right angle to bilateral "marginal" incisions—incisions made along the lower (caudal) margin of the lower lateral cartilage (LLC) (Fig. 86-2). Using a sharp wide two-pronged double hook, the surgeon everts the alar rim to expose the lower (caudal) border of the lateral crus of the LLC. The incision is made with a no. 15 blade, beginning laterally beneath the lateral crus (Fig. 86-3), curving medially beneath the dome of the LLC, and continuing alongside the lateral aspect of the columella (Fig. 86-4) adjacent to the caudal margin of the medial crus to meet the lateral extension of the previously outlined transcolumellar incision. The transcolumellar incision is made with a no. 15 blade while taking care to stay superficial so that the underlying medial crura are not inadvertently incised (Fig. 86-5).

Careful elevation of the columellar skin flap is carried out with fine scissors by passing from the marginal incision on one side of the columella completely through to the other side (Fig. 86-6). The scissors are

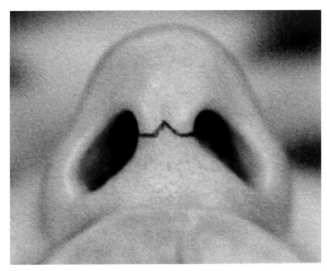

Figure 86-1. Five-cornered transcolumellar incision for an inverted-V external approach.

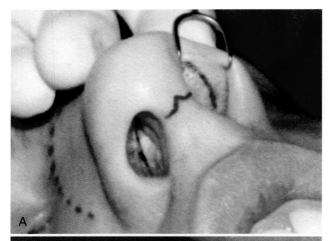
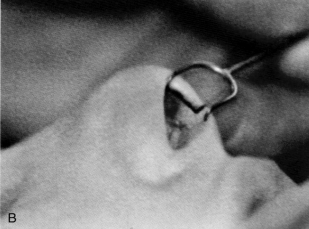

Figure 86-2. A, Marginal incision outlined along the caudal margin of the lateral crus. **B,** Marginal incision outlined along the caudal margin of the medial crus and joining the transcolumellar incision at a right angle.

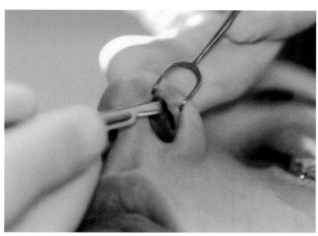

Figure 86-3. Marginal incision below the lateral crus of the lower lateral cartilage.

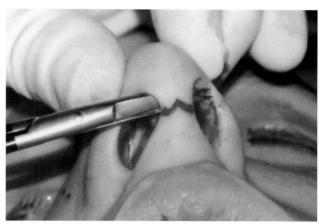

Figure 86-6. Elevation of the columellar skin flap is facilitated by first undermining from the marginal incision on one side through to the marginal incision of the opposite side.

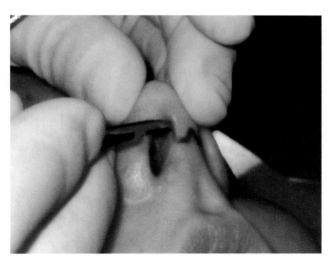

Figure 86-4. Marginal incision on the lateral aspect of the columella, below the medial crus of the lower lateral cartilage.

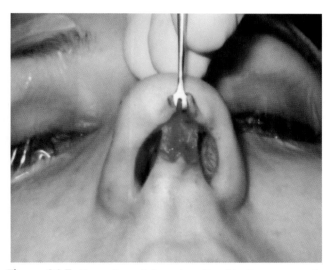

Figure 86-7. Retraction of the columellar skin flap exposes the underlying paired medial crura.

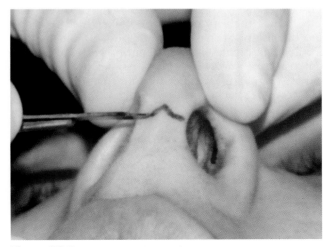

Figure 86-5. Trancolumellar incision.

then used to complete the transcolumellar incision and release any soft tissue attachments of the flap for exposure of the underlying medial crura (Fig. 86-7). A small double skin hook is placed beneath the columellar skin flap while a second such hook is placed beneath the alar cartilage to provide delicate counter-retraction (Fig. 86-8) as dissection of the skin–soft tissue envelope is carried anteriorly over the dome of the LLC and laterally over the lateral crura in a relatively avascular plane intimate to the overlying perichondrium. Precise and deliberate dissection is required to avoid inadvertent injury to or incision of the underlying cartilage.

Once the tip cartilage it exposed, it can be retracted inferiorly by a sharp medium-width two-pronged hook straddling the columella, with one hook beneath each dome (Fig. 86-9). The skin–soft tissue envelope that has already been elevated is retracted cephalically with a wide sharp double-pronged skin hook. The anterior septal angle (the most anterior and caudal point on the

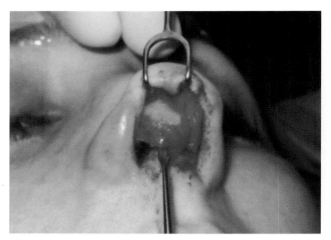

Figure 86-8. Retraction of the lateral crus of the lower lateral cartilage enables elevation of the overlying skin in a relatively avascular plane.

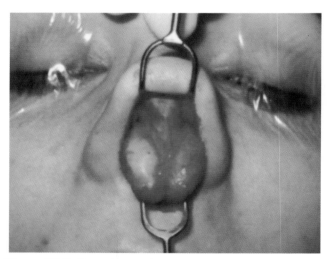

Figure 86-9. Retraction of the lower lateral cartilage caudally to expose the anterior septal angle for dissection superiorly along the nasal dorsum.

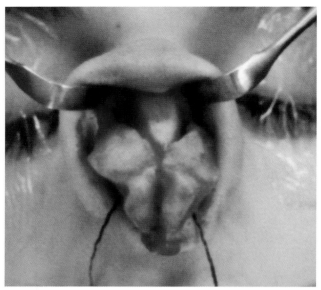

Figure 86-10. Complete exposure of the paired medial and lateral crura of the lower lateral cartilage and the cartilaginous nasal dorsum.

dorsal cartilaginous septum) is identified in the midline. The dissection is then carried superiorly along the dorsum in a plane intimate to the perichondrium overlying the dorsal septum to reveal the upper lateral cartilage (ULC) in the middle third of the nose (Fig. 86-10) and ultimately the nasal bones in the upper third, where one transitions to a subperiosteal plane. As the dissection moves cephalically, the best exposure is achieved with the use of an Aufricht dorsal nasal retractor.

Dorsal Reduction/Profile Alignment/Osteotomies

The use of life-size photographs will allow one to take precise measurements preoperatively to provide a more accurate guide to the amount of cartilaginous or bony reduction required intraoperatively. In general, the preference in men is for a stronger profile and a rela-tively straight nasal profile line from the nasion (root of the nose) to the nasal tip. In women, a slightly concave dorsal profile line that is 1 to 2 mm below the most anterior point of the projection of the nasal tip will yield an aesthetically pleasing feminine profile with a slight supratip break. In either case, extreme over-reduction or under-reduction is to be avoided.

Profile reduction is best done incrementally to arrive at the final level in a graduated fashion. The bulk of the reduction is carried out in the first pass, with fine-tuning and refinement thereafter. In most patients the osseocartilaginous hump is composed mostly of the cartilaginous vault, with a smaller contribution coming from the nasal bones themselves.

The cartilaginous dorsum is preferably reduced before septoplasty (if planned) to prevent inadvertent over-reduction of the dorsal septal strut that is to be preserved, which might otherwise occur if submucous resection of the septum is done before further reduction of the dorsal strut in the process of adjusting the profile. The cartilaginous reduction can be done with either a knife (no. 15 or 11 blade) or angled Fomon scissors (Fig. 86-11), with or without first separating the ULC from its attachment to the dorsal septum. If reduction of 3 mm or more is planned, submucosal separation of the ULC before dorsal reduction will preserve the support provided by the nasal mucosa below the ULC. When a smaller reduction is planned, it can generally be done without separating the ULC from its septal attachment yet still remaining extramucosal (i.e., without violating the nasal mucosa). Once the cartilaginous hump is removed, the height of the ULC relative to the dorsal septum is inspected and its medial borders lowered with a knife or fine scissors until they lie flush or level with the dorsal septum.

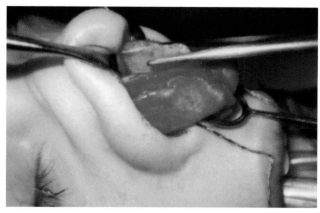

Figure 86-11. An angled (Fomon) scissors is used to reduce the height of the cartilaginous dorsum (note that the upper lateral cartilage has been separated from its attachment to the dorsal septum).

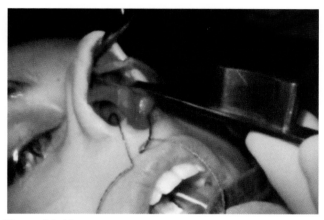

Figure 86-12. A Rubin osteotome is positioned for reduction of the bony dorsum. The incised portion of the cartilaginous dorsum to be resected is seen above the level of the osteotome.

The amount of bone to be removed is now defined by the height of the dorsal septum just below the caudal end of the nasal bones. Conservative reduction of the bony hump is carried out initially so that incremental refinement can be carried out as needed. The bony hump can be reduced with either nasal rasps or an osteotome.[7] Rasps allow more gradual reduction and are therefore recommended for a smaller bony hump and less experienced surgeons. For removal of a larger hump, a Rubin osteotome (a flat osteotome with a vertical fin to guide alignment and help keep the osteotomy level) is seated at the caudal end of the nasal bones (Fig. 86-12) and advanced toward the radix on a line parallel to the ideal dorsal line as the assistant strikes the back end of the osteotome with a mallet. Slight undercorrection is preferred, followed by final smoothing with a fine sharp nasal rasp.

When a large bony hump has been removed, an "open roof" deformity of the nasal bones is produced that requires closure with lateral osteotomies to mobilize and infracture the nasal bones. The osteotomies will also serve to narrow the bony nasal pyramid. A large

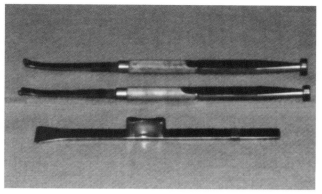

Figure 86-13. Curved right and left lateral osteotomes *(above)* and a Rubin osteotome *(below)*.

open roof deformity may not need medial osteotomies, but in many cases a short, fading medial oblique osteotomy will help establish a predictable, controlled location for the backfracture of the lateral osteotomy.

Five to 10 minutes before the osteotomies are carried out, the pathway of the proposed lateral osteotomies is reinjected with 1% lidocaine with 1:100,000 adrenaline to help minimize bleeding and therefore postoperative bruising.

Medial osteotomies[7] are carried out bilaterally with a straight osteotome—2, 3, or 4 mm wide, depending on the thickness of the nasal bones and the surgeon's preference. The osteotome is engaged at the cephalic end of the open roof deformity at the junction of the bony septum and nasal bone. As the assistant taps the back end of the osteotome with a mallet, the osteotome is advanced cephalically at first and then fades obliquely 15 to 25 degrees off midline to join with the medial end of the backfracture from the lateral osteotomy that follows. For thinner, delicate or shorter nasal bones in particular, medial osteotomies may not be necessary.

Lateral osteotomies are initiated through a stab incision at the base of the piriform aperture, just above the attachment of the inferior turbinate. Straddling the piriform aperture with a small or medium-size speculum will help bring the bone into relief and facilitate accurate placement of the stab incision. Through that incision a periosteal elevator is used to create a narrow tunnel through the soft tissue along the line of the proposed osteotomy to help diminish secondary soft tissue trauma and bleeding from the osteotomy itself.

A 4-mm curved guarded osteotome (Fig. 86-13) is initially directed laterally (as though aiming for the ipsilateral lateral canthus) to engage the osteotome in the ascending process of the maxilla. Once engaged, the osteotome is then directed cephalically while making certain to stay low in the nasofacial groove to avoid creating a visible or palpable step deformity on the bony nasal sidewall. Near the level of the infraorbital rim below the medial canthus, the osteotome begins to curve medially to meet the apex of the open roof deformity or the cephalic end of the medial osteotomy. The osteotome is then rotated medially to create a backfracture in the nasal bone for medialization and closure of the open roof deformity. The path of typical medial and lateral osteotomies is seen in Figure 86-14. A patient who underwent rhinoplasty with dorsal reduction and lateral osteotomies only is seen in Figure 86-15.

Nasal Tip Surgery

The range of surgical techniques described in the surgical literature to modify the nasal tip is a reflection of the complexity of nasal tip surgery and the evolution that has taken place to achieve better, enduring, and more consistent and predictable results while diminishing complication rates.

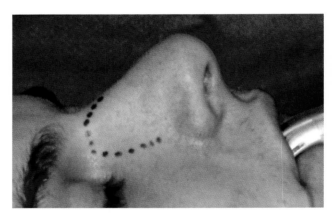

Figure 86-14. Typical path of fading medial and lateral osteotomies marked externally.

In most cases, the goals of nasal tip surgery are the same regardless of technique and include

- A natural looking, well-defined tip to address a broad or bulbous nose.
- Tip rotation appropriate to gender to address a drooping nasal tip (ideal nasolabial angle, 90 to 105 degrees in males and 100 to 115 degrees in females).
- Tip projection appropriate to the height of the nasal dorsum. In men, desirable tip projection creates a fairly straight profile from the root of the nose (the nasion or radix) to the tip, whereas in women the tip may project 1 to 2 mm above the level of the dorsum to yield a more feminine profile.

Nasal Tip Definition

As seen from the base of the nose, the ideal nasal tip contour will be more triangular in shape than broad, boxy, or trapezoidal. On a frontal view it should appear as a nasal tip lobule with two distinct tip-defining points closely approximating one another but without looking "pinched."

Enhancement of tip definition can be accomplished with suture techniques (more conservative) or with cartilage excision (more aggressive) to shape the cartilage at the lobular dome. The former is better suited to a patient with very thin skin, a tip in need of more limited refinement, or a surgeon with less experience, whereas the latter is best reserved for a patient with thicker skin and a surgeon more familiar with the nuances of excisional techniques.

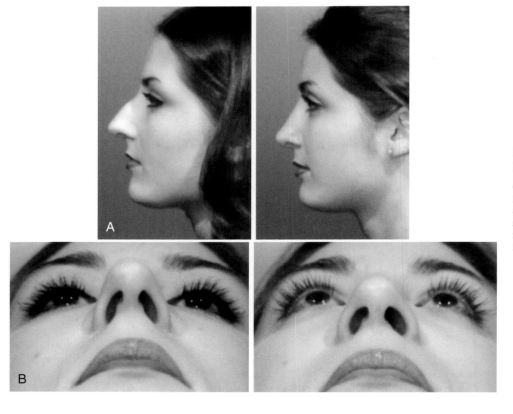

Figure 86-15. Preoperative and postoperative lateral (**A**) and base (**B**) views of a patient who underwent only dorsal reduction and lateral osteotomies. Note the deprojection of the nasal tip as seen on the base view that results from reducing the height of the nasal dorsum.

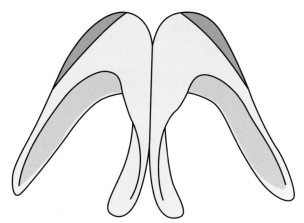

Figure 86-16. In a cephalic trim, the upper border (marked in red) of the lateral crus is excised to help improve definition of the nasal tip.

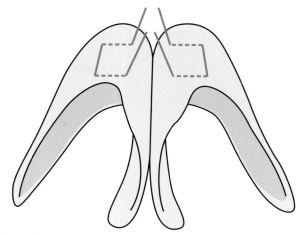

Figure 86-17. Bilateral horizontal mattress transdomal sutures will narrow the domal angle and reduce tip width as they are tightened. Suture ends from either side are then interlocked (interdomal suture).

1. *Cephalic trim.* Regardless of whether one is applying suture modification or excisional techniques at the dome of the LLC, both are frequently used in conjunction with a reduction in the overall height of the lateral crus known as a *cephalic trim* (Fig. 86-16). Volume reduction of the lateral crura will help address a tip that appears too bulbous. A cephalic trim is limited to the more medial aspect of the lateral crus. Trimming the cartilage more laterally does nothing to enhance definition more centrally in the lobule and may unduly risk alar collapse by compromising the strength and support that the lateral crura provide to the nasal ala.

    A minimum height of 6 to 7 mm of the lateral crus should be preserved to ensure adequate alar support and minimize the risk of alar collapse or retraction. A no. 15 blade is used to incise the lateral crura, and the cartilage to be removed is then dissected off the underlying vestibular mucosa with either fine scissors or the no. 15 blade. Care is taken to ensure that the height of the remnant of the lateral crus is symmetrical on the two sides.

2. *Tip suturing.* One method to narrow a broad or bulbous nasal tip uses permanent sutures[8] to modify the lower lateral crura at the tip (dome). This is a very effective and conservative (nondestructive) technique. By not actually excising any cartilage, one avoids having any incisional edges in the tip and thus diminishes the likelihood of visible irregularities.

    A 5-0 monofilament permanent suture is placed as a horizontal mattress stitch spanning the alar dome. The stitch is passed through cartilage only (superficial to the vestibular mucosa underneath) from a point medial to the dome; it exits the cartilage lateral to the dome and is then repassed back through the cartilage several millimeters below the first pass in a lateral-to-medial direction (Fig. 86-17). In this way the suture knot ends up between the two medial crura. This is known as a *transdomal* suture. As the suture is tightened, the domal angle is narrowed, thus reducing the width of the nasal tip. The

same maneuver is executed bilaterally. At the knot, one limb of the suture from each side is tied to that of the opposite side to unite the two domes from either side to one another (the *interdomal* suture). This adds stability to the new tip complex, helps ensure that the two tip-defining points rest at the same level, and minimizes the likelihood that as the nose heals, the effect of soft tissue contracture will draw the two domes apart from one another and lead to visible irregularities, asymmetry, or bossae (knuckling) of the cartilage. Finally, any sharp or prominent edges of the cartilage are shaved or beveled as necessary to yield a smooth final result. An example of tip narrowing with transdomal and interdomal sutures is seen in Figure 86-18.

3. *Vertical dome division.* Vertical dome division (VDD) refers to an excisional technique that involves interruption of the integrity of the LLC from its cephalic to its caudal border at or near the dome.[9] It has also been referred to as the *mobile tripod technique*[10] or *vertical lobule division.*[11] With this technique a cephalic trim is carried out in continuity with excision of either a cephalically based triangle (Fig. 86-19) or a wedge (Fig. 86-20) of cartilage at the chosen point of "division." The underlying vestibular mucosa is always preserved.

    Where the surgeon chooses to divide the cartilage will vary with what the surgeon is trying to achieve with respect to tip projection and tip rotation. Excision of a cephalically based triangle of cartilage (see Fig. 86-19) lateral to the dome will tend to increase both tip rotation and projection while simultaneously narrowing the tip. In such cases the medial border of the excised triangle should be no more than 2 to 3 mm lateral to the dome.[9] Alternatively, a wedge of cartilage can be excised right at the dome (Fig. 86-20), thus shortening the medial and lateral crura equally to effectively deproject and narrow the nasal tip.

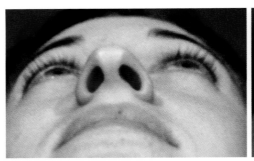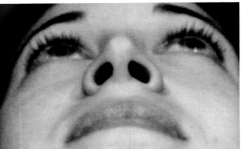

Figure 86-18. Preoperative *(left)* and postoperative *(right)* base views of a nasal tip refined with transdomal and interdomal sutures.

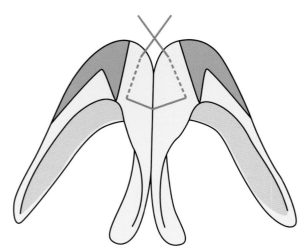

Figure 86-19. A vertical dome division (outlined in red, in continuity with a cephalic trim) carried out by excising a cephalically based triangle of cartilage 2 to 3 mm lateral to the dome will narrow the broad or boxy nasal tip while simultaneously increasing tip projection. The two medial crura are suture-united for stability of the medial complex.

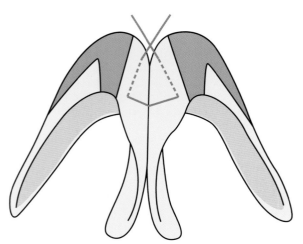

Figure 86-20. A vertical dome division (outlined in red, in continuity with a cephalic trim) carried out by excising a wedge of cartilage at the dome will reduce the medial and lateral crura equally. This will narrow the broad or boxy nasal tip while simultaneously decreasing tip projection. The two medial crura are suture-united for stability of the medial complex.

In either case, the two medial crura are then sutured to one another several millimeters proximal to the cut edge with 5-0 clear nylon mattress suture. This will stabilize the medial crural complex as natural scar contracture develops with healing and thereby help prevent migration or twisting of the cartilage, which might otherwise create visible irregularities. It is very important with VDD, especially in patients with thinner skin, to trim or round off any sharp or protruding edges of cartilage. Meticulous attention to such fine detail is essential when using this technique. An example of tip narrowing with VDD using the technique illustrated in Figure 86-19 is seen in Figure 86-21.

Nasal Tip Rotation

Elevation or increased rotation of the nasal tip (to address a drooping nose) may result from alterations to the LLC or as a by-product of other maneuvers that do not directly change the shape of the LLC. Some basic techniques that facilitate an increase in tip rotation are described.

1. ***Dorsal reduction.*** In patients in whom the dorsum is quite high and overprojected preoperatively, reduction of the nasal dorsum will promote upward rotation of the nasal tip. Whereas a more limited reduction (2 to 3 mm) may not effect a very significant change in nasal tip rotation, reductions of 4 mm or greater will often result in secondary rotation of the nasal tip.
2. ***Shortening the caudal septum.*** In patients with excessive columellar show (>4 mm on lateral view), shortening the overly long caudal septum is another effective means of promoting tip rotation. In such cases, a dorsally (anterior) based triangular wedge of cartilage is excised from the caudal end of the quadrangular cartilage together with the overlying septal mucosa. The septum can be stabilized with forceps in the nondominant hand while the cartilage is excised with a no. 15 blade.
3. ***Transdomal/interdomal sutures.*** Transdomal and interdomal sutures,[8] when applied as described earlier and illustrated in Figure 86-17, will provide a conservative and modest increase in tip rotation. A patient in whom a transdomal and interdomal suture technique was used is shown in Figure 86-22.

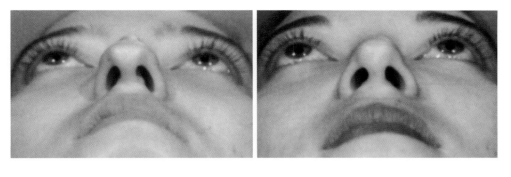

Figure 86-21. Preoperative *(left)* and postoperative *(right)* base views of the nasal tip refined via vertical dome division with excision of a cephalically based triangle of cartilage lateral to the dome.

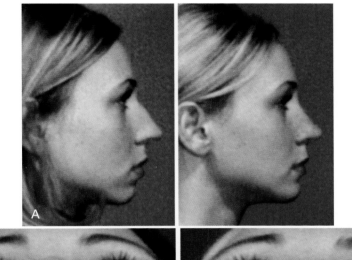

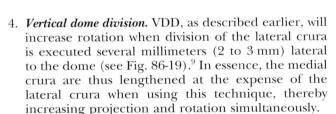

Figure 86-22. Preoperative and postoperative lateral (**A**) and base (**B**) views of a patient who underwent dorsal reduction and tip modification with transdomal and interdomal sutures (in addition to chin augmentation).

4. **Vertical dome division.** VDD, as described earlier, will increase rotation when division of the lateral crura is executed several millimeters (2 to 3 mm) lateral to the dome (see Fig. 86-19).[9] In essence, the medial crura are thus lengthened at the expense of the lateral crura when using this technique, thereby increasing projection and rotation simultaneously.

5. **Lateral crural overlay.** With this technique, vertical division of the lateral crura is carried out midway along the lateral crus, and the two segments are then overlapped and suture-fixated. A lateral crural overlay (also called a lateral crural flap) procedure[12,13] will rotate the tip upward while simultaneously deprojecting the tip (as the lateral crura are effectively shortened). When tip deprojection is desired together with tip rotation *and* the nasal tip itself is already narrow and well defined, maneuvers further out on the lateral crura that produce the desired changes are preferable to maneuvers exe-

cuted at the dome itself so that tip features that are already agreeable are not altered or disrupted.

It is helpful to first undermine the vestibular mucosa with fine scissors from beneath the lateral crus at the area to be divided and overlapped. Division of the cartilage is carried out with a no. 15 blade, and the two segments are then overlapped and secured with a 5-0 or 6-0 PDS mattress suture (Fig. 86-23). The greater the degree of rotation/deprojection desired, the greater the extent of the overlap.

Nasal Tip Projection

As is evident from the preceding sections on nasal tip surgery, many of the very procedures that are used to change either tip definition or tip rotation will have an effect on tip projection as well. There are many different options one may choose from to promote either an increase or a decrease in tip projection, and for this reason the surgeon needs to always consider the broader view of what one is trying to accomplish to select options that are best suited to each given patient. Some of the more commonly used techniques in tip projection are outlined.

1. ***Deprojection.*** As is the case with tip rotation, tip deprojection may occur directly as a result of alterations made to the LLC or as a secondary by-product of other maneuvers peripheral to the LLC. A smaller

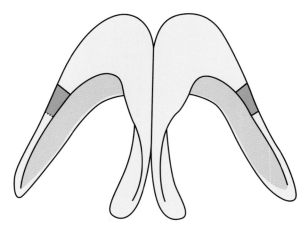

Figure 86-23. With a lateral crural overlay an incision is made in the lateral crus *(solid line)*. The cartilage medial to the incision is then overlapped with and sutured to the cartilage lateral to the incision to deproject and rotate the nasal tip. The area outlined in red illustrates an example of an area to be overlapped.

degree of tip deprojection will result naturally as tip support mechanisms are disrupted over the course of the operation, whereas greater deprojection will generally require some direct alteration of either the medial or the lateral crura.

Maneuvers that diminish tip support and thus deproject the nasal tip include significant *dorsal reduction* (described earlier; also see Fig. 86-15), *separating* the attachment of the LLC from the ULC (separation occurs as the scroll attachment of the two is eliminated with a cephalic trim), or a *full transfixion incision* along the caudal septum. For each of these maneuvers the degree of actual tip deprojection is limited. To make a full transfixion incision, a no. 15 blade is used to complete a through-and-through incision from the vestibular mucosa on one side of the caudal septum right through the vestibular mucosa on the opposite side. This severs the attachment of the medial crural feet to the caudal septum and thereby allows the tip to become retrodisplaced. Septocolumellar sutures (from the caudal septum to the columella) are used to resecure the tip in a new, deprojected position while at the same time closing the transfixion incision. Scar contracture will retrodisplace the tip toward the fixed nasal spine.

When more pronounced tip deprojection is required, changes will need to be directly made to the LLC. Shortening the lateral crura (the *lateral crural overlay*,[12,13] described earlier) will deproject and rotate the nose (Fig. 86-24). Alternatively, one could use exactly the same technical maneuver on

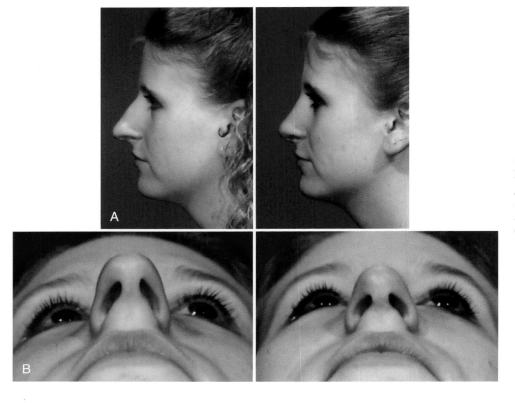

Figure 86-24. Preoperative and postoperative lateral (**A**) and base (**B**) views of a patient who underwent dorsal reduction, a complete transfixion incision, and lateral crural overlay to facilitate nasal tip deprojection and rotation.

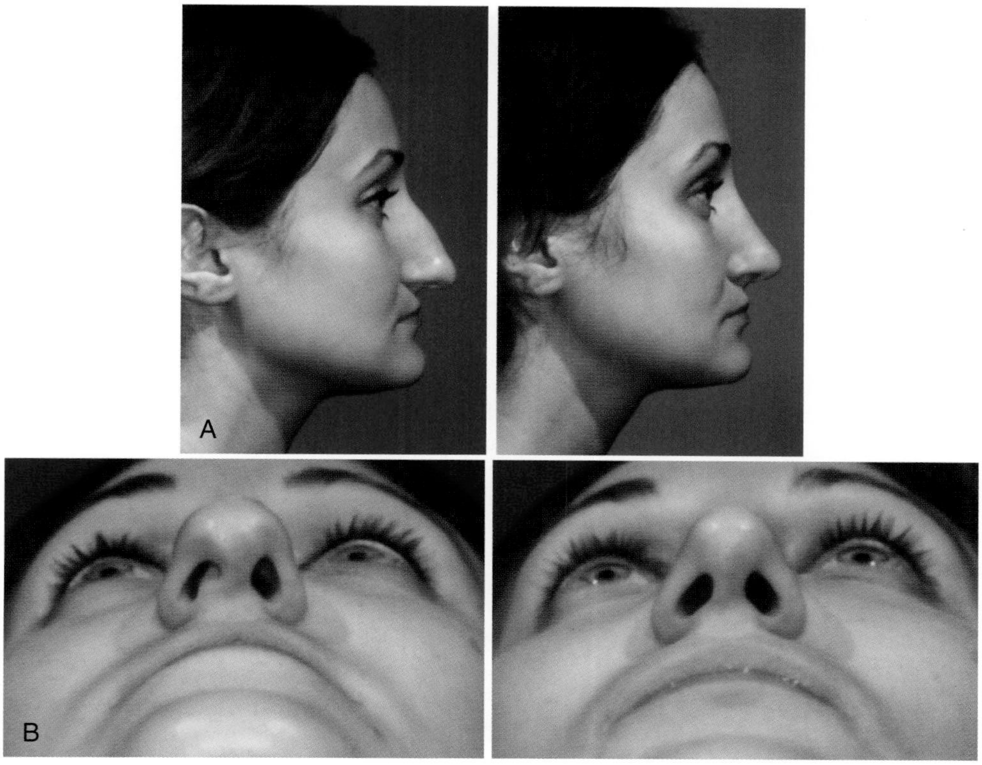

Figure 86-25. Preoperative and postoperative lateral (**A**) and base (**B**) views of a patient who underwent dorsal reduction, a complete transfixion incision, shortening of the caudal septum, and vertical dome division with excision of a domal wedge to facilitate nasal tip deprojection and rotation.

the medial crura to deproject and derotate (lengthen) a short nose by incising and overlapping the medial crural segments in a *medial crural overlay*.[13] Finally, one could also promote tip deprojection by shortening *both* the medial and lateral crura equally (which generally should not change tip rotation) either by combining the *lateral* and *medial crural overlay*[13] or by using the *dome division technique* (described earlier under tip definition), which involves resection of a wedge of cartilage right at the dome (see Fig. 86-19) to effectively shorten both the medial and lateral crura equally (Fig. 86-25).

2. *Increasing tip projection.* One of the more common techniques to increase tip projection is the use of *transdomal/interdomal sutures* (described earlier). The advantage of this method is that it is conservative, nondestructive, quick, and relatively easy to execute. Narrowing of the tip will also result, as will some modest tip rotation.

Another option is the use of *vertical dome division* (described earlier). To increase tip projection, the lateral crura are divided 2 to 3 mm lateral to the dome (see Fig. 86-19), and the medial elements are then brought together and suture-stabilized. What results is augmentation of the length of the medial crural complex at the expense of the lateral crura, thus increasing tip projection. At the same time the tip is narrowed and rotated cephalically. This technique requires fastidious attention to detail to reduce the likelihood of visible irregularities, particularly in a thinner-skinned patient. In these patients a thin tip

overlay graft of crushed cartilage can be used in addition to VDD as an added layer to smooth out the surface of the cartilage at the tip.

With the exposure provided by the external approach to rhinoplasty, a different alternative would be to isolate the caudal septum between the two medial crura and advance and resecure both medial crura on the caudal septum. These options have been referred to as *projection control sutures*[14] or a *tongue-in-groove technique*.[15]

Another means of augmenting tip projection is with the use of a cartilage *tip graft*, usually harvested and fashioned from septal or auricular cartilage. The edges of the graft must be beveled and thinned to minimize visibility, and the graft is then secured to the domes of the lower lateral crura with 6-0 PDS suture. This technique must also be used judiciously in a thin-skinned patient lest the graft edges become visible through the skin.

DRESSINGS AND POSTOPERATIVE MANAGEMENT

If a septoplasty was performed concurrently, Doyle splints may be secured intranasally to stabilize the septum. Some surgeons prefer packing with Telfa, Merocel sponges, or Vaseline gauze. All are acceptable. Packs are generally removed in 24 to 48 hours, whereas splints may stay in place from 4 to 7 days. Use of a prophylactic antibiotic is recommended as long as nasal packing remains in place.

If the ULC was separated from the dorsal septum before reducing the height of the nasal bridge, it should be resecured to the dorsal septum with a mattress 5-0 PDS suture. The marginal incisions are closed with absorbable suture (5-0 chromic or plain catgut), and the transcolumellar incision is closed with monofilament suture (6-0 nylon or Prolene). Meticulous realignment of skin edges will be rewarded with a very faint, well-camouflaged inconspicuous scar. An external dressing that consists of $\frac{1}{2}$-inch paper tape or Steri-Strips over the skin and a moldable splint over the tape is then applied.

Patients are advised to use saline spray frequently to keep intranasal splints clean. The inside of the nostril area and the transcolumellar incision should be cleaned several times daily with cotton-tipped applicators soaked in peroxide to remove dried blood and crust and then coated with an antibiotic ointment to help keep the tissue moist. Keeping the head elevated for the first 48 to 72 hours helps avoid postoperative edema, and ice packs or cool compresses are used over the eyes or a regular basis.

The patient is seen for suture and splint removal 5 to 7 days postoperatively. They are instructed at that time to avoid sunburn for 3 to 6 months with use of an appropriate sunblock and to avoid wearing glasses directly on the nose for the first 4 to 6 weeks while the edema continues to settle. Further follow-up appointments are usually made for 1, 3, 6, and 12 months postoperatively and annually thereafter.

COMPLICATIONS[16]

Patient Dissatisfaction

Managing expectations preoperatively is essential to minimizing the likelihood of having an unhappy patient.[17] Patients should be equally aware of the limitations of surgery and their own unique anatomy, as well as the difficulty that can sometimes arise in matching surgical outcomes to expectations. A patient who sets realistic goals and thoroughly understands the risks associated with rhinoplasty surgery will usually be a satisfied patient postoperatively.

Dorsal Over-reduction/Under-reduction

The use of life-size photographs from which one can make preoperative measurements is a useful guide to avoiding gross under- or over-reduction, particularly for a less experienced surgeon. Under-reduction, if significant, may require a revision procedure to further lower the dorsum. Gross over-reduction, on the other hand, will result in a "saddle" deformity[18] and necessitates a revision procedure to augment the dorsum, preferably with cartilage grafting.

Pollybeak Deformity

Over-reduction of the bony dorsum or under-reduction of the cartilaginous dorsum will result in a pollybeak deformity[19] in which the profile line appears high from the rhinion to the nasal tip. If caused by over-reduction of the bones, dorsal augmentation in that area is required. If secondary to under-resection of the cartilaginous dorsum, additional reduction of that part of the nasal bridge is then required.

Tip Asymmetry/Irregularities/Bossae

Meticulous attention to detail in planning and executing the surgery will help avoid such complications,[20] especially in a thin-skinned patient because tip irregularities are more likely to be camouflaged in patients with thicker skin. Nonetheless, scar contracture and shrinking of the soft tissue envelope can result in either asymmetry or visible irregularities despite vigilance of the surgeon intraoperatively. In such cases, targeted revision surgery (usually relatively minor) may be warranted.

Alar Retraction/Alar Collapse

Both these complications are typically caused by overly aggressive resection of the lateral crura and result in a deformity with both aesthetic and functional implications. For this reason, preservation of at least 6 mm of the height of the lateral crura is recommended. Both retraction and collapse will require structural grafting with cartilage (septal or auricular) to either replace or reinforce the overly resected lateral crura.[21,22]

PEARLS

- Complete and thorough analysis is a vital prelude to developing a successful surgical plan.
- Realistic goals must be established with the patient because patients with unattainable expectations are not good surgical candidates.
- Effort should be made to maintain dissection in tissue planes intimate to the underlying cartilage and bone to maximize the thickness of the soft tissue cover, which will minimize unnecessary bleeding and swelling.
- Conservatism is always warranted, and desirable preoperative features should be preserved.
- Many alterations to the lower lateral cartilage affect both tip projection *and* tip rotation.

PITFALLS

- Over-reduction of the nasal dorsum will produce an unnatural, scooped appearance and give the nose a telltale "surgical" look.
- Aggressive resection of tip cartilage will not yield better nasal definition but will set the stage for complications such as alar collapse or alar retraction.
- One cannot overcome thick skin by resecting more of the underlying cartilaginous support in search of better refinement.

- In patients with thin skin, inexact surgery at the tip-defining points will lead to visible prominences or bossae.
- Inattention to detail when closing the transcolumellar incision will result in visible notching or a wide unsightly scar.

References

1. Toriumi DM, Becker DG: Rhinoplasty analysis. In Toriumi DM, Becker DG (eds): Rhinoplasty Dissection Manual. Philadelphia, Lippincott Williams & Wilkins, 1999, pp 9-23.
2. Gunter JP, Hackney FL: Clinical assessment and facial analysis. In Gunter JP, Rohrich RJ, Adams WP (eds): Dallas Rhinoplasty: Nasal Surgery by the Masters. St. Louis, Quality Medical Publishing, 2002, pp 53-71.
3. Byrd HS, Burt JD: Dimensional approach to rhinoplasty: Perfecting the aesthetic balance between the nose and chin. In Gunter JP, Rohrich RJ, Adams WP (eds): Dallas Rhinoplasty: Nasal Surgery by the Masters. St. Louis, Quality Medical Publishing, 2002, pp 117-131.
4. Guyuron B: Dynamic interplays during rhinoplasty. Clin Plast Surg 23:223-231, 1996.
5. Guyuron B: Dynamics in rhinoplasty. Plast Reconstr Surg 105:2257-2259, 2000.
6. Davis RE: Proper execution of the transcolumellar incision in external rhinoplasty. Ear Nose Throat J 83:232-233, 2004.
7. Toriumi DM, Hecht DA: Skeletal modifications in rhinoplasty. Facial Plast Surg Clin North Am 8:413-431, 2000.
8. Toriumi DM, Tardy ME: Cartilage suturing techniques for correction of nasal tip deformities. Op Tech Otolaryngol Head Neck Surg 6:265-273, 1995.
9. Simons RL: Vertical dome division techniques. Facial Plast Surg Clin North Am 2:435-458, 1994.
10. Glasgold AI, Glasgold MJ, Rosenberg DB: The mobile tripod technique: The key to nasal tip refinement. Facial Plast Surg Clin North Am 8:487-502, 2000.
11. Constantinides M, Liu ES, Miller PJ, Adamson PA: Vertical lobule division in rhinoplasty: Maintaining an intact strip. Arch Facial Plast Surg 3:258-263, 2001.
12. Kridel RW, Konior RJ: Controlled nasal tip rotation via the lateral crural overlay technique. Arch Otolaryngol Head Neck Surg 117:411-415, 1991.
13. Soliemanzadeh P, Kridel RW: Nasal tip overprojection: Algorithm of surgical deprojection techniques and introduction of medial crural overlay. Arch Facial Plast Surg 7:374-380, 2005.
14. Tebbets JB (ed): Primary Rhinoplasty: A New Approach to the Logic and the Techniques. St. Louis, CV Mosby, 1999, pp 342-350.
15. Kridel RW, Scott BA, Foda HMT: The tongue-in-groove technique in septorhinoplasty. Arch Facial Plast Surg 1:246-256, 1999.
16. Simons RL, Gallo JF: Rhinoplasty complications. Facial Plast Surg Clin North Am 2:521-529, 1994.
17. Morehead JM: The dissatisfied patient. Facial Plast Surg Clin North Am 8:549-552, 2000.
18. Alsarraf R, Murakami CS: The saddle nose deformity. Facial Plast Surg Clin North Am 7:303-310, 1999.
19. Tardy ME, Kron TK, Younger R, Key M: The cartilaginous pollybeak: Etiology, prevention and treatment. Facial Plast Surg 6:113-120, 1989.
20. Perkins SW, Tardy ME: External columellar incisional approach to revision of the lower third of the nose. Facial Plast Surg Clin North Am 1:79-98, 1993.
21. Toriumi DM, Josen J, Weinberger M, Tardy ME: Use of alar batten grafts for correction of nasal valve collapse. Arch Otolaryngol Head Neck Surg 123:802-808, 1997.
22. Gunter JP, Friedman RM: Lateral crural strut graft: Technique and clinical applications in rhinoplasty. Plast Reconstr Surg 99:943-952, 1997.

Chapter **87**

Nasal Reconstruction

Frederic W.-B. Deleyiannis and Jayakar V. Nayak

The nose is of critical aesthetic and functional significance. Mastery of nasal reconstruction requires not only a knowledge of flaps and grafts but also an appreciation of facial aesthetics and functional rhinoplasty. A skin graft or local flap will close most nasal defects, but without a comprehensive evaluation of the nasal defect and the anticipated reconstructive outcome, re-establishment of facial balance and nasal breathing can be lost.

Nasal defects represent tissue loss, often the result of tumor resection or trauma. To reconstruct a nasal defect aesthetically and functionally, one must understand the layers and volumes missing from the defect, the nasal subunits involved, the cartilage support structures required, and the color and thickness of the proper skin replacement. This chapter describes the basic principles of nasal reconstruction as applied to acquired nasal defects.

PATIENT SELECTION

It is critical to define the extent and significance of an acquired nasal deformity to the patient. As in many aspects of plastic surgery, congruence between what is perceived by the patient and observed by the physician is essential. Discrepancies in form or function are best addressed before any consideration can be given to surgical intervention. Smoking will increase the risk of partial or total loss of a skin flap.[1] This risk should be discussed with the patient. The surgeon should insist that the patient stop smoking at least 3 weeks before surgery, and this should be documented in the patient's record. Preoperative counseling is also crucial to best define the anticipated cosmetic results and limitations. This might include demonstrating certain procedures to the patient by using a mirror and outlining schematic figures of the intended surgery. If multiple, staged surgical procedures are needed, the timing of the procedures should be emphasized.

Because of the importance of the nose for body image, most nasal defects are reconstructed. The patient's age is not generally a contraindication to nasal reconstructive procedures. However, a patient's general medical condition, as well as the extent of the procedure, may influence the decision for or against surgery. Sometimes a nasal prosthesis is a valuable and recommended option (Fig. 87-1). If the nasal defect is a result of tumor resection, the pathology, as well as the need and the timing of any adjuvant therapy (i.e., radiation therapy), should be discussed in the context of tumor surveillance, recurrence, and wound healing.

In children, reconstruction should be initiated and, if possible, completed before they have attained school age to avoid psychosocial repercussions.[2] The reconstructed nose, with skin, lining, and support, will grow with the child. However, additional surgical procedures to increase the nasal airway, to add cartilage grafts for enhancement of projection or contour, and to revise scars are expected.

PREOPERATIVE PLANNING

Analysis of the Defect by Adjacent and Underlying Facial Structures

Extended nasal defects are those that extend beyond the nose and involve the cheek, upper lip, underlying maxilla, or any combination of these structures. Large cheek and lip defects may require free tissue transfer before nasal reconstruction (Fig. 87-2) to replace missing volume and skin. Small defects of the medial part of the cheek and upper lip can be repaired with cheek advancement flaps or nasolabial flaps at the first stage. A foundation of skin and fat should exist or be reconstructed along the region of the piriform aperture (i.e., the nasal platform) to support the reconstructed alar bases and columella and to position the new nose anterior to the maxilla so that it does not extend beyond

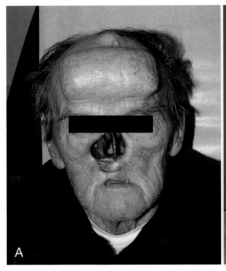
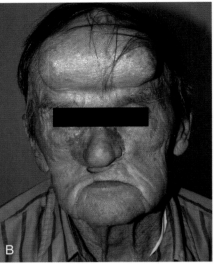

Figure 87-1. An 83-year-old man after total rhinectomy before (**A**) and after (**B**) coverage with a nasal prosthesis.

its normal borders and flow onto the cheek. Cheek advancement flaps can be used as a foundation for the nasal base before median forehead flap reconstruction and can be used for replacement of the nasal sidewall (Fig. 87-3). The nasal platform and base should be in harmony with the eyes (i.e., the width of the alar base should approximate the intercanthal distance).

Analysis of the Defect by Nasal Subunits

The nose is often divided into subunits (Fig. 87-4) that define areas of dissimilar skin texture and depth.[3-5] Borders between these areas are sites of shadow and highlights. The convex subunits of the nose are the tip, dorsum, alae, and columella. Application of the subunit principle is practical mainly for reconstruction of the convex subunits with flaps, not for the concave subunits—the nasal sidewalls and soft triangles. As skin flaps heal, they contract secondary to the collagen and myofibroblasts in the recipient bed. This contraction pulls the flap centripetally (i.e., trapdoors) into the convex shape of the unit that it covers. The subunit principle is not suitable for repair with skin grafts because skin grafts do not undergo trapdoor contraction. These grafts lie flat and do not bulge with wound contraction, probably because they lack a layer of subcutaneous fat. If more than 50% of the subunit is missing, the entire subunit (in particular, the tip or ala) should be replaced with a flap.

The nose in a young child is smaller, flatter, and less defined than in an adult.[6] The subunit borders are less distinct, but even in children the subunit principle can be used as a technique to hide scars and harness flap contraction.

Analysis of the Defect by Nasal Layers (Skin, Cartilage, and Mucosa)

Accurate analysis of the defect with regard to the component layers of the nose is essential. In general, when only skin is missing, reconstruction can be done reliably with local flaps, and if the underlying framework is deficient, cartilage grafts are needed. The difficulty of the reconstruction increases as the amount of nasal lining diminishes.

The nose has three distinct zones of skin thickness with differing degrees of subcutaneous fat, sebaceous gland content, and mobility (Fig. 87-5).[7,8] The skin of zone I is nonsebaceous and mobile and covers the upper dorsum and sidewalls of the nose. Zone II contains thick, sebaceous, nonmobile skin and covers the supratip area, tip, and alar lobules. Zone III skin is thin, nonsebaceous, and fixed to the underlying alar cartilage or fibrofatty structures of the alar margin, soft tissue triangles, infratip lobule, and columella.

SURGICAL APPROACH

Reconstruction of the nose begins with an analysis of the defect. With a diagnosis of the facial and nasal subunits involved and the nasal layers missing, one can now evaluate the various reconstructive options and plan the surgical approach.

Nasal Lining Options

Thin, vascular, and supple nasal lining remains the goal in reconstruction. Thick, bulky flaps, such as a nasolabial flap, will block the nasal airway.[9] Cartilage grafts placed on poorly perfused flaps will necrose and extrude. Lining flaps that are highly vascular and thin can be taken from multiple donor sites within the nose (Fig. 87-6).[9,10] Menick's technique of performing a folded forehead flap procedure in three stages offers a new, refined method of replacing nasal lining, and transfer of free fasciocutaneous flaps enables reconstruction of total or near-total defects.[11,12]

Turnover Flaps

Turnover flaps are small flaps of skin surrounding a defect that are turned over like the pages of a book into

Text continued on p. 827.

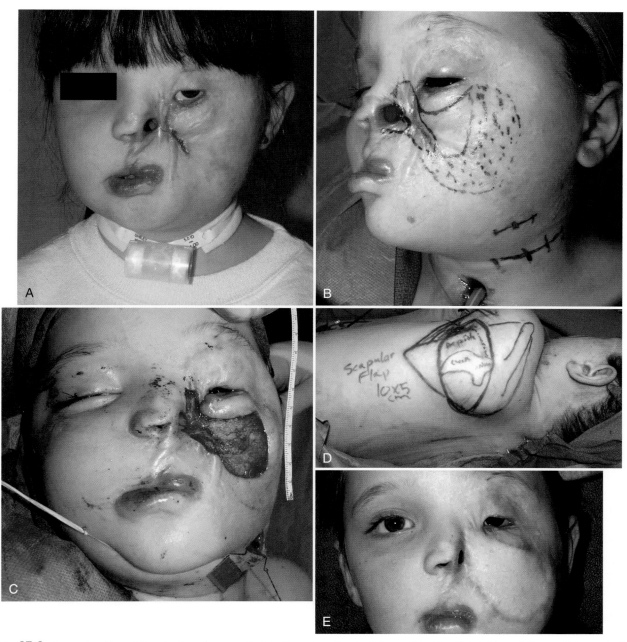

Figure 87-2. Reconstruction of the cheek and nose with free tissue transfer. **A,** A 4-year-old girl with total loss of the medial aspect of her left cheek (skin and underlying musculature) and heminose 1 year after an avulsion injury from a motor vehicle accident. **B,** Intraoperative plan—scar to be excised and reconstructed with a scapular flap. The *stippled* region is the area to be augmented with partial de-epithelization of the scapular flap. **C,** Cheek defect re-created. **D,** Design of the scapular flap. **E,** One year after reconstruction of the cheek with a scapular flap.

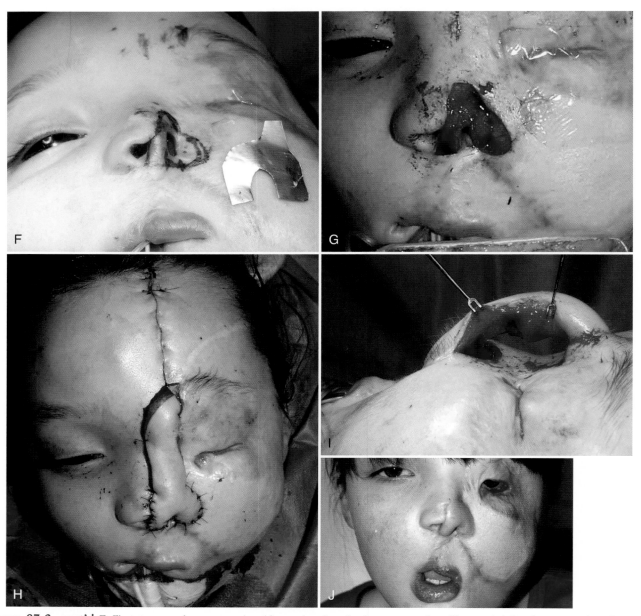

Figure 87-2, cont'd F, First-stage nasal reconstruction 16 months after cheek reconstruction. The nasal defect is re-created, and a nasal template is designed from the contralateral side of the nose. **G,** First-stage nasal reconstruction. The nasal lining is created with turnover flaps, and conchal cartilage is used for alar and tip grafting. **H,** Forehead flap for cutaneous covering. **I,** Second-stage nasal reconstruction, 4 weeks after the first stage. The forehead flap is bipedicled, and the flap was thinned of frontalis muscle and subcutaneous tissue. **J,** Appearance after division and inset of the forehead flap (after the third stage).

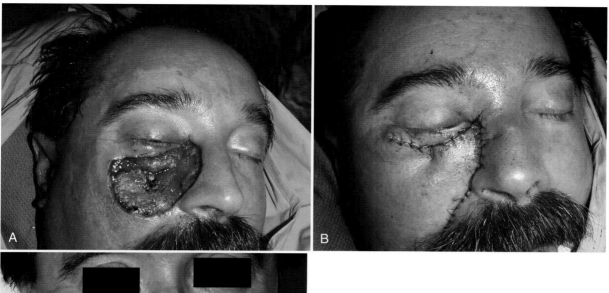

Figure 87-3. Reconstruction of the cheek and nose with a cheek advancement flap. **A,** Cheek and nasal defect (skin zone I, lateral nasal sidewall). **B,** Cheek flap. **C,** Appearance 19 months after surgery.

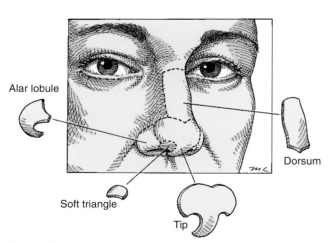

Figure 87-4. Nasal subunits. The surface of the nose can be segmented into distinct anatomic regions that correspond to sites of natural lines of shadow, curvature, and differing skin characteristics. The convex subunits of the nose are the tip, dorsum, alae, and columella. *(From Burget GC: Aesthetic restoration of the nose. Clin Plast Surg 12:463-480, 1985, with permission.)*

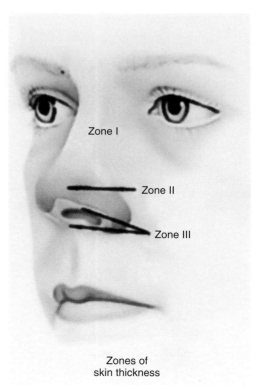

Zones of
skin thickness

Figure 87-5. Depiction of the three zones of nasal skin types. *(Reprinted from Burget GC: Modification of the subunit principle for reconstruction of nasal tip and dorsum defects [commentary]. Arch Facial Plast Surg 1:16-18, 1999, with permission.)*

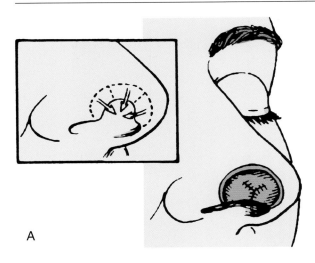

A

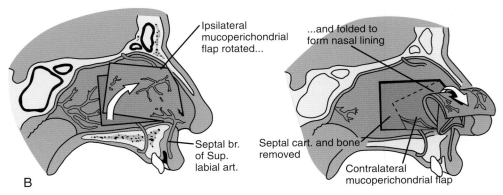

Ipsilateral
mucoperichondrial
flap rotated...

...and folded to
form nasal lining

Septal br.
of Sup.
labial art.

Septal cart. and bone
removed

Contralateral
mucoperichondrial flap

B

Figure 87-6. Nasal lining. Options for nasal lining include (**A**) the turnover/turn-in flap, (**B**) the septal mucoperichondrial flap, and (**C**) the bipedicled flap interposition. (*A and C, Reprinted with permission from Burget GC: Aesthetic reconstruction of the nose. In Mathes SJ [ed]: Plastic Surgery, vol 2. Philadelphia, Elsevier, 2006, p 578; and B, reprinted with permission from Burget GC, Menick FJ: Nasal support and lining: The marriage of beauty and blood supply. Plast Reconstr Surg 84:189-202, 1989.*)

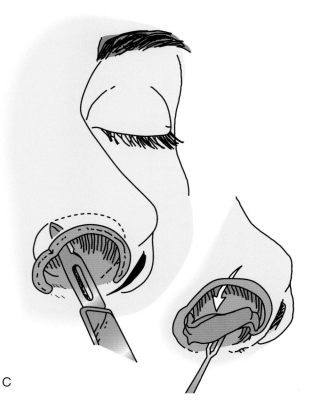

C

the nasal airway. Because they are based on scar, their blood supply can be tenuous and their length is limited. If their blood supply appears inadequate at the time of reconstruction, cartilage grafting should be done secondarily.

Septal Mucoperichondrial Flaps: Ipsilateral and Contralateral

An ipsilateral septal flap, based anteriorly on the septal branch of the superior labial artery, has been described by Burget and Menick.[9] The flap pivots on an anterior-inferior point near the nasal spine and folds outward to provide lining for the nasal domes. The exposed septal cartilage is either harvested as a graft or left to remucosalize.

A contralateral septal flap can be harvested with or without septal cartilage.[9,13] This technique involves harvesting the contralateral septal mucoperichondrium and swinging it like a trapdoor underneath the nasal dorsum through a dorsal perforation in the septum. The flap can reach the nasal sidewalls but not the alar margins.

Bipedicled Lining Flaps

The nasal lining of the alar margin can be successfully reconstructed with a bipedicled lining flap (Fig. 87-7).[13] The flap is based medially on the septum and laterally on the vestibule and is pulled down to the alar margin. The secondary lining defect made above the alar margin can be covered with a contralateral (or ipsilateral) septal mucoperichondrial flap.

Menick's Technique for Nasal Lining: The Folded Forehead Flap, Skin Grafts, and Three-Stage Nasal Reconstruction

To provide nasal lining, Menick has advocated folding the forehead flap on itself and insetting it into the defect (Fig. 87-8).[11,12] At a second operation 3 weeks later, the covering portion of the flap is separated from the nasal lining portion of the flap and lifted entirely off the nose. The nasal lining flap is now thinned by removal of the frontalis muscle and excess subcutaneous tissue. Cartilage grafts are placed at this second stage. The covering portion of the forehead flap is also

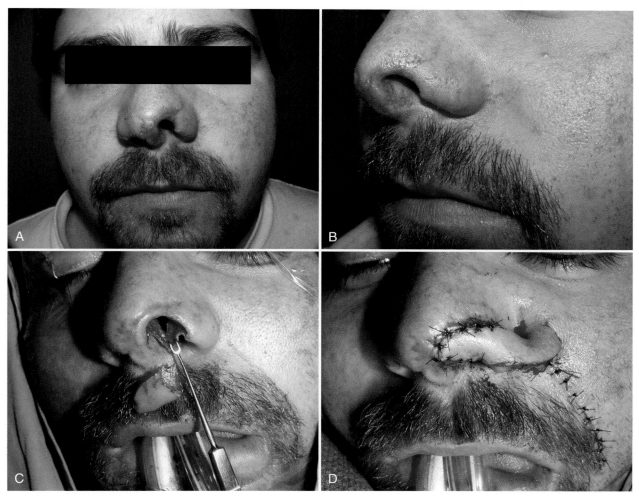

Figure 87-7. Superiorly based, two-stage nasolabial flap. **A,** Defect of the soft tissue triangle, frontal view. **B,** Oblique view. **C,** First stage: nasal lining reconstructed with a bipedicled lining flap (retracted downward with the skin hook, refer also to Figure 87-6C) and septal cartilage used to buttress the soft tissue triangle. **D,** Superiorly based nasolabial flap used for cutaneous coverage.

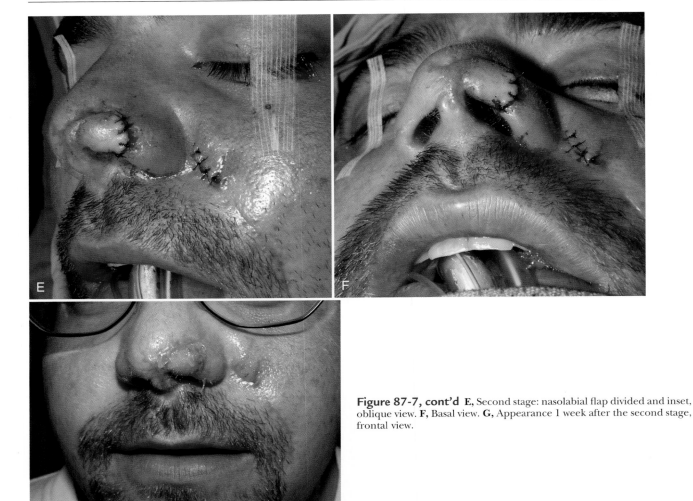

Figure 87-7, cont'd E, Second stage: nasolabial flap divided and inset, oblique view. **F,** Basal view. **G,** Appearance 1 week after the second stage, frontal view.

thinned and then reattached to the nose. At a third stage 3 weeks after the second stage, the pedicle is divided. For large nasal defects, a full-thickness skin graft can be sewn to the edges of the mucosal defect and to the frontalis muscle layer of the forehead flap in the first stage. Wound healing and contracture are not initiated until the subcutaneous and frontalis planes are surgically injured. Therefore, the reconstructed lining of the folded flap or skin graft remains supple and soft until supported by the delayed placement of cartilage grafts during the second stage. Reconstruction in three stages with a folded forehead flap or a forehead flap with a skin graft offers an excellent option for reconstructing a nasal defect with missing internal nasal lining.

Microvascular Free Tissue

Free tissue transfer of a fasciocutaneous flap, usually a radial forearm free flap, can be done to reconstruct the nasal lining vault for total or subtotal loss of the nose (Fig. 87-9).[14,15] However, a bulky free flap will obstruct the nasal airway unless supported on the nasal septum.

When the anterior nasal septum is present, Burget and Walton advocate rotating it forward as a septal pivot flap (Fig. 87-10).[16,17] This septal flap has the ability to support the length and projection of the nose without obstructing the airway. The raw external surface of the free flap is skin-grafted. At a second stage 5 to 6 weeks later, the skin graft and subcutaneous fat of the free flap are removed, and formal nasal reconstruction with cartilage grafting and a paramedian flap is carried out.

Without a septal pivot flap a single-paddle free flap will collapse against the piriform aperture. For correction of this problem, a double-paddle radial forearm free flap can be used to create double-vaulted nasal lining and columellar lining.

Skeletal Support

As the local flaps used for nasal reconstruction heal, the collagen and myofibroblasts within the flap and wound contract and pull the flap toward a center of centripetal contraction. Grafts of cartilage and bone support the skin flaps from contraction and after a few months show through the covering flap to give the reconstructed

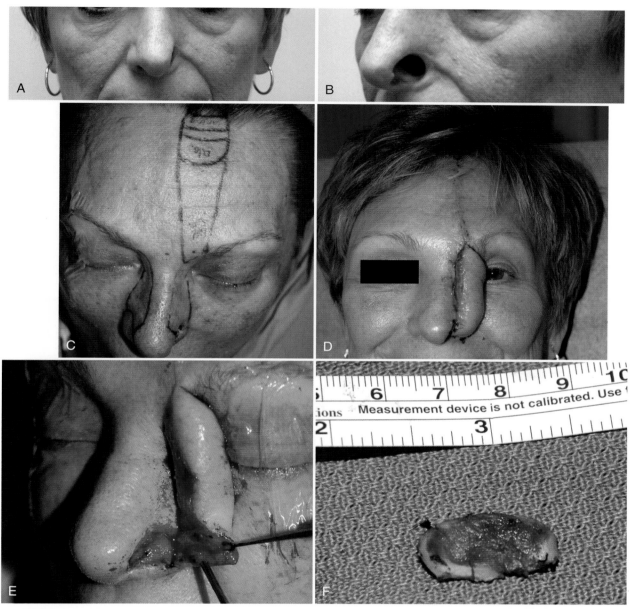

Figure 87-8. Three-stage nasal reconstruction with a forehead flap. **A,** Alar defect, frontal view. **B,** Oblique view. **C,** First stage: design of a folded forehead flap for nasal lining and cutaneous coverage. **D,** Immediate postoperative appearance. **E,** Second stage: flap divided along the alar margin and nasal and cutaneous flaps thinned of frontalis muscle and subcutaneous tissue. **F,** Conchal cartilage harvested.

nose a normal shape. Cartilage and bone from the septum, the concha of the ear, or the ribs (sixth through ninth ribs) are the best donor sites.[18] Because the septum is a possible growth center, the ear and costal cartilage are better options for sources of cartilage grafts in children. Grafts will survive only if placed on a well-vascularized bed, such as that provided by septal flaps. With use of the folded forehead flap or microvascular free flaps, secondary placement of grafts is preferred.

To provide midline nasal support, there are several well-accepted options. A cantilevered bone graft can be harvested either from the skull outer calvaria or from

rib as an osteochondral segment (Fig. 87-11).[18] A sturdy longitudinal segment can then be crafted to extend from the nasion to the superior aspect of the nasal lobule as an onlay or cantilevered graft. It can be secured in place by suture to the underlying cartilaginous dorsum or plated/wired to the frontal bone or nasal bones as needed. Smaller segments of calvarial bone, rib, or septal cartilage can be carved into longitudinal struts for more limited reconstructions, such as for the nasal sidewall.

For reconstruction of alar cartilage, strips of cartilage 4 to 5 mm in width and 1.5 to 2.0 cm long are harvested from the concha of the ear, septum, or rib

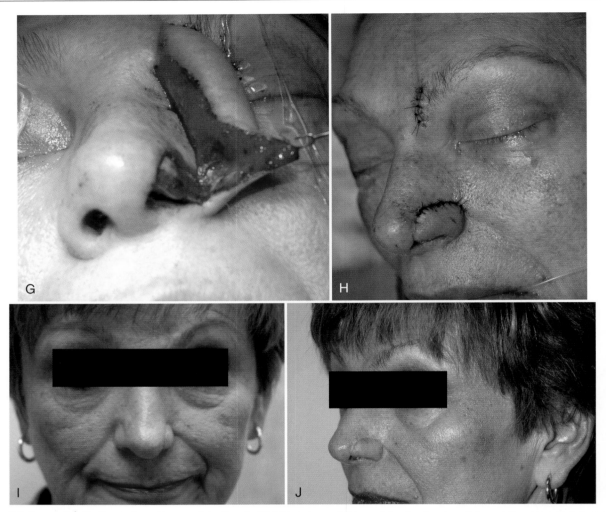

Figure 87-8, cont'd G, Conchal cartilage graft to the ala. **H,** Third stage: division of the forehead pedicle and flap inset. **I,** Appearance 4 months after pedicle division, frontal view. **J,** Oblique view.

(Fig. 87-12). To make an arch, one weakens or scores the cartilage in the area destined to be the lateral genu, and the cartilage is bent into a curve with one or two spanning mattress sutures. The intrinsic curves of conchal cartilage make it ideal for alar batten grafts, but conchal cartilage may be too weak to support a scarred nasal skin envelope. Septal and costal cartilage is stiffer than conchal cartilage and will better tolerate the compressive force of a contracted skin envelope. A separate cartilage graft should be used to brace the soft tissue triangle.

Nasal Skin Coverage

The size of the defect and the zone of nasal skin thickness can serve as a useful guide for selecting the appropriate skin cover. Because the skin of zone I is mobile, local rotation advancement flaps or primary closure can successfully reconstruct small defects (<1.5 cm). Zone II contains thick, sebaceous, nonmobile skin. The only donor skin that matches zone II is the remaining skin of zone II (i.e., transposed with a bilobed flap) or the forehead skin with its dense subcutaneous fat. Zone III skin is thin, nonsebaceous, and fixed to the underlying alar cartilage or fibrofatty structures. Composite grafts from the ear (<1.5 cm) and preauricular full-thickness skin grafts can blend well in zone III.

For large defects (>1.5 cm), a paramedian forehead flap is the preferred coverage for all zones. Columellar defects present a reconstructive challenge. A distal extension of the forehead flap provides an optimal solution when the columellar defect is a missing element of a larger defect. Other options, in particular for isolated columellar defects, include superiorly or inferiorly based nasolabial flaps.

Full-Thickness Skin Grafts

Because the skin of the upper two thirds of the nose (zone I) is thin with few sebaceous units, full-thickness skin grafts blend well in this area. Possible sites of harvest include the preauricular area, postauricular

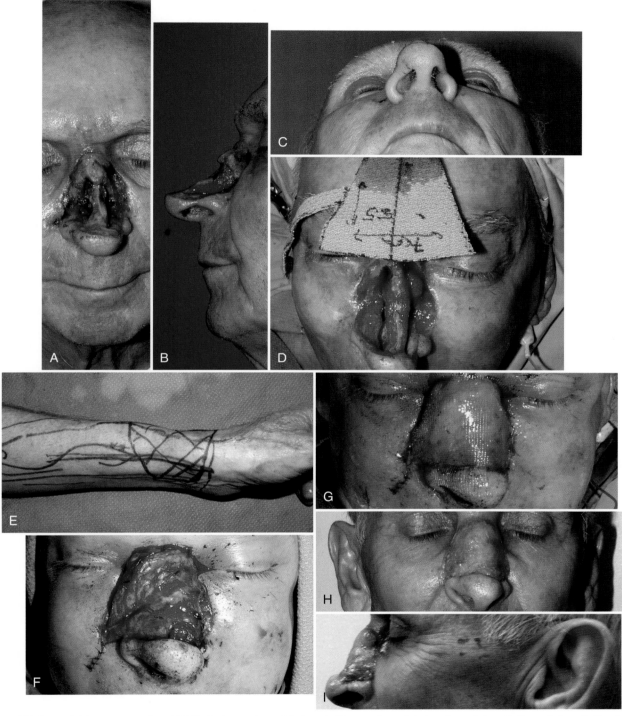

Figure 87-9. Radial forearm free flap (RFFF) for internal nasal lining. **A,** Near-total nasal defect, frontal view. **B,** Lateral view. **C,** Basal view. **D,** Template for the design of an RFFF for internal nasal lining. **E,** Harvest site and RFFF design. **F,** RFFF inset; forearm skin used for internal lining. **G,** Skin graft applied to the raw (i.e., external) surface of the RFFF. **H,** Postoperative appearance, frontal view. **I,** Lateral view. The patient will undergo removal of the skin graft, flap thinning, placement of a rib graft, and coverage with a forehead flap.

area, nasolabial fold, and supraclavicular area. The forehead has also been found to be an excellent site of graft donor skin. Skin and a few millimeters of subcutaneous fat can be transferred from the forehead for superficial defects of the alae and tip. A skin graft should not be harvested from an area that is a possible site for a forehead flap. Because of the temporary period of ischemia during wound healing, the melanocytes of a skin graft may be injured and cause the final graft to appear hypopigmented or hyperpigmented.

Composite Chondrocutaneous Grafts

A composite chondrocutaneous graft can be an option for reconstructing a nasal skeleton with defects that also include nasal skin or inner nasal lining, or both. Composite grafts can be harvested from the root of the helix or from the conchal bowl (Figs. 87-13 and 87-14).[9,18,19] Survival of the composite graft depends mainly on the size of the graft and the vascularity of the recipient bed. Diffusion from the recipient bed is the only source of nutrients for the composite graft in the early postoperative period. Several authors have reported complete healing of composite grafts after partial necrosis. In general, to minimize the possibility of necrosis, graft size should not exceed 1.5 cm, and if possible, composite grafts should be placed under or on well-vascularized tissue. Grafts may be harvested as two layers (skin-cartilage) or as three layers (skin-cartilage-skin). Composite grafts are used mainly for reconstruction of the alae and columella.

Bilobed Flaps

The bilobed flap as described by Zitelli[20] (Fig. 87-15) is the most suitable method to repair small (<1.5 cm), superficial defects of zone II (tip or ala, Fig. 87-16). It moves the nasal defect from the zone of thick, immobile skin (zone II) to the zone of thin, mobile skin (zone

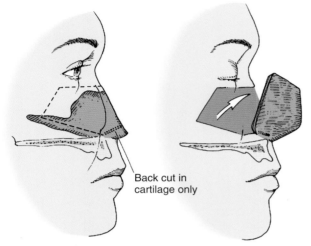

Figure 87-10. Septal pivot flap. To provide dorsal and caudal support, the central cartilaginous/bony septum can be pivoted or swung anteriorly. The blood supply of the septal pivot flap is centered over the septal branches of the superior labial arteries.

Back cut in cartilage only

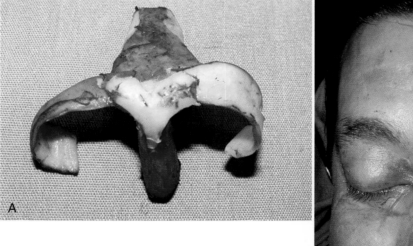
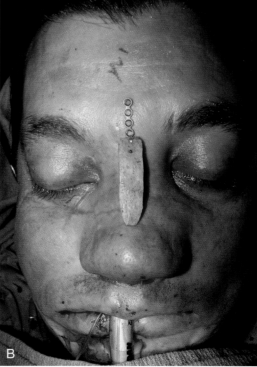

Figure 87-11. Structural support of the nasal midline/dorsum. **A,** Costochondral graft carved into a "L" strut with alar battens. **B,** Cantilevered cranial bone graft to be fixed to the frontal skull with a miniplate.

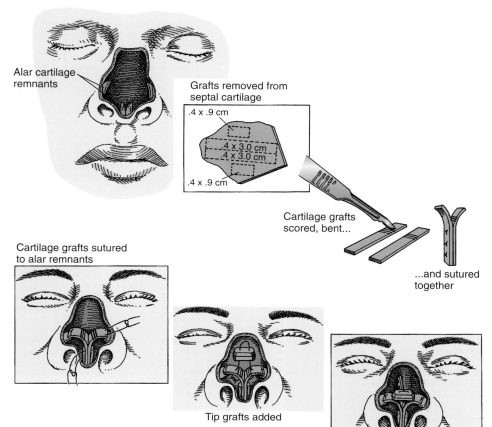

Figure 87-12. Reconstruction of cartilage support. If lining is created or preserved, cartilage from numerous sources (above: septum) can be tailored to restore the nasal contour and curvature. A cap graft or tip graft can be used to promote lobule projection. *(From Burget GC, Menick FJ: Nasal reconstruction: Seeking a fourth dimension. Plast Reconstr Surg 78:145-157, 1986, with permission.)*

Alar cartilage remnants

Grafts removed from septal cartilage

.4 x .9 cm
.4 x 3.0 cm
.4 x 3.0 cm
.4 x .9 cm

Cartilage grafts scored, bent...

...and sutured together

Cartilage grafts sutured to alar remnants

Tip grafts added

Flying buttress keeps tip from retracting

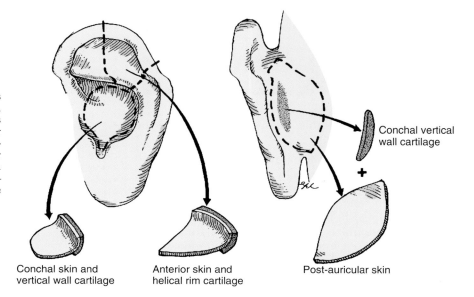

Figure 87-13. Composite graft. The ear is an ideal donor site for nasal reconstruction, including full-thickness chondrocutaneous grafts. Donor sites from the helical root or posterior aspect of the ear can be closed primarily with undermining. Anterior donor sites from the conchal bowl may require a skin graft for closure. *(From Barton FE Jr: Aesthetic aspects of partial nasal reconstruction. Clin Plast Surg 8:177-191, 1981, with permission.)*

Conchal vertical wall cartilage

+

Post-auricular skin

Conchal skin and vertical wall cartilage

Anterior skin and helical rim cartilage

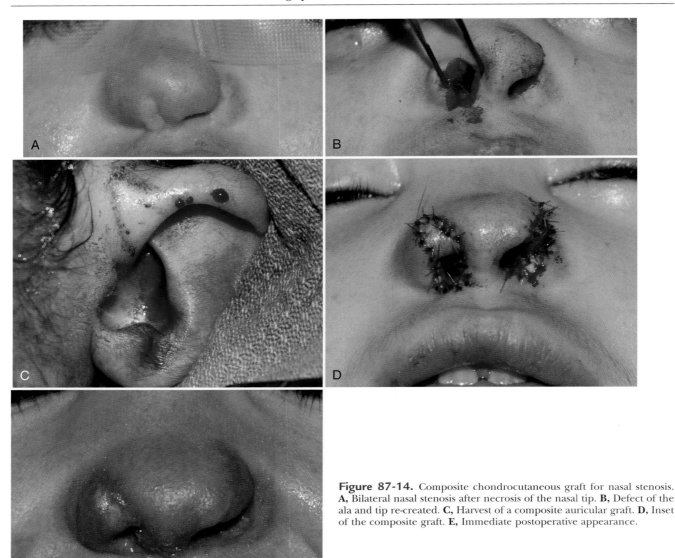

Figure 87-14. Composite chondrocutaneous graft for nasal stenosis. **A,** Bilateral nasal stenosis after necrosis of the nasal tip. **B,** Defect of the ala and tip re-created. **C,** Harvest of a composite auricular graft. **D,** Inset of the composite graft. **E,** Immediate postoperative appearance.

1). Fundamentals of this transposition flap are the following:

1. The arc of rotation can vary between 90 and 180 degrees, but it is generally designed to be between 90 and 100 degrees. The radius will usually approximate 1.5 diameters of the defect.
2. The first lobe should be the same size as the defect. The second lobe is smaller and just narrow enough to allow primary linear closure of the donor defect.
3. For medial defects, laterally based flaps should be designed.
4. Closure of secondary defects should not distort normal landmarks, such as the lower eyelid.

Potential disadvantages of the bilobed flap are trapdooring (convex bulging) and obliteration of the alar groove.

Nasolabial Flaps

Based either superiorly or inferiorly, the nasolabial flap relies on a random blood supply derived from facial artery perforators and takes advantage of the abundance of mobile, non–hair-bearing skin in the medial part of the cheek. Primary closure of the defect within the nasolabial fold creates a minimal postoperative deformity. Reconstruction involves first tracing an outline of the cutaneous defect on the donor site and then elevating the flap in a subcutaneous plane (Fig. 87-17; also see Fig. 87-7).[21-24] A superiorly based nasolabial flap is good for reconstruction of the entire alar subunit, the inferior aspect of the nasal sidewall, and the nasal platform on which the alar base rests. An inferiorly based nasolabial flap is most useful for defects of the upper lip, floor of the nose, and columella. A

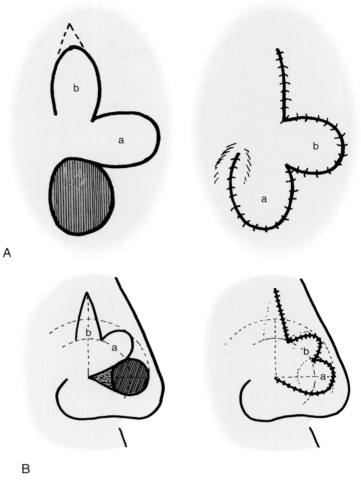

Figure 87-15. Zitelli modification of the bilobed flap. When compared with the original design of a 180-degree arc of rotation, which typically produces a dog-ear deformity at the rotational point (**A**), the modified transposition flap creates a smaller defect by using a 90-degree arc of rotation and minimizing dog-ear and trapdoor formation (**B**). *(From Zitelli JA: The bilobed flap for nasal reconstruction. Arch Dermatol 125:957-959, 1989, with permission.)*

nasolabial flap folded to create both internal and external lining produces a bulky alar rim that will require subsequent revision.

Forehead Flaps

A forehead flap transfers skin of ideal quality to reconstruct the nasal skin defect in patients of all ages. The forehead heals well with minimal scars even in donor sites left to heal secondarily. Midline or paramedian forehead flaps can be raised on either the supratrochlear or supraorbital vessels.[25] Most surgeons elevate a paramedian flap based on an ipsilateral, supratrochlear vascular pedicle that is located approximately 1.5 cm from the midline. Doppler ultrasound can be used to locate the pedicle, but even if no Doppler signal is found, a flap with a pedicle based almost anywhere along the midline of the forehead will probably survive. To avoid strangulation caused by twisting of a wide pedicle, the pedicle width of a paramedian flap should be about 1.5 cm. To gain length for a paramedian flap, one can extend the flap into the hair-bearing scalp or extend the flap 1.5 cm below the orbital rim, or both.

The pattern of the nasal defect should first be designed from the contralateral normal side of the patient's face as a model. If the contralateral side is also injured, a plaster or clay model of an ideal nose can serve as the template. Local anesthesia with epinephrine should not be injected into the forehead flap so that the blood supply can be evaluated intraoperatively. The forehead flap is elevated in a distal-to-proximal direction with all layers of the scalp (skin, subcutaneous tissue, and frontalis muscle) except periosteum. The forehead flap is thinned only at the columellar inset and along the alar rim. Closure of the donor site should be done over the periosteum with subgaleal undermining of the forehead. Any gaps that cannot be closed should be kept moist with antibiotic ointment, covered with Vaseline gauze, and allowed to heal secondarily. The pedicle of the paramedian forehead flap in the glabellar region is typically covered with a split-thickness skin graft to decrease bleeding and oozing.

Menick advises that only pristine, unexpanded forehead skin be transferred.[26] An expanded forehead flap can contract after the completion of nasal reconstruction and produce inferior aesthetic results. If necessary,

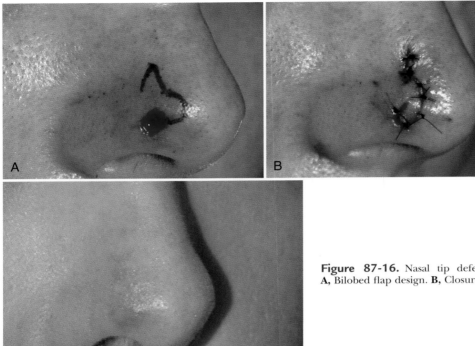

Figure 87-16. Nasal tip defect reconstructed with a bilobed flap. **A,** Bilobed flap design. **B,** Closure. **C,** Early postoperative appearance.

tissue expansion can be done secondarily after nasal reconstruction to close the forehead donor site or to perform forehead scar revision.

POSTOPERATIVE MANAGEMENT

Patients undergoing first-stage nasal reconstruction with a forehead flap should stay in the hospital overnight. Any blanching of the flap or signs of venous congestion can potentially be reversed with removal of sutures or reinsetting of the flap. Doyle splints or intranasal packs are not generally used unless there is concern for the formation of synechiae. Because external dressings may compromise flap circulation, they are not placed on a flap used for nasal reconstruction. Skin sutures, as well as any external bolster placed on a skin graft, are removed 5 to 7 day after surgery. Postoperative parenteral antibiotics are not routinely prescribed.

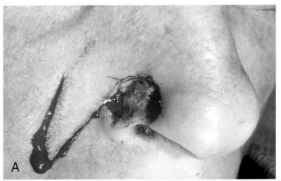

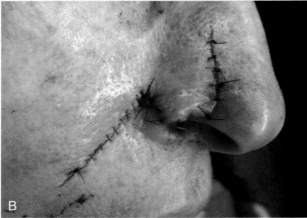

Figure 87-17. Superiorly based, single-stage nasolabial flap. **A,** Alar defect. **B,** Nasolabial flap inset.

PEARLS

- When designing a flap to reconstruct a defect or subunit, one should use a template based on the contralateral, uninjured side.
- If a forehead flap is to be used in a smoker, transfer of the flap should be delayed for 3 weeks by incising the perimeter without elevating the flap.

- Reconstruction with a forehead flap should be done in three stages, with secondary cartilage grafting and flap thinning performed during the second stage.
- Even though a normal alar lobule contains little cartilage, a reconstructed ala should contain a cartilage graft (i.e., in an nonanatomic position) that spans the entire lobule to prevent soft tissue contraction.
- Consideration of the subunit principle is useful only for reconstruction of the convex subunits of the nose (i.e., the tip, dorsum, alae, and columella) with local flaps because as a local flap heals, it contracts centripetally and pulls the flap into a convex shape.

PITFALLS

- If the first step in nasal reconstruction is not recreation of the defect (i.e., excising old scar and contractions), the final result will be a reconstruction and flap design that are too small.
- If nasal reconstruction is done at the same time as lip and cheek reconstruction, subsequent wound settling can shift the lip-cheek platform and cause a reciprocal shift in the position of the reconstructed nose.
- Reconstruction of missing nasal lining with bulky flaps, such as a nasolabial or free flap, can lead to nasal obstruction.
- When greater than 50% of a nasal convex subunit is missing, patching the nasal defect with a local flap without replacing the entire nasal subunit may worsen the aesthetic outcome.
- In a child, delaying nasal reconstruction until nasal growth is complete may lead to worsening psychosocial concerns.

References

1. Rees TD, Liverett DM, Guy CL: The effect of cigarette smoking on skin-flap survival in the face lift patient. Plast Reconstr Surg 73:911-915, 1984.
2. Bennett ME: Psychologic and social consequences of craniofacial disfigurement in children. Facial Plast Surg 11:76-81, 1995.
3. Burget GC, Menick FJ: The subunit principle in nasal reconstruction. Plast Reconstr Surg 76:239-247, 1985.
4. Singh DJ, Bartlett SP: Aesthetic considerations in nasal reconstruction and the role of modified nasal subunits. Plast Reconstr Surg 111:639-648, discussion 649-651, 2003.
5. Rohrich RJ, Griffin JR, Ansari M, et al: Nasal reconstruction—beyond aesthetic subunits: A 15-year review of 1334 cases. Plast Reconstr Surg 114:1405-1416, discussion 1417-1419, 2004.
6. Giugliano C, Andrades PR, Benitez S: Nasal reconstruction with a forehead flap in children younger than 10 years of age. Plast Reconstr Surg 114:316-325, discussion 326-328, 2004.
7. Shumrick KA, Campbell A, Becker FF, Papel ID: Modification of the subunit principle for reconstruction of nasal tip and dorsum defects. Arch Facial Plast Surg 1:9-15, 1999.
8. Burget GC: Modification of the subunit principle for reconstruction of nasal tip and dorsum defects [commentary]. Arch Facial Plast Surg 1:16-18, 1999.
9. Burget GC, Menick FJ: Nasal support and lining: The marriage of beauty and blood supply. Plast Reconstr Surg 84:189-202, 1989.
10. Barton FE Jr: Aesthetic aspects of partial nasal reconstruction. Clin Plast Surg 8:177-191, 1981.
11. Menick FJ: A 10-year experience in nasal reconstruction with the three-stage forehead flap. Plast Reconstr Surg 109:1839-1855, discussion 1856-1861, 2002.
12. Menick FJ: Nasal reconstruction: Forehead flap. Plast Reconstr Surg 113(6):100E-111E, 2004.
13. Burget GC: Aesthetic restoration of the nose. Clin Plast Surg 12:463-480, 1985.
14. Moore EJ, Strome SA, Kasperbauer JL, et al: Vascularized radial forearm free tissue transfer for lining in nasal reconstruction. Laryngoscope 113:2078-2085, 2003.
15. Winslow CP, Cook TA, Burke A, Wax MK: Total nasal reconstruction: Utility of the free radial forearm fascial flap. Arch Facial Plast Surg 5:159-163, 2003.
16. Walton RL, Burget GC, Beahm EK: Microsurgical reconstruction of the nasal lining. Plast Reconstr Surg 115:1813-1829, 2005.
17. Burget GC, Menick FJ: Nasal reconstruction: Seeking a fourth dimension. Plast Reconstr Surg 78:145-157, 1986.
18. Cervelli V, Bottini DJ, Gentile P, et al: Reconstruction of the nasal dorsum with autologous rib cartilage. Ann Plast Surg 56:256-262, 2006.
19. Gloster HM Jr, Brodland DG: The use of perichondrial cutaneous grafts to repair defects of the lower third of the nose. Br J Dermatol 136:43-46, 1997.
20. Zitelli JA: The bilobed flap for nasal reconstruction. Arch Dermatol 125:957-959, 1989.
21. Barton FE Jr: Aesthetic aspects of nasal reconstruction. Clin Plast Surg 15:155-166, 1988.
22. Guerrerosantos J, Dicksheet S: Nasolabial flap with simultaneous cartilage graft in nasal alar reconstruction. Clin Plast Surg 8:599-602, 1981.
23. Hollier HJ, Stucker FJ: Local flaps for nasal reconstruction. Facial Plast Surg 10:337-348, 1994.
24. Park SS, Cook TA: Reconstructive rhinoplasty. Facial Plast Surg 13:309-316, 1997.
25. Menick FJ: Aesthetic refinements in use of forehead for nasal reconstruction: The paramedian forehead flap. Clin Plast Surg 17:607-622, 1990.
26. Menick FJ: Facial reconstruction with local and distant tissue: The interface of aesthetic and reconstructive surgery. Plast Reconstr Surg 102:1424-1433, 1998.

Chapter **88**

Facial Reanimation

Barry M. Schaitkin

Rehabilitation of the patient with chronic facial paralysis must take into account the loss of form and function. When contemplating facial reanimation, the surgeon should consider all variables that might influence the choice of procedures, including the patient's age, prognosis, pathology, the extent of paralysis and functional deficit, the current status of the nerve and the likelihood of spontaneous recovery, other neural deficits, comorbidities, and patient expectations. Reanimation of the paralytic eyelid is usually required in addition to the procedures described in this chapter.

PATIENT SELECTION

Although each patient presents unique needs and challenges, experience has led to guidelines for caring for this group of patients.

1. The surgeon should reinnervate the facial muscles as soon as possible.
2. The eye and face should be reanimated separately to minimize mass movement.
3. A combination of static and dynamic procedures usually provides the best result.
4. Each procedure is individualized to the patient's deficit.

PREOPERATIVE PLANNING

Dynamic Reanimation Procedures

The dynamic procedures can be considered within four broad categories. One can think of the facial nerve nucleus as the proximal system and the facial nerve musculature as the distal system and look at the procedures based on what is surgically available. The procedures are then dictated by the integrity of those systems for use by the surgeon.

- Proximal system intact and distal system intact
- Proximal system intact and distal system not available

- Proximal system not available and distal system intact
- Neither system available

Patients with facial nerve disruption in the temporal bone are good examples of the proximal and distal system intact. These patients are ideally suited for having the facial nerve nucleus reconnected to the facial musculature by either primary neurorrhaphy or by use of a nerve graft. Reconstituting the nerve should be performed as soon as possible for the best results.[1]

Patients with extensive facial nerve invasion by cancer can create a situation without a distal nerve graft site. Ideally, the viable proximal facial nerve can then be used to innervate a microvascular free flap, or alternatively, these patients without a distal system can be helped by muscle transposition.

Patients who have lost the facial nerve as part of acoustic tumor surgery should have the nerve reconstituted immediately, if possible, by a nerve graft. However, this frequently is not possible, and patients are often reluctant to have a craniotomy for reestablishing nerve continuity. These patients are dynamically innervated by either a nerve substitution with a hypoglossal jump graft or by use of a cross-facial nerve graft. The jump graft works best if done in the first year of paralysis. A traditional hypoglossal to facial anastomosis causes a unilateral tongue paralysis as a tradeoff, but can be done as long as 2 years after facial nerve interruption with good results.

Finally, for those lacking both systems, two dynamic options are available: the temporalis muscle transposition and the innervated free flap based on another cranial nerve (V, the contralateral cranial nerve VII, XI, and XII have been used). This situation is characteristic of the patient who has undergone radical surgery for cancer of the parotid gland who presents years later for reanimation.

In this situation, if the patient is a candidate for and desirous of a dynamic procedure, and if that person understands the risks, options, and benefits, then another cranial nerve should be used to innervate a free muscle transfer. The free muscle (often the gracilis) is anchored to the modiolus to give an active smile. Some degree of static support should be provided at this setting to take away the gravitational effects. This offers immediate improvement because the nerve graft may not be completely functional before 18 months.

Static Procedures

These procedures can be combined with dynamic procedures or used independently depending on the desired outcome. The most common procedures to consider are the brow lift, nasal alar lateralization, suspension of the oral commissure, and digastric muscle transposition. Other minor static procedures for improvement of lip position and for providing a balanced smile can also be performed.

SURGICAL TECHNIQUE

Hypoglossal-Facial Jump Graft

Basic understanding of nerve repair is essential for many of the planned procedures. The hypoglossal-facial nerve jump graft will be described in detail to cover microscopic neural techniques essential to all of the procedures.

Surgical Principles

1. Neural repair, whether with a graft or directly, must be tension free.
2. The endoneurial surface of each end must match.
3. The ideal graft not only has the proper length but also a similar axon volume.
4. Nerve repair should always be performed under the operating microscope.

The patient is prepped and draped as for a parotidectomy, and a modified Blair incision is used. A nerve graft donor site must be prepped into the field if the preferred graft source, the greater auricular nerve, is not available. Alternatively, the facial nerve can be decompressed in the mastoid and transposed and directly anastomosed into the hypoglossal nerve.[2]

The facial nerve is found in its normal location in the parotid gland using the surgeon's preferred anatomic landmarks. The nerve may have undergone some atrophy depending on how long the paralysis has been present, but this does not make the nerve difficult to find.

If there has been previous parotid surgery and the surgeon is looking for nerve branches in a previously operated and/or irradiated bed, the surgery can be extremely difficult. The surgeon in this case must be comfortable finding the branches distal to the surgical site and working proximally. Even this may be quite difficult with the combination of nerve atrophy, scar tissue, and the inability of the nerve to respond to electrical stimulation.

Once the facial nerve is found, it is dissected to the level of the pes and meticulous hemostasis is performed to ease the microscopic nerve repair. The hypoglossal nerve is dissected to expose it just distal to the ansa cervicalis. In this way, the surgeon can be sure that voluntary tongue movement will stimulate all fibers being routed to the facial nerve.

The nerve graft is harvested and placed in a moist, saline-soaked gauze sponge for later use. The distance required is usually less than 8 cm, which is easily accomplished with the great auricular; alternatively, the medial brachial cutaneous or sural nerve can be used.

The hypoglossal nerve is elevated into the surgeon's view under the operating microscope and above the level of any blood by placing a Penrose drain under the nerve and gently elevating it with a self-retaining retractor. The hypoglossal nerve is larger in diameter than either the facial nerve or the great auricular nerve and ideally only a portion is used. The procedure requires less than half of the 11th nerve. Jack Kartush[2] has suggested passing an 8-0 nylon through a point representing one third of the neural diameter to allow the surgeon to know when this limit is reached. Sectioning the nerve under visual confirmation of serial stimulation with an electric stimulator also allows the surgeon to work with decreased risk of permanent tongue weakness. A beveled incision is made not more than one third of the way through the hypoglossal nerve, partially transecting the nerve and exposing a portion of the proximal endoneurial surface. The proximal end of the nerve graft is sutured to the proximal end of the endoneurial surface created in the 11th nerve. Two or three monofilament 8-0 or smaller nylon sutures will hold the graft in place. The Penrose drain is divided with scissors and gently removed without disrupting the graft.

Attention is then directed to the facial nerve site. The surgeon divides the nerve down to the epineurium on the posterior aspect. Preserving this epineurium will prevent the nerve from retracting into the parotid gland and greatly facilitates the repair. The nerve graft should be placed with a gentle S-curve to assure no tension on either anastomosis. Three 8-0 or 9-0 monofilament nylon sutures are adequate to prevent dehiscence.

Direct nerve repair and cross facial nerve repair is done with similar principles. If the nerve is disrupted intracranially, it is more difficult to repair because of the pulsations, cerebrospinal fluid, and lack of epineurium, but similar principles apply. One or two sutures are generally all that can be achieved.

The cross facial repair uses one or more branches of the facial nerve. The surgeon finds the desired branch, usually a distal midface branch, and with small incisions about the nasal ala the nerve is bluntly tunneled out to the pretragal region on the paralyzed side.

Static Procedures: Smile

Support of the modiolus is a valuable primary procedure (Fig. 88-1) or can be a useful adjunct to a dynamic

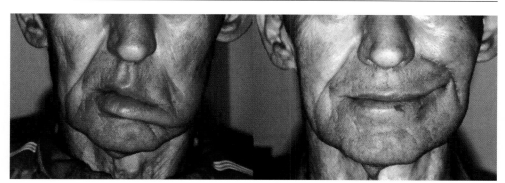

Figure 88-1. Patient with static suspension of nasolabial fold and lower lip wedge.

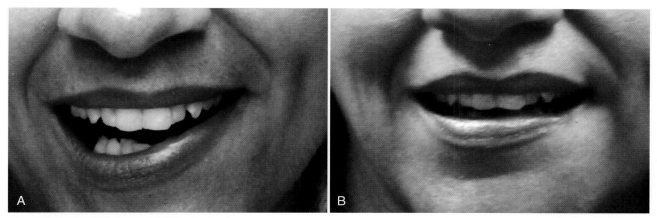

Figure 88-2. Patient before (**A**) and after (**B**) digastric muscle transposition after ramus mandibularis paralysis during parotidectomy.

procedure. Many materials have been used for this purpose, including permanent suture, fascia lata, palmaris longus tendon, and a variety of cadaver and collagen products. Autologous grafts have the disadvantage of donor site morbidity, but are still superior because of the decreased risk of infection, rejection, and extrusion.

Measurements are taken from the zygomatic arch to the modiolus. One half of the required length of fascia lata is used as the incision length on the lateral thigh. A 2.5-cm wide segment is taken and tunneled from the oral incision, which can be either in the proposed nasolabial fold or lip skin junction, to an incision in the hairline. Preoperative planning determines the vector of pull desired to mimic the contralateral side. Incisions in the nasolabial fold work best in older patients with deep folds on the normal side.

Static Procedures: Nasal Obstruction

Patients with loss of facial tone will shift the central upper lip filtrum and collapse the ipsilateral nasal ala. A portion of the suspension material used for the smile can be used to lateralize the nasal ala through an alar incision. If just the nasal ala is addressed, the procedure through an alotomy can be used to suspend the nasal ala to a lateral position of the front face of the maxilla using a surgical anchor.

Static Procedures: Lower Lip

Static procedures on the lower lip vary depending on the desired result and the presence of other facial nerve deficits. An isolated ramus mandibularis defect can be treated with a lip plication or a digastric muscle transposition (Fig. 88-2).

The procedure is performed through multiple small incisions in the neck to mobilize the digastric muscle from its posterior aspect. Leaving the anterior muscle belly fifth nerve intact rarely provides dynamic activity but does improve the missing inferior vector present with a normal smile.

Patients who have a total facial paralysis should not have a digastric muscle transposition because the inferior pull may decrease oral competence. These patients are best served with a lower lip wedge resection (Fig. 88-3). This procedure provides horizontal shortening of the lip, allowing for improved oral competence and speech as well as better symmetry from removal of the area that takes on a "fat lip" appearance.[3]

Less than one third of the lip is removed to avoid microstomia (Fig. 88-4).

POSTOPERATIVE CARE

Patients require very little specific postoperative care after the majority of these procedures, and most are

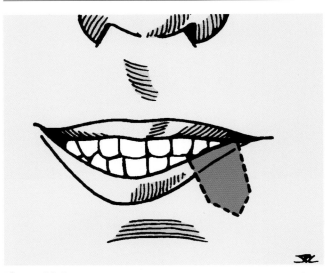

Figure 88-3. Left lip wedge excision planning. *(Reprinted with permission from May M, Schaitkin BM: The Facial Nerve, May's 2nd Edition. New York, Thieme, 2000.)*

discharged on the day of surgery. However, there are a few precautions one should take.

1. The patient with surgery that abuts the oral cavity should be covered with prophylactic antibiotics.
2. Patients with muscular or facial attachments near the modiolus should be placed on a soft diet to avoid dehiscence.
3. No pressure dressings are used over nerve grafts or muscle flaps.
4. Lower extremity fascia and nerve graft sites are treated with pressure dressings.

COMPLICATIONS

The main complication of the nerve graft procedures is the lack of recovery of nerve function at all or to the extent anticipated. Patients should be counseled about the possibility of dehiscence of the nerve or failure of the nerve to reach the target muscle. All patients who have recovery from a neural procedure will have synkinesis.

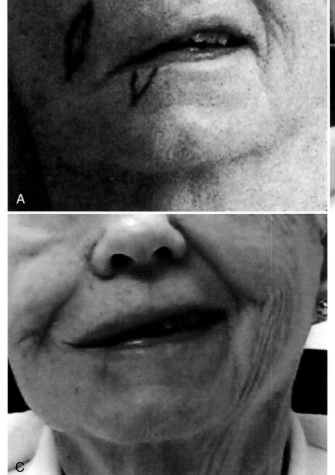

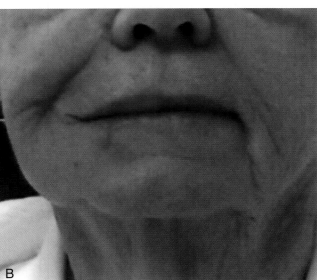

Figure 88-4. A, Preoperatively, patient with complete right facial paralysis demonstrating surgical planning. **B,** Patient at rest. **C,** Patient smiling after lower lip wedge excision and fascia lata suspension only.

Likewise the static procedures are mostly subject to the possible dehiscence of the tissues providing support. Most of these issues are actually easier to remedy through revision surgery because the scar from the first procedure provides a better means of attachment.

The use of foreign material for reanimation is subject to the formation of granuloma, extrusion, and infection.

PEARLS

- Great results begin with careful evaluation of the patient's history and desired outcome.
- Realistic expectations are necessary for patient satisfaction. Preoperative and postoperative photos from other patients are very helpful.
- Combined procedures with multiple levels of eye, static, and dynamic reanimation provide the best results.
- Hypoglossal jump grafting avoids tongue paralysis.

PITFALLS

- Avoiding donor sites for graft material can lead to long-term infection and extrusion.
- Pulling down a paralyzed lower lip for symmetry may exacerbate oral competence problems.
- It is important to have a variety of procedures in one's armamentarium to avoid trying to place all patients into the same procedure.

References

1. May M: Regional reanimation: Nose and mouth. In May M, Schaitkin BM (eds): The Facial Nerve, May's 2nd Edition. New York, Thieme Medical, 2000, pp 775-796.
2. May M: Nerve substitution techniques. In May M, Schaitkin BM (eds): The Facial Nerve, May's 2nd Edition. New York, Thieme Medical, 2000, pp 611-634.
3. Glenn MG, Goode RL: Surgical treatment of the "marginal mandibular lip" deformity. Otolaryngol Head Neck Surg 97:462-468, 1987.

Chapter 89

Face Lift (Rhytidectomy)

Grant S. Gillman

Society places a high premium on a youthful appearance, yet there is no way to stop the natural effects of gravity, sun exposure, and dermal atrophy associated with aging on one's appearance. These facts have led to a growing demand for reversal of the visible effects of aging. Furthermore, these requests now come from younger and younger patients—both male and female. In addition, there is ever-increasing interest in preventive measures, minimally invasive procedures, shorter recovery times, reduced risk, and a more natural postoperative appearance.

Although the fundamental goals of face-lift surgery are similar in most patients, there exists a wide array of surgical techniques and many procedural variations among surgeons. Issues to be considered include placement of the incision, the length of the incision (short scar or limited incision face lift versus traditional incision face lift), the extent of skin undermining, the depth of dissection, management of the superficial musculoaponeurotic system (SMAS), treatment of the neck and vector of the SMAS, and skin redraping, to name a few. Indeed, if a single technique were clearly superior, it would be adopted by all surgeons. In all cases, preoperative analysis, clinical judgment, and individualizing care based on the patient's present state of aging, expectations, and ability to tolerate and accept each contemplated procedure and its postoperative recovery and potential complications should be combined to direct surgical choices.

PREOPERATIVE PLANNING

Preoperative evaluation begins by having patients highlight their specific areas of concern and outlining for the surgeon what bothers them most. In this way not only can one begin to formulate a surgical plan, but equally important, one can also begin to get a sense of how realistic the patient's expectations are, as well as the motivation for having surgery. Proper patient selection cannot be overstated as an important determinant of postoperative patient satisfaction.

A medical history is obtained and should cover all past medical problems, with special emphasis on hypertension, diabetes, thyroid disease, facial muscle weakness, previous facial surgery, cardiovascular disorders, smoking, and the use of any anticoagulant medications (including products containing warfarin [Coumadin], aspirin, or ibuprofen and any herbal products). A general medical consultation is obtained if there is any concern about the patient's past or present state of health. Smokers must be forewarned of the increased risk of complications such as hematoma, skin sloughing, and poor healing. Ideally, they should stop smoking at least 2 weeks before surgery and for 2 weeks afterward.

A complete physical evaluation of the patient's entire head and neck is performed. For most patients considering facial rejuvenation surgery, this will require attention to forehead rhytides, brow position, and the upper and lower eyelids, in addition to issues relevant to face-lift surgery in particular.

For face-lift surgery, physical evaluation begins with an overall assessment of the facial structure, shape, and contour. Patients with good underlying bone structure, prominent facial features, and a thin face are likely to have more dramatic improvement and are therefore better candidates for a face-lift than those with poor facial skeletal structure and a rounder heavy face.

Skin texture—the quality, thickness, laxity, and degree of wrinkling of the patient's skin—is noted and recorded. Older, thicker, less elastic skin with more obvious actinic changes cannot be expected to hold the contour as well as younger, thinner, more elastic skin with less sun damage.

The examination continues with an evaluation of the degree of sagging in the midface and cheek, jowls, and submental region. The neck is examined for overall contour, laxity of the platysma, and the presence or absence of platysmal bands. One should ask the patient to clench the teeth tightly to accentuate the platysmal bands. Chin position should be assessed as well because relative microgenia may be an indication for chin augmentation, which will help facilitate improvement in overall neck definition.

The hairline is evaluated to enable decisions regarding placement of incisions.[1] Whereas a patient with a low sideburn or temporal tuft may tolerate some superior shift of the hairline (and therefore a temporal incision that extends upward from the helical root), a patient with a high sideburn or temporal hairline will not tolerate any hairline shift (and should therefore have an incision that follows the temporal hairline).

Decisions also need to be made regarding a pretragal or post-tragal incision. Although a post-tragal incision is better camouflaged, it is balanced against the risk of a tragus that then looks unnatural postoperatively. In patients with a deep preauricular crease, a pretragal incision in front of the ear is a reasonable option. In general, a pretragal incision is preferred in men to avoid moving hair-bearing skin (the beard) all the way back to the posterior edge of the tragus, as would happen with a post-tragal incision. It is wise to discuss all incision options and the rationale for the various choices with the patient preoperatively and to engage the patient in the decision-making process.

A thorough discussion with the patient should follow regarding realistic expectations for outcome, the typical intraoperative and postoperative course, and potential complications and their relative frequency.

A complete set of photographs is important for documentation and planning. At a minimum, frontal, right and left oblique, and lateral views should be included. Additional views that are frequently helpful include three-quarter views from each side and a frontal view with the patient's teeth clenched to highlight platysmal banding.

Anesthesia

The patient and physician must decide together on the most appropriate anesthesia for that particular patient. Local anesthesia, supplemented by intravenous sedation, is adequate for many aesthetic surgical procedures on the face. The choice of intravenous sedation with local anesthesia versus general anesthesia should take into consideration the surgeon's comfort level, the patient's preference, the anesthesiologist's preference, the duration of the procedure, and any tendency or predisposition of the patient to obstruction of the airway when sedated. Even with a general anesthetic, local anesthesia with epinephrine is used for its hemostatic effect and postoperative pain relief. Limiting the combined operative procedures to be performed on the same day to a maximum of 6 hours will lead to fewer complications and will be better tolerated by the patient and surgeon.

When intravenous sedation is chosen, in all circumstances it should be managed by the anesthesiologist/nurse anesthetist rather than the operating surgeon to maximize safety and allow the surgeon to focus only on the procedure at hand. During infiltration of the local anesthetic the sedation is deepened, and then patients can be allowed to "come up" from the sedation and it can be titrated to a level at which they can respond to commands, breathe on their own, and express any discomfort.

Injections of local anesthetic are not performed until all markings have been made. A mix of 50 mL of 1% lidocaine with 1:100,000 epinephrine combined with 30 mL of 0.5% bupivacaine (Marcaine) with 1:200,000 epinephrine is used for the face and neck. Typically, the neck is injected together with one side of the face at the outset. The other side of the face is injected when the first operative side is being closed. In this way one can distribute the total amount of lidocaine and Marcaine injected over a longer interval to avoid toxicity.

Markings

Skin markings are made with the patient in a semi-upright or sitting position preoperatively. Markings include those for skin incisions, the planned extent of undermining, the topographic location of the facial nerve (a line from 0.5 cm below the inferior attachment of the earlobe to 1.5 cm above lateral brow), the inferior border of the mandible, the angle of the mandible, the specific location of the sagging jowls, and platysmal banding when present.

In the temporal area, if the patient's sideburn is low enough to tolerate some hairline shift without looking unnatural, the planned incision can extend superiorly from the helical root in curvilinear fashion into the temporal hair, where it will be well camouflaged (Fig. 89-1). If any doubt exists about whether the patient can tolerate a shift of the sideburn tuft or if the patient already has a higher sideburn, the temporal incision is designed to follow the hairline, several millimeters within the hair, extends anteriorly from the helical root, and then curves superiorly along the hairline for an additional 1 to 2 cm (Fig. 89-2). By placing this incision several millimeters within the hairline one can bevel the incision to preserve the hair follicles below the incision. Over time hair will then grow back through the incision and render it less conspicuous.

A pretragal or post-tragal continuation of the incision is marked as determined preoperatively. A post-tragal incision is made right along the free posterior margin of the tragus. A pretragal incision follows the crus of the helix into the incisura anteriorly before it curves slightly forward in front of the tragus and travels inferiorly in a natural skin crease to the base of the earlobe.

In a female the incision is designed to curve around the earlobe at its junction with the cheek, whereas in males, a small cuff (several millimeters) of skin is maintained below the earlobe to prevent advancing bearded skin right into the junction of the earlobe with the cheek. The incision continues along the posterior auricle, where it is carried 2 to 3 mm onto the posterior surface of the conchal cartilage (i.e., lateral to the post-auricular sulcus) because this incision will ultimately generally settle into the sulcus rather than drift onto a more visible area of postauricular skin. As with the infralobular incision, in men the postauricular incision is made either in or several millimeters behind the postauricular sulcus to avoid drawing bearded skin up onto the auricle.

The postauricular incision is drawn superiorly to a point where the helical rim crosses the hairline (usually 1 to 1.5 cm above the level of the tragus) before turning horizontally and posteriorly. From here the incision may extend back into the occipital hair for several centimeters (see Fig. 89-1) or may follow the hairline inferiorly (several millimeters within the hairline) and gently curve further into the hair for 1.5 to 2 cm at its inferior extent (Fig. 89-2). The length of this incision depends on the amount of redundant skin that is to be excised; it must be long enough to allow the skin to redrape without leaving a posterior scalp "dog-ear" or a fold in the neck. Placing the incision along the hairline will make it easier to prevent any step-off deformity along the postauricular hairline, particularly if one anticipates removing a significant amount of skin in this region as the skin of the neck is lifted and redraped. An example of intraoperative skin markings is presented in Figure 89-3.

It is not necessary to shave or cut the patient's hair, but after parting the hair, segments of twisted hair in front and behind the planned incisions are wrapped with rubber bands or paper tape. Lacri-Lube ointment is combed into the hair on each side of the part to further prevent hair from interfering with the wound closure.

Once all markings are complete, injections of local anesthetic are carried out with a 22- or 25-gauge spinal needle in the subcutaneous dissection plane. Appropri-ate infiltration facilitates subsequent dissection. To prevent injection of excessive amounts of lidocaine/bupivacaine, only the first region to be dissected is injected at the outset of the operation, with each successive region injected intraoperatively 10 to 15 minutes before transitioning to that part of the surgery.

SURGICAL TECHNIQUE

As alluded to earlier, there are multiple variations on face-lift surgery—a skin-only lift, skin dissection with some modification of the SMAS,[2-6] deep-plane face-lifts,[7] composite face-lifts,[8] subperiosteal face-lifts,[9] and others.[10,11] In general, the more extensive the dissection or the deeper the plane of dissection, the greater the risk of postoperative complications and facial nerve injury. Furthermore, from surgeon to surgeon there will be differences in incision preference, degree of liposuction, extent of undermining, and methods of treating the SMAS and platysma. With that in mind, what is described herein is an outline of a safe, basic, generic procedure with elaboration of some variations.

Preoperative evaluation of the neck and platysmal banding will help identify patients who will require direct submental fat resection, liposuction, or medial plication of the platysmal bands. In a patient with a good cervicomental angle without excessive submental fat or platysmal banding it may not be necessary to do any direct submental dissection or flap elevation at all. If it is thought that liposuction is warranted (a particularly heavy neck with excessive subcutaneous fat) or there are platysmal bands that need to be addressed, this part of the surgery is done first.

The operation begins with infiltration of local anesthetic into the neck. The incision is placed in the submental area several millimeters behind (posterior to)

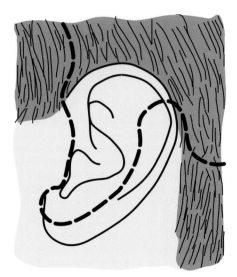

Figure 89-1. Schematic of a face-lift incision extending superiorly from the helical root into the temporal hair anteriorly. It can be used in patients with a low temporal hairline tuft and extended posteriorly behind the ear into the occipital hair.

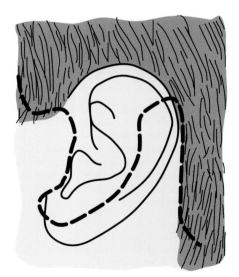

Figure 89-2. Schematic of a face-lift incision extending anteriorly within the temporal hairline. This incision is preferred in patients with a low temporal hairline to prevent posterior shift of the hairline. Posteriorly, an incision along the occipital hairline is illustrated.

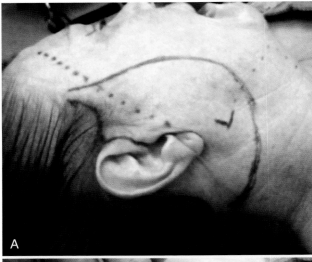

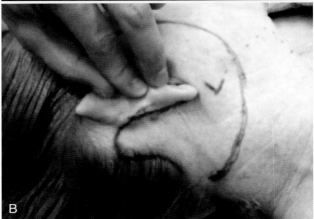

Figure 89-3. **A**, Preoperative skin markings along the temporal hairline and post-tragally. The topographic location of the facial nerve is outlined *(dashed line)*, as is the extent of the proposed undermining, the angle, and inferior border of the mandible. **B**, The postauricular markings, which extend superiorly on the posterior auricle several millimeters from the postauricular sulcus, traverse the scalp above the level of the tragus, and extend inferiorly just within the occipital hairline.

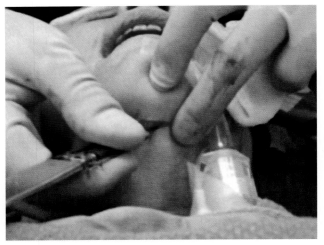

Figure 89-4. The submental incision used for access to elevate the neck skin flap.

the submental crease (Fig. 89-4). This incision provides the access necessary for submental liposuction if planned or, alternatively, for elevation of neck skin flaps for better redraping or platysmal plication. Bear in mind that the surgery will draw this incision anteriorly and superiorly, so consideration must be given to ensuring that it remains well concealed in the submental region. If only liposuction is planned, a smaller incision is sufficient (0.5 to 1 cm), whereas if a skin flap is to be elevated and the platysma plicated, a slightly longer incision will be needed for optimal visualization.

For liposuction, one can pretunnel with the liposuction cannula off suction to initiate elevation of the neck skin flap.[12] A 3- or 4-mm three-hole blunt bullet-tipped cannula is used initially while taking care at all times to keep the aperture in the cannula directed deep, away from the overlying skin, to prevent injury to the dermis and minimize the potential for postopera-

tive irregularities or unevenness in the skin. The cannula is then attached to suction and the liposuction is carried out with care taken to maintain an even contour (to palpation) across the entire area suctioned.

An alternative is to elevate the skin flap over the neck first with face-lift scissors and maintain an even 2- to 3-mm cuff of fat on the undersurface of the skin. "Open" liposuction is then conducted under more direct vision. Boundaries for safe liposuction extend from the inferior border of the mandible down to the thyroid cartilage while remaining between the anterior borders of the sternocleidomastoid muscles from either side.

After using the 3- to 4-mm blunt cannula, a 5- to 6-mm single-hole spatula-tipped cannula is passed over the same area to smooth out, sculpt, and contour the area. Care is taken to avoid overaggressive resection, which may lead to cutaneous depressions and contour irregularities postoperatively.

At this point it is helpful to inject local anesthetic into the first side of the face to be operated on. Next, if not already done, the skin flap is elevated through the submental incision over the neck (Fig. 89-5). Dissection across the entire neck is needed in patients who require substantial fat excision or redraping of significant excesses of skin. Plication of the medial borders of the platysma is then carried out if indicated for platysmal banding. Either a lighted retractor is placed in the submental incision or two Senn retractors can be used with headlight illumination. The medial edge of the platysma muscle from either side is identified. The medial edges are then sutured together from the level of the thyroid notch up to the incision with buried 3-0 or 4-0 Vicryl or PDS suture. In selected cases in which it is thought that there is a great redundancy of platysma muscle, it may be necessary to resect a strip of the medial margin of muscle from either side before suturing the medial borders to one another. Hemostasis should be ensured beneath the neck flaps before moving to the next step.

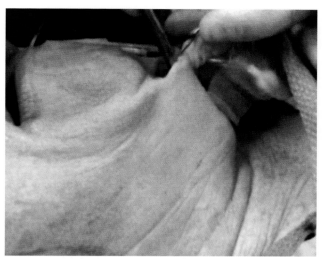

Figure 89-5. Elevation of the neck skin flap.

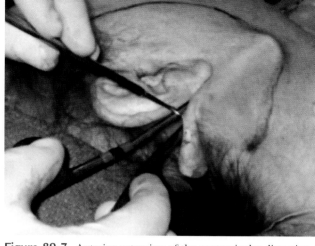

Figure 89-7. Anterior extension of the postauricular dissection to join the neck flap dissection.

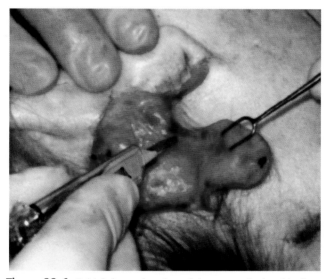

Figure 89-6. Initial sharp elevation of the postauricular skin flap.

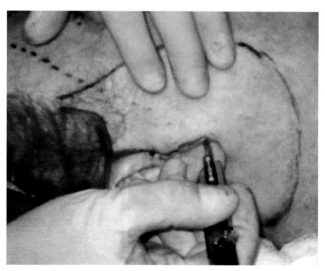

Figure 89-8. The preauricular skin incision.

The postauricular and occipital incisions are then made and the flaps elevated with scalpel dissection for the first 2 to 3 cm (Fig. 89-6). Care is required initially to maintain a thick flap over the mastoid region (because this is some of the thinnest skin elevated in the entire operation and therefore most at risk for necrosis or skin sloughing). As one transitions down into the neck below the mastoid, the flap must be superficial to the fascia overlying the sternocleidomastoid muscle to protect the integrity of the greater auricular nerve as it crosses the midportion of the muscle 6.5 cm below the external auditory meatus. Once beyond the mastoid region, further dissection is carried out with face-lift scissors, and the flap is retracted with one or two sharp double hooks and counter-traction provided by the assistant distal to the point of elevation. The dissection is carried forward within the plane of the sub-

cutaneous fat until one joins the dissection of the neck skin already elevated (Fig. 89-7).

Attention is then turned to elevation of the facial skin flaps. The incision is begun in the temporal region along the predetermined markings and continues to the base of the earlobe (Fig. 89-8). Dissection in the temporal region can be either in the subcutaneous plane or right on the deep temporal fascia—the former being superficial to the frontal branch of the facial nerve, the latter deep to the nerve. In either case, awareness of the depth of dissection relative to the facial nerve is critical to prevent injury.[13]

Having completed the incision with a no. 15 blade, dissection along the deep temporal fascia can generally be done quickly and bluntly with the back end of the knife handle or even with finger dissection to the level of the lateral orbital rim and the lateral aspect of the forehead while always staying above the level of the zygomatic arch. It is important to recognize that a sub-cutaneous soft tissue bridge or mesentery from the deeper tissues up to the skin must be preserved at the level of the zygomatic arch and lateral canthus to separate the deeper temporal dissection from the subcutaneous dissection of the preauricular cheek skin flap because the frontal branch of the facial nerve lies in this soft tissue. When the temporal dissection is in the subcutaneous plane (as opposed to being right on the deep temporal fascia), it is contiguous with the plane in which the facial skin is elevated and superficial to the nerve at all levels. In this case it is not necessary to preserve a soft tissue bridge at the level of the zygomatic arch.

Subcutaneous dissection of the facial skin (and temporal skin when that plane is chosen) is initiated with either a no. 15 blade or sharp serrated iris scissors and a sharp double-hook retractor for the first 1 to 2 cm because the deep tissues in this region are more adherent to the overlying skin than the skin further forward over the cheek.

Once the proper plane of dissection is identified, after the first 1 to 2 cm, subsequent elevation of the preauricular facial skin flap is performed with face-lift scissors under direct vision (Fig. 89-9). The flap should be elevated while leaving a thin, even layer of fat on the undersurface of the skin to protect the subdermal plexus. Having the assistant apply constant countertraction on the skin medially and using the operating room lights to backlight or transilluminate the flap will help one identify and maintain the proper plane of dissection and an even thickness of the skin flap. The flap is undermined out to the limits that were marked preoperatively (usually about 5 to 6 cm). Preliminary hemostasis is achieved at this point with bipolar cautery for maximal safety. A moist sponge can then be placed beneath the flap as attention is turned to the postauricular area.

Once the preauricular cheek flap is elevated, the dissection is connected with the postauricular skin flap and continues into the neck to bring this flap into continuity with the neck skin previously undermined (Fig. 89-10). With the neck and cheek skin thus elevated, hemostasis is once again addressed.

SMAS suspension is carried out next. Suspension may be in the form of SMAS plication (suture suspension whereby the SMAS is folded on itself) or imbrication (either as a lateral SMAS-ectomy or by elevation and trimming of a SMAS flap, with suture fixation of the margins of the excision). Because SMAS plication can lead to bunching of soft tissue beneath the skin, SMAS imbrication is favored and will be discussed here.

One method of SMAS imbrication involves formal SMAS flap elevation,[2] redraping of the SMAS along a superolateral vector, trimming of the excess, and suspension with 3-0 PDS or Vicryl suture to reapproximate the edges after excision of redundant SMAS. Alternatively, SMAS imbrication can be carried out by way of a lateral SMAS-ectomy (without actual elevation of the SMAS flap).[5,6,12] In the latter method, a J-shaped, 1.5- to 2-cm strip of SMAS is excised (the "SMAS-ectomy") in the preauricular area down to the parotid fascia (Fig. 89-11), with extension superiorly and anteriorly from below the lobule of the ear up toward the malar eminence (Fig. 89-12). The SMAS excision should not go higher than the zygomatic arch to prevent injury to the frontal branch of the facial nerve.

Approximation of the edges of the SMAS defect that results from SMAS-ectomy will create the SMAS suspension needed to elevate the jowl, neck, and nasolabial fold. The direction of SMAS suspension is not simply posterior, but rather primarily superior and slightly posterior. Multiple 3-0 PDS or Vicryl sutures are used to close the two exposed edges of the SMAS-ectomy defect (Fig. 89-13).

The advantage of SMAS-ectomy over SMAS flap dissection is that it can be done quickly and with less risk to the facial nerve if one remains over the parotid fascia. Furthermore, less tissue elevation/dissection

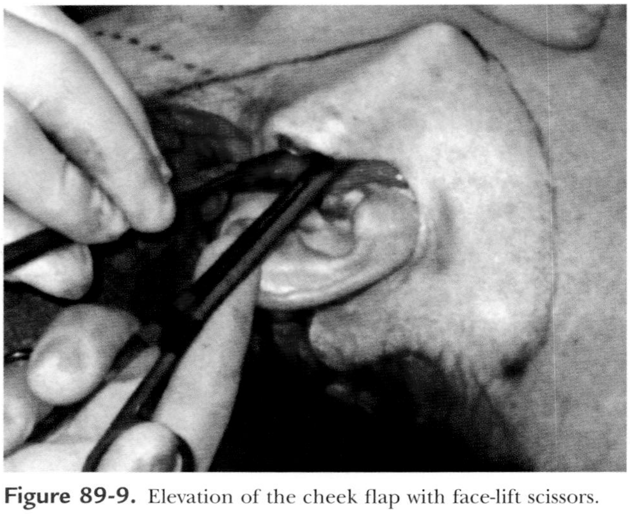

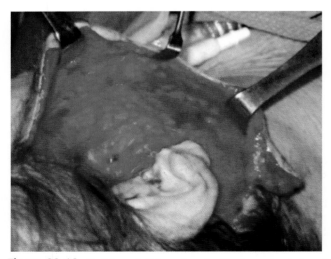

Figure 89-9. Elevation of the cheek flap with face-lift scissors.

Figure 89-10. Facial, occipital, and neck skin flaps elevated and joined in continuity.

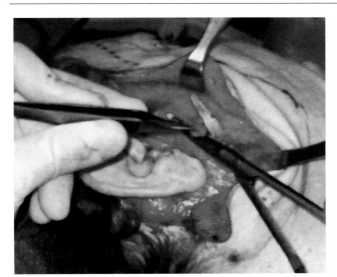

Figure 89-11. Initiation of the SMAS-ectomy by gently retracting the SMAS while engaging the face-lift scissors to resect the SMAS tissue down to the parotid fascia.

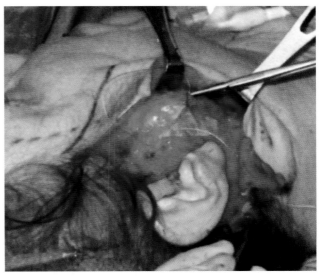

Figure 89-13. Initiation of imbrication of the edges of the SMAS defect with 3-0 Vicryl. The tension placed on the SMAS closure relieves the tension on the skin closure.

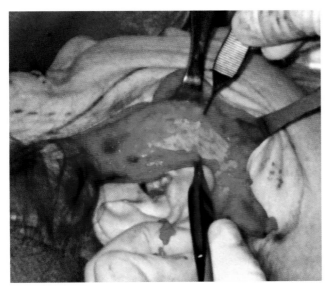

Figure 89-12. The completed SMAS-ectomy. Parotid fascia is visible between the edges of the SMAS defect, which are being grasped with forceps.

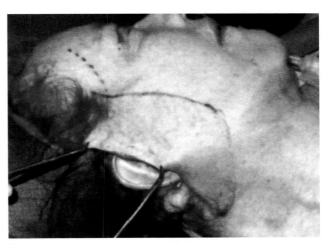

Figure 89-14. Redraping of the cheek flap along a posterior superior vector.

should theoretically help reduce the risk for postoperative hematoma.

Once the SMAS suspension is complete, the redundant skin will be overlapping the ear. Redraping and excision of the excess skin follow. If there are any irregularities, dimpling, or bunching of skin as a result of the SMAS suspension, further undermining of the skin flap will resolve these problems and is carried out before the skin excision.

For skin redraping, the anterior (preauricular) skin flap is retracted along a superior and slightly posterior vector while the posterior (postauricular) skin flap is drawn superiorly and slightly anteriorly (if the postauricular incision extends straight back into the hair) to enable one to realign the hairline and thus avoid any step-off in that area. If the postauricular incision was designed to follow the hairline, the skin flap can be redraped in a more superior and posterior direction.

The flap is tailored with two key tension sutures. The key sutures placed during closure of a face-lift assume the greatest degree of tension on the closure and also serve as guides for the direction of pull of the facial skin. The anterior skin flap (preauricular cheek skin) is first "lifted" in a superior and posterior direction (Fig. 89-14). An incision is made in the flap down to the helical root (Fig. 89-15). The first tension or tacking suture of 4-0 Prolene (or staple) is placed at this point to effectively separate the temporal skin excess from the preauricular skin excess (Fig. 89-16). The excess temporal skin above the first tension suture is

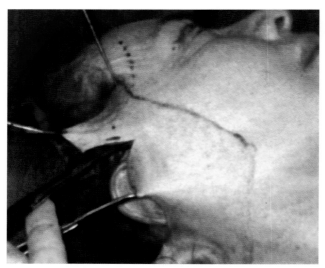

Figure 89-15. Incision in the facial flap down to the helical root.

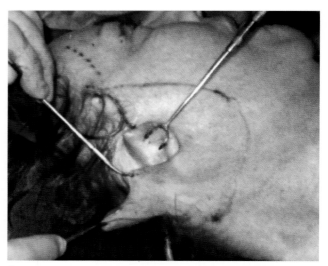

Figure 89-17. The postauricular skin flap is redraped to facilitate skin excision and closure without tension. In this case, because the incision was just inside the hairline, the skin flap is retracted along a posterior and superior vector. Note also that the anterior temporal skin excess has been excised and sutured without tension.

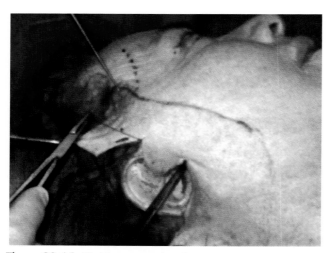

Figure 89-16. Tacking suture placed to separate the temporal skin excess from the cheek skin excess.

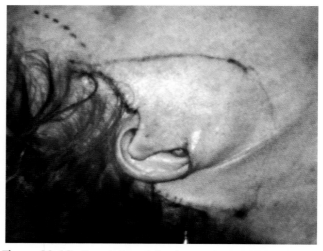

Figure 89-18. Completion of the closure along the occipital hairline leaves only the skin excess that cradles the auricle.

then excised. Skin closure in this area is achieved with staples if in the hair or with 5-0 or 6-0 Prolene if along the temporal hairline. If much tension is encountered, a deep layer of 5-0 PDS sutures is used.

The postauricular skin flap is then redraped (Fig. 89-17). The second tension suture is next placed in the postauricular incision at the level of the postauricular hairline by cutting into the flap posteriorly at the point where the hairline needs to be realigned. This effectively separates the occipital portion of the skin flap from the more immediate postauricular portion of the flap.

The excess occipital skin behind the second tension suture can then be excised and closure carried out in a fashion similar to that in the temporal area—staples if the occipital incision heads into the hair or running 5-0 or 6-0 Prolene or staples if the incision follows the hairline (Fig. 89-18). A flat closed suction drain is

brought out through a separate stab wound in the occipital hair (behind the incision) and laid in the neck before closing the occipital incision.

Moving from the hairline over the premastoid skin to the superior aspect of the incision along the postauricular sulcus, the redundant skin is trimmed and the skin edges closed with 5-0 plain or fast-absorbing catgut suture.

Skin now overlies the ear and only the trim around the ear remains to be completed. Scissors are used to cut the skin overlying the ear down toward the earlobe along a line parallel to the auricular helix or postauricular sulcus (Fig. 89-19). The incision should not come all the way down to the lower pole of the earlobe but rather stop approximately 0.5 to 1 cm above the base of

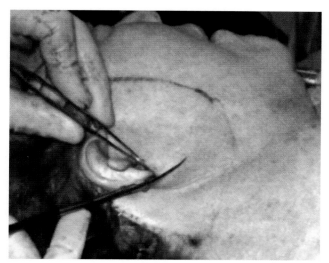

Figure 89-19. Skin is incised along the line of the auricular helix toward the lower pole of the ear; the incision stops 0.5 to 1 cm above the base of the earlobe to allow the skin to be tucked under the earlobe without any inferior pull or tension at closure.

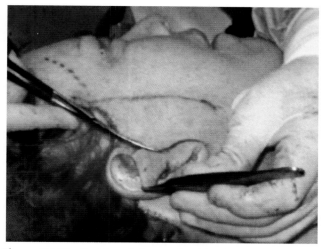

Figure 89-21. Excision of the anterior (cheek) skin redundancy.

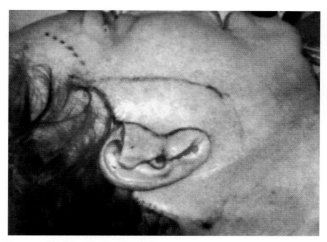

Figure 89-20. The earlobe position has been secured and the excess skin along the postauricular sulcus excised and closed.

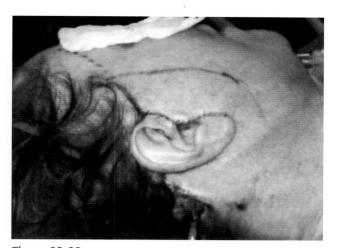

Figure 89-22. Appearance on completion of skin closure.

the earlobe. This preserves more skin below the earlobe to cradle the earlobe at closure rather than risking closure under tension and inferior retraction of the earlobe with healing. The earlobe is then sutured in place (Fig. 89-20), and any excess skin overlying the postauricular sulcus incision line is trimmed. Postauricular closure is with 5-0 plain or fast-absorbing catgut.

The excess preauricular skin is then tailored to facilitate an exacting tension-free closure (Fig. 89-21) with running 6-0 Prolene (Fig. 89-22).

Ten to fifteen minutes before completing closure on the first side, the second side of the face should be injected with local anesthetic. The second side of the face-lift proceeds in the same way as the first side. The submental incision is closed at the completion of surgery with either 5-0 fast-absorbing gut or 6-0 Prolene suture.

Dressings

The end of the operation is the best time to comfortably clean the patient's hair. Saline and a large-toothed comb are used to remove all loose hair, dried blood, and debris. Bacitracin ointment is next applied to all incisions, which are then covered with either Xeroform gauze or a nonadherent dressing (Telfa).

A lightly compressive dressing of open fluffed 4 × 4-inch gauze is applied to provide padding over the periauricular area, around the lower part of the face, and over the neck. The dressing is then secured with a 3- or 4-inch Kerlix gauze wrap and either an elastic bandage or a 3-inch roll of Coban self-adhesive tape to hold the dressing in place. The goal is a snug but comfortable dressing.

POSTOPERATIVE MANAGEMENT

The patient is instructed to keep the head of the bed elevated 30 degrees, avoid bending over, and not undertake strenuous activities for the first week. Most patients are kept overnight in a unit capable of caring for face-lift patients unless they have made appropriate arrangements for home care. Ice-cool compresses are applied to the face during the first 24 to 48 hours. Many patients have found small bags of frozen peas to be an excellent source of cool compresses over these moist dressings. The peas are in plastic bags, conform well to the face and eyes, and hold the cool temperature for a prolonged period. In addition, they can be refrozen and reused for this purpose. Patients are told preoperatively that they will swell and bruise during the first few postoperative days.

Patients are evaluated on the first postoperative morning for any evidence of hematoma and to test the integrity of the facial nerve. The drains are removed, and a clean, lighter dressing is secured. Patients are told to remove the dressing the following day (postoperative day 2) and may then begin to gently wash their hair and care for their own face. They are instructed to be careful with the temperature of the water and their blow dryer because of temporary alterations in scalp and facial sensation. In addition, patients should wait 3 to 4 weeks before undergoing hair coloring or a permanent. A nylon or spandex elasticized facial support dressing is supplied to the patient, who wears it full-time (aside from bathing) for the first week. Patients are told to gently clean the visible incisions with hydrogen peroxide and then reapply an antibacterial ointment three times daily.

The preauricular sutures are removed on the fifth or sixth postoperative day. Scalp staples are removed 7 to 10 days postoperatively. The absorbable postauricular sulcus stitch is allowed to dissolve.

Representative preoperative and postoperative patient photos are seen in Figure 89-23.

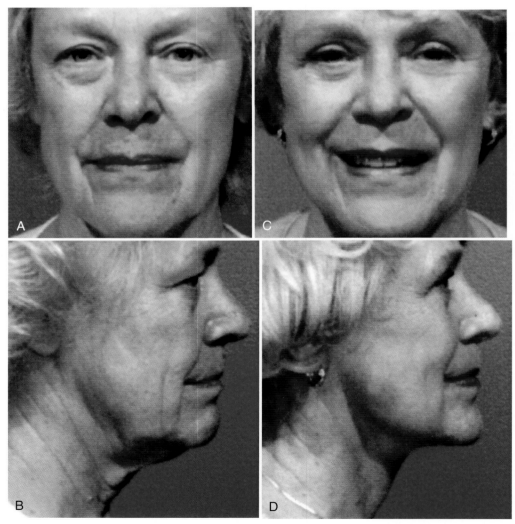

Figure 89-23. **A** and **B**, Preoperative frontal and lateral views of a patient before a face-lift and blepharoplasty. **C** and **D**, Postoperative frontal and lateral views of the patient who underwent a face-lift and blepharoplasty.

COMPLICATIONS[14-16]

Hematoma

Small hematomas are one of the most common and troublesome complications. If identified immediately postoperatively, they can often be aspirated with an 18-gauge needle. However, when a small hematoma is camouflaged by swelling, one must wait 7 to 14 days before the hematoma will liquefy and allow removal by aspiration. Residual hematomas may cause some dimpling and firmness beneath the facial skin. Larger hematomas (incidence of approximately 3% in females and up to 9% in males) are generally apparent within the first 24 hours and mandate return to the operating room for evacuation, hemostasis, and reclosure. Failure to identify or address a more substantial hematoma puts the patient at increased risk for skin necrosis, infection, and dimpling or irregularities in the overlying skin.

Facial Nerve Injury

Most immediate postoperative facial nerve paralysis will resolve spontaneously within 6 weeks and is due to the effects of the local anesthetic, stretch, local crush injury, inflammation, or compression by a support suture. Occasionally, permanent paralysis will occur as a result of complete transection of the frontal, marginal mandibular, or buccal branch or injury induced by electrocautery. If the injury is identified intraoperatively, immediate repair is indicated; otherwise, treatment is expectant in the hope that the deficit will resolve or diminish. Ultimately, prevention of such injuries is paramount, and if the dissection is maintained in the proper plane and the surgeon is cognizant of the depth of the facial nerve relative to the depth of dissection, facial nerve injuries are avoidable.

Skin Necrosis

The incidence of significant skin necrosis is between 1% and 3%. It is most common in the mastoid region because the skin flap is the thinnest there, tension is greatest, and it is farthest away from the blood supply. The usual causes of more extensive skin necrosis are some combination of the following: delayed recognition of a significant hematoma, excess tension on the closure, excessive superficial dissection (overly thin skin flaps), a history of impaired circulation secondary to smoking or diabetes, excessive pressure from the dressing, infection, or traumatic handling of tissues. All sloughing should be treated by observation, reassurance, and wound care. A lot of personal attention is required to help these patients deal psychologically with this unexpected sequela. An eschar will eventually form at sites with full-thickness skin loss, and the scars are usually satisfactory. Scars that heal unacceptably can be revised later.

PEARLS

- Attention to detail in the preoperative evaluation will help establish realistic patient expectations and guide decisions to optimize surgical results.
- Careful consideration should be paid to the position of the hairline, and incisions should be chosen to avoid excessive shift or misalignment of the hairline, which can result in telltale signs of surgery.
- Incisions in males should be modified to avoid shifting bearded skin all the way back to the posterior margin of the tragus or right up to the attachment of the earlobe.
- The surgeon should always be conscious of the location and depth of the facial nerve relative to the plane of dissection to avoid inadvertent injury.
- Suspension of the SMAS, whether by plication, imbrication, or SMAS-ectomy, is fundamental to minimize skin closure tension and improve the longevity of the face-lift.

PITFALLS

- Tobacco smokers are at much higher risk for complications and must be counseled appropriately preoperatively; heavy smokers should not be considered candidates for this procedure.
- Dissection deep to the fascia overlying the sternocleidomastoid muscle in the neck may injure the greater auricular nerve.
- Overaggressive surgery must be avoided to prevent an unnatural, pulled, "surgical" look.
- Excessive tension on the skin closure will increase the risk for skin necrosis and widened scars, both of which are largely preventable.
- Disproportionate, particularly unilateral facial pain may be indicative of a hematoma and mandates immediate examination of the patient.

References

1. Kridel RW, Liu ES: Techniques for creating inconspicuous face-lift scars: Avoiding visible incisions and loss of temporal hair. Arch Facial Plast Surg 5:325-333, 2003.
2. Stuzin JM, Baker TJ, Baker TM: Refinements in face lifting: Enhancing facial contour using Vicryl mesh incorporated into SMAS fixation. Plast Reconstr Surg 105:290-301, 2000.
3. McCullough EG, Perkins SW, Langsdon PR: SASMAS suspension rhytidectomy: Rationale and long term experience. Arch Otolaryngol Head Neck Surg 115:228-234, 1989.
4. Mittleman H, Newman J: SMASectomy and imbrication in face lift surgery. Facial Plast Surg Clin N Am 8:173-182, 2000.
5. Baker DC: Lateral SMASectomy. Plast Reconstr Surg 100:509-513, 1997.
6. Baker DC: Minimal incision rhytidectomy (short scar face lift) with lateral SMASectomy: Evolution and application. Aesthetic Surg J 21:14-26, 2001.
7. Hamra ST: The deep-plane rhytidectomy. Plast Reconstr Surg 86:53-61, 1990.
8. Hamra ST: Composite rhytidectomy. Plast Reconstr Surg 90:1-13, 1992.

9. Psillakis JM, Rumley TO, Camargos A: Subperiosteal approach as an improved concept for correction of the aging face. Plast Reconstr Surg 82:383-392, 1988.

10. Baker SR: Triplane rhytidectomy: Combining the best of all worlds. Arch Otolaryngol Head Neck Surg 123:1167-1172, 1997.

11. Saylan Z: The S-lift for facial rejuvenation. Int J Cosmetic Surg 7:18-24, 1999.

12. Williams EF, Lam SM: Lower facial rejuvenation. In Williams EF, Lam SM (eds): Comprehensive Facial Rejuvenation. Philadelphia, Lippincott Williams & Wilkins, 2004, pp 105-151.

13. Larrabee WF Jr, Makielski KH, Cupp C: Facelift anatomy. Facial Plast Surg Clin N Am 1:135-152, 1993.

14. Ahn MS, Kabaker SS: Complications of face lifting. Facial Plast Surg Clin N Am 8:211-221, 2000.

15. Adamson PA, Moran ML: Complications of cervicofacial rhytidectomy. Facial Plast Surg Clin N Am 1:257-271, 1993.

16. Baker DC: Complications of cervicofacial rhytidectomy. Clin Plast Surg 10:543-562, 1983.

Chapter 90

Blepharoplasty

Grant S. Gillman

As our population continues to grow older, society's emphasis on a more youthful appearance continues to increase and has led to rising interest in reversing the visible signs of aging. The periorbital region is usually the first area of the face to show significant signs of aging. Correction of this imperfection can significantly "turn back the clock" of aging and has thus led to the popularity of aesthetic surgery on the eyelids.

PATIENT SELECTION

Appropriate candidates for upper eyelid blepharoplasty are patients who objectively have redundant skin of the upper eyelids (dermatochalasis). Although in most cases the motivation is purely cosmetic, other patients with more significant excess skin and hooding of the upper lids may have functional visual field restriction. In the latter patients, automated visual field testing is necessary for proper documentation to justify the medical necessity so that reimbursement by third-party payers is facilitated.

Appropriate candidates for lower eyelid blepharoplasty will generally have pseudoherniation of the orbital fat ("bags"), either with or without a vertical excess of skin.

In all cases patients must be well motivated and have realistic expectations regarding the surgical outcome.

PREOPERATIVE PLANNING

All patients are asked to describe their particular area of concern. A thorough history of any ocular problems is then elicited, including any history of periorbital surgery, previous blepharoplasty, visual difficulties, glaucoma, and "dry eye" symptoms such as frequent blinking, tearing, dryness, red eyes, itching, burning, or crusting of the lid margins.

A medical history is obtained and should cover all past medical problems with special emphasis on hypertension, diabetes, thyroid disease, facial muscle weakness, cardiovascular disorders, and the use of any anticoagulant medications (including aspirin products, warfarin, nonsteroidal anti-inflammatory drugs, vitamin E, multivitamins, and over-the-counter oral herbal preparations). If the surgeon has any concerns regarding other ophthalmic conditions (e.g., dry eyes, glaucoma, ptosis), the patient should be evaluated preoperatively by an ophthalmologist for clearance before making plans for surgery.

Whether one is planning upper or lower eyelid surgery, the surgeon must be familiar with the anatomy of the eyelid and periorbital area[1] to make the best preoperative decisions, in addition to performing well-executed surgery.

In assessing the upper eyelid area, the position of the brow is first evaluated to determine the extent to which brow ptosis might be contributing to the apparent skin excess of the upper eyelids. In men, a youthful brow position rests at the level of the superior orbital rim, whereas in women, the brow should rest at a level about 1 cm above the orbital rim. Significant brow ptosis should prompt a conversation with the patient about the merits of a brow-lift or a combination of brow-lift and blepharoplasty.

The size, shape, and configuration of the bony orbit, as well as the size, shape, and symmetry of the palpebral aperture, are then evaluated. Complete eye closure preoperatively is naturally critical—any pre-existing lagophthalmos is a definite contraindication to upper eyelid blepharoplasty because it will undoubtedly increase if upper lid surgery is performed. It is important to look at the position and symmetry of the upper lid folds and supratarsal creases, the amount of scleral show, and the position of the globe in the orbit. Any asymmetry should be pointed out to the patient preoperatively. A patient with eyelid ptosis must understand that blepharoplasty alone will not correct eyelid ptosis and that ptosis repair is necessary in addition.

The appearance of aging in the periorbital area can be due to an excess of periorbital skin, protuberant fat, and hypertrophic orbicularis muscle. It is important to correctly diagnose and record the contribution of each to the patient's deformity. One should record the degree of excess skin in each eyelid and fat in each fat compartment (upper medial and central; lower medial, central, and lateral). Any orbicularis oculi muscle hypertrophy is also recorded.

The patient is asked to look straight at the surgeon with the eyes open, then with the eyes closed, and finally in upward gaze without moving the head. During these maneuvers, the upper and lower eyelids are closely evaluated for the relative amount of excess skin and fat. The excess fat in the lower lid compartments is highlighted in the upward gaze position. Applying pressure to the patient's globe while the eyelids are closed helps exaggerate and delineate the locations of excess fat in both the upper and lower eyelid compartments.

Lower eyelid tone is assessed with a "snap test" (also called the lid distraction test) whereby the lid is drawn anteriorly outward from the globe with the thumb and forefinger. More than 10-mm movement of the lid margin is considered abnormally lax. In addition, one watches how long it takes for the lower lid to return to its pretest position. A normal, youthful lid will snap back immediately. In the lid retraction test, the lower lid is drawn inferiorly toward the orbital rim, and once again one observes for abnormally slow return of the lid to its normal position. Poor lower lid tone should lead the surgeon to consider alternative techniques to standard skin-muscle lower lid blepharoplasty or a concomitant canthoplasty or canthopexy.

Finally, the visual acuity of each eye should be tested individually with an eye chart or by having the patient read fine print with one eye.

Preoperative photographs are important for documentation and planning. A complete set would include a full facial view (vertically oriented, 1:7 or 1:8 ratio) and close-up (1:4 ratio, horizontally oriented) frontal, oblique, and lateral views of the eyes. The close-up frontal view should include a photo with the eyes closed and one with the eyes gazing upward. Consistent preoperative and postoperative focal length, lighting, background, patient positioning, and subject-to-lens distance are essential.

The patient and physician must decide together on the most appropriate anesthetic for each patient. Local anesthesia, supplemented by intravenous sedation, is usually adequate for all aesthetic surgical procedures on the eyelids. Patients who require only resection of skin of the upper eyelids often do well with local anesthesia alone. In some cases the patient or anesthesiologist may feel most comfortable with general anesthesia.

Patient comfort should be the ultimate goal for maximal surgical safety.

SURGICAL TECHNIQUES

Upper Lid Blepharoplasty

For upper eyelid blepharoplasty, the amount of skin resected depends on the amount of excess as determined by preoperative examination.[2] It is again emphasized that one should ensure that the brow is not ptotic and that it is held in correct position during marking of the upper eyelid resection.

Markings

The incisions are marked preoperatively with the patient in the sitting position and the brow held in proper position before injection of local anesthetic. The level of the inferior incision is usually between 8 and 12 mm from the lash line in the midpupillary line and 5 to 6 mm above the medial and lateral canthi. The inferior incision is generally marked in the patient's natural upper eyelid crease, which lies at the upper edge of the tarsal plate, unless the crease is less than 8 mm from the lash line centrally. In such cases the central marking should be measured to lie 8 to 10 mm above the lashes. The incision is planned such that it lies in the upper eyelid crease and the skin resected is from the preseptal region, not the pretarsal area. The natural supratarsal crease may or may not be symmetrical from one side to another. One can choose to use the patient's natural crease regardless or adjust one side to ensure symmetry. This decision is best made with the patient preoperatively.

At the lateral canthus the marking should sweep gently laterally and upward toward the tail of the brow, as much as needed to excise the skin that accounts for any lateral hooding. It rarely needs to extend beyond the lateral aspect of the lateral orbital rim. Medially, the incision marking should not extend more than 1 to 2 mm beyond the punctum of the eyelid. Extending the incision too far nasally into the concavity at the medial orbit increases the risk of creating a webbed scar across this area. In patients with significant excess skin, the medial extension is curved upward in a W pattern to avoid a dog-ear and keep the scar from coinciding with the epicanthal fold.

It is important to hold the patient's brow in its correct anatomic position when determining the amount of skin to be resected from the upper lid. A "skin pinch" technique is then used to determine the amount of excess skin to be resected. Conservatism is always recommended. The middle of the excess skin is gently grasped with fine forceps and lifted until slight eversion of the lashes occurs. The upper incision is marked at the point where the lower incision meets the upper limit of the excess skin. This is done in at least four positions across the upper eyelid. The marks are then connected to outline the upper incision line (Fig. 90-1). This resection is tested at multiple levels by pinching the upper and lower incision lines together (before

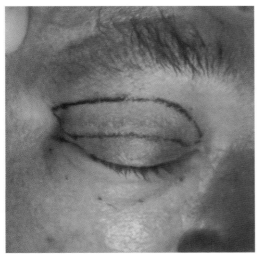

Figure 90-1. Outline of an upper eyelid blepharoplasty incision.

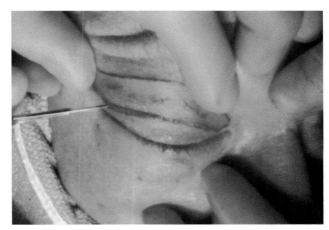

Figure 90-3. Skin incision with a no. 15 blade for upper eyelid blepharoplasty.

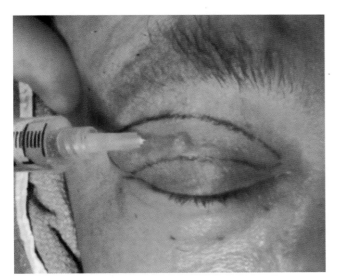

Figure 90-2. Injection of local anesthetic.

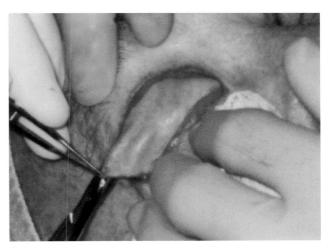

Figure 90-4. Skin excision with scissors undermining superficial to the orbicularis oculi.

injecting the local anesthetic) and checking for excess eversion of the lid margin.

Infiltration of the local anesthetic is accomplished with a 30-gauge, $1\frac{1}{2}$-inch needle (Fig. 90-2). Injecting just below the skin and superficial to the underlying orbicularis oculi will minimize hematoma formation. Total volume per lid is generally about 1 to 1.5 mL. After allowing adequate time for the hemostatic effect of the local anesthetic to commence, the skin is incised along the markings (Fig. 90-3). A skin-only resection is first performed with either a no. 15 scalpel, a needle-tipped cautery, or sharp scissors (Fig. 90-4). Hemostasis is obtained with a needle-tipped electrocautery (Fig. 90-5).

In patients in whom the supratarsal crease needs to be accentuated, excision of a 3-mm strip of orbicularis muscle is done separately with fine forceps and fine,

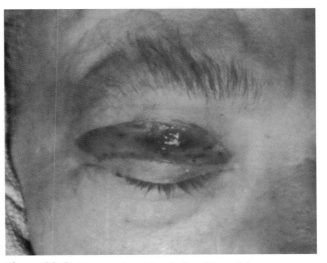

Figure 90-5. Hemostasis achieved after skin excision.

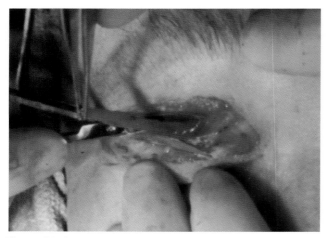

Figure 90-6. Excision of a thin strip of orbicularis oculi muscle in the midportion of the upper eyelid wound.

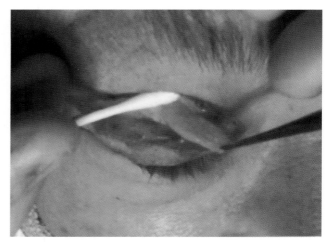

Figure 90-8. Teasing orbital fat through the orbital septum (upper eyelid lateral compartment).

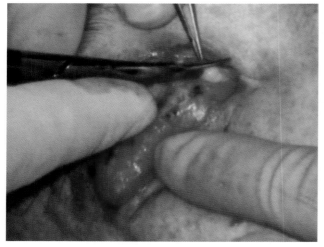
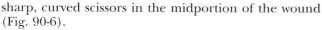

Figure 90-7. Opening of the orbital septum over the medial upper eyelid fat compartment.

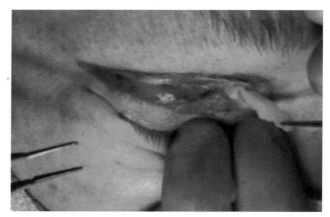

Figure 90-9. Bipolar cautery (seen at the corner of the photo) is used to cauterize across the base of the fat pad, which is then carefully excised.

sharp, curved scissors in the midportion of the wound (Fig. 90-6).

If it was determined preoperatively that excision of orbital fat is necessary, one proceeds with that step at this time. Preoperative evaluation of each compartment will help one determine the amount of excess fat to be excised and avoid under-resection. With finger pressure on the globe, the excess fat in the orbital compartments can be seen bulging through the orbital septum. A small opening is made through the orbital septum over the top of the fat compartments to be addressed (Fig. 90-7). The excess fat is then teased through the opening in the septum with fine forceps and a cotton swab (Fig. 90-8).

Before fat excision, a small amount of local anesthetic should be injected into the base of the fat pedicle because the excision can be uncomfortable for the patient. A small, curved hemostat is then placed at the base of the excess fat to be removed. To avoid over-resection, excess traction is not placed on the fat, and

only the fat that is *easily* delivered through the orbital septum is resected. Small, curved scissors are used to excise the fat while leaving a small cuff above the hemostat. The cut edge is cauterized before releasing the hemostat. As an alternative, one can slowly cauterize across the base of the fat (bipolar cautery) *without* clamping across the base of the pedicle (Fig. 90-9), thereby minimizing the risk of excess traction on the posterior orbital vessels that might result from manipulation of the hemostat.

Simple interrupted sutures can be placed in the incision lateral to the lateral canthus (Fig. 90-10) to better manage tension at the closure line in this part of the wound. The remainder of the upper lid incision is closed with running 6-0 monofilament pullout subcuticular suture (Fig. 90-11). Any gaps in the closure should be addressed with an additional simple stitch of interrupted 6-0 fast-absorbing gut suture. Mastisol and small Steri-Strips are used to anchor the medial and lateral extent of the suture.

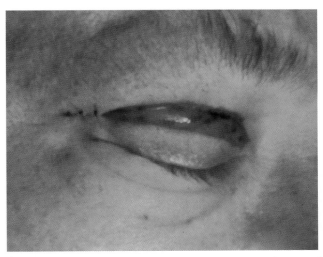

Figure 90-10. Interrupted stitches are used to close the wound lateral to the lateral canthus.

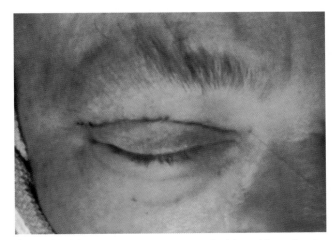

Figure 90-11. Closure of the remaining incision with a subcuticular stitch.

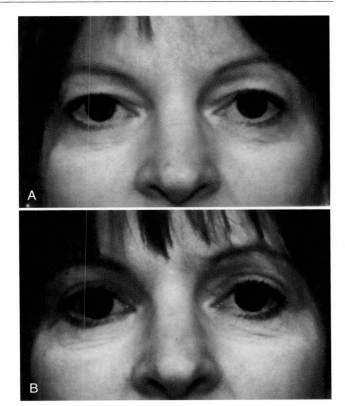

Figure 90-12. Preoperative (**A**) and postoperative (**B**) views of an upper eyelid blepharoplasty patient.

Postoperative Management

The patient applies ice-cool compresses to the eyes during the first 24 to 48 hours. Many patients have found small bags of frozen peas to be an excellent source of cool compresses. The frozen peas are in plastic bags, they conform well to the face and eyes, and they hold the cool temperature for a prolonged period. In addition, they can be refrozen and reused for this purpose.

Patients are told preoperatively that their eyes will swell and bruise during the first few days postoperatively. Liquid tears are used for daytime dryness of the eyes if needed, and Lacri-Lube ointment can likewise be used for nighttime protection if required. An ophthalmic antibiotic ointment is applied over the incisions three times daily after gently cleaning the incisions with a cotton swab soaked in hydrogen peroxide.

The subcuticular suture is removed at a follow-up appointment about 5 days postoperatively. A representative preoperative patient photo and postoperative result are seen in Figure 90-12.

Lower Lid Blepharoplasty

Preoperative evaluation of the lower lids is essential in determining the type of operation most appropriate for each patient. One should evaluate and record the amount of excess fat in each of the lower lid compartments (medial, central, and lateral), the amount of excess skin of the lower lids, the presence or absence of orbicularis hypertrophy, the extent of fine skin wrinkling, and the degree of lower lid laxity.

In patients with minimal excess skin, the transconjunctival approach[3] to the lower lids is preferred. The transconjunctival approach eliminates the "rounding" deformity often found in the lateral aspect of the lower lid after the traditional transcutaneous approach. It also minimizes the chance of lower eyelid retraction developing (scleral show and frank ectropion). A mild trichloroacetic acid (TCA) chemical peel can be used as an adjunct to transconjunctival blepharoplasty. In patients with significant excess skin of the lower lid or those who already have lower lid deformities secondary to lid laxity that require correction, a transcutaneous approach[4] is used with a subciliary incision and elevation of a skin-muscle flap.

Transconjunctival Approach

Although this operation can be done under general anesthesia, it is typically performed under local anesthesia with intravenous sedation. Once the depth of sedation is adequate, the conjunctivae are anesthetized with 0.5% topical ophthalmic tetracaine or proparacaine hydrochloride solution, and corneal shields (green contacts) are lubricated with ophthalmic ointment and used to protect the cornea.

Lidocaine (1%) with 1:100,000 epinephrine is injected via a 27- or 30-gauge needle in the conjunctiva beneath the planned incision (Fig. 90-13) and percutaneously deep to the orbicularis overlying the orbital septum of the lower lid to anesthetize and hydrodissect the plane of dissection.

A wide double hook is then used to retract the lower lid margin (Fig. 90-14). A conjunctival incision is made with a needle-tipped cautery at a level 1 to 2 mm

below the tarsal plate (Fig. 90-15) and deepened to divide the attachment of the lower lid retractors to the inferior tarsus. Medially, the incision should stop short of the punctum of the lacrimal duct to avoid inadvertent injury to the lacrimal canaliculi, and laterally the incision is carried as far as necessary to provide adequate exposure of the lower lid fat compartments.

A 5-0 silk or nylon traction suture is then placed through the inferior conjunctival incision margin, with a hemostat on the free ends of the suture. The hemostat is passed over the patient's forehead to retract the conjunctiva and inferior retractors up over the cornea. This provides countertraction for the dissection and protects the underlying cornea as well. An assistant then uses a wide double hook or a Desmarres retractor to retract the lid side of the conjunctival incision (the superior incision margin). Preseptal dissection (Fig. 90-16) is then carried out to elevate the overlying skin and muscle off the orbital septum down to the orbital rim with a combination of sharp and blunt dissection. The orbicularis can easily be separated from the septum by pushing the muscle anteriorly and inferiorly with a cotton swab. The dissection should be relatively quick and avascular.

Once the flap is elevated, orbital fat should be readily apparent behind the orbital septum (Fig. 90-17). Pressure on the globe will cause the orbital fat to bulge forward; a small opening is then made in the septum overlying the fat compartments to be addressed.

The fat from each compartment is dealt with separately. The fat is teased free from the surrounding fascia and attachments with fine forceps in one hand and a cotton-tipped swab in the other (Figs. 90-18 and 90-19; lateral fat dissection not shown). Once the orbital fat has been mobilized, one can resect the excess fat. As with upper lid fat removal, a small amount of local anesthetic should be injected into the base of the fat pedicle before excision.

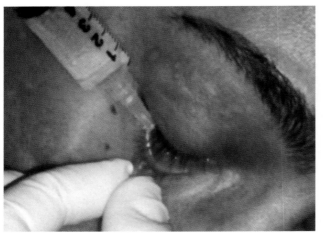

Figure 90-13. Injection of the lower eyelid conjunctiva (right eye).

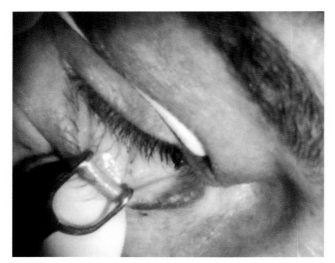

Figure 90-14. Eversion of the lower eyelid with a blunt double hook to expose the conjunctiva before making an incision (right eye).

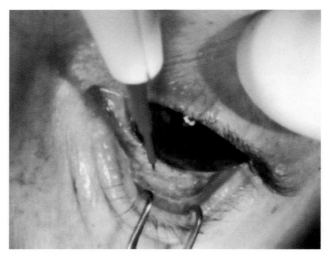

Figure 90-15. Conjunctival incision (with needle-tipped electrocautery) just below the inferior edge of the tarsal plate (left eye). Note the corneal protector in place.

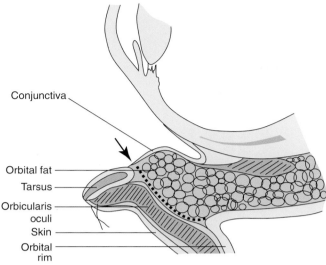

Figure 90-16. Sagittal schematic view of the plane of dissection for preseptal transconjunctival blepharoplasty. The *arrow* indicates the level of the conjunctival incision, just below the inferior edge of the tarsal plate. The dissection then proceeds *(dashed line)* toward the inferior orbital rim in the plane between the orbicularis oculi and the orbital septum overlying the orbital fat compartments.

Labels: Conjunctiva, Orbital fat, Tarsus, Orbicularis oculi, Skin, Orbital rim

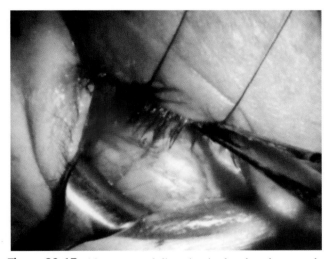

Figure 90-17. After preseptal dissection in the plane between the orbicularis oculi and the orbital septum, a Desmarres retractor placed deep to the muscle exposes the orbital septum, through which one can see the underlying orbital fat compartments (right eye). A bridle suture is in place to retract the conjunctiva superiorly for corneal protection.

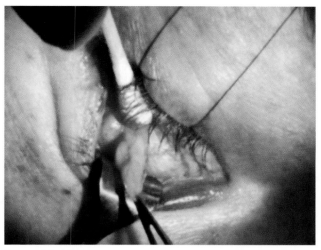

Figure 90-18. Central compartment fat being teased though an opening in the orbital septum with the aid of a cotton-tipped applicator (right eye).

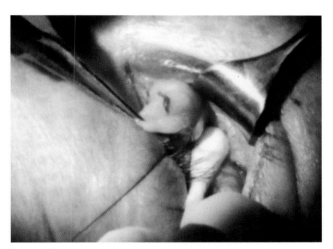

Figure 90-19. Medial compartment fat teased through an opening in the orbital septum before removal (right eye).

A fine curved hemostat is placed at the base of the mobilized fat, and small curved scissors are used for sharp resection while leaving a small cuff of fat above the hemostat. A cautery device is then used to coagulate the cut edge of the fat. Alternatively, one can use bipolar cautery across the base of the fat without a hemostat and fine scissors to incise the cauterized stump and excise the fat. With this technique one works slowly and incrementally across the base of the fat to maximize control and minimize the risk of bleeding. Adequate resection is achieved by removing only the fat that extends above the plane of the inferior orbital rim without traction; at this level one minimizes the risk of injuring the inferior oblique muscle, which lies between the medial and central fat compartments.

It is important to address each compartment individually to avoid missing any of the fat pads. The medial fat pad is distinguished from central or lateral fat by its paler color. After adequate resection has been performed, one should evaluate the resection by replacing the lower lid in its anatomic position and examining the lower lid with and without pressure on the globe. It is important to re-explore any area that continues to look prominent and to pay particular attention to bilateral symmetry. With the patient in the supine position, a slight concavity of the overall contour of the lid will generally ensure a good result.

It is not absolutely necessary to close the conjunctival incision. It will heal without problem even if left unsutured. Alternatively, a single suture can be placed

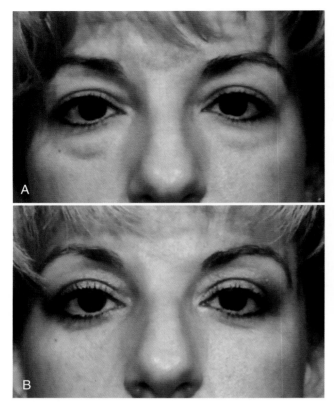

Figure 90-20. Preoperative (**A**) and postoperative (**B**) views of a lower eyelid transconjunctival blepharoplasty patient.

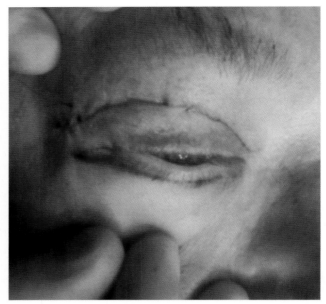

Figure 90-21. The subciliary incision is marked approximately 2 mm below the lash margin and extends 5 to 7 mm beyond the lateral canthus.

in the incision to properly align the conjunctival wound, but it should be placed lateral or medial to the corneal limbus (corneal-scleral junction) to avoid any direct corneal irritation from the suture. Fast-absorbing 6-0 catgut suture is used with an inverted buried knot. Preoperative and postoperative photos of a lower eyelid transconjunctival blepharoplasty patient are seen in Figure 90-20.

As one becomes more comfortable with the procedure, small amounts of excess skin can be removed by subciliary "pinch" excision at the same time if only a minor amount of skin resection is needed, or a mild 35% TCA peel of the periorbital area can be used to treat fine wrinkles.

Transcutaneous Approach

Transcutaneous lower lid blepharoplasty is reserved for patients with large amounts of excess skin or hypertrophy of the orbicularis muscle that needs to be addressed, as well as those with lower lid deformities secondary to laxity that would benefit from a lower lid suspension procedure.

In patients with a significant disparity in the amount of excess skin and muscle, separate skin and muscle flaps are raised to the level of the infraorbital rims, and the appropriate excesses are dealt with individually. This is less common and probably accounts for no more than 2% to 3% of all blepharoplasty patients. All other transcutaneous blepharoplasty patients are treated with the standard skin-muscle flap technique that is described later.

Markings

The lower eyelid incision parallels the lash line and is placed 1.5 to 2 mm below it (Fig. 90-21). Adequate access can often be achieved with an incision extending medially only as far as the medial limbus of the cornea and lengthening the incision further only if need be. Beyond the lateral canthus, the incision angles slightly downward and lateral, parallel to or in a lateral periorbital skin crease (crow's foot), and extends about 5 to 7 mm. It is important to make this extension only as long as needed to remove the redundant skin. The distance between the designed lateral extents of the upper and lower incisions should be at least 5 to 7 mm.

Procedure

Although this operation can be done under general anesthesia, it is typically performed under local anesthesia with intravenous sedation. Once the depth of sedation is adequate, the eyes are lubricated with ophthalmic ointment. Lidocaine (1%) with 1:100,000 epinephrine is injected along the proposed incision, as well as deep to the preseptal orbicularis oculi, with a 27-gauge, 1½-inch needle.

A no. 15 blade is then used to incise through the skin of the small extension beyond the lateral canthus or along the entire subciliary incision, through skin only. The incision lateral to the canthus is next deepened to a submuscular (preseptal) plane (Fig. 90-22). One can then blindly predissect or elevate inferiorly and medially down to the orbital rim deep to the muscle to separate the muscle from the septum beneath it with fine scissors in a blunt spreading motion (Fig. 90-23).

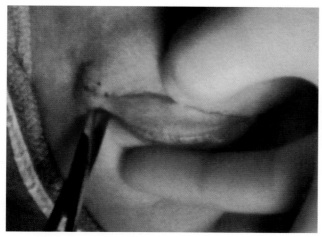

Figure 90-22. On completion of the subciliary skin-only incision, the segment beyond the lateral canthus is deepened to a submuscular plane.

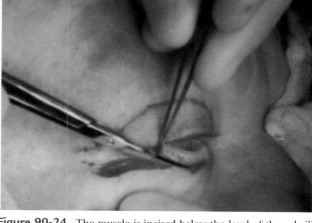

Figure 90-24. The muscle is incised below the level of the subciliary incision with a "blade-in, blade-out" maneuver to connect the skin-only pretarsal dissection with the submuscular elevation below the tarsus.

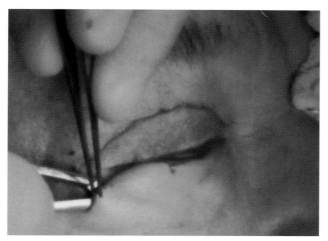

Figure 90-23. The initial blind submuscular dissection should proceed easily, without encountering any resistance, through the relatively avascular plane between the orbicularis oculi and the orbital septum deep to it. The dissection is carried toward the inferior orbital rim.

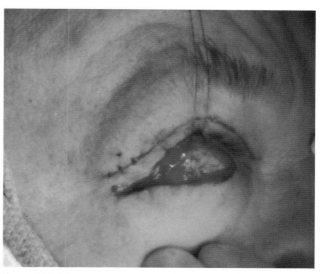

Figure 90-25. A bridle suture is placed to retract the tarsus and conjunctiva superiorly for corneal protection.

Small, sharp curved scissors are then tunneled medially under the skin in the pretarsal area, superficial to the orbicularis oculi, and the subciliary incision is completed through skin only.

At this point the dissection has involved skin only in the pretarsal area, and the pretarsal orbicularis muscle is left intact and not elevated. It is important to leave the pretarsal orbicularis muscle intact to act as a hammock and help support the lower lid to decrease the likelihood of ectropion. The dissection in the preseptal area has thus far been deep to the orbicularis.

The planes of the skin-only elevation (pretarsal) and the skin-muscle flap dissection (preseptal) are then connected by incising the muscle below the tarsus, approximately 3 to 5 mm from the lash line (Fig. 90-24). A bridle suture is placed through the superior incision margin or the gray line to retract the conjunc-

tiva cephalically for corneal protection (Fig. 90-25). The skin-muscle flap is then elevated down to the level of the infraorbital rim, and the entire orbital septum is exposed. The flap can be retracted by an assistant with a wide blunt double-ball hook (Fig. 90-26).

Small openings are made through the orbital septum to facilitate dissection of fat from each compartment (central, medial, and lateral) as needed (Figs. 90-27 and 90-28 show removal of fat from the central and medial compartments, respectively). Fat removal proceeds as previously described for preseptal transconjunctival lower lid blepharoplasty.

The skin-muscle flap is then redraped over the lower lid lashes in an upward and slightly lateral direction (Fig. 90-29). If sufficiently responsive at this point, the patient is asked to open the mouth and to look toward the top of the head. A cut is then made in the

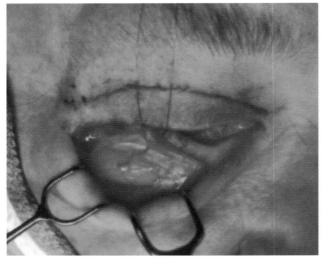

Figure 90-26. The skin-muscle flap is elevated and retracted toward the inferior orbital rim to expose the orbital septum and the underlying orbital fat compartments.

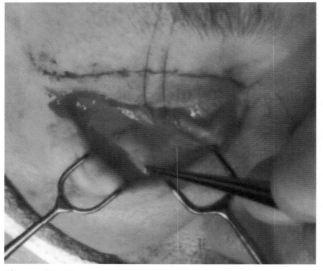

Figure 90-27. Delivery of fat from the central compartment.

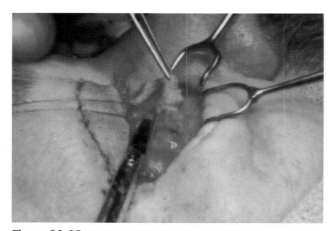

Figure 90-28. Delivery of fat from the medial compartment.

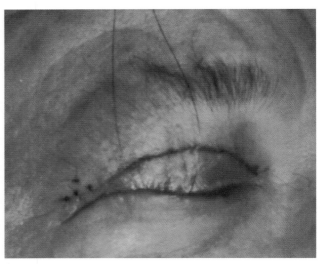

Figure 90-29. The skin-muscle flap is redraped over the infraciliary incision.

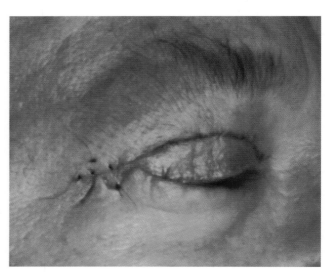

Figure 90-30. An incision is made in the flap at the lateral canthus as far as the edge of the infraciliary incision, and that point is secured with 6-0 Prolene suture, thereby effectively dividing the skin excess into two separate triangles—one medial and one lateral to the canthus.

skin-muscle flap at the level of the lateral canthus to the point at which the excess skin meets the cut edge of the infraciliary margin. That point is sutured with 6-0 Prolene, and the excess skin is effectively divided into two triangles of excess skin—one medial and one lateral to the canthus (Fig. 90-30). The surgeon next excises the extra skin, first the lateral triangle (Fig. 90-31) and then the medial triangle (Fig. 90-32), so that there is no tension on the skin closure. It is imperative that the surgeon be conservative with skin excision from the lower eyelid to minimize the risk of lid malposition. A strip of orbicularis (several millimeters) is then excised from beneath the upper margin of the skin-muscle flap (Fig. 90-33)—failure to do so would result in overlap-

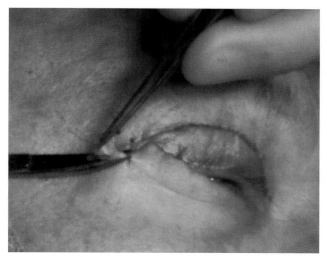

Figure 90-31. Excision of excess skin lateral to the lateral canthus.

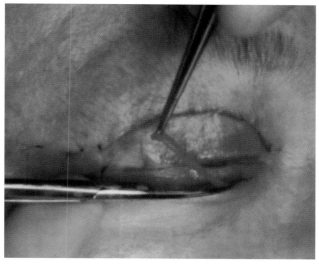

Figure 90-33. Excision of a thin strip of orbicularis muscle from beneath the skin-muscle flap edge to prevent muscle beneath the flap from overlapping the pretarsal muscle, which was preserved.

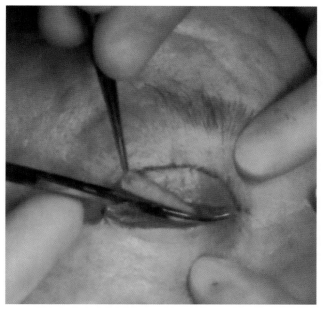

Figure 90-32. Excision of the excess triangular skin medially.

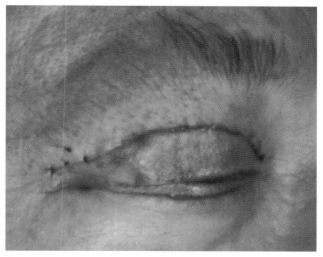

Figure 90-34. Skin-muscle flap blepharoplasty, just before skin closure with easy tension-free approximation of skin edges.

ping of this muscle over the pretarsal orbicularis that was not elevated.

After hemostasis is verified, a flap suspension suture of 5-0 PDS is placed to support the position of the lower lid through the healing period.[5] The orbicularis under the skin-muscle flap is grasped medial to and below the lateral orbital tubercle (Whitnall's tubercle) and suspended with a buried inverted suture to the periosteum at the lateral orbital tubercle. It is important to get a good bite of periosteum and also to ensure sufficient purchase on the muscle *without* dimpling the overlying skin. The skin edges at this point should lie in easy approximation (Fig. 90-34) to allow closure without tension. The wounds are then closed with interrupted 7-0 Prolene suture lateral to the canthal angle and inter-

rupted or running 6-0 fast-absorbing gut suture along the subciliary portion of the incision. Preoperative and 4-month postoperative photos of a patient who underwent a lower eyelid skin-muscle flap blepharoplasty are seen in Figure 90-35.

Postoperative Management

Postoperative management of a patient after lower lid blepharoplasty is similar whether done via the transconjunctival or the transcutaneous approach and not unlike that of the upper lids. The only difference is that if a transconjunctival approach is used for the lower lids, an ophthalmic antibiotic drop with steroid (e.g., Tobra-Dex) is applied for the first 5 days postoperatively. Patients are instructed to not wear contact lenses for at least 1 week after surgery.

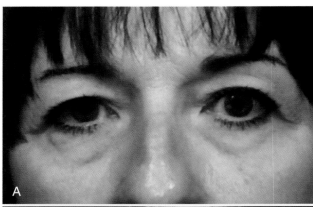
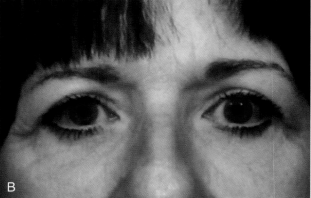

Figure 90-35. Preoperative (**A**) and postoperative (**B**) views of a lower eyelid skin-muscle flap blepharoplasty patient.

COMPLICATIONS[6]

Corneal Injury

The best treatment of corneal injuries is prevention. Lubrication should be placed in the eyes to prevent desiccation during surgery. Shields can be worn during blepharoplasty to protect the cornea, and the surgeon should be cautious about the use of abrasive gauze near the cornea.

Pain in the eye is a warning sign of a corneal injury. If any concern exists postoperatively regarding possible corneal injury, evaluation by an ophthalmologist is recommended. Fluorescein staining can be used for diagnosis, and treatment includes ophthalmic antibiotic ointment and maintenance of the eye at rest with an occlusive dressing until healing is complete.

Wound Separation

Sutures are typically removed on or before the fifth postoperative day. Infrequently, the lateral aspect of the wound may begin to separate, and this should be corrected with Steri-Strips or the wound should be resutured if necessary.

Asymmetries

Not uncommonly, postoperative asymmetries will reflect unrecognized preoperative asymmetries in excess lid skin or asymmetric preoperative brow position. Noting such asymmetries and discussing them with the patient *preoperatively* will often make minor postoperative asymmetries acceptable. If a brow procedure is not indicated, asymmetric skin excision may be necessary in an attempt to avoid postoperative differences between the two sides. Asymmetry in fat excision can also be apparent postoperatively. Again, attention to detail intraoperatively will help avoid such problems. If asymmetry persists after several months postoperatively, revision surgery will be necessary.

Dry Eyes

Possible causes of dry eyes include an unrecognized preoperative condition, injury to the lacrimal gland (uncommon), excessive skin resection, and edema. By far postoperative edema is the most common cause and should settle over a 1- to 3-week period postoperatively. The interim use of artificial tears and lubricating ointments is important to help prevent keratitis. Excessive skin resection will ultimately require repair with a full-thickness skin graft replacement.

Epiphora

Excess tearing from the eyes is common during the first 48 hours postoperatively. It is usually due to edema of the skin or temporary muscular atony, which can then impair the function of the tear drainage system. The epiphora usually resolves as the swelling subsides. Intermittent episodes may persist with changes in weather. Other possible causes include eversion of the punctum (secondary to either edema or ectropion—see later) or, less commonly, injury to the canaliculus.

Lagophthalmos

Patients are often unable to completely close their eyes because of edema in the immediate postoperative period. Most commonly, lagophthalmos is due to immediate postoperative edema. It is treated with lubricating ointments and time. If this condition is secondary to over-resection of upper lid skin, desiccation can lead to corneal injury. In such cases, release of the upper lid along with skin grafting must be considered. Again, the best treatment is prevention, which is why it is imperative to measure the amount of skin to be resected (via the aforementioned pinch technique) several times before making any skin incisions.

Ptosis

Temporary "pseudoptosis" secondary to swelling is not uncommon in the first postoperative week. Persistent ptosis suggests injury to the levator expansion during opening of the orbital septum. The levator apparatus is most at risk in the inferior portion of the wound where the surgeon is closest to the upper border of the tarsal plate, the point at which the levator fuses with the orbital septum. Any excision of muscle or opening of the septum is safest if one stays away from the lower portion of the wound after excision of skin. Persistent ptosis should be corrected by reinsertion of the levator into the tarsus or dermis.

Extraocular Muscle Injury

The inferior oblique muscle lies in a vulnerable position between the medial and central fat compartments of the lower lid. It should be looked for in every case, although it is not always seen. Being alert to the location of the muscle, however, will help avoid inadvertent injury. Care must be taken to avoid clamp, Bovie, or sharp injury to this muscle during fat dissection and resection. If immediately identified, the transected ends should be approximated. Diplopia on upward lateral gaze is indicative of injury to the muscle. Persistent postoperative diplopia that lasts longer than 1 or 2 weeks should be evaluated by an oculoplastic surgeon for appropriate care.

Lower Lid Malposition

Temporary excess "scleral show" in the immediate postoperative period may be due to edema and temporary paresis of the orbicularis oculi muscle. It will often resolve in the perioperative period as the edema lessens and the muscle reinnervates. Treatment of any chemosis includes topical steroids and prevention of exposure keratitis. Massage of the lower lid in an upward and outward direction will also help. Often, tape support of the lower lid during the early postoperative period will lessen the degree of scleral show.

Unrecognized preoperative lower lid laxity may also contribute to postoperative ectropion. In such cases, secondary canthopexy or canthoplasty may be required. If the ectropion is due to overaggressive skin resection, secondary surgery to correct the deformity with scar release and full-thickness skin grafting may be necessary after several months of observation and conservative management.

The best means of treatment is prevention. The transconjunctival approach avoids the contraction associated with healing of the skin and muscle incisions used for the infraciliary approach. In addition, patients with any degree of laxity who require skin excision via an infraciliary approach should be considered for prophylactic lateral canthopexy.

Retrobulbar Hematoma/Visual Loss

Retrobulbar hematoma is the most feared complication after routine blepharoplasty. The most likely cause is a vascular injury with retraction of the bleeding vessel into the retrobulbar space. The eye becomes firm, chemotic, and progressively more proptotic. The lids cannot close as the globe continues to bulge outward. Progressively increasing intraocular pressure can lead to ophthalmoplegia, ischemia of the optic nerve, and visual loss. A retrobulbar hematoma generally develops within the first 4 to 6 hours postoperatively, and prompt diagnosis and management are critical to prevent permanent visual loss.

Initial treatment involves opening of incisions; iced saline compresses; 20% mannitol (2 g/kg) as an osmotic agent to decrease intraocular pressure; acetazolamide (Diamox) 500 mg intravenously; dexamethasone (Decadron) 10 mg intravenously; control of hypertension (if present); head elevation; and correction of any coagulopathies. Visual acuity should be evaluated frequently.

Any deterioration in visual acuity is an urgent sign and, when coupled with elevated intraocular pressure, signifies potential optic nerve ischemia. In this situation, in addition to removal of all external sutures, lateral canthotomy and inferior cantholysis are indicated on an emergency basis to facilitate orbital decompression. Emergency ophthalmic consultation is necessary but should not delay performance of canthotomy and cantholysis if faced with visual compromise.

PEARLS

- A well-considered preoperative evaluation of the upper and lower eyelids, including assessment of orbital fat, skin, lid laxity/tone, and brow position, and a general medical and ophthalmic history are essential for guiding decisions regarding the surgical approach and extent of surgery.
- Conservatism is always warranted with eyelid surgery. It is always easier to do more at a later date if necessary, but complications resulting from overaggressive eyelid surgery can be very difficult to correct.
- For upper eyelid surgery, preoperative skin markings should be checked and rechecked to avoid excessive excision of skin.
- Absolute hemostasis is necessary to minimize the possibility of postoperative retrobulbar hematoma.
- The risk of lower eyelid malposition is much lower with a transconjunctival approach.

PITFALLS

- Failure to consider brow position as it relates to any apparent excess of upper eyelid skin may still leave patients with a somewhat hooded appearance or "crowded" upper periorbital region. In patients in whom the primary problem is brow ptosis, it should be addressed either instead of or in addition to upper blepharoplasty.
- Opening the orbital septum low toward the tarsal plate in the upper eyelid increases the risk for injury to the levator aponeurosis and iatrogenic ptosis.
- Overaggressive surgery or fat removal, whether from the upper or lower eyelids, can create a hollowed, gaunt appearance in addition to functional complications such as lagophthalmos and eyelid malposition.

- Patients with a very prominent, protrusive globe ("pseudoproptosis") in which the corneal plane lies anterior to the inferior orbital rim on lateral view—the so-called negative vector—are at high risk for postoperative eyelid malposition with lower lid transcutaneous approaches.
- Lack of attention to hemostasis through every step of the operation may result in injury to important structures (e.g., levator aponeurosis, lacrimal gland, tarsal plate, inferior oblique muscle) or worse, retrobulbar hematoma.

References

1. Kontis TC, Papel ID, Larrabee WF: Surgical anatomy of the eyelids. Facial Plast Surg 10:1-5, 1994.
2. Pastorek N: Upper lid blepharoplasty. Facial Plast Surg Clin N Am 3:143-157, 1995.
3. Perkins SW: Transconjunctival lower lid blepharoplasty. Facial Plast Surg Clin N Am 3:175-187, 1995.
4. Smullen SM, Mangat DS: Cosmetic lower eyelid surgery: Transcutaneous approach. Facial Plast Surg Clin N Am 3:167-174, 1995.
5. Pastorek NJ: Blepharoplasty update. Facial Plast Surg Clin N Am 10:23-27, 2002.
6. Adamson PA, Constantinides MS: Complications of blepharoplasty. Facial Plast Surg Clin N Am 3:211-221, 1995.

Chapter **91**

Soft Tissue Trauma

Bernard J. Costello and John F. Caccamese, Jr.

Facial injuries account for a significant number of emergency department visits each year, with 50% to 70% of these injuries having a soft tissue component.[1,2] Repair plus reconstruction of facial injuries is a highly specialized endeavor best treated by those with experience and a comprehensive understanding of the mechanism of injury, the complex anatomy of the region, and the physiologic and psychosocial impact that some injuries have. Most patients have a high level of expectation that after treatment their appearance will be largely unchanged from their preinjury state. Unfortunately, regardless of the skill of the surgeon, this is sometimes not the case because of the severity of the injury. A recent survey prioritized cosmetic outcome, more so than function, as the single most important factor to patients with facial lacerations.[3] This chapter reviews the basic concepts important in the repair and reconstruction of soft tissue injuries of the face.

EVALUATION

Evaluation of soft tissue injuries of the face begins much the same as for any injured state. The primary and secondary surveys are performed, at which time other injuries might be recognized. At times, airway protection is needed because of the complexity of the injury or massive bleeding involving the airway. Tracheotomy or cricothyrotomy is considered for patients with severe injuries that prohibit intubation or when extensive edema is anticipated, such as with severe avulsion or blast injuries of the oral cavity.

Initial stabilization occasionally requires control of hemorrhage. In the facial region, pressure dressings usually suffice for such purposes; however, larger vessel and arterial bleeding will require ligation. Blind application of clamps is discouraged because there are multiple structures of importance, such as the facial nerve, within the deep tissues.

After stabilization, a detailed examination of the craniofacial skeleton and soft tissues is performed. In addition, the superficial structures of the face (e.g., eyelids, nose, ears), deep structures such as the parotid gland and duct, facial nerves, and the lacrimal gland and its drainage system must be carefully examined in a systematic fashion. Imaging is then used to further delineate the injuries, because facial fractures are common in patients who have sustained soft tissue trauma to the face. Injuries may then be managed definitively, as in simple lacerations, or expectantly, as in crush and blast injuries. Severe crush or blast injuries are often subject to further soft tissue necrosis and leave a more significant wound than that seen at initial examination.

PREPARATION

Preparing the sites for repair and reconstruction is important for both defining the extent of injury and preventing complications. Most facial wounds should be closed within 24 hours to avoid an increased risk for infection. The rich vascular supply of the region affords the surgeon some latitude in the management of these injuries that is not seen with extremity wounds or other less vascularized regions. Perioperative intravenous antibiotics should be considered for contaminated wounds and those exposed to sinus and oral flora.

In preparation for closure, wounds should be thoroughly cleansed with sterile saline, and pulsatile irrigation systems should be considered if the wound is grossly contaminated with debris. Most wounds will be clean or clean-contaminated with little chance for infection if irrigated appropriately and empirical perioperative antibiotics are selected according to the expected contaminants. However, for grossly contaminated wounds, consideration should be given to a prolonged course of antibiotics.

After thorough preparation, the wound should be rendered hemostatic, again using local measures, suture ligation, and electrocautery when appropriate. Bipolar cautery is helpful in areas where motor nerves may be present. Débridement of the wound is accomplished when necessary, and hemostasis is achieved again. Removal of debris that is both large and small is important for healing, as well as for cosmesis of the area. Fine particles left embedded in the epidermis and dermal layers may cause tattooing, which is more difficult to manage secondarily. Aggressive removal of these particles with a nail brush, individually with a no. 11 blade, or by primary dermabrasion is recommended in most cases because secondary removal tends to be less successful and may be more damaging.

CLASSIFICATION OF INJURY AND MANAGEMENT TECHNIQUES

Types of Injury

Lacerations

Lacerations of the superficial and deep soft tissues of the face occur in an assortment of patterns and with varying complexity. The term *laceration* implies that all tissues are present but disrupted, so primary closure is usually uncomplicated. However, lacerations vary greatly, depending on the mechanism of injury. The shearing action involved in a dog bite injures the tissues in a much different manner than does the clean cut of a sharp blade. Moreover, the mechanism and severity of injury have implications with regard to the final aesthetic result. Planning closure of the laceration requires consideration of the patient's healing capabilities, tissue quality, and orientation of the laceration in relation to the relaxing skin tension lines (RSTLs).

Simple linear lacerations are easily repaired if particular attention is paid to reapproximation of the deep layers, obliteration of dead space, and orientation of the wound to the RSTLs. In simple lacerations, revision is not usually necessary unless excessive scarring occurs or if the wound directly opposes the RSTLs, which may benefit from reorientation. Stellate lacerations are generally the result of shearing, blunt, or explosive forces that crush and break the skin in multiple directions and thus naturally violate the RSTLs with multiple flaps of varying depth and irregularity. The force often results in contused and necrotic wound edges, which at times culminates in further tissue loss. A combination of blood, clot, edema, and elastic retraction of the skin edges often gives the appearance of an avulsion injury. However, after meticulous cleansing the true extent of the wound can be appreciated. Débridement of these wounds should be sparing but complete because the vascular supply is generally good and aesthetic results are best with minimal débridement.

Repair of lacerations requires precision and attention to detail when they are present in such a conspicuous place as the face. A variety of techniques are used when closing lacerations of the facial tissues (Fig. 91-1). Several basic concepts warrant discussion when considering selection of the repair technique:

1. *Tension-free closure.* A tension-free closure minimizes scarring and is achieved by ensuring that the deeper layers of the closure provide enough tensile strength to allow reapproximation of the epidermis without undue tension. Suture marks are more likely to occur when a wound is closed under tension at the epidermal level. Precisely placed sutures are helpful in preventing this problem. A well-performed deep closure will also allow early removal of skin sutures, thereby further preventing epithelialization of the suture tract, which leads to suture marks.

2. *Wound eversion.* Placement of sutures to evert the superficial layers is important in obtaining an aesthetic result. Eversion should be explained to patients so that they will understand that flattening should occur with time. Repairs that are neutral or inverted have a tendency to contract and invert further during the initial healing phases. Scarring that is depressed is much more noticeable.

3. *Anatomic placement of sutures.* Attention to anatomic layers with symmetry and precise placement contributes to a wound that heals in a more predictable and aesthetic manner.

Contusions

Contusions exhibit bruising and swelling, as well as hematoma formation when subcutaneous vessels rupture. Contusions may indicate an underlying fracture, such as on the chin (e.g., subcondylar mandible fractures), and spectacle hematomas of the periorbital tissues (e.g., orbitozygomatic fractures). Most contusions require no treatment other than for symptomatic relief of pain and swelling, such as the application of ice, elevated head positioning, and analgesics. However, severely contused laceration edges should also be sharply débrided if it is likely that these areas may break down later because of the extent of the trauma.

Abrasions

Abrasions are superficial wounds of the skin and mucosa and involve loss of superficial epithelium with exposure of the underlying dermis or submucosa. Injuries of greater depth tend to be grouped with avulsions. Healing occurs by rapid re-epithelialization (0.5 mm/day) and typically requires only supportive care. Initial débridement and tissue cleansing may be of benefit when the skin is embedded with road debris or has been subject to powder burns. Failure to cleanse the wound may potentiate traumatic tattooing, which occurs when wound healing takes place with embedded debris. Thorough cleansing with a brush usually accomplishes this quite well, but primary or secondary dermabrasion is sometimes necessary. Other adjuvant materials can be used to facilitate the healing process and prevent the accumulation of fibrinous plaque, such as antibiotic ointments, nonadherent dressings, and silicone gel sheeting. It should be noted that to date, few data have demonstrated significant aesthetic improvement with the use of these materials; however, in the author's experience, for large abrasions, these dressings decrease crusting and make wound care less painful.

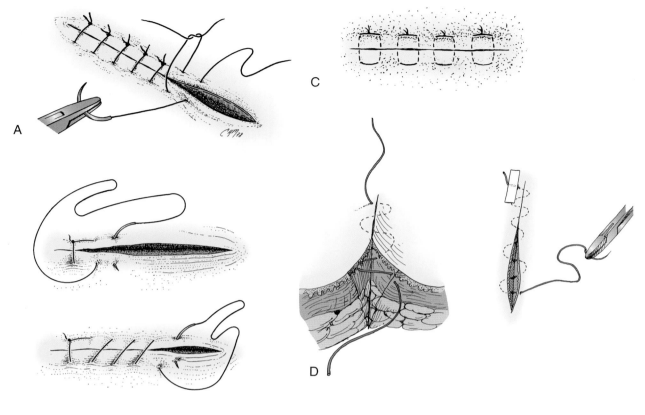

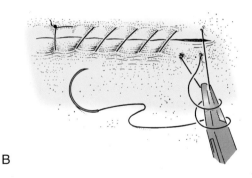

Figure 91-1. **A,** Simple interrupted sutures should be placed evenly and far enough away from the laceration edge that eversion of the skin edge is achieved. **B,** A simple continuous suture may be used for lacerations that are easily approximated. **C,** Horizontal mattress sutures are rarely used on skin but may be used for wounds that require extra strength, such as avulsions or gunshot wounds, and are expected to require revision. The surgeon must remember to avoid tying the sutures too tight or the blood supply to the margins of the laceration will be constricted. **D,** Running subcuticular sutures may be used in wounds that are well approximated and cleanly lacerated. A very aesthetic closure can be achieved if the wound edges are everted appropriately. (*Redrawn from Laskin DM [ed]: Oral and Maxillofacial Surgery, vol 1. St Louis, CV Mosby, 1980, pp 277-280.*)

Burns

Facial burns range from superficial to full thickness, depending on the cause and duration of the exposure. Facial burns occur in approximately one half of all patients admitted to the burn unit. Although most facial burns are superficial, deep partial-thickness or full-thickness burns do occur, and the facial anatomy is inexorably altered. Primary reconstructive efforts are focused on preservation of function with the understanding that achieving an aesthetic preinjury result is challenging. Large areas of skin loss are sometimes replaced with split-thickness skin, but it is a poor substitute for facial skin and specialized structures such as the eyelids and lips. Serial excision, local flaps, and free tissue transfer are also options, depending on the burn site.[4]

Trapdoor and Circular/Pedicled Lacerations

"*Trapdoor*" *lacerations* result in a soft tissue flap that presents healing dilemmas because of the beveled nature of the flap, which then results in a pincushion deformity. The traumatic event creates varied wound depth that often requires additional undermining of the opposing side of the laceration to properly layer the closure and evert the edges. Freshening of the edges is also commonly needed to provide opposing parallel surfaces in the same tissue plane to better distribute contractile force during the healing period. Small Z-plasties along the circumference of a trapdoor wound may be helpful in avoiding less than ideal contraction, scarring, and contour deformities; however, this technique should be attempted only when one is sure that the injury does not have a significant contusive element.

Bite Wounds

Treatment of bite wounds merits separate discussion because they are often complex wounds with features of lacerations, avulsions, and contusions concomitant with polymicrobial contamination. The crushing force delivered by the dog's jaw often results in widespread tissue injury that is grossly contaminated with up to 64 species of bacteria.[5] Antibiotics are always considered in the management of bite wounds because the contamination is usually polymicrobial in nature. Penicillins and cephalosporins are generally effective in treating the predominantly gram-positive flora.

Children younger than 10 years are most frequently the victims of facial dog bites, largely because dogs have easy access to a child's face.[6,7] The lips, nose, and cheeks are the most commonly injured structures and some the most challenging to reconstruct.[8,9] Conservative débridement and aggressive cleansing should be undertaken promptly, followed by primary closure when appropriate. Definitive reconstruction with local or distant tissue can be carried out once the zone of necrosis has become evident and the wound is sufficiently clean (Fig. 91-2). Puncture wounds are often left unclosed.

Though uncommonly encountered in the United States, rabies must always be considered with animal bites, especially with unprovoked attacks or bites from high-risk animals. Raccoons and bats carry the disease with the greatest frequency in the United States, although foxes, skunks, and wild dogs are also considered high risk. Human rabies immune globulin and vaccine are recommended for bites and exposures, irrespective of the time between exposure and treatment, unless the individual has previously been vaccinated and rabies antibodies can be detected. The vaccine takes 7 to 10 days to induce an immune response, and immunity lasts approximately 2 years. The vaccine is injected into the deltoid region at a dose of 1 mL on days 0, 3, 7, 14, and 28. Rabies immune globulin (20 IU/kg) is administered with as much of the dose as possible infiltrated in and around the wound (location permitting) and the rest given intramuscularly in the gluteal region with a needle of sufficient length to ensure intramuscular injection. The syringes and needles used for vaccine and immune globulin should be different. The tetanus vaccination status of the patient should also be ascertained, and appropriate administration of either tetanus vaccine or tetanus immune globulin should be completed (Table 91-1).[10]

Avulsions

Avulsions occur as a result of a high-energy or shearing injury, such as motor vehicle trauma, a gunshot, or an animal bite. For small wounds, adjacent tissue can be mobilized and advanced for primary closure. However, these injuries can be some of the greatest challenges to the facial trauma surgeon. Flaps that can be revascularized should be replanted when possible. When tissue loss is imminent because of the severity of trauma or delay in treatment, avulsive injuries may benefit from a period of observation with serial débridement and dressing changes to ensure adjacent tissue viability before definitive reconstruction. Typically, wound necrosis is evident within a few days to weeks and reconstruction can then be completed. Avulsion of special structures such as the ear and scalp may require salvage with microvascular replantation techniques. Other large defects may call for the recruitment of distant pedicled or microvascular flaps after a period of observation and expectant wound management (Fig. 91-3). Finally, primary skin grafting, followed by secondary revision (i.e., tissue expansion with local flap rotation, serial graft excision, free flap reconstruction), continues to remain a good option in many complex wounds rather than depending on healing by secondary intention, which can lead to extensive scar contraction.

Gunshot Wounds

Firearm injuries are common in countries that do not have strict gun control laws. A detailed discussion of the complexities of gunshot wounds is beyond the scope of this chapter, but the basic concepts presented here are important to recognize. A variety of injury patterns can be expected depending on the type of projectile. Low-velocity weapons such as pellet guns may cause limited local damage, whereas high-velocity projectiles may disrupt tissue along a defined vector. Various projectiles are designed with differing degrees of soft and hard tissue damage capability. Most of these injuries depend on how the projectile passes through tissue, including tumble, yaw, and other physical properties. Projectiles with higher velocity and a propensity to twist, fragment, and turn through tissue will produce more significant damage. Additionally, bone and tooth fragments become secondary projectiles that tend to increase the field of injury. The blast injury that occurs with the initial trauma varies according to these projectile characteristics but is often not apparent for days after the injury. The greater the injury capability of the projectile, the longer the surgeon should wait to consider definitive reconstruction. A certain degree of additional tissue necrosis will occur in a delayed fashion, depending on these characteristics, and expectant wound management is advisable. The ultra high-velocity weapons used in combat may cause particularly devastating injury to the facial soft tissues and skeleton. Reconstruction may include local, regional, or free tissue flaps, depending on the degree of injury. Revision may be expected in more significant injury.

Several key concepts are important to remember when closing complex wounds such as gunshot wounds:

- Layered closure prevents tension on the wound at the epidermal level, which will decrease scarring potential. All dead space should be closed with an anatomically layered closure. This is particularly important for the random-pattern flaps that may be developed as rotation or advancement flaps for local closure of small to medium-sized defects.
- Débridement is important for successful healing of the wound, but the surgeon should remember that

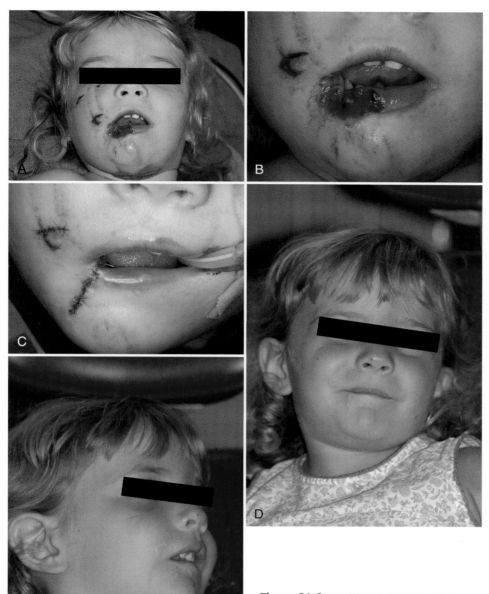

Figure 91-2. A, Clinical photo showing a young girl after being bitten multiple times by her dog. **B,** Magnified view showing that 50% of the superficial lip was avulsed to the commissure. **C,** Layered closure yields an aesthetic repair by closing muscle, mucosa, and skin independently. **D** and **E,** One year after the injury.

because the face is very vascular, aggressive débridement is often not necessary. Tissues that are minimally contused do not generally need to be débrided. Small irregular edges should be excised and simplified in most cases.

- RSTLs are helpful in planning local flap recruitment. A more aesthetic result is obtained when the flaps can be designed to allow incisions, backcuts, and dog-ear repairs to fall within the RSTLs.

Anesthesia

In most instances, local anesthesia, when appropriately applied, is sufficient to allow complete closure of the wounds typically seen in the emergency department.

Table 91-1	PROTOCOL FOR PROPHYLAXIS OF WOUNDS FOR TETANUS			
	Clean and Minor Wounds		**All Other Wounds**	
Tetanus Toxoid Vaccination Status	**Td**	**TIG**	**Td**	**TIG**
Unknown or less than 3 doses	Yes	No	Yes	Yes
3 or more doses	No*	No	No†	No

*Yes if more than 10 years since the last dose.
†Yes if more than 5 years since the last dose.
Td, tetanus and diphtheria toxoids; TIG, tetanus immune globulin.
Adapted from Diphtheria, tetanus, and pertussis: Recommendations for vaccine use and other preventive measures. Recommendations of the Immunization Practices Advisory Committee (ACIP). MMWR Recomm Rep 40(RR-10):1-28, 1991.

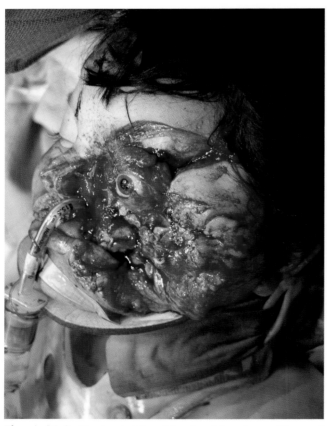

Figure 91-3. Massive facial avulsion involving the eyelids, nasal complex, upper and lower lips, and check after a motor vehicle crash in which this young child was not restrained. It is important to note damage to the globe, lacrimal system, facial nerve, salivary glands, and nasal drainage system for the sinuses in such complex injuries. Composite soft tissue grafting with microvascular techniques can be used either immediately or as a staged procedure.

Particularly complicated wounds or wounds in small children will often require sedation or general anesthesia. The benefits of general anesthesia in the operating room are evident when caring for complicated wounds because better instrumentation and lighting are readily available.

It is helpful to be proficient in local anesthetic blocks of the trigeminal system when repairing wounds of the face. Frequently, large areas can be profoundly anesthetized when blocking the region with a precisely placed local anesthetic. Generally, 1% lidocaine with 1:100,000 epinephrine is used and provides profound anesthesia in the area of repair. One must consider the maximal allowable dose in individuals who require other procedures concurrently or have extensive lacerations requiring multiple injections. Such consideration is particularly important in small children because it is not difficult to reach the maximal allowable dose with what seems to be a small volume of anesthetic. Nerve blocks can be helpful in these patients inasmuch as less volume is required to achieve profound anesthesia. One must also make sure that facial nerve function has been thoroughly evaluated when anesthetizing lateral face wounds, because exploration and primary repair may be warranted before wound closure.

Suture Materials

A variety of sophisticated materials are available to the surgeon for repair and reconstruction of soft tissue injury, and understanding their capabilities and handling characteristics is important (Table 91-2). Both nonresorbable and resorbable materials are available in a variety of sizes and with a variety of needle types. Deeper layers are best reapproximated with longer-lasting resorbable suture that is braided. Suture strength and the rate of degradation should anticipate forces placed on the wound particular to the anatomic locale and provide enough tensile strength to support the wound and allow complete healing. Subcutaneous and deep dermal sutures are best placed with the knot buried and the use of resorbable suture. Skin is best reapproximated with nonresorbable monofilament suture at least 5-0 or smaller in size. It is often convenient to consider resorbable material in pediatric patients because they may require an additional anesthetic or involuntary restraint to remove simple sutures. These materials may have slightly more reactivity and cause additional inflammation at the healing site. Staples may be used in less cosmetic areas such as scalp wounds.

Needles come in a variety of shapes and sizes as well. The skin is best sutured with a cutting needle to minimize trauma to skin during placement. Most deep tissues and mucosa are best approximated with tapered or combination needles to minimize trauma to tissues. Keratinized mucosa such as the palate or gingiva may be closed with a cutting needle.

Adequate instrumentation and lighting are essential for accurate surgical closure. Delicate needle holders and fine pickups are helpful to approximate tissue in a detailed and atraumatic fashion. Fastidious tissue handling is also crucial for an aesthetic closure. Excessive epidermal handling with tissue forceps can result in crush injury to the skin edges. Picking up tissue in the deep and subcutaneous planes minimizes trauma to the epidermis and improves superficial healing. The surgeon should be comfortable with all forms of hand and instrument ties, as well as suture-placing techniques. Mastering these techniques is essential to providing a superior closure.

Cyanoacrylate Tissue Adhesives

When applied carefully, the use of tissue adhesives for closure of wounds is both cost-effective and efficient. Their efficacy for strength of closure and cosmesis has been demonstrated in the literature.[11,12] Two main cyanoacrylate-based tissue adhesives are available for traumatic wound closure, butyl-2-cyanoacrylate (Histoacryl, Braun, Germany) and 2-octylcyanoacrylate (Dermabond, Ethicon, Somerville, NJ). The 2-octyl polymer was created to avert some of the shortcomings of its predecessor. Butyl-2-cyanoacrylate maintains only 10% to 15% of the wound strength of 5-0 monofilament on closure day 1; however, its strength was equivalent on days 5 to 7. 2-Octylcyanoacrylate, in contrast, has roughly three times the three-dimensional breaking strength of butyl-2-cyanoacrylate, which compares more favorably with conventional wound closure.

Cyanoacrylate tissue adhesive can be used topically to close skin lacerations on its own, or it can be used along with deep sutures. Deep dermal sutures can be placed to obtain proper wound edge eversion. As with suture techniques, everting the wound edges is essential to the cosmetic success of skin closure with tissue adhe-

sives, because eversion helps alleviate the effects of scar widening. Skin apposition should be maintained with forceps or fingers regardless of whether deep sutures are used during the application. For optimal results, multiple thin layers should be applied over the epidermis and allowed to dry for approximately 10 to 30 seconds. This technique prevents pooling and running of the tissue adhesive, which can lead to significant complications in certain areas of the face (i.e., eyes, ears), and it also diminishes the heat transferred to tissues during polymerization.[12-14] It should be noted that this material is not recommended around the eyelid tissues because unintended adhesion of the eyelid or other critical structures has occurred. Tissue adhesive materials are not viscous and tend to run quite easily. For this reason, moist gauze should be present to remove excess when necessary.

Postoperative Wound Care

A carefully crafted dressing is important both for protection of the wound from contaminants and for care of the wound. In most instances, a minimal dressing is used that may consist of small bandage strips or antibiotic ointment placed several times a day for 1 week. Complex wounds may require extensive dressings, retention sutures, or temporary bolsters. Pressure dressings may be helpful in certain types of scalp wounds to avoid hematoma formation, or drains may be used in areas of potential dead space. Ear lacerations often require the placement of bolster dressings to help avoid hematoma formation. Tarsorrhaphy and Frost sutures may be placed in eyelids to prevent unwanted contraction and disruption of certain repairs.

After the acute healing phase has passed and a small amount of intrinsic strength has developed in the wound, early suture removal is possible, and meticulous

Table 91-2	COMMONLY USED SUTURE MATERIALS FOR FACIAL REPAIR AND RECONSTRUCTION WITH SOME OF THEIR IMPORTANT CHARACTERISTICS			
Suture	**Absorbable**	**Common Site of Use**	**Pearls**	
Polyglycolic acid	Yes	Deep layers of closure such as fascia	Excellent handing characteristics because it is a braided suture; moderate reactivity; offered with antibiotic treatment; smaller suture may lose tensile strength at about 2 weeks; bury the knots	
Polyglecaprone	Yes	Deep and subcuticular closure; fine suture may be used for skin	Good handing characteristics for a monofilament suture; moderate reactivity; very small sizes such as 5-0 can be used for key sutures on skin because resorption is rather quick	
Chromic gut	Yes	Mucosal repair; very fine suture may be used for skin closure	More reactivity and less desirable handing characteristics; monofilament suture; very useful for mucosal closure because it is resorbed quickly	
Nylon	No	Skin closure or subcuticular pull-out suture	Monofilament suture that requires removal; minimal reactivity; easily seen for removal because of its black color	
Polypropylene	No	Skin closure or subcuticular pull-out suture	Monofilament suture that requires removal; excellent handing characteristics; minimal reactivity; easily seen for removal because of its blue color	

care of the wound continues. Sutures can generally be removed in 5 to 7 days for most facial wounds. Early removal prevents hatchmarking, although wounds that are under some tension may require a longer retention period. Alternatively, every other suture can be removed at an early visit. Additional adhesive bandaging may be used to reinforce and protect the wound for an additional week or two. Once the sutures are removed, the wound may be gently massaged several times daily to help hasten maturation and soften any hypertrophic or uneven subcutaneous scarring. Supplemental material such as vitamins, silicone gels, or lotions may help improve scarring in some instances, but positive outcome data are lacking. Use of sunblock is encouraged because excessive exposure to ultraviolet radiation can alter the pigmentation and leave the scar more visible. Sunblock that is nonirritating to the eyes is important for upper facial wounds.

Revision

Secondary reconstruction of soft tissue injuries of the face is beyond the scope of this chapter, but it is important to discuss the likelihood of secondary surgery with patients who have endured trauma. Scar revision is inevitable in some patients who either do not exhibit optimal healing or have scarring as a result of a more severe injury. In general, most revisions are best performed after 1 year unless extremely unfavorable aesthetics or functional concerns are present. Scar maturation continues beyond the initial months of healing and will continue to improve the appearance of many scars without significant intervention in the first year. A long-term follow-up schedule should be discussed with patients to ensure the best result, as well as their own personal satisfaction.

SPECIAL CONSIDERATIONS

Periocular Injury

When evaluating periocular soft tissue trauma, one must first exclude underlying globe injury and cranio-orbital fractures. In addition, when evaluating the upper and lower eyelids, one should consider the location, depth, tissue loss, function, and presence of foreign bodies. Measurements of canthal distances and symmetry are important to assess medial or lateral canthus detachment. Primary reconstruction of these specialized orbital injuries is usually more successful than secondary reconstruction.

If the injury is linear in nature, repair consists of anatomic reapproximation of the tissue layers. The eyelid margin, the eyelash line, the gray line, and the meibomian glands are conventionally used as landmarks to direct the operative repair. The first sutures are placed along the lid margin or gray line to initiate proper alignment, as well as to provide traction for the remainder of the closure. Size 6-0 silk or nylon is used for this purpose, with the ends cut long and tied down under adjacent skin sutures to avoid corneal abrasion. The tarsal plate and pretarsal muscles are closed with

6-0 Vicryl, and the skin is closed with 6-0 nylon. The conjunctiva may be left unclosed if the wound edges are well apposed. It is essential to ensure proper alignment of the tarsus and eversion of the lid margin to avoid a notched appearance of the lid.

Complex lacerations and eyelid avulsion injuries may appear to have what seems to be significant tissue loss; however, once cleaned and thoroughly evaluated, they can usually be closed primarily. Should the cornea become exposed, *immediate* attention is required to keep it moist until definitive lid repair has been accomplished (Fig. 91-4). It is important to reposition the injured tissues so that the canthi, orbital septum, and levator aponeurosis are restored to the best positions possible (Fig. 91-5). When tissue loss has occurred, every effort should be made to preserve existing structures, even when their appearance is marginal. Avulsed tissues can often be used as composite or full-thickness grafts for the reconstruction of partial-thickness defects. Full-thickness defects of up to one half the eyelid may be closed primarily with the use of releasing incisions. Tissue loss of greater than one half the eyelid may require a cheek advancement flap, lid switch procedure, or skin graft.

Any disturbance in the lacrimal system can lead to an excess or deficit of tear availability, which may then result in corneal damage or visual changes. Both the secretory and excretory aspects of the lacrimal system are vulnerable to injury. The secretory component consists of the lacrimal gland, the conjunctiva, and the minor glands of the eyelid. A tear film is produced and distributed over the cornea primarily by the action of the eyelids and then drains medially. Drainage occurs via the lacrimal canalicular system, the lacrimal sac, and the nasolacrimal duct. The canaliculi are absolutely crucial for normal tear drainage and are the most frequently injured structures of the lacrimal system.[15]

Injury to the lacrimal canaliculi should be suspected with any laceration medial to the puncta. The wound should be evaluated by direct inspection, probing, or direct or indirect instillation of visible fluids into the canalicular system. This should allow thorough evaluation of the patency and continuity of the canaliculi by the presence or absence of injected fluid in the wound versus the nose. Fluorescein is most commonly used for this purpose.

Injuries to the superior canaliculus rarely cause epiphora; however, most transections of the inferior system should be repaired, because the inferior canaliculus is responsible for the majority of normal tear drainage. Primary repair of canalicular injuries includes careful probing and intubation of the canaliculi under magnification. The proximal canaliculus is often difficult to identify and may be localized by probing the uninjured punctum and then passing the probe medially. The probe can then be passed through the wound into the distal aspect of the canaliculus and through the injured punctum. Intubation is frequently performed with either a monocanalicular or bicanalicular silicon tube, which is left in place for 3 months until re-epithelialization of the canaliculus has occurred and the peri-

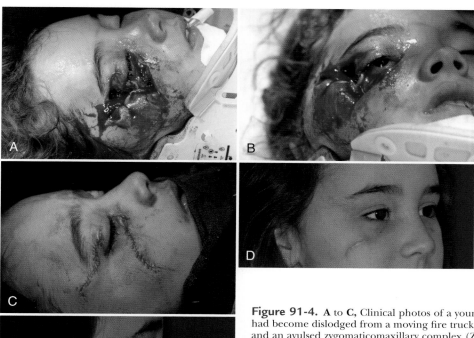

Figure 91-4. **A** to **C,** Clinical photos of a young girl who was struck by a fire hose that had become dislodged from a moving fire truck with disruption of the periorbital tissues and an avulsed zygomaticomaxillary complex (ZMC) fracture. After plating the ZMC on the back table, the wound was closed and all the periorbital structures were repositioned with minimal débridement. **D** and **E,** Three months after the repair, the wound has the typical erythema associated with ongoing tissue remodeling, and all her orbital and periorbital structures are functioning well.

canalicular inflammation has resolved.[15,16] Once this is complete, pericanalicular sutures are placed and the lid margin is closed.

Facial Nerve Injury

Traumatic injury to the extracranial facial nerve should be suspected when lateral facial lacerations and parotid injuries are recognized. When possible, it is important to obtain an accurate examination of the cranial nerves before the administration of local anesthetic, sedative medications, or paralytics. Unfortunately, this may be difficult in patients who have suffered multisystem trauma or significant neurologic injury. Focal deficits in facial tone and expression may help localize the damaged segment. This also facilitates appropriate exploration at the time of wound closure. As a general rule, facial nerve injuries distal to a vertical line dropped from the lateral canthus of the eye are not repaired because they are too small for successful coaptation. Microsurgical repair of the nerve can be successfully performed within 2 to 3 weeks of the original injury. However, immediate repair may be easier for the surgeon because stimulation of the distal axons before wallerian degeneration aids in identification of the nerves. Should the repair be delayed as a result of severe systemic injuries, the nerve endings should be marked with suture at the time of débridement (Fig. 91-6).

Options for repair of extracranial facial nerve injury include primary neurorrhaphy, graft neurorrhaphy, and nerve transposition. Occasionally, superficial parotidectomy must be performed to adequately mobilize the proximal and distal nerve branches for an optimal tension-free repair. Concomitant gland and duct injuries should be addressed at this time to avoid the formation of a sialocele, tissue inflammation, and impaired healing, which may adversely affect the outcome of the nerve repair. Regardless of the procedure chosen, the repair is best performed under magnification. In preparation for the repair, excision of the proximal and distal nerve stumps to provide healthy fascicles should be undertaken.

Common nerve donor sites for reconstruction of the facial nerve include the great auricular nerve, the sural nerve, and the median antebrachial cutaneous nerve. Selection of the donor site should be based on the graft dimensions needed for the particular repair and the patient's acceptance of the notion that anesthesia will be experienced at the donor site. Finally, nerve transposition of the hypoglossal nerve or an intact branch of the ipsilateral facial nerve has proved useful in select cases. One drawback of this technique includes mass movement of the face rather than detailed individual muscle group movement.[17,18]

Parotid Gland and Duct Injuries

Lacerations of the gland parenchyma are managed by layered closure (to include the capsule of the gland) whenever possible. Sialocele is an infrequent

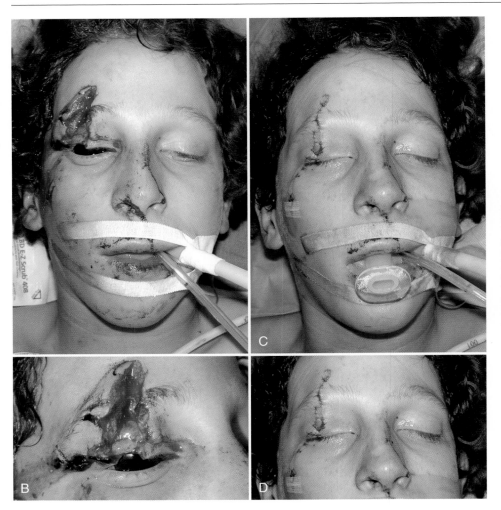

Figure 91-5. A and **B,** Preoperative photos of an Amish boy with a chainsaw injury to the right upper lid and brow. The orbital musculature and septum are disrupted, the tarsus is intact, and there is minimal tissue loss. **C** and **D,** Primary débridement and closure are achieved with anatomic repositioning of the components of the upper eyelid. Prompt lubrication is important to keep the cornea moist and avoid abrasion.

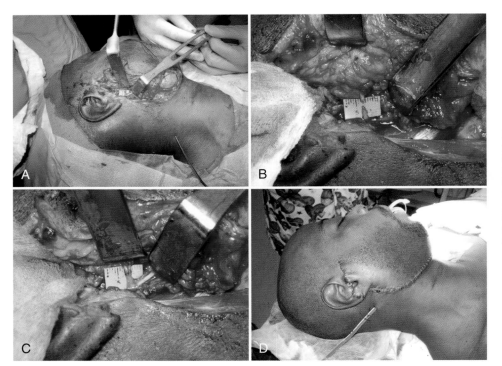

Figure 91-6. A, A stab injury has severed the superior division of the facial nerve. **B** and **C,** Isolation of the nerve under high-power magnification allows excellent visualization of the proximal and distal stumps and primary repair of the nerve. **D,** Closure over a suction drain helps avoid hematoma, seroma, and sialocele formation.

complication, especially when the drainage mechanism of the gland is intact. Persistent sialocele should alert one to the possibility of a missed duct injury and warrants re-exploration. In addition to the facial nerve, the parotid gland and Stenson's duct are particularly susceptible to lateral facial injuries and present special management challenges. Causes of parotid injury are numerous but frequently involve slash or stab wounds to the cheek, glass injuries from bottle fragments or automobile windows, and avulsive and blast injuries. Failure to recognize and appropriately manage significant gland and duct injuries may result in a sialocele or salivary-cutaneous fistula.

The anatomic course of the duct can be approximated externally by a line extending from the tragus of the ear to the midpoint of a vertical line drawn from the alar base of the nose to the vermilion of the upper lip. Thorough exploration should be undertaken and both ends of the severed duct identified. Retrograde cannulation of the duct may confirm the presence of injury, as well as identify the distal stump. The proximal portion may be identified by milking saliva from the gland. The proximal duct is large, thus making it amenable to identification with loupe magnification. When possible, the duct should be repaired primarily over a stent. The stent is then left in place for several weeks to encourage re-epithelialization. Should there be a continuity defect involving the duct, a vein graft may be used in an attempt to re-establish continuity. Another approach is to divert the remaining proximal duct posteriorly in the oropharynx to develop a new drainage site. Alternatively, the proximal stump may be tied off in the hope that the gland will eventually atrophy. Pressure dressings and antisialagogue medications may be useful as adjuncts.

External Ear Injury

The ear is highly vascular and will often survive on a narrow pedicle despite severe trauma. Therefore, the surgeon should be conservative when débriding tissue in this area. For simple lacerations, the ear has the advantage of well-defined landmarks that are easily reapproximated (Fig. 91-7). Layered closure with fine, undyed, slowly resorbable suture to approximate and support the cartilage framework and with fine monofilament suture to close skin is appropriate in this situation. Auricular hematomas secondary to blunt trauma are commonplace and should be drained acutely lest the patient be left with a "cauliflower ear" deformity. The incision for drainage should be placed in a recessed portion of the pinna over the hematomas. A bolster dressing is placed with transauricular sutures to obliterate the resultant dead space and assist in redraping the soft tissue.

Avulsed segments that are no greater than 1.5 cm may be suitable as composite grafts. If the segment is not available, wedge excision and primary closure may be performed. Avulsions of the entire ear may be reattached with the use of an operative microscope if the time until replantation is short and the vessels are minimally damaged. Alternatively, the cartilage can be de-epithelialized and buried within the dermis to preserve the tissue for secondary reconstruction. Rarely do buried cartilage replantations or total auricular reconstructions live up to the cosmetic expectations of the patient, except in the hands of exceptionally skilled

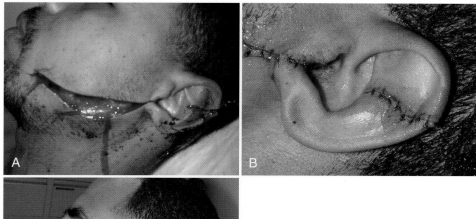
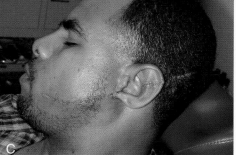

Figure 91-7. A, Slash injury with disruption of the facial, ear, and scalp tissues. Only the superficial layers were affected. No parotid duct or facial nerve injury occurred. **B,** Primary repair of the laceration in anatomic layers. **C,** One week after repair once the sutures were removed. (*Courtesy of Domenick Coletti, DDS, MD, Baltimore, MD.*)

surgeons with considerable experience. Implant-supported prostheses are very aesthetic but may induce chronic irritation associated with the abutment-skin interface.

Nasal Injuries

Injuries to the nose range from simple lacerations to avulsions and may involve the underlying bone, cartilage, and mucosa. The injury frequently occurs at the junction of the bony and cartilaginous skeleton and is often much more extensive than apparent on the surface. As with other structures of the face, tissues that appear somewhat questionable should be preserved and used as pedicled flaps or composite grafts. Significant partial nasal avulsions may survive, provided that one of the multiple vascular pedicles remains intact (Fig. 91-8). Mucosa should be closed when possible, and nasal cartilage should be carefully repositioned and sutured to preserve the tip projection and support. The skin envelope is closed to protect the underlying cartilage. For avulsion injuries and full-thickness nasal skin injuries, composite grafts and full-thickness skin grafts

from the ear and periauricular skin may be considered. Before entertaining primary reconstruction (e.g., local flaps and grafts), one must ensure a clean viable wound bed with minimal risk of infection.

Scalp Injuries

The scalp encompasses the area from the supraorbital rims anteriorly to the occiput posteriorly and is composed of five distinct layers. The total area of the scalp is quite substantial and the tissue highly vascular. Significant blood loss can occur in association with scalp injuries and should be replaced aggressively with isotonic fluids or blood products. Hemostasis is often of primary concern when managing scalp wounds and can largely be achieved with the judicious use of clamps and hemostatic sutures. Acutely, digital pressure and large-volume sterile saline injection directly applied to the wound can achieve temporary hemostasis until the proper instrumentation is available for definitive surgical control.

Primary closure of the scalp is easily accomplished when there is no significant tissue loss. The scalp should

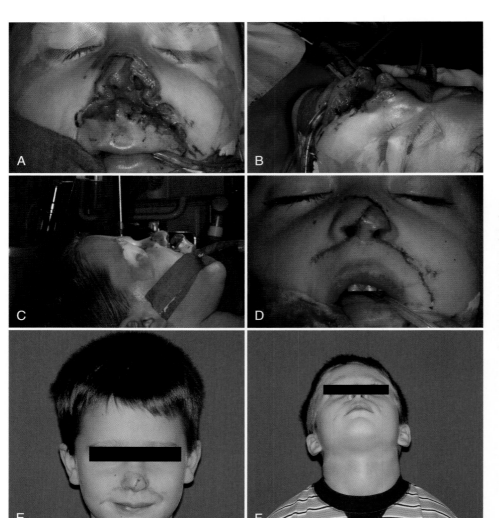

Figure 91-8. A to **C,** Preoperative views of a young boy who sustained a dog bite injury to the nasal complex with near avulsion of the external nose and upper lip. The upper lip is pedicled on the superior labial arteries and the injury has penetrated through the oral cavity to the maxillary vestibule. **D,** After reconstruction. **E** and **F,** Three weeks after the repair, the child is shown with the typical erythema of the wounds and excellent healing.

be closed in two layers: 2-0 or 3-0 Vicryl sutures for the galea, followed by 3-0 monofilament or staples for skin closure. The galea is firmly affixed to the more superficial tissues and, when closed properly, provides appropriate scalp contour, relieves tension, and aligns the skin edges. A suction drain is recommended for large wounds or when significant undermining has taken place.

The tissues of the scalp, in addition to being highly vascular, are quite thick and equally inelastic. Mobilization of local flaps requires wide undermining and galeal scoring (Fig. 91-9). Care must be taken to preserve the more superficial subcutaneous vessels when extensive scoring is necessary. Just as challenging is the recruitment of hair-bearing tissue to reconstruct larger avulsion defects. Free tissue transfer or pedicled flaps must often be used to provide adequate surface coverage while keeping in mind that future tissue expansion and local flap reconstruction may be necessary to provide optimal cosmesis. Smaller defects may be reconstructed with local hair-bearing flaps or skin grafting (or both), followed by serial excision. One issue to be considered is the presence of intact periosteum. When periosteum is present, a defect can simply be skin grafted and reconstructed at a later date; however, if periosteum is lost, the exposed cranium should be covered with local tissue raised in the supraperiosteal plane or with distant tissue. When local or free tissue is not an option, multiple burr holes can be placed in the diploic space to encourage the formation of granulation tissue and subsequent outer table coverage. This wound bed is then maintained and optimized with dressing changes until it is ready to accept a split-thickness skin graft.

Lip Injuries

The lips are a key focal point in the central portion of the face and require meticulous repair to avoid the obvious stigmata of traumatic injury. It is crucial that a layered anatomic closure be performed to ensure proper function and maximize aesthetics (see Fig. 91-2). Like other facial structures, there are anatomic landmarks to guide precise repair of the lips, including the wet-dry line, the white roll, Cupid's bow, and the commissure. For injuries in which the vermilion has been lacerated, tattooing these landmarks with methylene blue may help ensure appropriate repositioning, especially because edema and hemorrhage make identification of these structures more difficult. In addition to proper repositioning of the external lip, it is also imperative to achieve realignment of the muscle. If the muscle is not properly repaired, bulging may be evident on either side of the repair, as well as shortening and notching of the lip.

In cases in which a portion of the lip has been avulsed, reconstruction varies greatly, depending on the size of the defect and which aspects of the lip are involved. For instance, if only a portion of the vermilion is missing, consideration should be given to whether an improved aesthetic result will be gained by excising a wedge of the lip and performing primary closure or repairing the lip as it is. The best results and ease of anatomic alignment are usually obtained when the laceration is oriented at 90 degrees to the lip margin. For defects of one third to one half the width of the lip, primary closure is possible but may result in microstomia. Options include a variety of advancements, rota-

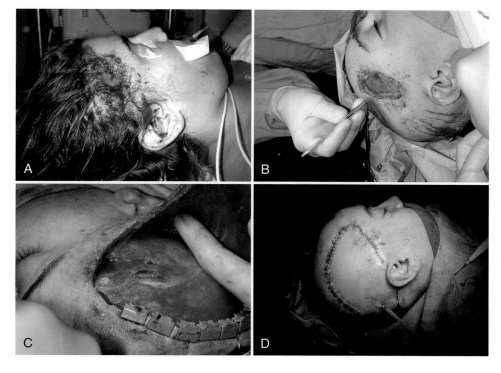

Figure 91-9. A, Preoperative view of a scalp wound with a significant crush and avulsive injury to a portion of the temporal scalp. **B,** The wound is shown after excision and débridement of nonviable tissue. **C,** A local advancement flap is mobilized, and galeal scoring assists in advancement of the scalp. **D,** Closure of the wound with minimal tension and a suction drain minimizes complications and achieves complete reconstruction in one stage. (*Courtesy of Domenick Coletti, DDS, MD, Baltimore, MD.*)

tions, and local flaps that are beyond the scope of this chapter. As with all facial injuries, the choice of primary versus secondary reconstruction is based on the extent and the mechanism of the injury. If primary reconstruction is not possible, mucosa can be closed to skin until definitive reconstruction is performed.

SUMMARY

Management of soft tissue trauma can be challenging and requires a firm understanding of the common mechanisms of injury, biologic principles of healing, and the most successful reconstructive techniques. Careful planning for each repair and precise execution of technique ensure the best possible result in even the most devastating of injuries. Patients should be made aware at the initiation of treatment that some injuries will benefit from revision or secondary reconstruction even after appropriate primary surgical correction has been performed.

PEARLS

- Copious irrigation, conservative débridement, a hemostatic field, and careful preparation set the stage for successful wound closure.
- Precise suturing with everted wound edges yields the most predictable healing and the best aesthetic results.
- Planning closure and local flaps to respect the RSTLs optimizes aesthetic healing.
- Discuss revision possibilities at the initial repair by highlighting the likelihood of revision in severe wounds.

PITFALLS

- Do not consider performing very complex closures in the emergency department setting because patient cooperation, optimal lighting, and quality instrumentation will probably improve the outcome.
- Do not perform definitive closure of an extensive gunshot wound at the first visit because most will require additional débridement.
- Inspect areas with complex anatomy carefully because injury to specialized structures is much better managed definitively at the initial repair than at a secondary procedure.
- Postoperative wound care and protection are important to avoid complications and to discuss the expectations of healing or revision.

References

1. Hollander JE, Singer AJ, Valentine S, et al: Wound registry: Development and validation. Ann Emerg Med 25:675-685, 1995.
2. Gassner R, Tuli T, Hachl O, et al: Cranio-maxillofacial trauma: A 10 year review of 9,543 cases with 21,067 injuries. J Craniomaxillofac Surg 31:51-61, 2003.
3. Singer AJ, Mach C, Thode HC Jr, et al: Patient priorities with traumatic lacerations. Am J Emerg Med 18:683-686, 2000.
4. Eppley BL, Sood R: Facial burns. In Booth PW, Eppley B, Schmelzeisen R (eds): Maxillofacial Trauma and Esthetic Reconstruction. Edinburgh, Churchill Livingstone, 2003, pp 429-444.
5. Callaham M: Controversies in antibiotic choices for bite wounds. Ann Emerg Med 17:1321-1330, 1988.
6. Morgan JP 3rd, Haug RH, Murphy MT: Management of facial dog bite injuries. J Oral Maxillofac Surg 53:435-441, 1995.
7. Sacks JJ, Sattin RW, Bonzo SE: Dog bite–related fatalities from 1979 through 1988. JAMA 262:1489-1492, 1989.
8. Lackmann GM, Draf W, Isselstein G, Tollner U: Surgical treatment of facial dog bite injuries in children. J Craniomaxillofac Surg 20:81-86, 1992.
9. Palmer J, Rees M: Dog bites of the face: A 15 year review. Br J Plast Surg 36:315-318, 1983.
10. Diphtheria, tetanus, and pertussis: Recommendations for vaccine use and other preventive measures. Recommendations of the Immunization Practices Advisory Committee (ACIP). MMWR Recomm Rep 40(RR-10):1-28, 1991.
11. Osmond MH, Klassen TP, Quinn JV: Economic comparison of a tissue adhesive and suturing in the repair of pediatric facial lacerations. J Pediatr 126:892-895, 1995.
12. Toriumi DM, O'Grady K, Desai D, Bagal A: Use of octyl-2-cyanoacrylate for skin closure in facial plastic surgery. Plast Reconstr Surg 102:2209-2219, 1998.
13. Quinn J, Wells G, Sutcliffe T: Tissue adhesive versus suture wound repair at 1 year: Randomized clinical trial correlating early, 3-month, and 1-year cosmetic outcome. Ann Emerg Med 32:645-649, 1998.
14. Maw JL, Quinn JV, Wells GA, et al: A prospective comparison of octylcyanoacrylate tissue adhesive and suture for the closure of head and neck incisions. J Otolaryngol 26:26-30, 1997.
15. MacGillivray RF, Stevens MR: Primary surgical repair of traumatic lacerations of the lacrimal canaliculi. Oral Surg Oral Med Oral Pathol Oral Radiol Endod 81:157-163, 1996.
16. Hartstein ME, Fink SR: Traumatic eyelid injuries. Int Ophthalmol Clin 42:123-134, 2002.
17. Blanchaert RH Jr: Surgical management of facial nerve injuries. Atlas Oral Maxillofac Surg Clin North Am 9(2):43-58, 2001.
18. Myckatyn TM, Mackinnon SE: The surgical management of facial nerve injury. Clin Plast Surg 30:307-318, 2003.

Chapter **92**

Fractures of the Mandible

Mark W. Ochs

The mandible is the second most commonly fractured bone in patients sustaining facial trauma.[1] When a mandibular fracture is detected, additional fractures of the mandible or midface should be sought out. Failure to do so will inevitably result in an incomplete or undesirable treatment outcome. The mandible is the thickest bone of the maxillofacial complex. Therefore, with panfacial fractures, adequate mandibular restoration to full continuity often serves as the reference and pillar to re-establishing normal facial contours and projection.

Mandibular fractures are classified by their anatomic location (Fig. 92-1): symphysis/parasymphysis, anterior (between the canine teeth), body (between the canine and second molar), angle (in the third molar region up to the level of the lower occlusal plane), and ramus (at the posterior mandibular vertical component, excluding the condylar process and coronoid). Condyle fractures are further subdivided into subcondylar—below the sigmoid notch (the U-shaped junction of the condyle and the coronoid) and coursing down into the ramal area, the condylar neck (at or above the sigmoid notch), and intracapsular—the condylar head, or articular surface. Dentoalveolar fractures are confined to a tooth or a segment of teeth and their surrounding bone but do not extend down or through the inferior border of the mandible.

These same fractures are also classified as open or closed. By definition, any fracture in a tooth-bearing area is an open fracture. Mandibular fractures will often course along or parallel the tooth roots in the anterior region, thereby resulting in a new gap between the adjacent teeth, a gingival tear, or a heavier radiodense line along the tooth root. With multirooted posterior teeth, the fracture can traverse along a mesial or distal root surface or involve the tooth itself. Generally, fractures of the ramus, condyle, and coronoid are closed

unless severe displacement or a penetrating-type injury has occurred. Edentulous mandible fractures, particularly the body, can be open because of an intraoral tear of the thin overlying mucosa.

Fractures of the posterior body, the angle, and the ramus can be classified as favorable or unfavorable based on the direction (the orientation) of the fracture line and the net effect of the masseteric muscle pull under function (Fig. 92-2). Favorable fractures are angled such that with masseteric closing force, the fracture is further reduced or supported. Unfavorable fractures are further distracted by this same force.

General knowledge of the dentition and occlusion is necessary to adequately access and treat mandible fractures. The full adult dentition consists of 32 teeth, including the third molars and wisdom teeth (Fig. 92-3). The teeth are numbered sequentially, starting with the maxillary right third molar (no. 1) and moving forward to the other molars, bicuspids, canines, and incisors and all the way across to the left maxillary third molar (no. 16). The left mandibular third molar is next (no. 17), and numbering continues forward and across the midline to the right mandibular third molar (no. 32). It is prudent practice to routinely "count teeth" and assess for any missing or splayed teeth with concomitant open sockets, gingival tears, or bleeding. These are all telltale signs suggestive of a fracture. The primary dentition also has a nomenclature that uses capital letters (Fig. 92-4).

When discussing a particular surface or a relationship to a tooth, a set of terms is used: mesial refers to the anterior surface (in front of or toward the midline), distal refers to the posterior surface (or away from the midline), lingual identifies the inner surface or tongue side, and buccal/labial/facial all refer to the outer surface or the cheek side.

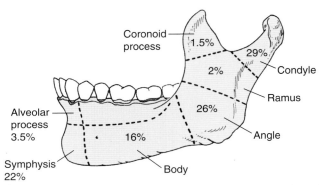

Figure 92-1. Anatomic classification and percent distribution of mandibular fractures in dentate adult patients.

The most widely used classification system for describing maxillary and mandibular intraoral bite relationships is the Angle system. An Angle class I occlusion is characterized by the maxillary canine being just distal to or behind (half a tooth) the mandibular canine, and the mesial buccal (front) cusp of the maxillary first molar is slotted in the buccal groove of the mandibular first molar (Fig. 92-5).

Although Angle class I is the most common and desirable occlusal relationship, it is not present in all patients before injury. Classification may be different on the right versus the left side. When evaluating a patient with a mandibular fracture, it is important to ask the patient or family whether a preexisting malocclusion was present, specifically, "Were your upper teeth in the front overlapping your lower teeth?" (class I). Additionally, one may ask, "Was your lower jaw

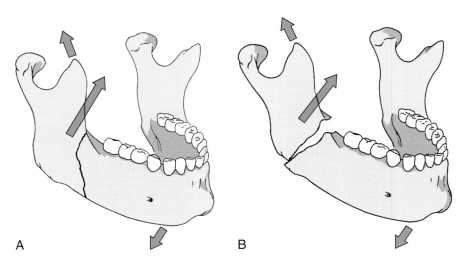

Figure 92-2. A, Favorable mandibular angle fracture. With the muscular pull of the temporalis and masseter and the minor influence of the digastrics and suprahyoid musculature, there is a tendency toward further fracture reduction or stabilization. **B,** Unfavorable mandibular angle fracture. With these same muscular forces there is a tendency toward gapping at the superior border and rotation of the proximal or angle segment upward. This bony step can also be palpated intraorally.

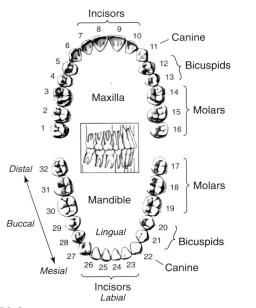

Figure 92-3. Adult/permanent dentition with numbering system and descriptors that help accurately describe the relationship of an injury or abnormality relative to the dentition.

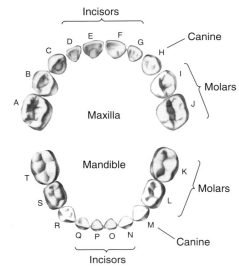

Figure 92-4. The pediatric/primary dentition with alphabetic designations.

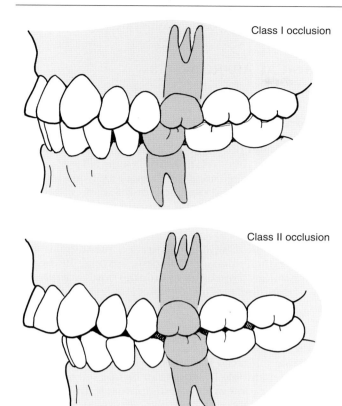

Class I occlusion

Class II occlusion

Class III occlusion

Figure 92-5. Angle's classification of occlusion. In class I occlusion, the mesial buccal cusp of the maxillary first molar fits into the buccal groove of the mandibular first molar. In class II occlusion, the mandibular first molar is distal relative to the maxillary first molar, a consequence of mandibular retrusion. If the mandible is prognathic (class III occlusion), the mandibular first molar is completely in front of the maxillary first molar.

recessive/receding or did it jut out?" (class II or class III, respectively). Finally, ask "Did your front teeth not come all the way together or were they gapped vertically?" (indicating an anterior open bite). These queries, along with appropriate radiographs, help avoid surprises and struggles in the operating room when attempting to align the fractures and re-establish the habitual occlusion. Wear facets on the teeth and interdigitation of the bite are useful aids in determining more precise fracture alignment.

PATIENT SELECTION

Patients with mandibular fractures may have the classic signs and symptoms: pain, trismus (difficulty opening), swelling, malocclusion, gingival tear, ecchymosis of the floor of the mouth, bony crepitus on functioning, and paresthesia or anesthesia of the lower lip and chin (cranial nerve V_3 distribution).[2] The most common initial complaints are pain and malocclusion. The paresthesia or anesthesia is generally due to swelling or a direct injury to the inferior alveolar nerve cable somewhere along its course through the mandibular canal from the lingula/medial midramus to the mental foramen (exiting below and between the apices of the mandibular bicuspid teeth). This would be indicative of fracture of the body, angle, or ramus. Focal preauricular pain during active jaw motion or palpation is suggestive of a condylar or subcondylar fracture. Floor of the mouth ecchymosis is typically seen with symphyseal fractures, especially in edentulous elderly patients.

Unless there is gross fracture displacement in a thin individual, it is difficult and painful to palpate a bony step. A more productive maneuver is to gently flex the mandible across the suspected fracture site to detect mobility, gapping of teeth, or widening of a gingival/mucosal tear.

PREOPERATIVE EVALUATION AND PLANNING

Once a clinical diagnosis of a mandibular fracture is established, it is important to query the patient about any preexisting malocclusion; any previous fractures, injuries, or surgery involving the jaws or the temporomandibular joints; and any previous orthodontic treatment (generally indicates a class I or more favorable occlusion, but not always). After the initial clinical examination and history, selective radiographs can be obtained to determine the specific location, extent, and characteristics of the fracture. The radiographic studies must fully evaluate the entire mandible because multiple fractures are fairly common. A parasymphyseal or body fracture will often have an associated contralateral subcondylar fracture. The two best initial radiographic studies are a panoramic tomogram (Panorex) and an open-mouth reverse Towne view to further assess condylar fractures.[3] If the findings are equivocal or the study is not diagnostic, it can be repeated or additional mandibular views can be taken, such as posteroanterior (best for the symphyseal area), lateral (images the body and angle well), or oblique (visualizes the body, angle, and ramus well and the condylar neck less reliably). The quality and diagnostic accuracy of the mandible series can be diminished if a portable study is performed or the patient is in a cervical collar, which hampers positioning and leads to structural overlap. In any event, if more definitive imaging is required, a computed tomography (CT) scan with axial cuts ranging from 5 to 1.5 mm is indicated. Intravenous contrast enhancement is not indicated and provides no additional information in the acute trauma setting. Direct coronal views can be helpful in ascertaining the exact pattern and alignment of condyle fractures, particularly intracapsular ones. Three-dimensional reformatting is generally unnecessary and adds further expense. If there is any suspicion of maxillary, midfacial, or skull fractures, the axial CT scan should be continued through these regions as well.

Once all the radiographic studies have been reviewed, it is often helpful to re-examine the patient so that issues such as suitability and number of teeth for arch bars, soft tissue swelling, and associated lacerations can be incorporated into the surgical treatment plan and the approaches to be used.

The timing of treatment of mandibular fractures depends on many factors, but in general it is better to treat a fracture as soon as possible. Evidence shows that the longer an open or a compound fracture is left untreated, the greater the incidence of infection.[4] Antibiotics have been shown to decrease the risk of wound infection in patients with mandible fractures.[5] Antibiotics with appropriate activity against oral bacteria can be initiated upon diagnosis and administered for several doses after surgery. Grossly contaminated wounds or open defects may warrant longer therapy. In addition, delay of several days or weeks makes ideal anatomic reduction of a given fracture difficult, if not impossible, particularly for condylar and subcondylar fractures. Furthermore, progressive edema 2 or 3 days after surgery frequently makes surgical access and soft tissue dissection more difficult.

However, treatment of facial fractures is frequently delayed for several reasons. In many cases, other more serious or life-threatening injuries are present, and the patient is not neurologically or hemodynamically stable enough to undergo general anesthesia and a surgical procedure. Moreover, it is highly desirable to have the cervical spine cleared of any injury and to have the cervical collar removed before surgery, especially with any extraoral approaches and open treatment of condyle fractures. Infrequently, excessive soft tissue edema or anticoagulation requires a 3- to 4-day delay in surgical treatment.

The primary goals of treatment of mandibular fractures are to restore continuity of the mandible and return to the patient's habitual functioning occlusion. In addition, consideration should be given to maintaining acceptable facial and dental aesthetics and minimizing neurosensory or facial nerve impairment. During the treatment and healing phases it is also important to maintain adequate nutritional status and minimize patient discomfort and inconvenience. Therefore, patients with neurologic injuries, preexisting mental disabilities, or seizure disorders may not be suitable candidates for closed treatment and the use of postoperative maxillomandibular fixation (MMF). Finally, preoperative assessment of the patient's nasopharyngeal airway should be undertaken because nasoendotracheal intubation and intraoperative interdental fixation are almost always necessary for treatment of a dentate mandibular fracture. Septal deviation, turbinate hypertrophy, bleeding, and coagulopathies are several factors to be considered.

SURGICAL APPROACHES

Fractures of the mandible can be treated in either closed or open fashion. The surgeon needs to consider the adequacy of the teeth with regard to number, the amount of decay or periodontal disease present, extensive crown and bridge work, and opposing dentition to maintain the bite relationship. Generally, a patient must have the majority of teeth in all four quadrants of the mouth for closed treatment and 6 weeks of MMF to be effective. Circumdental wiring and arch bars may only add further stress to an already compromised dentition.

The decision whether to treat a mandibular fracture by either open or closed means may be heavily influenced by concomitant injuries and fractures at other mandibular sites or associated facial bones.[6,7] More extensive concomitant facial injuries may prompt opening and rigid plating of all mandible fractures to restore facial proportions and projection or to assist in closed reduction or a period of postoperative MMF for less stable midfacial fractures.

Most mandible fractures can be opened and plated from an intraoral or extraoral approach. In general, it is easiest to approach and plate parasymphyseal fractures transorally. Condyle fractures, when opened, are best approached extraorally via a modified submandibular or retromandibular dissection and, very infrequently, via a preauricular dissection. The decision to open a mandibular body, angle, or ramus fracture, either intraorally or extraorally, should be based on a specific fracture pattern, soft tissue swelling, ease of access, and the surgeon's preference. Surgical planning should take into account these factors and the possibility of combined approaches such as an intraoral vestibular incision and percutaneous drilling and screwing through a cannula.

Arch Bar Application

Proper treatment of mandibular fractures in dentate patients usually begins with the application of prefabricated arch bars. The teeth are gently brushed with a preparative solution and rinsed to clear any clots or debris. A moist throat pack is then inserted to prevent loss of any wire trimmings into the hypopharynx. It is helpful to infiltrate a local anesthetic with 1:100,000 epinephrine throughout the maxillary and mandibular vestibule because annoying oozing can occur in patients with preexisting gingival inflammation. The segment of arch bars is cut to appropriate length for at least first molar–to–first molar engagement (preferable to include the second molars) around the arch. The arch bar is gently bent into a curve and preadapted to the dental arch at the level of the necks of the teeth and the free gingival margin (Fig. 92-6). Usually, posterior teeth (bicuspids and molars) are ligated to the arch bar with 24-gauge stainless steel wire, and anterior teeth are secured circumdentally with 26-gauge wire. It is easiest

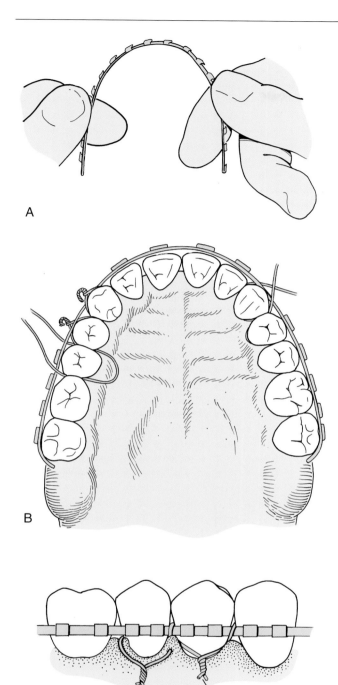

Figure 92-6. Technique of placement of arch bars and maxillo-mandibular fixation (MMF). **A,** The arch bar is cut and bent to the appropriate length and shape of the dentition, including all stable teeth, for fixation. **B,** The arch bar is fixed to the posterior teeth with 24-gauge circumdental wire and to the anterior teeth with 26-gauge circumdental wire. It is often helpful to start in the bicuspid regions because these teeth have undercuts that engage the circumdental wires well and seat the arch bar at the cervical margin of the teeth. The wires pass above the bar on one side of the tooth and below the bar on the other side and are then twisted in a clockwise direction. **C,** The wires should pass between the tooth and the interdental papilla to avoid strangulation of these structures.

to start with the first bicuspids because they have a bulbous shape that is favorable for seating of the wires below the height of contour. As the wires are tightened, the arch bars should be held in proper anteroposterior alignment and snug against the cervical margins of the anterior teeth. One limb of the wire is passed under the bar and one over the bar on return from the lingual pass and twisted in a clockwise direction while fully seating the wire around the neck of the tooth with a forked wire director (see Fig. 92-6B). This is most important for canine and anterior teeth, which are slender and have minimal undercuts to resist dislodgement when the MMF wire loops are tightened to bring the patient into full occlusion.

The wires should lie on the surface of the teeth and not pass through or around the interdental papillae (see Fig. 92-6C). When fractures of the mandibular body or parasymphyseal region are present, a wire may be looped around the teeth adjacent to the fracture site and gently tightened until proper fracture alignment has been achieved (see Fig. 92-6D). Placement of the arch bar can then continue distally to the site of the fracture; the fracture must be properly reduced at the superior mandibular surface. If the arch bar interferes with reducing a fracture, it can be sectioned at the fracture site to allow proper alignment. After the arch bars have been placed in stable fashion on both the maxillary and mandibular dentition, MMF is performed (see Fig. 92-6E). It is important to not overtighten the MMF wires, especially with fractures of the parasymphyseal region, because the inferior fracture gap will widen (see Fig. 92-6F and G) and result in "lingual version" of the mandibular dentition.

When the dentition is inadequate to completely stabilize an arch bar, the arch bar may be further secured with circum-mandibular wiring for the mandibular arch bar and wiring of the piriform aperture or circumzygomatic wires for the maxillary arch bar (Fig. 92-7). The skeletal fixation wires provide added stability.

Several important considerations must be kept in mind for proper placement of arch bars. A circumdental wire should not pass through the interdental papilla of the gingiva because necrosis of this important structure can occur. The wires should be carefully positioned directly adjacent to the tooth and slid beneath the gingiva to avoid gingival necrosis. Before tightening the wires around the bars, the two ends of the circumdental loop should be adjusted so that they are of equal length and form an isosceles triangle. If the ends of the wire are of equal length, they will firmly anchor the arch bar to the teeth as the wires are carefully twisted under tension. Wire twisting is always performed in a clockwise direction so that other surgeons will know which direction to twist for tightening or removal postoperatively.

Dental and Dentoalveolar Fractures

Teeth can be individually fractured through the crowns at various levels. Management of fractures of the teeth is individualized according to the severity of the injury.[8]

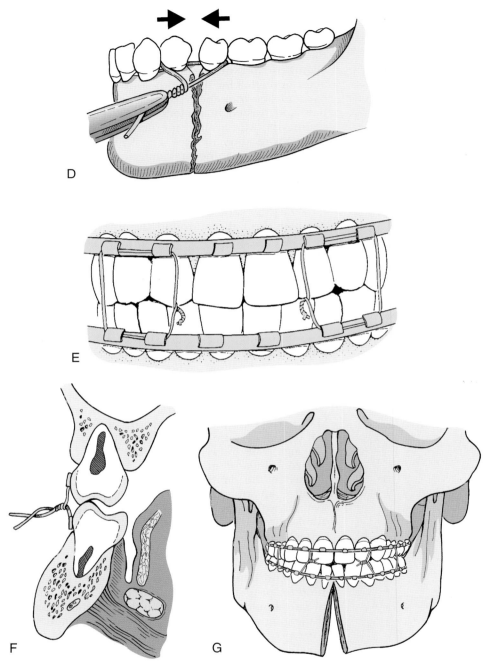

Figure 92-6, cont'd D, A bridal wire is passed around the first and second bicuspids with a left mandibular body fracture to aid in reduction and stabilization. This is done before fixation of the arch bar and allows the arch bar to be secured to the mandible in an already reduced position. **E,** MMF, or wire loops, are placed between the upper and lower arch bars to maintain dental occlusion during fixation of the fracture. **F** and **G,** Overtightening the MMF wires in the presence of a symphyseal or parasymphyseal fracture will cause the inferior border of the fracture to splay apart with accompanying lingual version of the occlusal surface. If this is not detected, adequate reduction of the fracture is not possible.

Even if the pulp is exposed and the tooth is fractured off at the base of the crown, these teeth should be maintained and can be restored with endodontic treatment (root canal) and crowns. Teeth that have been subluxated or dislodged should be manually repositioned within the socket and dental arch. It is usually best to secure the injured tooth or segment of teeth to the adjacent dentition with a braided wire and bonding agents (such as cured resins, which are used by orthodontists to apply brackets to the teeth). If a dental specialist is not available for assistance, temporary sta-

bilization with less tightly applied arch bars can suffice until more definitive treatment is rendered. Overtightening the circumdental wires merely serves to extrude and extract the injured or subluxated teeth. Large dentoalveolar fracture segments (four or more teeth) are more amenable to arch bar stabilization or miniplating (or both). Totally avulsed teeth need to be reimplanted within 1 hour for a reasonable prognosis. The tooth should be bonded to the adjacent teeth. Teeth that have sustained root fractures are not usually salvageable and should be removed.

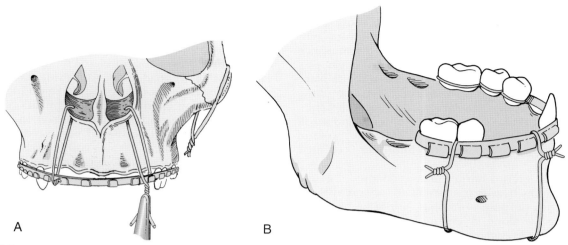

Figure 92-7. A, When the maxillary dentition is inadequate for fixation, suspension wires can be passed through the piriform aperture and tied directly to the arch bar, or circumzygomatic wires can be passed and an intermediate loop of wire can engage the lower arch bar or be secured to a circum-mandibular wire (**B**), which can also help retain a lower arch bar with inadequate dentition. Generally, 24-gauge wire is used for skeletal fixation wires, and lighter wire (26-gauge) is used for any intermediate loops that lock the skeletal fixation wires to each other.

Symphyseal and Parasymphyseal Fractures

Either an intraoral or an extraoral approach can be used for symphyseal and parasymphyseal fractures. The intraoral approach requires less tissue stripping and is quicker. Once the arch bars are in place, fairly snug but not overtightened MMF should be instituted to avoid splaying of the inferior border. The MMF is secured before soft tissue dissection and the mandible supported, which offers resistance when undermining the periosteum and mentalis muscle. Dissection should be carried out to the inferior border. A toe-up Obwegeser or symphyseal retractor aids in stabilization and retraction. With the lip retracted and stretched slightly, the vestibular mucosal incision should be 1 cm away from the mucogingival junction. This will allow stronger multilayered closure of both muscle and the mucosa and will also help avoid postoperative oral dehiscence with plate exposure. In addition, the incision heals more comfortably within the depth of the vestibule. Once adequate exposure is gained for plating (usually a 3- to 4-cm incision), the fracture can be gently splayed by inserting a Freer or periosteal elevator and twisting lightly. The fracture margins should be irrigated and gentle curettage performed to remove all debris, trapped muscle, small bone fragments, clot, or fibrin. This is especially important for fractures that are being treated more than 48 hours after injury. The MMF is then snugged and tightened while placing gentle inward extraoral pressure on the bilateral angle or body regions. Inward bilateral angle pressure helps prevent inferior and labial bone gapping. Generally, a superior four- to six-hole tension band plate (2.0-mm system) is adapted and secured with monocortical screws (4 to 5 mm in length) (Fig. 92-8). Before fixating the plate, the occlusion and fracture alignment should be checked. A previously placed bridal wire (see Fig. 92-6D) can assist

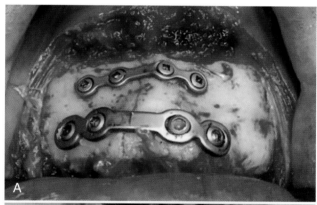

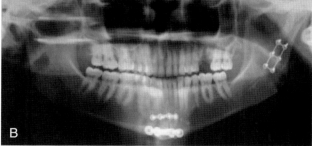

Figure 92-8. A, Transoral approach and plating of a symphyseal fracture. A superior monocortical tension band plate (2.0-mm system) and a heavier inferior border fracture plate (2.7-mm system, bicortical screws) can be used. **B,** The patient was treated with arch bars, was maintained in maxillomandibular fixation (MMF) during fracture reduction plating, and underwent an extraoral approach for the treatment of a left subcondylar fracture. On the release of the MMF wires, the occlusion was checked and found to be stable and reproducible. The arch bars were then removed and soft tissue closure performed.

in gaining firm interdental contact. The superior mono-cortical plate should be placed below the roots of the incisor and canine teeth. The outline of the roots may be visible, or placement of the plate 22 to 24 mm (incisors) or 26 mm (canine) below the incisal edges provides safe clearance. Generally, an ideal and safe place for plating is at the level of the greatest concavity of the mandible, where the alveolar process meets the chin. The screw holes should be carefully centered and a drill guide used. The circumdental and MMF wires will not resist displacement caused by improper eccentric drilling.

When an inferior border plate is adapted, I generally use a slightly heavier fracture plate (or compression plate) for this purpose—one that cannot be bent with finger pressure alone. Slight judicious contouring of any gross bony irregularities (preexisting irregularities, not improperly reduced fracture margins) facilitates plate adaptation and optimal contact with the facial cortical bone. A four- or six-hole plate with a small center span is ideal because most fractures have some degree of obliquity. It is best to avoid traversing the fracture line with the bicortical screws. With the MMF secure and the superior tension band plate in place, the fracture is stationary and maintains its position while adapting and securing the heavier inferior border plate, which will more readily resist movement and masticatory and functional force during healing. Once adapted and flush to the bone, it is helpful to overbend the heavier fracture plate slightly in the central portion so that it is raised 0.5 mm off the bone surface.[9] During screw tightening, this will help minimize unfavorable lingual gapping and posterior flaring or widening of the mandible (see Fig. 92-6). These heavier plates are generally secured with 2.3- to 2.7-mm-diameter screws systems. It is important to use drill guides because eccentric hole placement will cause a shift in the bone fragments and malocclusion. It is sound surgical practice to place at least two screws on each side of the fracture line within each plate (i.e., a minimum of four screws per plate). This prevents pivoting and rotational movement. A single, nonrigid 2.0-mm plate can be used for fracture stabilization if the patient is being maintained in MMF for 6 weeks because of other facial fractures. In addition, some surgeons prefer to use 2.0-mm plates for both the superior tension band and the inferior bicortical plate. It is possible to use a lag screw technique without a plate for oblique fractures of the symphysis, but this method is rather technique sensitive, and any minor drilling malalignment will result in a noticeable and unforgiving malocclusion, usually with a step in the dental arch.

After rigidly fixating the fracture, if there are no other mandibular fractures to treat, the MMF wires (not the circumdental wires) can be cut and removed and the occlusion checked. It is best to push upward on the bilateral angles externally to gently seat the condyles during closure. If the result is satisfactory and stable, muscular closure is performed with several 4-0 Vicryl (braided polyglactin) sutures, and the mucosa is closed with 3-0 or 4-0 chromic suture in a running horizontal mattress stitch. If the arch bars are not to be maintained, they should be removed before soft tissue closure. In general, I do not leave arch bars on postoperatively unless the patient is to be maintained in MMF or if there is some need for elastic guidance. Arch bars without MMF are inadequate to provide stability at the alveolar level and should not be relied on to serve as a superior tension band or to provide "fixation."

If an extraoral approach is to be used, the 4- to 5-cm curvilinear incision line should be placed in the submental region so that it is not visible from the frontal view. The incision should be centered around the point at which the fracture crosses the inferior border of the mandible.

Body Fractures

Fractures of the mandibular body are readily exposed via an intraoral mucosal approach. There are scant muscle attachments and little tissue thickness to traverse during dissection. The mucosa and deeper tissues are infiltrated with local anesthetic and a vasoconstrictor to minimize bleeding and optimize visualization. Reinjection during surgery is more advisable than cautery, especially in proximity to the mental nerve. As previously described, the 5- to 6-cm mucosal incision is made 1 cm lateral or inferior to the mucogingival junction. Along the anterior extent a mucosal-only incision is made, and blunt dissection with small curved hemostats helps identify and free the mental nerve from the anterior or labial flap of soft tissue. The mental nerve exits the mandible between the root tips of the bicuspid teeth. This nerve should be preserved and protected throughout the procedure. It is best to perform dissection with the teeth in MMF because MMF allows more lateral and inferior posterior retraction of the lip, cheek, and commissure of the mouth. A toe-up Obwegeser retractor beneath the inferior border of the mandible helps provide excellent retraction and visualization. Excessive torquing on the obwegeser retractor or body retractor can cause the fracture segments to splay laterally. A single heavier fracture plate can be readily adapted along the typically flat, broad surface of the body's inferior border. The lower edge of the plate should be even with the lowest edge of the mandibular inferior border (Fig. 92-9) to allow proper drilling and bicortical screw placement and avoid injury to the inferior alveolar nerve. Generally, the anterior screws are easily placed transorally, and because of the limits of cheek and lip retraction, added safety is provided by angling slightly inferiorly as one proceeds medially. If necessary, a trocar, cannula, and guard can be used to percutaneously drill and place screws in the posterior plate holes. These are done last because the plate is already stabilized and held in place with the anterior screws. Therefore, the surgeon can concentrate on centering the hole with the aid of a drill guide within the cannula and create a perpendicular path for screw insertion. In most instances there is adequate room above the inferior alveolar canal and below the tooth root apices for a monocortically fixated tension band plate (Fig. 92-9B). If the fracture is located more toward

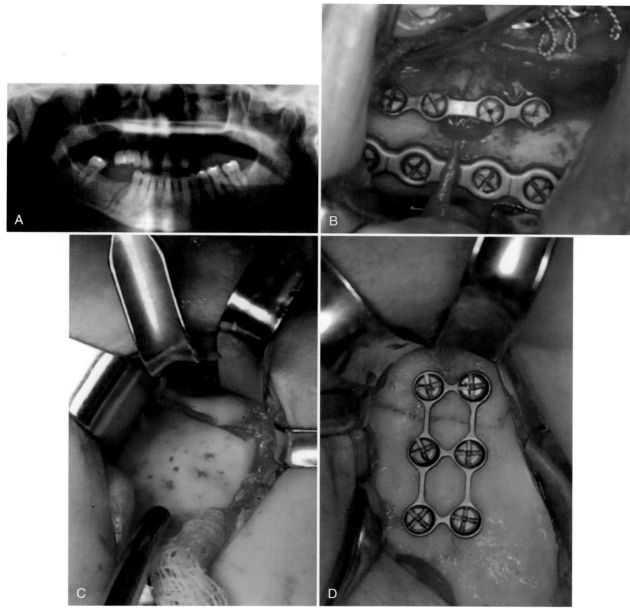

Figure 92-9. Right body and left subcondylar fracture of the mandible. **A,** Panoramic radiograph demonstrating a slightly oblique fracture of the right mandibular body with mild displacement and vertical overlap of the left subcondylar segment. Note that there is inadequate dentition, particularly in the left posterior maxilla, to re-establish a proper vertical dimension through maxillomandibular fixation (MMF) alone. **B,** A transoral approach to the right body fracture was made after placing the patient in MMF. A superior monocortical tension band, four-hole miniplate was applied above the mental nerve, and a four-hole heavier fracture plate was applied at the inferior border, with the distal screws angled inferiorly to avoid the inferior alveolar nerve canal. **C,** Left submandibular/retromandibular approach to the displaced subcondylar fracture. Note that the inferior edge of the proximal segment is laterally displaced. This is quite classic because the pull of the lateral pterygoid on the condylar head displaces it forward and medially. When dissecting subperiosteally, this segment often falls underneath the dissection and must be palpated and retrieved from the superior flap. **D,** The reduced left subcondylar fracture, which was fixated with a ladder plate and a locking 2.0-mm system. Intraoperatively, the MMF and arch bars were removed, and the patient was allowed to ingest a soft diet.

the anterior body region, the monocortical superior plate must "straddle" it above the mental foramen. Remember that the mental nerve has a genu as it exits the mandible. The nerve courses upward and posteriorly several millimeters as one proceeds anteriorly. Therefore, the inferior alveolar canal and nerve are slightly below the level of the mental foramen. A pan-

oramic radiograph is invaluable in assessing this relationship and clearance relative to the nerve canal and root apices. The occlusion should be checked frequently during fracture reduction and fixation to help ensure restoration of preinjury alignment.

If the extraoral approach is chosen, a transverse incision is made at least two finger breadths below the

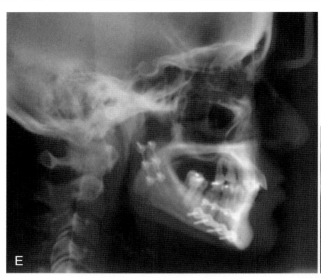
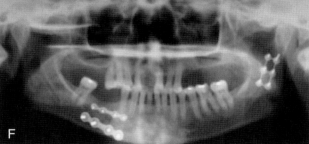

Figure 92-9, cont'd E, A lateral cephalogram taken the first postoperative day shows good preservation of the posterior vertical dimension and projection of the mandible. **F,** Panoramic radiograph demonstrating postoperative reduction and fixation of the right body and left subcondylar fractures.

inferior border of the mandible and carried down through the platysma and then the fascia overlying the submandibular gland to protect the marginal mandibular branch of the facial nerve. It is usually helpful to have a nonparalyzed patient and a nerve stimulator to test any questionable branches or nerve-like structures. The mandible is then exposed by excising the periosteum on its inferior border. Elevation of the periosteum allows wide exposure of the mandible and placement of mandibular reduction clamps when necessary. The extraoral approach may provide better exposure if the mandibular body is comminuted. After the mandible is plated, the MMF is again released, the occlusion is checked, and the arch bars are removed before tissue closure.

Angle Fractures

Mandibular angle fractures are often associated with an impacted or partially erupted third molar (wisdom tooth). Nondisplaced fractures can be treated in closed fashion with 6 weeks of MMF. No MMF plus a soft diet as the sole treatment is not recommended because malunion or unfavorable occlusal changes will develop in a significant proportion of patients. Completely impacted third molars that do not interfere with fracture reduction may be left in place. In fact, removal may cause excessive distraction of the segments and a significant bony void. If a tooth is partially erupted or fractured or interferes with reduction, it should be removed completely. Removal may include vertical sectioning of the tooth with a fine (1.5 mm) fissure burr and high-speed (100,000 rpm) drill with copious irrigation. The tooth fragments can then be split and elevated out independently. Either intraoral or extraoral exposure can be used. Arch bars are placed before soft tissue surgery. The intraoral approach is similar to that described for a body fracture, except that it is located

somewhat more superior along its posterior extent and overlies the external oblique ridge (Fig. 92-10). If a partially erupted third molar is being removed, the incision should course along the lateral exposed crown (the sulcus) and fade back out to the lateral oblique ridge posteriorly to allow primary closure of the tooth socket. Wider tissue dissection with subperiosteal stripping is needed to facilitate lateral retraction and visualization. It is sometimes easier to perform the soft tissue dissection and fracture reduction before placing the patient in MMF. A straight or gently curved monocortical miniplate is usually placed along the lateral aspect just beneath the external oblique ridge (see Fig. 92-10B). Screws can be inserted either transorally or percutaneously, depending on soft tissue stretch and access. Another miniplate or heavier fracture plate is typically applied along the inferior border, often angling upward at the posterior extent but still below the inferior alveolar nerve canal. When placing the cannula and trocar percutaneously, it is best to first sound the proposed skin puncture site with a long anesthetic needle and see whether it corresponds to the fracture line or the center of the planned percutaneous screw placement (Fig. 92-11). Sounding helps avoid the necessity of making additional stab incisions and replacing the cannula at a different site. I do not prefer to use preformed mandibular angled fracture plates transorally. They are difficult to adapt, and any eccentric drilling of the screw holes within the plate tends to create exaggerated unfavorable vectors and displacement of the bony segments.

If the angle fracture is approached extraorally, a skin incision is made approximately 2 to 2.5 cm below the inferior border of the angle and carried slightly upward toward the earlobe at the posterior extent (Fig. 92-12). The incision should be of adequate length (5 cm) to allow retraction and exposure while plating.

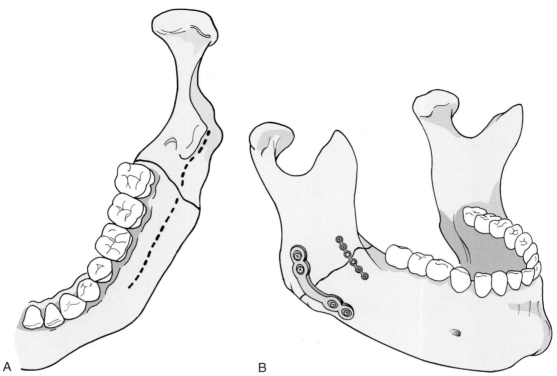

Figure 92-10. Left angle fracture of the mandible. **A,** Incision line for a transoral approach to the fracture. **B,** A six-hole tension band plate is adapted along the external oblique line. There is no center span in this plate and the central plate holes were too close to the fracture line, so no screws were placed in them. Doing so may have caused crazed lines or the screws may have traversed into the fracture line itself. The inferior border angle plate is usually applied via a percutaneous approach with cannula and a drill guide.

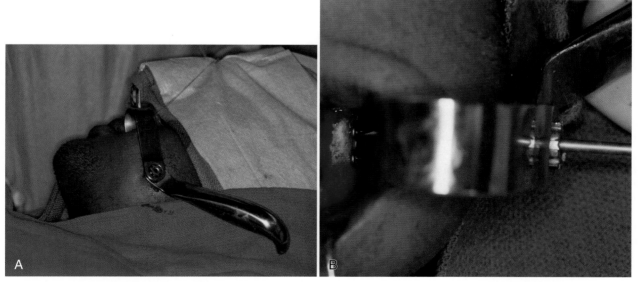

Figure 92-11. Left mandibular angle fracture. **A,** After intraoral dissection and placing the patient in maxillomandibular fixation, a 25-gauge anesthetic needle was used to sound the proposed percutaneous stab incision site, which was then stretched slightly with a small hemostat and a cannula with a trocar was inserted and a cheek guard placed. **B,** The operator is then able to view the fracture and plate transorally while using the percutaneous access to drill and, as seen here, to place screws along the lateral cortex of the mandible.

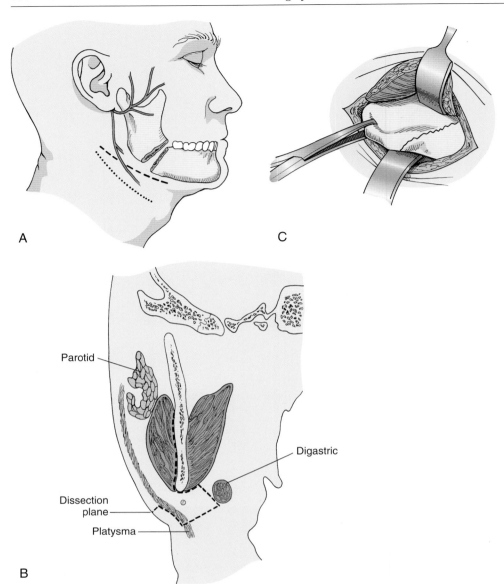

Figure 92-12. External approach to a mandibular angle fracture. **A,** The skin incision is centered around the fracture and designed so that it is just inferior to the angle of the mandible, parallel or within cervical skin creases *(dashed line).* By making the skin incision high in the neck, the length of the incision can be minimized (approximately 4 to 5 cm). The platysma muscle will be cut more inferiorly in the neck at the traditional level *(dotted line)* to preserve the marginal mandibular branch of the facial nerve. **B,** Cross section through the region of the mandibular angle showing the avascular plane of dissection that allows easy access to the mandibular angle. The facial nerve branches are protected by initially dissecting inferiorly into the neck. The dissection then proceeds to the digastric muscles, where the point of dissection is deep to the facial nerve. The mandibular periosteum is incised on the inferior border of the mandible. **C,** Exposure of a reduced fracture through an extraoral approach.

Blunt dissection with slight undermining of the deep subcutaneous layers is performed. The platysma is divided at the lower extent of the dissection, as is the superficial layer of the deep cervical fascia, while testing for the marginal mandibular branch of the facial nerve (Fig. 92-12B). This branch is just inferior to the tail of the parotid gland. The incised layers and skin flaps are retracted superiorly to expose the pterygomasseteric muscle sling and the periosteum of the mandible. This is incised and widely dissected subperiosteally. The fracture is then gently débrided, irrigated, and reduced while placing the patient in MMF. A four- or six-hole straight or gently curved monocortical (2.0 mm) plate is applied superiorly just below and along the external oblique lines. A four- or six-hole heavier mandibular plate is then applied bicortically along the inferior border and below the inferior alveolar canal (see Fig. 92-10B). After all fractures are plated, the MMF should

be released and the occlusion checked. The wound is then irrigated and closure performed with continuous locking 4-0 Vicryl in the platysma and interrupted buried sutures subcutaneously. The cuticular layer is closed with interrupted or continuous 5-0 or 6-0 nylon. Suction drains are rarely indicated, and a gentle pressure dressing or facial support helps prevent postoperative hematoma formation.

Ramus, Condyle, and Coronoid Fractures

Coronoid fractures are uncommon and usually associated with a zygomatic complex fracture that has been driven inward. Coronoid fractures do not require closed or open treatment. They heal uneventfully on their own, except if an overlying zygomatic complex is not properly reduced and is in close proximity, thereby risking fibro-osseous union of the entire coronoid and zygomatic complex fracture.

Ramus fractures can be treated satisfactorily by closed reduction and 6 weeks of MMF. Transoral approaches for plating are difficult. The external skin incision plus approach for ramus fractures is similar to that for angle fractures but with more extension superiorly and with subperiosteal dissection and retraction. Y plates, L plates, and "box" or "ladder" plates allow several screws to be placed in the proximal superior segment closer to the fracture line and decrease the need for further superior dissection and retraction (see Fig. 92-9E and F).

Condylar and subcondylar fractures can be treated with 2 to 4 weeks of MMF. If the fracture is intracapsular (head of the condyle), 2 weeks is appropriate to limit the risk for ankylosis.[10] When a unilateral subcondylar fracture is associated with other mandibular fractures, open reduction with rigid fixation of the coexisting mandibular fractures is indicated so that the subcondy-

lar fracture can be mobilized and returned to function at 2 to 4 weeks (Fig. 92-13).

Open reduction and plating of condyle fractures may be indicated[11] and is necessary in the following situations:

1. Displacement of the condylar head into the middle cranial fossa
2. When condylar displacement prevents re-establishment of proper occlusion
3. With lateral or severe displacement of the condylar head out of the fossa
4. When a foreign body, such as a bullet or bone fragment, is lodged within the temporomandibular joint capsule
5. Open fractures with extensive soft tissue injuries (gunshot wounds) in which early function can help minimize fibrosis

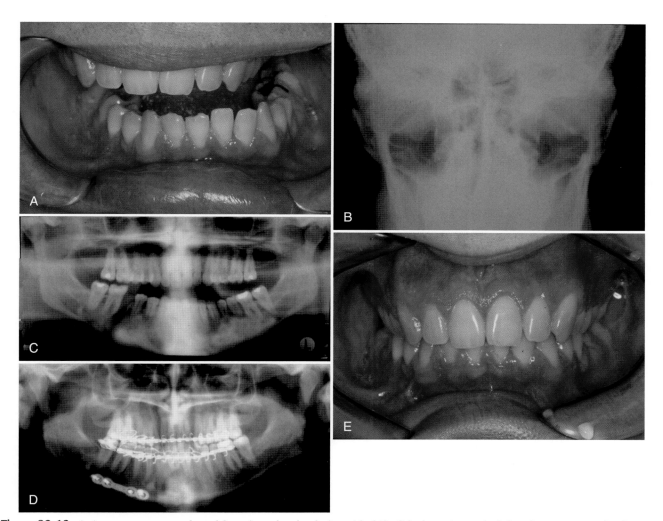

Figure 92-13. A, A young man was evaluated for pain and malocclusion with shift of the lower jaw to the left and premature occlusal contact on the right posterior teeth. An open-mouth reverse Towne view (**B**) and a Panorex view (**C**) demonstrate the left condyle fracture with overlap and a right body fracture gapping between the second bicuspid and first molar. **D,** The patient underwent placement of arch bars, maxillomandibular fixation (MMF), and a transoral approach to the right body fracture with placement of a heavy fracture plate along the inferior border. Adequate reduction and posterior vertical dimension were re-established by keeping the patient in 2 weeks of MMF. **E,** Postoperative occlusion at 6 weeks. The bars were removed at week 4. Between weeks 2 and 4, some light box elastics were placed on the right side and anterior arch bar regions to help guide the occlusion.

Other relative indications include bilateral condyle fractures associated with midfacial fractures or bilateral condyle fractures in an edentulous patient. In these situations, open reduction of one or both condylar fractures greatly aids re-establishment of proper facial dimensions. When significant displacement has resulted in the loss of posterior vertical height, open reduction with rigid fixation is usually recommended (see Fig. 92-9). Severely comminuted intracapsular condyle fractures are not amenable to plate-and-screw fixation and result in only more soft tissue trauma. These patients should be treated with 2 weeks of MMF and then guided (elastic) function as necessary for several more weeks.

When open reduction of a condyle fracture is performed, it is generally through a skin incision similar to that for angle fractures, with a posterior tail that is within 2 cm of the ear lobe. Infrequently, condyle fractures are exposed through a preauricular incision to allow retrieval of a medially displaced condylar head. The preauricular incision is usually performed in conjunction with the submandibular/retromandibular angle approach so that reduction and plating of the fracture are possible without excessive inferior retraction and stretch from above, which might place the facial nerve and superior branches at risk. Condyle fractures (adult or pediatric) should not be approached intraorally. Careful planning and multiple techniques are often needed, even with extraoral approaches. Treatment of mandible fractures should be undertaken by surgeons familiar with the surgical approaches, and it is beneficial to have another surgeon assisting. Judicious stripping and muscular reflection for 1 to 1.5 cm on the medial surface of the inferior angle will greatly improve the ability to retract superiorly. In addition, a channel or toe-up Obwegeser retractor placed in the sigmoid notch will enhance visualization and access to the condyle fracture. Plate configurations that allow several screws to be inserted within the condylar segments close to the fracture line will facilitate plating (see Fig. 92-9D).

Endoscopically assisted reduction plus plating of condyle fractures has been advocated by several authors, but it has limitations and has not been shown to be more efficacious or to have less risk than traditional approaches.

Pediatric mandible fractures (≤6 years of age) are usually best treated with closed techniques involving the use of skeletal fixation wires and sometimes acrylic interocclusal splints (Fig. 92-14). Because of immature bone, limited bone stock, and developing permanent tooth buds, children's mandibles are difficult to plate effectively,[12] especially condyle fractures.

Multiple Fractures

With comminuted mandible fractures, I find it easier to piece together the larger, more stable fragments with miniplates and then consolidate and rigidly fixate the entire complex with a larger spanning fracture or reconstruction plate (Fig. 92-15). Locking screws that engage the plate itself help improve stability and minimize distraction of segments during screw tightening because it is virtually impossible to adapt the large plate in full passive contact with all the bony segments.

When deciding whether to use an intraoral versus an extraoral approach for plating, the surgeon should take into consideration several factors. More posterior fracture locations, any comminution, and edentulous fractures are better suited to extraoral approaches.

Thin edentulous bilateral body fractures are best treated via an extraoral approach.[13] After the chin segment is dissected at the inferior extent of the mandibular border, a portion of the mentalis is stripped and a single bicortical screw is inserted in the midpoint of the chin with 3 to 4 mm exposed beneath the head. A large Kelly clamp is then used to grasp the screw shaft and retract anteriorly to make the tissue planes more identifiable and the posterior subperiosteal dissection easier. A long-span rigid plate with three to four screws in the symphysis and three to four screws in the angle provides more reliable rigid fixation and predictable healing without any secondary procedures (Fig. 92-16).

When treating comminuted or edentulous mandible fractures or when drilling at an angle to avoid vital structures, locking screw systems help prevent displacement of the segments and provide excellent rigidity. When drilling screw holes for these or any rigid plating systems (>2-mm external thread diameter, 1.5-mm burr), the drill guide should be used to properly align the bony hole within the plate hole and thus prevent deflection with screw tightening (see Fig. 92-16E).

POSTOPERATIVE MANAGEMENT

Patients treated by open reduction and plating of mandibular fractures should be placed on a soft diet that does not require chewing for several weeks and then advanced to a normal diet only after 6 weeks. Even then, tough foods such as raw carrots, bagels, and the like should be avoided for several more weeks.

If the fracture has been treated in closed fashion and the patient is in MMF, oral hygiene is especially important. The patient should be instructed to brush the teeth and arch bars daily and to perform oral saline rinses. Soft dental wax can be given to the patient to place over any sharp or prominent areas. Wire tails should be bent inward to minimize lip and cheek irritation. Wire cutters should be given to the patient at the bedside and on discharge from the hospital so that the MMF (the vertical wires) can be cut in the event of an airway emergency. Nutrition consultation should be considered for patients with planned periods of 4 to 6 weeks of MMF. The MMF and circumdental wires can be removed in the office under local anesthesia, sometimes supplemented with intravenous sedation. The MMF wires should be released first, before intravenous sedation, in case airway access or support is needed. Patients with open mandible fractures are usually placed on antibiotics at the time of diagnosis, through surgery, and for several postoperative doses. Prolonged antibiotic therapy or broad-spectrum antibiotics are not indicated and have not been shown to provide any benefit.

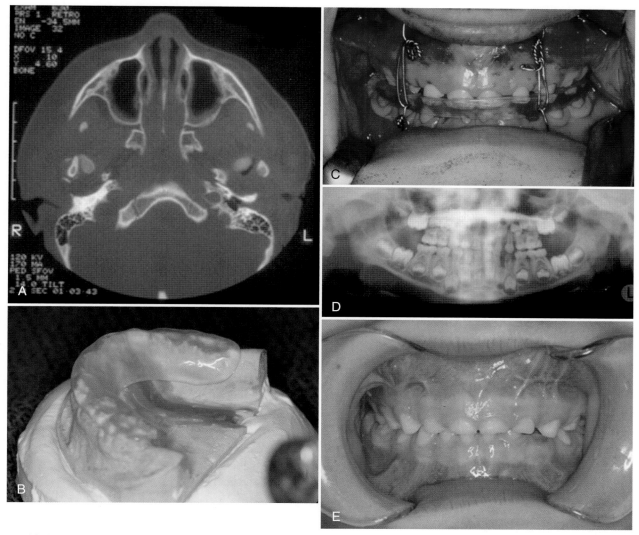

Figure 92-14. A 5-year-old patient was an unrestrained passenger in a motor vehicle accident. **A,** Non–contrast-enhanced axial computed tomography scan demonstrating multiple intracapsular fractures of the bilateral condyles. Additional lower cuts also revealed a right symphysis fracture through the developing permanent canine tooth bud. **B,** After nasally intubating the patient in the operating room, dental molds were taken and stone casts poured. The lower cast, seen here, was sectioned at the displaced fracture line of the right parasymphysis and reduced relative to the maxillary dentition. **C,** An acrylic splint was then fabricated to index these adjustments. The acrylic splint was inserted after placing bilateral 24-gauge skeletal wires at the piriforms and circum-mandibularly. Care was taken to not pass the right circum-mandibular wire within the fracture line of the right parasymphysis. The patient was maintained in skeletal and maxillomandibular fixation for 2 weeks. The intermediate 26-gauge wires were then cut and the patient allowed to function. **D,** A panoramic radiograph taken 2 weeks after removal of the skeletal suspension wires shows good maintenance of the entire dentition and no developing open bite. Both condyles are beginning to re-form. **E,** Occlusion 6 months after surgery showing vertical overlap and good interdigitation.

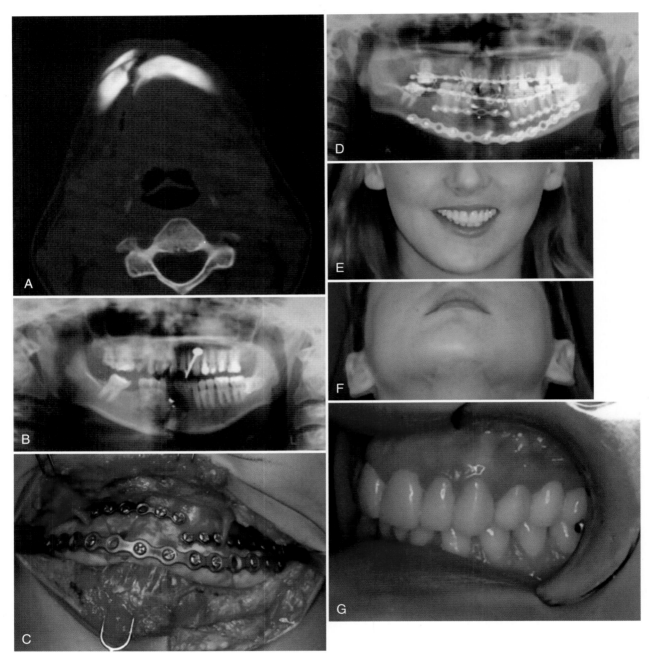

Figure 92-15. Twenty-four-year-old woman involved in a motor vehicle accident. **A,** Non–contrast-enhanced axial computed tomography (CT) scan showing comminution of the inferior border of the mandible. **B,** A panoramic radiograph obtained before the CT scan shows comminution of the right parasymphysis, a left body fracture, and a right condyle fracture with numerous craze lines. **C,** The patient had a large laceration of the chin and submental region that was extended 2 to 3 cm along the left mandibular angle region. First, monocortical miniplates and a locking screw system were used to piece the bony fragments together. The larger spanning rigid plate was then adapted to the inferior border and locking screws inserted. **D,** Postoperative panoramic radiograph showing maxillomandibular fixation, which was maintained for 2 weeks to treat the right condyle fracture in closed fashion. **E,** Three months' postoperative facial appearance. **F,** Submental view of the healed laceration. The patient declined to have any revision surgery for this. **G,** Left lateral view of the final occlusion.

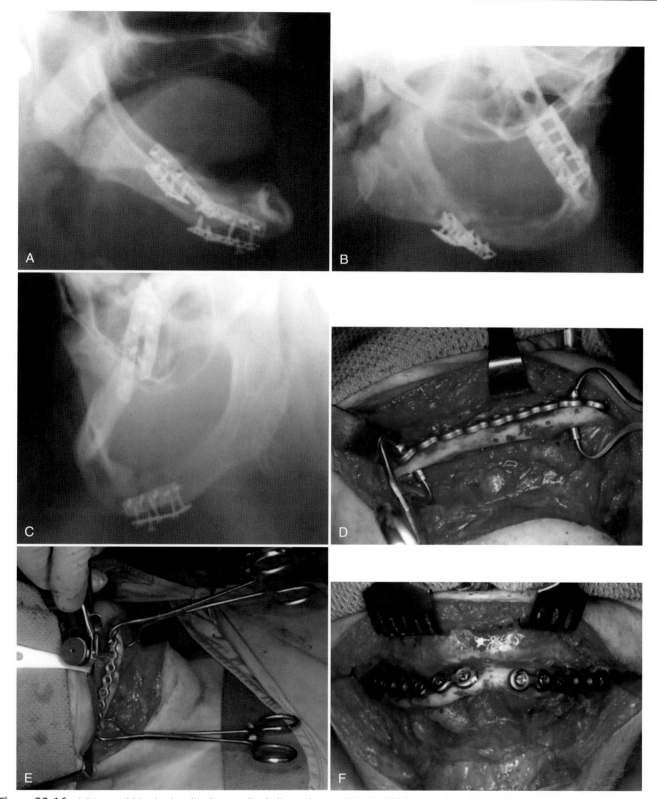

Figure 92-16. A 54-year-old institutionalized, mentally challenged man with spina bifida was referred for nonhealing and infection of bilateral edentulous body fractures. **A,** A lateral mandibular radiograph shows that the patient had previously undergone open reduction and internal fixation of the fractures and that miniplates had been applied to the lateral surface and the inferior border. The plates were fairly short in span and placed in an unfavorable compression zone, so during function the fracture would tend to gap superiorly. **B,** Right oblique view showing complete loss of fixation and osteolysis. **C,** Left oblique view demonstrating similar findings and screws backing out. **D,** The patient underwent wide extraoral exposure and débridement of the fibrous and granulation tissue on all bony margins. The right body fracture is seen reduced and a rigid reconstruction plate (2.3-mm system) was positioned and held with self-retaining clamps. **E,** A drill guide was used and locking screws inserted in the sound bone at least 4 to 5 mm away from the fracture site. **F,** Frontal view of the fully fixated mandible.

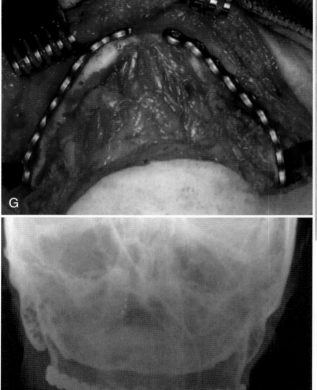

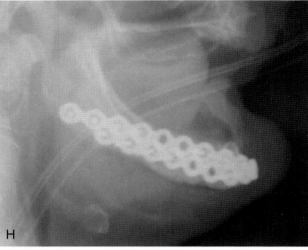

Figure 92-16, cont'd. G, Submental view. **H,** Postoperative lateral mandibular radiograph showing excellent projection and contours. **I,** Anteroposterior radiograph demonstrating symmetry and normal contours.

PEARLS

- Use drill guides with the more rigid plating systems to help prevent subtle shifting of segments.
- During application of rigid fixation, continuously recheck the occlusion to make sure that tightening of the last screw did not distract the bony segments.
- Mandible fractures in the pediatric age group are often best treated with closed techniques.
- Place the patient in maxillomandibular fixation before plating any fractures.
- Remove arch bars at the end of surgery unless they are necessary for postoperative interdental fixation or elastic guidance.

PITFALLS

- Lack of copious irrigation while drilling screw holes may result in overheated or necrotic bone that does little to stabilize fixation screws and can result in microscopic or gross mobility of the fixation and fracture before healing.
- If a tooth is left in the line of fracture or if the tooth itself is fractured or grossly decayed, it may limit bony reduction or result in a postoperative infection.

- Plates that are not placed perpendicular to the fracture line can cause vertical deflection during screw tightening and may be less stable.
- Mucosal incisions that are less than 1 cm away or close to the mucogingival junction do not allow suturing of the muscle layer, which is a risk for wound dehiscence and plate exposure.
- Intraoral approaches to condylar, subcondylar, and ramal fractures often result in a prolonged frustrating attempt at plating and lead to suboptimal alignment.

References

1. Thaller SR: Management of mandibular fractures. Arch Otolaryngol Head Neck Surg 120:44-47, 1994.
2. Chacon GE, Larsen PE: Principles of management of mandibular fractures. In Miloro M (ed): Peterson's Principles of Oral and Maxillofacial Surgery, 2nd ed. Hamilton, Ontario, BC Decker, 2004, pp 401-443.
3. Chacon GE, Dawson KH, Myall RW, Beirne OR: A comparative study of two imaging techniques for the diagnosis of condylar fractures in children. J Oral Maxillofac Surg 61:668-672, 2003.
4. Zallen RD, Curry JT: A study of antibiotic usage in compound mandibular fractures. J Oral Surg 33:431-434, 1975.
5. Chloe RA, Yee Y: Antibiotic prophylaxis for facial fractures. A prospective, randomized clinical trial. Arch Otolaryngol Head Neck Surg 114:1114-1122, 1988.

6. Ellis E, Moos KF, El-Attar A: Ten years of mandibular fractures: An analysis of 2,137 cases. Oral Surg 59:120-129, 1985.
7. May M, Tucker HM, Ogura IH: Closed management of mandibular fractures. Arch Otolaryngol 95:53-57, 1972.
8. Leathers RD, Gowans RE: Management of alveolar and dental fractures. In Miloro M (ed): Peterson's Principles of Oral and Maxillofacial Surgery, 2nd ed. Hamilton, Ontario, BC Decker, 2004, pp 383-400.
9. Tucker MR, Ochs MW: Basic concepts of rigid internal fixation: Mechanical considerations and instrumentation overview. In Tucker MR, Terry BC, White RP, Sickels JV (eds): Rigid Fixation for Maxillofacial Surgery. Philadelphia, JB Lippincott, 1991, pp 30-53.
10. Mathog RH, Rosenberg Z: Complications in the treatment of facial fractures. Otolaryngol Clin North Am 9:533-552, 1976.
11. Zide MF, Kent JN: Indications for open reduction of mandibular condylar fractures. J Oral Maxillofac Surg 41:89-98, 1983.
12. Amaratunga NA: Mandibular fractures in children—a study of clinical aspects, treatment needs, and complications. J Oral Maxillofac Surg 46:637-640, 1988.
13. Marciani RD: Invasive management of the fractured atrophic edentulous mandible. J Oral Maxillofac Surg 59:792-795, 2001.

Chapter 93

Fractures of the Upper Facial and Midfacial Skeleton

Mark W. Ochs

Depending on the point of impact and the degree of force, the upper facial and midfacial bones can sustain isolated or characteristic fracture patterns. A single blow from a fist to the midface often results in a displaced nasal fracture, the most common midfacial fracture, or in a tripod fracture of the zygomatic complex (ZMC). The midfacial bones tend to fracture in areas where they are thin and weak, such as the nasal bones, the anterior maxillary sinus wall, the orbital floor, the medial walls, and the nasal-orbital-ethmoid (NOE) complex. Suture lines also provide a natural cleavage plane for fractures to occur. If the facial bones are struck in strong thicker areas, the force is transmitted to the suture lines or thinner bony areas.

When severe or multiple midfacial fractures occur or when such fractures are associated with lacerations or penetrating injuries, significant hemorrhage can occur. Patients are often brought by emergency medical personnel on spine boards and in cervical collars. These restraints can lead to airway compromise, so measures to suction and control hemorrhage are essential. A significant number (>5%) of patients with frontal sinus or multiply displaced midfacial fractures will have an injury to the cervical spine.[1] When the airway needs to be secured, emergency tracheostomy or cricothyrotomy is generally the safest and most predictable course of action. It is difficult to perform direct laryngoscopy while maintaining in-line cervical spine traction. Fiberoptic intubation (either nasally or orally) is usually hampered by blood obstructing the view. Attempts at "blind nasal intubation" should be undertaken only by skilled individuals once a fracture of the NOE complex and possible fracture of the cribriform plate (with their potential for false passage into the anterior cranial fossa) have been excluded.

Control of hemorrhage can be accomplished by injection of local anesthetic containing vasoconstrictors, tacking sutures, localized packing, and less frequently, direct clamping of vessels. Blind clamping or electrocautery should not be undertaken in injured areas along the course of the facial nerve. Some blood loss during facial fracture surgery is unavoidable, but the use of injected vasoconstrictors and topical agents with nasal packing will greatly reduce oozing throughout the surgical procedure. Local infiltration may be repeated as often as necessary if the vasoconstrictors wear off. Bleeding vessels should be ligated or cauterized. The patient must be kept warm and the proper coagulation mechanism should be evaluated. The anesthesiologist must make every effort to maintain normotension or a systolic blood pressure of 110 mm Hg or lower. This should be done only when appropriate and neurologically and systemically tolerated by the patient.

Before general anesthesia, a gross visual acuity check of both eyes and assessment of facial motion must be made. This information is invaluable when correlated with computed tomography (CT) during treatment planning.

Goals of treatment of facial fractures are to restore the patient to the preinjury facial form with normal function. Re-establishment of the proper anterior facial projection without abnormal widening of the face is essential.[2] There is a tendency for a broad, flat face to occur as a result of blunt force and the direction of displacement. Severe midfacial fractures are often associated with multiple fractures of the mandible, which further compounds this situation.

Precise repositioning plus fixation prevents malocclusion and shortening of the midface. Horizontal relationships are maintained by buttresses at several levels, including the supraorbital rims and frontal bone, the zygomatic arch, the infraorbital rims, the nasal bones, and the maxillary alveolus. These horizontal relationships determine facial width, malar projection, occlusal relationships of the maxillary dentition, orbital position, and the width of the base of the nasal pyramid.

In addition to anatomic repositioning of the facial skeleton, surgical treatment must also consider the importance of restoring function, including an intact blood-brain barrier; mucociliary clearance of the frontal, maxillary, and ethmoid sinuses; nasal breathing; lacrimal drainage; dental occlusion; and conjugate movement of the extraocular muscles. The latter depends on establishing proper orbital volume and position of the globe.

PATIENT SELECTION AND PREOPERATIVE EVALUATION

Although each anatomic entity will be discussed separately, the surgeon should bear in mind that midfacial fractures are frequently multiple, have associated soft tissue injuries, and may be accompanied by neurologic injuries.

Maxilla

Direct blunt force trauma to the maxilla results in several classic fracture patterns that are designated by a Le Fort classification (Fig. 93-1). A Le Fort I fracture is a horizontal maxillary fracture of the horseshoe-shaped dentoalveolar complex (above the tooth roots) through the midmaxillary sinus and base of the lateral nasal walls. A Le Fort II fracture is a pyramidal break of the nasomaxillary complex with separation at the fron-

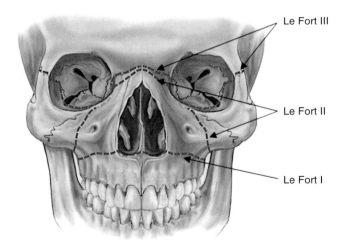

Figure 93-1. Le Fort classification of midfacial fractures. A Le Fort I fracture courses along the base of the nasal septum and floor or the midmaxillary sinus walls with separation at the pterygoid plates. A Le Fort II fracture traverses along the anterior maxillary wall and through the medial orbital rim, coupled with the nasal complex. A Le Fort III fracture has breaks at the zygomatic frontal sutures, frontonasal junction, zygomatic arches, and pterygoid plates. In essence, the entire midface is separated from the cranium (craniofacial dysjunction).

tonasal junction, through the inferior orbital rims, and then laterally along the anterior maxillary sinus wall, below the zygomatic buttresses. To clinically differentiate a Le Fort I from a Le Fort II fracture, the examiner should grasp the anterior maxillary teeth and alveolar ridge while stabilizing the forehead with the opposite hand. Anterior-posterior, or side-to-side, force should be applied to the anterior maxilla while observing for symmetrical motion of the entire maxilla (Le Fort I versus an isolated dentoalveolar fracture) or the maxilla and nasal complex together (Le Fort II). Complete craniofacial dysjunction is termed a Le Fort III fracture. Here, the entire facial complex, including the zygomatic buttresses, moves with applied maxillary force. Generally, Le Fort fracture patterns are not "pure" and have additional lines of fracture (i.e., dentoalveolar component), comminution, combinations (such as Le Fort I and III levels), or associated midfacial fractures (i.e., ZMC or orbit). Typically, the direction of the force fracturing the maxilla displaces the maxilla upward and back. This results in an anterior or lateral open bite and malocclusion. The face is flattened and elongated.

Patients sustaining Le Fort fractures demonstrate malocclusion, severe bilateral facial and periorbital edema, epistaxis, and ecchymosis (especially in the maxillary vestibule). These patients will often have paresthesia of the midface because of edema and pressure on the infraorbital nerves. Palpation of the maxillary vestibule, orbital rims, and nasal complex can reveal bony steps or detect motion while manipulating the maxilla. Edema and pain while palpating can readily mask these deformities. Tears in the gingiva or palatal mucosa should be sought because they are indicative of segmental fractures of the dentoalveolar complex and may alter the treatment plan. Traumatic open gaps in the dental arch should be accounted for either by an avulsed and missing tooth or by displacement or splaying of the fractured maxillary segments. Any watery or clear rhinorrhea should be collected and sent for β_2-transferrin assay to determine whether a cerebrospinal fluid (CSF) leak is present.

If there is strong clinical suspicion of a maxillary fracture, fine-cut (1.5 mm) axial CT scans through the entire facial complex offer the best imaging information for surgical planning and have replaced plain radiographs such as a Waters view, which offer little precise information. It is advisable to carry the CT scan through the mandible because there are invariably mandibular injuries such as condylar fractures that can be difficult to diagnose clinically or with plain films. Intravenous contrast material in the setting of acute facial trauma does not provide any additional detail and is not indicated.

Zygoma

Fractures of the ZMC are the second most commonly occurring facial fracture. They typically occur as a result of lateral blunt force, such as a blow to the face with a fist. These fractures are also termed "tripod" fractures because they are breaks along the zygomaticofrontal and zygomaticomaxillary junction (infraorbital rim and anterior sinus wall) and the zygomatic arch.[3] Usually, the zygomatic buttress is driven medially inward, inferior, and slightly posterior. There will be flattening of the malar projection, but this can be masked by edema. Frequently, clinical signs and symptoms include inferior displacement of the lateral canthus, tenderness of the frontozygomatic suture (located 1 cm above the lateral canthus), lateral subconjunctival hemorrhage, pain or limitation while opening the mouth, paresthesia of the cheek/lip, midfacial edema, and limited range of ocular motion (secondary to an orbital floor component). Palpation of the inferior orbital rim may reveal a step at the mid or medial half of the rim. Visual acuity should be assessed to rule out the possibility of a retrobulbar hematoma. Limited opening of the mouth is generally mild and due to the pain associated with masseteric muscle pull. However, with severe displacement of the ZMC, there can be direct impingement of the coronoid process and marked limited opening (1 cm interincisally). In anticipation of oral intubation for surgical repair, it is helpful to ask the patient to deviate the mandible to the contralateral side of the ZMC fracture and to assist the individual with opening. This often clears the path for the ipsilateral coronoid and allows adequate opening.

Isolated fractures of the zygomatic arch are usually due to a focused blow, such as with an elbow or a hardball, directly to the midarch. Typically, there are three separate vertical fracture lines with inward displacement in a V- or W-shaped pattern (Fig. 93-2). An indentation and tenderness in the area directly over the fracture may be noted or camouflaged by edema. Mild limited opening because of muscular pain is often present.

Radiographic imaging of fractures of the ZMC can initially include a Waters view to look for opacification or an air-fluid level in the maxillary sinus or a teardrop sign in the maxillary sinus caused by sagging of the periorbital contents through the orbital defect. Separation or widening of the zygomaticofrontal suture line is often difficult to ascertain except with extreme displacement. Axial CT offers the best views to determine the direction and degree of displacement of the ZMC. Direct coronal views or, less ideally, reformatted images can provide additional details of the orbital floor component if repair of this area is contemplated. Minimally displaced or nondisplaced fractures of the ZMC will heal uneventfully with sinus precautions, decongestants, and antibiotics, if indicated. In patients with minimally displaced or nondisplaced isolated fractures of the ZMC, orbital floor, or anterior maxillary wall, one should not operate for V2 paresthesia alone. The infraorbital nerve does not need to be decompressed, and "surgical exploration" will only further traumatize the nerve and not hasten recovery. Surgical repair is directed toward realignment, restoration of midface form, and unrestricted motion of the globe and mandible.

Isolated zygomatic arch fractures can be imaged with a submental vertex or "jug-handle" view. These inexpensive plain radiographs are adequate for planning surgical treatment. If further images are to be obtained, an axial CT scan is the image of choice. Isolated arch fractures are usually treated by open reduction through limited incisions in the temporal area, lateral aspect of the brow, or transorally and then not plated. Therefore, early operative intervention (preferably within the first 24 to 72 hours) is desirable to improve stability of the reduction and prevent the fragments from sagging back inward.

Orbit

Isolated fractures of the orbit constitute 10% of all facial fractures. If one includes fractures of the orbit that extend outside the confines of the orbit into the facial skeleton, the incidence approaches 40% to 55%. Fractures involving the orbit can be classified as ZMC, NOE, or internal orbital fractures.[4] Internal fractures of the orbit can occur in numerous patterns and can be described as *linear, blowout,* and *complex.* Linear fractures maintain periosteal attachments and do not generally result in a defect, but they can cause entrapment or impingement of the extraocular muscles or the capsulopalpebral fascia (Tenon's capsule). This most commonly occurs with linear fractures of the orbital

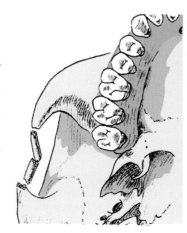 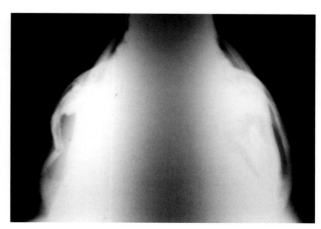

Figure 93-2. Isolated fracture of the right zygomatic arch. The *diagram* shows an inferior view of a classic fracture pattern with three breaks that typically occurs after a focused blow with a blunt object. The submental vertex radiograph reveals an inwardly displaced fracture of the right zygomatic arch and a normal left zygoma.

floor, especially in pediatric patients, whose facial bones are more pliable and momentarily expand or displace open at the time of impact and then snap back closed and entrap soft tissue. These patients will have firm, fixed limitation on upgaze or, more commonly, on downgaze. The patient may exhibit head tilting, nausea, and episodic bradycardia. Early repair (within 24 hours) and freeing of entrapped tissue are essential to prevent ischemia and fibrosis of the tissues with long-term restriction. Any equivocal entrapment or ocular restriction can be assessed by topically anesthetizing the globe and performing forced duction by grasping the insertion of the inferior rectus muscle through the lower eyelid fornix and attempting to move the globe superiorly and inferiorly.

Blowout fractures of the orbit are the most commonly occurring orbital injury and are limited to one wall, with the defect being less than 2 cm in diameter. Blowout fractures most frequently occur in the anterior or medial part of the orbital floor; however, they can occur in the medial wall or orbital roof, where they can be manifested as *blow-in* fractures. Orbital floor blowout fractures occasionally cause entrapment and limited ocular motility, but they more commonly result in expansion of the orbital volume with sagging of the orbital contents into the maxillary sinus. Initially, enophthalmos may not be apparent, but with clearance of hemorrhage and resolution of edema, the condition may become evident.

The decision to undertake surgical repair or reconstruction of these defects is based on functional limitations or cosmetic deformity.[5] Defects of 25% or less of the surface area without entrapment generally heal uneventfully without any intervention. Repair of intermediate defects involving 25% to 50% of the surface area is based on the degree of displacement, the amount of volume expansion, and any coexisting enophthalmos, even with edema. Larger or comminuted defects (>50%) with significant disruption are best treated by early repair (within 7 days) because some degree of enophthalmos or diplopia is the norm when left unrepaired. Fractures of the lateral wall rarely result in entrapment or volume changes since this area is well supported laterally by the bulky temporalis muscle. The lateral wall is most frequently fractured at the junction of the zygoma and greater wing of the sphenoid (one third of the way back from the rim), and it is usually a component of a ZMC fracture. Medial wall fractures rarely cause entrapment but can result in significant volume changes with a shift of orbital content into the ethmoid air cell spaces. In this instance, repair and reconstruction are usually indicated.

Exploration, repair, or reconstruction of fractures of the orbital roof (or any combination of such procedures) may be indicated if a dural tear is suspected or to prevent the development of a "pulsatile globe." This inward and outward movement of the eye is due to the arterial pulsations and respiratory fluctuations that occur in the overlying cerebral hemisphere. The *pulsatile globe* phenomenon often becomes apparent after resolution of edema and hematoma in unrepaired

defects of the roof of the orbit and causes persistent blurred or double vision.

Complex fractures consist of extensive fractures that affect two or more orbital walls; they often involve the posterior orbit and may involve the optic canal. Superior orbital fissure syndrome or orbital apex syndrome can occur.[6] The former consists of dysfunction of cranial nerves III, IV, V, and VI as a result of compression by bone fragments or hematoma. Orbital apex syndrome consists of superior orbital fissure findings with the addition of injury to the optic nerve. High-dose systemic steroids, blood pressure control, and elevation of the head of the bed can be palliative. Surgical intervention with decompression is based on correlation of CT with physical findings, the degree of optic nerve compromise, and the patient's neurologic, hemodynamic, and systemic stability. Retrobulbar hematoma can be treated on an emergency basis by performing a lateral canthotomy or inferior cantholysis (or both) and evacuating the clot by inserting a small curved hemostat along the lateral orbital wall and spreading it. A small Penrose drain can then be inserted.

Fractures of the orbital complex are usually associated with fractures of the facial skeleton outside the orbital framework (Le Fort II or III fractures or frontal sinus fractures) and are classified as *combined fractures*. A systematic approach to assessment of both orbits will further define the functional and anatomic defects associated with injuries to the orbit. The initial ophthalmic evaluation should include a periorbital examination and testing of visual acuity, ocular motility, pupil responses, and visual fields, as well as a funduscopic examination. The eyelids and periorbital areas should be inspected for edema, ecchymosis, lacerations, ptosis, asymmetric lid droop, injury to the canaliculus, and disruption of the canthal tendon.

Once the clinical assessment is complete, fine-cut (1.0 to 1.5 mm) axial CT images can be correlated with abnormalities or deficits. Direct coronal images are beneficial in evaluating defects of the walls of the sinus, and three-dimensional reformatting can be useful in patients with complex facial trauma or in instances of delayed or secondary repair. Magnetic resonance imaging has been used to identify wood or nonmetallic foreign bodies in penetrating injuries. These objects can be misdiagnosed by CT as intraorbital air and should be suspected when the apparent air collection within the post-traumatic orbit does not resorb rapidly.

The timing of any orbital repair is based on the urgency of the clinical findings (optic nerve compromise or muscle entrapment), the extent of the defects, associated facial fractures, or the patient's medical condition and health (Fig. 93-3). Early repair (within 5 to 7 days) offers the best results. Interval repair (within 7 to 14 days) can be undertaken once the edema and hematoma have resolved, a clear functional or cosmetic reason to intervene exists, and the patient is stable enough to undergo surgery with general anesthesia. Late repair (after 14 days) generally yields suboptimal

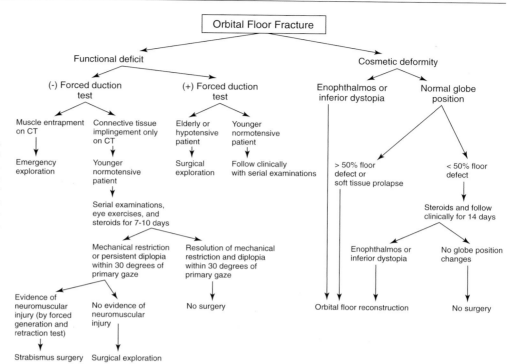

Figure 93-3. Management of a fracture of the orbit floor. The two primary indications for surgical intervention are to restore normal function of the globe and extraocular muscles and to repair a cosmetic deformity that would be noticeable. CT, computed tomography.

outcomes because of malunion and unfavorable soft tissue adaptation.

Nose

Fractures of the nose are the most common fracture of the face and are usually due to blunt force trauma. Lateral or oblique blows to the nose cause inward depression of the area of impact and lateral bowing of the contralateral side. A concomitant fracture of the nasal septum may accentuate the C-shaped deformity of the nasal dorsum. The degree of displacement can be masked by soft tissue swelling. Direct anterior force to the nasal bridge creates a depression of the nasal bridge and splaying of the nasal bones overlapping the frontal process of the maxilla (Fig. 93-4). Higher-energy impacts in this area can result in fracture of the ethmoid sinuses and NOE fractures. Frontal sinus and anterior basilar skull fractures are commonly associated with NOE fractures.

Fractures of the nose are primarily diagnosed by clinical examination. Patients sustaining a nasal fracture typically have epistaxis, nasal airway obstruction, localized pain, and an altered appearance of the nose. Physical examination requires proper lighting, suction, and intranasal application of vasoconstrictors by either aerosol spray or cotton pledgets. External signs of trauma such as lacerations, ecchymosis, or deviation of the nasal bridge should be noted. Edema often masks more subtle nasal fractures, and follow-up examination in 3 to 5 days is advisable if there are equivocal signs of nasal fracture. All areas of the nasal bones and cartilage should be palpated lightly to detect any bony crepitus, steps, focal tenderness, or loss of support. Once the

internal nares have been adequately cleared of clots and the vasoconstrictor has taken effect, speculum examination may reveal mucosal tears, septal deviation and hematoma, and protrusion of fractured bony segments or displaced cartilage intranasally.

The patient should be questioned regarding any preexisting nasal trauma, deformity, or septal deviation because many of these patients will have previously sustained a fracture. Significant or obstructive nasal septal deviation with pink, firm, normal overlying mucosa is suggestive of chronic septal deviation and not an acute injury. The point of attachment of the upper lateral cartilage to the nasal bones should be carefully assessed for disruption or detachment.

Plain radiographs of the nasal bones are seldom useful in the diagnosis or treatment decision making related to isolated nasal fractures. Normal suture lines and old healed fracture lines may be indistinguishable from acute fractures. In addition, fractured or displaced cartilaginous structures are not visualized by plain radiographs. If the need for a radiographic diagnosis exists, CT is the preferred imaging modality. CT scans clearly delineate the hard and soft tissue nasal structures, and signs such as lack of mucosal edema or asymmetric inferior turbinate size and shape suggest a previous injury or chronic nasal septal deformity.

Acute nasal bleeding is best managed by topical measures: vasoconstrictors, external pressure, ice compresses, and elevation of the head of the bed. More severe bleeding is managed by nasal packing.

The need for reduction of nasal fractures and stabilization is based on the patient's cosmetic appearance and the patency of the nasal airway. Nasal fractures elevated and reduced within the first 48 hours are

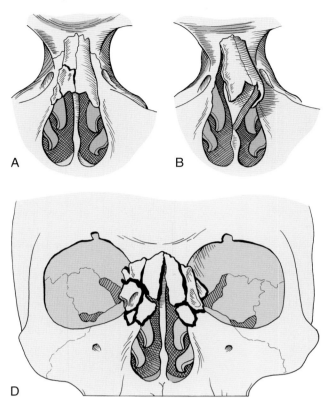
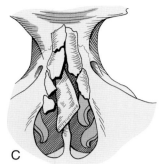

Figure 93-4. Patterns of fractures of the nose. **A,** Bowing or C-shaped deformity caused by direct lateral force. The ipsilateral nasal bones are depressed. **B,** Greater force causes fractures of the nose and deviation of the septum with lateralization of the contralateral nasal bones. **C,** Comminution secondary to more midline and heavy force with fracture of the septum results in loss of anterior projection and dorsal support. **D,** Fracture of the nasoethmoid complex caused by an extreme anterior impact. The fractures extend posteriorly to involve the medial orbital walls with typical splaying of the medial canthal tendons.

generally very stable. However, it may be necessary to wait 3 to 5 days to allow resolution of edema so that evaluation and proper alignment can be achieved. Most simple nasal fractures can be reduced with closed techniques under local anesthesia or intravenous sedation in an ambulatory setting.

Nasal-Orbital-Ethmoid Complex

Impacts of higher force to the nasal complex can result in fractures of the nasal bones, splaying, and posterior displacement into the ethmoids (Fig. 93-4C). Clinical signs of a fracture of the NOE complex are severe edema, telecanthus, lack of nasal projection, persistent epistaxis, occasionally CSF rhinorrhea, and periorbital ecchymosis. Blurred or altered vision may be present and is usually due to the edema and not to ocular restriction.

Fine-cut (1.0 to 1.5 mm) axial CT scans should be obtained to fully evaluate fractures of the NOE complex. Even with overlying lacerations, the medial canthal tendons are still usually attached to the bony anterior lacrimal crest.[7] The telecanthus is due to lateral displacement of the central portion of the frontal process of the maxilla. These segments are typically rotated outward and inferiorly displaced. The canaliculi should be evaluated for possible disruption.[8] If uncertainty exists, exploration of the wound plus repair under general anesthesia is warranted. Any copious, watery, or clear drainage should be collected and sent for β_2-transferrin assay to determine whether CSF rhinorrhea

has resulted from fracture of the cribriform plate or anterior basal skull.

Open nasal fractures and coexisting septal fractures are best treated under general anesthesia because of patient comfort, the degree of manipulation required for reduction, and the possibility of excessive bleeding during instrumentation. An oropharyngeal pack is helpful to have in place so that clots do not pool in the hypopharynx. NOE fractures require open reduction, internal fixation, and often transnasal wiring under general anesthesia.

Frontal Sinus

Fractures of the frontal sinus occur almost exclusively in adults. The frontal sinuses are two separate bony cavities formed either by invagination of the nasal cavity into the frontal bone or by extension of superior ethmoidal air cells into the same area. The frontal sinus is not radiographically evident until 6 years of age and becomes fully formed around the age of 15 years. The frontal sinus drains into the middle meatus of the nasal cavity via a foramen or ostium (85%) and less frequently through the frontal nasal ducts. Five percent of the adult population have either a unilateral frontal sinus or almost no frontal sinus. The anterior sinus wall, or outer table, is relatively thick and resistant to fracture. The posterior table is thin membranous bone with adherence to the surrounding dura and periorbita. The frontal sinus wall and ducts are lined with cuboidal respiratory epithelium that invaginates into small bony depressions. These depressions (foramina of Breschet) allow venous drainage of the sinus mucosa. After trauma or incomplete removal of the mucosa, mucocele formation may arise from these remnants.

Fractures of the frontal sinus require high-impact force such as that experienced by passengers in a motor vehicle accident without safety restraints. Fractures of the frontal sinus account for less than 15% of fractures of the mid and upper portion of the face. The majority of the time these fractures are associated with overlying lacerations of the forehead. Palpation and inspection through an open laceration of the forehead can reveal a depressed deformity or bony ledge indicating a fracture of the frontal sinus. It is common to have associated nasal, NOE, and orbital and maxillary fractures. Intracranial injuries such as cerebral contusion, subdural hematoma, epidural hematoma, dural tear, intraparenchymal bleeding, pneumocephalus, and CSF leak are also often associated. A hyperextension injury or a fracture of the cervical spine should be considered in this high-risk group.

When fracture of the frontal sinus is suspected, an axial CT scan (1.5- to 3.0-mm cuts) should be obtained to assess the fracture and the degree of displacement of the anterior and posterior tables. Displacement of a frontal sinus fracture is defined as overlap by the amount of thickness of the adjacent cortical bone. Intermediate distinctions such as *mild* or *moderate* are confusing and have no clinical relevance. Both the anterior and posterior tables should be categorized as fractured or not involved and displaced or nondisplaced. A displaced posterior table (overlapped fracture margins) is often associated with tears of the dura or cerebral injury requiring neurosurgical intervention.

Management of fractures of the frontal sinus should follow a logical decision-making process, as outlined in Figures 93-5 and 93-6. Open fractures of the frontal sinus require emergency exploration and treatment. Open fractures can be treated by primary cutaneous repair and delayed treatment of the injury to the frontal sinus, if necessary. A fractured frontal sinus usually fills with blood and mucus after trauma. Prophylactic antibiotics that cover most sinus microorganisms (ampicil-

lin with clavulanate) or a first-generation cephalosporin is generally recommended. Patients with involvement of the posterior table and displacement are often administered a broader-spectrum antibiotic that can cross the blood-brain barrier. Cervical immobilization should be maintained until cervical spine injury can be definitively excluded. Sinus decongestants are of potential benefit and should be considered in patients with frontal sinus trauma.

Definitive treatment of fractures of the frontal sinus depends on the extent of the fracture.[9] If the drainage system of the sinuses is significantly compromised, obliteration or cranialization is generally recommended. If only the anterior table is fractured and nondisplaced, surgical treatment is not usually necessary. A displaced fracture of the frontal sinus that is extensive enough to create a cosmetic deformity can be accessed directly through the fracture or via a liberal sinusotomy. The mucosal lining is then completely removed by curettage and drilling to deter formation of a mucocele, typically years later. The nasofrontal ducts can then be obliterated with fascia or bone grafts and the frontal sinus can be obliterated with autologous fat, bone, pericranium, or alloplastic material.

If only the anterior table is displaced without involvement of the nasofrontal ducts, primary repair without obliteration can be performed. Significant involvement or displacement of the posterior table usually requires direct exploration, with repair or cranialization depending on the degree of damage.[10] Smaller frontal sinuses in young patients can be cranialized by simply removing the posterior wall of the sinus, smoothing the edges, removing the mucosal lining, and obliterating the frontonasal ducts. Such treatment in

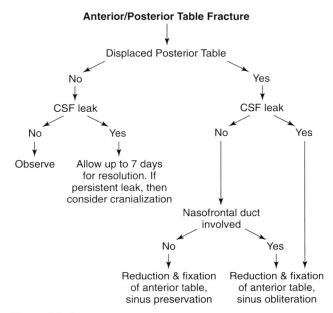

Figure 93-6. Fracture of the frontal sinus involving the posterior table requires further evaluation, and more treatment options exist, depending on the alignment of the posterior table and whether a cerebrospinal fluid (CSF) leak is present.

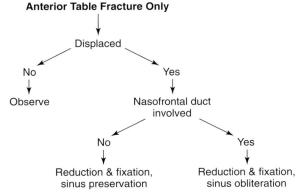

Figure 93-5. Fracture of the frontal sinus with appropriate management.

older patients and those with large frontal sinuses may predispose to the development of chronic subdural fluid accumulations. With displaced fractures of the posterior table, the presence of associated tears of the dura requiring neurosurgical management is the rule rather than the exception.

SURGICAL APPROACHES

Airway Management

Special consideration should be given to secure the airway when repair of midfacial and panfacial fractures is undertaken.[11] A coordinated strategy and discussion of issues that affect the airway, such as the complexity of the injury, the length of the procedure, the surgical approach, the use of intraoperative or postoperative maxillomandibular fixation (MMF), and the route and method of intubation, should take place between the surgeon and anesthesiologist. Cervical collars, Mayfield head holders, and the direction of the anesthetic tube, including the method of securing it, should also be considered. Patients with isolated nasal or zygomatic fractures should be orally intubated. Patients with Le Fort I–level fractures can be safely intubated nasally with a standard tube or nasal RAE tube. Cervical spine precautions may necessitate that intubation be performed fiberoptically. Patients with Le Fort II, Le Fort III, and NOE fractures may not be suitable for nasal intubation as a result of the need to repair or manipulate the nasal bones and septum. Oral intubation is often not possible because of full dentition and the need for MMF during surgery to re-establish the occlusion and align the fracture segments. If adequate edentulous space exists for insertion of the oral endotracheal tube between the teeth in MMF, this is an option. The tube can be secured to the sound adjacent teeth with 26-gauge circumdental wire. Passing the tube distal to the second molars in a fully dentate patient is often not satisfactory because of kinking of the tube, interference with surgical access, or potential displacement during surgical manipulation and turning of the head. In this instance or when concern for violation of the cribriform plate exists, a tracheostomy should be performed at the start of the procedure and a reinforced cuffed endotracheal tube placed, its position confirmed, and the tube secured with suture.

Sequencing of Treatment

Generally, arch bars are first applied to the maxillary and mandibular dentition as described in the previous chapter.

An intact mandible provides an excellent reference for re-establishing proper midfacial projection and transverse alignment with the use of MMF. It is often preferable to then open all fracture sites that require reduction and plating. It is usually easiest to start plating around points of broad, solid bony contact such as the frontozygomatic sutures, frontal sinus, zygomatic arches, and zygomatic buttresses along the posterior maxilla. The thinner piriform rims, anterior maxilla, and nasal

bones are fixated last. If the mandible is fractured, it is still best to place arch bars first, apply MMF, and then re-establish mandibular continuity by anatomic reduction and plating of the more anterior fractures (symphysis) and progressively working to the more posterior fractures, with condyles treated last. If both condyles are fractured, it is beneficial to open and plate at least one side to help re-establish proper posterior vertical dimension and a stable hinge axis point. When a patient is edentulous in one or both arches, best-fit anterior reduction plating is practical. If dentures exist, they can be secured to their respective arch by circum-mandibular wiring or screwing to the palate through holes pre-drilled in the lateral palatal shelves of the denture itself. In most instances, dentures interfere with surgical access, are ill-fitting or unstable, and do not greatly aid in fracture reduction. Repair or reconstruction of internal orbital fractures and defects is generally performed last because stable and aligned orbital rims help guide and stabilize the repair.

Maxillary/Le Fort Fractures

Le Fort I fractures are approached through a maxillary vestibular incision placed 1 cm from the outstretched mucogingival junction from first molar to first molar. Distal extension beyond this point invites herniation of the buccal fat pad and additional bleeding. Subperiosteal dissection is then accomplished with minimal stripping and soft tissue reflection on the inferior (or dental-bearing) segment that will just permit plate and screw placement. Infiltration of the maxillary vestibule with local anesthetic containing a vasoconstrictor minimizes oozing, and placing the patient in MMF before incision helps stabilize the maxillary segment and facilitates soft tissue dissection. Subperiosteal placement of toe-up Obwegeser retractors along the lateral maxillary "pockets" provides excellent "hands-free" exposure. Once the entire anterior maxillary fracture line is exposed with adequate areas for plating, the MMF is rechecked and tightened slightly, if needed, because of stretching of the wire. Any debris or small free-floating piece of bone is removed, and the fracture is reduced by applying upward vertical pressure on the mandibular angles bilaterally. Digital pressure in the submental region or chin often provides what appears to be improved reduction of the fracture, but at the expense of slight distraction of the condylar heads from the fossae. Plating in this position results in an immediate anterior open bite on release of the MMF wires, or it can occur postoperatively when the patient's masticatory muscles seat the mandibular condyles. Therefore, it is best to plate and fixate the maxilla with slight anterior wall contact irregularities because the fractured heavier posterior maxilla and pterygoid regions may not allow complete vertical reductions either. With the condyle seated by applying constant pressure to the angle region, the maxilla is fixated with 1.7- or 2.0-mm miniplates in the piriform and zygomatic buttress regions.[12] Generally, four plates are applied, and L shapes seem to work the best because two screws can be

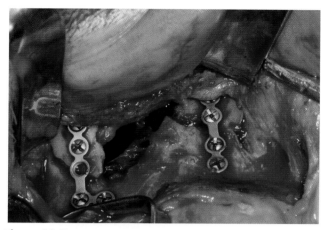

Figure 93-7. Le Fort I fracture repair. The right maxillary vestibular incision was made 1 cm above the mucogingival junction. Arch bars were secured and the patient placed in maxillomandibular fixation. The anterior maxillary bony reductions appear slightly off, but this is typical because it is usually impossible to fully reduce a fractured posterior maxilla with the condyles seated by pressure at the angles of the mandible. The maxilla is fixated with miniplates and 2.0-mm screws in the areas of heaviest bone: the buttress *(left)* and the piriform rim *(right)*. No attempt is made to "reconstruct" the anterior maxillary wall defect, and it should heal uneventfully. Any free bone fragments should be removed from the sinus.

placed in the inferior segment of each plate without violating any tooth roots (Fig. 93-7). Irrigation should be used during drilling to prevent overheating of the thin maxillary bone. Placing the anterior plates 2 to 3 mm laterally from the edge of the piriform rims and slightly medially inward allows engagement of both the anterior maxillary and lateral nasal walls and thus provides improved stability.[13] Screws 4 to 5 mm in length are the norm. Once all plates are placed, the MMF wires (not the arch bars and circumdental wires) are cut and removed, and the occlusion is checked by applying intermittent mild pressure on the mandibular angles. The circumdental wires and arch bars are removed only after adequate fracture reduction and fixation are confirmed and the surgeon is confident that there will be no need for a period of postoperative MMF or elastic guidance.

For closure, a nasal cinch suture that engages the underside or inner aspects of the alar bases is placed and secured to draw the ala together to the preinjury/presurgical position. Closure of the muscular layer is then performed on each side with several interrupted 4-0 Vicryl sutures (braided polyglactin suture, Ethicon). The maxillary mucosal incision is closed with 3-0 or 4-0 chromic suture in a running horizontal mattress stitch. The pack should be removed from the throat and an orogastric tube passed. The area should be suctioned and then the tube withdrawn before extubation.

Treatment of a Fort II fracture is similar to treatment of a Le Fort I fracture but usually requires higher medial dissection for plating. Generally, plating of the frontonasal or high medial nasomaxillary fracture lines is unnecessary. However, if comminution or lack of stability dictates the need to fixate in this region, access via a coronal incision is preferred over an "open-sky"

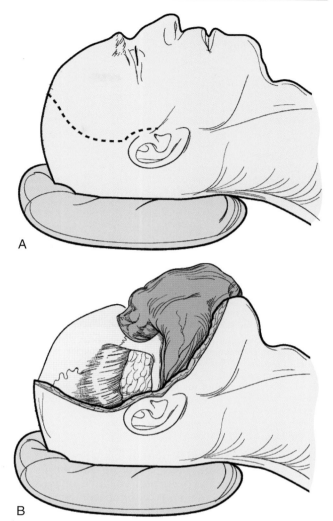

Figure 93-8. Design of a coronal flap. **A,** The preauricular incision is not extended below the lower edge of the tragus. Going below and deep to this invites injury to the main trunk of the facial nerve. At the superior extent of the auricular attachment the incision is curved posteriorly for about 0.5 cm to help avoid cutting the superficial temporal artery (STA). The STA can generally be left intact and reflected forward with the coronal flap. **B,** A soft wavy line rather than a straight side-to-side incision allows ease in turning the flap over.

approach (H shaped; combined medial brow and glabellar and lateral nasal incisions). Sometimes an existing laceration can be accessed and extended slightly for plating. Fixation of the frontonasal junction with bilateral smaller plates along the lateral nasal/medial orbital rim contours is less palpable than fixation with a miniplate directly over the midforehead and nasal dorsum.

Le Fort III fractures generally require both a maxillary vestibular incision (because there are usually additional maxillary lines of fracture) and a coronal approach to access and fixate the frontonasal, zygomaticofrontal, and zygomatic arch fractures. The coronal incision is a wavy line that is placed approximately 2 cm posterior to the hairline (midline) and extended posteriorly and then inferiorly in the preauricular region (Fig. 93-8). The wavy line facilitates "turning the flap

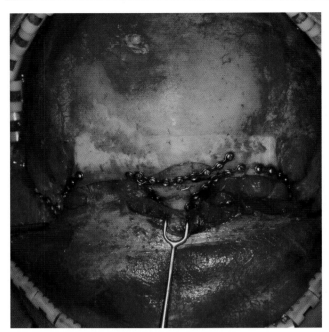

Figure 93-9. Frontal view of a reflected bicoronal flap. The pericranium is cut horizontally 2 to 3 cm above the superior orbital rims. The supraorbital nerves were in notches (not foramina) and were freed for full exposure of the nasal complex and superior medial orbital walls. Reduction of the fractures of the nose and orbit completely reduced the telecanthus, and therefore transnasal wiring was unnecessary.

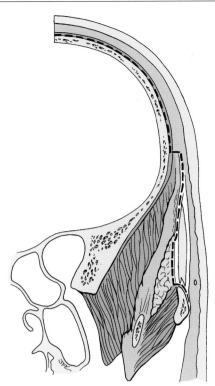

Figure 93-10. Left coronal view of the incision through the superficial layer of the deep temporal fascia just below the temporal line. The dissection should be deep to this layer to protect the frontal branch of the facial nerve and be confluent and deep to the periosteum of the zygomatic arch to protect the superior division of the facial nerve.

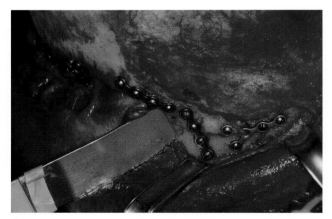

Figure 93-11. Left lateral view of a bicoronal dissection and plating of the arch and lateral orbital rim. Note that clean reflection of the superficial temporal fascia along with the arch periosteum led to a safe and dry field.

over" and has the added benefit of being less noticeable when the hair is wet, such as during swimming, and when mild hair loss has occurred. The incision is carried through skin, subcutaneous connective tissue, galea aponeurotica, and loose areolar tissue in the midline and extended laterally in the supraperiosteal plane to the superior temporal line bilaterally.

The subgaleal plane of dissection is contiguous with a plane deep to the parietotemporal fascia in the area of the temporalis muscle. Dissection is carried anteriorly to the frontal bone, and a horizontal incision is made through the periosteum approximately 2 to 3 cm superior to the orbital rim (Fig. 93-9). This incision is carried laterally to the superior temporal line and is joined with the preauricular area inferiorly through the superficial layer of the deep temporal fascia to protect the temporal branch of the facial nerve (Fig. 93-10). The frontal branch or superior division of the facial nerve courses in a plane superficial to the deep temporal fascia approximately 1 to 2.5 cm from the tragus along the zygomatic arch. This approach provides access to the entire medial, lateral, and superior orbital frame. Closure may include suspension of the cut temporal fascia over the temporalis muscle and should include deep closure of the galea aponeurotica, subcutaneous tissue, and skin. Miniplates secured with 3- to 4-mm-length screws are adequate for fixation (Fig. 93-11). It is desirable to use burrs with drill stops (ledges that prevent drilling beyond predetermined depths) when working around the orbital rims. The lateral canthal

attachments to the internal orbit (Whitnall's tubercle) should not be disturbed during dissection and therefore do not require reattachment.

Skeletal suspension wires from the intact portion of the facial bones (frontal or circumzygomatic) can aid in stabilizing the maxillary fractures or can be used as a sole means for accomplishing closed reduction by securing them through intermediate wires to the

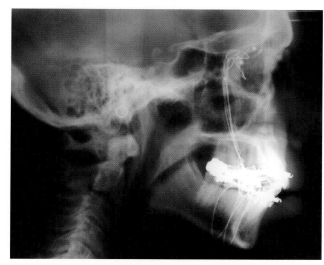

Figure 93-12. Skeletal suspension wires as seen on a lateral cepha-logram. Bilateral frontal suspension wires (24- and 26-gauge "pullout wires") and circum-mandibular wires (24 gauge) were passed with awls and secured to arch bars to support and immobilize a Le Fort I fracture. The frontal and circum-mandibular suspension wires were secured to each other with a 26-gauge intermediate wire loop. Open treatment was not performed because of cervical spine injury and the patient's critical status. A tracheostomy had been performed previously to secure the airway.

mandibular arch bar or circum-mandibular wires (Fig. 93-12).

After repair of any Le Fort fracture (I, II, or III), the nasal septum should be inspected to make sure that it is not subluxated or laterally displaced. The nasal septum can be repositioned or slightly trimmed at the inferior aspect, if necessary, to allow positioning in the midline. Once the fractures are reduced and fixated, a forced duction test of both eyes should be performed to rule out entrapment of muscle because the majority of these fractures have an orbital component.

Zygomatic Fractures

Isolated fractures of the zygomatic arch are best repaired within 72 hours of the injury. In this time frame the arch tends to reduce easily, with excellent indexing and stability and no need for internal fixation or external splints. Fractures of the arch can be approached through a limited lateral brow incision with blunt dissection down to the supraperiosteal plane or via a Gillies (2.5-mm oblique temporal hairline) incision and avoid-ance of the superficial temporal artery.[14] The temporal fascia is exposed, and a Freer elevator is used to create a small pocket between the fascia and temporalis muscle. With either approach, a blunt stout instrument (curved Kelly clamp, urethral sound, or Rowe zygomatic eleva-tor) is inserted beneath the arch. It is often helpful to palpate with the opposite hand intraorally in the poste-rior buccal sulcus to detect a slight deflection from the tip of the instrument. The arch is then elevated with lateral and superior force while taking care to not lever off any other facial bones. An audible crack or pop

indicates that the fracture has been reduced, and palpa-tion of a convex contour confirms the reduction. The subcutaneous and skin layers are closed, and the patient is advised to avoid contact to the area for several weeks. A maxillary vestibular (buccal sulcus) approach can be used, but it might be accompanied by bleeding from the masseter muscle and has the risk of inferior/lateral orbit violation if the arch elevator is overinserted beneath a moderately depressed arch fracture.

Fractures of the ZMC can be approached by a variety of incisions: lateral brow, modified blepharo-plasty, hemicoronal, transconjunctival, infraciliary, and maxillary-vestibular. The degree of injury and the dis-placement often dictate which areas of the ZMC must be accessed and fixated.[15,16] Although a single miniplate at the frontozygomatic suture may suffice for healing, it may not provide absolute rigidity to maintain malar projection and ideal contours. Typically, at least two points of fixation and plating are used to achieve rigid-ity. We generally prefer plating at the frontozygomatic suture because it is easily indexed and has heavy bone stock for fixation. The second area of fixation can be either across the zygomatic buttress (maxillary vestibu-lar incision) or at the infraorbital rim. The latter is chosen when exploration of the orbital floor or recon-struction is anticipated (Fig. 93-13). These approaches and materials for repair are fully discussed in the next section.

Before plating any fracture lines, all sites are exposed, and the ZMC is reduced to satisfaction in each area.[17] The ZMC is then fixated with miniplates (1.7- to 2.0-mm systems) while taking care to maintain the plates several millimeters away from the orbital rim so that they will not be visible or palpable. If associated facial fractures (Le Fort, frontal sinus) or comminution exists, it may be necessary to obtain direct access to the entire zygomatic arch for fixation and stabilization.[18] This is accomplished via a coronal or hemicoronal approach. Care should be exercised to not "overele-vate" the arch at its midpoint. The zygomatic arch has a slight curve at its anterior and posterior extents but is flat in the middle. Overprojection of the arch should be avoided because it causes a tumor-like protrusion postoperatively that will persist.

Orbit

Once it has been determined that a patient requires surgical intervention for a fracture of the orbit, several factors must be considered when selecting the surgical approach and method of reconstruction. The primary consideration is to determine which walls need to be repaired. Associated facial fractures, lacerations, and surgeon preference are other important factors.

Three basic incisions provide access to the orbital floor: infraorbital, subciliary, and transconjunctival (Fig. 93-14). The subciliary and transconjunctival inci-sions, because of their superior aesthetics, are the most commonly used today.[19,20] In the subciliary approach, the skin is incised several millimeters below the lid margin in a skin crease and dissected from the

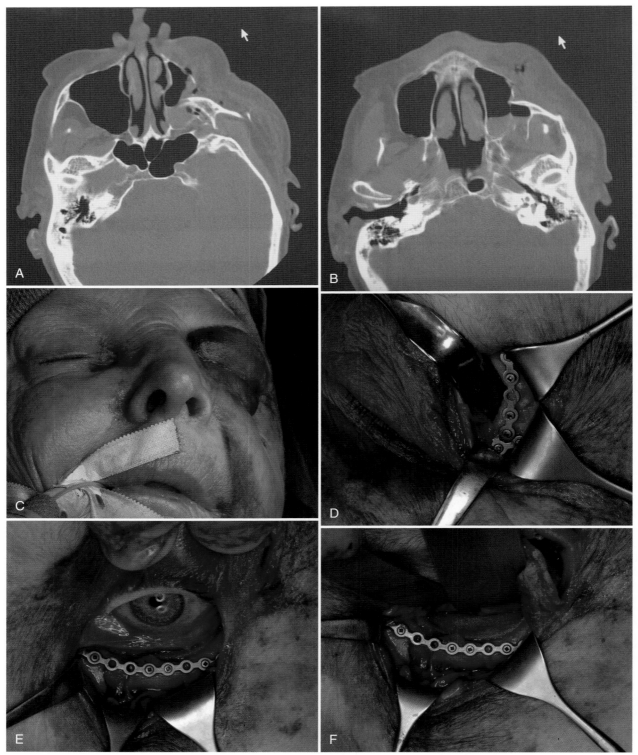

Figure 93-13. Severely displaced fracture of the left zygomatic complex. **A,** Axial computed tomography (CT) scan showing the buttress driven inward to the posterior maxillary sinus and approaching the pterygoid plates. The *cursor arrow* overlies the area of impact, and a depression is seen despite tremendous soft tissue swelling. **B,** Slightly inferior CT scan demonstrating the fractured posterior zygomatic arch component with probable mechanical impingement on the tip of the coronoid process. Difficulty opening the mouth for oral intubation should be anticipated and evaluated. The soft tissue swelling "masks" the degree of bony displacement. **C,** Facial appearance as the patient was prepared for surgery urgently because of a tense left periorbita and decreased vision in the left eye. She was taking warfarin (Coumadin) for atrial fibrillation and suffered significant localized bleeding and in essence "a compartment syndrome" of the orbit. **D,** The left lateral brow incision was first undertaken and the entire zygomatic complex grossly reduced. A miniplate was fixated with 1.7-mm-diameter, 3 mm-long screws after the inferior orbital rim and zygomatic buttress were exposed and reduced. **E,** Orbital rim plated after transconjunctival retroseptal dissection and inferior cantholysis. The rim was stabilized with a miniplate and 1.3-mm-diameter screws. **F,** The floor of the orbit had been almost completely destroyed. It was reconstructed with a 0.85-mm-thick sheet of Medpor (high-density porous polyethylene) that was fixated inferolaterally to the intact floor ledge with a single 5-mm-long, 1.7-mm-diameter screw to prevent migration or "unflexing" of the gently curved Medpor. Forced duction of the globe should be performed at this stage to ensure that none of the orbital contents have become entrapped or tethered by the repair or fixation.

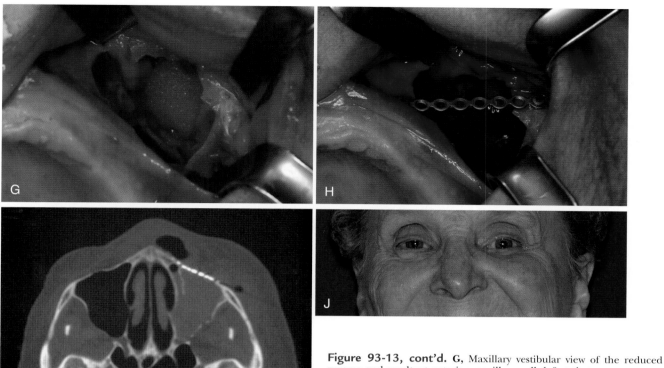

Figure 93-13, cont'd. G, Maxillary vestibular view of the reduced zygoma and resultant anterior maxillary wall defect that was not reconstructed. The Medpor orbital floor repair is visible from below. The patient's edentulous maxillary ridge can be seen in the lower left area. **H,** The zygomatic buttress was fixated with a miniplate and 1.7-mm-diameter screws. **I,** Postoperative axial CT scan obtained the following day showing symmetrical alignment. **J,** Facial view 1 month after surgery.

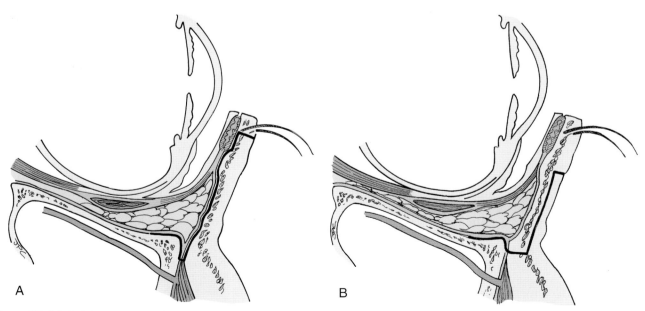

Figure 93-14. Inferior lid approaches. **A,** Subciliary dissection with the initial skin incision just below the lash line through orbicularis oculi muscle and staying anterior to the orbital septum and carried inferiorly to the rim. The periosteum is incised several millimeters below the rim (level of the arcus marginale and orbital septum attachment) and then reflected to gain access to the orbital floor. **B,** Lower eyelid skin crease approach to the inferior orbital rim and floor. After incising the skin, the inferior dissection is performed anterior to the orbicularis oculi muscle.

orbicularis oculi for a few millimeters before splitting the muscle fibers down to and anterior to the orbital septum. Division of skin and muscles at different levels helps prevent direct scarring and retraction of the eyelid. The dissection is then carried down to the orbital rim, the periosteum is incised 2 mm below the orbital rim (below the arcus marginale), and the dissection is extended posteriorly along the orbital floor to elevate the orbital contents and reduce the floor fractures. One can safely dissect 30 mm back along the floor because the optic canal is 40 mm from the anterior lacrimal crest and is superiorly and medially located. After repair is complete, several tacking sutures can be placed in the periosteum at the rim, and only the skin is closed with cutaneous 6-0 nylon suture.

The transconjunctival approach has two variations: retroseptal and preseptal. The retroseptal approach is a more direct approach to the orbital floor, but it exposes the extraconal fat, which can obstruct the surgeon's view. For this reason the preseptal approach is preferred. To avoid excessive tension and stretching of the lower eyelids, many surgeons prefer to start by performing a lateral canthotomy (3-mm skin incision in a crow's foot line) and inferior cantholysis, which consists of division and release of only the inferior leaflet of the lateral canthus (Fig. 93-15). The lid is then held out and forward with fine forceps, and the palpebral conjunctiva and inferior lid retractors (smooth muscle that is an extension of the capsulopalpebral fascia) are undermined and incised 2 to 3 mm below the inferior edge of the tarsus. If one undermines and incises at the depth of the fornix and aims toward the caruncle (small yellow mound of tissue) medially, injury to the tarsus and inferior canaliculus can be avoided.

The dissection is then carried inferiorly along the plane superficial to the septum (to avoid herniation of fat) down to the orbital rim, and the periosteum is incised on the facial aspect. After orbital repair the periosteum is approximated with several fine interrupted sutures. The conjunctiva is closed with several 6-0 fast-absorbing gut sutures. If there is any uncertainty in reapproximating the correct layers, do not suture. Tacking the orbicularis oculi to the periosteum of the orbital rim will result in acute ectropion, lid retraction, and a "hound dog eyes" appearance. If this occurs, have the patient vigorously massage the area to stimulate its release. If the situation does not resolve within several weeks, reopen the site and release it. It may be advisable to place a reverse-Frost (modified tarsorrhaphy suture) for 24 hours. Reattachment of the inferior leaflet of the lateral canthus is accomplished with 4-0 Mersilene double-armed suture on an S-2 needle. The needles are passed internally to externally along the lateral orbital rim (cut margins) to ensure proper insetting of the lid.

Access to the superior orbital rim and the frontozygomatic suture can be achieved with an eyebrow incision, an upper blepharoplasty incision, or coronal dissection. The eyebrow and blepharoplasty incisions, because of their excellent aesthetics, are most often used. The coronal incision is used when extensive facial or skull fractures are present. The eyebrow incision is placed on the lateral aspect (1.5 cm) above the brow and parallel to the hair follicles. Sharp dissection with electrocautery can be carried down through the subcutaneous tissue, orbicularis oculi muscle, and periosteum. This provides excellent access to the lateral rim and plating at the frontozygomatic suture, which is 1 cm above the lateral canthus. The upper blepharoplasty incision is similar to the brow incision, but slightly more inferior and more horizontal. It is placed in one of the skin creases of the upper eyelid and carried through the subcutaneous tissue, orbicularis oculi, and periosteum. A 1.0- to 1.5-cm incision is all that is necessary because of the mobility and laxity of the lid tissues. Closure requires suturing of the periosteum and skin.

Access to the medial orbital rim and superior aspect of the medial orbital wall can be obtained through a coronal (see Fig. 93-9) or a lateral nasal incision. Access to the inferior medial orbital wall can be achieved via a transconjunctival approach. The lateral nasal approach involves a vertical, 1.5-cm curvilinear incision approximately 0.5 to 1.0 cm anterior to the medial canthus. Care must be taken to not place the incision too close to the medial canthus, which can result in scar contracture and "webbing." Dissection is carried through the skin, subcutaneous tissue, orbicularis oculi, and periosteum. The periosteum can then be reflected posteriorly and superiorly to the medial orbital rim and wall. The medial canthal tendon, which envelopes the lacrimal sac, lies posterior and inferior to the incision. A single subcutaneous suture and multiple interrupted skin sutures are all that is required for closure.

The goal of primary reconstruction of internal fractures of the orbit is restoration of mobility and function of the globe, re-establishment of normal volume, and elevation of prolapsed soft tissues from the paranasal sinuses.[21] Isolated linear fractures are reduced, and any entrapped soft tissues are freed. No grafting is required, but a piece of Gelfilm or fine (0.85 mm) Medpor (porous polyethylene, Porex Surgical) can be laid over the site if the surgeon is concerned about impingement or risk of re-entrapment.[22]

Blowout and larger defects can be reconstructed with a variety of materials: split calvarial bone, Medpor, and titanium mesh. The graft should not extend all the way to or over the inferior orbital rim. This creates a posterior ramping effect on the globe and does not restore the normal contours of the orbital floor. The orbital floor dips down several millimeters immediately behind the inferior rim and has a gentle concave curve from side to side and anterior to posterior. Overgrafting with excessive reduction of orbital volume or placing the graft too anterior with posterior sloping tends to prop the globe too far superiorly and creates a vertical dystopia with the possibility of persistent enophthalmos. Attempts should be made to rest the graft on intact bony ledges and to position the graft beyond the equator of the globe posteriorly. The grafts can be secured with screws or sutures, depending on the nature of the reconstruction (Fig. 93-16). Unsecured grafts can

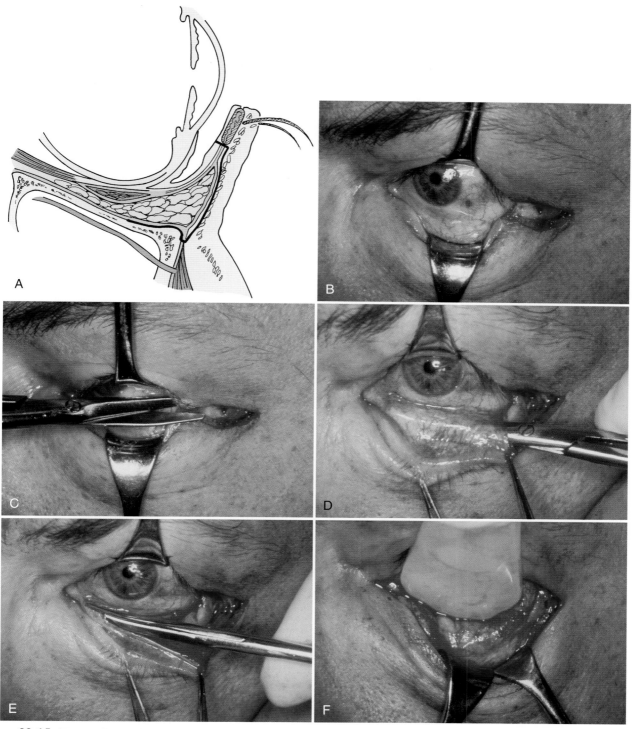

Figure 93-15. Transconjunctival preseptal approach. **A,** The palpebral conjunctiva and inferior lid retractors are incised below the inferior edge of the tarsal plate. The inferior dissection is anterior to the septum to avoid herniation of orbital fat into the operative field. **B,** Left lateral canthotomy incision. Generally, it is only 5 to 7 mm in length and carried through the orbicularis oculi muscle. **C,** Inferior cantholysis performed with tenotomy or iris scissors. It is helpful to angulate the tips of the scissors slightly downward to ensure division of only the inferior canthal tendon and leaving the superior leaflet intact. The tips of the scissors are just superficial to the periosteum of the rim when the cut is performed. The cut lateral edge of the lid is grasped with 0.5-mm pickups, and additional "snipping" of the canthal attachments is performed until the lid can be adequately mobilized for the following step. **D,** The lid is gently held outward at two points by the assistant while the surgeon undermines the palpebral conjunctiva and inferior lid retractors (smooth muscle). This is toward the depth of the fornix, and the tip of the blunt scissors is pointed medially toward the caruncle. **E,** These same layers are then divided. **F,** Desmarres retractors are used to reflect the lower lid inferiorly. A Lucite lid plate or malleable retractor rests on the inner edge of the rim to retract the septum and orbital contents inward during incision of the facial periosteum several millimeters below the rim.

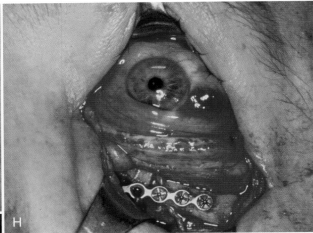

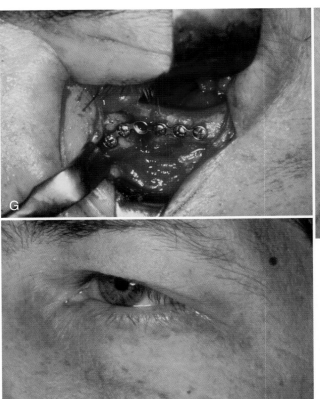

Figure 93-15, cont'd. G, The fracture of the zygoma has been reduced and the rim aligned and fixated with a miniplate and 1.7-mm screws. **H,** Generous access as a result of inferior cantholysis and a clean field secondary to the preseptal approach. **I,** Postoperative appearance at 6 weeks.

migrate forward to the rim and be palpable or angle and protrude into the paranasal sinuses.

Fractures of the orbital floor should not be overtreated. If there are no firm findings—entrapment, greater than a 50% floor defect with orbital herniation, acute enophthalmos—allow the edema to resolve, reevaluate the wound, and intervene only if a functional deficit or cosmetic deformity warrants repair.

Nose

Nasal and septal fractures should be repaired as soon as possible but can be delayed 7 to 10 days to allow resolution of edema and reassessment. Closed reduction is all that is required for most nasal and septal fractures. It can be accomplished under topical anesthesia, local anesthesia, intravenous sedation, or general anesthesia. Topical anesthesia and vasoconstriction are achieved with the insertion of cottonoids (0.5 × 3 inches) or cotton pledgets saturated with 2% to 4% lidocaine and the vasoconstrictor of choice (1 : 50,000 epinephrine, 1 : 10 dilution of 0.25% phenylephrine [Neo-Synephrine], 0.05% oxymetazoline). These objects are inserted high into the nasal vault between the nasal bones and septum, at the base of the septum, and at the lateral inferior turbinates.

It is beneficial to inject local anesthetic at each site (0.5 mL) along the lateral nasal bones, at the infraorbital nerve externally, and at the base of the anterior septum. Even if general anesthesia is used, the local anesthetic with vasoconstrictor facilitates direct vision and minimizes bleeding and postoperative pain. After waiting a full 10 to 15 minutes for the vasoconstrictive action, the pledgets are removed. A blunt elevator (Goldman elevator, knife handle) is inserted a predetermined amount with the thumb pressed against the external skin overlying the nasal bone to be elevated. Slight thumb pressure allows rotational or twisting motion as the nasal bone is elevated and aligned (Fig. 93-17). The nasal bones and dorsum are then inspected and palpated for midline alignment, projection, and symmetry. In general, the nasal bone fractures are reduced first, and then the nasal septum is inspected with a speculum and aligned as needed. Asch forceps are inserted bilaterally into the nasal cavity; they can be placed higher in the nasal vault to provide additional anterior force and elevation of the nasal bones or, more commonly, along the base and midseptum to bring the structures into midline. The reduced septum should provide support to the overlying nasal bones and allow a patent bilateral nasal airway. After final inspection of the nasal bones and septum, internal silicone splints can be placed bilaterally along the septum, and a 3-0 silk transfixion suture should be passed through both splints and the anterior septal cartilage to secure them.

The nasal skin is then dried and "defatted" with alcohol wipes and a small amount of topical adhesive

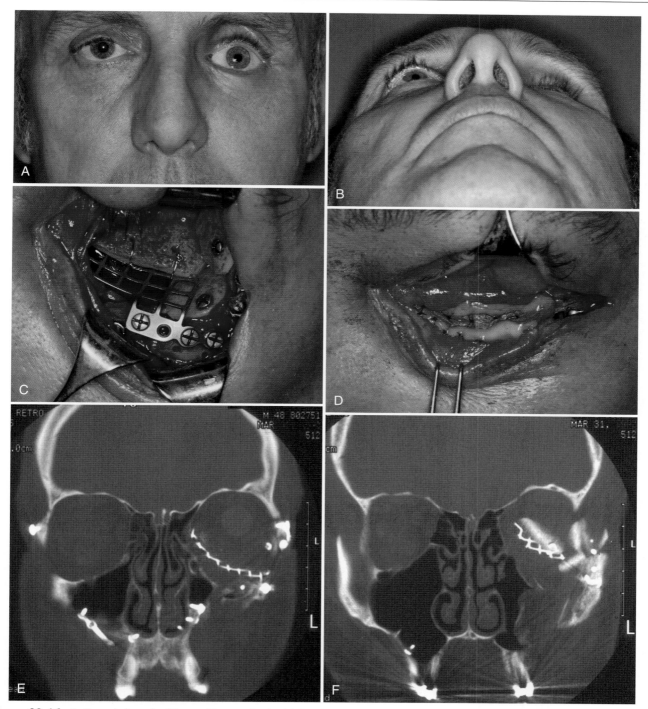

Figure 93-16. A, Frontal view of a 53-year-old man who had fallen from a tree and sustained a fracture of the zygomatic complex (ZMC) and a ruptured left globe. He had been treated at another center by open reduction and internal fixation of the left ZMC, enucleation of the globe, and insertion of a 12-mm hydroxyapatite (HA) sphere. He complained that his prosthesis would dislodge and that his left "eye" appeared sunken in and down. **B,** Submental view showing significant left enophthalmos (>10 mm). The HA implant sphere was too small and the orbital volume was too large. **C,** The left orbit was reconstructed with a titanium mesh plate that served as a scaffold for multiple calvarial split-thickness grafts. The grafts were placed posteriorly and laterally behind the equator of the HA globe. **D,** To restore lower lid length and reconstruct the fornix, a free mucosal graft was harvested from the buccal aspect of the mouth and inset and the form supported by 6-0 Prolene sutures and a Telfa bolster. **E** and **F,** Postoperative coronal computed tomography scans demonstrating the reduced orbital volume with mesh and grafts in place.

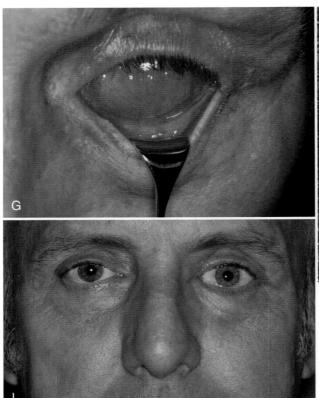

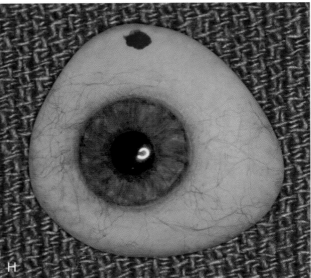

Figure 93-16, cont'd G, Fornix and anterior projected mucosalized HA sphere 6 weeks after surgery. **H,** New and thinner prosthesis (eye contact lens) with a red dot that helps the patient orient it for insertion. **I,** Facial appearance 2 months after the procedure.

solution applied, followed by porous paper tape or Steri-Strips. A thermoplastic splint can then be trimmed, heated, and adapted to the external nasal contours and secured with adhesive tape. These coverings are generally left in place for 1 week. Compound nasal fractures should be repaired earlier. Direct access to the bones through the laceration may allow wiring or plating for stabilization if necessary. Closed reduction is accomplished with a similar sequence and protocol. External splinting, even over sutured lacerations, is acceptable. Attempts should be made to close mucosal lacerations over the nasal and septal cartilage with absorbable 5-0 suture.

Nasal-Orbital-Ethmoid Complex

NOE injuries result in significant aesthetic deformities. Injuries to the nasal airways and lacrimal system can also occur. Injuries to the lacrimal system can be managed by placing small silicone tubes (Crawford tubes) within the superior and inferior canaliculi down through the lacrimal sac, retrieving them intranasally with a Crawford hook below the inferior turbinate, and then tying them together. Repair of NOE injuries is recommended within the first week after injury because soft tissue collapse and readaptation cause permanent thickening of this region. Medial rectus entrapment with NOE injuries is uncommon. The primary defects that occur with NOE injuries are splaying of the nasal bones, posterior displacement with lack of support, and lateral canthal displacement.

Isolated medial orbital wall defects are best approached directly through lateral nasal incisions. Approaches to the inferior orbital rim and floor, such as the subciliary or transconjunctival approaches, are often necessary for fixation of displaced segments of bone or fixation of graft material (alloplastic or autogenous bone) to stable bone. Coronal approaches may be necessary when there are associated frontal sinus fractures; however, these approaches offer limited access for isolated NOE fractures.[23] Access through any combination of overlying laceration, coronal incision, or lateral nasal incision is generally required to adequately treat these injuries (Fig. 93-18).

Traumatic telecanthus should be treated by direct fixation techniques with 1.0- to 1.7-mm plating systems. External splinting rarely yields satisfactory results. With NOE fractures, the medial canthal tendons usually maintain their attachments to the bony segments. Proper reduction plus fixation of the bony skeleton to the surrounding stable bone (maxillary, orbital, or frontal) often corrects the telecanthus deformity. With more severe injuries it is often necessary to perform transnasal fixation. A fine stainless steel wire (30 gauge) can be directly secured or sutured to the canthal tendon for this purpose (Fig. 93-19). The wire is inserted just posterior and superior to the lacrimal fossa by a wire-passing burr or curved needle. The two limbs of the wire can then be twisted gradually around a short section of plate in the opposite orbit to adjust and "fine-tune" the canthal position. Avoid nasal packing to

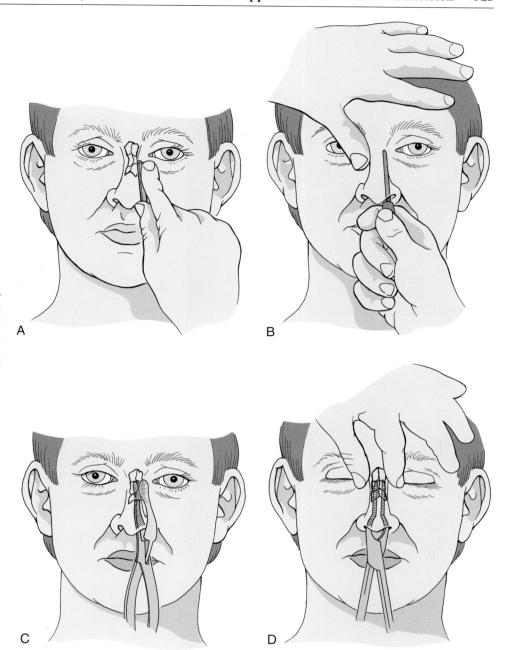

Figure 93-17. Reduction of a fracture of the nose. **A** and **B,** The bowed or C-shaped deformed nasal complex is reduced with a blunt elevator. **C** and **D,** Reduction of fractures of the nose that are telescoped is accomplished with Walsham and Asch forceps.

stabilize or align the nasal septum. The packing tends to bow the nasal bone reduction out and creates a permanently full and broad-appearing nose. If the septum is not in the midline, realign the septum surgically or trim the base and stabilize with thin Silastic internal splints bilaterally. Inadequate narrowing of the nasal bones when treating NOE fractures leads to persistent telecanthus and lack of nasodorsal projection. Transnasal wiring during the initial repair avoids this complication, which is extremely difficult to correct later.

If nasal dorsal strut grafts, such as split calvarial bone or alloplast, are being contemplated, the health and adequacy of the overlying soft tissue and skin must be assessed. If maceration or significant soft tissue devi-

talization is present, secondary reconstruction of the nasal dorsum is advisable (Fig. 93-20). The decision whether to perform immediate reconstruction or delay grafting is made on an individual case basis. Before undertaking any secondary reconstruction of an NOE injury, it is helpful to obtain a CT scan with three-dimensional reformatting. This aids greatly in surgical planning, preparation, and selection of graft materials (Fig. 93-21).

Frontal Sinus

The coronal approach provides the best access for repair of fractures of the frontal sinus. Only extensively large and degloving lacerations permit adequate direct

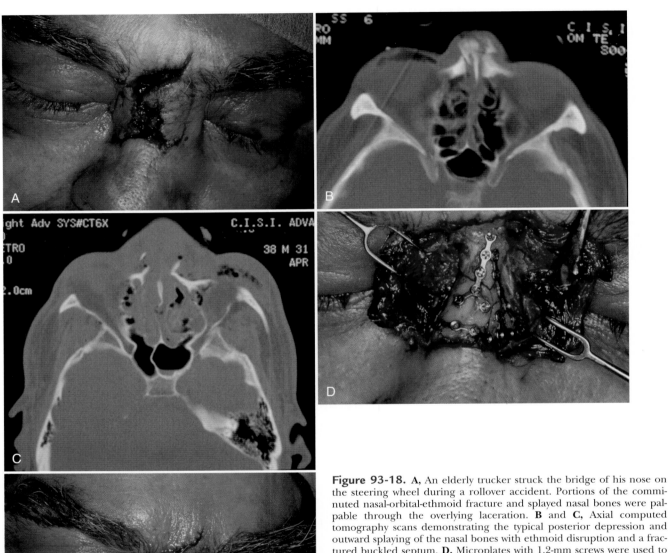

Figure 93-18. A, An elderly trucker struck the bridge of his nose on the steering wheel during a rollover accident. Portions of the comminuted nasal-orbital-ethmoid fracture and splayed nasal bones were palpable through the overlying laceration. **B** and **C,** Axial computed tomography scans demonstrating the typical posterior depression and outward splaying of the nasal bones with ethmoid disruption and a fractured buckled septum. **D,** Microplates with 1.2-mm screws were used to meticulously piece all the fragments into place. No transnasal wiring was necessary because the medial canthal tendons remained attached to the bony lacrimal crests and were reduced with the fracture repair. **E,** Sutured laceration and narrowed canthi at the end of the procedure.

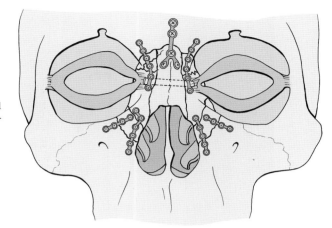

Figure 93-19. Fracture of the nasal-orbital-ethmoid complex repaired with miniplates and the medial canthi reduced and narrowed with trans-nasal 30-gauge wires sutured to the tendons.

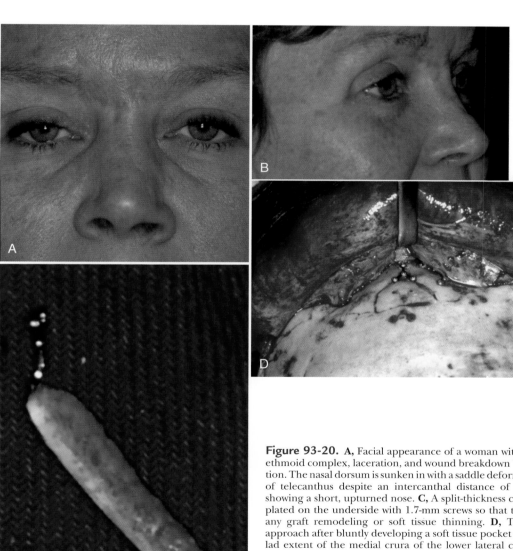

Figure 93-20. A, Facial appearance of a woman with a fracture of the nasal-orbital-ethmoid complex, laceration, and wound breakdown because of a postoperative infection. The nasal dorsum is sunken in with a saddle deformity, and there is the appearance of telecanthus despite an intercanthal distance of 29 mm. **B,** Right oblique view showing a short, upturned nose. **C,** A split-thickness calvarial graft was contoured and plated on the underside with 1.7-mm screws so that they would not be palpable with any graft remodeling or soft tissue thinning. **D,** The graft is inset via a coronal approach after bluntly developing a soft tissue pocket that extends down to the cephalad extent of the medial crura of the lower lateral cartilages. This length is beyond the native nasal bones, and it is necessary to adequately restore proper projection of the dorsum and tip without the nares being fully visible from the frontal view.

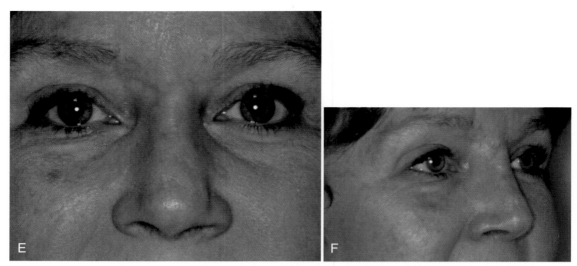

Figure 93-20, cont'd. E, Facial view 6 weeks after surgery. No canthopexy or scar revision was performed, yet the scars are less noticeable because they are stretched over a smooth convex framework and the canthi appear narrower as a result of proper anterior projection and volume of the nasal dorsum. **F,** Right oblique view.

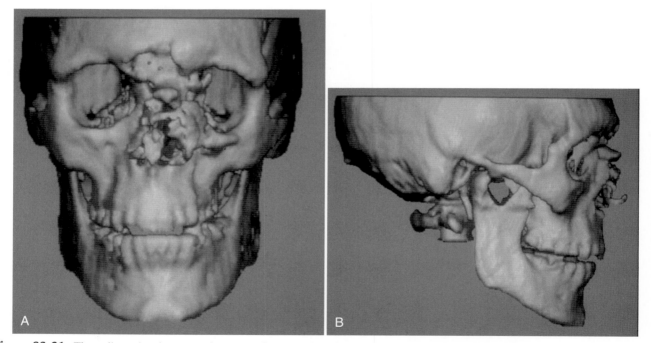

Figure 93-21. Three-dimensional computed tomography scans. **A** and **B,** Reformatted frontal and lateral views of a young man who was assaulted with a pipe and sustained a fracture of the nasal-orbital-ethmoid complex that was not repaired at his local hospital because of severe brain injury and a questionable chance for survival. These images greatly aid in preoperative planning for secondary reconstruction. The healed fracture edges have remodeled and smoothed, so osteotomizing or attempting to "reduce" the segments generally leads to a poor result. Reduction and recontouring of any excess or full areas and grafting onto stable areas for projection and contour with debulking of scarred soft tissue yield a better result. Several revision procedures should be anticipated.

exposure. Smaller lacerations should be repaired and a coronal approach undertaken. During reflection of the coronal flap, any free or loose anterior bone fragments should be preserved on the back table and oriented for later replacement and reconstruction. Displaced fractures of the anterior table should be elevated and the sinus floor, ostia, and posterior wall inspected. Patency of the nasofrontal ducts or foramen may be difficult to discern visually. Saline or methylene blue can be irrigated into the openings with an 18-gauge angiocatheter and then observed to emerge from the middle turbinate or collect in the posterior pharynx, thereby confirming patency. If the posterior table and nasofrontal ducts are free of injury, the anterior table can be reassembled and fixated with low-profile miniplates (1.0- to 1.7-mm systems) or titanium mesh. Mesh is useful in covering noncritical defects (<1.0 cm in diameter).

With larger defects, though rarely necessary, consideration should be given to harvesting split calvarial grafts and recontouring.

If the posterior table is fractured, one should determine radiographically and clinically whether the fracture is *displaced*. Displacement is defined as a discrepancy that is equal to or greater than the thickness of the adjacent fractured bony edges. The fracture is either displaced or nondisplaced. Intermediate terms, such as mildly displaced or angulated, are confusing and do not help direct clinical decision making. Displaced fractures warrant neurosurgical consultation. Oftentimes an osteotomy of a larger section of the frontal bone or the entire frontal bar (including the supraorbital rims) must be carried out and removed to permit adequate visualization and access for management of cerebral injuries and dural repair (Fig. 93-22). Care should be

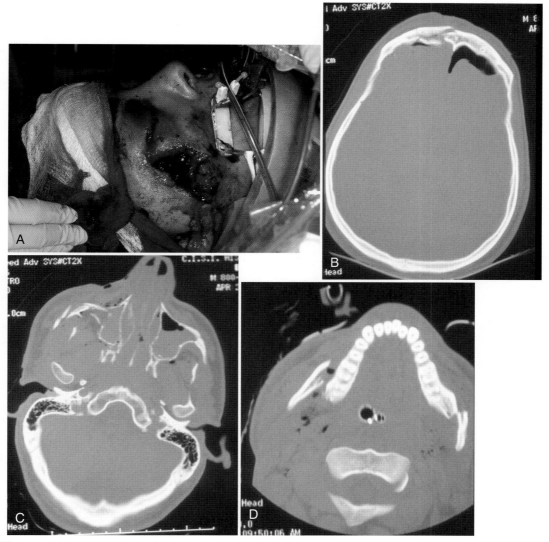

Figure 93-22. A, Lateral view of a young man whose left face was impaled by a crane hook and who then fell several stories from a steel building frame. His cervical spine was stabilized and he was orally intubated. A tracheostomy was performed. **B,** Computed tomography scan revealing a displaced frontal bone fracture with intracranial air. **C,** The maxilla and arches are fractured with comminution of the right maxilla. **D,** There are bilateral displaced angle fractures of the mandible and a right subcondylar fracture not seen on this lower cut.

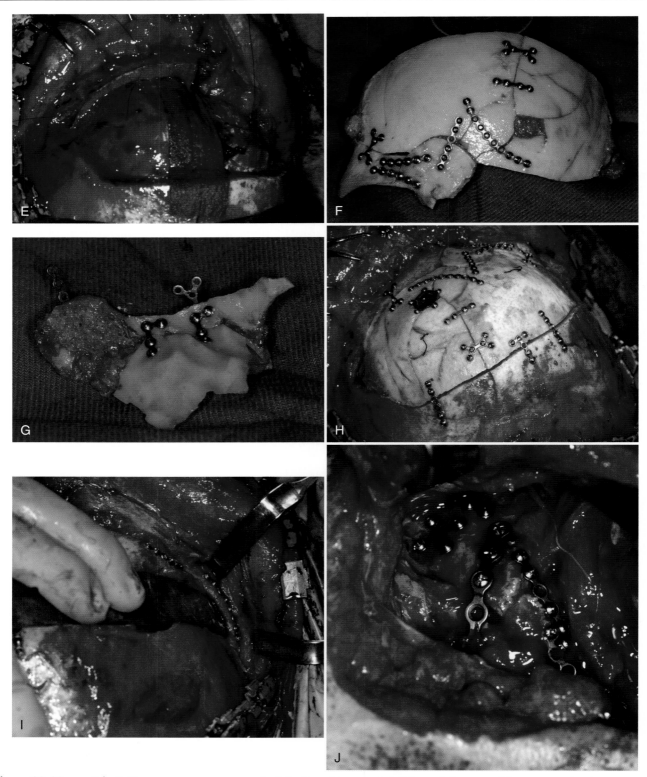

Figure 93-22, cont'd. E, The neurosurgeon osteotomized the frontal bone and skull beyond the areas of fracture to gain adequate access for dural repair without excessive retraction on the injured frontal lobes, which could lead to further edema. A lyophilized dural patch was inset over the torn right frontal area and the margins sealed with fibrin glue. **F,** The skull vault was pieced back together and plated ex situ with a 1.7-mm system. The right superior orbital rim is in the right lower corner of the field. **G,** A large portion of the anterior cranial fossa was free floating. It was retrieved during dural inspection and repair, "preplated" so that it could be slid between the frontal lobes and right orbit, and then fixated to the reconstituted skull when it was placed back in position. **H,** Cranial vault fixated and burr holes covered. Note that several small holes (1.5 mm) were made bilaterally to aid in the suspension of dural tacking sutures to discourage epidural blood accumulation. **I,** Fixated right zygomatic arch as viewed from above. **J,** The right zygoma and orbit were repaired through the gaping cheek exit wound with 1.7- and 1.3-mm miniplates. The right canaliculi were intubated before conservative excision of devitalized tissue margins and deep repair of the eyelid and cheek wound.

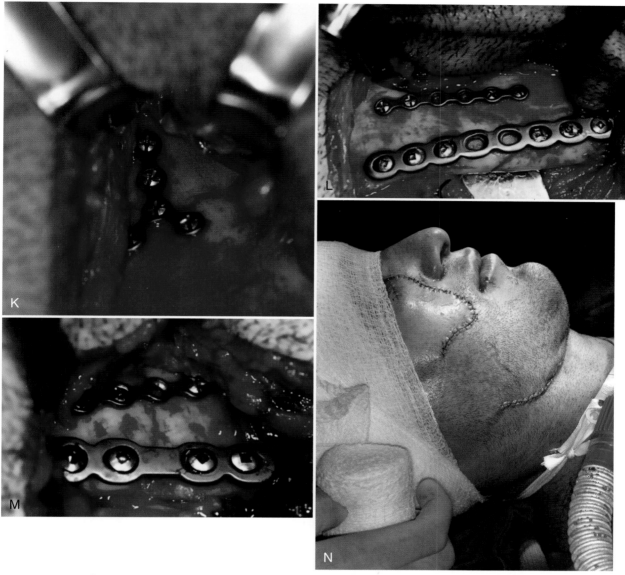

Figure 93-22, cont'd. K, Inferior view of the plated right subcondylar fracture, which was accomplished through the submandibular entry wound after placing arch bars and wiring the patient into maxillomandibular fixation. **L,** Next, the oblique fracture of the right angle and posterior body is fixated with a 2.0-mm tension band plate and a bicortical inferior border plate. **M,** An extraoral approach was used to plate the left angle. **N,** Intraoperative appearance of the revised entrance and exit wounds and a head wrap being placed.

taken to avoid entry into and damage to the sagittal sinus, which will result in severe hemorrhage. In cases in which there is severe cerebral contusion with anticipated postoperative edema or a moderate or small frontal sinus, cranialization of the frontal sinus is preferred. Cranialization involves complete removal of the posterior wall of the sinus, removal of all sinus mucosa, and smoothing of the bony margins (Fig. 93-23). Any dural tear is repaired primarily or patched with fascia, lyophilized dura, synthetic patch, or pericranium. Tissue sealants such as fibrin glue can be used to help reinforce the repair. Dural tacking sutures to the overlying reconstructed anterior table can help prevent acute or chronic subdural fluid accumulation. Before reas-

sembling and plating the anterior table, the sinus mucosa in the nasofrontal ducts should be reflected downward into the nasal cavity and the orifice obliterated with local bone fragments, harvested temporalis muscle, or free pericranium.

If the nasofrontal ducts are fractured or obstructed, the patient is at risk for the development of sinusitis, meningitis, or osteomyelitis.[24] If the ducts are injured or if the frontal sinus is to be obliterated with grafted fat (harvested from the abdomen), bone, pericranium, or acceptable alloplastic material, or cranialized, the ducts should be obstructed and sealed off as described. Obliteration of the nasofrontal duct is necessary to seal off the frontal sinus or intracranial space from nasal

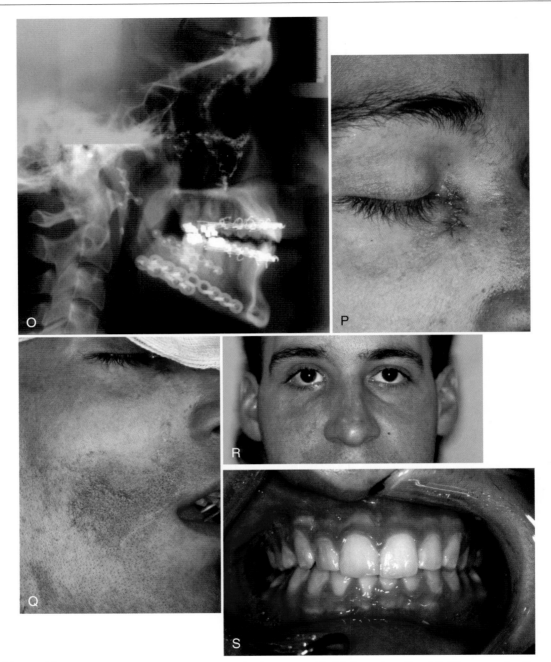

Figure 93-22, cont'd. O, Postoperative lateral cephalogram showing restored facial dimensions. **P** and **Q,** Three months after repair, Z-plasty of the medial canthal scar and mechanical dermabrasion of the cheek wound were performed. **R,** Facial appearance 6 month after injury. He had returned to full-time construction work without disability. **S,** Occlusion.

contamination. Sinus obliteration is undertaken to eliminate dead space, discourage fluid accumulation, and provide an additional barrier between the nasal cavity and the brain.

When obliteration of the nasofrontal duct and sinus and cranialization are undertaken, it is critical to remove all remnants of sinus membrane and mucosa. Vigorous use of the curette and sometimes curettage with a round diamond burr are required for complete removal.

Mucosal remnants can lead to mucocele formation and infection many years later. With more limited unilateral sinus injuries or with limited access through a laceration via endoscopic visualization to ensure that no free fragments are located within the sinus, lateral nasal incisions (Lynch) and elevation of the anterior fractures can be performed. This should be attempted only by an individual skilled in functional endoscopic surgical techniques and only for mild unilateral injury.

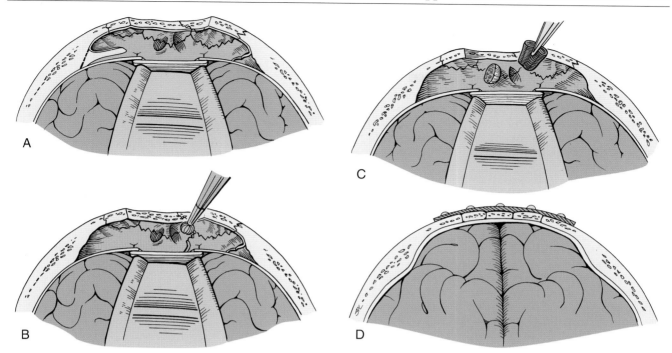

Figure 93-23. Steps in cranialization of a fractured frontal sinus. **A,** The dura is repaired and the posterior sinus wall is removed through a bicoronal approach. **B,** Mucosal remnants are removed by burring the anterior wall and floor. **C,** The nasal frontal ostia are plugged. **D,** The anterior table is reconstructed with microplates, and the brain accommodates and fills the space.

POSTOPERATIVE MANAGEMENT

The postoperative course and regimen are dependent on the variety and severity of the facial fractures. Routine orders include cold compresses for the face, elevation of the head of the bed, decongestant nasal sprays, and wire cutters at the bedside if the patient is maintained in MMF. Instructions on how to cut the wires in case of emergency are useful. However, if the arch bars are left in place, soft wax can be given to the patient to place over any wire causing irritation, and nutrition consultation is also advisable. For patients not in MMF but who have undergone repair of Le Fort fractures, a soft diet that does not require chewing is recommended for 4 to 6 weeks. The patient should be instructed in oral hygiene and saline rinses. Perioperative steroids administered intravenously can greatly aid in reduction of soft tissue swelling. Methylprednisolone (125 mg intravenously every 6 hours) is preferable over dexamethasone (8 mg intravenously every 8 hours). This regimen should not be confused with the high-dose steroids that are given to patients with traumatic optic neuropathy and visual compromise. In these instances, intravenous methylprednisolone (3 mg/kg) and subsequent doses of 1.5 mg/kg every 6 hours are administered to reduce edema and optic nerve compression.[25] Evaluation of visual acuity should be performed frequently within the first 24 hours after any orbital surgery. Even with significant periorbital edema the eyelids should be separated and pupillary reactivity and adequate vision confirmed. Any equivocal or worrisome findings should prompt an emergency ophthalmic con-

sultation. Occasionally, proptosis or chemosis of the bulbar conjunctiva with exposure develops. Lubrication of the eye should be applied frequently (every 2 hours) to avoid desiccation or ulceration. Any lid retraction or ectropion should be assessed and managed by direct massage, steroid injection, or surgical revision. Paresthesia and dysesthesia of the supraorbital and infraorbital nerves are common after injury and repair. Unless surgically transected, most will recover fully within 3 to 6 months.

Blurred vision and mild diplopia are common after fractures of the orbit and usually resolve when the edema subsides. Marked diplopia or decreased vision should be evaluated on an emergency basis by an ophthalmologist. Evacuation of a retrobulbar hematoma, high-dose steroids, and other sight-preserving maneuvers can be performed as indicated. Serial examinations are important for early detection of decreased vision.

Any persistent clear or watery fluid from the nose should be evaluated with a β_2-transferrin assay to rule out CSF rhinorrhea. Radionuclide studies can be performed to localize the source of the CSF rhinorrhea, and transnasal endoscopic patching of the CSF leak along with placement of a lumbar drain for 3 to 5 days is usually successful.

Perioperative antibiotics are frequently used in the care of patients treated for facial fractures. Intravenous antibiotics are usually given before and for 24 hours after surgery. Beyond this time, there is no proven benefit of intravenous antibiotics. Antibiotics should provide gram-positive and staphylococcal coverage. Amoxicillin with clavulanate and clindamycin are good first-line choices. Sinus precautions should be instituted in patients who have undergone repair of maxillary or ZMC fractures. Early wound infections are often due to nonviable bone, breakdown of soft tissue, retained tooth fragments in the line of fracture, or mobility across fracture lines. Attempts should be made to ascertain the cause and direct therapy toward the same. Simply administering antibiotics fails to completely resolve the infection and delays the necessary inevitable treatment of débridement, surgical drainage, or refixation of fractures.

Late infections (>6 weeks) are usually due to paranasal sinus obstruction and possibly a devitalized maxillary tooth requiring extraction or root canal therapy. Clinical examination, local sensitivity, and radiographic imaging can help identify the source, and appropriate treatment can be rendered.

Pressure dressings can be applied to suit the patient's needs, particularly with coronal flaps, or when extensive soft tissue stripping has been performed. Suction drains can be placed beneath the coronal flaps and maintained for 24 hours. Generally, drains are unnecessary, except in the presence of excessive oozing during closure.

Postoperative radiographs can be useful in assessing the adequacy of reduction, alignment of fixation, and skeletal relationships. They also serve as a baseline if future occlusal changes, shift in segments, or infection or loosening of hardware occurs. These radiographs can include Panorex, a posteroanterior or lateral cephalogram, a Waters view, or skull films. Follow-up CT scans are generally required for complex orbital repairs and frontal sinus repairs with intracranial injury. Patients should avoid strenuous physical activity for 6 weeks and avoid contact sports for an additional period if warranted by the injury.

Malocclusion discovered immediately after surgery or within the first week is usually due to improper reduction of the fractures and fixation in that position. The most common postoperative malocclusion is an anterior open bite deformity caused by upward pressure on the chin with displacement of the condyles while plating midfacial fractures. If the anterior open bite is slight (less than 2 mm), vertical elastic traction on the arch bars may resolve the situation satisfactorily. A large open bite must be addressed by revision surgery with plating in the correct anatomic position while seating the mandibular condyles. Excessive amounts of box elastics to close malocclusions can lead to loss of fixation, nonunion, and damage to the teeth.

Malocclusion that occurs later (during the healing phase) is usually due to loss of fixation, use of plates with inadequate rigidity, or backing out of screws because of overheated bone at the time of surgery or infection. The patient may also be overactive and eating a normal diet, or infrequently the patient sustains additional facial trauma and may not report it to the surgeon. Grasping the maxillary complex to detect mobility and comparing current radiographs with ones taken immediately postoperatively may reveal loss of fixation or shift of the bony segments. Generally, reoperation plus reapplication of fixation is required to address this situation. Meticulous passive plate adaptation and the use of locking screw systems can help avoid torquing segments and misalignment.

PEARLS

- A thorough preoperative evaluation with a logically sequenced treatment plan helps avoid complications and unfavorable outcomes.
- The patient's imaging studies must be reviewed personally by the surgeon, who should correlate any radiographic fractures with the physical findings.
- When grafting defects of the orbital floor, reconstitute the defect and restore the normal orbital floor contour, which is not flat.
- Do not operate on nondisplaced ZMC, isolated anterior maxillary wall, or orbital floor fractures for the purpose of improving V_2 paresthesia or anesthesia.
- When treating moderate or severely displaced ZMC fractures, accessing at least two fracture points and fixating them along both areas aids in reduction and helps ensure proper alignment and adequate postoperative stability.

PITFALLS

- Nasal and zygomatic arch fractures treated after 48 hours of injury do not reduce as precisely and tend to be less stable and drift back into the injured position.
- When closing eyelid incisions, either infraciliary or transconjunctival, improper reapproximation and suturing unlike layers will result in lid tethering and possibly ectropion.
- Serial perioperative visual acuity checks or patient complaints indicating decreased vision must be taken seriously and should prompt immediate evaluation and appropriate treatment.
- Early postoperative malocclusion (<24 hours) is usually due to fixation of fracture segments that were improperly aligned.
- Later postoperative malocclusion is probably due to nonunion or shift of bony segments secondary to inadequate fixation, infection, or excessive use.

References

1. Turvey TA: Midfacial fractures: A retrospective analysis of 593 cases. J Oral Surg 35:887-891, 1977.
2. Cunningham LL, Haug RH: Management of maxillary factures. In Miloro M (ed): Oral and Maxillofacial Surgery, 2nd ed. Hamilton, Ontario, BC Decker, 2004, pp 435-444.

3. Ellis E, El-Attar A, Moos KF: An analysis of 2,067 cases of zygomatico-orbital fracture. J Oral Maxillofac Surg 43:417-428, 1985.

4. Hammer B: Orbital Fractures: Diagnosis, Operative Treatment, Secondary Corrections. Seattle, Hogrefe & Huber, 1995, pp 7-41.

5. Hartstein ME, Roper-Hall G: Update on orbital floor fractures: Indications and timing for repair. Facial Plast Surg 16:95-106, 2000.

6. Ochs MW, Buckley MJ: Anatomy of the orbit. Oral Maxillofac Surg Clin North Am 5:419-429, 1993.

7. Markowitz BL, Manson PN, Sargent L, et al: Management of the medial canthal tendon in nasoethmoid-orbital fractures: The importance of a central fragment in classification and treatment. Plast Reconstr Surg 87:843-853, 1991.

8. Gruss JS, Hurwitz JJ, Nik NA, Kassel EE: The pattern and incidence of nasolacrimal injury in naso-orbital-ethmoid fracture: The role of delayed assessment and dacryocystorhinostomy. Br J Plast Surg 38:116-121, 1985.

9. Rohrich RJ, Hollier LH: Management of frontal sinus fractures. Changing concepts. Clin Plast Surg 19:219-232, 1992.

10. Donald PJ: Frontal sinus ablation by cranialization. Arch Otolaryngol 108:142-146, 1982.

11. Manson PN, Clark N, Robertson B, et al: Comprehensive management of pan-facial fractures. J Craniomaxillofac Trauma 1:43-56, 1995.

12. Manson PN, Clark N, Robertson B, et al: Sub-unit principles in midface fractures: The importance of sagittal buttresses, soft-tissue reductions, and sequencing treatment of segmental fractures. Plast Reconstr Surg 103:1287-1306, 1999.

13. Haug RH, Jenkins WS, Brandt MT: Advances in plate and screw technology: Thought on design and clinical applications. Semin Plast Surg 16:219-227, 2002.

14. Zingg M, Laedrach K, Ceen J, et al: Classification and treatment of zygomatic fractures: A review of 1025 cases. J Oral Maxillofac Surg 50:778-790, 1992.

15. Ellis E, Kittidumkerng W: Analysis of treatment of isolated zygomaticomaxillary complex fractures. J Oral Maxillofac Surg 54:386-400, 1966.

16. Manson PN: Discussion: Analysis of treatment for isolated zygomaticomaxillary complex fractures. J Oral Maxillofac Surg 54:400-401, 1996.

17. Makowski GJ, Van Sickels JE: Evaluation of results with three-point visualization of zygomaticomaxillary complex fractures. Oral Surg Oral Med Oral Pathol 80:624-628, 1995.

18. Zingg M, Chowdhury K, Ladrach K: Treatment of 813 zygoma–lateral orbital complex fractures. Arch Otolaryngol Head Neck Surg 11:611-620, 1991.

19. Converse JM: Two plastic operations for repair of the orbit following severe trauma and extensive comminuted fracture. Arch Ophthalmol 31:323-325, 1944.

20. Baumann A, Ewers R: Use of preseptal transconjunctival approach in orbital reconstruction surgery. J Oral Maxillofac Surg 59:287-291, 2001.

21. Mathog RH, Hillstrom RP, Nesi FA: Surgical correction of enophthalmos and diplopia: A report of 38 cases. Arch Otolaryngol Head Neck Surg 115:169-178, 1989.

22. Berghaus A: Porous polyethylene in reconstructive head and neck surgery. Arch Otolaryngol Head Neck Surg 111:154-160, 1985.

23. Ellis E: Sequencing treatment for naso-orbito-ethmoid fractures. J Oral Maxillofac Surg 51:543-588, 1993.

24. Wilson BC, Davidson B, Corey JP, Haydon RC III: Comparison of complications following frontal sinus fractures managed with exploration with or without obliteration over 10 years. Laryngoscope 98:516-520, 1988.

25. Spoor TC, Hartel WC, Lensink DB, Wilkinson M: Treatment of traumatic optic neuropathy with corticosteroids. Am J Ophthalmol 110:665-669, 1990.

Chapter **94**

Fractures of the Orbit

S. Tonya Stefko

Because the orbit is made up in part by two of the horizontal beams of facial structure and two of the vertical buttresses, orbital fractures are common, and proper repair of such fractures is key to restoring normal facial appearance and function. Complicating evaluation and treatment are the vital and complex structures contained within: the eye and optic nerve, extraocular muscles, and the lacrimal secretory and excretory systems. Understanding the classes of fractures involving the orbit is critical to their evaluation and prediction of other possible associated injuries. These categories will suggest a systematic approach to their treatment and repair.

The bony orbit is shaped like a pyramid with its apex directed posteromedially (Figs. 94-1 and 94-2). The medial walls are approximately parallel, and the lateral walls diverge at roughly 90 degrees. The normal volume of an adult orbit is 30 mL. The periosteum of the orbit is also known as the periorbita, and it surrounds the orbital contents in a continuous sheet except over the various foramina and fissures.

Most fractures involving the bones of the orbit occur as a consequence of blunt trauma to the face. Penetrating trauma, such as that caused by a projectile, is less common. Consideration of the probable velocity (momentum and direction) of the inciting object will often give clues to the likely location and severity of the bony involvement. For example, true blowout fractures are frequently the result of low-velocity trauma to the orbit, such as a thrown baseball, whereas a motor vehicle collision or being struck by a baseball bat in the face (high-velocity trauma) may cause a displaced zygomaticofacial complex (ZMC) or Le Fort–type fracture.

PATIENT SELECTION

Most orbital fracture repairs can be delayed for 7 to 10 days, so consideration of the status of the rest of the patient must be undertaken immediately. The usual trauma evaluation, including establishment of the airway, breathing, and circulation, is performed first. A secondary survey will then uncover less urgent issues, including facial fractures. Delayed repair allows stabilization of the patient, full evaluation of the impact of the injury, and attention to more urgent issues (e.g., decompression craniotomy). However, in some instances fracture repair will be undertaken more urgently because of intercurrent issues, such as an intractable cerebrospinal fluid leak.

Evaluation of the severity of the fracture must include attention to the orbital contents. A basic eye examination can be performed on even a comatose patient by using a penlight and pair of toothed forceps. In most major trauma centers, an ophthalmologist is available on call to evaluate the eye and periocular area, the safest way to ensure that no occult injury is overlooked. In other emergency rooms, the otolaryngologist will need to document at least vision, if possible, pupillary reactions, eye movements, and appearance of the eye.

Types of Orbital Fractures

Force applied to the lower midface region produces variations of the classic fracture patterns described by Le Fort. Rarely do Le Fort fractures occur precisely as he described or symmetrically; however, these divisions help guide repair and provide an orderly and predictable approach. Le Fort II fractures, discussed in more detail in Chapter 93, traverse the maxillary sinus, orbital floor, medial wall, and nasal bones. Le Fort III fractures, also called craniofacial dysjunction, involve the zygomatic bones in the lateral orbital walls, the floor and medial orbital walls, and the nasal bones. Although an air-fluid level noted on computed tomography (CT) in one maxillary sinus suggests a sinus or orbital fracture, when this sign is present in both maxillary sinuses, one must assume a Le Fort II or III fracture until careful

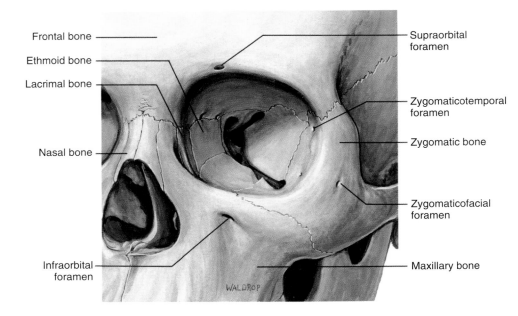

Frontal bone

Ethmoid bone

Lacrimal bone

Nasal bone

Infraorbital foramen

Supraorbital foramen

Zygomaticotemporal foramen

Zygomatic bone

Zygomaticofacial foramen

Maxillary bone

WALDROP

Figure 94-1. Orbital bones, frontal view. *(From Dutton JJ: Atlas of Clinical and Surgical Orbital Anatomy. Philadelphia, WB Saunders, 1994.)*

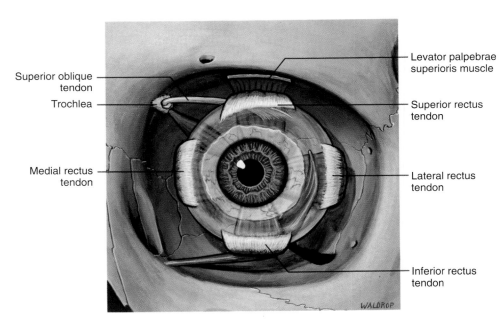

Superior oblique tendon

Trochlea

Medial rectus tendon

Levator palpebrae superioris muscle

Superior rectus tendon

Lateral rectus tendon

Inferior rectus tendon

WALDROP

Figure 94-2. Extraocular muscles, frontal composite view. *(From Dutton JJ: Atlas of Clinical and Surgical Orbital Anatomy. Philadelphia, WB Saunders, 1994.)*

examination has proved otherwise. All Le Fort fractures also cause some measure of malocclusion.

Application of significant force to the upper midface area can lead to telescoping nasal fractures and naso-orbito-ethmoidal fractures. The hallmark of these injuries is traumatic telecanthus, with the normal intercanthal distance being about 35 mm or less. Fracture lines generally travel posteriorly through the medial orbital walls. The most urgent issues with these fractures involve possible leakage of cerebrospinal fluid with associated meningitis and trauma to the brain, as well as the possibility of involvement of the optic canals posteriorly. Careful consideration must be given to the urgent need for decompression. When repairing these fractures, it will also be necessary to re-establish the normal anatomic relationships of the medial canthi. These injuries are discussed further in Chapter 93.

ZMC fractures involve force directed posteriorly over the malar eminence or zygomatic arch. They were formerly referred to as "tripod" fractures, but this term is not entirely accurate because this bone articulates in five places, even though two of the five generally do not require fixation during reduction. The characteristic facial deformity of a displaced ZMC fracture is flattening of the malar eminence, with or without apparent enophthalmos, and difficulty opening the mouth completely.

The remaining fractures involving the orbit are referred to as blowout fractures. They were first described by Smith and Regan in 1957[1] after observing a patient who had been hit in the periorbital area by a hurling ball. With a Waters view on plain films, the characteristic opacification of the maxillary sinus was observed, and the patient complained of diplopia. Surgical exploration via a Caldwell-Luc approach allowed visualization of the inferiorly displaced orbital floor (maxillary sinus roof) and prolapse of the orbital contents. Repair was undertaken by packing of the maxillary sinus to elevate its roof, and further cadaver experiments were carried out by the authors.

A classification of orbital fractures was described in 1967 and consisted of separating the fractures into "pure" blowout and "impure" blowout fractures.[2] Impure blowout fractures referred to those associated with other orbital rim fractures, mainly those mentioned earlier and the occasional unclassifiable rim fracture with a floor component. The term was expanded to include fractures of the orbital roof unassociated with frontal sinus fractures, which occur almost exclusively in children. The definition of a blowout fracture has come to mean an orbital floor, medial wall, or roof fracture not associated with a rim fracture.

The hydraulic theory suggests that the orbital contents are deformable and that a blow to the soft tissues causes rapid expansion beyond what the elastic modulus of the surrounding bone can tolerate. Thus, the weakest areas of the orbital structures fracture outward, often lacerating the periorbita and intraorbital tissues, and allow prolapse into the adjacent sinus. Younger patients merit special consideration because they often suffer greenstick-type orbital wall fractures, during which the orbital contents can herniate and become trapped by rapid recoil of the partially fractured orbital wall (so-called trapdoor fractures). A second explanation, the "buckling" theory, instead explains fracture of the orbital walls by the application of a load to the thick orbital rim, which deforms somewhat and causes the orbital wall posterior to it to bend.[3] As the tougher orbital rim returns to its original position, the thin and brittle bones of the associated wall have less elasticity and consequently break. It is likely that some combination of these mechanisms explains most blowout fractures.

Determination of Need for Repair

The initial symptoms of the patient will provide the first clue to the need for and timing of repair. Many patients with ZMC fractures complain of pain or numbness in the cheek (or both) and notice deformity of their cheek. The deformity may be obscured in the early stages by edema. If the zygomatic arch is involved, the patient may have symptoms of pain with attempted opening of the mouth. Because this fracture only rarely causes significant orbital injury or airway compromise, the approach to repair is most often elective and based on the amount of cosmetic deformity or the presence of symptomatic bony fragments in the temporomandibular joint space. Earlier repair is preferable to obviate the need for osteotomy. If the fragments are nondisplaced and stable, surgery is unnecessary.

Patients with blowout fractures of the floor may have the classic triad of enophthalmos, hypoesthesia of the cheek, and a deficit of upgaze. Hypoesthesia of the cheek is common to most patients with blowout fractures of the floor because the fracture occurs medial to the infraorbital canal and often involves it. Young patients with significant deficiency of upgaze, particularly if accompanied by nausea and vomiting,[4] require careful evaluation to determine whether a trapped inferior rectus muscle is present. These so-called white-eyed blowout fractures are the most critical, and repair should proceed within 24 hours if possible.

Clues to muscle entrapment include age of the patient, small fracture size, severe pain on attempted duction, severe limitation of upgaze, and nausea and vomiting (Figs. 94-3 to 94-5). Traction on the inferior rectus is thought to activate the oculocardiac reflex (bradycardia, hypotension, and vomiting) and could theoretically be fatal. In addition, the muscle is compressed and quickly becomes ischemic, thereby rapidly

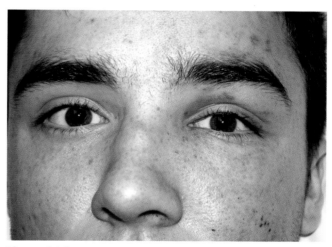

Figure 94-3. Patient 1: 16-year-old with a blowout fracture of the left orbit.

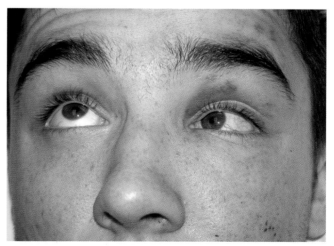

Figure 94-4. Patient 1: attempted upgaze.

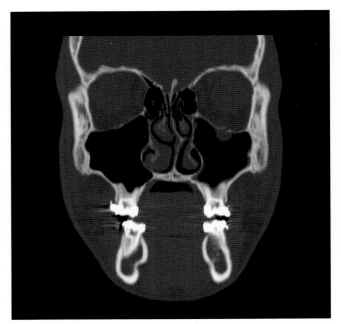

Figure 94-5. Coronal scan of a trapdoor fracture of the left eye; note the "hanging drop" sign and small, nondisplaced fracture.

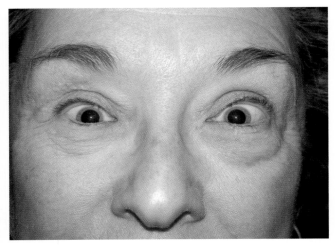

Figure 94-6. Patient 2: $4\frac{1}{2}$ months after fracture of the orbital floor and medial wall. Diplopia and 6 mm of enophthalmos are evident in the right eye.

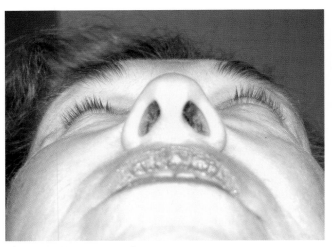

Figure 94-7. Patient 2: $4\frac{1}{2}$ months after a blowout fracture.

leading to irreversible scarring and permanent double vision.[5]

Decisions regarding the suitability and timing of repair of other blowout fractures may be undertaken with less urgency. Factors affecting such decisions include the size of the fracture, injury to other adjacent structures, associated symptoms, and characteristics of the particular patient.

Symptoms associated with blowout fractures most commonly include pain, hypoesthesia of the cheek, diplopia, and enophthalmos. The former two nearly always resolve without intervention, and thus only diplopia and enophthalmos remain as possible indications for repair. Putterman and colleagues[6] showed that the natural history of most uncomplicated blowout fractures (i.e., those without entrapped muscle) is resolution of the diplopia over a period of days to weeks. Early enophthalmos (immediate or within the first week) bodes poorly for cosmetic outcome because this sign generally portends a large and displaced fracture. With the advent of CT scanning and more precise measurement of the size and location of these injuries, it became possible to predict which patients will suffer long-term consequences, including cosmetic deformity and permanent double vision.

It is generally accepted that fractures involving more than 50% of the orbital floor are likely to cause later enophthalmos. Displaced fractures with an area of 2 cm^2 or greater are most significant: approximately 1 cm^2 produces about 1 mm of enophthalmos,[7] and at a 2-mm or greater difference in projection of the globes, an aesthetic defect is noticed. The area of the medial wall fractured must be accounted for when making this rough calculation; although the medial wall is repaired less frequently, it contributes to later enophthalmos (Figs. 94-6 to 94-8).

The risk of diplopia after repair of a blowout fracture is difficult to quantify without a randomized, controlled prospective trial. A small retrospective trial of 54 patients who underwent surgical repair found that approximately a third of the patients continued to have diplopia more than 6 months after repair.[8] However, approximately two thirds of these patients had combined floor and medial wall fractures, thus making the risk greater than after floor fracture alone, for which it is about 10% to 12%.

In considering the general health of the patient, it is best to frankly discuss with the patient that the repair to be undertaken is for aesthetic reconstruction and occasionally to prevent double vision, not to treat abnormal cheek sensation or pain. Nor, in most instances, is it necessary to undergo surgery to prevent double vision from persisting. Thus, a patient in her 80s in a nursing home would be a less likely candidate for

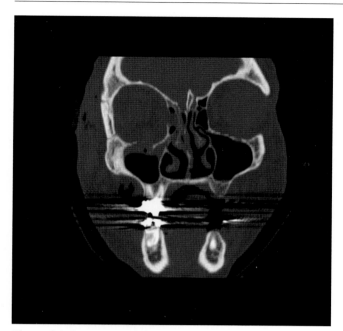

Figure 94-8. Blowout fracture of the floor and medial wall of the orbit.

intervention than a 22-year-old student with a similar-appearing fracture.

PREOPERATIVE EVALUATION

Evaluation of Orbital Contents

The most complete evaluation of a patient with an orbital fracture occurs when the otolaryngologist and ophthalmologist work together to manage the case. Ensuring the integrity of the eye is of utmost importance. Open globe injuries, particularly in the case of penetrating trauma, are occasionally seen in association with orbital fractures. A high index of suspicion must be maintained in patients with decreased vision, obvious globe deformity, opacification of areas of the cornea, an irregularly shaped pupil, and areas of hemorrhagic conjunctival chemosis. Although subconjunctival hemorrhage is common in the setting of any orbital fracture, chemosis (significant edema of the conjunctiva) associated with hemorrhage is quite worrisome for occult rupture. In such instances, structural integrity of the eye must be established first, with repair of any significant orbital fracture undertaken with caution at a much later time. A retrospective study of open globe injuries recently found 26% to be associated with orbital or adnexal trauma (or both), and conversely, a review of orbital injuries found approximately the same proportion with significant injury to the globe.[9,10]

The second instance in which orbital fracture repair ought not be undertaken immediately is in patients with traumatic optic neuropathy. The sine qua non of this injury is a relative afferent pupillary defect, except in those with bilateral neuropathy. A relative afferent pupillary defect (Marcus Gunn pupil) is observed by noting a difference in the reactivity of one pupil versus the other by transferring a bright light rapidly from one eye to the other. It is important that the patient not focus on the examiner during the examination because this will cause constriction of both pupils and render the examination more difficult. The patient should be asked to focus on a distant object such as a light switch. The patient will usually note that the light is brighter in the unaffected eye than in the affected one. Several caveats attend this examination: a decrease in reactivity of a pupil can also be caused by third nerve injury, accompanied by ptosis of the upper eyelid and deficit of upgaze, downgaze, and adduction, or by direct pupillary trauma, in which case hyphema will often be present.

If the patient is thought to have traumatic optic neuropathy, consideration should be given to surgical decompression of the optic nerve, particularly when bony fragments are obviously present in the canal or posterior orbit on CT scan. Associated findings are frontal sinus fractures, blood in the posterior ethmoid air cells and sphenoid sinus, and sphenoid sinus fractures. No established treatment of traumatic optic neuropathy exists. The International Optic Nerve Trauma Study attempted to determine whether observation, treatment with corticosteroids, or surgical intervention made any difference in outcome for patients with indirect (i.e., nonpenetrating) trauma to the optic nerve.[11] The trial was changed to an observational one because of low enrollment, and no clear benefit was found for either treatment.

Small case series have suggested that unroofing the bony canal may be of benefit. Complicating factors in these reports have been a lack of standardization of timing or technique of surgery, lack of definition of visual "improvement," and poor understanding of the natural history of the disease (a significant number of patients will improve without treatment). In any case, repair of orbital fracture in this setting is fraught with uncertainty and could presumably make the situation worse.

The third contraindication to early exploration of orbital fractures is the presence of hyphema (bleeding into the anterior chamber of the eye). Hyphema is often visible grossly as a red layer between the cornea and iris, but more subtle cases may go undetected without slit-lamp examination. The highest chance of rebleeding in these patients occurs during the first 5 days after injury, during which the patient must remain at bed rest and keep the eye shielded. Any further trauma to the eye (e.g., retraction of the orbital contents during surgery) is to be strictly avoided. If the hyphema is small and resolves entirely within the 5-day period, it is probably safe to proceed with repair of the fracture the following week. If the hyphema is large and remains unresolved, it is most prudent to defer surgery on the orbit until a later date.

Examination of ocular motility is easily done by asking the patient to move the eyes to all extremes of gaze. Edema of muscle or periorbita or patient discomfort is a very common cause of limitation of duction, so in instances in which there is doubt about the nature of the limitation, forced ductions should be performed. This is done by instilling anesthetic drops into the eye and then holding a cotton-tipped applicator soaked in these drops over the conjunctiva at the 6-o'clock position for at least 90 seconds. Toothed forceps can then be used to firmly grasp the conjunctiva and underlying connective tissue and rotate the eye in each direction. Resistance to forced movement suggests either entrapment of tissues in a fracture site or decreased compliance of the extraocular muscle (e.g., by hematoma).

If possible, a dilated fundus examination should be performed to rule out or document any intraocular hemorrhage or retinal pathology before exploration of the fracture.

Associated Soft Tissue Injuries

Any associated soft tissue injuries should be noted at the time of initial examination. This will guide repair of any lid or lacrimal injury, and a preexisting laceration can often be used for good surgical access. If the repairs are to be performed at the same surgery, the fractures should be repaired before any eyelid repair to avoid undoing the reconstruction already performed. However, during exploration and repair, the tissue must be kept hydrated and treated as gently as possible to avoid further damage. A laceration, no matter how small, between the lacrimal punctum and medial canthus usually means avulsion of the canalicular system and should be repaired within 72 hours with a silicon stent. Most injuries, excluding dog bites and motor vehicle collisions with sharp laceration, leave the bulk of the periorbital tissue intact. The blood supply in this area is excellent, so every attempt should be made to complete the original repair with the available tissue. Extreme caution should be exercised during any attempt at débridement of apparently devitalized soft tissue in the area. A laceration at the orbital rim is particularly helpful to the surgeon because it provides direct access to the ZMC and orbital floor.

Imaging

CT scanning with fine cuts through the orbit and direct coronal projections if possible is the best study for evaluation of orbital fractures. Most modern coronal reconstructions are more than adequate for evaluation of the size of the fracture and the orbital contents. Intravenous contrast material is not necessary, and magnetic resonance imaging of the orbits is of little use in the evaluation of bony injury.

When evaluating an orbital fracture, attention must be paid to the size of the fracture. Tiny trapdoor fractures may be missed on an initial look by radiology, so if clinically suspected, scrutiny of the film for the position and size of the inferior rectus and surrounding tissue is important. The rough area of the fracture may be calculated by measuring its width and length on the scan while keeping in mind that a fracture approximately 1 cm^2 will produce about 1 mm of enophthal-

mos. The normal aesthetics of the orbit allow up to a 2-mm difference in the projection of the eyes.

Access to the scans during surgery, if at all possible, can be extremely helpful in orientation within the orbit.

SURGICAL APPROACHES

Zygomaticomaxillary Complex Fractures

By combining the approaches described later with a buccal sulcus incision, most ZMC fractures can be reduced and plated. If the arch is involved and displaced medially, a Gillies maneuver may suffice for repair. If, however, the arch is badly comminuted and displaced outward, it is likely that a coronal incision will be required. This is described in more detail in Chapter 93.

When reduction plus fixation of the zygomatic and maxillary bones has been accomplished, it is necessary to examine the state of the orbital floor. Most often, repair of the floor will also be required lest a large defect be left and place the patient at risk for a suboptimal cosmetic result.

Blowout Fractures of the Orbital Floor

Surgical access for repair of blowout fractures depends on the patient's associated injuries. If a laceration is present along the inferior orbital rim, it is acceptable to expose the fracture site by way of this laceration. Most frequently, however, there is no associated laceration, and blowout fractures of the floor should be approached via a transconjunctival incision. Subciliary, mideyelid, and rim incisions all provide good exposure but leave the patient with a risk of eyelid malposition because of scarring within the delicate lamellae of the lower eyelid. A transconjunctival incision as described here is rapid and provides wide access to the floor and very little risk of entropion or ectropion (Fig. 94-9). This incision can also be combined with a lateral canthotomy for access to the zygomaticofrontal suture and lateral wall and with a transcaruncular incision for access to the medial wall.

The patient is placed under general anesthesia for the surgery. An antibiotic such as cephalexin and a steroid such as dexamethasone should be administered intravenously during surgery. The opposite eye usually need not be left exposed in the surgical field unless late repair of enophthalmos is being performed and comparison of projection is necessary.

Before placement of a lubricated corneal protective lens, forced ductions should be performed with toothed forceps and any limitation noted (Fig. 94-10). Although the goal of the surgery is to improve any limitation of duction, at the end of surgery the excursion of the eye must be at least as good as at the beginning.

An assistant uses a Desmarres or similar retractor to reflect the lower eyelid down anterior to the rim, and a malleable retractor is used to hold the orbital contents back, with both retractors compressing the tissue somewhat over the rim (Fig. 94-11). A Colorado needle–

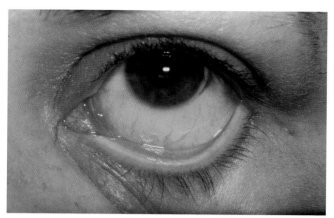

Figure 94-9. Inferior conjunctival fornix 3 weeks after repair of a blowout fracture via a transconjunctival approach.

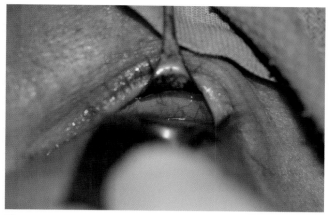

Figure 94-11. Retraction of the lower eyelid and orbital contents.

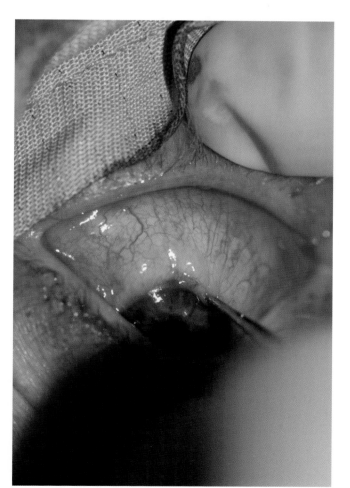

Figure 94-10. Forced duction.

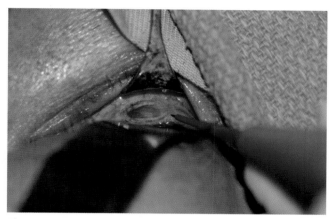

Figure 94-12. Transconjunctival incision with a Colorado needle.

tipped Bovie or similar insulated electrocautery device is used to palpate the rim of the orbit and then cut down directly on it. This will place the incision roughly in the inferior conjunctival fornix, well below the lower extent of the tarsus and well away from the globe (Fig. 94-12). If it is necessary to carry the incision fairly far

medially, care should be taken to stay anterior to the origin of the inferior oblique muscle and avoid the lacrimal system.

A Cottle or similar small sharpened periosteal elevator is then used to cut the periosteum of the rim and lift the periorbita in one continuous layer back to the fracture site (Fig. 94-13). The medial shelf of the fracture, the lateral shelf, and later, the posterior shelf must all be accessible and free of periosteum for proper implant placement. As the fracture site is exposed, gentle elevation of the orbital contents from the maxillary sinus should proceed in a hand-over-hand manner by using the elevator and malleable retractor (Fig. 94-14). The maxillary sinus may be débrided of bone fragments and clot. Care is taken to disturb the infraorbital neurovascular bundle as little as possible. A small orbital branch of the infraorbital vessels may be encountered and should be divided with cautery.

When all orbital tissue has been freed and brought superiorly, the posterior limit of the fracture should be located. This is done by bringing the elevator around from the medial or lateral fixed bone or, in some cases, by drawing the elevator superiorly along the posterior wall of the sinus until the upper aspect is reached.

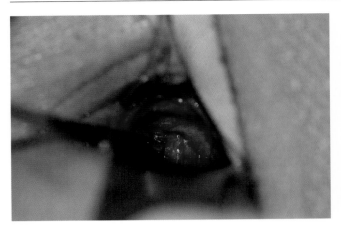

Figure 94-13. Anterior extent of the fracture with herniation of orbital fat into the sinus.

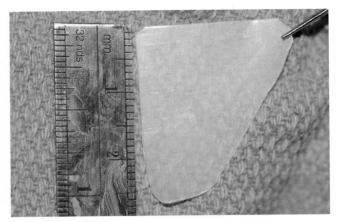

Figure 94-15. Measurement of a nylon implant.

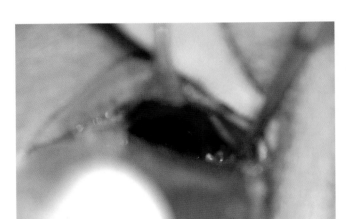

Figure 94-14. Exposure of the floor fracture.

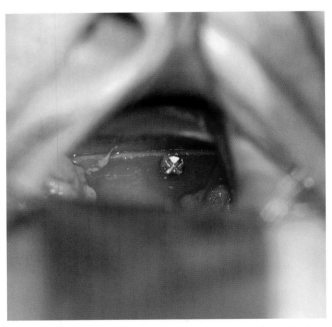

Figure 94-16. Fixation of the nylon implant with a titanium screw.

At intervals of several minutes during the surgery, it is wise to withdraw the retractors from the orbit and allow the tissues to reperfuse.

A suitable implant is now cut to size, dipped in antibiotic solution, and placed in the orbit to support the tissue (Fig. 94-15). It is critical that the implant rest firmly on the posterior edge of the fixed bone around the fracture or the fracture will remain incompletely reduced. A small unrepaired area at the anterior extension of the fracture is acceptable if necessary. When the implant is properly placed, it will remain in position when the retractors are gently removed. It must be placed several millimeters posterior to the rim or it will be palpable postoperatively. Inspection of the tissue surrounding the implant ensures that no orbital contents are trapped beneath the plate, and forced ductions are again performed to confirm the absence of trapping.

A small pilot hole is drilled in the anteromedial corner of the implant, and the plate is fixed with a titanium microscrew (Fig. 94-16). It is not necessary that the screw be perpendicular to the implant because it is not providing structural support (placement of the implant firmly on the medial, lateral, and posterior shelves ensures support), but it does prevent rotation or migration of the material. If insufficient bone is present medially, the plate may be fixed with hardware placed laterally, but great care must be taken to not place the screw through the infraorbital canal. Usually, one point of fixation is sufficient.

A Penrose or similar drain may be placed in the wound to emerge at its lateral extreme. The drain is placed superior to the implant and sutured to the lid with a 5-0 nylon loose drain stitch. The end is cut to approximately 5 mm beyond the lid margin. A 5-0 nylon modified Frost stitch is then placed through the skin and orbicularis in the center of the lid just inferior to the lashes. It is taped to the brow under tension and serves to extend the conjunctival edges and obviate the need for closure of the wound (Fig. 94-17). The stitch

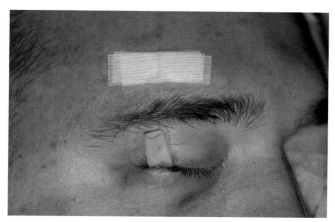

Figure 94-17. Postoperative view of a patient with a drain and traction stitch in place.

and drain are removed the following morning before the patient is discharged home. Before closure of the lid, ophthalmic antibiotic-steroid ointment is placed on the eye. A light absorbent dressing is placed so that perception of light may be checked by the nursing staff through the patch.

Blowout Fractures of the Medial Wall of the Orbit

Repair of medial blowout fractures is similar in principle, but the incision used is either a Lynch incision or a conjunctival incision placed between the plica semilunaris and the caruncle.[12] A Desmarres retractor is used to retract the caruncle medially, and a Colorado needle again makes the incision through the conjunctiva, with the eye protected by a narrow malleable retractor and corneal shield. Tissue is then gently divided with blunt Stevens scissors in a posteromedial direction to avoid the lacrimal system. The periosteum is again incised and elevated posteriorly to expose the fracture site. It is likely that at least the anterior and, possibly, the posterior ethmoid arteries will require cautery and division. If the posterior ethmoid artery is reached, dissection must proceed with great care because the optic foramen will be found 3 to 8 mm posterior to this artery. Frequently, a less robust allograft is needed, such as 0.4-mm nylon. Caution is required to avoid driving the fixation screw above the frontoethmoidal suture.

The incisions may be joined to provide wide exposure of the floor and medial wall.

Fractures of the Roof of the Orbit

Fractures of the roof of the orbit associated with intracranial injury may be approached via a coronal incision to provide wide access for examination and repair of possible dural injury. Other fractures without intracranial involvement may be exposed endoscopically by way of the frontal sinus. The bony fragment may be reduced and, if necessary, fixated. If associated outer table frac-

tures are to be repaired, they may then be plated through the same sub-brow incision while taking care to preserve the supraorbital neurovascular bundle. Most commonly, however, roof fractures that need to be repaired require neurosurgical consultation and a combined approach.

Choice of Implant Material

In the current era, alloplastic materials have advanced enough that surgeons can often avoid the use of autografts, thereby precluding donor site morbidity and resorption. Titanium mesh has been a common choice for reconstruction of the orbit because it is readily shaped and cut. However, tissue adheres strongly to this mesh, thus making it less desirable in such situations.

A variety of plastic materials have been designed for reconstructive use. Silicon is an older implant that causes no adhesions but is quite soft. Porous polyethylene is a popular choice for floor and medial wall fractures and is particularly useful when barrier coated on the side facing the orbit. It is available in numerous sizes and shapes and is easily shaped with scissors or scalpel. Although no fixation is theoretically required, the periosteum over the implant must be closed with interrupted sutures.

Our group uses nylon foil implants. This material is easily shaped, has some memory, and rarely becomes infected. The 0.6-mm thickness is malleable enough to bend for insertion but stiff enough to support the orbital contents. A 0.4-mm thickness is useful for repair of medial wall fractures, where less strength is necessary and the ability to temporarily deform the plate is desirable. No tissue adhesion occurs, and because the implant is fixed to bone, closure of periosteum is unnecessary.

A relatively new alloplastic material has also been found to be well suited to repair of these fractures: a titanium mesh–reinforced thin porous polyethylene sheet. It has the advantages of tissue ingrowth and excellent memory with easy intraoperative shaping, and the barrier coating on the side placed toward the orbit prevents adherence of tissue.

POSTOPERATIVE MANAGEMENT

Our group admits patients overnight for observation and pain control after fracture repair. If orbital hemorrhage occurs, the most serious complication of the surgery, it will be noted quickly and may be drained as soon as possible. Placement of a drain and lack of conjunctival closure are intended to help prevent buildup of significant orbital pressure in the event of bleeding, but occasionally, opening of the wound, evacuation of hematoma, and possibly removal of hardware may be necessary. Oral narcotic/acetaminophen combinations generally suffice for control of pain. The patient rests with the head of the bed elevated and is instructed to not bend below the waist, lift greater than 5 lb, or strain for 3 days. Nose blowing is not allowed for the following

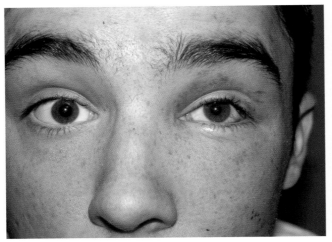

Figure 94-18. Trapdoor fracture of the left eye 24 hours after repair.

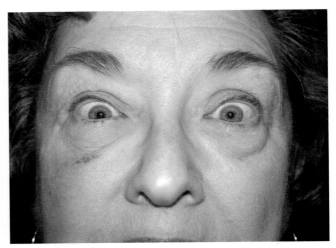

Figure 94-20. Patient 2, 1 week postoperatively—the diplopia has resolved.

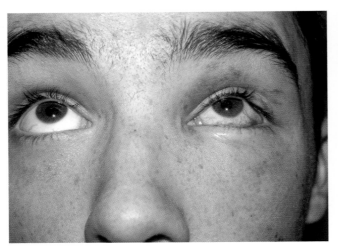

Figure 94-19. Upgaze.

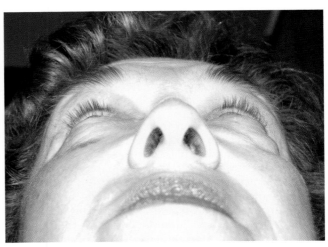

Figure 94-21. Patient 2, 1 week postoperatively.

4 weeks. Nausea is treated with an antiemetic because vomiting might cause a severe increase in orbital pressure. An antibiotic such as cephalexin and a steroid are administered intravenously while in the hospital. Antibiotics are taken orally for 7 days postoperatively to prevent infection of the allograft, along with rapidly tapering doses of oral steroid.

The patient is seen in the office 1 week and 1 month postoperatively and as needed after that. In the event of entrapped muscle, it is wise to prepare the patient and family for the probable subsequent temporary paresis of the involved muscle and to reassure them that when the patch is removed, the abnormal eye position is expected and almost certainly temporary (Figs. 94-18 to 94-21).

PEARLS

- Documentation of the condition of the eye before and after surgery is critical.
- Young patients with small floor fractures, particularly when experiencing severe pain or nausea, must be suspected of having an entrapped inferior rectus muscle.
- Muscle entrapment does not occur in large fractures, but muscle herniation (not an emergency) does.
- Floor implants should be placed far enough posterior to the orbital rim that they are not palpable.
- Approximately 1 cm^2 of fracture will allow the eye to move posteriorly about 1 mm.

PITFALLS

- Failure of the implant to rest on the posterior shelf of bone may cause continued enophthalmos.
- Manipulation of the orbit in the presence of significant globe injury or traumatic optic neuropathy must be avoided.
- Failure to check and document that forced ductions at the conclusion of the procedure are as free as or better than those at the beginning may allow orbital tissue trapped under the implant to go unnoticed.

References

1. Smith B, Regan WF Jr: Blow-out fracture of the orbit; mechanism and correction of internal orbital fracture. Am J Ophthalmol 44:733-739, 1957.
2. Converse JM, Smith B, Obear MF, et al: Orbital blowout fractures: A ten-year survey. Plast Reconstr Surg 39:20-36, 1967.
3. Fujino T, Makino K: Entrapment mechanism and ocular injury in orbital blowout fracture. Plast Reconstr Surg 65:571-576, 1980.
4. Bansagi ZC, Meyer DR: Internal orbital fractures in the pediatric age group: Characterization and management. Ophthalmology 107:829-836, 2000.
5. Smith B, Lisman RD, Simonton J, et al: Volkmann's contracture of the extraocular muscles following blowout fracture. Plast Reconstr Surg 74:200-216, 1984.
6. Putterman AM, Stevens T, Urist MJ: Nonsurgical management of blow-out fractures of the orbital floor. Am J Ophthalmol 77:232-239, 1974.
7. Fan X, Li J, Zhu J, et al: Computer-assisted orbital volume measurement in the surgical correction of late enophthalmos caused by blowout fractures. Ophthal Plast Reconstr Surg 19:207-211, 2003.
8. Biesman BS, Hornblass A, Lisman R, et al: Diplopia after surgical repair of orbital floor fractures. Ophthal Plast Reconstr Surg 12:9-16, discussion 17, 1996.
9. Hatton MP, Thakker MM, Ray S: Orbital and adnexal trauma associated with open-globe injuries. Ophthal Plast Reconstr Surg 18:458-461, 2002.
10. Ioannides C, Treffers W, Rutten M, et al: Ocular injuries associated with fractures involving the orbit. J Craniomaxillofac Surg 16:157-159, 1988.
11. Levin LA, Beck RW, Joseph MP, et al: The treatment of traumatic optic neuropathy: The International Optic Nerve Trauma Study. Ophthalmology 106:1268-1277, 1999.
12. Graham SM, Thomas RD, Carter KD, et al: The transcaruncular approach to the medial orbital wall. Laryngoscope 112:986-989, 2002.

ORBITAL SURGERY

Chapter 95

Orbital Decompression

S. Tonya Stefko and Carl H. Snyderman

Decompression of the orbit may be considered for the treatment of space-occupying lesions causing compromise of function as a result of expansion of the orbital contents or a decrease in the rigid orbital confines. The volume of the orbit averages about 30 mL, and only anteriorly is it not bound by bone. By far the most common indication for decompression is Graves orbitopathy, but similar surgical techniques are applied to infectious, traumatic, neoplastic, and iatrogenic complications (e.g., orbital hematoma after sinus surgery) (Figs. 95-1 and 95-2).

The incidence of Graves disease in the general population is about 1% to 3%. Females are affected about five times as often as men, but older men who experience orbitopathy often have a more fulminant course. About a third of patients with Graves disease will have orbitopathy, often asymmetrical and usually mild or moderate. Approximately 85% of patients evaluated primarily for orbitopathy will be found to have a dysthyroid state. In adults, Graves disease is the most common cause of unilateral and bilateral proptosis. The first report of decompression for this condition occurred in 1911.[1]

The pathogenesis of Graves orbitopathy remains only partially understood. Serum levels of antibodies to the thyroid-stimulating hormone (TSH) receptor and collagen XIII seem to correlate with orbital disease activity.[2] TSH receptors are found on orbital fibroblasts, which may differentiate into adipocytes, and are more sensitive to TSH receptor antibodies than dermal fibrocytes are. The proptosis is due to an increase in retrobulbar glycosaminoglycan deposition and edema, as well as to a later increase in retrobulbar fat. Smoking is thought to affect this either by creating increased oxygen-reactive species or by causing local tissue hypoxia, both of which lead to increased chemokines recruiting T cells from the bloodstream. TH_2 cells are the predominant type involved in the orbital disease.[3]

The acute phase of the disease, which consists of orbital congestion, inflammatory cell infiltrate, and forward movement of the globe, generally lasts between 6 and 24 months. After this phase, the disease is characterized pathologically by increased fibrosis of the tissues. A second acute phase may occasionally affect the patient later in life. Asymmetrical involvement of the orbits is frequent.

The only external factor proved to affect Graves orbitopathy is cigarette smoking. Current smoking outweighs previous smoking as a predictor of disease severity. Patients in whom orbital disease develops are four times as likely to smoke, and discontinuation of smoking appears to lessen the severity, as well as protect patients from the development of further symptoms.[4] Pretibial myxedema, acropachy, and female sex are also associated with more severe orbital disease.[5]

Symptoms of Graves orbitopathy include eyelid retraction, proptosis, diplopia, dryness of the eyes, a sensation of pressure behind one or both eyes, and

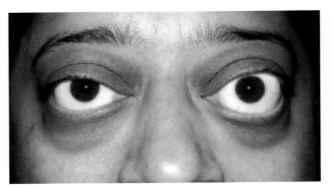

Figure 95-1. Patient with Graves orbitopathy preoperatively.

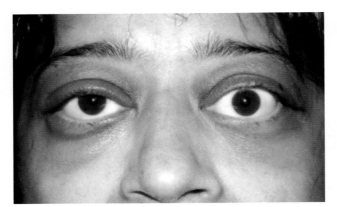

Figure 95-2. Patient with Graves orbitopathy 6 days after balanced decompression of both eyes.

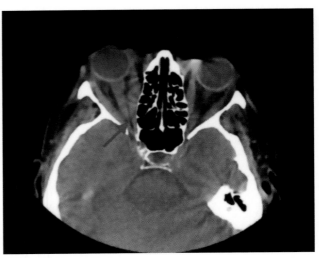

Figure 95-3. Patient with Graves orbitopathy, optic neuropathy in the right eye, visual acuity of 20/50 in the right eye, and Ishihara color vision of 1.5 of 11 plates. Note the apical crowding.

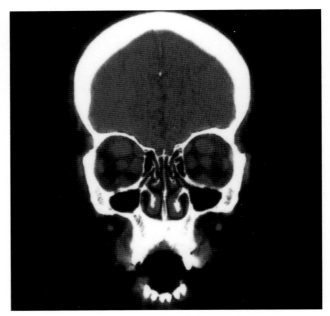

Figure 95-4. Coronal view of the patient from Figure 95-3.

swelling of the lids and conjunctiva (chemosis). Signs consists of eyelid retraction more than 1 mm from the limbus, eyelid lag on downward gaze (failure of the upper eyelid to descend properly when the patient looks down), unilateral or bilateral proptosis, restriction of extraocular movements (particularly upward gaze and abduction), hyperemia over the insertions of the horizontal rectus muscles, and corneal staining with fluorescein observed with a cobalt filter (Figs. 95-3 and 95-4).

The course of the orbital disease and the course of any associated thyroid disease in Graves disease are independent. Euthyroid patients may have severe orbitopathy causing optic neuropathy or corneal perforation, whereas severely hyperthyroid patients may have no signs or symptoms. Treating the thyroid abnormalities is essential to the patient's general health, but it is unlikely to help the eye disease. Exceptions are removal of a large goiter, which may lessen the orbital symptoms, and treatment with radioactive iodine, which sometimes acutely worsens the condition of the orbits (ameliorated by concurrent treatment with oral steroid).[6]

Orbital decompression is sometimes undertaken for other causes of proptosis: infection with abscess, tumor, trauma to the optic nerve, or hematoma (such as might occur after endoscopic sinus surgery). Abscesses located along the lamina papyracea in the orbit or medially along the roof or floor are most amenable to endoscopic drainage. In the setting of head trauma and a new optic neuropathy, traumatic optic neuropathy is assumed. If the optic canal is fractured, the fragments may be removed endoscopically, but authors disagree about the benefits of this procedure.[7-9] Occasionally, an orbital apex tumor causing compressive optic neuropathy may be successfully treated by decompression when resection of the tumor is inadvisable.[10]

ANATOMY

The orbit is bounded by four walls: superior, medial, inferior, and lateral. The medial wall of the orbit extends

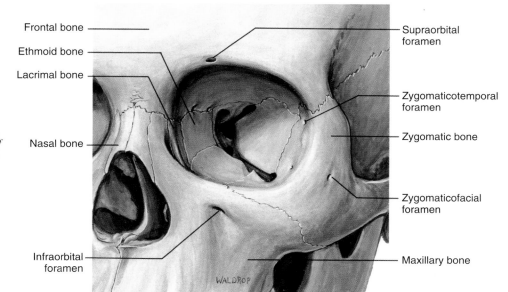

Figure 95-5. Orbital bones, frontal view. *(From Dutton JJ: Atlas of Clinical and Surgical Orbital Anatomy. Philadelphia, WB Saunders, 1994.)*

Frontal bone
Ethmoid bone
Lacrimal bone
Nasal bone
Infraorbital foramen
Supraorbital foramen
Zygomaticotemporal foramen
Zygomatic bone
Zygomaticofacial foramen
Maxillary bone

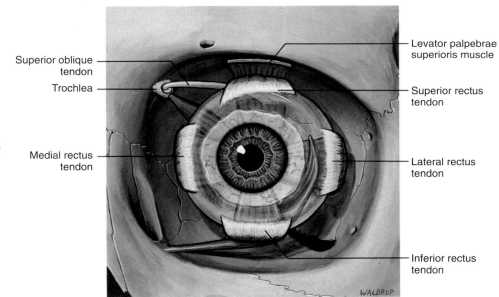

Figure 95-6. Extraocular muscles, frontal composite view. *(From Dutton JJ: Atlas of Clinical and Surgical Orbital Anatomy. Philadelphia, WB Saunders, 1994.)*

Superior oblique tendon
Trochlea
Medial rectus tendon
Levator palpebrae superioris muscle
Superior rectus tendon
Lateral rectus tendon
Inferior rectus tendon

from the ethmoidal roof superiorly to its junction with the inferior wall inferiorly. Posteriorly, it is continuous with the medial surface of the optic canal. Anteriorly, it is bounded by the thicker bone of the lacrimal fossa and ascending process of the maxilla. The inferior wall of the orbit is thicker than the medial wall and is divided by the infraorbital neurovascular bundle. The bulge of the canal is often visible, and the vessels can be visualized through the thinned bone. The lateral wall of the orbit is bounded laterally by the temporalis muscle (Figs. 95-5 and 95-6).

PATIENT SELECTION

By the time that a patient with Graves disease has reached the otolaryngologist for consultation, the patient will most likely have been evaluated by an ophthalmologist. A frank conversation between the two physicians will establish the urgency with which surgery should proceed: a patient with severe exposure keratitis may require decompression within the week, whereas another patient with inactive disease and strictly cosmetic concerns may be scheduled when convenient for surgeon and patient. If the patient has not undergone a complete ophthalmologic examination, including evaluation of optic nerve function, extraocular movement, and ocular surface, one must be conducted before planning surgery. Documentation of preoperative visual function is critical.

Occasionally, other disease processes will necessitate surgical decompression of the orbits, including infection, tumor, hemorrhage, and trauma. Usually, these cases will develop more rapidly than dysthyroid orbitopathy, and the decision regarding timing and the approach for surgery will be more urgent. Surgical approaches are the same; however, each of these cases will have its attendant challenges. In all these situations, the anatomy will be obscured and great care must be taken to avoid harm to vital structures that the surgeon seeks to protect.

In the case of an orbital abscess causing proptosis, particularly in children younger than 9 years, it is often prudent to wait 24 to 48 hours for a response to intravenous antibiotics. In adults, particularly when the abscess is associated with concurrent sinus disease, the decision to proceed with endoscopic drainage of the cavity (when located medially) or external drainage (when located superiorly or laterally) should be made earlier (Fig. 95-7). In the case of optic neuropathy, surgery should proceed as soon as safely possible.

Orbital hematoma, whether traumatic, iatrogenic, or rarely, spontaneous, should also be approached with urgency. If optic neuropathy is present and lateral canthotomy/cantholysis has failed, decompression of the orbit is necessary. Endoscopic decompression of the medial wall is particularly helpful because a fairly posterior decompression of the optic nerve is possible.

Frequently in cases of trauma with fracture of the orbit, the orbit will have decompressed itself. In some instances, however, bone fragments may impinge on orbital structures and require urgent removal or reduction. This occurs again in the presence of optic neuropathy or with an intractable increase in intraocular pressure (Fig. 95-8).

In cases of Graves orbitopathy, communication between the ophthalmologist, otolaryngologist, and patient will determine how best to serve the patient. Patients may be divided into two groups: those who require urgent surgery during an active phase of disease and those who seek cosmetic and functional improvement later in the course of the disease. Whenever possible, it is best to defer patients from the first group into the second. If the patient has active orbitopathy characterized by inflammatory signs and evolution and can be treated by nonsurgical means, this should be pursued first. Temporization may often be accomplished with the use of oral (1 mg/kg/day) or intravenous pulse prednisone or by radiation treatment of the orbits (up to 2000 cGy, below the threshold for causing optic neuropathy). Retinopathy rarely occurs late after radiation treatment, but nearly always in diabetic patients, and cataract formation appears only as frequently as it does when patients are treated with steroids.[11] Surgery is both more technically challenging and more likely to be complicated by excessive bleeding in the setting of active inflammation. However, some patients will require immediate surgery, particularly when an impending corneal perforation or severe optic neuropathy is present.

Patients who have passed the active stage and entered the cicatricial phase are good candidates for decompression, either for improvement in appearance or for maximization of residual function. Endoscopic decompression of the medial wall combined with removal of the medial floor and lateral wall offers the most significant decrease in proptosis, up to 6 to 10 mm. The degree of improvement depends partly on the increase in volume, but also on the rigidity of the tissues (periorbital tissues that are more densely fibrotic relax poorly into the newly created space). Decompression of

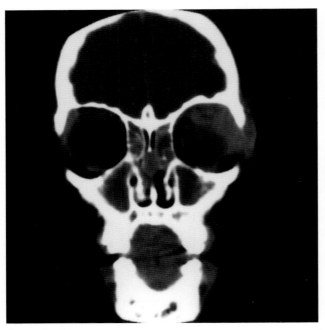

Figure 95-7. Twelve-year-old patient with a superior subperiosteal orbital abscess that improved after endoscopic ethmoidectomy and percutaneous drainage of the abscess.

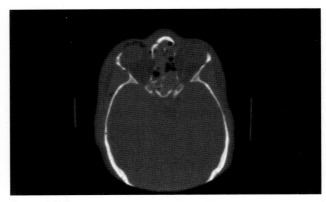

Figure 95-8. Patient with bone fragments in the optic canal and right optic neuropathy after closed head injury.

the orbital roof is seldom performed. Unilateral or bilateral orbital decompression may be performed at the same time.

PREOPERATIVE EVALUATION

All patients undergoing orbital decompression require a comprehensive preoperative ophthalmologic examination. A computed tomography (CT) scan of the orbit is helpful to identify any anatomic abnormalities before surgery.

It is helpful for the otolaryngologist to see the patient preoperatively to obtain a history of sinonasal problems and evaluate the anatomy of the nasal cavity. The CT scan should be reviewed to assess for occult disease and anatomic variations that may pose problems: low cribriform plate, Onodi cells, Haller cells, or nonpneumatization of sinuses. Active sinusitis should be treated and completely resolved before proceeding with elective orbital decompression. Severe deviations of the nasal septum can interfere with surgical access and may need to be corrected at the same time. Coexistent sinus problems such as chronic sinus obstruction or nasal polyposis can also be addressed. Informed consent includes the usual discussion of risks from endoscopic sinus surgery: visual loss, diplopia, cerebrospinal fluid (CSF) leak, hemorrhage, sinusitis, loss of olfaction, and intranasal synechiae.

PREOPERATIVE PLANNING

Preoperative counseling is particularly important so that the patient understands that this procedure, when performed for Graves disease, is likely to be the first in a series of surgeries. New-onset or worsened postoperative diplopia will occur in about a third of patients undergoing decompression of three walls,[12] but it has been observed in retrospective series that a "balanced decompression" consisting of only the medial and lateral walls is associated with only about a 10% incidence of new-onset diplopia.[13] Strabismus surgery may be performed for unresolved diplopia, and eyelid surgery (either correction of retraction or blepharoplasty) may be required after that.

SURGICAL APPROACHES

Over the years a number of different operations have been described for decompression of the orbit, which may include anywhere from one to four walls. The amount of decompression that can be achieved increases with the number of walls removed. Removal of the superior wall is not usually performed because of its minimal additional benefit and the added morbidity. The medial wall may be decompressed from an external ethmoidectomy approach, a transantral approach, or a transnasal approach. The inferior wall may be decompressed from a transconjunctival approach, a transantral approach, or a transnasal approach. With the advent of endoscopic sinus surgery techniques, most surgeons prefer a transnasal endoscopic approach for decom-

pression of the medial and inferior orbital walls. Removal of bone lateral to the infraorbital nerve provides minimal additional decompression and risks injury to the infraorbital nerve. The lateral orbital wall is decompressed from an external approach.

Medial Wall

The nose is decongested with pledgets soaked in 0.5% oxymetazoline. If a septoplasty is necessary for access, it is performed first. The inferior aspect of the middle turbinate is resected to provide greater access and room for the orbital tissues to expand. The uncinate process is removed and the antrostomy is maximally enlarged posteriorly and superiorly. The bulla ethmoidalis is opened for removal of ethmoid air cells in an anterior-to-posterior direction. The sphenoid sinus is opened and the sphenoidotomy is maximally enlarged with Kerrison rongeurs. Residual septations are then removed in a posterior-to-anterior direction along the skull base. The nasofrontal recess is exposed, but further dissection of the frontal sinus is unnecessary.

The medial wall of the orbit is palpated and the thin bone of the lamina papyracea is fractured anteriorly. Bone fragments are carefully elevated from the underlying periorbita with a Cottle elevator or ball-tipped probe. Removal of bone continues posteriorly to the anterior face of the sphenoid sinus. Superiorly, bone is removed to within 2 mm of the skull base while being careful to not fracture the skull base. Removal of bone continues inferiorly to the junction of the medial and inferior orbital walls. Examination of the maxillary sinus with an angled endoscope usually reveals the neurovascular bundle of the infraorbital nerve running across the roof of the maxilla. The floor of the orbit is then removed with angled Kerrison rongeurs to the medial aspect of the neurovascular bundle. Removal of additional bone does not contribute to decompression and risks injury to the nerve.

If the decompression is being done for proptosis, decompression of the orbital apex beyond the anterior wall of the sphenoid sinus is not necessary.[14] If the patient is undergoing decompression for visual loss, additional bone is removed posteriorly. Landmarks within the sphenoid sinus are first identified: the carotid canal, optic canal, and optic-carotid recess.[15] The bone is carefully thinned with a diamond drill over the optic canal until it can be fractured and elevated with a small elevator. Drilling of bone should be along the axis of the optic canal to avoid injury to the carotid artery.

A sickle blade is then used to incise the periorbita of the medial orbit, starting posteriorly and superiorly and proceeding anteriorly. Multiple parallel incisions are made from the ethmoid roof to the floor of the orbit. The medial rectus muscle is often infiltrated and enlarged and is susceptible to injury if the incisions are too deep. Intervening strands of periorbita are transected to allow complete herniation of the orbital contents. Gentle external pressure on the orbit with the hand facilitates herniation of orbital fat into the ethmoid defect (see Video 95-1).

Silastic nasal splints are placed to prevent intranasal synechiae. Nasal packing is not used.

Lateral Wall

The lateral wall of the orbit is approached via a lateral canthotomy incision. The incision created is approximately 2 cm in length and extends posteriorly from the lateral canthal angle in a crow's foot crease. Stevens or similar scissors are used to cut the lateral canthal ligament and deepen the incision to bone. Bleeding is controlled with electrocautery. The periosteum is incised vertically along the apex of the rim with a scalpel or needle-tipped electrocautery. A Cottle elevator is then used to clear the periosteum from the lateral orbital wall while keeping the periorbita intact as much as possible. The periosteum must be elevated from both the interior and exterior surfaces of the lateral wall of the orbit. The bone should be identified as far superiorly as the fossa of the lacrimal sac and inferiorly to just above the level of the zygomatic arch. Careful elevation along the exterior surface proceeds in a posterior direction and then turns medially in the temporal fossa.

Once the periosteum has been elevated from the bone, a wide ribbon retractor is inserted between the periorbita and bone by an assistant. A Desmarres vein retractor is placed over the cut surface of the skin. An oscillating bone saw is used to cut through the lateral wall, perpendicular to the bone. Frequent pauses to assess position and adequacy of protection of the orbital contents are essential. It is only necessary to make an osteotomy posteriorly through the vertical zygomaticofrontal buttress. A parallel osteotomy is made inferiorly above the zygomatic arch, again through the triangular thick bone of the rim.

A rongeur is now used to grasp the vertical strut, which is rocked medially and laterally until the bone breaks free posteriorly. It will be necessary to elevate the remainder of the temporalis muscle from the posterolateral surface of the bone with electrocautery. Bone wax is applied as needed, and any remaining small fragments of bone are removed with the same instrument. The sharp surfaces of the remaining zygomatic and frontal bones are smoothed with a burr or rongeur.

A short-bladed knife, such as a sickle knife, is now applied to the periorbita in a very superficial manner, directed posteriorly to anteriorly, to slit the fibrous septa and allow the orbital contents to prolapse into the temporal fossa. Care is taken to place no traction on the orbital fat and to remain superficial so that the lacrimal gland and lateral rectus muscle are not damaged. Bipolar cautery is used to obtain hemostasis.

Careful closure of the wound is accomplished by precise realignment of the upper and lower gray lines of the eyelid with a single horizontal stitch of 6-0 absorbable material, such as polyglactin, buried laterally. The deep tissues are reapproximated with inverted 6-0 suture and the skin closed carefully with running 7-0 nylon or interrupted chromic gut suture. Before complete closure, a longitudinal strip of 0.25-inch Penrose

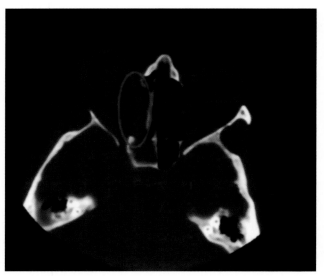

Figure 95-9. Postoperative axial view of the patient from Figure 95-3 with right optic neuropathy secondary to Graves orbitopathy. One week after balanced decompression, visual acuity in the right eye was 20/25 and Ishihara color vision was normal (17/18 plates). Note the herniation of the enlarged medial rectus into the bony defect.

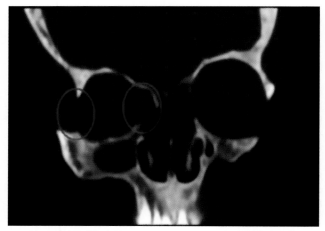

Figure 95-10. Postoperative coronal view of the patient from Figure 95-3. Note the bony defects with herniation of the orbital contents.

drain is placed into the wound to emerge between suture bites. A patch is placed loosely over the eye to absorb drainage. The patient is admitted for observation overnight, both for pain control and to monitor for any hemorrhage (Figs. 95-9 and 95-10).

POSTOPERATIVE CARE

Patients are administered a steroid pulse intravenously while undergoing surgery and observation (8 to 12 mg of dexamethasone during the procedure, and 4 to 8 mg every 8 hours thereafter while in the hospital). A rapid taper of oral steroid medication is adequate for most patients; those decompressed in an acute setting require a much more aggressive regimen and longer taper.

Patients are instructed to not blow their nose for 1 month after the procedure, and a steroid/antibiotic ointment is applied to the sutures twice a day for a week. Nonabsorbable sutures are removed in 5 to 7 days. Intranasal splints are removed at 1 week, and a saline spray is used as necessary to minimize crusting. Mucosalization of the orbital tissues is usually complete by 2 months. Patients are counseled to expect some initial diplopia and that the final appearance is often not reached for at least 3 months.

Patients are observed for at least 6 months after surgery before consideration of extraocular muscle or eyelid surgery.

COMPLICATIONS

The risks associated with endoscopic medial and inferior orbital decompression are similar to those after any endoscopic sinus surgery. Excessive or aggressive removal of bone superiorly can fracture the skull base and cause a CSF leak. Injury to the ethmoidal arteries can occur and result in a retro-orbital hematoma. Posteriorly, the optic nerve and carotid artery are at risk for injury. The medial rectus muscle is often enlarged and is susceptible to injury when the periorbita is incised. Postoperatively, the exposed orbital fat is at greater risk for infection, but this is a rare occurrence. Positive pressure ventilation after extubation or nose blowing by the patient postoperatively can force air into the orbital tissues and result in subcutaneous emphysema. Injury to the infraorbital nerve can lead to loss of sensation of the midface.

The lateral rectus muscle is susceptible to injury during decompression of the lateral orbital wall. Ecchymosis of the periorbital tissues is common but may be associated with a hematoma.

As discussed previously, unbalanced decompression of the orbit can result in significant diplopia. The diplopia is often transient but may require corrective surgery if it persists beyond 6 months.

SUMMARY

Decompression of the orbit is considered for the treatment of Graves ophthalmopathy and other mass lesions of the orbit (abscess, hematoma, and neoplasm). Maximal decompression can be achieved with endoscopic decompression of the medial and inferior orbital walls and external decompression of the lateral wall. Balanced decompression minimizes the risk for postoperative diplopia.

PEARLS

- Balanced decompression (medial and lateral orbital walls) minimizes the likelihood of postoperative diplopia.
- Careful realignment of the lateral commissure of the eyelids is necessary for an optimal cosmetic result.

- In patients with compressive optic neuropathy, it is vital to perform posterior medial wall decompression to relieve pressure on the optic nerve in the orbital apex.
- When decompressing the optic canal, the optic nerve sheath should be opened cautiously in the superonasal quadrant to minimize the risk of injury to the ophthalmic artery.
- Any removal of intraconal fat must be done with a minimum of traction and from the inferotemporal quadrant (between the lateral and inferior rectus muscles) to decrease the risk of retrobulbar hematoma and injury to orbital structures.

PITFALLS

- The medial and lateral rectus muscles are often enlarged and just deep to the periorbita and may be injured by aggressive sharp dissection.
- Bony decompression without adequate division of the periorbital septa is ineffective.
- Aggressive endoscopic removal of bone superiorly may be associated with fractures of the skull base and CSF leak.
- Unrecognized injury to the ethmoid arteries may cause retro-orbital hematoma, a risk that is increased when the patient coughs or struggles when emerging from anesthesia.
- Monopolar cautery should be avoided near the apex of the orbit.

References

1. Dollinger J: Die Druckenlastung der Augenhöhle durch Entfernung der äusseren Orbitalwand bei hochgradigem Exophthalmus (Morbus basedowii) und konsekutive Hornhauterkrankung. Dtsch Med Wochenschr 37:1888-1890, 1911.
2. El-Kaissi S, Frauman AG, Wall JR: Thyroid-associated ophthalmopathy: A practical guide to classification, natural history and management. Intern Med J 34:482-491, 2004.
3. Ludgate M, Baker G: Unlocking the immunological mechanisms of orbital inflammation in thyroid eye disease. Clin Exp Immunol 127:193-198, 2002.
4. Cawood T, Moriarty P, O'Shea D: Recent developments in thyroid eye disease. BMJ 329:385-390, 2004.
5. Fatourechi V, Bartley GB, Eghbali-Fatourechi GZ, et al: Graves dermopathy and acropachy are markers of severe Graves ophthalmopathy. Thyroid 13:1141-1144, 2003.
6. Bartalena L, Marcocci C, Bogazzi F, et al: Relation between therapy for hyperthyroidism and the course of Graves ophthalmopathy. N Engl J Med 338:73-78, 1998.
7. Goldenberg-Cohen N, Miller NR, Repka MX: Traumatic optic neuropathy in children and adolescents. J AAPOS 8:20-27, 2004.
8. Kountakis SE, Maillard AA, El-Harazi SM, et al: Endoscopic optic nerve decompression for traumatic blindness. Otolaryngol Head Neck Surg 123:34-37, 2000.
9. Levin LA, Beck RW, Joseph MP, et al: The treatment of traumatic optic neuropathy: The International Optic Nerve Trauma Study. Ophthalmology 106:1268-1277, 1999.

10. Kloek CE, Bilyk JR, Pribitkin EA, Rubin PA: Orbital decompression as an alternative management strategy for patients with benign tumors located at the orbital apex. Ophthalmology 113:1214-1219, 2006.

11. Wakelkamp IM, Tan H, Saeed P, et al: Orbital irradiation for Graves ophthalmopathy: Is it safe? A long-term follow-up study. Ophthalmology 111:1557-1562, 2004.

12. Russo V, Querques G, Primavera V, Delle Noci N: Incidence and treatment of diplopia after three-wall orbital decompression in Graves ophthalmopathy. J Pediatr Ophthalmol Strabismus 41:219-225, 2004.

13. Graham SM, Brown CL, Carter KD, et al: Medial and lateral orbital wall surgery for balanced decompression in thyroid eye disease. Laryngoscope 113:1206-1209, 2003.

14. Snyderman C, Hobson S: Endoscopic orbital decompression. In Myers E (ed): Operative Otolaryngology. Philadelphia, WB Saunders, 1997, pp 796-806.

15. Snyderman C, Hobson S: Endoscopic orbital decompression for endocrine ophthalmopathy. In Myers E, Bluestone C, Brackmann D, Krause C (eds): Advances in Otolaryngology–Head and Neck Surgery. St Louis, CV Mosby, 1996, pp 205-215.

Chapter **96**

Optic Nerve Decompression

Allan D. Vescan, Ricardo L. Carrau, Carl H. Snyderman, and Amin B. Kassam

Optic nerve injury with loss of vision is a devastating event.[1-10] Optic nerve injury can be classified in various ways, including but not limited to the anatomic region and pathophysiologic mechanisms. Anatomic classification includes intraorbital, intracanalicular, and intracranial sites of injury. Pathophysiologic classification includes traumatic and nontraumatic mechanisms of injury. Traumatic optic nerve injury can be further subclassified as either direct or indirect injury. Direct injury includes penetrating injury to the orbit or optic nerve canal as a result of a foreign body or fracture of the lesser wing of the sphenoid. Indirect injury is generally the result of blunt head trauma. The exact mechanism of injury is not well understood, however, but may include hematoma, neural edema, and disruption of the microvascular circulation and axonal transport. Nontraumatic causes of optic nerve injury include compressive effects from benign or malignant tumors, inflammatory conditions such as Graves' disease, and fibro-osseous lesions. The most effective treatment of traumatic optic neuropathy (TON) remains controversial. Options for treatment include observation, intravenous corticosteroids, and surgical decompression. In 1999 the International Optic Nerve Trauma Study (IONTS) attempted to answer the question of which therapeutic modality was most efficacious in treating indirect TON. It attempted to randomize patients to "megadose" steroids alone or in conjunction with extracranial optic nerve decompression. Because of patient recruitment factors, however, this was abandoned and the investigators proceeded to a comparative nonrandomized interventional study with concurrent treatment groups. They concluded that there was no clear benefit of corticosteroid therapy over optic canal decompression and that treatment should be tailored to the individual patient. Subsequent to IONTS, several retrospective series have been published that both support and refute the use of optic nerve decompression in addition to corticosteroid use for the treatment of indirect optic neuropathy.

Despite the controversy regarding TON, optic nerve decompression to alleviate compressive effects is widely accepted. Its technique, indications, and complications are the focus of this chapter, although the concepts apply to most situations.

PATIENT SELECTION

Patient selection is dictated by the cause of the visual loss.[6,11-14] In the scenario of TON, a diagnosis must first be secured. The diagnosis of TON is a clinical diagnosis supported by a history of direct or indirect injury to the head or face. The level of consciousness of the patient can make the situation fairly straightforward or make it a challenge. Features of TON include an afferent pupillary defect, monocular or binocular involvement, impairment of color vision, visual field defects, loss of visual acuity (ranging from mild to no light perception), and delayed development of optic atrophy in the weeks after the injury. In the setting of compressive optic neuropathy secondary to benign or malignant tumors, chronic inflammatory processes, or fibro-osseus lesions, many of the same features will be present; however, their onset will be much more insidious, and careful and detailed ophthalmologic assessment will be required to quantify the visual deterioration. Once compressive neuropathy is ascertained, the underlying pathology and degree of compression will dictate the need for surgical decompression.

PREOPERATIVE PLANNING

Before embarking on endoscopic decompression of the optic nerve, imaging studies of the paranasal sinuses and skull base are critical (Figs. 96-1 to 96-4). Understanding the close relationship of the optic nerve to the paracavernous internal carotid artery is fundamental before proceeding to surgery (Figs. 96-5 and 96-6). In the setting of benign tumors and fibro-osseus lesions leading to compressive neuropathy, the sphenoid sinus

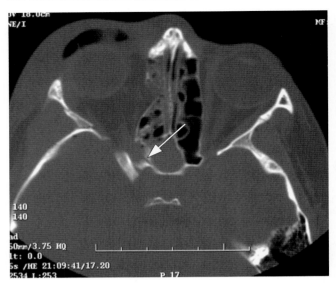

Figure 96-1. Axial computed tomography scan demonstrating a fracture of the right optic nerve canal *(arrow)* in a patient involved in a motor vehicle accident.

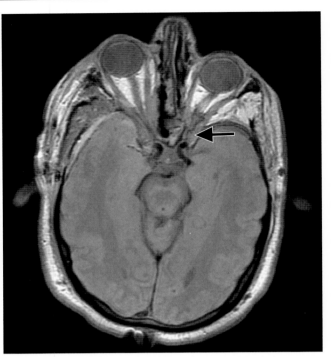

Figure 96-3. Axial magnetic resonance image demonstrating perineural extension of adenoid cystic carcinoma *(arrow)* along the left optic nerve.

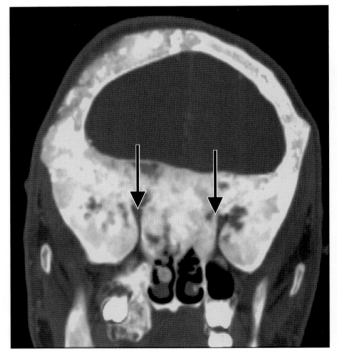

Figure 96-2. Coronal computed tomography scan demonstrating severe fibrous dysplasia with bilateral compression of the optic nerves *(arrows).*

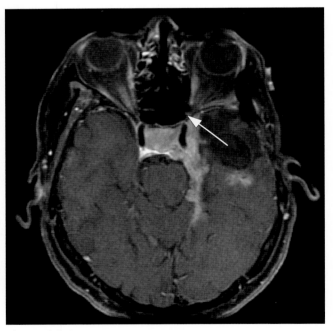

Figure 96-4. Axial magnetic resonance image demonstrating a recurrent meningioma *(arrow)* compressing the optic nerve within its canal and intracranially.

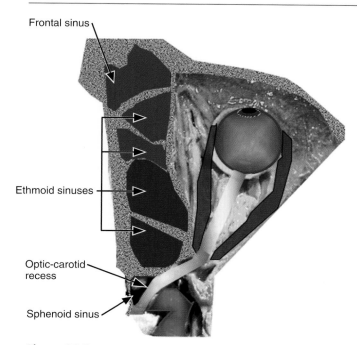

Figure 96-5. Diagrammatic representation in an axial plane demonstrating the lateral-to-medial direction of the optic nerve as it is followed in an anteroposterior direction and the relationship of the optic canal and internal carotid artery.

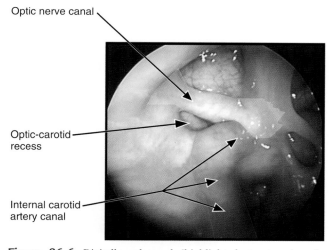

Figure 96-6. Digitally enhanced (highlighted structures) endoscopic view of the right sphenoid demonstrating the relationship of the optic nerve canal and the internal carotid artery. In this patient, pneumatization of the optic strut resulted in a deep optic carotid recess. Pneumatization of the anterior clinoid forms the recess superior to the optic canal.

and nasal anatomy may be distorted and almost impossible to predict (see Fig. 96-2). Image guidance becomes a valuable tool to assist the endoscopic surgeon in safely approaching the optic nerve and skull base. We prefer a fine-cut computed tomography (CT) scan of the sinuses and skull base with contrast enhancement before proceeding to optic nerve decompression. In situations in which there may be a soft tissue mass causing compression, magnetic resonance imaging (see

Figs. 96-3 and 96-4) can be added and fused with the CT scan to give further assistance in preoperative planning and navigation. Thorough ophthalmologic assessment, including all the issues mentioned in the previous section, is a prerequisite.

INDICATIONS

There are numerous indications for optic nerve decompression, including but not limited to optic neuropathy secondary to a compressive effect from either benign or malignant tumors, inflammatory processes such as Graves' disease, or fibro-osseous lesions such as fibrous dysplasia. Direct or indirect TON that has not responded to conservative or medical management is likewise an indication.

SURGICAL TECHNIQUE

The patient is positioned supine on the operating table and an orotracheal airway is secured. We insert cottonoids soaked in 0.05% oxymetazoline as a topical decongestant. Image guidance or intraoperative navigation systems are useful, if not critical for the surgery. If an optical tracking navigation system is available, we fix the head in a slight turn toward the surgeon's side with a three-pin head holder. We then obtain appropriate image guidance registration via surface fiducial markers (placed before imaging), a light-emitting diode–based face mask, or a laser surface registration device. For electromagnetic navigation systems, the helmet is placed and a straight probe is used for registration. Once this has been completed, the middle turbinate, lateral nasal wall, and posterior nasal septum are then sequentially infiltrated, in a posterior-to-anterior direction, with 0.5% lidocaine (Xylocaine) with 1:100,000 epinephrine. Resection of the right middle turbinate may be necessary, albeit rarely, to improve visualization and widen the space for instrumentation. In addition, outfracturing of the inferior turbinates widens the nasal corridor.

We use a 0-degree rod-lens endoscope to provide visualization throughout most of the procedure and reserve the use of an angled endoscope for visualization of the superior ethmoid sinuses or skull base. An uncinectomy is completed with back-biting rongeurs and a straight-blade microdébrider. Its superior aspect is spared because the frontonasal recess does not need to be exposed. We then complete anterior and posterior ethmoidectomies with a microdébrider or Tru-cut rongeurs (Fig. 96-7). This exposes the skull base (fovea ethmoidalis) and lamina papyracea. In patients who suffer trauma to the optic canal and orbit, the surgeon should be attentive to the possibility of exposed periorbita or orbital fat, or both. Via a transmeatal approach we remove the inferior aspect of the superior turbinate. The superior turbinate forms the medial aspect of the posterior ethmoids, and removal of it exposes the natural ostium of the sphenoid sinus. The ostium is enlarged in an inferior and medial direction until the endoscope can be inserted inside the sphenoid sinus

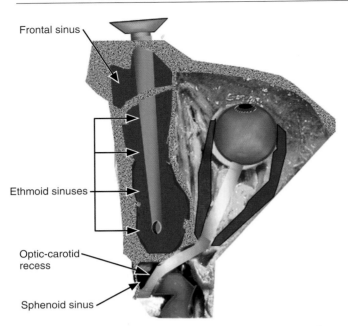

Figure 96-7. Diagrammatic representation in an axial plane demonstrating complete ethmoidectomy and sphenoidotomy to expose the lamina papyracea and skull base.

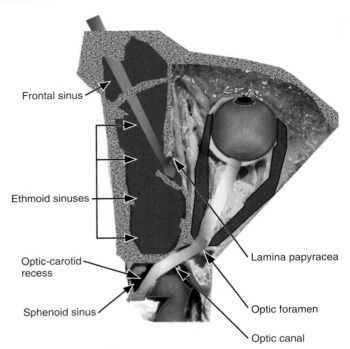

Figure 96-8. Diagrammatic representation in an axial plane demonstrating removal of the posterior aspect of the lamina papyracea. The periorbita is preserved to avoid herniation of orbital fat.

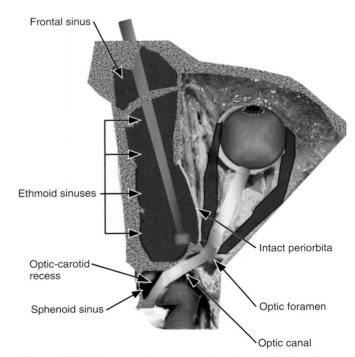

Figure 96-9. Diagrammatic representation in an axial plane demonstrating drilling of the optic foramen (pterygoid process).

for close visual inspection. Herniation of intracranial structures or an exposed internal carotid artery may be associated with trauma to the skull base. After these possibilities are discarded, the rest of the rostrum of the sphenoid is removed with up- and down-biting 2-mm Kerrison rongeurs. The rostrum must be removed until the roof and lateral wall of the sphenoid sinus are in plane with the roof of the posterior ethmoid sinuses and the lamina papyracea, respectively. Inferiorly, the posterolateral septal artery runs 1 cm above the posterior choana, and it is best to avoid injury to it. It can easily be controlled with bipolar or suction electrocautery. Use of suction electrocautery posterior to the rostrum or over the lamina papyracea is best avoided. Next, the posterior aspect of the lamina papyracea is removed to expose the periorbita covering the orbital apex (Fig. 96-8). Any injury to the periorbita will result in herniation of orbital fat, thereby impeding visualization. Cauterizing the fat with bipolar electrocautery may control limited herniation of this fat. The position of the optic nerve is at the top of the orbital apex, and it follows a lateral-to-medial and caudal-to-cephalad direction. The posterior ethmoidal artery is 4 to 6 mm anterior to the nerve.

If the foramen and optic canal are fractured, they can often be removed with a small Cottle elevator or 1- to 2-mm bone curette to displace the fractured fragments medially. Otherwise, the medial aspect of the foramen and canal has to be thinned with a 3-mm burr mounted on a high-speed drill (Fig. 96-9). It is critical to provide continuous irrigation to avoid thermal injury to the nerve or ophthalmic artery. The canal is decompressed back to the optic carotid recess because this marks the optic strut and the point where the nerve is intradural (Figs. 96-10 and 96-11). The decompression

should include the medial 120 degrees. More extensive decompression may be achieved if the optic strut (below the nerve) and anterior clinoid (above the nerve) are pneumatized (see Fig. 96-6). The optic nerve sheath is not opened because this does not contribute to the

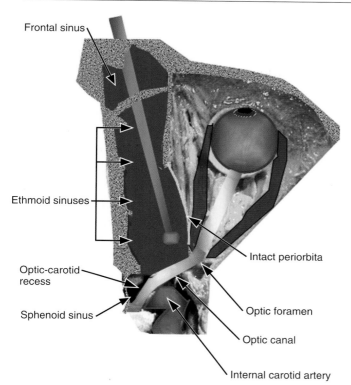

Frontal sinus

Ethmoid sinuses

Optic-carotid recess

Sphenoid sinus

Intact periorbita

Optic foramen

Optic canal

Internal carotid artery

Figure 96-10. Diagrammatic representation in an axial plane demonstrating complete decompression of the optic canal.

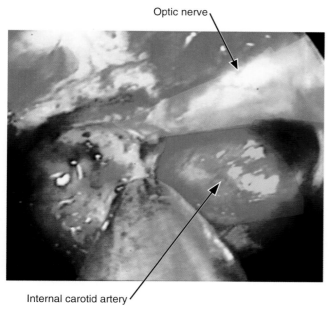

Optic nerve

Internal carotid artery

Figure 96-11. Digitally enhanced (highlighted structures) endoscopic view of a decompressed left optic nerve.

decompression. Furthermore, opening the sheath may cause leakage of cerebrospinal fluid (CSF) by opening the meningeal sleeve that often accompanies the optic nerve extracranially.

Subsequent to the decompression, copious irrigation is performed and Silastic splints are sutured to the nasal septum to prevent synechia formation. A small amount of packing can be used if hemostasis is an issue; however, one must be cautious because of the exposed optic nerve.

POSTOPERATIVE MANAGEMENT

Typically, patients are kept in the hospital overnight after optic nerve decompression. We routinely administer systemic steroids before, during, and after endoscopic decompression. Nasal saline sprays are started before discharge home. We routinely use silicone splints to prevent the formation of synechiae between the nasal septum and turbinate. Generally, they remain in place for 10 to 14 days. Nasal débridement is usually carried out biweekly for the first few postoperative visits, followed by monthly intervals. We recommend switching to a nasal saline douche after the first week to assist in remucosalization. We do not perform routine postoperative imaging after optic nerve decompression. Patients are monitored with serial visual examinations postoperatively, in addition to formal visual field testing in the first 24 hours.

COMPLICATIONS

Cerebrospinal Fluid Leak

In a patient with postoperative rhinorrhea, testing of the fluid for β_2-transferrin or β-trace protein is prudent to confirm a CSF leak. Accumulation of irrigation fluid in the sinonasal tract, with subsequent drainage, can mimic a CSF leak in the immediate postoperative period.[15,16]

A postoperative CSF leak is best managed by immediate re-exploration and surgical repair.

Postoperative Sinonasal Bleeding

Significant postoperative nasal bleeding most commonly arises from a branch of the internal maxillary or anterior ethmoidal arteries, which are amenable to endoscopic control. Angiography with embolization is reserved for patients who are not surgical candidates. Care must be taken with this complication because blind nasal packing in the setting of a dehiscent, decompressed optic nerve may lead to a decrease in vision.

Subcutaneous Emphysema

Because of a dehiscence in the medial orbital wall and optic canal, vigorous nose blowing or sneezing can result in significant subcutaneous air collection and facial swelling. Patients should be forewarned about appropriate nasal precautions. Observation and potential use of antibiotics if any signs of infection are present are all that is required.

Visual Deterioration

Vision can worsen after optic nerve decompression. Such deterioration can be related to heat injury to the optic nerve as a result of inadequate irrigation during thinning of the optic canal or a vascular event affecting the ophthalmic artery. In addition, small bony fragments can lead to impingement of the optic nerve during outfracture of the optic canal with a curette.

PEARLS

- Thorough review of preoperative imaging is necessary to account for variations in anatomy such as Onodi cells.
- Image guidance is an extremely valuable tool in cases in which normal anatomy is distorted, such as by fibrous dysplasia and skull base neoplasms.
- Removal of the posterior 1 cm of the lamina papyracea facilitates identification of the optic foramen and optic canal decompression.
- Copious irrigation must be used during drilling over the optic canal to prevent thermal injury.
- One hundred twenty-degree medial decompression can be achieved to alleviate compressive symptoms.

PITFALLS

- Failure to bring all septations and air cells in plane with the lateral orbital wall will make decompression more difficult.
- Breach of the periorbita will lead to herniation of fat and poor visualization.
- Incision of the nerve sheath is contraindicated because it may produce a CSF leak.
- Care must be taken with postoperative packing to not cause iatrogenic compression of the exposed optic nerve.
- A high-speed drill shaft can cause alar burns if left in the same position for a prolonged period.

References

1. Kountakis SE, Maillard AA, El-Harazi SM, et al: Endoscopic optic nerve decompression for traumatic blindness. Otolaryngol Head Neck Surg 123:34-37, 2000.
2. Cook MW, Levin LA, Joseph MP, et al: Traumatic optic neuropathy: A meta-analysis. Arch Otolaryngol Head Neck Surg 122:389-392, 1996.
3. Levin LA: Mechanisms of optic neuropathy. Curr Opin Ophthalmol 8:9-15, 1997.
4. Luxenberger W, Stammberger H, Jebeles JA, Walch C: Endoscopic optic nerve decompression: The Graz experience. Laryngoscope 108:873-882, 1998.
5. Levin LA, Joseph MP, Rizzo JF III, Lessell S: Optic canal decompression in indirect optic nerve trauma. Ophthalmology 101:566-569, 1994.
6. Levin LA, Beck RW, Joseph MP, et al: The treatment of traumatic optic neuropathy: The International Optic Nerve Trauma Study. Ophthalmology 106:1268-1277, 1999.
7. Jiang RS, Hsu CY, Shen BH: Endoscopic optic nerve decompression for the treatment of traumatic optic neuropathy. Rhinology 39(2):71-74, 2001.
8. Rajiniganth MG, Gupta AK, Gupta A, Bapuraj JR: Traumatic optic neuropathy: Visual outcome following combined therapy protocol. Arch Otolaryngol Head Neck Surg 129:1203-1206, 2003.
9. Yang WG, Chen CT, Tsay PK, et al: Outcome of traumatic optic neuropathy—surgical versus nonsurgical treatment. Ann Plast Surg 52:36-42, 2004.
10. Anderson RL, Panje WR, Gross CE: Optic-nerve blindness following blunt forehead trauma. Ophthalmology 89:445-455, 1982.
11. Acheson JF: Optic nerve disorders: Role of canal and nerve sheath decompression surgery. Eye 18:1169-1174, 2004.
12. Chen C, Selva D, Floreani S, Wormald PJ: Endoscopic optic nerve decompression for traumatic optic neuropathy: An alternative. Otolaryngol Head Neck Surg 135:155-157, 2006.
13. Thakar A, Mahapatra AK, Tandon DA: Delayed optic nerve decompression for indirect optic nerve injury. Laryngoscope 113:112-119, 2003.
14. Lubben B, Stoll W, Grenzebach U: Optic nerve decompression in the comatose and conscious patients after trauma. Laryngoscope 111:320-328, 2001.
15. Pletcher SD, Sindwani R, Metson R: Endoscopic orbital and optic nerve decompression. Otolaryngol Clin North Am 39:943-958, 2006.
16. Metson R, Pletcher SD: Endoscopic orbital and optic nerve decompression. Otolaryngol Clin North Am 39:551-561, 2006.

Chapter 97

Orbital Exenteration

S. Tonya Stefko

PATIENT SELECTION

The radical surgery of orbital exenteration is occasionally necessary in the management of head and neck cancer. Most frequently for the otolaryngologist, it will be due to spread of malignant tumor from adjacent paranasal sinuses or the skull base. Some cancers arising in the skin will also require total or subtotal removal of the orbital contents. Invasive fungal infections are indications for aggressive débridement, sometimes including orbital exenteration. Rarely, a benign but locally aggressive tumor or intractable pain will be an indication.

The most clear-cut indications for orbital exenteration are those involving malignant tumors with no hope of salvaging vision in the affected eye (Fig. 97-1). These situations most often include squamous cell carcinoma and other epithelial malignancies. In the largest reported series of orbital exenteration, squamous cell carcinoma (originating in the sinus, skin, or conjunctiva) accounted for one third of exenterations.[1] A more recent series found basal cell carcinoma to be the most frequent diagnosis, followed by melanoma and sebaceous cell carcinoma.[2] Conversely, a review of 70 consecutive cases of maxillectomy found that 40% of these patients required concurrent orbital exenteration.[3] Imaging is likely to underestimate the extent of tumor invasion into the orbit, and the decision to proceed may need to be made in the operating room. The recent trend, particularly with squamous cell carcinoma, has been preservation of the orbit except in instances of proven invasion of the periorbita (by frozen section at the time of surgery). In several retrospective series there has been no difference in disease-free survival between patients treated with orbit-sparing procedures and those whose surgery included orbital exenteration.[4]

Malignant tumor of the orbit or eyelids, although not strictly invading the eye or periorbita itself, may require removal of the orbital contents because of insufficiency of the remaining tissue for protection of the globe (Figs. 97-2 and 97-3).

Surgical decision making in the setting of aggressive infection is difficult. Most fungal infections of the orbit spread from adjacent sinuses, and two main types occur. *Aspergillus* affects both immunocompromised and immunocompetent hosts. In the former patients, the prognosis is extremely poor if immune status cannot be improved and if intracranial involvement is present.[5] In the latter setting, exenteration is likely to be necessary in cases of apical involvement, but not when the infection is confined to the anterior, inferomedial orbit,[6] where limited débridement may suffice.

Rhino-orbital-cerebral mucormycosis is a rare but serious infection caused by *Rhizopus* species (occasionally *Mucor* or *Absidia*). It affects immunocompromised patients, most often those with a concurrent metabolic acidosis. These patients require aggressive surgical débridement to the level of bleeding tissue. This has frequently included orbital exenteration in the presence of orbital signs, but one series showed no difference in survival between patients with orbital involvement who underwent exenteration and those who did not.[7] However, the overall mortality in patients with orbital involvement was higher (33% versus 14%). The operation may be followed by hyperbaric oxygen therapy, which improves survival.[8]

Three percent to 17% of patients requiring exenteration have benign orbital disease.[1,9-12] The various associated diagnoses include inflammatory disease, Stevens-Johnson syndrome, lymphangioma, meningioma, and others. These diseases are either painful,

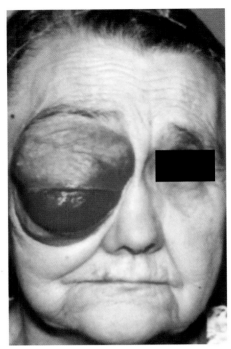

Figure 97-1. Patient with malignant melanoma destroying the globe, adnexa, and orbital contents.

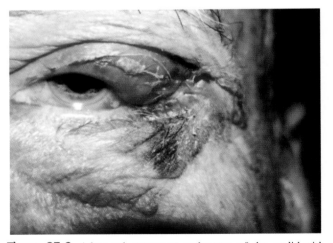

Figure 97-2. Advanced cutaneous melanoma of the eyelid with orbital extension.

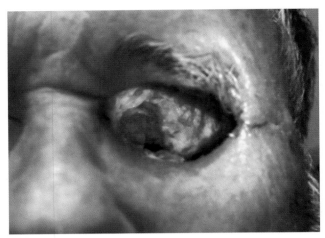

Figure 97-3. Patient from Figure 97-2, 12 days after exenteration with a split-thickness skin graft in the orbit.

inadequately controlled medically, and "grossly disfiguring" or, although histologically benign, tend to invade adjacent tissue.[13] The pain associated with the disease most often resolves immediately after surgery.

PREOPERATIVE EVALUATION

Patients who may be candidates for orbital exenteration should, at the very least, be evaluated by computed tomography or magnetic resonance imaging (or both) of the orbits, sinuses, and brain. In the majority of cases that involve malignancy, positron emission tomography is also indicated. When neck dissection is anticipated, preoperative imaging of the neck and scintigraphy may be considered. The choice of imaging will be guided by the patient's diagnosis. In patients with malignancies contiguous with the orbit, it is likely that imaging will underestimate the extent of disease and intraoperative histopathologic monitoring will be necessary.

Before the operation, coagulation studies, a complete blood count with platelets, and typing and cross-matching of two units of packed red blood cells should be performed.

In many instances, given the radical nature of the surgery, pathology of the lesion should be independently confirmed by pathologists experienced in the field of head and neck or orbital disease.

Before scheduling surgery, a complete ophthalmologic examination of the remaining eye is indicated both to guide surgical decision making and to maximize the remaining vision.

In most otolaryngologists' practices, exenteration will be undertaken in conjunction with maxillectomy or during aggressive sinus débridement (e.g., for invasive fungal infection). During the informed consent process, if the decision whether to exenterate the orbit will be made at surgery, it must be made very clear to the patient and family that although every effort will be made to preserve the orbit and eye, this goal will not preclude complete eradication of disease.

SURGICAL APPROACHES

Total or subtotal exenteration should be planned. Subtotal exenteration most often means a partially lid-sparing technique (Fig. 97-4A), which is appropriate in most cases of benign disease and with tumors that primarily affect the posterior or deep portions of the orbit. It is inappropriate in any tumors affecting the skin, conjunctiva, or lacrimal gland. Lid-sparing exenteration gives an excellent color match to surrounding skin and heals relatively quickly. Globe-sparing exenteration has been described, with purported advantages of easier prosthetic fitting later.[14]

Primary Reconstructive Options

Reconstructive options should be considered before surgery. The simplest option is healing by secondary intention, or granulation. The advantages of such healing are shorter operating time, good color match to surrounding tissue, excellent visibility for monitoring of possible recurrence of disease, and a tendency to produce a shallow socket (easier for eventual patient care).[15] Disadvantages include a long healing time and the necessity for several painful dressing changes.

Split-thickness skin grafts, most commonly from the thigh, are frequently used to line the orbital cavity when total exenteration with removal of periosteum is performed (see Fig. 97-3). Although this leads to shorter recovery time and excellent visual monitoring for recurrence, a deeper cavity is formed, for which care and prosthetic fitting are somewhat more difficult. The pain encountered after this reconstructive option is generally from the donor site.

Local or free tissue flaps are most commonly performed at our institution, particularly for defects resulting from concurrent partial or complete maxillectomy. Temporalis flaps,[16] with or without cervicofacial,[17] radial forearm,[18] and rectus abdominis flaps, are most frequently mentioned. These flaps have the advantage of ample tissue and good vascularity, which is desirable in a field likely to require radiation therapy. Disadvantages of longer operating time, donor site morbidity/disfigurement, and a requirement for highly specialized microsurgical techniques (in the case of free flaps) discourage their use in very sick patients. These options also render monitoring for local recurrence of disease more difficult.

It has been reported that most patients are likely to wear an occlusive eye patch regardless of attempts at reconstruction.[19] Prostheses may be fashioned by a prosthodontist and may be affixed by topical adhesive. Alternatively, prostheses may be fixed magnetically to osseointegrated dental implants.[20,21]

Surgical Procedure

The patient is placed under general anesthesia, and the surgical margins are marked (see Fig. 97-4A); in the case of concurrent maxillectomy, that procedure is performed first. A suture tarsorrhaphy is usually helpful. If the exenteration is to be a lid-sparing technique, an incision line several millimeters proximal to the eyelid margins and parallel to them is marked. A knife is used to cut through skin and orbicularis, and blunt dissection in the pretarsal/preseptal plane is then carried out to the level of the orbital rim. Periosteum is incised, and the surgery proceeds as described in the following text.

If the skin is to be included in the resection, the excision margins are drawn at the orbital rim and at least 1 to 2 cm from the cutaneous lesion. The marked areas may be infiltrated with local anesthetic with epinephrine to help with hemostasis. A no. 15 scalpel is used to cut through skin to the periosteum. Bleeding should be expected at the supraorbital vessels. The periosteum is elevated with a Cottle or Freer elevator, beginning at the superotemporal portion of the orbit where the bone is thickest. Dissection in this plane continues circumferentially and posteriorly, with cautery of the zygomaticofacial and zygomaticotemporal vessels encountered in the lateral wall. Resistance will occur in the area of the trochlea (superomedially) and at the canthal ligaments and may require sharp dissection in these areas. The posterior limb of the medial canthal tendon should be elevated from bone, and the lacrimal sac should be divided at its junction with the nasolacrimal canal. The inferior oblique muscle originates just

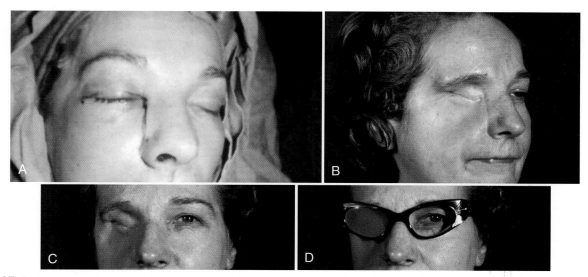

Figure 97-4. A, Patient with mucoepidermoid cancer of the maxillary antrum who underwent orbital exenteration and radical maxillectomy. A lid-sparing incision is outlined. **B,** Postoperative appearance with the lids sewn together, thus eliminating view of the open orbit. **C,** Oblique view. **D,** Patient wearing special glasses that obscure view of the orbit.

lateral to the sac and should be elevated with the periosteum.

Dissection proceeds posteriorly toward the orbital apex, with special care directed to the following areas: first, elevation of the periosteum over the lamina papyracea must be carried out very gently to not create dehiscences in the bone. The ethmoidal vessels must be divided and bleeding controlled with bipolar cautery and bone wax if needed. Second, areas of the roof, particularly posteromedially, are often quite thin or contain frank dehiscences. It is here that an iatrogenic cerebrospinal fluid leak may be created, either by direct trauma or by the use of monopolar cautery, which may travel through emissary foramina or dehiscences.[22] Monopolar cautery should be avoided except in the anterior-most portion of the orbit.

The contents of the superior and inferior orbital fissures and the apical stump must now be divided, which may be accomplished with a curved knife, curved enucleation scissors, or a snare. The latter is tightened to a soft stop and tightened sequentially over a period of several minutes to assist with hemostasis. The snare may then be tightened completely to transect the apical stump, or curved scissors may be used to cut just anterior to it. The orbit should immediately be packed with gauze and pressure applied for 5 to 10 minutes. The apex should then be explored cautiously with suction and bipolar cautery to localize and control any bleeding.

If the orbit is to heal by granulation, it should now be lined with a nonadherent dressing such as Telfa followed by Xeroform gauze, packed with fluffed gauze, and bandaged tightly. A small pledget of cellulose (Surgicel) or other hemostatic agent may be placed over the apical stump.

It may be possible in some patients to preserve the eyelids. After a skin graft has been placed in the orbit, the margins of the eyelid are sewn together to provide a good appearance or at least a better appearance than if the orbit were open to view (see Fig. 97-4B to D).

If the lid skin has been spared, it is draped over the rim and spread posteriorly as far as possible. The remainder of the orbit may be left to granulate or may be covered with a split-thickness skin graft. If a split-thickness graft is used, it is harvested from a non–hair-bearing area of the inner surface of the thigh or the abdomen and the donor site covered with an adherent dressing. Dimensions of the graft are approximately 5 × 10 cm before meshing. The graft is carefully draped into the orbital cavity, with care taken to ensure that the epithelial side remains exterior. The graft is sutured in place at the rim with interrupted 7-0 chromic gut or silk suture. The wound is then dressed as discussed earlier.

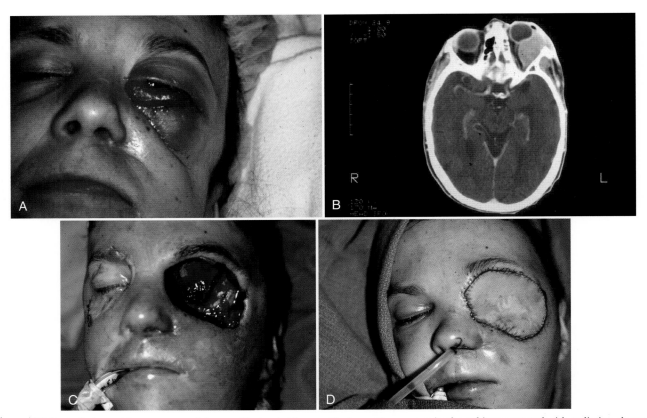

Figure 97-5. A, Patient with a sarcoma of the maxilla treated by maxillectomy. Recurrence in the orbit was treated with radiation therapy. The tumor recurred once again and destroyed the orbital contents. **B,** Computed tomography scan demonstrating invasion of the orbit and destruction of the bony orbital wall. **C,** Defect after orbital exenteration. **D,** Reconstruction with a rectus abdominis free tissue transfer.

If a local or free flap is to be used for reconstruction, it is prepared and placed as dictated by the specific procedure. The patient in Figure 97-5A underwent maxillectomy for sarcoma of the maxilla. A recurrence was treated with radiation therapy. The tumor recurred once again and destroyed the orbital contents and the orbital wall (see Fig. 97-5B). The orbital defect (see Fig. 97-5C) was reconstructed with a rectus abdominis free tissue transfer (see Fig. 97-5D).

When flap reconstruction is not used, the pressure dressing remains undisturbed for 3 to 5 days. During this time the patient should have antibiotic coverage. After this time, the pressure dressing is gently removed, and the area is soaked with saline. After 5 to 10 minutes, the lining layer (nonadherent dressing such as Telfa or Xeroform) may be gently loosened from the underlying tissue. Minimal débridement should occur at this stage because areas of skin that appear devitalized may heal surprisingly well. The area is coated lightly with antibiotic ointment, and the patient and family are instructed to repeat the application of ointment twice daily. Ointment should also be applied to the light dressing placed over the orbit to prevent adherence. Vigorous cleaning of the area should be avoided.

The patient is examined in the office 1 week postoperatively and then at regular intervals afterward as dictated by disease process. Weekly or biweekly visits are appropriate in the first 4 to 6 weeks for cleaning of the socket and monitoring for infection. In most cases in which radiation therapy is not necessary, the patient is ready for prosthesis fitting in 3 months (Fig. 97-6).

COMPLICATIONS

Possible complications of the operation include intraoperative bleeding, postoperative hematoma, postoperative infection, and dehiscence of the surgical wound. Intraoperative bleeding is treated by packing and pressure, prothrombotic agents applied to the orbital apex, and transfusion of packed red blood cells if necessary. Postoperative hematoma requires therapy if it occurs under a skin graft or in a free flap. The former may be drained by making a small incision in the graft, gently evacuating the hematoma, and then replacing the pressure dressing for 2 to 5 days. Free flaps must be monitored carefully by Doppler ultrasound to ensure patency of the artery and vein, and a pressure dressing is contraindicated. Postoperative infection must be vigorously treated with intravenous and then oral antibiotics, with judicious surgical débridement of devitalized tissue or drainage of purulent collections as needed. Dehiscence of the surgical wound should raise suspicion of infection, which must be treated aggressively before considering secondary repair.

Fistulas resulting from orbital exenteration may communicate with either the sinuses or dura. If a bone or dural defect is noted intraoperatively, it should be repaired. If the orbit is to heal by granulation or a skin graft is used, a small flap of extraocular muscle and fat may be spared and used to cover either the bone window or the dural repair.[23]

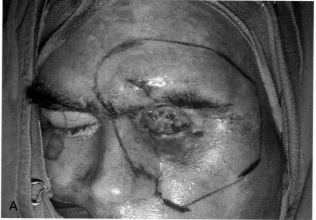
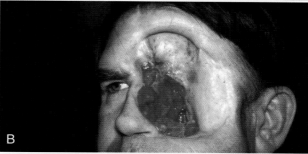
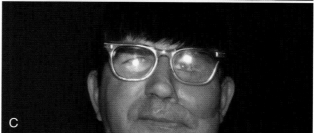

Figure 97-6. A, Patient with recurrent basal cell carcinoma in a previously exenterated orbit. **B,** Postoperative defect. **C,** Postoperative appearance with a prosthesis and glasses.

PEARLS

- Orbital exenteration is appropriate for patients with tumor invasion of periorbita proved by frozen section examination.
- Patients with invasion of orbital bone only will probably have comparable survival if the orbital contents are spared.
- In patients with malignant tumors of the lacrimal gland, exenteration is the procedure of choice.
- Aggressive débridement of skin grafts early in the postoperative period is to be avoided.
- Postoperative infection must be treated early and completely.

PITFALLS

- Sino-orbital fistulas are most easily created over the lamina papyracea and result in chronic discharge.
- Use of monopolar cautery in the deep or superior aspect of the orbit is to be avoided because cerebrospinal fluid leak may result.
- Resection of most of the orbital floor frequently leads to loss of integrity of the eye because of dystopia, diplopia, or ocular surface problems. This may be compounded by postoperative radiation effects on the eye.[24]

References

1. Levin PS, Dutton JJ: A 20-year series of orbital exenteration. Am J Ophthalmol 112:496-501, 1991.
2. Rahman I, Cook AE, Leatherbarrow B: Orbital exenteration: A 13 year Manchester experience. Br J Ophthalmol 89:1335-1340, 2005.
3. Yucel A, Cinar C, Aydin Y, et al: Malignant tumors requiring maxillectomy. J Craniofac Surg 11:418-429, 2000.
4. Carrau RL, Segas J, Nuss DW, et al: Squamous cell carcinoma of the sinonasal tract invading the orbit. Laryngoscope 109:230-235, 1999.
5. Kraus D, Bullock J: Orbital infections. In Pepose J, Holland G, Wilhelmus K (eds): Ocular Infection & Immunity. St Louis, Mosby–Year Book, 1996, pp 1321-1340.
6. Dhiwakar M, Thakar A, Bahadur S: Invasive sino-orbital aspergillosis: Surgical decisions and dilemmas. J Laryngol Otol 117:280-285, 2003.
7. Peterson KL, Wang M, Canalis RF, Abemayor E: Rhinocerebral mucormycosis: Evolution of the disease and treatment options. Laryngoscope 107:855-862, 1997.
8. Yohai RA, Bullock JD, Aziz AA, Markert RJ: Survival factors in rhino-orbital-cerebral mucormycosis. Surv Ophthalmol 39:3-22, 1994.
9. Naquin HA: Exenteration of the orbit. AMA Arch Ophthalmol 51:850-862, 1954.
10. Bartley GB, Garrity JA, Waller RR, et al: Orbital exenteration at the Mayo Clinic. 1967-1986. Ophthalmology 96:468-473, 1989.
11. Mohr C, Esser J: Orbital exenteration: Surgical and reconstructive strategies. Graefes Arch Clin Exp Ophthalmol 235:288-295, 1997.
12. Rathbun JE, Beard C, Quickert MH: Evaluation of 48 cases of orbital exenteration. Am J Ophthalmol 72:191-199, 1971.
13. Rose GE, Wright JE: Exenteration for benign orbital disease. Br J Ophthalmol 78:14-18, 1994.
14. Catalano PJ, Laidlaw D, Sen C: Globe sparing orbital exenteration. Otolaryngol Head Neck Surg 125:379-384, 2001.
15. Putterman AM: Orbital exenteration with spontaneous granulation. Arch Ophthalmol 104:139-140, 1986.
16. Menon NG, Girotto JA, Goldberg NH, Silverman RP: Orbital reconstruction after exenteration: Use of a transorbital temporal muscle flap. Ann Plast Surg 50:38-42, 2003.
17. Cuesta-Gil M, Concejo C, Acero J, et al: Repair of large orbito-cutaneous defects by combining two classical flaps. J Craniomaxillofac Surg 32:21-27, 2004.
18. Tahara S, Susuki T: Eye socket reconstruction with free radial forearm flap. Ann Plast Surg 23:112-116, 1989.
19. Ben Simon GJ, Schwarcz RM, Douglas R, et al: Orbital exenteration: One size does not fit all. Am J Ophthalmol 139:11-17, 2005.
20. Nerad JA, Carter KD, LaVelle WE, et al: The osseointegration technique for the rehabilitation of the exenterated orbit. Arch Ophthalmol 109:1032-1038, 1991.
21. Konstantinidis L, Scolozzi P, Hamedani M: Rehabilitation of orbital cavity after total orbital exenteration using oculofacial prostheses anchored by osseointegrated dental implants posed as a one-step surgical procedure. Klin Monatsbl Augenheilkd 223:400-404, 2006.
22. Wulc AE, Adams JL, Dryden RM: Cerebrospinal fluid leakage complicating orbital exenteration. Arch Ophthalmol 107:827-830, 1989.
23. Bartley GB, Kasperbauer JL: Use of a flap of extraocular muscle and fat during subtotal exenteration to repair bony orbital defects. Am J Ophthalmol 134:787-788, 2002.
24. Stern SJ, Goepfert H, Clayman G, et al: Orbital preservation in maxillectomy. Otolaryngol Head Neck Surg 109:111-115, 1993.

Chapter **98**

Dacryocystorhinostomy

S. Tonya Stefko and Carl H. Snyderman

External dacryocystorhinostomy (DCR) was first described by Toti in the early 20th century.[1] The technique is applicable to patients complaining of tearing and demonstrating obstruction of the lacrimal outflow system. The procedure consists of creating a fistula for egress of tears directly from the lacrimal sac into the nose and bypassing the nasolacrimal duct (Figs. 98-1 and 98-2). Description of endonasal DCR took place even before report of external DCR.[2]

PATIENT SELECTION

Patients may complain of tearing for one of three reasons: hypersecretion of tears, impaired drainage of tears, or a combination of both. Primary hypersecretion of tears is uncommon, but secondary hypersecretion is a frequent cause of tearing. It may be due to a variety of ocular surface disorders, some as benign in nature as seasonal allergy. Associated symptoms and signs will help in making these diagnoses, and their proper treatment should proceed before surgical repair. For example, a patient with itching may have hypersecretion because of seasonal allergy and may be treated with antihistamine drops. Reflex hypersecretion in patients with ocular surface dryness (as in those with Graves' disease) must be addressed by referral to an ophthalmologist. Abnormal eyelid position can cause reflex tearing by rubbing of lashes against the cornea or by desiccation of the cornea as a result of inadequate blinking or closure. Patients' complaints will assist in making the diagnosis inasmuch as those with surface disorders causing reflex hypersecretion will complain of burning and a foreign body sensation. Fluorescein drops instilled into the conjunctival cul-de-sac will highlight defects in the corneal epithelium when viewed with a cobalt blue filter on a penlight in patients with dry eye.

Impaired drainage of tears can occur at any level of the lacrimal outflow system. In newborns and infants, the most common site of obstruction is distally at the valve of Hasner, where canalization is often incomplete at the time of birth. In most patients, congenital nasolacrimal duct obstruction will resolve by the age of 6 to 12 months, so probing of the lacrimal system should be delayed until the end of the first year of life. Probing of the lacrimal system is most often curative at this age.[3]

In adults, tearing secondary to insufficient lacrimal drainage is common and may be due to functional or physical obstruction. Functional obstruction includes poor function of the medial canthal lacrimal pump, usually secondary to eyelid malposition or aberrant anatomy. Physical obstruction may occur at the level of the punctum, canaliculus, common canaliculus, lacrimal sac, or nasolacrimal duct. The latter two account for about 74% of lacrimal outflow obstructions[4] and are treated with greater than 90% success by external DCR surgery.[5]

Patients may have acute dacryocystitis and complain of tearing, discharge, swelling, and pain over the lacrimal sac. Some cases proceed to periorbital cellulitis before diagnosis, so a high index of suspicion in this setting must be maintained. Pressure over the sac produces purulent reflux from the punctum, which is often quite painful for the patient. Probing or irrigation at this time is useless and may complicate the situation. About two thirds of acute infections grow gram-positive organisms in culture, and about 7% are anaerobic.[6] Treatment of acute infection consists of at least 3 weeks of oral antibiotic, antibiotic-steroid drops, and warm compresses. An abscess in the area necessitates prompt percutaneous drainage, often possible in the office under local anesthesia. The sac may then be irrigated with antibiotic solution. Occasionally, poor response to oral therapy will necessitate intravenous antibiotic treatment and prompt surgery.

Endonasal DCR has enjoyed renewed interest since the 1980s but is less preferred because of lagging success

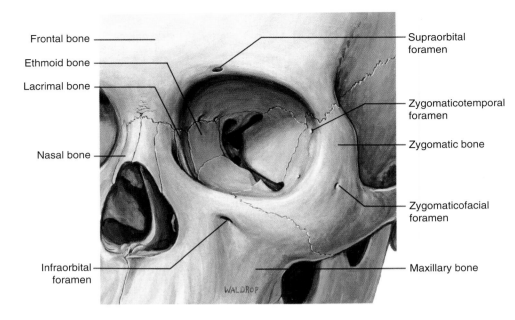

Figure 98-1. Orbital bones, frontal view. *(From Dutton JJ: Atlas of Clinical and Surgical Orbital Anatomy. Philadelphia, WB Saunders, 1994.)*

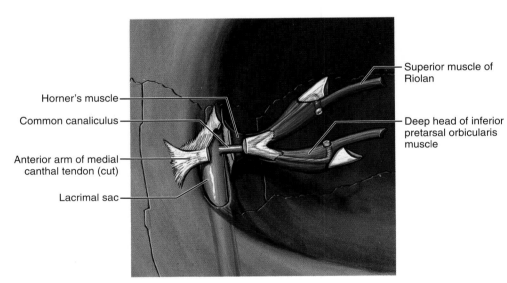

Figure 98-2. Lacrimal drainage system, superficial anatomy. *(From Dutton JJ: Atlas of Clinical and Surgical Orbital Anatomy. Philadelphia, WB Saunders, 1994.)*

rates and expense. Recent reports suggest that the technique is becoming more successful.[7]

Successful DCR requires a functional upper outflow system. Treatment of upper system (punctum, canaliculus, and common canaliculus) obstruction must be undertaken either separately or in the setting of surgical DCR. Punctal stenosis may be treated by various punctoplasty techniques. Canalicular stenosis may be treated with silicon intubation, generally only in the setting of incomplete obstruction. Common canalicular stenosis may sometimes be treated in the setting of DCR by silicon intubation. If intractable upper system obstruction is present, primary conjunctivodacryocystorhinostomy with placement of a Jones tube is necessary.

In 8% to 14% of DCR surgeries, dacryoliths composed of precipitated organic material will be found.[8,9] Affected patients may complain of intermittent tearing and pain and demonstrate distended, tender lacrimal sacs but minimal or no inflammation. Alternatively, the dacryolith may mimic complete obstruction and occasionally cause acute dacryocystitis.

In the presence of any suspicion of a mass in the lacrimal system, external DCR with biopsy is mandatory. The symptom of bloody tears is particularly worrisome for tumor. If intraoperative frozen sections are available, it may be possible to complete the DCR if the sections are benign. If malignancy is found, however, dacryocystectomy with appropriate margins should be performed and creation of an ostium into the nose avoided.

PREOPERATIVE EVALUATION

Most patients referred to an otolaryngologist with complaints of tearing will already have been evaluated by an ophthalmologist and treated for ocular surface disorders causing hypersecretion. If not, ophthalmologic workup should proceed before any consideration of lacrimal surgery for correction of tearing.

Complete endonasal examination, with particular attention paid to the distal end of the nasolacrimal duct beneath the inferior turbinate, should be performed in the office. Occasionally, physical obstruction of the ostium is visible and readily treated. Significant rhinitis should also be treated before surgical correction because it also rarely causes functional obstruction. Note of any septal defects or deviation is important, particularly if an endonasal approach is selected.

Dilatation and irrigation of the lacrimal system in the office can be used to localize the outflow blockage. Probing of the lacrimal system, however, has no place in adult patients. This procedure is rarely if ever curative and will cause significant patient discomfort. In addition, there is a risk of trauma to the delicate mucosa-lined canalicular system, which is a considerably more difficult problem to treat than nasolacrimal duct obstruction. Quick, easy passage of saline into the nasopharynx after topical anesthesia and gentle injection into the canaliculus may call into question the diagnosis of lacrimal obstruction. However, this will often occur in the setting of a dacryolith because the liquid will drain around the object. It is also sometimes possible to open the nasolacrimal duct with forceful injection, but resistance will be palpable and indicates that the system is probably functionally obstructed. The physician should note the speed and volume of flow, in addition to the presence of resistance or frank reflux of fluid. Reflux in the presence of resistance to flow indicates obstruction. If reflux occurs from the canaliculus being injected or if resistance to easy passage of a 22-gauge or smaller cannula is felt, canalicular obstruction is present. Reflux of fluid from the opposite lid suggests obstruction distal to the common canaliculus, and DCR is likely to be curative.

Computed tomography of the orbits and sinuses may be ordered in some situations to evaluate sinus and nasal anatomy and whenever a mass is suspected. It is particularly helpful in the setting of previous facial trauma.

A complete medical history is necessary, with particular attention directed to bleeding/clotting disorders and hypertension-related pathology. If the patient will be under general anesthesia, evaluation by the primary physician is frequently necessary.

SURGICAL APPROACHES

External DCR is performed under local anesthesia with sedation or under general anesthesia. Our preference is general anesthesia because control of the airway in the presence of nasopharyngeal blood is desirable. Before sterile preparation and draping, a local anesthetic with epinephrine is injected transcutaneously over the anterior lacrimal crest and intranasally just anterior to the middle turbinate. The patient may be administered nasal decongestant before anesthesia, or cottonoids soaked in decongestant may be placed.

A no. 15 scalpel blade is used to create an approximately 1.5-cm skin incision over the anterior lacrimal crest by cutting in one stroke down to periosteum (Fig. 98-3). A Cottle or similar instrument is used to elevate the periosteum over the maxillary bone. Elevation proceeds posteriorly and superiorly and includes the lacrimal sac fused to the periosteum (Fig. 98-4).

A small dehiscence of bone is often encountered at the junction of the maxillary and lacrimal bones and is useful for insertion of a Kerrison punch to begin bone

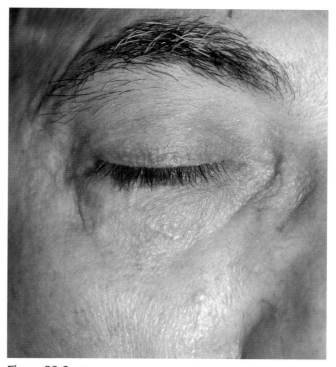

Figure 98-3. Anterior lacrimal crest. The incision will be hidden in the lower eyelid crease.

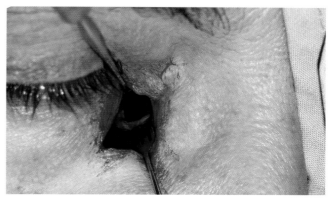

Figure 98-4. Lacrimal sac elevated from the fossa (medial).

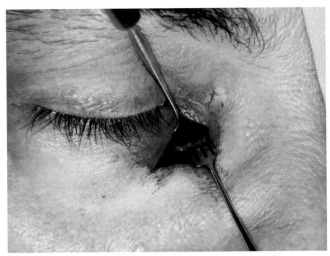

Figure 98-5. Lacrimal sac reflected and bone partially removed from the fossa.

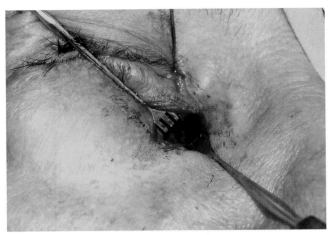

Figure 98-6. Probe in the lacrimal punctum emerging in the wound from the opened lacrimal sac.

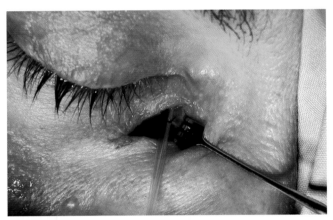

Figure 98-7. Silicon stents emerging from wound are tied together with suture (to rest in the area of the sac).

removal. If this dehiscence is not present, the bone may often be cut with a small osteotome. Only rarely is it necessary to drill to gain access to the nose, although drilling is more frequent in patients with duct obstruction in the setting of inflammatory diseases such as sarcoid or Wegener's granulomatosis. If the anterior lacrimal crest obstructs visualization, it may be partially resected with the bone punch.

A wide area of bone removal facilitates working in the nose (Fig. 98-5). The patient's upper punctum is gently dilated, and a 0 or 00 Bowman or similar probe is inserted. The probe is immediately turned medially, and gentle lateral traction is placed on the lid to straighten the canaliculus. When the probe is in the sac, it is rotated up over the medial aspect of the brow and visualized through the wound to be distending the sac. The sac is opened over the probe, and the incision is extended as completely superiorly and inferiorly as possible (Fig. 98-6). The sac may be incised with an angled crescent blade, an angled needle-tipped cautery, or a radiofrequency dissector. Extension of the incision in the sac anteriorly at its upper and lower limits is helpful for inspection of the interior of the sac. Any foreign bodies should be removed, and a low threshold for biopsy should be maintained. The probe is removed from the lacrimal punctum.

The nasal packing is now removed. An oval or round opening into the nasal mucosa is created with a needle-tipped cutting/cautery device. One probe of a silicon intubation system (such as a Guibor tube) is passed through the upper canaliculus, into the sac, and through the fistula and retrieved in the nose with the appropriate device (such as a grooved director). The second probe is passed through the lower canaliculus and retrieved in the same manner. Both tubes are then elevated from the lacrimal sac with a small blunt hook, and 6-0 silk suture is tied around both at about the level of the skin incision (Fig. 98-7). It should be tied in a single square knot to facilitate later removal via the

punctum. The hook should then be used to check tension of the tubes at the medial canthal angle: the loop should prolapse no farther than the medial limbus (Fig. 98-8). The ends of the suture are trimmed to 3 mm.

Approximately 4 cm of a 12F red rubber straight catheter is cut. One end may be beveled with drape scissors if desired. It is passed, beveled end first, over both wire probes, into the naris, and up into the wound. The catheter is retrieved in the wound with sturdy forceps, such as Adson's. Double-armed 4-0 chromic gut suture is passed across the lumen of the tube approximately 4 mm from its end while taking care to not cut the silicone stents with the needle (Fig. 98-9). The tube is retracted into the nose, and both ends of the suture are passed through the anterior wall of the lacrimal sac. The tube is pulled up into the sac, the sutures are tied in a series of six to eight overhand knots, and the ends are cut (Fig. 98-10).

The lacrimal sac area is now irrigated with an antibiotic solution. The three tubes are cut approximately 1 cm proximal to the naris, and a 5-0 nylon loose stitch

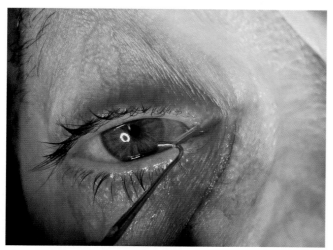

Figure 98-8. Silicon stents should be loose enough to prolapse only as far as the medial limbus.

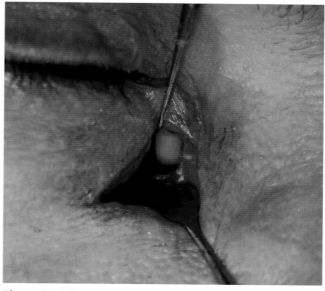

Figure 98-10. Rubber catheter sewn into the anterior of the sac remnant and tied to rest in a fistula.

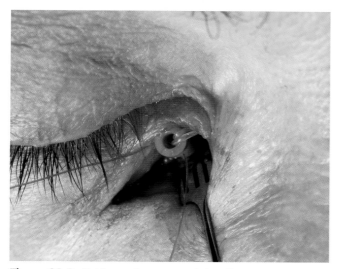

Figure 98-9. Rubber catheter around the silicone stents and gut suture passed across the lumen (for fixation into the sac remnant).

is fashioned to secure the catheter to the nasal mucosa. The ends are cut short and rotated into the lumen of the tube so that they do not irritate the patient. Skin is closed with running 8-0 nylon suture or interrupted 7-0 chromic suture, and antibiotic-steroid ointment is applied (Fig. 98-11). This may be followed by a pressure bandage if significant hematoma is expected.

POSTOPERATIVE MANAGEMENT

Patients are discharged from surgery on a regimen of oral antibiotic, topical antibiotic-steroid drops, and nasal steroid spray. Topical antibiotic-steroid ointment is applied to the stitches until they are removed in 5 to 7 days. Patients are instructed to not blow or pick their noses for 3 weeks. The first three medications are maintained until removal of the red rubber catheter 3 weeks postoperatively, at which time the drops are tapered

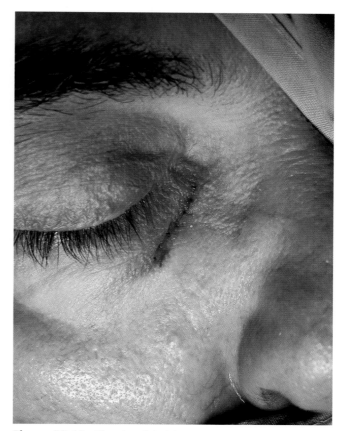

Figure 98-11. The closed incision will be hidden in the lower eyelid crease.

Table 98-1	POSTOPERATIVE MANAGEMENT SCHEDULE AFTER DACRYOCYSTORHINOSTOMY	
One week postoperatively	Remove skin sutures	Discontinue ointment
Three weeks postoperatively	Remove rubber catheter	Discontinue oral antibiotic Taper antibiotic-steroid drops
Two months postoperatively	Remove silicone stent	

from four times a day to twice a day and then discontinued 1 week later, and the oral antibiotic is discontinued. The nasal steroid is continued until removal of the silicon stents, 2 months postoperatively.

The patient is seen in the office 1 week postoperatively for removal of the skin sutures. Two weeks after this visit (3 weeks after surgery) the nylon stitch in the naris is cut and the catheter is withdrawn from the nostril in the office. The chromic gut suture holding the proximal end will have dissolved by this time. Two months postoperatively, the silicon tubes are removed either from the naris after cutting at the medial canthal angle or from the punctum by rotating the tube until the silk suture emerges from one punctum, cutting between them, and pulling the end with three lengths of tubing from the punctum (Table 98-1).

PEARLS

- A functional upper lacrimal drainage system must be present for dacryocystorhinostomy to be effective.
- The rubber catheter stent must be sewn securely up into the body of the lacrimal sac.
- Gentle handling of the puncta and canaliculi is essential to avoid injury.
- Any suspicion of a mass in the lacrimal sac area must be approached externally.

PITFALLS

- Too much tension on the silicone stent (placing the silk suture too deep) will cause erosion of the lacrimal puncta.
- Failure to put lateral traction on the eyelid (i.e., straightening the canaliculus) while passing a lacrimal probe will cause damage to the canalicular mucosa.
- Using an unfamiliar absorbable suture (i.e., one that will not predictably break down at 2 to 3 weeks) may cause difficulty in removal of the rubber stent.

References

1. Toti A: Nuovo metodo conservatore di cura radicale delle suppurazioni croniche del sacco lacrimale (dacriocistorinostomia). Clin Mod Firenze 10:385, 1904.
2. Caldwell G: Two new operations for obstruction of the nasal duct with preservation of the canaliculi. Am J Ophthalmol 10:189, 1893.
3. Kashkouli MB, Kassaee A, Tabatabaee Z: Initial nasolacrimal duct probing in children under age 5: Cure rate and factors affecting success. J AAPOS 6:360-363, 2002.
4. Mullner K, Bodner E, Mannor GE: Endoscopy of the lacrimal system. Br J Ophthalmol 83:949-952, 1999.
5. Kashkouli M, Parvaresh M, Modarreszadeh M, et al: Factors affecting the success of external dacryocystorhinostomy. Orbit 22:247-255, 2003.
6. Coden DJ, Hornblass A, Haas BD: Clinical bacteriology of dacryocystitis in adults. Ophthal Plast Reconstr Surg 9:125-131, 1993.
7. Ben Simon GJ, Joseph J, Lee S, et al: External versus endoscopic dacryocystorhinostomy for acquired nasolacrimal duct obstruction in a tertiary referral center. Ophthalmology 112:1463-1468, 2005.
8. Hawes MJ: The dacryolithiasis syndrome. Ophthal Plast Reconstr Surg 4:87-90, 1988.
9. Iliadelis E, Karabatakis V, Sofoniou M: Dacryoliths in chronic dacryocystitis and their composition (spectrophotometric analysis). Eur J Ophthalmol 9:266-268, 1999.

Chapter 99

Eye Reanimation in Patients with Facial Paralysis

Barry M. Schaitkin

One of the most important aspects in caring for patients with facial paralysis is eye care. Inattention to this detail can lead to corneal exposure, ulceration, and permanent scarring with loss of vision. Patients who have a concomitant fifth cranial nerve deficit are at particularly high risk and should be managed in conjunction with a corneal specialist. For patients without a sensory deficit, primary treatment is the use of topical drops and lubricants. A wide variety of products are available, and the otolaryngologist should work closely with an ophthalmologist if uncomfortable with this field to ensure optimal care of the patient.

Topical preparations in the form of drops and ointments are available in a wide range of viscosity, depending on the scope of the exposure problem. Attention should also be paid to the presence or absence of a preservative because some patients are intolerant of these chemicals.[1]

Other extremely important nonsurgical therapies include the use of clear moisture chambers, taping the eyelids closed at night, manual blinking, and external lid loading. The use of an opaque patch over the eye should be discouraged because it can lead to corneal irritation if the eye opens beneath it.

PATIENT SELECTION

Abnormal eyelid position and disorders of the lacrimal apparatus are the usual ocular symptoms in patients with paralysis of the eyelids. The surgeon must evaluate the entire effect of the facial nerve paralysis on the eye, including brow position, lagophthalmos, lid laxity, lid position, and epiphora. Most patients can be managed without surgery indefinitely, and the decision to operate is therefore generally elective. Careful assessment of the lid preoperatively will lead to more satisfactory outcomes.

The patient's history, including the cause of the paralysis and the patient's likelihood of spontaneous nerve recovery or recovery after neural reanimation procedures, is vitally important in surgical planning. The age of the patient plays a role, and the contralateral eye should be observed for age-related changes in the eyelids and brow.

Detailed physical examination of these patients includes evaluation of visual fields and acuity. The conjunctiva is examined for signs of inflammation with topical fluorescein and ideally with a slit lamp. The level of the brows, eyelid approximation with involuntary blink and voluntary effort, tear production, extraocular muscle function, and pupillary size and response should be noted.

A systematic evaluation of the eyelids before reanimation surgery as suggested by Moe is very useful. Moe's Ectropion Grading Scale ranks the lower eyelid on a I to V scale with predominantly medial and lateral determinations. Likewise, upper eyelid function can be objectively compared with the normal side by using medial and lateral measurements of the distance between the eyelids in the closed position.[2]

Factors favoring successful medical management of paralyzed eyelids include an expectation of early recovery, residual facial function, preservation of static lid tone, normal tear function, normal Bell's phenomenon, intact corneal sensation, young age, and the ability to have close follow-up appointments.

SURGICAL TECHNIQUE

Interested readers will find much more extensive writings on this subject, including in May and Schaitkin's *The Facial Nerve,* where 100 pages are devoted to eye reanimation. This chapter will therefore consider only the most common procedures used in eyelid reanimation. Partial tarsorrhaphy is mentioned only to be condemned, except in very rare situations, because of its limitations: restriction of vision, cosmetic disfigurement, and in some cases, failure to provide protection.

BROW-LIFT

Patients with brow ptosis have asymmetry as a cosmetic problem. They will often have visual field deficits superiorly as a result of redundant skin from the upper brow. Symmetry can be improved by injection of a small dose of botulinum toxin (Botox) into the normal side. A brow-lift can provide more definitive resting symmetry but should never be undertaken at the expense of corneal protection. Manual distraction of the brow with the patient sitting upright can indicate the effect of a brow-lift on lid closure. A direct brow-lift allows the surgeon to better control the shape and position of the brow but unfortunately leaves a visible scar.

Skin removal is usually necessary in an older patient. The procedure is easily accomplished under local anesthesia with mild sedation. The ellipse of skin taken should be larger laterally to mimic the shape of the normal brow. Removal of only the skin and subcutaneous tissue protects the supraorbital neurovascular bundle. Once the excision is accomplished, the inferior aspect is sutured with two or three permanent 4-0 clear monofilament sutures. If necessary, a portion of the orbicularis muscle and soft tissue can be included in this suture to improve drooping of the supratarsal fold. In general, a man's brow lies close to the orbital rim and a woman's above the rim, although the normal side should be used for comparison. Beveling the incision to parallel the hair follicles can reduce scar visibility. The incision should be kept central for maximal concealment, and meticulous wound closure is necessary.

An endoscopic brow-lift, which has been introduced more recently, is also an alternative technique.[3]

Upper Eyelid Procedures

A number of methods can be used to improve upper eyelid closure, but lid loading with gold is the method most commonly performed (Fig. 99-1). Jobe, in 1974, was the first American to place a gold weight and is responsible for popularizing the procedure.[4] This tech-

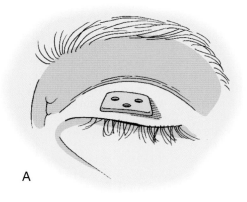

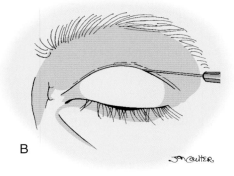

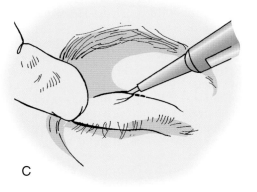

Figure 99-1. Insertion of a gold weight. **A,** Gold weights are tried as external lid loads preoperatively. **B,** Minimal local anesthesia is required. **C,** A corneal protector is always used. The incision is made along the tarsal-supratarsal fold with an ophthalmic knife. (*Reprinted from May M, Levine RE, Patel BCK, Anderson RL: Eye reanimation technique. In May M, Schaitkin BM [eds]: The Facial Nerve. New York, Thieme Medical, 2000, p 708.*)

nique remains appealing because of its high success, simplicity, low complication rate, and cosmetic acceptability.

Several aspects, emphasized by Jobe, must be adhered to:

1. Preoperative fitting of the prosthesis involves finding a weight that closes the eye, with the lower lid in neutral position, without causing significant ptosis at rest. One millimeter of ptosis is considered acceptable. Ideally, the patient wears the prosthesis for 24 hours to evaluate its function during fatigue and in different head positions. Less expensive sizing prostheses are available for this purpose.
2. The prosthesis works best when it is placed medial to the midpupillary line. Such placement overcomes the wider area of exposure between the eyelids medially.
3. The prosthesis should be placed in a pocket just lateral to the tarsal plate to minimize visibility of the plate through the soft tissues and decrease the risk of exposure.
4. The weight is fixed with three 8-0 monofilament permanent sutures 3 mm above the lash line. This area is easily appreciated surgically inasmuch as a vascular arcade is noticed below this level in the tissue pocket.
5. The soft tissues are closed with 7-0 chromic suture and the skin with absorbable plain gut.
6. Patients with gold sensitivity can have platinum weights or chains inserted.

The procedure can be performed under local anesthesia with or without sedation and combined with other reanimation procedures. The patient's midpupillary line is marked before applying topical anesthesia to the eyelid and placing a corneal protector. Under loop magnification, an incision is made through the skin along the tarsal-supratarsal fold. With gentle forceps traction, Westcott scissors are used to divide the soft tissues overlying the orbicularis muscle and levator aponeurosis and expose and identify the tarsal plate as a dense white structure (Fig. 99-2). The dissection continues above the tarsal plate inferiorly to within 3 mm of the lash line (Fig. 99-3).

Two sutures are used for fixation inferiorly. Although some authors prefer to suture to the levator aponeurosis,[1] suturing to the soft tissues overlying the tarsus is also acceptable.[5] Kao and Moe have described a retrograde implantation technique that has certain advantages but may produce a more apparent surgical scar[5] (see Video 99-1).

Lower Eyelid Procedures

Many procedures have been described for lower eyelid reanimation, including the Bick procedure (Fig. 99-4), lateral tarsal strip, medial and lateral canthopexy, cartilage grafting, precaruncular medial canthopexy, and transorbital canthopexy.

The surgeon should have intimate knowledge of the anatomy of the eyelids before performing lower eyelid reanimation, including the orbicularis oculi muscle, the medial and lateral canthal tendons and

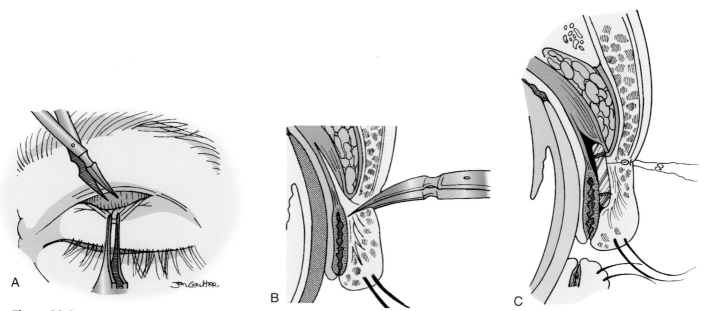

Figure 99-2. Surgical dissection and fixation for the gold weight procedure. **A,** Double-action scissors are used to sharply dissect a pocket to the tarsal plate noted as a white plane. **B,** Further dissection divides the orbicularis muscle and levator aponeurosis. The lowest point of dissection is 3 mm from the lash line, often noted surgically as the position of the vascular arcade. **C,** The gold weight is centered at the medial and central third of the lid to improve coverage medially. Three-point fixation is necessary to avoid extrusion, and the levator and orbicularis are closed with 6-0 absorbable suture. (*Reprinted from May M, Levine RE, Patel BCK, Anderson RL: Eye reanimation technique. In May M, Schaitkin BM [eds]: The Facial Nerve. New York, Thieme Medical, 2000, p 709.*)

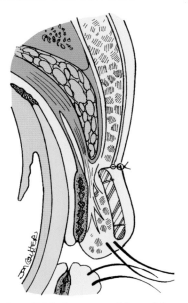

Figure 99-3. Superficial placement of the weight or dissection too close to the lash line will produce cosmetic disfigurement and increase the risk of extrusion. *(Reprinted from May M, Levine RE, Patel BCK, Anderson RL: Eye reanimation technique. In May M, Schaitkin BM [eds]: The Facial Nerve. New York, Thieme Medical, 2000, p 710.)*

their attachment sites, the tarsal plate, and the lacrimal system.[6] Preoperative assessment, in addition to upper eyelid and brow recommendations, should include notation of eyelid position relative to the limbus, position of the punctum, results of a snap test, and medial and lateral distances between the upper and lower eyelids.

The Bick procedure or any of its modifications allow tightening of the lower lid and suspension at a higher position to the lateral orbital rim. Patient who do not require skin excision to achieve this result may best be served with a lateral transorbital canthopexy.[7] The procedure begins with a 1.5-cm lateral canthotomy and cantholysis to expose the periosteum of the lateral orbital rim. The lid is tightened to achieve the desired snap without significant displacement of the punctum of the lower lid. A full-thickness wedge resection is then designed and executed with fine scissors. This creates a free edge of tarsal tissue that can be resuspended with 5-0 nonabsorbable suture to the lateral orbital periosteum. The soft tissues require minimal absorbable sutures for reapproximation.

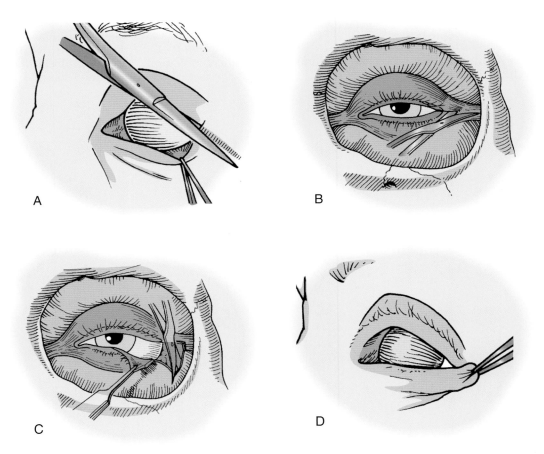

Figure 99-4. Lower lid tightening procedure (modified Bick). **A,** The procedure is performed under local anesthesia with a corneal protector. The lateral canthal incision follows the relaxed skin tension lines. **B,** The anatomy of the lateral canthal tendon is key to understanding the procedure. **C,** Scissors complete the lateral canthotomy and inferior cantholysis. **D,** The lower eyelid is pulled laterally to achieve shortening without distorting placement of the punctum, which would lead to epiphora.

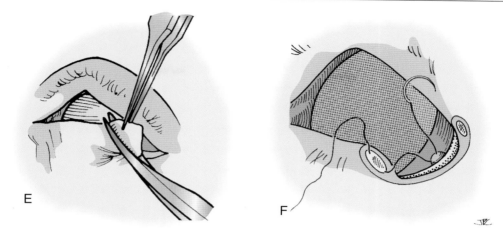

Figure 99-4, cont'd. **E,** The excess skin is resected. **F,** Absorbable 4-0 suture is used to reattach the new lateral margin of the tarsus to the orbital rim. *(Reprinted from May M, Levine RE, Patel BCK, Anderson RL: Eye reanimation technique. In May M, Schaitkin BM [eds]: The Facial Nerve. New York, Thieme Medical, 2000, p 739.)*

PEARLS

- The otolaryngologist must acquire familiarity with this anatomy.
- Preoperative weight selection is important to avoid ptosis or incomplete closure.
- Gold weights must be sutured in place.
- Neglect of the position and function of the lower eyelid will lead to imperfect results.

PITFALLS

- Surgically corrected brow position can make eye closure difficult.
- Patients without eventual neural recovery will undergo atrophy over time, which can make upper lid loads more apparent.
- Patients who are allergic to gold can be transitioned to platinum.
- If the lower eyelid is tightened too much, it will ride underneath the equator of the globe and provide a poor cosmetic and functional result.

References

1. May M, Levine RF, Patel BCK, Anderson R: Eye reanimation techniques. In May M, Schaitkin BM (eds): The Facial Nerve. New York, Thieme Medical, 2000, pp 676-774.
2. Moe KS, Linder T: The lateral transorbital canthopexy for correction and prevention of ectropion. Arch Facial Plast Surg 2:9-15, 2000.
3. Ducic Y, Adelson R: Use of the endoscopic forehead-lift to improve brow position in persistent facial paralysis. Arch Facial Plast Surg 7:51-54, 2005.
4. Jobe RP: A technique for lid loading in the management of the lagophthalmos of facial palsy. Plast Reconstr Surg 53:29-31, 1974.
5. Kao C, Moe KS: Retrograde weight implantation for correction of lagophthalmos. Laryngoscope 114:1570-1575, 2004.
6. Fedok F: Restoration of lower eyelid support in facial paralysis. In Schaitkin BM (ed): Facial Plastic Surgery: Facial Paralysis. New York, Thieme Medical, 2000, pp 337-343.
7. Moe KS, Kao C: Precaruncular medial canthopexy. Arch Facial Plast Surg 7:1-6, 2005.

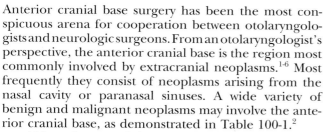

SECTION **11**

CRANIAL BASE SURGERY

Chapter **100**

Surgery of the Anterior Cranial Base

Ricardo L. Carrau, Carl H. Snyderman, Allan D. Vescan, and Amin B. Kassam

Anterior cranial base surgery has been the most conspicuous arena for cooperation between otolaryngologists and neurologic surgeons. From an otolaryngologist's perspective, the anterior cranial base is the region most commonly involved by extracranial neoplasms.[1-6] Most frequently they consist of neoplasms arising from the nasal cavity or paranasal sinuses. A wide variety of benign and malignant neoplasms may involve the anterior cranial base, as demonstrated in Table 100-1.[2]

Although some of these neoplasms have been associated with exposure to environmental carcinogens, the cause of the majority of neoplasms involving the anterior cranial base is unknown. Squamous cell carcinomas arising in the nasal cavity or paranasal sinuses, unlike those arising in other areas of the upper aerodigestive tract, are not associated with the use of alcohol or tobacco products. Squamous cell carcinoma of the paranasal sinuses, however, has been associated with exposure to nickel refining, softwood dust, leather tanning processing, chromium, soldering and welding, radium dial painting, and isopropyl oils. Hardwood workers have an increased incidence of adenocarcinoma.[4,6]

The symptoms and signs of neoplasms involving the anterior cranial base are nonspecific and are not useful in predicting a histologic diagnosis. These symptoms and signs do, however, reflect the location of the tumor and may be predictive of the extent of involvement of adjacent anatomic structures. Nonetheless, the clinical manifestations of the tumor may be identical to those of inflammatory sinus disease. Common symptoms include unilateral or bilateral nasal obstruction, recurrent epistaxis, rhinorrhea, and anosmia. Diplopia may be associated with invasion of orbital structures. Intracranial extension with significant involvement of the frontal lobes may occur without the production of any particular symptoms (Fig. 100-1). Because of this "silent" area of the brain, the first indication of invasion of the brain may be symptoms associated with elevated intracranial pressure, such as headache. On further questioning, patients and family members may relate subtle alterations in personality with disinhibition of emotions and inappropriate responses.

As a result of the location of these tumors there may be no external manifestations until the tumor reaches a large size. With slow-growing benign and malignant neoplasms, remodeling of bone with widening of the nasal dorsum may be seen (Fig. 100-2). Extension laterally into the orbit may result in periorbital swelling, proptosis, or restriction of extraocular movement and diplopia.[7] Visual loss is a late occurrence and is seen more often with tumors that originate close to the optic chiasm or orbital apex. Intracranial extension may be associated with signs of elevated intracranial pressure, such as papilledema. Evidence of frontal lobe involvement may be suggested by detecting abnormal reflex responses associated with frontal lobe release (glabella blink response, palmar-mental reflex).

Table 100-1	TUMOR DIAGNOSIS AND PATIENT STATUS				
		Disease Status (Follow-up: Months)			
Tumor	Total	NED	AWD	DOD	DOC
Benign Lesions					
Meningioma	4	2 (48)	1 (31)	—	1 (36)
Ossifying fibroma	2	2 (27)	—	—	—
Cranial defect	2	1 (30)	—	—	1 (1)
Chondroblastoma	1	1 (45)	—	—	—
Fibrous dysplasia	1	—	1 (18)	—	—
Inverted papilloma	1	1 (22)	—	—	—
Pituitary adenoma	3	1 (44)	2 (26)	—	—
Subtotal	14	8	4	0	2
Low-Grade Malignancies					
Chordoma	7	4 (32)	2 (13)	1 (29)	—
Esthesioneuroblastoma	6	4 (27)	1 (13)	—	1 (22)
Adenoid cystic carcinoma	4	3 (31)	—	—	1 (24)
Chondrosarcoma	2	2 (27)	—	—	—
Subtotal	19	13	3	1	2
High-Grade Malignancies					
Squamous cell carcinoma	7	3 (33)	1 (23)	3 (7)	—
Undifferentiated carcinoma	2	—	1 (24)	1 (36)	—
Adenocarcinoma	2	1 (33)	—	1 (12)	—
Osteogenic sarcoma	2	2 (36)	—	—	—
Melanoma	1	—	1 (43)	—	—
Rhabdomyosarcoma	1	—	—	1 (10)	—
Malignant fibrous histiocytoma	1	1 (16)	—	—	—
Subtotal	16	7	3	6	—
Grand total	49	28	10	7	4

AWD, alive with disease; DOC, dead of other causes; DOD, dead of disease; NED, no evidence of disease.

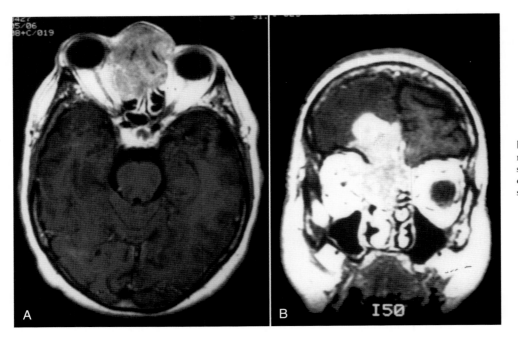

Figure 100-1. **A** and **B,** Magnetic resonance images demonstrating extensive neoplasm with erosion of the skull base and invasion of the right frontal lobe.

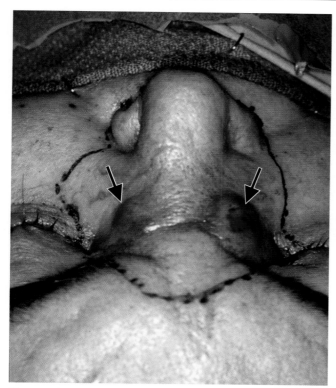

Figure 100-2. Widening of the nasal dorsum is evident with this neoplasm extending to and involving skin *(arrows).*

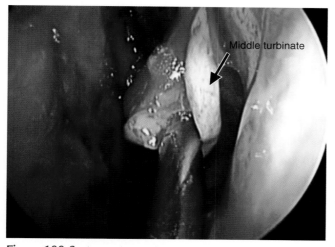

Figure 100-3. A mass is noted arising medial to the attachment of the middle turbinate in the left nasal cavity *(arrow).* Biopsy confirmed an esthesioneuroblastoma.

Intranasal examination may be hindered because of deviations of the nasal septum, mucosal edema, or obstructing nasal polyps. Examination is greatly facilitated with the use of flexible or rigid fiberoptic endoscopes. The appearance and location of the tumor may suggest a histologic diagnosis. Origin of a tumor from the nasal vault, medial to the attachment of the middle turbinate, suggests an esthesioneuroblastoma (Fig. 100-3). Extension of a neoplasm from the maxillary

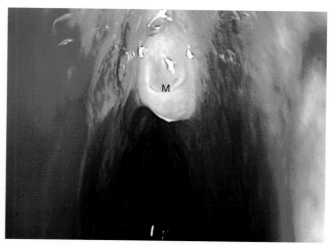

Figure 100-4. This patient had a history of unilateral nasal obstruction. Endoscopic examination revealed a meningocele (M) in the region of the cribriform plate.

sinus to the anterior cranial base may be evident. Posteriorly, involvement of the eustachian tube may be detected. This is important in explaining an associated middle ear effusion, as well as being a potential route of spread of tumor to the infratemporal skull base or carotid canal.

PATIENT SELECTION

Some aspects of the physical examination have already been addressed. Endoscopic visualization of the nasal cavity and nasopharynx is considered a routine part of the examination that may provide useful information regarding the origin, extent, and vascularity of the tumor. Additional preoperative testing may include assessment of olfactory function with "scratch-and-sniff" panels and neuro-ophthalmologic examination, including visual acuity and visual field testing. Biopsy samples are not usually obtained in the office setting because of concern for bleeding and possible communication with cerebrospinal fluid (CSF) (Fig. 100-4). Additionally, biopsy may alter the magnetic resonance imaging (MRI) characteristics of the tumor. However, large fungating tumors that are easily visualized in the nasal cavity may undergo biopsy with minor risk in the office setting.

Radiologic imaging is an essential part of the evaluation of these patients. Involvement of the orbit and intracranial extension may not be clinically apparent. Computed tomography (CT) of the paranasal sinus with contrast enhancement is the preferred initial examination. Images through the skull base are obtained at 1-mm intervals to achieve maximal resolution. CT provides excellent bone detail and is superior to MRI in detecting bony erosion of the anterior cranial base and paranasal sinuses. A contrast agent provides assessment of the overall vascularity of the tumor (Fig. 100-5). Coronal images of the anterior cranial base are superior to axial images in demonstrating intracranial extension. MRI provides much greater detail of soft tissue

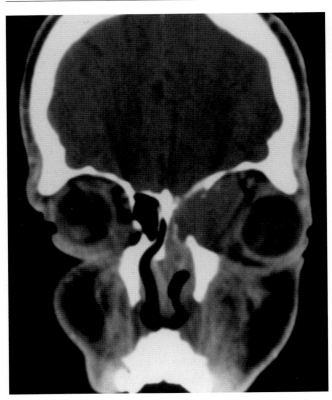

Figure 100-5. Computed tomography scan demonstrating bone erosion of the anterior cranial base resulting from rhabdomyosarcoma of the left orbit.

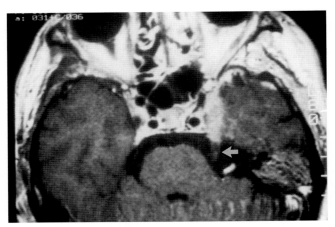

Figure 100-6. In this patient with a malignant neoplasm, magnetic resonance imaging demonstrates tumor involvement of the left cavernous sinus and perineural extension along the route of the trigeminal nerve *(arrow)*.

structures and is complementary to CT scanning in most patients. Bone detail is poorly visualized, however. MRI is particularly valuable for demonstrating dural involvement and invasion of the brain. MRI is also superior for demonstrating perineural extension of tumor (Fig. 100-6). Highly vascular tumors may be associated with flow voids within the tumor. When a sinus is opacified, a CT scan may not be able to differentiate tumor

Table 100-2	CHOICE OF TREATMENT OF TUMORS OF THE ANTERIOR CRANIAL BASE
Neoplasm	**Treatment**
Benign	Surgery
Low-grade malignancy	Surgery ± radiotherapy
High-grade malignancy	Surgery + radiotherapy ± chemotherapy Radiotherapy + chemotherapy ± salvage surgery

from retained secretions. In this case, the use of MRI with T1- and T2-weighted images allows differentiation of tumor and secretions (Fig. 100-7). When the sinus contains fungus, however, a signal void indistinguishable from air may give a false impression of a normal examination on T2-weighted images (Fig. 100-8).

Angiography is not necessary for neoplasms involving the anterior cranial base unless there is neoplastic involvement of the cavernous sinus or extensive extracranial involvement with extension of tumor to the infratemporal skull base. CT or MR angiography is usually adequate to establish the status of the vasculature in these areas. If the neoplasm is suspected to be highly vascular based on CT or MRI characteristics, angiography with preoperative embolization may be considered. Nevertheless, preoperative embolization is rarely necessary because the vascular supply to these tumors is usually accessible at the time of surgery.

The choice of therapy is dependent on the histology of the tumor and its expected biologic behavior, the tumor site, and involvement of critical anatomic structures. Surgical excision is the preferred treatment modality for the majority of benign and malignant tumors involving the anterior cranial base (Table 100-2). Complete removal of the tumor can be achieved in the majority of cases with contemporary surgical techniques. Because regional or distant metastases are unusual at the time of initial evaluation, the critical problem is that of local control. Rhabdomyosarcomas, melanomas, and adenoid cystic carcinomas, which are known to disseminate hematogenously, are an important exception to this concept. Sarcomas are not considered operable until the absence of distant metastases is confirmed by CT scanning of the lungs and liver and a bone scan.[8-10] We prefer the use of a fused positron emission tomography (PET)/CT study to evaluate for metastasis.

Cytologic examination of the spinal fluid is recommended for some tumors with intracranial extension, such as sarcomas or other high-grade malignancies. Positive cytology may indicate the need for combined therapy to prevent intracranial dissemination. The role of preoperative chemotherapy in the treatment of high-grade malignancies with intracranial extension has not been adequately addressed in the adult population. Strong consideration should be given, however, to the use of chemotherapy postoperatively in these patients.

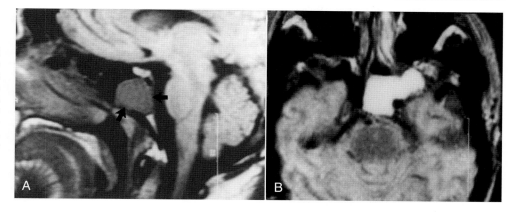

Figure 100-7. A, A T1-weighted magnetic resonance image demonstrates a sphenoid sinus mass *(arrows)* that is consistent with either a tumor or secretions. **B,** A T2-weighted image, however, demonstrates high signal intensity consistent with secretions from obstruction of the ostium of the sinus.

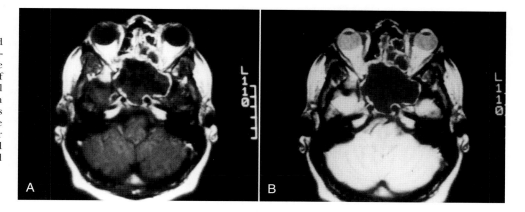

Figure 100-8. A, A T1-weighted magnetic resonance image demonstrates an extensive lesion of the sphenoid sinus with remodeling of bone and erosion of the cranial base. The variable-density pattern is consistent with fungal sinus disease. **B,** A T2-weighted image gives a false impression of a clear sinus. This patient was treated endoscopically for allergic fungal sinusitis.

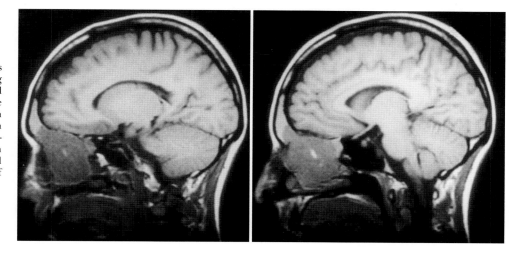

Figure 100-9. This patient has an extensive neoplasm involving the nasal cavity and paranasal sinuses. Magnetic resonance imaging demonstrates protrusion of tumor into the inferior portion of the frontal sinus. There is evidence of tumor extension through the bone of the anterior cranial base with possible involvement of the dura.

Orbital involvement by a malignant neoplasm may require orbital exenteration to achieve complete tumor removal. Orbital exenteration is recommended when there is soft tissue involvement of the orbit by malignant neoplasms.[7] Surgical therapy may be contraindicated in patients with malignant neoplasms invading the soft tissue of the orbit who adamantly refuse orbital exenteration. The orbit can usually be spared when there is involvement by benign neoplasms.

Intracranial extension of malignant neoplasms is not necessarily a contraindication to surgery. If it appears that the neoplasm is extradural, the dura may be excised as the margin (Fig. 100-9). Adequate surgical margins may also be obtained if there is minimal involvement of the frontal lobes (Fig. 100-10). However, when dealing with aggressive neoplasms such as squamous cell carcinoma or adenoid cystic carcinoma, which have a predilection for extending great distances beyond the observable margin of the tumor, the likelihood of achieving local control with surgery is slim. Significant palliation, however, may be achieved with the addition of postoperative chemoradiotherapy. Additionally,

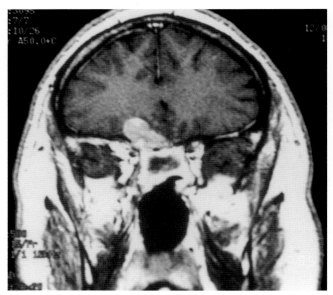

Figure 100-10. In this patient, squamous cell carcinoma developed in an inverting papilloma. Magnetic resonance imaging demonstrates minimal tumor invasion of the right frontal lobe.

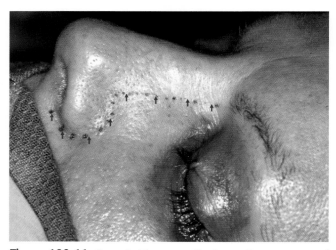

Figure 100-11. Lateral rhinotomy affords excellent exposure of the ipsilateral nasal cavity and paranasal sinuses.

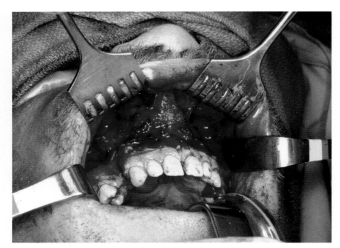

Figure 100-12. A midfacial degloving approach is useful for tumors involving the sinonasal cavity bilaterally.

given the insidious natural history of adenoid cystic carcinoma, tumor recurrence may not become evident for 5 to 10 years despite incomplete tumor excision.

Adequate exposure of the anterior cranial base for excision of neoplasms traditionally requires a combined intracranial and extracranial approach. The choice of an extracranial approach depends on the site and extent of the tumor and aesthetic considerations, as well as the experience of the surgeon with particular approaches. For most neoplasms arising from the nasal cavity or paranasal sinuses, lateral rhinotomy provides excellent exposure when combined with an intracranial approach (Fig. 100-11). This approach allows complete resection of the medial wall of the maxilla and the orbit and nasal septum. Excellent exposure of the ipsilateral

nasopharynx is also possible. Access to lesions that extend bilaterally, however, is limited. In addition, patients object to the facial scars. A midfacial degloving approach avoids external scarring and provides improved access to bilateral lesions (Fig. 100-12). It is also possible to resect some tumors limited to the cribriform plate and superior ethmoid air cells through an intracranial approach exclusively. Most tumors that were previously managed by lateral rhinotomy combined with a transcranial approach or by a degloving approach may be removed by endoscopic or endoscopic-assisted resection. Endoscopic or endoscopic-assisted approaches will obviate the need for facial scars and have been our favored approaches for the past 10 years.

Preoperative informed consent includes discussion of the various treatment options, as well as the sequelae and potential risks associated with the surgery. For patients undergoing anterior craniofacial resection, standard discussion of risks includes possible brain injury, hemorrhage, infection, CSF leak, stroke, and visual loss. Patients are informed that anosmia is a sequela of the operation.

PREOPERATIVE PLANNING

Special consideration must be given to perioperative and intraoperative management of these patients. As a result of the prolonged nature of the surgery, these patients are at risk for the development of deep venous thrombosis (DVT). Since anticoagulation is contraindicated in these patients because of the risk of intracranial hemorrhage, DVT prophylaxis is best achieved with sequential pneumatic compression stockings intraoperatively and in the postoperative period until ambulation is possible.

Anterior craniofacial surgery necessarily results in contamination of the intracranial space by bacterial flora of the upper aerodigestive tract. These are considered clean-contaminated cases, and perioperative antibiotic prophylaxis is indicated. Broad-spectrum antibiotics are recommended to provide adequate coverage of the flora of the sinuses *(Streptococcus pneumoniae, Haemophilus influenzae, Branhamella catarrhalis)* and skin *(Staphylococcus aureus).* Previous studies have demonstrated that the use of a single agent such as a broad-spectrum cephalosporin may provide adequate protection. Antibiotic prophylaxis is instituted at least 2 hours before the skin incision and is continued through the second postoperative day. Antibiotic prophylaxis for 24 hours or less is associated with a significant increase in local infections.[11,12] Such infections may be due to transient CSF leaks postoperatively with potential contamination of the intracranial cavity. Antibiotic prophylaxis for more than 48 hours may be associated with an increased risk for infection by resistant organisms.

To minimize the need for retraction of the brain, which may lead to contusion and the development of encephalomalacia, it is desirable to minimize intracranial pressure with various anesthetic techniques, including removal of CSF by lumbar puncture, as well as using a balanced anesthetic technique to maintain adequate cerebral perfusion while minimizing intracranial pressure. Hyperventilation to produce hypocapnia usually provides adequate relaxation of the frontal lobes. If significant frontal lobe retraction is necessary, a lumbar spinal drain is placed preoperatively and approximately 50 mL of spinal fluid is removed. Because these drains tend to malfunction intraoperatively, it is best to remove additional CSF at the time of catheter placement. Additional CSF may be removed intraoperatively or postoperatively to minimize intracranial pressure and decrease the risk for a postoperative CSF leak. In most cases, the spinal drain can be removed in the recovery room after surgery. Relaxation of the brain may be enhanced intraoperatively with the use of osmotic diuretics such as mannitol. The surgical approach is designed to minimize frontal lobe retraction through the use of a subfrontal approach.

The patient is positioned on a Mayfield horseshoe head holder to improve access to the face and scalp areas. Because frequent repositioning of the face and head is necessary with a combined intracranial and extracranial approach, head tongs or pins are not generally used. Since access to the airway is limited intraoperatively, the endotracheal tube is additionally secured by placement of a wire around a mandibular or maxillary molar. Wiring of the tube to the maxilla is preferred, when feasible, because such wiring provides greater stability. If the patient is edentulous, a circummandibular wire is placed for anchoring of the endotracheal tube.

An additional concern for the anesthesiologist is the development of an air embolus intraoperatively. This risk is minimized by operating with the patient in a supine position. A precordial Doppler probe is used to detect significant air embolism. A central line is also placed preoperatively to allow advancement into the right atrium for aspiration of an air embolus should it occur.

Most approaches to the anterior cranial base require exposure of the intracranial structures via frontal craniotomy. Before proceeding with the skin preparation, the eyes are protected by suturing the lids closed with 6-0 silk suture. This allows inclusion of the eyes within the surgical field and decreases the risk of corneal abrasion. The tarsorrhaphy suture may be placed through the lids at the tarsal line. Pledgets soaked in 0.05% oxymetazoline nasal solution are placed intranasally with the strings attached. To allow adequate time for the vasoconstrictive effects of a local anesthetic, the proposed incision line is infiltrated with 0.5% lidocaine (Xylocaine) with 1 : 200,000 epinephrine at this time. On average, approximately 20 mL of local anesthetic is infiltrated. The skin is then prepared with a povidone-iodine solution. It may be used around the eyes, although it is advisable to rinse the eyes with balanced saline solution to prevent chemical irritation. The povidone-iodine solution should be allowed to dry for it to be most effective.

SURGICAL TECHNIQUES

Open Technique

To provide access to the right and left frontal areas, a bicoronal scalp incision is made over the vertex of the scalp. Laterally, the incision extends to the superior attachment of the auricle. When additional lateral exposure is necessary, the incision is extended into a preauricular crease. The incision may be extended as necessary with a parotidectomy incision (Fig. 100-13). If lateral exposure is not necessary, small anterior

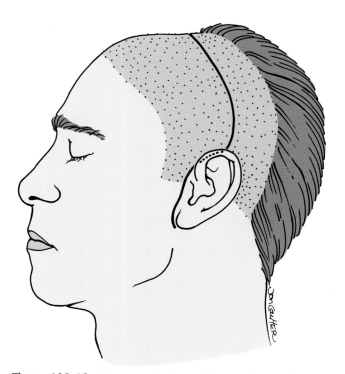

Figure 100-13. The coronal scalp incision may be extended in a preauricular skin crease to provide additional lateral exposure.

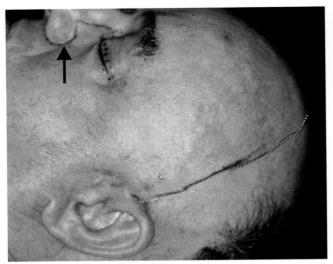

Figure 100-14. As an alternative to extending the incision inferiorly, a short angulation of the incision anteriorly increases the arc of rotation of the scalp flap and provides adequate frontal exposure. This patient has also been marked for a lateral rhinotomy.

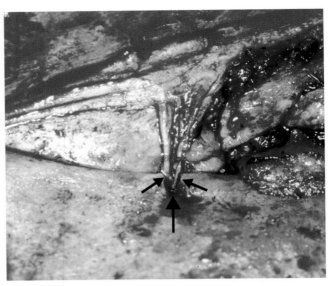

Figure 100-15. Subperiosteal elevation of the frontal scalp reveals the supraorbital nerve exiting from a completely enclosed bony foramen *(arrows)*.

backcuts are made at the ends of the incision in the temporal hair-bearing scalp (Fig. 100-14). This increases the arc of rotation of the scalp flap without the need for extending the incision inferiorly. The incision is made over the vertex of the scalp to maximize the length of any potential scalp flaps used for reconstruction. For this reason, incisions that follow the hairline or that have a V-shaped peak projecting anteriorly in the midline are to be avoided. Because of placement of the incision high over the vertex of the scalp, an acceptable cosmetic result is achieved even in bald persons. If there is any loss of hair along the incision line, it is well hidden.

Superiorly, the incision extends through all layers of the scalp, including the pericranium. Laterally, the incision extends to the level of the deep temporalis fascia. The lateral dissection is more meticulous to avoid injury to the superficial temporal artery. The branching pattern of this artery is variable, but in 85% of patients it divides into major anterior and posterior branches. By placing the scalp incision in line with the ear, the posterior branches are divided with preservation of the anterior branch. Preservation of the superficial temporal artery is not essential for viability of the scalp in most patients, but it may be important in patients who previously have undergone surgery or who have received radiation therapy. Additionally, if a galeal-pericranial scalp flap is used for reconstruction, collaterals from the superficial temporal artery are important to provide adequate circulation to the overlying skin.

The edges of the scalp are elevated with a broad periosteal elevator, and Raney clips are placed along the skin margins of the incision to provide hemostasis. The pericranium is not separated from other layers of the scalp at this time to prevent desiccation of the flap during a prolonged procedure. The scalp is then elevated, deep to the pericranium, with a periosteal eleva-

tor and blunt dissection with gauze. Laterally, this requires separation of the pericranium from the deep temporalis fascia at the origin of the temporalis muscle. The thin fascial layers overlying the deep temporalis fascia are easily elevated with a wide periosteal elevator. Bleeding from perforating veins of the frontal bone is controlled with bone wax or electrocautery.

As the scalp is elevated and reflected inferiorly, care is taken to avoid injury to the supraorbital and supratrochlear vessels. The supraorbital vessels and nerve are usually found in a notch along the medial half of the superior orbital rim (Fig. 100-15). With a sharp elevator such as a Cottle instrument, the vessels and nerve can usually be elevated from the bony notch without injury. Occasionally, however, the nerve and vessels may be completely encompassed by a bony foramen. In such cases, the inferior portion of the foramen can be mobilized with a 2- to 3-mm osteotome (Fig. 100-16). If the neurovascular bundle is found to exit through a foramen more than 1 cm from the orbital rim, it may be sacrificed. If a bifrontal craniotomy is performed without a subfrontal approach, it is not necessary to elevate the periorbita. A basal subfrontal approach is generally preferred, however, to provide additional exposure of the anterior cranial base posteriorly and to minimize retraction of the frontal lobes.

The periorbita is then elevated from the medial, superior, and lateral walls of the orbit with an Adson, Freer, or Penfield elevator. The supraorbital nerve runs along the surface of the orbital tissues. The globe is retracted with a malleable ribbon retractor to provide adequate visualization. Pressure on the globe may result in an ocular reflex, with resultant bradycardia and hypotension. This usually recovers quickly once pressure is released. Violation of the periorbita frequently occurs and results in herniation of orbital fat. Though a nuisance for visualization, it is not necessary to repair

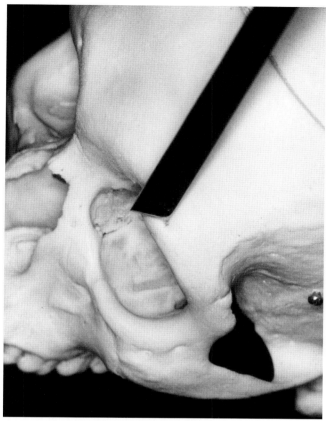

Figure 100-16. When the supraorbital nerve is enclosed by bone, it may be released by making angled bone cuts with an osteotome on both sides of the nerve through the supraorbital rim.

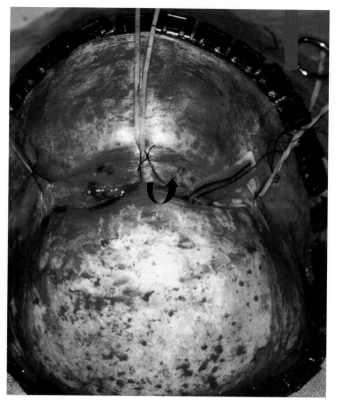

Figure 100-17. The scalp over the frontal bone has been rotated inferiorly *(curved arrow)*. The periorbita has been elevated from the superior and medial orbital walls. The anterior attachments of the temporalis muscles have been released.

the periorbita. Medially, elevation of the periorbita continues as far inferiorly as the anterior ethmoid artery and the frontoethmoid suture.

During elevation of the scalp laterally, it is important to avoid injury to the temporal branches of the facial nerve. Injury to these nerves is unlikely with a strictly anterior approach because dissection to the level of the zygomatic arch is not usually necessary. The temporal branches of the facial nerve are found in the superficial temporal fascia layer (superficial muscular aponeurotic system [SMAS], galea). These branches can be elevated with the scalp flap and protected from injury by developing a plane of dissection deep to the outer layer of the deep temporal fascia. The deep temporal fascia splits into superficial and deep layers 1 to 2 cm above the zygomatic arch. This space contains fatty tissue that can be elevated from the deep temporal fascia and muscle by blunt dissection with a broad periosteal elevator (see Chapter 101).

The anterior origin of the temporalis muscle is then elevated from the temporal fossa by electrocautery. A 3- to 4-mm margin of fascia is left intact to allow resuturing of the muscle after replacement of the craniotomy bone flap. Alternatively, the muscle may be sutured to holes drilled at the temporal line or to a titanium plate placed over the temporal line. Traction

sutures are placed along the anterior border of the temporalis muscle and in the scalp anteriorly, and rubber bands are used to facilitate exposure of the operative site (Fig. 100-17). The rubber bands are looped over Allis clamps, which are then attached to the surgical drapes. A unilateral or bifrontal craniotomy is then performed. The lateral burr hole is placed in the region of the pterion where the temporalis muscle is elevated. Small burr holes may be placed on each side of the sagittal sinus to facilitate dissection of the sinus from the calvaria and avoid laceration of the sinus (Fig. 100-18). After elevation of dura from the cranium with Adson elevators, the craniotomy bone flap is removed with a craniotome (Fig. 100-19). The inferior osteotomy is placed just superior to the prominence of the supraorbital rims and glabella. The anterior and posterior walls of the frontal sinus are frequently transgressed by the craniotomy. After removal of the bone, dural "tack-up" sutures are placed through drill holes at the margin of the craniotomy to prevent postoperative epidural dissection by blood or fluid. In older individuals, the dura is very thin and adherent to bone, and lacerations of the dura frequently result. They may be repaired primarily or with the use of a pericranial graft. If pericranium is used, it is harvested from the posterior aspect of the scalp incision to preserve anteriorly based scalp flaps for later reconstruction.

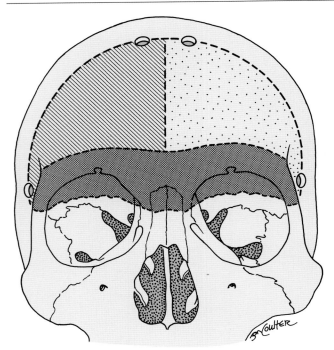

Figure 100-18. Various segments of the frontal bone and supraorbital rims may be removed to provide adequate exposure of the anterior cranial base.

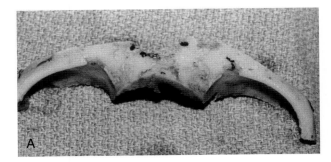

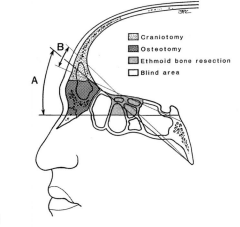

Craniotomy
Osteotomy
Ethmoid bone resection
Blind area

Figure 100-20. A, The superior orbital rims and nasion may be removed as a single bone unit to provide additional subfrontal exposure. **B,** This provides additional access to the limits of the anterior cranial base (arc A) with decreased need for frontal lobe retraction (arc B).

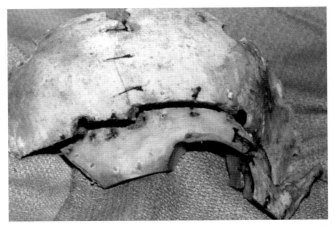

Figure 100-19. This patient required a bifrontal and left temporal craniotomy. The left orbital rim and zygomatic arch were removed as a single unit to provide additional subfrontal and anterolateral exposure.

The frontal lobe dura is then carefully elevated from the roof of the orbits and the crista galli and cribriform plates. Because of perforations of the olfactory nerves, multiple dural lacerations in the region of the cribriform plate necessarily result. It may be necessary to incise the dura along the crista galli. If there is intracranial extension of tumor with potential involvement of dura, a patch of dura is incised and left attached to the tumor specimen. In rare instances it may be necessary to resect a portion of one or both frontal lobes to obtain an adequate tumor margin. To maximize additional exposure while minimizing frontal lobe retraction, the supraorbital rims and nasion are removed as a single bone segment (Fig. 100-20). While the brain and orbit are protected by malleable retractors, a reciprocating saw with a long blade is used for osteotomies through the orbital rims at approximately the supraorbital notch. The cuts are beveled laterally to allow greater stability of the bone segment at the time of closure. Osteotomies through the orbital roof are made with reciprocating or oscillating blades (Fig. 100-21). An attempt is made to remove a large portion of the orbital roof as a single unit to avoid postoperative problems with enophthalmos because of loss of the orbital walls or pulsating exophthalmos because of contact of the brain with the soft tissues of the orbit. Near the midline, the osteotomy is necessarily directed to the anterior margin of the cribriform plate. A horizontal osteotomy is then made through the nasion superior to the level of the frontoethmoid suture line. The tip of the saw blade is placed approximately 2 cm deep to the nasion for this cut. This osteotomy usually transgresses the nasofrontal ducts superior to the ethmoid labyrinth. The entire bone segment, including both orbital rims and orbital roofs, can then be further mobilized, if necessary, with an osteotome.

Additional elevation of frontal lobe dura can then be performed with minimal brain retraction. After iden-

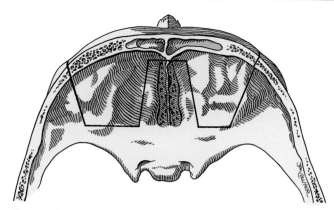

Figure 100-21. The sphenoid sinus is opened in the region of the planum sphenoidale. Osteotomies are then made anteriorly and laterally through the roof of the orbit or fovea ethmoidalis. Anteriorly, an osteotomy is made anterior to the crista galli.

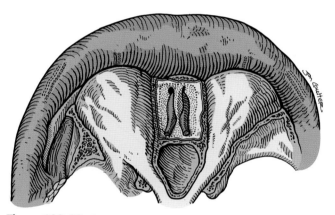

Figure 100-22. Depending on the extent of the tumor, the medial wall of the orbit may be included with the ethmoid sinus to provide an adequate tumor margin.

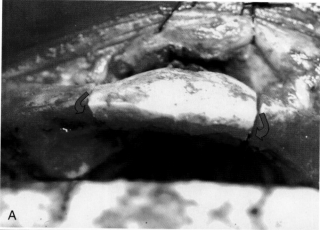

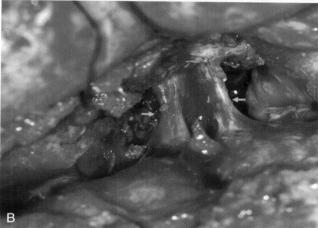

Figure 100-23. A, In this patient with a malignant neoplasm of the nasal cavity, it was necessary to remove only a short segment of the nasion *(curved arrows)*. **B,** After removal of this bone segment, additional osteotomies were made through the fovea ethmoidalis bilaterally and across the roof of the sphenoid sinus posteriorly *(arrows)*.

tification of the planum sphenoidale posterior to the crista galli and cribriform plates, the anterior clinoid processes and optic canals are identified bilaterally. In patients with tumor in proximity to the orbital apex, the optic canal is carefully decompressed with Kerrison rongeurs. Decompression is performed to prevent an entrapment syndrome postoperatively as a result of edema of the optic nerves. An opening is next made through the planum sphenoidale into the sphenoid sinus with cutting burrs. The sinus may then be inspected for evidence of tumor involvement. Bone removal from the roof of the sphenoid sinus continues anterolaterally on both sides toward the orbit (Fig. 100-22). If tumor does not involve the ethmoid sinus, the bone cut extends through the ethmoid air cells. When there is involvement of the sinus, the medial orbital wall is included to provide an adequate resection margin (Fig. 100-23).

Extracranial exposure of the neoplasm is now obtained with a lateral rhinotomy or midfacial degloving approach or with an endoscopic-assisted approach (see Chapter 10). Resection of the medial orbital wall

is facilitated with this approach. The intracranial exposure allows en bloc removal of the anterior cranial base with direct visualization of the optic nerves and the lateral walls of the sphenoid sinus with the internal carotid artery. An osteotome, drill, or Mayo scissors may be used to transgress the anterior wall of the sphenoid sinus, thus separating the specimen from its attachment inferiorly. Transection of the nasal septum from below is necessary to mobilize the specimen. This cut extends from the nasion anteriorly and superiorly to the posterior edge of the nasal septum inferior to the rostrum of the sphenoid.

After removal of the specimen, the defect is examined and additional bone or soft tissue margins can be obtained under direct visualization from above. A large defect frequently results in direct communication between the cranial cavity and the nasopharynx (Fig. 100-24).

Open Reconstruction

Every attempt should be made to attain a watertight closure of the dura to minimize the risk of a postopera-

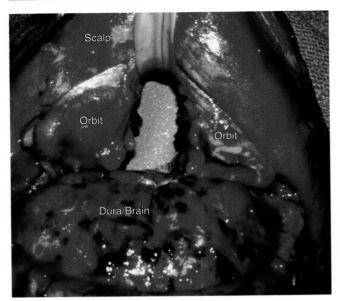

Figure 100-24. After resection of the neoplasm, a large defect of the anterior cranial base remains and communicates with the paranasal sinuses.

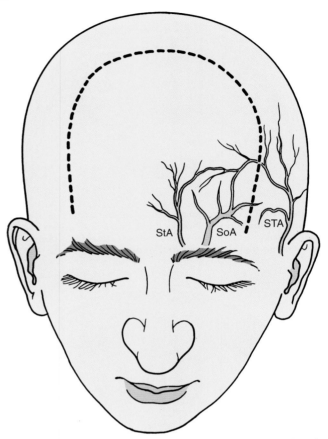

Figure 100-25. An anteriorly based pericranial flap receives its blood supply from the supratrochlear (StA) and supraorbital (SoA) vessels. The superficial temporal artery (STA) also contributes to the vascular supply of the galeal layer.

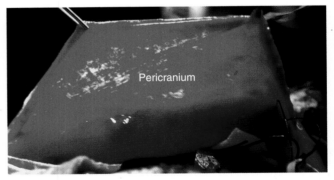

Figure 100-26. The pericranial flap is dissected from the galea by sharp dissection to the level of the orbital rim.

tive CSF leak and resultant meningitis. Small lacerations of the dura may be closed primarily. Larger defects of the dura may require the use of a fascial graft. Suitable materials include fascia lata harvested from the lateral aspect of the thigh or cadaveric dura. It is not necessary to remove all the mucosa from the sphenoid sinus unless a pericranial flap is used to obliterate the sinus.

Defects of the anterior skull base, including the cribriform plate, planum sphenoidale, and roof of the sphenoid sinus, can be reconstructed with a vascularized pericranial scalp flap. The flap is designed as an inverted U based on the supraorbital neurovascular bundles (Fig. 100-25). The primary blood supply of the flap comes from the supraorbital and supratrochlear vessels, although the anterior branches of the superficial temporal artery can also be included. The pericranial layer is easily dissected from the galea, beginning at the edge of the bicoronal scalp flap. The layer is elevated with tenotomy scissors down to the level of the supraorbital rim (Fig. 100-26). It is important to dissect close to the undersurface of the galea to maximize the thickness of the pericranial flap. As one approaches the base of the flap, it becomes more difficult to separate the galeal and pericranial layers, and extra care is needed to avoid injury to the vessels at this point. If necessary, the arc of rotation of the flap can be increased by incising its base on one side. A unilateral blood supply has proved to be adequate for survival of the flap.

The pericranial flap may be transferred into the defect above or below the supraorbital bone graft. The latter is preferred to increase the reach of the flap and to separate the supraorbital bone graft from the nasal cavity. The distal edge of the pericranial flap is sutured to the dura at the posterior limit of the cranial base defect (Fig. 100-27). In elderly patients with thin dura, this may be quite difficult because of tearing of the dura. In such cases it may be necessary to place small drill holes at the posterior margin of the defect for suturing of the pericranial flap. Laterally, the pericranial flap is sutured to the periorbita.

A galeal-pericranial flap is preferred for larger defects or when the vascularity or integrity of the pericranium is in question. The flap requires dissection of

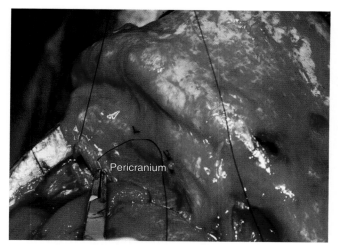

Figure 100-27. The pericranial flap is rotated posteriorly and sutured to bone, mucosa, or dura at the posterior margin of the surgical defect. Laterally, the pericranial flap is sutured to the orbital tissues to provide watertight separation of the nasopharynx from the cranial cavity. This step is performed before replacement of the supraorbital and craniotomy bone flaps.

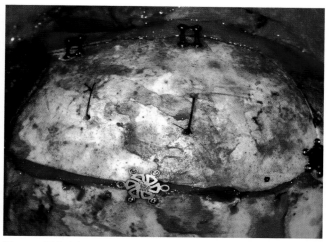

Figure 100-28. Bone defects may be covered with titanium burr hole covers to prevent a postoperative deformity.

the galeal-pericranial layer from the skin at a plane between the frontalis muscle and the hair follicles. The thickness and vascularity of this flap are superior to that of the pericranial flap, but at the expense of the vascularity and thickness of the bicoronal scalp flap. In cases in which the pericranium is not available, the galea may still be used as a flap. Rarely, the galeal and pericranial flaps may be used separately to cover different defects.

The use of free bone grafts in conjunction with these flaps does not appear to contribute to support of the brain and is associated with a higher incidence of infection and osteoradionecrosis. The use of nonvascularized tissue is avoided as much as possible to decrease the risk of wound infection. Placement of a nonvascularized fat or bone graft against a nonvascularized dural graft may interfere with vascularization of the dura. The pericranial flaps are rapidly mucosalized on the nasal surface. Therefore, skin grafting is not recommended. (For anterolateral defects, see Chapter 101.)

Before replacement of the bone flaps, it is necessary to remove all mucosal remnants from the frontal sinus to prevent postoperative mucocele formation. The frontal sinus is cranialized by removing the posterior table of the frontal sinus with rongeurs or a saw. The mucosa is then stripped from the sinus with an elevator. Removal of mucosal remnants in deep crevices is facilitated by the use of a cutting burr. The mucosa is also stripped from the nasofrontal ducts, and the ducts are obliterated with Surgicel or soft tissue plugs.

The craniotomy and supraorbital bones are then replaced superior to the pericranial flap. Care is taken to avoid compression of the vascular supply of the flap by the bone. It may be necessary to remove an additional 2 to 3 mm of bone in the midline to prevent compression. The bones are held in place with multiple 2-0 braided nylon sutures through drill holes in the margins of the bone or with microplates. Titanium microplates are currently preferred because of greater stability of the bone flap, rapid repair, and the ability to cover small bone defects. This affords adequate stabilization of the bones with excellent healing and bony union. Steel wire and nontitanium plates are not generally used because of the potential for scatter artifacts on postoperative radiologic imaging. Bone dust and chips are used to fill defects surrounding the craniotomy bone flap. Titanium burr hole covers may also be used to cover burr holes when adequate autologous bone is not available (Fig. 100-28). Alternatively, the inner cortex of the bone flap or the posterior wall of the frontal sinus may be used for bone reconstruction. Larger defects may be covered with titanium mesh.

A Jackson-Pratt drain is use for drainage of the wound. The exit wound is placed posterior to the incision line to avoid potential compromise of the vascular supply to the anterior portion of the scalp. Whenever there is the potential for a CSF leak, the drain is placed to empty by gravity with the use of a bile bag. There are potential risks of excessive CSF drainage or sudden cardiac arrest as a result of changes in intracranial pressure if high suction is applied to the drains. The anterior margins of the temporalis muscle are then sutured to the cranium to prevent a cosmetic defect, and the scalp incision is closed with interrupted 2-0 Vicryl or Dexon sutures. Staples are used for skin closure. Telfa coated with povidone-iodine ointment is applied to the suture line, and a standard neurosurgical gauze compressive dressing is applied. It is important to make sure that there are no compressive points anteriorly that might compromise anterior scalp vascularity.

Endoscopic Technique

We have described several endoscopic "modules" based on exposure and control of key anatomic structures. Although this chapter addresses resection of the anterior skull base for the specific indication of sinonasal tract malignancies, we consider this approach to be part of an encompassing modular system that provides endoscopic exposure of the entire anatomy of the sinonasal tract and the anterior and middle skull base and clival region.[13-18]

Patients are positioned supine on the operating table with the head in neutral position and fixed by a three-pin head holder with the neck slightly rotated to the right side. If exposure of the frontal sinus (endoscopic Lothrop or Draf III procedure) will be required, the head is extended mildly. Video monitors are positioned directly in front of the surgeons.

The nasal cavity is decongested with cottonoids soaked in 0.05% oxymetazoline and then examined with 0- and 45-degree endoscopes. One percent lidocaine with 1 : 100,000 epinephrine may be infiltrated into the lateral nasal wall, middle turbinates, posterior nasal septum, and rostrum of the sphenoid sinus for additional hemostasis. Infiltration must be avoided in areas involving the vascular pedicle for a nasoseptal flap if one is to be harvested. The operation begins with debulking of the tumor or with exenteration of the anterior paranasal sinuses, depending on the origin, extent, position, and bulk of the tumor. The tumor is debulked with a microdébrider to increase exposure of the skull base. Dissection of the paranasal sinuses follows a technique similar to that used for the management of inflammatory disease. The dissection can be unilateral or bilateral, depending on the extent of the tumor. Uncinectomy is followed by identification and widening of the natural ostium of the maxillary sinus in a posterior and inferior direction. A wide middle meatal antrostomy helps define the inferior and medial walls of the orbits and exposes the posterior wall of the antrum, thereby facilitating control of the sphenopalatine and posterior nasal arteries. Completion of anterior and posterior ethmoidectomies and exposure of the nasofrontal recess will define and expose the paramedian anterior skull base, including the fovea ethmoidalis, the vertical and horizontal lamellae of the cribriform plate and its olfactory fila, and the anterior and posterior ethmoidal artery canals. The middle turbinates may also be removed to create more room for intranasal instrumentation.

At this point, if a vascularized nasoseptal flap is required for reconstruction and the oncologic principles of resection can be respected, it is harvested from the nasal septum. Until recently, options for endoscopic reconstruction of the skull base were limited to the use of nonvascularized tissue. This resulted in CSF leak rates of 20% to 30% and became a major obstacle to widespread acceptance of these techniques. Recently, the Haddad-Bassagasteguy flap (HBF), or nasoseptal flap, has proved to be a versatile, robust vascularized flap for the reconstruction of expanded endonasal approaches defects.[19] Since adopting this technique, our CSF leak rates have dropped to numbers that compare with those of traditional techniques (around 5%). The advantage of this flap as a reconstructive option is that a second approach or incision is not necessary and the flap can be harvested endoscopically. The major drawback of the HBF is that its need must be anticipated before embarking on resection because

the vascular pedicle to this flap is frequently compromised during the sphenoidotomy and posterior septectomy portion of the procedure. In addition, if a revision procedure is necessary, the flap may have been used previously or the pedicle previously damaged.

Design of the flap should be based on the expected size of the defect. This point is counterintuitive to most reconstructive surgeons because the flap is harvested before the resultant defect is created; thus, one can be left with a flap that is inadequate. As a result of this potential flaw, we tend to harvest a larger flap. The first incision is the most critical and involves the use of electrocautery along the free edge of the choana from the lateral nasal wall toward the nasal septum. This incision is exceedingly difficult to perform once the flap has been elevated, so extra time and patience are warranted to ensure a full incision down to the level of the sphenoid floor. Two longitudinal incisions are then created in a posterior-to-anterior direction. The most inferior incision is placed along the maxillary crest; however, it can be extended inferiorly and laterally to harvest the mucoperiosteum of the nasal floor. The superior incision is created 1.0 to 1.5 cm inferior to the cribriform plate to preserve olfactory function. It then crosses the rostrum of the sphenoid at the level of the sphenoid sinus os. This leaves approximately a 1- to 2-cm width of pedicle across the anterior face of the sphenoid. Both these incisions are joined anteriorly with a vertical incision at the level of the anterior end of the inferior turbinate. Once all the incisions are completed, the flap is elevated in a subperichondrial and subperiosteal plane back to its pedicle on the sphenopalatine foramen. The flap can then be "stored" for the duration of the resection in the nasopharynx or inside the antrum through a wide maxillary antrostomy.

In the event that a flap cannot be harvested because of oncologic margins or because the blood supply has been compromised from previous procedures, the nasal septum is separated from the sphenoid rostrum via a transfixion incision with a Cottle elevator. A similar vertical transfixion incision is performed at a level just posterior to the nasofrontal recess (this is modified to include the anterior extent of the tumor). A third septal transfixion incision, horizontal and parallel to the floor of the nose, connects these two vertical transfixion incisions and leaves the bony nasal septum attached to the cribriform plate. Bilateral wide sphenoidotomies to remove the entire rostrum help define the posterior limit of the tumor (planum sphenoidale) and further delineate the position of the skull base. At this point in the surgery the skull base from orbit to orbit and from frontal sinus to sella turcica, as well as the base of the tumor, is completely exposed and the resection can begin. The lamina papyracea may be removed as a lateral margin or as part of an endoscopic medial maxillectomy (unilaterally or bilaterally according to the necessary resection), with care taken to preserve the periorbita while identifying the anterior and posterior ethmoidal arteries at their entry into their respective canals at the skull base. Gentle curettage or drilling helps remove the bone over the canal, thereby exposing the arteries, which can then be dissected and controlled with clips or bipolar electrocautery.

Using a high-speed drill with a 2- to 3-mm coarse diamond hybrid burr, a horizontal osteotomy is made at the planum sphenoidale, parallel and anterior to the sphenoid rostrum. Another horizontal osteotomy is made just posterior to the frontal sinus posterior wall. These osteotomies are then connected by bilateral osteotomies performed lateral to the cribriform plate and running parallel to the superomedial wall of the orbits, thereby forming a rectangle surrounding the tumor and adjacent structures such as the nasal septum, the entire cribriform plate, and the planum sphenoidale. The resection then proceeds in an anterior-to-posterior direction. The olfactory nerves are identified and transected after bipolar cauterization. If the tumor extends to the dura, its anterior surface is coagulated with bipolar cautery and then incised. Dural incisions that match the previously described osteotomies facilitate removal of the specimen with adequate control of the dural margins. It is critical to establish the completeness of the resection with the use of intraoperative frozen section analysis. Any positive margin mandates additional resection.

The crista galli is most often fractured from the rest of the resected skull base. It must nonetheless be removed to improve visualization and facilitate the reconstruction. It should be noted that the crista galli can extend for a variable depth into the intracranial cavity, so removal of it involves drilling internally until it becomes eggshell thin so that it can be fractured. Meticulous hemostasis completes resection of the anterior cranial base.

This resection may be combined with other approaches such as a Draf III or endoscopic Lothrop, with or without endoscopic medial maxillectomy. As previously stated, the resection can be unilateral to preserve the contralateral turbinates and possibly the olfactory fibers.

Endoscopic Reconstruction

Currently, we use a subdural inlay graft (between the brain and dura) of collagen matrix (Duragen, Integra Life Sciences) to help obliterate the dead space.[15,17,19] Its pliability and texture allow manipulation around neurovascular structures. This subdural graft should extend beyond the dural margins, ideally by 5 to 10 mm in all directions. Closely adherent skull base and dura around the resection margins are dissected. A subsequent inlay graft of acellular dermis is placed in the epidural space (between the dura and skull base). Occasionally, the bony ledges are not adequate to support an inlay graft; in this case the acellular dermis graft is placed extracranially (at the nasal side of the defect) as an onlay graft (Fig. 100-29). All the edges of the defect should be denuded of mucosa to allow revascularization of the graft and avoid the formation of mucoceles. Alternatively, this graft can be sutured to the dura with nitinol U-clips (Medtronic U-Clips, Memphis, TN).

Although this is an off-label indication for acellular dermal grafts, we found that its handling characteris-

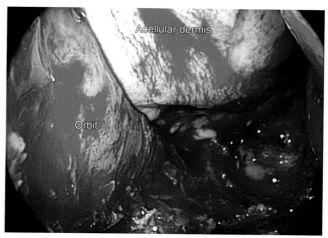

Figure 100-29. Endoscopic appearance of acellular dermis used for skull base reconstruction after endoscopic anterior craniofacial resection.

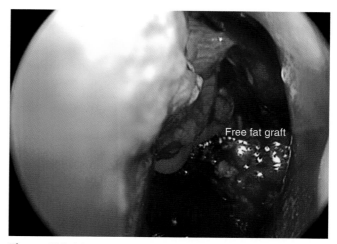

Figure 100-30. Endoscopic appearance of a free fat graft used to support the endonasal skull base reconstruction.

tics, its availability (i.e., no need for harvesting from a distant site), ingrowth of the patient's own tissue, and rapid epithelialization are advantages that outweigh its cost. It is important that a single graft with dimensions that will extend beyond the defect margins in all direction be used and that the graft be adequately hydrated in normal saline solution before insertion. It is our experience that medium-thickness grafts (0.30 to 0.70 μm) offer the best combination of tissue handling and "take."

According to the contour of the skull base and how anterior the extent of the resection is, the acellular matrix is supported by free abdominal fat or nasal packing (Fig. 100-30). An abdominal free fat graft harvested through a periumbilical incision acts as a biologic dressing and applies pressure to reduce any early brain herniation that may lead to migration of the underlying grafts and a subsequent CSF leak. Nasal packing ($\frac{1}{2}$-inch strip gauze impregnated with Bacitracin ointment) is preferred if the resection involves the convexity of the posterior wall of the frontal sinus because the packing can accommodate for this curvature better than the globular shape of a free fat graft can. Another alternative is to harvest the fat in a wedge or teardrop shape that will match the contour of the skull base more effectively. Recently, we have adopted the use of a pedicled vascularized flap based on the posterior nasoseptal artery. The technique for harvest was described earlier. When a vascularized nasoseptal flap is available for reconstruction, it is used as an onlay flap over top of the inlay collagen matrix and acellular dermis graft. It is critical to separate the grafts from the packing with some type of nonadherent material such as Gelfoam or Gelfilm because this will prevent traction on the grafts when the packing is removed. In addition, shifting of the underlying inlay/onlay grafts may occur during placement of the fat graft or the packing, so the surgeon must be vigilant and the graft should be placed under direct visualization with the endoscope. Fibrin sealants are applied only after the final tissue barrier has been placed.

We then use the balloon of a 12F Foley catheter to splint the fat graft or packing, which in turn will stabilize the inlay/onlay grafts and thus further prevent early brain herniation. The balloon is fixed in position by threading the Foley catheter through a Doyle splint, advancing it to the desired position, and then securing the Doyle splint to the septum with 4-0 nylon. Placement plus inflation of the balloon catheter with 5 mL of saline is also performed under endoscopic vision. Overinflation may result in compressive effects over the intracranial structures. Any nasal packing or balloons are removed 3 to 5 days after resection.

POSTOPERATIVE MANAGEMENT

Most patients can be extubated in the recovery room. After extubation, it is important to avoid external mask ventilation because air may be forced intracranially through the anterior cranial base defect. Similarly, all instrumentation of the nose, including passing of tubes, should be avoided. A nasal dressing is useful to absorb any drainage and also to prevent the patient from nose blowing.

If the patient has a spinal drain and watertight closure of the dura was achieved intraoperatively, the spinal drain is usually removed in the recovery room. This avoids excessive CSF drainage and decreases the risk of infection. If closure of the dura is tenuous, physiologic drainage of CSF is generally continued for 3 to 5 days. Intermittent drainage of CSF is performed (approximately 50 mL every 8 hours). This is preferable to leaving the lumbar drain open to gravity because excessive CSF drainage may occur with changes in patient position. Intermittent clamping of the drain also allows the patient to begin early ambulation.

On the first or second postoperative day, a follow-up CT scan of the head without contrast enhancement is obtained to acquire information about any intracranial complications such as hemor-rhage or pneumocephalus. This scan also serves as a basis for future examinations should neurologic symptoms develop.

Early ambulation is encouraged, and an oral diet can usually be instituted on the first postoperative day. Patients are instructed to not blow their nose. A saline nasal spray may be used to gently irrigate the nasal cavity during hospitalization. This spray is continued after discharge from the hospital. Most patients can be discharged within 5 to 10 days.

During the month after surgery, excessive instrumentation of the nasal cavity is avoided. Gentle suctioning of the nasal cavity under endoscopic visualization is performed while taking care to avoid instrumentation of the reconstructed cranial base defect. Mucosalization of the pericranial flap occurs within 6 to 8 weeks. Depending on the original pathology, patients are seen at periodic intervals to screen for recurrent disease or complications of surgery. For any patient with a malignant neoplasm, baseline CT or MRI is performed at approximately 3 months after surgery to allow adequate time for healing of the surgical site and resolution of edema or fluid collections. It serves as a baseline for future examinations to look for recurrent disease. Patients may require lifelong nasal hygiene to remove excessive crusts, especially after radiation therapy. Patients are instructed to irrigate the nasal cavity with saline solution via a Water-Pik with a nasal adaptor. An Alkalol solution may be helpful in loosening crusts. Because of the loss of olfactory function, patients should be counseled about the need for in-home monitors to detect natural gas leaks. Similarly, the home should be equipped with smoke detectors.

COMPLICATIONS

Metabolic

The fluid and electrolyte balance of patients undergoing skull base surgery should be monitored closely. Postoperative hyponatremia is generally the result of inappropriate fluid balance in the operating room, but the syndrome of inappropriate antidiuretic hormone (SIADH) secretion may develop in patients with cerebral edema or contusion. Excessive antidiuretic hormone (ADH) secretion leads to water retention with a serum sodium concentration of usually less than 130 mg/dL. The syndrome is generally self-limited and may be treated by restriction of fluid to less than 1000 mL/day. If the patient shows signs of disorientation, seizures, or muscle irritability, 3% saline solution is administered intravenously.

In contrast, ischemia or trauma to the hypothalamus may lead to insufficient production of ADH and result in diabetes insipidus. During diabetes insipidus the patient loses the ability to concentrate urine, which leads to increased free water loss and hypernatremia/hypovolemia. Serum sodium is usually higher than 145 mg/dL, and urine specific gravity is less than 1.002. Careful replacement of fluids is necessary because urine output can be greater than 2 L/hr. Aqueous ADH may be replaced initially (2.5 units intramuscularly every 4 hours). Iatrogenic SIADH, through overuse of parenteral ADH, should be avoided.

Hyperglycemia is very common in patients receiving steroids and should be ruled out in any patient with increased diuresis and hypernatremia. It is treated by a sliding scale of regular insulin titrated to glycemia. Other electrolyte disorders such as hypomagnesemia (<1.8 mg/dL), hypophosphatemia (<2 mg/dL), and hypocalcemia (<8.0 mg/dL) are common in patients after skull base surgery, especially if the patient requires replacement of significant blood loss (>5 units of packed red blood cells). These disorders can add to the postoperative delirium and diminished mental state. Hypocalcemia and hypomagnesemia increase muscle irritability and can lead to confusion. Calcium is replaced as 10% calcium gluconate administered intravenously at a rate slower than 1 mL/min. Phosphates are replaced intravenously as a solution containing 10 to 15 mmol phosphate in 250 mL of 5% dextrose solution administered over a period of 6 hours. Magnesium may be replaced intravenously as 4 g in 100 mL normal saline solution given over a 30-minute period.

Vascular

DVT is prevented with the use of sequential compression stockings. Heparin is contraindicated because of the risk of postoperative intracranial bleeding. If DVT occurs, an inferior vena cava filter is recommended to prevent pulmonary embolism. In selected patients at high risk for DVT or pulmonary embolism, the filter is placed preoperatively.

Coagulopathies may be induced by rapid bleeding and blood replacement temporarily exhausting the coagulation factors. This is treated by replacing the coagulation factors with fresh frozen plasma.

Central Nervous System/Skull Base

Seizures secondary to frontal lobe trauma are rare. Nevertheless, in the presence of significant brain contusion or when parenchymal resection is necessary, seizure prophylaxis in the form of phenytoin (Dilantin) is recommended. Treatment of a grand mal–type seizure consists of diazepam (Valium), 10 mg intravenously, and ventilatory support, followed by phenytoin in a 15-mg/kg loading dose and 5-mg/kg/day maintenance dose. It is essential to rule out electrolyte or acid-base imbalances, as well as an intracranial space-occupying lesion or inflammation as a cause of the seizures.

CSF leaks that occur in the immediate postoperative period are managed with a lumbar spinal drain. The drain bag is kept at shoulder level, and 50 mL is drained every 8 hours. This approximates the physiologic production of CSF in 24 hours. Overdrainage may lead to pneumocephalus. High-flow or persistent CSF leaks (beyond 1 week) require surgical repair. The site of the leak may be identified by means of a CT-cisternogram. Repair of the leak usually involves repair of the dural defect and the use of a vascularized flap to separate the leak from the upper aerodigestive tract. Patients

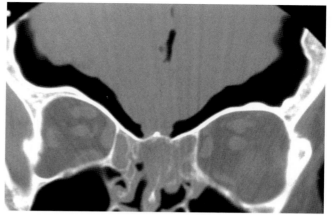

Figure 100-31. Mental status changes developed in the postoperative period. Computed tomography demonstrated a tension pneumocephalus that required aspiration to relieve frontal lobe compression.

in whom hydrocephalus develops require a ventriculoperitoneal shunt.

A small amount of pneumocephalus is frequently seen in the early postoperative period. It generally resolves spontaneously over about 1 week. Persistent or substantial pneumocephalus implies a CSF leak and may be managed conservatively, as described previously. Tension pneumocephalus, which is the accumulation of intracranial air under pressure, may compress brain tissue and cause impairment of the sensorium or focal neurologic deficits (Fig. 100-31). Although the mechanism of the increased air pressure is poorly understood, it may result from forceful expiration through the nose when there is an incompletely sealed defect in the anterior cranial base. The pneumocephalus is treated by needle aspiration when neurologic changes or evidence of increasing pressure is noted. Recurrent tension pneumocephalus may require repair of the dura. A tracheotomy may be used to bypass ventilation.

Wound infection and meningitis are rare complications of anterior cranial base surgery and are usually the result of faulty surgical technique. An epidural dead space often results from cranialization of the frontal sinus and may increase the risk for a postoperative wound infection. Antibiotic therapy is directed by Gram stain or culture and the ability to achieve adequate CSF penetration. Involvement of bone grafts by the infection may require their removal. If the bones are not mobile (repaired with rigid fixation), they can be salvaged by using a suction irrigation system for the delivery of local antibiotics. It is essential that separation of the cranial cavity from the upper aerodigestive tract be achieved. When bone flaps are removed because of infection, the soft tissues are allowed to collapse onto the underlying tissues (dura or flap). Reconstruction is typically delayed for 6 months to avoid the risk of osteomyelitis.

Dissection of a galeal-pericranial or galeal scalp flap may compromise the vascularity of the superficial scalp layers, especially in patients who have previously received radiation therapy. A constrictive head dressing should be avoided because it may compromise the remaining vascularity. With thinning of the scalp, bone irregularities may become more apparent. Reabsorption of bone chips may result in depressions at the site of burr holes. Patients who require postoperative radiation therapy may also experience additional bone reabsorption.

Encephalocele and pulsatile exophthalmos rarely occur as late postoperative complications. They are corrected by reoperation and reconstruction of the dural and bone defects. Loss of medial orbital support and imprecise realignment of the medial canthus may result in ocular asymmetry and a disconjugate gaze. Whenever possible, large orbital defects should be reconstructed.

PEARLS

- Because of the location of anterior cranial base pathology, the initial clinical symptoms may be subtle and are often very similar to chronic inflammatory sinus symptomatology.
- Preoperative confirmation of histopathology is critical because of the wide variety of pathology of the anterior cranial base and the treatment options available.
- Care must be taken when raising a bicoronal flap to not compromise the blood supply from the supraorbital and supratrochlear vessels to the pericranial flap.
- A basal subfrontal approach is preferred to avoid excessive retraction of the frontal lobe.
- If undertaking endoscopic resection of anterior cranial base pathology, oncologic principles should never be compromised and the same resection must be achieved endoscopically as would be through a traditional technique.

PITFALLS

- Elevation of the bicoronal flap must occur in a plane deep to the superficial layer of the deep temporal fascia to avoid injury to the frontal branch of the facial nerve.
- Failure to preserve the superficial temporal vessels may forfeit the use of a temporoparietal flap for reconstruction.
- All frontal sinus mucosa should be drilled away to avoid late complications related to retained mucosal function.
- Lack of a watertight barrier separating the intracranial contents from the paranasal sinuses may lead to CSF leakage or infection.
- Early postoperative manipulation of endonasal reconstruction could lead to an iatrogenic CSF leak.

References

1. Snyderman CH, Costantino PD, Sekhar LN: Anterior approaches to the cranial base. In Apuzzo MLJ (ed): Brain Surgery. Complication Avoidance and Management. New York, Churchill Livingstone, 1993, pp 2265-2281.
2. Snyderman CH, Sekhar LN, Sen CN, Janecka IP: Malignant skull base tumors. Neurosurg Clin N Am 1:243-259, 1990.
3. Janecka IP, Sekhar LN: Anterior and anterolateral craniofacial resection. In Sekhar LN, Janecka IP (eds): Surgery of Cranial Base Tumors. New York, Raven Press, 1993, pp 147-156.
4. Carrau RL, Snyderman CH, Nuss DW: Surgery of the anterior and lateral skull base. In Myers EN, Suen JY, Myers JN, Hanna EYN (eds): Cancer of the Head and Neck, 4th ed. Philadelphia, WB Saunders, 2003, pp 207-228.
5. Snyderman CH, Carrau RL: Anterior cranial base. In Myers EN (ed): Operative Otolaryngology–Head and Neck Surgery. Philadelphia, WB Saunders, 1997, pp 808-834.
6. Carrau RL, Zimmer L, Myers EN: Neoplasms of the nose and paranasal sinuses. In Bailey B (ed): Head and Neck Surgery–Otolaryngology, 2nd ed. Philadelphia, Lippincott-Raven, 2006, pp 1481-1500.
7. Carrau RL, Segas J, Nuss DW, et al: Squamous cell carcinoma of sinonasal tract invading the orbit. Laryngoscope 109:230-235, 1999.
8. Carrau RL, Segas J, Nuss DW, et al: Role of skull base surgery for local control of sarcomas of the nasal cavity and paranasal sinuses. Eur Arch Otorhinol 251:350-356, 1994.
9. Crist WM, Anderson JR, Meza JL, et al: Intergroup Rhabdomyosarcoma Study-IV: Results for patients with nonmetastatic disease. J Clin Oncol 19:3091-3102, 2001.
10. Baker KS, Anderson JR, Link MP, et al: Benefit of intensified therapy for patients with local or regional embryonal rhabdomyosarcoma: Results from the Intergroup Rhabdomyosarcoma Study IV. J Clin Oncol 18:2427-2434, 2000.
11. Carrau RL, Snyderman CH, Janecka IP, et al: Role of antibiotic prophylaxis in cranial base surgery. Head Neck Surg 13:311-317, 1991.
12. Kraus DH, Gonen M, Mener D, et al: A standardized regimen of antibiotics prevents infectious complications in skull base surgery. Laryngoscope 115:1347-1357, 2005.
13. Kassam A, Snyderman CH, Mintz A, et al: Expanded endonasal approach: The rostrocaudal axis. Part II. Posterior clinoids to foramen magnum. Neurosurg Focus 19(1):E4, 2005.
14. Kassam A, Snyderman CH, Mintz A, et al: Expanded endonasal approach: The rostrocaudal axis. Part I. Crista galli to the sella turcica. Neurosurg Focus 19(1):E3, 2005.
15. Kassam A, Carrau RL, Snyderman CH, et al: Evolution of reconstructive techniques following endoscopic expanded endonasal approaches. Neurosurg Focus 19(1):E8, 2005.
16. Cavallo LM, Messina A, Cappabianca P, et al: Endoscopic endonasal surgery of the midline skull base: Anatomical study and clinical considerations. Neurosurg Focus 19(1):E2, 2005.
17. Snyderman CH, Kassam AB, Carrau R, Mintz A: Endoscopic reconstruction of cranial base defects following endonasal skull base surgery. Skull Base 17:73-78, 2007.
18. Carrau RL, Kassam AB, Snyderman CH, et al: Endoscopic transnasal anterior skull base resection for the management of sinonasal malignancies. Op Tech Otolaryngol Head Neck Surg 17:102-110, 2006.
19. Hadad G, Bassagasteguy L, Carrau RL, et al: A novel reconstructive technique after endoscopic expanded endonasal approaches: Vascular pedicle nasoseptal flap. Laryngoscope 116:1882-1886, 2006.

Chapter **101**

Surgical Approaches to the Infratemporal Fossa

Ricardo L. Carrau, Allan D. Vescan, Carl H. Snyderman, and Amin B. Kassam

The anatomy of the infratemporal fossa (ITF), otherwise known as the *pterygoid fossa,* is confusing for both neurosurgeons and head and neck surgeons. Although its anatomic description varies, the most accepted boundaries are shown in Table 101-1.

The first report in the English literature of a surgical approach to the ITF is attributed to Fairbanks-Barbosa, who in 1961 described his approach for advanced tumors of the maxillary antrum.[1] Subsequently, others reported different surgical techniques or modifications of the Fairbanks-Barbosa approach (Table 101-2).[1-8]

PATIENT SELECTION

Tumors may arise in the ITF or may invade it by direct extension from the upper aerodigestive tract, the parotid gland, the temporal bone, the skull base, or the cranial cavity. It is fundamental that the origin and extension of the tumor be established to offer the patient the most effective treatment.

Selection of the surgical approach depends on the characteristics of the patient, the biologic behavior of the tumor, and the experience of the surgeon. In most instances, these tumors require a multidisciplinary approach to properly stage, diagnose, and extirpate the tumor and to provide an acceptable cosmetic and functional reconstruction.

Clinical Evaluation

The history and physical examination must emphasize neurologic deficits, especially those resulting from dysfunction of the cranial nerves. These deficits are an important consideration in the development of a surgical plan, as well as postoperative care, because they have

a significant impact on recovery and functional rehabilitation of the patient. As a result of the location of these tumors, considerable growth may occur before obvious clinical findings develop and the patient seeks medical care. The initial symptoms are diverse and are usually secondary to dysfunction of the masticatory muscles or cranial nerve deficits.

Symptoms and signs that are attributable to deficits of the trigeminal nerve are frequently evident. Pain may be present in the distribution of any of the divisions of the trigeminal nerve and may be exacerbated by jaw movement, jaw clenching, or head position. Sensory losses characterized by hypoesthesia or paresthesia of the divisions of the trigeminal may be present, and the pattern of deficits provides clues to the location and extent of the tumor. Pain may be referred to the ear because of sensory innervation of the external auditory canal (EAC).

Physical examination focuses on sensory and motor deficits. In addition to assessing cutaneous sensation, corneal sensation is tested with a cotton swab. In the presence of a concomitant facial nerve palsy, protective measures to prevent corneal injury may need to be instituted preoperatively or postoperatively. Trigeminal motor function is assessed by palpation of the masticatory muscles (masseter and temporalis) during jaw clenching. Deviation of the jaw laterally with jaw opening reflects dysfunction of the pterygoid musculature. Trismus may be due to mechanical restriction of the jaw as a result of infiltration of tumor into the pterygoid muscles or temporomandibular joint (TMJ), or it can be due to pain. The extent and cause of the trismus are important considerations in the perioperative management of the airway. Trismus secondary to pain will disappear with general anesthesia and allow safe oral

Table 101-1	ANATOMIC BOUNDARIES OF THE INFRATEMPORAL FOSSA				
	Superior	**Medial**	**Lateral**	**Anterior**	**Posterior**
Bone	Greater wing of the sphenoid, temporal bone	Lateral pterygoid plate, pterygopalatine fissure	Mandible Zygoma		Articular tubercle of the temporal bone, glenoid fossa and condyle, styloid process
Muscle		Superior constrictor, pharyngobasilar fascia	Masseter temporalis	Lateral and medial pterygoid, masseter	Prevertebral fascia
Foramina	Carotid canal Jugular foramen Foramen ovale Foramen spinosum Foramen lacerum Soft tissue Muscles				
Nerves	Foramen ovale (V3), jugular foramen (pars nervosa)				IX-XI Sympathetic plexus
Vessels	Internal carotid artery	Internal maxillary artery			Internal carotid artery
	Internal jugular vein	Pterygoid venous plexus			Jugular vein
Other			Parotid		

Table 101-2	SURGICAL APPROACHES TO THE INFRATEMPORAL FOSSA: HISTORICAL BACKGROUND	
Authors*	**Year**	**Technique**
Fairbanks-Barbosa[1]	1961	Extracranial resection of advanced tumors of the antrum
Terz et al.[2]	1969	Craniofacial resection of tumors of the SNT with invasion of the ITF
Fisch[3]	1979	ITF approaches for tumors of the upper aerodigestive tract or intracranial tumors invading the ITF
Biller et al.[4]	1981	Median mandibulotomy
Sekhars et al.[5]	1987	Subtemporal-preauricular approach
Cocke et al.[6]	1990	Extended maxillotomy/ maxillectomy approach
Janecka et al.[7]	1990	Facial translocation approach
Catalano and Biller[8]	1993	Vascularized facial translocation

*Many other authors have contributed immensely to the advancement of surgery of the ITF. This table is intended to present an overview of what we consider novel approaches and is by no means comprehensive.

ITF, infratemporal fossa; SNT, sinonasal tract.

endotracheal intubation. Awake nasotracheal intubation may be performed in patients with constant trismus if it is anticipated that surgery will correct the trismus. Otherwise, awake tracheostomy should be performed at the beginning of surgery.

Facial nerve deficits may be manifested as facial weakness, epiphora, hyperacusis, hyperkinesis, and dysgeusia. The motor function of all divisions of the facial nerve is assessed. It is important to remember, however, that significant involvement of the facial nerve by tumor may occur before any facial weakness is clinically apparent. Deficits of the facial nerve or first division of the trigeminal nerve (V1), or both, may result in corneal exposure. Insertion of a gold weight in the upper eyelid or tightening of the lower lid may be necessary to protect the cornea and prevent future complications.

Hearing loss may be either conductive or sensorineural. Conductive hearing loss is usually a result of eustachian tube dysfunction with accumulation of fluid in the middle ear space. Sensorineural hearing loss may result from tumor involvement of the temporal bone or posterior cranial fossa. The presence of hearing loss may be helpful in localizing the tumor, especially when it is observed in combination with other cranial nerve deficits. Because hearing loss impairs effective communication with the patient during the perioperative period, the use of a hearing aid or other amplification device may be required for communication. It should be anticipated that extensive surgery involving the infratemporal skull base will result in a conductive hearing loss that may compound a previous sensorineural hearing loss.

Deficits of the lower cranial nerves (IX, X, XI, and XII) are seen with tumors that arise high in the parapharyngeal space near the jugular foramen. Patients may exhibit varying degrees of hypernasal speech, nasal regurgitation, dysphagia, aspiration, and dysphonia. Findings on physical examination include decreased elevation of the palate, decreased mobility of the tongue with deviation to the involved side on protrusion, pooling of secretions in the hypopharynx, decreased supraglottic sensation, ipsilateral vocal cord paralysis, and decreased prominence and strength of the sternocleidomastoid and trapezius muscles. In patients with incomplete lower cranial nerve deficits, surgical therapy can be expected to increase nerve dysfunction with resultant increased risks of dysphagia and aspiration. Consequently, a tracheostomy is often necessary in the perioperative period. Laryngeal framework surgery (thyroplasty) may be considered at the same time to improve glottic closure and decrease the risk of aspiration. Strong consideration should also be given to placement of a gastrostomy (percutaneous or open) to facilitate postoperative feeding and decrease the risk of aspiration. Palatal dysfunction may be ameliorated by a palatal lift prosthesis to push the soft palate against the posterior pharyngeal wall. Alternatively, a pharyngeal flap or surgical fixation of the palate to the pharyngeal wall (palatopexy) may be necessary.

Because of the relative inaccessibility of the infratemporal space to physical examination, radiologic imaging is an essential part of the evaluation. Both computed tomography (CT) and magnetic resonance imaging (MRI) provide valuable information and are performed with a standard skull base protocol. CT scanning provides adequate resolution of most tumors and is superior for demonstrating enlargement of neural foramina or erosion of bone. For most tumors involving the ITF, MRI provides better resolution of soft tissue planes and tumor invasion along neural and vascular structures (Fig. 101-1). CT and MRI are often complementary in the evaluation of cranial base tumors.

A critical question in the evaluation of tumors in this area is the relationship of the neoplasm to the internal carotid artery (ICA). Magnetic resonance angiography (MRA) may be used in selected cases to provide a noninvasive assessment of the ITF and intracranial vasculature. If preoperative embolization of the tumor is warranted, as is the case for many juvenile angiofibromas, paragangliomas, or other highly vascularized tumors, angiography is preferable to MRA because the tumor can be embolized during the initial angiogram (Fig. 101-2). In addition to yielding information about tumor vascularity and involvement of the ICA, angiography provides important information on the intracranial circulation and collateral blood supply. Neither study is adequate, however, to reliably assess the adequacy of collateral intracranial circulation in the event that manipulation or sacrifice of the ICA is necessary. Whenever manipulation of the ICA is likely, evaluation of collateral cerebral blood flow with angiography–balloon occlusion–xenon computed tomography (ABOX-CT) is recommended (Fig. 101-3).

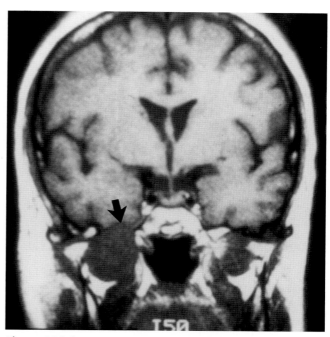

Figure 101-1. Magnetic resonance image demonstrating a neurilemmoma arising from the mandibular division of the trigeminal nerve (*arrow*). Although there is intracranial extension of the tumor, it is extradural. Tumors in this location may reach a large size before they are visible or palpable on physical examination. Such tumors may cause facial numbness, pain, or difficulty with mastication.

Briefly, ABOX-CT consists of the introduction of a nondetachable balloon into the ICA. The balloon is inflated for 15 minutes, and the awake patient is monitored for sensory, motor, or higher cortical function deficits. The balloon is deflated and the patient is transferred to a standard CT suite. The balloon is then reinflated and a mixture of 32% xenon and 68% oxygen is administered to the patient via facial mask for 4 minutes. The CT scan will demonstrate the distribution of xenon within cerebral tissue, which reflects blood flow (Fig. 101-4). This study provides a quantitative assessment of millimeters of blood flow per minute per 100 g of brain tissue. This test accurately predicts patients at risk for a cerebrovascular accident when blood flow through the ICA is compromised (Table 101-3).[9] It should be recognized that patients can still suffer ischemic brain injury despite negative ABOX-CT findings because of embolic phenomena or the loss of collateral vessels, which are not assessed by balloon occlusion testing. For these reasons, every attempt is made to preserve or reconstruct the ICA when feasible. Other techniques that provide similar information regarding collateral cerebral blood flow include single-photon emission computed tomography (SPECT) with balloon occlusion and transcranial Doppler monitoring.

Biopsy

Histologic confirmation is mandatory before subjecting the patient to any major extirpative surgery. Tissue is usually obtained by incisional or punch biopsy. Occa-

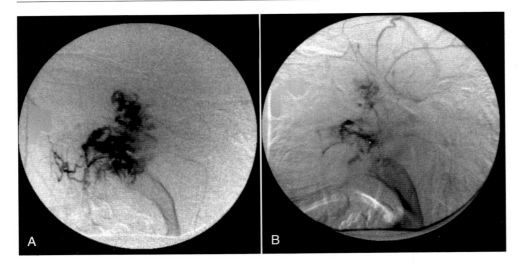

Figure 101-2. Angiography of the left internal maxillary artery in a patient with an angiofibroma demonstrates an extensive tumor blush (**A**) that is markedly decreased after embolization (**B**).

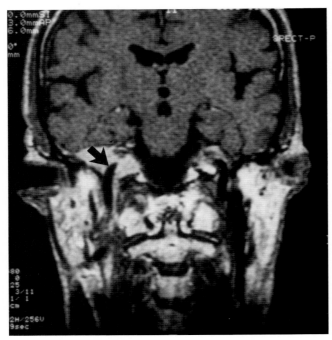

Figure 101-3. Magnetic resonance image demonstrating a neoplasm of the right infratemporal skull base that is encasing the petrous portion of the internal carotid artery (ICA) *(arrow)*. Preoperative evaluation of collateral cerebral blood flow with angiography–balloon occlusion–xenon computed tomography is recommended because of the increased risk of injury to the ICA with attempted removal of this tumor.

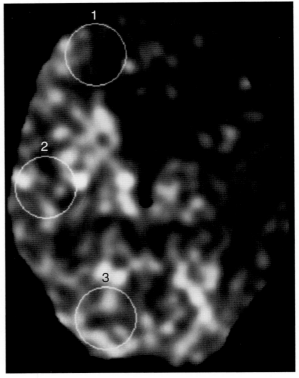

Figure 101-4. After balloon occlusion of the left internal carotid artery (ICA), a significant reduction in blood flow was noted in the distribution of the left anterior and middle cerebral arteries (1-3). This patient is at high risk for development of a stroke after permanent occlusion of the left ICA.

sionally, fine-needle aspiration biopsy under CT or MRI guidance is required for tumors arising in deep locations. Biopsy of many cranial base tumors can be performed with minimally invasive endoscopic approaches through the paranasal sinuses.

The surgeon should consider the possibility of metastasis to the cranial base when the tumor appears to originate from the bone and is in an unusual location. In such cases, a thorough history and physical examination will usually provide evidence of a primary

tumor elsewhere (breast, prostate, lung, or gastrointestinal system). Although the cost-effectiveness of an extensive search in asymptomatic patients is questionable, a screening test such as a mammogram or serum prostate-specific antigen level may be revealing. The search for a primary tumor or other metastases should be intensified when a biopsy reveals an adenocarcinoma that is not originating from a major salivary gland. "Intestinal-type" adenocarcinomas of the nasopharynx,

Table 101-3	XENON COMPUTED TOMOGRAPHY	
Cerebral Blood Flow (mL/min/ 100 g Tissue)	Risk	Implication
<20	High	Patient will not tolerate occlusion of the internal carotid artery
21-35	Moderate	Patient will tolerate occlusion under controlled circumstances; reconstruction is recommended
>35	Low	Carotid may be sacrificed

Table 101-4	STANDARD ANESTHETIC MONITORING
Electrocardiogram Pulse oximeter Capnometer Arterial line Central venous catheter*	
*In selected cases, a pulmonary artery catheter may be necessary.	

in particular, can be confusing and may necessitate thorough evaluation of the lower gastrointestinal tract.

Metastatic Workup

The extent of the evaluation to rule out regional or distant metastasis is dictated by the suspected histologic type and stage of the tumor. CT or MRI of the neck is considered more sensitive than physical examination for the detection of regional metastases. Patients with tumors showing a predilection for hematogenous metastasis (sarcomas, melanoma) should undergo a CT scan of the chest and abdomen and a bone scan. A positron emission tomographic (PET) scintigram may aid in identifying both the primary and metastatic tumors. A lumbar puncture for cerebrospinal fluid (CSF) cytology is reserved for patients with tumors invading the dura or with symptoms of "drop metastasis" to the spinal cord. Consultation with an experienced neurosurgeon is recommended for tumors invading the skull base or for tumors that require resection of the skull base for margins.

Reconstructive/Rehabilitation Considerations

Finally, the reconstructive requirements of oncologic surgery should be anticipated. In most cases, a temporalis muscle transposition flap is adequate to separate the cranial cavity from the upper aerodigestive tract and obliterate the dead space. Nevertheless, the use of microvascular free flaps such as the rectus abdominis flap (for soft tissue defects), latissimus dorsi flap (for myocutaneous or massive defects), or iliac and scapular composite flaps (for defects requiring bone reconstruction) is recommended when the temporalis muscle or its blood supply will be sacrificed, when the patient requires complex resection involving composite tissue flaps with skin or bone, or when the extirpative surgery produces a massive soft tissue defect and dead space.

Attention should also be directed to functional and cosmetic deficits created by the tumor and surgery. Facial rehabilitation may be achieved during the primary surgery. When a temporary facial palsy is anticipated, corneal protection with lubricants or a temporary lateral tarsorrhaphy is generally adequate. When grafting of the facial nerve is necessary and a longer period of recovery of facial nerve function is expected, implantation of a gold weight into the upper eyelid is performed. If reconstruction of the facial nerve is not feasible, static fascial slings or muscle transpositions are appropriate. Lower cranial nerve deficits may be ameliorated by laryngeal framework surgery, tracheotomy, or laryngotracheal separation.

PREOPERATIVE PLANNING

The patient is premedicated with a short-acting benzodiazepine. Narcotics may be used in the absence of elevated intracranial pressure. Preoperative steroids are administered if manipulation of the brain or motor cranial nerves is anticipated. H_2-blockers or proton pump inhibitors are given perioperatively to decrease the incidence of gastroesophageal reflux and stress ulcers. If retraction of the temporal lobe is necessary, prophylactic anticonvulsants are administered during surgery and in the postoperative period.

Preoperatively, the patient's blood is typed and cross-matched for 4 to 6 units of packed red blood cells or cryoprecipitate. A Cell Saver/autotransfusion device may be used when the tumor is benign and there is no contamination by flora of the upper aerodigestive tract.

Perioperative antibiotic prophylaxis that provides coverage against the flora of the skin and upper aerodigestive tract and exhibits good penetration of the blood-brain barrier is administered 2 hours before surgery and continued for 48 hours after the surgery is completed. The use of a broad-spectrum cephalosporin with good CSF penetration (e.g., ceftriaxone) appears to be as effective as multiple antibiotic regimens.

The patient is taken to the operating room, and all standard monitoring electrodes and lines are placed and secured (Table 101-4). The choice of anesthetic agent depends on the extent of intracranial dissection and the potential for brain injury, systemic hemodynamics, the need for monitoring of cortical and brain stem functions (e.g., brain stem evoked response, somatosensory evoked potentials, electroencephalography), and the need for cranial nerve monitoring (7th and 10th through 12th cranial nerves). Somatosensory evoked potential monitoring using the median nerve is indicated whenever surgical manipulation of the ICA is anticipated.

When changes in head position during surgery are anticipated, the endotracheal tube is secured with a circumdental or circum-mandibular wire ligature (no. 26 stainless steel wire). The operating table is positioned perpendicular and away from the anesthetic equipment. If significant brain retraction or intradural dissection is expected, a spinal drain is placed and secured with sutures and adhesive dressing (e.g., Tegaderm, Op-Site). Other measures to diminish intracranial pressure, such as hyperventilation, osmotic diuresis, or steroids, are used as needed throughout surgery. A nasogastric tube and Foley catheter are passed and secured after adequate placement is corroborated. Antiembolic sequential compression stockings are mandatory to diminish the risk for deep venous thrombosis. Heparin is not recommended because of the potential for increased intracranial bleeding.

The head of the patient is positioned on a Mayfield horseshoe head holder or, if necessary for intracranial neurovascular work, on Mayfield pins. When the horseshoe is used, it is important that additional "egg crate" foam padding be used, because scalp ischemia may result from the hard rubber pads during prolonged surgery. The head should be positioned in slight extension to provide access to the neck for proximal control of the ICA. Monitoring electrodes are carefully placed and secured with sutures or staples. A baseline recording is obtained for intraoperative reference. Tarsorrhaphy sutures are placed for protection of the eyes. Ribbon gauze or pledgets soaked in oxymetazoline (0.05%) solution may be inserted intranasally at this time for additional hemostasis if communication with the nasal cavity is anticipated. The proposed incision lines are infiltrated with local anesthetic containing epinephrine (1:200,000). The hair is parted with a comb and held in place with staples. Standard skin preparation with povidone-iodine (Betadine) solution is performed.

SURGICAL TECHNIQUE

Preauricular (Subtemporal) Approach

This approach is suited for tumors arising in the ITF and intracranial tumors arising in boundaries of the anterior temporal bone or greater wing of the sphenoid bone and extending into the ITF.[10-13] The preauricular approach does not allow safe resection of any portions of the tympanic bone or control of the infratemporal facial nerve or jugular bulb.

A hemicoronal or bicoronal incision across the vertex of the scalp and posterior to the hairline is extended through the subcutaneous tissue, galea, and pericranium over the cranium (Fig. 101-5A). In the temporal area, the incision extends down to the deep layer of the temporal fascia overlying the temporalis muscle. Ipsilateral to the tumor, the incision is extended into the preauricular area. A separate incision may be made in the neck for proximal control of the carotid arteries (see Fig 101-5B).

The scalp flap is elevated anteriorly in a subpericranial plane to separate attachments of the pericranium

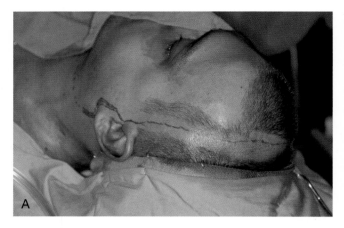

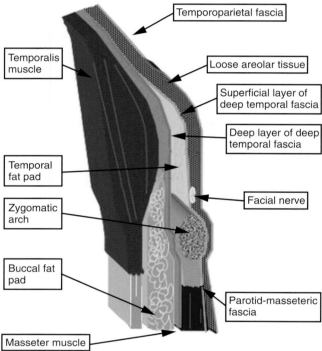

Figure 101-5. **A,** A hemicoronal scalp incision is made posterior to the hairline in the temporal area and extended along a preauricular skin crease, similar to a parotidectomy incision. It may be continued into the upper cervical region, or a separate cervical incision may be made for exposure of the vessels and nerves. **B,** The different tissue planes of the temporal area are illustrated. The frontal branch of the facial nerve is found in the superficial layer of the deep temporal fascia. Safe dissection must occur deep to this plane.

to the deep layer of the temporal fascia at the margin of the temporalis muscle down to the level of the superior orbital rim. The anterior branches of the superficial temporal artery are preserved to ensure adequate blood supply to the scalp flap. The scalp flap is easily elevated from the deep temporal fascia with a broad periosteal elevator. Approximately 1 to 2 cm above the zygoma the fascia splits into superficial and deep layers that attach to the lateral and medial surfaces of the zygomatic arch, respectively. This creates a triangular

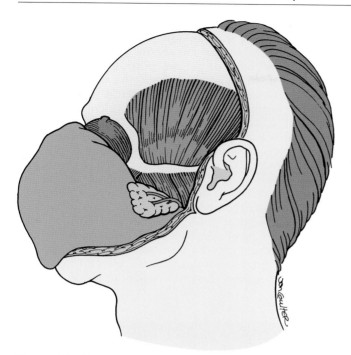

Figure 101-6. The scalp flap is elevated from the underlying cranium, deep temporal fascia, lateral orbital rim and zygomatic arch, and masseteric fascia. The plane of dissection is deep to the parotid gland and the temporal branches of the facial nerve. *(Redrawn from Sekhar LN, Janecka IP [eds]: Surgery of Cranial Base Tumors. New York, Raven Press, 1993.)*

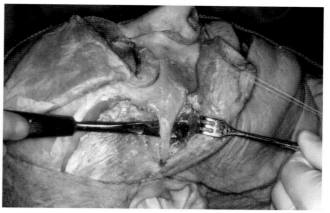

Figure 101-7. In this cadaver dissection, the masseteric fascia and other fascial attachments to the zygomatic arch are separated after elevation of the facial soft tissues from the superficial surface of the masseteric fascia. This frees the zygomatic arch for performance of the osteotomy.

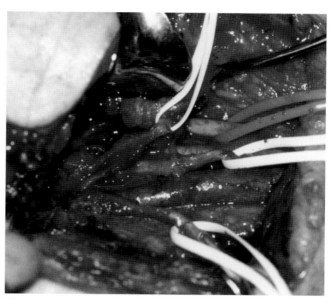

Figure 101-8. The nerves and vessels of the right upper cervical region have been isolated in this patient (left superior). White vessel loops are placed around the hypoglossal, vagus, and spinal accessory nerves. A dark vessel loop is placed around the internal carotid artery.

space filled with adipose tissue. The superficial layer of the deep temporal fascia is incised obliquely above the level of the superior orbital rim toward the zygomatic root. Dissection is then carried deep to this plane, and the superficial layer of the deep temporal fascia and the adipose tissue are elevated off the zygomatic arch and reflected anteriorly with the flap. The orbitozygomatic complex is exposed by subperiosteal dissection. This maneuver protects the frontal branches of the facial nerve that are superficial to the superficial layer of the deep temporal fascia (Fig. 101-6). Periosteum is elevated from the lateral surface of the zygomatic arch and malar eminence. The periorbita is elevated from the lateral orbit with a Freer or Adson elevator to expose the area from the roof of the orbit to the inferior orbital fissure. It is helpful to separate the masseteric fascia from the overlying parotid gland with a broad periosteal elevator before detaching the masseter muscle from the zygomatic arch (Fig. 101-7). The masseteric fascia is transected at its insertion into the zygomatic arch, and the periosteal elevator is then used to separate it from the muscle while leaving it attached to the deep surface of the parotid.

All soft tissue anterior to the temporal bone can be transected to the level of the facial nerve pedicle to increase the arc of rotation of the flap. The facial nerve is identified and preserved with a standard technique (see Chapter 62). It is helpful to leave a pedicle of soft tissue around the facial nerve trunk to prevent excessive traction injury to the facial nerve with retraction of the

facial flap. The attachments of the temporalis and masseter muscles to the zygomatic arch are transected with electrocautery. Using the caudal limb of the incision, the sternocleidomastoid muscle is dissected laterally and the carotid sheath is exposed. The internal, common, and external carotid arteries, as well as the internal jugular vein, are exposed, dissected, and controlled. Cranial nerves X through XII are identified and preserved. Vessel loops are placed around the structures and secured with hemoclips rather than hemostats to avoid inadvertent traction on a hemostat (Fig. 101-8).

The attachments of the temporalis muscle to the pericranium are transected with electrocautery, and the muscle is elevated off the temporal fossa. If the muscle will be returned to its original position at the completion of surgery, a few millimeters of fascia may be left attached to the cranium at the margin of the muscle to facilitate suturing of the muscle. The temporal muscle is then reflected inferiorly until the infratemporal crest is fully visualized. Bleeding from underlying bone is usually encountered and controlled by the application of bone wax. Care should be exercised when dissecting on the deep surface of the temporalis muscle near its attachment to the mandible because the blood supply to the muscle (deep temporal arteries from the internal maxillary artery) may be injured. Dissection of soft tissue from the infratemporal skull base is associated with troublesome bleeding from the pterygoid plexus. It can be controlled with bipolar electrocautery and the application of hemostatic materials. A subtemporal craniectomy is performed at this time to aid in identification and exposure of the neural and vascular foramina. The coronoid process can be fractured or removed to increase the inferior arc of rotation of the temporal muscle. It is important to protect the soft tissue at the sigmoid notch to prevent accidental injury to the internal maxillary artery at the point where it travels on the medial surface of the mandibular ramus.

The orbitozygomatic bone graft is freed by osteotomies at the zygomatic root posteriorly, the zygomaticofrontal suture superiorly, and the zygomaticomaxillary buttress at the level of the zygomaticofacial nerve medially (Figs. 101-9 and 101-10). A reciprocating saw is used to make beveled and V-shaped bone cuts to maximize exposure and facilitate replacement of the bone graft at the completion of surgery. If there is tumor involvement of the orbit, the bone cut through the lateral wall of the orbit may include only the orbital rim to avoid violation of the tumor. For lesions that do not involve the temporal bone or petrous portion of the ICA, this approach provides adequate exposure to the infratemporal skull base. If dissection of the ICA throughout its petrous portion is necessary, the glenoid fossa is removed as part of the bone graft. It is first necessary to perform a temporal craniotomy for exposure of the superior aspect of the glenoid fossa (Fig. 101-11). The capsule of the TMJ is dissected free from the fossa and displaced inferiorly. If possible, the capsule and meniscus are preserved. If additional exposure is necessary, the mandibular condyle can be transected at the level of the sigmoid notch and removed (Fig. 101-12). Using a reciprocating saw, a V-shaped cut is then made through the bone of the glenoid fossa to incorporate approximately the lateral two thirds of the glenoid fossa (Fig. 101-13). This avoids potential injury to the ICA, which

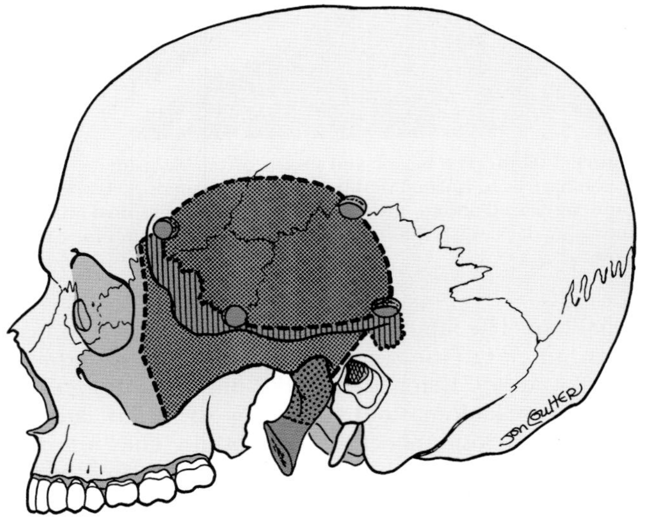

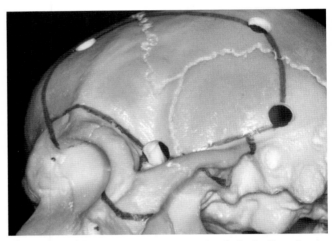

Figure 101-10. In this plastic model of a skull, the lines for the craniotomy and orbitozygomatic osteotomy are marked. If it is not necessary to remove the glenoid fossa, the zygomatic arch is transected posteriorly at its attachment to the cranium.

Figure 101-9. The areas of bone removal are noted *(dark stippled area).* A temporal craniotomy is performed in conjunction with an orbitozygomatic osteotomy. This illustration demonstrates transection of the zygomatic arch anterior to its posterior attachment and preservation of the lateral orbital rim. Additional exposure of the infratemporal skull base may be achieved by removal of the subtemporal cranium *(striped area)* and resection of the mandibular condyle *(light stippled area).*

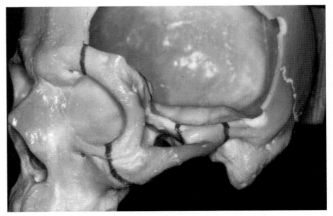

Figure 101-11. A temporal craniotomy has been performed to provide adequate exposure for osteotomies through the glenoid fossa and orbital walls.

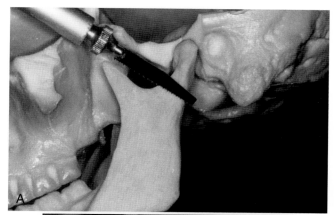

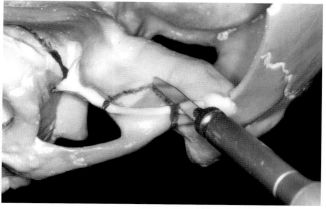

Figure 101-13. The lateral two thirds of the glenoid fossa is removed by performing osteotomies with a reciprocating saw. Care is taken to avoid injury to the internal carotid artery medially and the cochlea posteriorly.

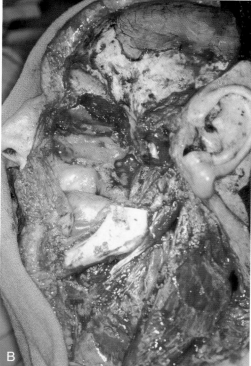

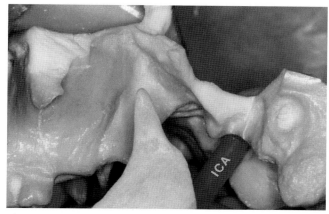

Figure 101-14. The location of the internal carotid artery (plastic tube) is noted in this model to be medial to the mandible and the glenoid fossa.

Figure 101-12. A, An osteotomy of the mandibular condyle is performed with a reciprocating saw to provide additional exposure. **B,** Removal of the coronoid process in conjunction with the condyle provides further exposure and facilitates rotation of the temporalis muscle.

is located medial to the glenoid fossa (Fig. 101-14). If the bone cut is made too posteriorly, there is risk of injury to the cochlea. This modification provides better stability for the mandibular condyle after reconstruction.

Elevation of the periorbita from the lateral and inferior walls of the orbit is necessary to identify the inferior orbital fissure and complete the orbitozygomatic osteotomies (Fig. 101-15). The tip of the reciprocating saw is placed in the most lateral aspect of the inferior orbital fissure along the orbital floor, and an osteotomy through the malar eminence is performed (Fig. 101-16). This separates the zygoma from the lateral

wall of the maxilla. On occasion, violation of the maxillary sinus may occur, especially if the maxilla is well pneumatized. If this happens, the mucosal remnant attached to the zygoma is removed. Adequate closure of the maxillary defect is achieved after replacement of the orbitozygomatic bone segment at the completion of surgery. It is not necessary to strip the mucosa from the remainder of the sinus. Using both intracranial and extracranial approaches, osteotomies are made through the superior and lateral orbital walls to completely free the orbitozygomatic bone segment (Fig. 101-17). This provides excellent access to the infratemporal skull base, orbital apex, and lateral maxilla (Fig. 101-18).

Several anatomic relationships are useful for identification of infratemporal skull base structures (Fig. 101-19). After completion of the temporal craniotomy, additional bone is removed from the inferior margin of the defect with rongeurs (see Fig. 101-9). The origin of the lateral pterygoid plate from the skull base is identified anteriorly. The curve of the lateral pterygoid plate

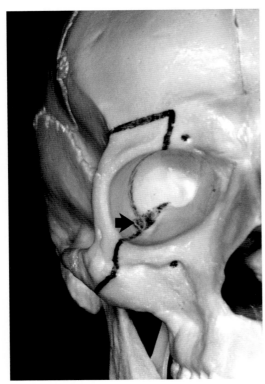

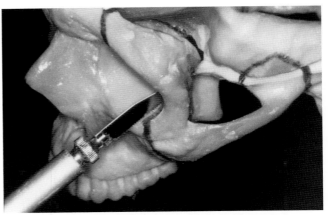

Figure 101-16. An osteotomy is made from the inferior orbital fissure across the malar eminence and lateral to the maxilla.

Figure 101-15. The osteotomies communicate with the lateral aspect of the inferior orbital fissure *(arrow).*

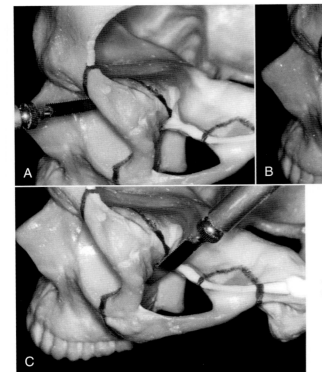

Figure 101-17. With the use of intracranial and extracranial approaches, osteotomies of the superior orbital roof (**A** and **B**) and lateral orbital wall (**C**) are performed.

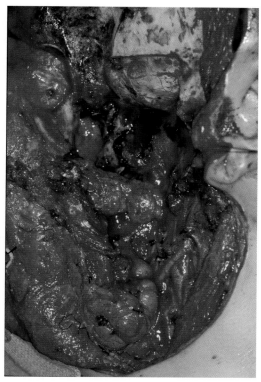

Figure 101-18. Extent of exposure after a temporal craniotomy and orbitozygomatic osteotomy.

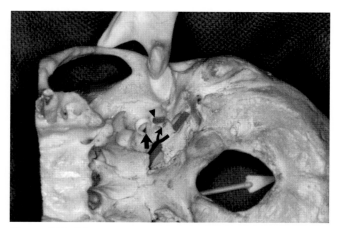

Figure 101-19. Skull demonstrating the anatomic relationships of the internal carotid artery (ICA) and carotid canal. The foramen ovale (*straight arrow;* white vessel loop) and foramen spinosum (*arrowhead;* short dark vessel loop) are in a direct line from the lateral pterygoid plate to the spine of the sphenoid. The ICA (long dark vessel loop) courses through the carotid canal medial to the eustachian tube (*curved arrow*) and the glenoid fossa. The mandible has been disarticulated to reveal the glenoid fossa.

is followed posteriorly to identify the foramen ovale, foramen spinosum, and the spine of the sphenoid bone. These structures lie in a straight line and are all lateral to the ICA. The middle meningeal artery is cauterized with bipolar electrocautery and transected. Bleeding from venous communications through the foramen

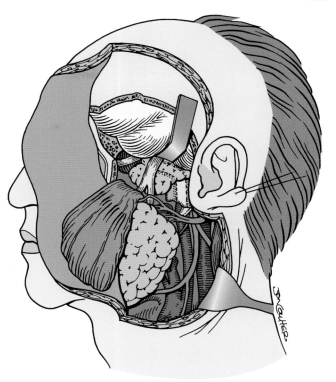

Figure 101-20. Illustration demonstrating a tumor medial to the mandibular division of the trigeminal nerve and in close proximity to the petrous portion of the internal carotid artery (ICA). Additional exposure of the ICA and removal of the tumor often necessitate transection of the mandibular division of the trigeminal nerve. *(Redrawn from Sekhar LN, Janecka IP [eds]: Surgery of Cranial Base Tumors. New York, Raven Press, 1993.)*

ovale may be controlled with Surgicel packing. If complete dissection of the petrous portion of the ICA is required, it is usually necessary to transect the mandibular division of the trigeminal nerve at the foramen ovale for additional exposure (Fig. 101-20). The lateral aspect of the sphenoid sinus may be accessed by removal of bone between the second and third divisions of the trigeminal nerve (Fig. 101-21). Extirpation of the tumor can now proceed, including the involved soft tissue and bone (Fig. 101-22). For tumors invading the mandible, partial mandibulectomy is essential to obtain negative margins. In the pediatric age group, the distance from the body of the mandible to the infratemporal skull base is greatly foreshortened. Adequate exposure of the infratemporal skull base can often be achieved from a transcervical approach with superior displacement of the facial nerve (Fig. 101-23).

After extirpation of the tumor, it is necessary to close any defects that are communicating with the upper aerodigestive tract (Fig. 101-24). If the blood supply to the temporalis muscle is preserved, transposition of the temporalis muscle provides obliteration of the dead space, as well as protection of the ICA (Fig. 101-25). Because of the branching pattern of the blood supply to the temporalis muscle, the anterior one half

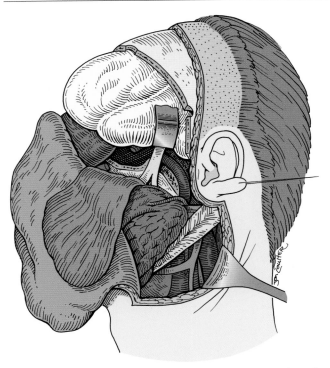

Figure 101-21. Illustration demonstrating an opening into the sphenoid sinus medial to the transected second division of the trigeminal nerve. A segment of the petrous portion of the internal carotid artery has been exposed. *(Redrawn from Sekhar LN, Janecka IP [eds]: Surgery of Cranial Base Tumors. New York, Raven Press, 1993.)*

or lateral portion of the muscle may be transposed with its blood supply intact (Fig. 101-26). The remaining portion of the muscle is used to fill in the anterior portion of the temporal defect. Defects of the orbit may be obliterated by temporalis muscle transposition with skin grafting (Fig. 101-27). In some circumstances, anteriorly or posteriorly based pericranial scalp flaps may be elevated to provide protection of the infratemporal skull base. In the absence of the temporalis muscle, large soft tissue defects are best reconstructed with microvascular free tissue transfers (Fig. 101-28). The orbitozygomatic bone graft is then replaced and held in position with titanium microplates. If resection of the mandibular condyle is necessary for exposure of the petrous ICA, reconstruction of the TMJ is not attempted. Reconstruction has not been shown to improve postoperative function and may actually contribute to scarring and postoperative trismus. Standard closure of soft tissues is performed.

Postauricular (Transtemporal) Approach

The postauricular approach is ideal for lesions involving the temporal bone and extending into the ITF.[10,11] A "question mark" or C-shaped incision is started in the temporal area, extended postauricularly into the mastoid region, and curved down to follow one of the midneck horizontal skin creases (Fig. 101-29). If middle ear function is going to be sacrificed as part of the approach or tumor resection and there is a risk of a postoperative CSF leakage, the EAC is closed permanently to prevent CSF otorrhea. The EAC is divided

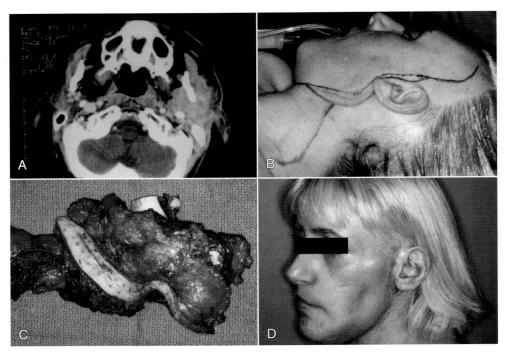

Figure 101-22. A, Computed tomography scan demonstrating recurrent adenocarcinoma of the left infratemporal fossa that is encasing the mandible and extending to the lateral aspect of the internal carotid artery (ICA). **B,** A left infratemporal skull base approach was used with excision of the previous scar. **C,** The resected specimen included the ramus and condyle of the mandible, the parotid gland and associated soft tissue, the pterygoid musculature, and the left neck contents. The medial limit of the resection was the extracranial portion of the ICA. **D,** Excellent healing of the surgical site is noted after completion of postoperative neutron beam therapy. Some permanent hair loss has occurred secondary to the radiation therapy.

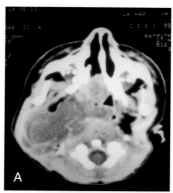

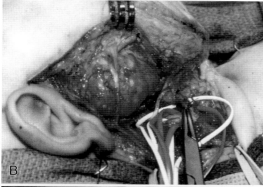

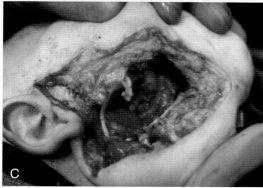

Figure 101-23. A, A 4-month-old infant had a large teratoma of the right parapharyngeal space with extension to the skull base and into the cervical region. **B** and **C,** The tumor was successfully removed via a transcervical approach, with preservation of facial nerve function.

procedure (Fig. 101-31). An incision within the EAC is not used because it is difficult to suture and obtain a watertight closure and there is a risk of postoperative stenosis. A Penrose drain can be inserted through the defect in the skin flap to provide gentle retraction (Fig. 101-32). The remaining conchal bowl and tragus may be sutured together temporarily to provide better exposure of the operative field.

The cervicofacial flap is elevated in a subplatysmal plane in the cervical area, lateral to the plane of the superficial aponeurotic system (SMAS) over the parotid area, and along the deep layer of the deep temporal fascia over the cranium. It is then reflected anteriorly (Fig. 101-33).

Dissection continues anterior to the EAC to identify the main trunk of the facial nerve, as done during parotidectomy (see Chapter 62). If the facial nerve does not need to be mobilized, a cuff of soft tissue is left around the facial nerve to minimize direct traction on the nerve when the facial flap is retracted anteriorly. In select cases, an inferior superficial parotidectomy ("tail parotidectomy") may enhance exposure of the retromandibular area. Attention is then directed to the neck to identify and obtain proximal control of the common, internal, and external carotid arteries, as well as the internal jugular vein. Cranial nerves X through XII are identified and preserved. The sternocleidomastoid and digastric muscles are transected at their insertion into the mastoid bone. The stylohyoid and stylopharyngeus muscles are transected and the styloid process is removed. The ninth cranial nerve can usually be identified at this time as it crosses lateral to the ICA.

Mastoidectomy and dissection of the vertical portion of the facial nerve allow superior translocation of the nerve to provide wider access to the ITF (Fig. 101-34). It also permits access to the jugular bulb and lower cranial nerves. Completion of the infratemporal skull base approach, including a temporal craniotomy and orbitozygomatic osteotomy, is performed as described in the previous section. At this time, the anterior, superior, medial, and posterior boundaries of the ITF are well exposed, and all major vessels are "controlled" (Fig. 101-35). Extirpation of the tumor can now proceed, including the involved soft tissue and bone. Reconstruction of the defect is performed as discussed previously.

Anterior Transfacial Approach (Facial Translocation)

This approach is best used for lesions invading the ITF, the masticator space, or the pterygomaxillary fossa and for tumors of the nasopharynx extending into the ITF[10,11] (Fig. 101-36) (see Chapter 105). A bicoronal incision with an ipsilateral preauricular extension is performed and extended through the subcutaneous tissue (see "Preauricular [Subtemporal] Approach" earlier in this chapter). A Weber-Fergusson incision is completed and extended down to the periosteum. A

at the bony–cartilaginous junction and then closed with everting stitches. This closure is reinforced with a myoperiosteal U-shaped flap based on the posterior margin of the EAC. Occasionally, closure of the EAC may be necessary in patients with a preexisting tympanotomy tube. Alternatively, the canal may be preserved by placing the incisions in the conchal area (Fig. 101-30). The incision follows the margin of the conchal bowl and tragus so that the scar will be camouflaged. In the conchal area, the skin, cartilage, and perichondrium are incised to communicate with the retroauricular plane of dissection. These incisions allow anastomosis of the EAC to the pinna at the end of the extirpative

Text continues on page 1014.

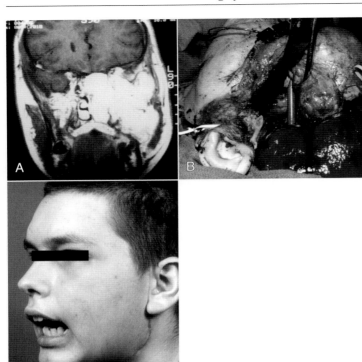

Figure 101-24. A, Preoperative magnetic resonance image demonstrating a large angiofibroma extending from the nasopharynx to the left infratemporal skull base. **B,** This tumor was completely excised by subtemporal craniectomy from a left infratemporal skull base approach. A marking pen has been inserted through the nasal cavity to show the extent of the communication with the nasopharynx. **C,** Excellent healing of the surgical site is noted postoperatively with no cosmetic deformity. Moderate trismus with mild deviation of the jaw is present.

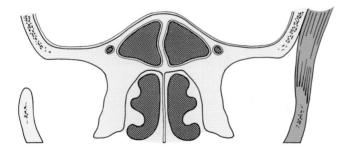

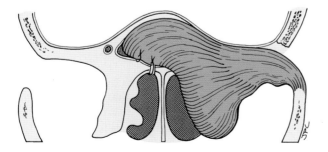

Figure 101-25. The entire temporalis muscle is available for obliteration of a defect in the orbit or infratemporal skull base. *(Redrawn from Sekhar LN, Janecka IP [eds]: Surgery of Cranial Base Tumors. New York, Raven Press, 1993.)*

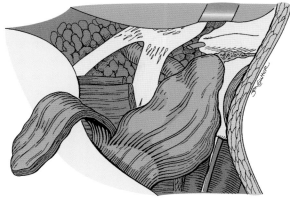

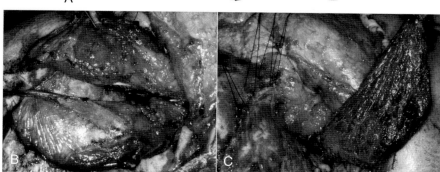

Figure 101-26. A, The anterior portion of the muscle may be transposed to fill an infratemporal skull base defect, as illustrated with this left temporalis muscle. **B,** The right temporalis muscle has been split vertically with preservation of its axial blood supply. **C,** The posterior one half of the muscle is sutured to the fascia or bone bordering the superior temporal line and lateral orbital rim to prevent a cosmetic defect.

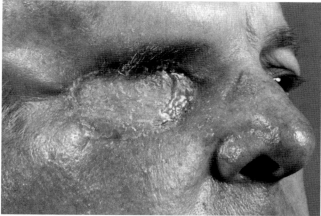

Figure 101-27. This patient required orbital exenteration and resection of the lateral orbital wall for recurrent squamous cell carcinoma. The defect was reconstructed by temporalis muscle transposition and a skin graft.

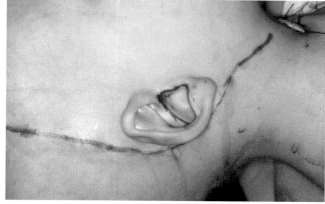

Figure 101-29. A curvilinear incision is made from the temporal area to the mastoid bone and upper cervical region. The flap is elevated superficial to the deep temporal fascia, deep to the mastoid periosteum, and deep to the platysma muscle. A conchal incision is preferable to incision of the external auditory canal when permanent obliteration of the ear is not indicated.

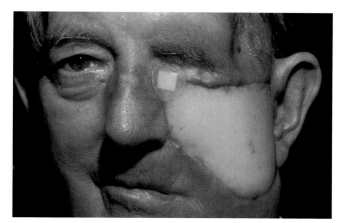

Figure 101-28. Large soft tissue defects are best reconstructed by microvascular free tissue transfer, most commonly the rectus abdominis muscle.

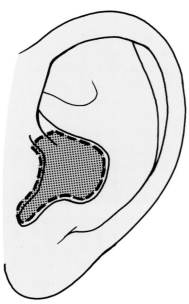

Figure 101-30. The conchal incision is made at the margins of the conchal bowl to facilitate closure and provide an optimal cosmetic result.

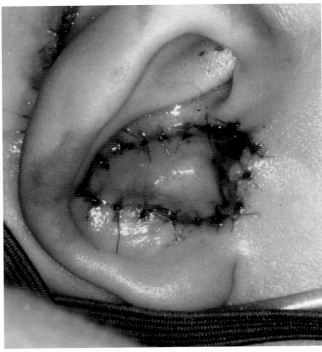

Figure 101-31. The auricle is repaired by double-layer closure of the perichondrium and skin. A watertight closure is achieved to prevent cerebrospinal fluid otorrhea.

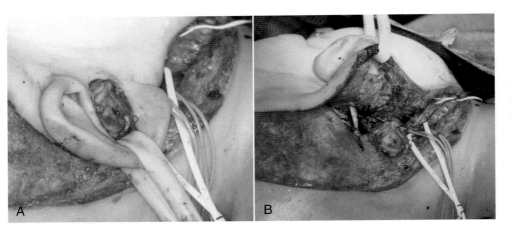

Figure 101-32. The conchal incision communicates with the postauricular incision (**A**), and a Penrose drain is used to retract the auricle and facial flap anteriorly (**B**).

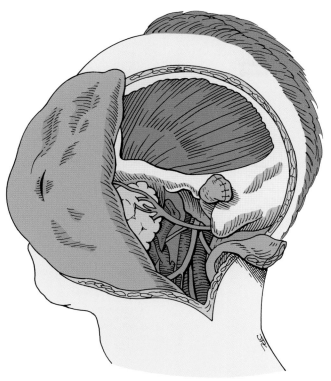

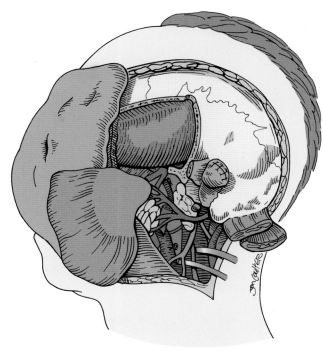

Figure 101-33. The facial flap is reflected anteriorly with exposure of the temporalis muscle, orbitozygomatic bone, masseteric fascia, mandible, parotid gland and facial nerve, and cervical vessels and nerves. The conchal tissues of the auricle are temporarily sewn together to maximize operative exposure.

Figure 101-35. The extent of surgical exposure is demonstrated after temporal craniotomy and reflection of the temporalis muscle inferiorly.

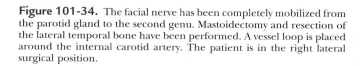

Figure 101-34. The facial nerve has been completely mobilized from the parotid gland to the second genu. Mastoidectomy and resection of the lateral temporal bone have been performed. A vessel loop is placed around the internal carotid artery. The patient is in the right lateral surgical position.

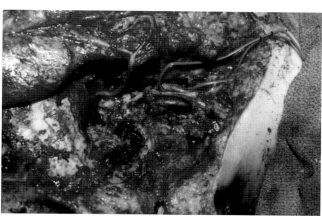

Figure 101-36. A and **B,** Computed tomography scans demonstrating a large ameloblastic fibrosarcoma of the left maxilla with extension into the infratemporal fossa. The anterior transfacial approach is ideally suited for excision of such lesions.

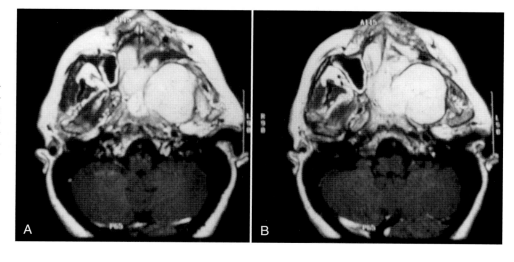

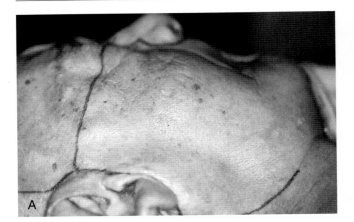

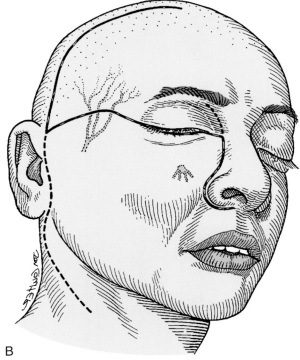

Figure 101-37. A and B, A hemicoronal incision is combined with an extended Weber-Fergusson incision in the anterior transfacial approach. The incision may be made through the conjunctiva or through the skin several millimeters inferior to the ciliary line.

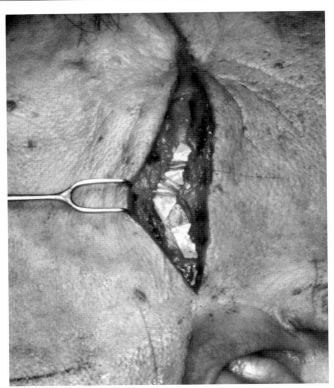

Figure 101-38. Multiple temporal branches of the facial nerve are identified and entubulated with silicone tubes before transection. This facilitates anastomosis of the nerves at the end of the procedure.

horizontal incision is carried over the superior edge of the zygomatic bone and extended into the lateral canthus to meet the Weber-Fergusson incision (Fig. 101-37). The frontal branches of the facial nerve are identified and dissected as they cross over the zygomatic arch. They are then entubulated with silicone tubing and transected. These nerve branches will be reanastomosed at the end of the procedure with an entubulation technique (Fig. 101-38). An inferiorly based flap that includes the upper third of the upper lip, the entire cheek, the lower eyelid, the parotid gland, and the facial nerve is reflected inferiorly. The infraorbital nerve is transected and tagged to facilitate reanastomosis at the end of the procedure. The frontotemporal

scalp flap is elevated in a subpericranial plane. This flap is reflected anteriorly to expose the superior orbital rims (Fig. 101-39).

Orbitozygomatic osteotomies are performed and joined with unilateral maxillary Le Fort II or Le Fort III osteotomies to free the anterior face of the maxilla en bloc with the orbitozygomatic complex. Alternatively, this bone graft can be elevated as a vascularized graft attached to the cheek flap, as described by Catalano and Biller.[8] The temporal and masseter muscles are dissected from the zygomatic bone with electrocautery. Osteotomies are completed, and the bone graft is removed (Fig. 101-40). The temporalis muscle is reflected inferiorly. An osteotomy or removal of the coronoid process increases the caudal arc of rotation of the temporalis muscle. At this time, the anterior, medial, and lateral boundaries of the ITF are well exposed (Fig. 101-41). In select cases, the pterygoid plates can be excised to provide further access to the medial ITF or nasopharynx. A temporal-subtemporal craniotomy provides additional exposure superiorly and allows dissection of intracranial structures (Fig. 101-42). After tumor resection, the temporalis muscle may be transposed to obliterate the surgical defect and provide separation of the cranial cavity from the upper aerodigestive tract (Fig. 101-43).

The incisions are closed in a multilayer technique. The conjunctiva is repaired with running 6-0 mild

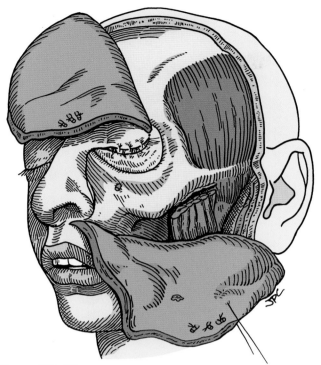

Figure 101-39. The scalp and facial flaps are elevated from the underlying bone and muscle fascia to expose the facial skeleton. The inferior orbital nerve is transected but tagged for later reconstruction.

chromic suture. The lacrimal canaliculi are stented with Crawford silicone tubing secured in the nasal cavity. The eye is closed with a temporary tarsorrhaphy for 10 to 14 days to prevent lower lid ectropion.

Transorbital Approach

In select cases, a transorbital approach may be used for optimal exposure of the orbital apex and cavernous sinus. This approach consists of transection of the orbital tissues posterior to the globe with preservation of the attachments of the superficial orbital structures, including the globe, to the scalp flap.

The tissues of the orbital apex and surrounding bone are then removed to provide direct anterior access to the cavernous sinus and cavernous ICA. This approach is reserved for patients with benign tumors of the orbital apex and cavernous sinus who have already lost vision as a result of tumor growth (Fig. 101-44). It may also be used for limited malignant neoplasms with minimal involvement of the orbital tissues. More extensive involvement of the orbital tissues requires orbital exenteration. The advantages of this approach are an improved cosmetic result with preservation of the globe and excellent anterior and lateral exposure of the cavernous sinus and its associated structures.

A preauricular infratemporal skull base approach is used. After elevation of the scalp flap (Fig. 101-45), an orbitozygomatic osteotomy is performed (Fig. 101-46).

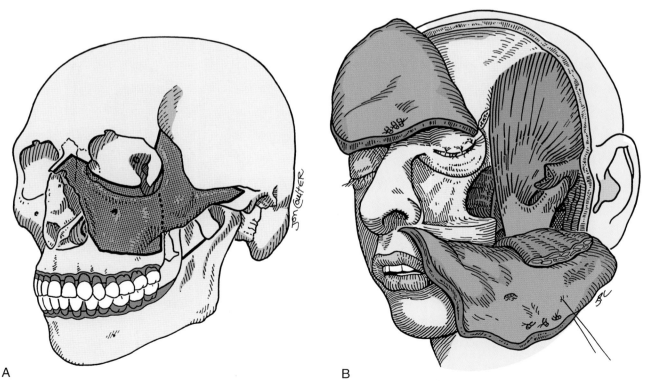

A   B

Figure 101-40. A, Segments of the facial skeleton that are removed en bloc with the anterior transfacial approach. **B,** Exposure provided by this approach.

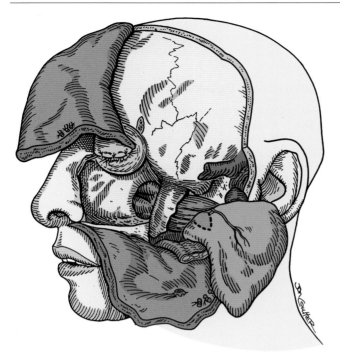

Figure 101-41. After transection of the coronoid process of the mandible and reflection of the temporalis muscle inferiorly, the infratemporal skull base, maxilla, and nasopharynx are well exposed.

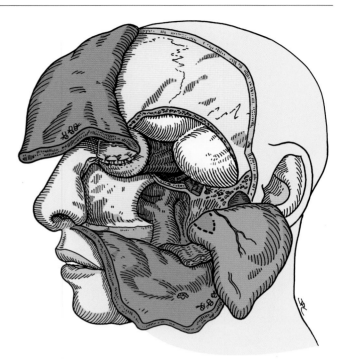

Figure 101-42. A subtemporal craniectomy is performed to provide additional exposure and an adequate resection margin of extracranial tumors. Maximal exposure of the infratemporal and central skull base is achieved.

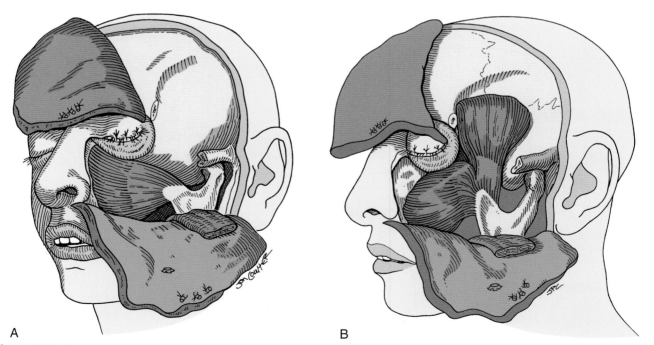

A   B

Figure 101-43. The entire temporalis muscle (**A**) or the anterior one half of the muscle (**B**) may be transposed to obliterate the surgical defect and provide separation of the cranial cavity from the upper aerodigestive tract. If the temporalis muscle is not available because of loss of its blood supply, microvascular free flap reconstruction is indicated.

Figure 101-44. Magnetic resonance image **(A)** and computed tomography scan **(B)** demonstrating a meningioma involving the lateral wall of the orbit with extension to the orbital apex and middle cranial fossa. If the patient has permanent visual loss as a result of such a tumor, a transorbital approach may be used.

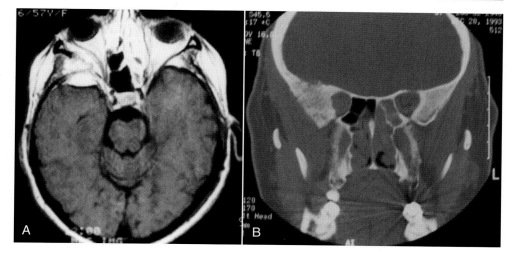

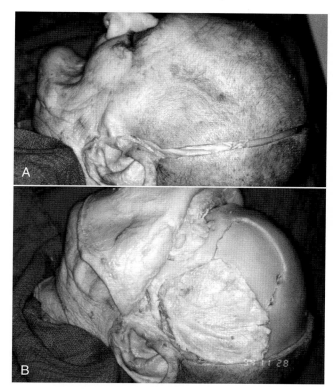

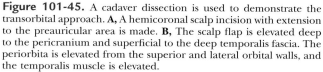

Figure 101-45. A cadaver dissection is used to demonstrate the transorbital approach. **A,** A hemicoronal scalp incision with extension to the preauricular area is made. **B,** The scalp flap is elevated deep to the pericranium and superficial to the deep temporalis fascia. The periorbita is elevated from the superior and lateral orbital walls, and the temporalis muscle is elevated.

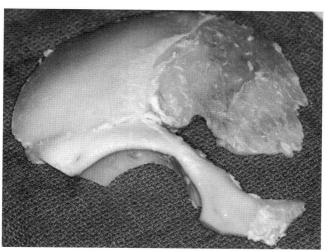

Figure 101-46. A frontotemporal craniotomy and orbitozygomatic osteotomy are performed to provide direct lateral access to the orbital tissues and cavernous sinus region.

The periorbita is elevated from the superior, lateral, and inferior walls of the orbit. The periorbita is then incised, and orbital tissues are transected posterior to the globe with bipolar electrocautery and sharp dissection. A cuff of tissue remains at the orbital apex to provide an adequate tumor margin. The remaining periorbital attachments are then elevated medially to allow complete displacement of the globe from the

orbital cavity (Fig. 101-47). Using rongeurs, bone is removed from the lateral wall of the orbit to the superior orbital fissure. The contents of the superior orbital fissure and the optic canal are then transected to provide additional exposure of the orbital apex (Fig. 101-48). Further removal of bone and dissection of intracranial structures are performed in conjunction with the neurosurgeon.

Because of loss of orbital support, enophthalmos results unless the orbital defect is reconstructed with bone grafts or soft tissue is interposed. A temporalis transposition or free tissue transfer provides excellent soft tissue augmentation and protection of the carotid artery.

Endoscopic Approaches

Select benign tumors originating at the ITF and select benign and malignant tumors of the sinonasal tract extending to the ITF are amenable to resection by

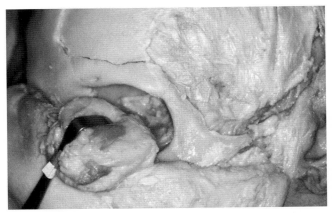

Figure 101-47. The orbital tissues are transected posterior to the globe.

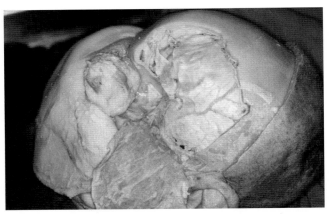

Figure 101-48. Additional bone is removed from the orbit and infratemporal skull base to provide exposure of the contents of the superior orbital fissure and cavernous sinus region.

endoscopic transnasal or transantral techniques (or both).[14-17]

The patient's head is usually fixed in a three-pin fixation system to facilitate navigation with a line-of-sight optical system. The nose is decongested with 0.05% oxymetazoline. Both sides of the nose are used for the surgical corridor, which is augmented by resection of the posterior septum. Because a bimanual technique is necessary for surgical dissection in this area, a two-surgeon, four-hands technique is recommended. Access to the ITF is gained by removing the medial and posterolateral walls of the antrum. Depending on the need for further exposure, the pterygoid plates, the torus tubarius, and the medial eustachian tube may be removed. To increase lateral exposure, the piriform aperture may also be removed to increase the angle of exposure. The basic steps include removal of the middle turbinate ipsilateral to the lesion; posterior septectomy; creation of a wide middle nasoantral window (may be extended inferiorly by removing the posterior one half of the inferior turbinate); removal of the posterior and lateral walls of the antrum; control of the neurovascular structures of the pterygopalatine fossa by ligation of the sphenopalatine and posterior nasal arteries; and, if necessary, removal of the pterygoid plates, the torus tubarius, and the middle one third of the eustachian tube.

POSTOPERATIVE MANAGEMENT

The patient is transferred to an intensive care unit for continuous cardiovascular and neurologic monitoring. Laboratory tests are ordered to rule out postoperative anemia and electrolyte abnormalities. Patients requiring multiple blood transfusions should be screened for transfusion-induced coagulation disorders. Mild narcotic analgesia is provided, but strong narcotic or sedative medications are avoided to prevent interference with accurate neurologic assessment.

If surgical manipulation, ligation, or grafting of the ICA has been performed, close monitoring of the patient's hemodynamic status is essential. Blood transfusions are considered when the hematocrit is less than 27% or the patient shows heart or brain disfunction. Fluid balance is carefully monitored to prevent hypotension. Strict bed rest is maintained for several days until the patient is hemodynamically stable to prevent hypotension. A CT scan of the head without contrast enhancement is performed on the first or second postoperative day to screen for intracranial complications, such as cerebral contusions, significant edema, hemorrhage, fluid collections, or pneumocephalus. When grafting of the ICA is performed or after surgical injury, an angiogram is obtained in the early postoperative period to assess the patency of the graft and detect pseudoaneurysm formation.

A compressive dressing is maintained for 24 to 72 hours. Once the dressing is removed, the wound is cleaned with normal saline solution and covered with antibiotic ointment three to four times a day. The scalp and other wound drains are kept on suction (80 mm Hg) until the amount of drainage is less than 20 mL/day. If the cranial cavity is entered, suction drainage is not used because of the risk of direct negative pressure on the central nervous system, and the drains are left to gravity drainage.

In most cases, the spinal drain is needed only during surgery and is removed on completion of the procedure. If there is a significant risk of postoperative CSF leak, the spinal drain is kept at the level of the patient's shoulder and 50 mL are removed every 8 to 12 hours. The spinal drain is removed 3 to 5 days after surgery. The lumbar puncture site is closed with an encircling stitch (e.g., 2-0 nylon) placed at the time of surgery.

Inadequate closure of the eye because of weakness or paralysis of the facial nerve may lead to exposure keratoconjunctivitis. Initially, an exposed eye can be protected with artificial tears every 1 to 2 hours, lubrication ointment at bedtime, eye patching, or a moisture chamber. Taping or a temporary tarsorrhaphy is advised if rapid recovery is anticipated. If prolonged paralysis is expected, the authors prefer a gold weight implant. Implantation of a 0.1- to 0.12-g weight (no. 10 or 12) can be performed at the time of the original surgery, or it may be performed days later. Except in select cases, the authors favor the latter because it provides the advantage of being able to insert the exact weight needed by the patient.

In the vast majority of cases, the airway can be secured with a short-term endotracheal tube (high-volume/low-pressure cuff). Nevertheless, for patients in whom significant edema of the upper aerodigestive tract or prolonged intubation is anticipated, the authors recommend a tracheotomy. In patients with an ineffective cough or severe aspiration, tracheotomy also provides better access to the airway for pulmonary toilet.

Patients with high vagal lesions or any combination of deficits of cranial nerves IX, X, or XII will suffer severe swallowing difficulty and aspiration. These patients can be assisted with a thyroplasty type I/arytenoid adduction procedure with or without cricopharyngeal myotomy. Patients who continue to aspirate are managed with a laryngotracheal separation procedure (see Chapter 69).

COMPLICATIONS

Most of the morbidity associated with conventional cranial base surgery for neoplasms involving the ITF is related to deficits of the trigeminal nerve. Sacrifice of the third and sometimes the second division of the trigeminal nerve may be necessary for surgical exposure or adequate tumor margins. Facial anesthesia may predispose the patient to self-inflicted injuries. On rare occasions, neurotrophic ulcers may develop as a result of repeated self-inflicted trauma. Loss of corneal sensation, especially in someone with paresis of the facial nerve, greatly increases the risk of corneal abrasion or exposure keratitis. Loss of motor function of the mandibular nerve causes asymmetry of the jaw opening and decreased force of mastication on that side (Fig. 101-49). Mastication may be further impaired by resection of the TMJ or mandibular ramus. Whenever feasi-

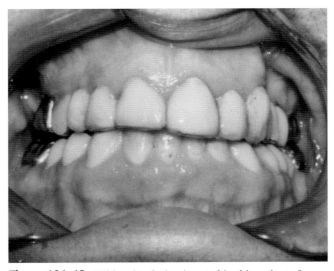

Figure 101-49. Mild malocclusion is noted in this patient after an infratemporal skull base approach. A posterior open bite and deviation of the mandible to the right side are noted.

ble, the sensory and motor divisions of the trigeminal nerve are repaired after transection for surgical exposure.

Accidental injury to the facial nerve with subsequent permanent paralysis is uncommon, although possible with the approaches described here. The temporal branches of the facial nerve are at risk for injury with elevation of the scalp flap. Injury is usually a result of dissection in a plane superficial to the superficial layer of the deep temporal fascia. The main trunk of the facial nerve is susceptible to traction injury with retraction of the facial flap anteriorly. For this reason, a pedicle of soft tissue is preserved around the facial nerve when a preauricular approach is used. Temporary paresis of the facial nerve is to be expected with mobilization of the mastoid segment of the facial nerve. Close attention to postoperative eye care must be observed in patients with combined deficits of the trigeminal and facial nerves.

Postoperative trismus is a common occurrence because of postoperative pain and scarring of the pterygoid musculature and TMJ (see Fig. 101-24C). Less trismus is noted six months postoperatively if patients regularly perform stretching exercises by opening the jaw. Devices such as the Therabite appliance are helpful in stretching the scar tissue and forcefully opening the mouth. In severe cases, a dental appliance that is gradually opened with a screw may be fabricated. Surgical resection of the TMJ does not appear to be a major factor in the development of postoperative trismus or difficulties with mastication. Rather, mastication appears to be most affected by loss of function of the mandibular division of the trigeminal nerve. Nevertheless, every attempt is made to preserve the TMJ. If resection of the glenoid fossa is necessary, the capsule of the TMJ is displaced inferiorly. If resection of the TMJ is necessary, no attempt is made to reconstruct the joint.

Infectious complications are rare. Predisposing factors include communication with the nasopharynx, seroma or hematoma, and a CSF leak. In general, all dead spaces should be obliterated to prevent collection of fluid. The use of vascularized tissue flaps is preferred, especially when dissection of the ICA or resection of dura has been carried out.

Necrosis of scalp flaps is an uncommon occurrence because of the excellent blood supply of the scalp. Poorly designed incisions, however, may result in areas of hypovascularity, particularly around the auricle (Fig. 101-50).

Vascular complications are a great concern with surgery in this area. Surgical dissection of the ICA can result in injury to the wall with either immediate or delayed hemorrhage. The artery is particularly vulnerable to injury at the point where it enters the cranial base. Injuries to the ICA should be repaired primarily. An angiogram is obtained in the early postoperative period to assess adequacy of the repair and to detect early pseudoaneurysm formation. In the event that repair of the artery is not possible, permanent occlusion of the artery by ligation or placement of a detachable latex balloon or vascular coil may be performed. There

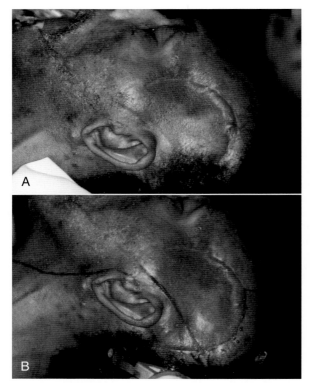

Figure 101-50. This patient had previously undergone surgery that used a question mark–shaped left temporal incision. **A,** There is an additional scar anterior to the auricle. These incisions are cosmetically unfavorable, may violate the underlying temporalis muscle, and greatly increase the risk of injury to the temporal branches of the facial nerve. **B,** It was necessary to use segments of the original scars on reoperation to prevent further compromise of the vascularity of the scalp and auricle.

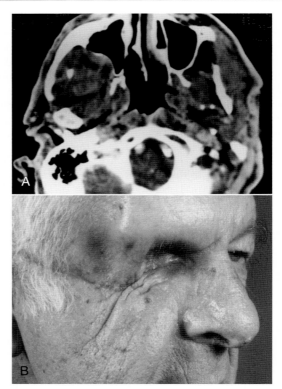

Figure 101-51. A, Computed tomography scan demonstrating hemangiopericytoma of the right temporal area with involvement of the temporalis muscle, orbitozygomatic bone, and orbit. **B,** Resection of the temporalis muscle, lateral orbital wall, zygomatic bone, and orbit was necessary to achieve clear tumor resection margins but resulted in a significant cosmetic deformity.

is a significant risk of immediate and delayed stroke, however, in patients who do not have greater than 35 to 40 mL of blood flow/min/100 g brain tissue by ABOX-CT testing.

Postoperative cerebral ischemia may result from surgical occlusion of the ICA, temporary vasospasm, and thromboembolic phenomena. When the artery is permanently occluded, the occlusion is performed as distal as possible near the origin of the ophthalmic artery. It is believed that there is less potential for thrombus formation with a short column of stagnant blood above the level of occlusion. After reconstruction of the ICA with a vein graft, there is a risk of postoperative occlusion secondary to thrombus formation at the suture line, as well as torsion or kinking of the graft. Pseudoaneurysm formation and delayed blowout of the graft are also risks, especially in the presence of infection. For this reason, reconstruction of the ICA is not usually performed in a contaminated field in which there is communication with the upper aerodigestive tract. In such cases, permanent occlusion of the ICA or rerouting of a vein graft posterior to the surgical field is performed. An extracranial-intracranial bypass graft to the middle cerebral artery may be performed before tumor resection when sacrifice of the ICA is anticipated. Patients who undergo surgical manipulation of the ICA are also sus-

ceptible to cerebral ischemia in watershed areas, at the margins of the vascular territories of the cerebral vessels. This is of particular concern when extracranial-intracranial collateral blood vessels, which are not routinely assessed by ABOX-CT, have been sacrificed as part of the surgical approach. Decreased oxygen delivery because of postoperative anemia or hypotension can result in cerebral infarction in these watershed areas.

Watertight dural closure may be difficult to achieve with large infratemporal skull base defects, particularly around nerves and vessels. An epidural fluid collection may result. In most cases, it is contained by the soft tissues and slowly resolves without further intervention. Occasionally, the CSF collection may communicate with the outside through the EAC or along the eustachian tube to the nasopharynx. Most CSF leaks can be managed nonsurgically by placement of a spinal drain to lower CSF pressure and an external pressure dressing. If the CSF leak does not resolve within 1 week, surgical exploration and repair of the dural defect may be necessary. A middle ear effusion is often apparent after infratemporal skull base approaches as a result of dysfunction or interruption of the eustachian tube. Tympanostomy tubes are not placed for at least 6 weeks postoperatively because there is always a risk of CSF communication. The authors have encountered a few patients with profuse unilateral rhinorrhea in the post-

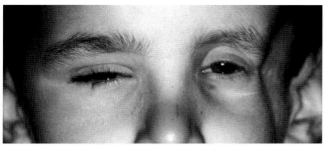

Figure 101-52. This 8-year-old boy underwent a left infratemporal skull base approach for excision of a large angiofibroma that involved the infratemporal skull base. The infratemporal skull base was reconstructed via temporalis muscle transposition, and a significant depression was left in the temporal area. This depression was later reconstructed with a custom-made alloplastic implant.

operative period that was misinterpreted as a CSF leak. These cases were all associated with surgical manipulation of the ICA and were probably due to loss of sympathetic fibers to the nasal mucosa that travel along the ICA. This represents a form of iatrogenic vasomotor rhinitis and may be treated similarly with the use of anticholinergic nasal sprays. Testing of the fluid for β_2-transferrin may be necessary to rule out a CSF leak.

Cosmetic deformities may result from the loss of soft tissue and bone (Fig. 101-51). Transposition of the temporalis muscle results in a depression in the temporal area (Fig. 101-52). It can be lessened by placement of a free fat graft at the time of surgery or at a later date. If the temporalis muscle is not transposed, the anterior margin of the muscle should be resutured anteriorly to prevent a slight depression lateral to the orbital rim. The use of free muscle flaps for reconstruction may necessitate sacrifice of the zygomatic arch. With atrophy of the muscle, a significant depression may occur. Large lateral muscle flaps, such as a latissimus dorsi flap, may also compress the brain if the underlying cranium is not reconstructed.

PEARLS

- Establishment of the origin and extension of tumors involving the ITF is critical to provide optimal surgical management.
- Subtle lower cranial nerve symptoms are often the first sign of ITF/skull base pathology.
- Postoperative stretching and physical therapy will facilitate improved TMJ range of motion and reduce the extent of trismus at 6 months.
- Because of wide variability in histopathology of the ITF, preoperative pathologic confirmation is necessary before proceeding to major ablative surgery.
- Large soft tissue and bone defects are best reconstructed with composite free tissue transfer.
- Partial resuspension of the temporalis muscle to the lateral orbital rim will minimize cosmetic deformity postoperatively.

PITFALLS

- Despite preoperative carotid balloon test occlusion with CT xenon flow testing, some patients will still suffer ischemic brain injury because of loss of collateral vessels and nonphysiologic conditions during testing.
- Dissection superficial to the superficial layer of the deep temporal fascia will put the frontal branch of the facial nerve at risk.
- After resection of the condyle, reconstruction of the TMJ may lead to more scarring and trismus than would occur with no reconstruction.
- Large composite defects of bone and soft tissue are best reconstructed with a free tissue transfer that includes bone to minimize postoperative cosmetic morbidity.
- Unilateral rhinorrhea may be misinterpreted as a CSF leak when in fact it is related to manipulation of the sympathetic supply to the nose during carotid artery dissection.
- Patients with lower cranial nerve deficits will have significant impairment of speech and swallowing function that will necessitate aggressive rehabilitation, if not surgical correction and augmentation.

References

1. Fairbanks-Barbosa J: Surgery of extensive cancer of paranasal sinuses. Presentation of a new technique. Arch Otolaryngol 73:129-138, 1961.
2. Terz JJ, Young HF, Lawrence W Jr: Combined craniofacial resection for locally advanced carcinoma of the head and neck. II. Carcinoma of the paranasal sinuses. Am J Surg 140:618-624, 1980.
3. Fisch U: The infratemporal fossa approach for the lateral skull base. Otolaryngol Clin North Am 17:513-552, 1984.
4. Biller HF, Shugar JMA, Krespi YP: A new technique for wide-field exposure of the base of the skull. Arch Otolaryngol 107:698-707, 1981.
5. Sekhar LN, Schramm VL, Jones NF: Subtemporal-preauricular infratemporal fossa approach to large lateral and posterior cranial base neoplasms. J Neurosurg 67:488-499, 1987.
6. Cocke EW Jr, Robertson JH, Robertson JT, Crooke JP Jr: The extended maxillotomy and subtotal maxillectomy for excision of skull base tumors. Arch Otolaryngol Head Neck Surg 116:92-104, 1990.
7. Janecka IP, Sen CN, Sekhar LN, Arriaga M: Facial translocation: A new approach to the cranial base. Otolaryngol Head Neck Surg 103:413-419, 1990.
8. Catalano PJ, Biller HF: Extended osteoplastic maxillotomy. A versatile new procedure for wide access to the central skull base and infratemporal fossa. Arch Otolaryngol Head Neck Surg 119:394-400, 1993.
9. Snyderman CH, D'Amico F: Outcome of carotid artery resection for neoplastic disease: A meta-analysis. Am J Otolaryngol 13:373-380, 1992.
10. Johnson JT, Derkay CS, Mandell-Brown MK, Newman RK (eds): AAO-HNS Instructional Courses, vol 6. New York, Mosby-Year Book, 1993, pp 341-346.
11. Nuss DW, Janecka IP, Sekhar LN, Sen CN: Craniofacial disassembly in the management of skull-base tumors. Otolaryngol Clin North Am 24:1465-1497, 1991.

12. Sekhar LN, Sen C, Snyderman CH, Janecka IP: Anterior, antero-lateral, and lateral approaches to extradural petroclival tumors. In Sekhar LN, Janecka IP (eds): Surgery of Cranial Base Tumors. New York, Raven Press, 1993, pp 157-223.

13. Mansour OI, Carrau RL, Snyderman CH, Kassam AB: Preauricular infratemporal fossa surgical approach: Technique and surgical indications. Skull Base 14:143-151, 2004.

14. Bilsky MH, Bentz B, Vitaz T, et al: Craniofacial resection for cranial base malignancies involving the infratemporal fossa. Neurosurgery 57(4 Suppl):339-347, 2005.

15. Kassam AB, Gardner P, Snyderman C, et al: Expanded endonasal approach: Fully endoscopic, completely transnasal approach to the middle third of the clivus, petrous bone, middle cranial fossa, and infratemporal fossa. Neurosurg Focus 19(1):E6, 2005.

16. Robinson S, Patel N, Wormald PJ: Endoscopic management of benign tumors extending into the infratemporal fossa: A two-surgeon transnasal approach. Laryngoscope 115:1818-1822, 2005.

17. Hartnick CJ. Myseros JS, Myer CM 3rd: Endoscopic access to the infratemporal fossa and skull base: A cadaveric study. Arch Otolaryngol Head Neck Surg 127:1325-1327, 2001.

Chapter **102**

Petrosal Approaches

Trevor Hackman and Elizabeth H. Toh

Several surgical approaches can be used to provide access to the petrous apex and lateral skull base for resection of tumors within the middle and posterior cranial fossae. The most common tumors of the skull base include petroclival meningiomas, chordomas, and chondrosarcomas. The most common lesions in the petrous apex include mucoceles, epidermoids, cholesterol granulomas, and arachnoid cysts. Petroclival meningiomas are the predominant lesions requiring petrosal approaches for surgical resection.

Multiple surgical approaches have been developed over the years to provide access to tumors in the petroclival region. Central to all these approaches is the ability to develop exposure through which the tumor can be visualized and spare important neural and vascular structures within the petroclival region. In the past, morbidity and mortality rates in patients treated surgically for petroclival tumors was high, probably because of lack of knowledge of petrous temporal bone anatomy and therefore a tendency to attempt surgical approaches through the more familiar suboccipital and pterional approaches. Transpetrosal approaches through the lateral skull base offer more direct surgical exposure for resection of tumors in the petroclival region and less risk to neurovascular structures lateral and anterior to the brain stem.

Current transpetrosal approaches encompass a variety of surgical exposures through the petrous portion of the temporal bone to provide access to the cerebellopontine angle, the petroclival region, the basilar artery, and the brain stem (Table 102-1). Abdel Aziz and colleagues in 2000 grouped transpetrosal approaches into anterior and posterior categories and then subclassified them into individual approaches based on the spectrum of bone resection and exposure of the posterior fossa.[1] The anterior transpetrosal approaches to the posterior fossa, also known as subtemporal approaches, are a continuum of the basic middle fossa approach. The addition of anterior petro-

sectomy and opening of the temporal lobe dura mater enhances visualization of the posterior fossa. The posterior transpetrosal approaches include the retrolabyrinthine, translabyrinthine, transcochlear, and total petrosectomy approaches, use of which depends on the location and extent of the tumor.

The location and extent of cranial base tumors within the middle and posterior fossae often necessitate a combination of petrosal approaches, such as a subtemporal middle fossa approach along with a transpetrosal approach, to enhance surgical exposure and thereby limit neurovascular morbidity. The extent of temporal bone resection required for adequate exposure is dependent on the approach and tumor location. Anterior, posterior, combined, and complete petrous bone resections must be tailored to each case.

Advantages of transpetrosal approaches include (1) minimal retraction of the cerebellum and temporal lobe; (2) reduced operative distance of the clivus (3 cm shorter than with the suboccipital approach); (3) superior angle of surgical exposure with regard to the anterior and lateral aspects of the brain stem; (4) preservation of the vein of Labbé and the transverse and sigmoid sinuses; (5) anatomic preservation of all critical neural and otologic structures, including the cochlea, vestibule, and facial nerve; (6) availability of multiple angles and routes for tumor resection within the same surgical exposure; and (7) early vascular control of the tumor, thus making subsequent tumor resection easier.[2-4]

The development of newer microsurgical and skull base surgery techniques, along with improvements in anesthesia, neuroradiology, and monitoring, have significantly reduced surgical morbidity. Recently, newer techniques, including stereotactic radiation therapy and surgical resection through expanded endoscopic nasal approaches, have been used to treat these lesions with relatively low complication rates. Stereotactic radiation therapy offers a nonsurgical option for controlling tumor growth. The expanded endoscopic nasal

Table 102-1	PETROSAL APPROACHES TO THE CRANIAL BASE

Anterior petrosal approaches (middle fossa)
    Classic subtemporal approach
    Middle fossa approach to the internal auditory canal
    Middle fossa approach to the petrous carotid artery
    Petrous apicectomy	

Posterior petrosal approaches
    Retrolabyrinthine approach
    Partial labyrinthine approach
    Translabyrinthine approach
    Transcochlear approach
    Total petrosectomy	

Combined anterior and posterior transpetrosal approaches	
Expanded endoscopic nasal approaches	

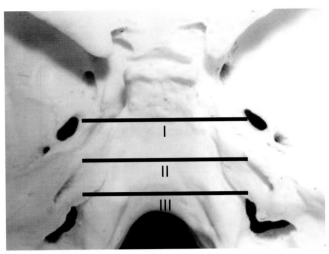

Figure 102-1. Zoning classification of lateral skull base lesions used to select the surgical approach for resection.

approach is used for removal of lesions in the middle third of the clivus, petrous internal carotid artery, cavernous sinus, and medial infratemporal fossa, which are located centrally with the surrounding neurovascular structures displaced laterally.[5]

PATIENT SELECTION

Factors found to be important in determining selection of the approach for surgery include the size, location, and extent of the tumor; anatomic variations in temporal bone anatomy; location of the sigmoid sinus; and the patient's hearing status. Larger tumors and those with involvement of critical neurovascular structures are more likely to require a combination of approaches for optimal surgical exposure. The approach selected should be tailored to fit the individual patient and maximize access while limiting morbidity. Abdel Aziz and colleagues developed a zoning classification for lateral skull base lesions to guide selection of the surgical approach (Fig. 102-1). Zone I (upper zone) extends from the dorsum sellae to the upper border of the internal auditory canal (IAC) and represents the exposure provided via the anterior petrosal approaches. Zone II (middle zone) extends from the IAC to the upper border of the jugular tubercle and represents the exposure provided via the posterior petrosal approaches. Zone III (lower zone) extends from the upper border of the jugular tubercle to the lower edge of the clivus and represents the exposure provided via a transcondylar approach. Zone III is essentially the anterior lip of the foramen magnum.[1]

Anterior Petrosal Approaches

Based on the standard middle fossa approach, anterior petrosal approaches can provide exposure for resection of zone I lesions extending from the oculomotor nerve anterosuperiorly down to the IAC posteroinferiorly. They also provide the advantage of optimal exposure and vascular control of the petrous carotid artery and superior visualization of the upper clivus. Their relative

disadvantages include the risk of facial nerve injury, necessity for temporal lobe retraction, and limited access to the posterior fossa.

Middle Fossa Approach to the Internal Auditory Canal

Indications for the use of this approach and the surgical technique are described in detail in Chapter 124.

Middle Fossa Approach to the Petrous Carotid Artery

Anatomic identification of the petrous carotid artery is paramount for successful surgical outcomes in skull base surgery, especially when intraoperative hemorrhage is anticipated or when the tumor directly involves the carotid artery or cavernous sinus (or both). Tumors with extensive invasion of the temporal bone, such as squamous cell carcinoma, paraganglioma, and high-grade chondrosarcoma, or tumors of the cranial base, such as meningioma, chondrosarcoma, and chordoma, present such an extirpative dilemma. The middle fossa approach was initially popularized by William House for surgical removal of small acoustic neuromas in patients with aidable hearing in the affected ear. It was subsequently adapted by Glasscock for exposure of the petrous carotid artery and used for surgical removal of skull base tumors in 1975 by Bochenek and Kukwa, who termed the approach the anterior petrosal approach.[2-4] The approach provides ideal surgical exposure of the horizontal segment, vertical segment, and genu of the petrous carotid artery, as well as for resection of petroclival lesions. With tumors involving the carotid artery, the carotid artery may be mobilized and controlled proximally and distally with this approach to allow improved exposure, more controlled surgical resection, and the ability to repair the carotid artery or perform carotid artery bypass when indicated. Preoperative assessment of these tumors with computed tomography (CT), magnetic resonance imaging (MRI), angiography, and balloon occlusion testing is essential for preoperative planning.

Petrous Apicectomy

Depending on the size, location, and neurovascular involvement of the tumor, the standard middle fossa approach may need to be expanded to include a petrous apicectomy. When used alone, this approach affords access to the midclivus, anterior cerebellopontine angle, Meckel's cave, the lateral wall of the cavernous sinus, and the petroclival synchondrosis for resection of small meningiomas, chondrosarcomas, and chordomas. The petrous apicectomy approach can also be used to manage aneurysms of the vertebrobasilar junction. The expanded surgical field also allows better vascular control of larger petroclival tumors, thereby leading to more complete and safer resection.

The increased labor associated with more extensive bony resection of the petrous temporal bone in this approach is well balanced by the improved surgical vector and field of exposure afforded to the clivus and even the ventral portion of the posterior fossa. This reduces the need for temporal lobe retraction, thus minimizing the risk for neurologic sequelae caused by prolonged temporal lobe retraction, such as seizures and cerebrovascular events. For larger petroclival tumors extending far into the posterior fossa, additional exposure via a posterior petrosal approach is often needed. In such cases, the anterior and posterior petrosal approaches are used in combination.

Posterior Petrosal (Transpetrosal) Approaches

Posterior petrosal approaches include the retrolabyrinthine, partial labyrinthine, translabyrinthine, transcochlear, and total petrosectomy approaches, for which a mastoidectomy is the surgical foundation. The progressive degrees of bone resection anteriorly via the retrolabyrinthine, translabyrinthine, and transcochlear approaches, respectively, provide graduated exposure of the posterior fossa within zone II (IAC to the jugular tubercle).[1] The retrolabyrinthine, translabyrinthine, and transcochlear approaches, when combined with temporal craniotomy and release of the tentorium, are best suited for mid and upper petroclival lesions located in the lateral, anterolateral, and anterior portions of the brain stem, respectively.

Retrolabyrinthine Approach

The retrolabyrinthine approach is ideally suited for patients with good hearing and medium to large tumors of the midclivus and anterior cerebellopontine angle. The approach may be combined with a middle fossa approach for removal of larger lesions lateral to the brain stem and over the clivus, with preservation of hearing and facial nerve function and minimal morbidity. The retrolabyrinthine approach hinges on the ability to mobilize the sigmoid sinus posteriorly for access to the posterior fossa through the presigmoid space. Although the approach can provide lateral expo-

sure from cranial nerve IV to the upper border of the jugular tubercle, the vestibular labyrinth anteriorly limits access to the ventral (anterior) surface of the brain stem and clivus, also known as the paramedian portion of zone II (or the central clival depression).[1,6] Therefore, tumors with dural attachment in the central clival depression cannot be totally resected with this approach.

The retrolabyrinthine approach is also limited by the variable anatomy of the temporal bone. A contracted mastoid or a far-forward sigmoid sinus can limit the anteroposterior extent of bony exposure provided through this approach. Similarly, a high-riding jugular bulb or low-lying tegmen mastoideum can reduce the superoinferior limits of surgical exposure. Tumor involvement of the cavernous sinus or lower clivus often necessitates additional exposure via a frontotemporal orbital–zygomatic approach or transcondylar approach, respectively. Alternatively, exposure of tumors in the central clival depression may be accomplished via the translabyrinthine or transcochlear approach with posterior mobilization of the facial nerve and sacrifice of hearing in that ear.[1,6]

Partial Labyrinthectomy Approach

The partial labyrinthectomy approach is an extension of the retrolabyrinthine approach that provides additional ventral exposure while preserving hearing in the operated ear. The principle of the partial labyrinthectomy approach involves removal of only a portion of the vestibular labyrinth, thereby attempting to conserve hearing. Specifically, removal of the posterior and superior semicircular canals can provide an additional 6 to 10 mm of posterior exposure and 10 to 15 mm of superior exposure, which significantly reduces temporal lobe retraction and increases the angle of exposure up to 30 degrees. The anterior limit of resection is the IAC. Tumors extending only to the medial half of the IAC can be removed through this exposure. Tumors extending into the lateral portion of the IAC require a translabyrinthine approach if there is no useful hearing or an anterior petrosal approach if hearing preservation is being attempted. The partial labyrinthectomy approach is typically reserved for large neoplastic and vascular lesions in the midportion of the clivus between the trigeminal and vagus nerves.[2]

Translabyrinthine Approach

Patients with poor hearing or those with lesions extending into the IAC are considered suitable candidates for the translabyrinthine approach. Removal of the vestibular labyrinth provides added exposure to the anterolateral aspect of the clivus and brain stem but sacrifices any residual hearing. The anterior limit of the approach is the facial nerve, which is not mobilized with this approach.

Transcochlear Approach

When additional access to the ventral aspect of the clivus and brain stem is required and hearing is poor, the translabyrinthine exposure can be extended into a transcochlear exposure by continuing the bony dissection anteriorly and drilling out the cochlea. The approach provides superior lateral exposure and ventral access to the brain stem, which aids in resection of tumors in the central clival depression. The surgical approach requires posterior mobilization of the facial nerve with resultant facial dysfunction. Therefore, this approach is used primarily for tumors involving the petrous temporal bone, for large petroclival tumors extending to the lateral clivus, for patients with preexisting facial nerve dysfunction, and for those with no serviceable hearing.

Total Petrosectomy

Total petrosectomy provides the widest and most complete field of exposure for the petroclival region. The approach involves extending the transcochlear approach to include exposure and anterior mobilization of the petrous carotid artery. This approach allows complete resection of the petrous temporal bone and clivus when these bones are involved with tumor, as well as removal of giant petroclival tumors with significant involvement of the carotid artery. Total petrosectomy also gives the widest possible access to the mid and upper clivus and the entire zone II.[1-6] Disadvantages of this approach include extended operative time, complete hearing loss in the operated ear, and significant risk of injury to the facial nerve and internal carotid artery. This approach does not provide adequate exposure of zone III and the lower clivus. Small lesions located in these areas may be resected through a retrosigmoid approach, whereas larger lesions will require a transcondylar approach. Upper clival lesions resected through this approach may require retraction of the temporal lobe or partial resection of the inferior gyrus.

Expanded Endoscopic Nasal Approach

Recently, the expanded endoscopic nasal (endonasal) approach has been proposed for removal of centrally based lesions in the middle third of the clivus, petrous internal carotid artery, and cavernous sinus when the neurovascular structures are displaced laterally.[5] The principle of endonasal approaches to the skull base centers around the anatomy of the sphenoid sinus, which provides the gateway to the middle and posterior cranial fossae. Also known as the transsphenoidal approach, the expanded endonasal approach has many advantages over lateral approaches, including improved access and reduced morbidity. Traditional microscopic transsphenoidal surgery was limited by the conical exposure to the skull base and therefore a narrow working field. The advent of endoscopes has revolutionized this approach. Endoscopes provide magnified and unparalleled visualization of key structures, thereby allowing better preservation of uninvolved structures.[7]

When compared with lateral approaches and microscopic approaches, endoscopic approaches provide superior lighting, the ability to see around corners with angled rigid telescopes, excellent maneuverability, and a magnified, comprehensive view of the surgical field.[4,7] The endoscopic approach also affords expanded visualization in both the transverse and vertical dimensions from the sella turcica to the foramen magnum. The addition of three-dimensional image guidance technology has allowed surgeons to extend approaches into the middle and posterior skull base for resection of tumors previously only approachable via traditional petrosal approaches. From a cosmetic perspective, endonasal approaches have a significantly reduced burden of healing and provide superior cosmesis by eliminating external incisions and soft tissue retraction. From a morbidity standpoint, the endonasal approach avoids complications related to temporal lobe retraction and injury to neurovascular structures typically encountered with lateral approaches, thus decreasing the rate of postoperative lower cranial neuropathy. Finally, the reduced surgical morbidity allows patients with advanced tumors to proceed with adjuvant radiation therapy in timely manner.[5,7]

Endoscopic approaches come with some inherent disadvantages. First and foremost, expanded endonasal approaches require advanced endoscopic surgical skills, which take significant time to acquire. Second, because of the relative infancy of expanded endonasal approaches, only a few centers are using them. Third, the endonasal approach does not usually permit en bloc resection of the tumor. For the most commonly encountered skull base neoplasms, this is not likely to affect the long-term prognosis, especially if surgical decompression is the primary goal of treatment. Conversely, the magnified endoscopic view often provides an enhanced view of tumor margins and attachment of tumor to surrounding normal tissue. If complete tumor resection is the treatment goal, additional tissue margins may be sent for pathologic examination after the tumor has been resected. Fourth, the incidence of cerebrospinal fluid (CSF) leakage is increased, and it may at times be difficult to control endonasally. Finally, control of bleeding during surgery requires considerable technical expertise and careful planning.[5,7]

PREOPERATIVE PLANNING

Preoperative evaluation of patients with petroclival lesions includes an extensive history and physical examination. The history should focus on the onset and duration of symptoms, including visual disturbances, auditory changes, weakness, paresthesias, and voice and swallowing abnormalities. Patients should have a complete head and neck and neurologic examination, including gait testing, cranial nerve examination, otologic evaluation, and sensory and motor testing of the extremities. Ancillary preoperative testing should include a complete audiogram and imaging studies of the skull base. Contrast-enhanced CT of the skull base, including the temporal bone, and gadolinium-enhanced MRI of the brain are essential for determining the extent and location of the lesion and for selecting the appropriate surgical approach or combination of approaches. If symptoms of swallowing dysfunction are detected preoperatively, videofluoroscopic evaluation of swallowing function should be performed. Preoperative cranial nerve function should be carefully documented because the risk for postoperative cranial neuropathy is significant. Patients should be counseled regarding the risk for potential postoperative cranial neuropathy, temporal lobe injury, seizures, CSF leakage, bleeding, and the possible need for additional surgery to address these complications.

SURGICAL APPROACHES

Anterior Petrosal Approaches

Middle Fossa Approach to the Petrous Carotid Artery

The patient is positioned supine with the head turned so that the operated ear is facing up. The ipsilateral shoulder is elevated to decrease tension on the cervical musculature, stretching of the brachial plexus, and torsion of the jugular veins. Intraoperative facial nerve monitoring is established at the beginning of the procedure. Paralytic agents are not used after induction of general anesthesia. Brain stem auditory evoked responses are also monitored routinely because hearing preservation is desired. Perioperative medications administered include broad-spectrum antibiotics with good CSF penetration (Ceftriaxone, 2 g); furosemide (Lasix, 20 mg); mannitol, 0.5 mg/kg; and dexamethasone, 10 mg. Bacitracin (50,000 U/L of saline solution) is used in the irrigation fluid. Lumbar drainage is not routinely performed.

When the goal of surgery is complete removal of a petroclival lesion or isolation of the petrous carotid artery, the standard skin incision used for the conventional middle fossa approach (Fig. 102-2) must be adapted to provide increased anterior and inferior exposure (Fig. 102-3). The incision can be combined with a modified Blair incision to allow complete exposure of the petrous carotid artery. The planned incision is marked and then infiltrated with a solution of 1% lidocaine with 1 : 100,000 epinephrine 10 to 15 minutes before elevation of the skin flaps to provide hemostasis. The incision is typically carried down through epidermis and dermis with a scalpel and then continued through subcutaneous tissue with electrocautery. As the skin flap is developed anteriorly, care should be taken to avoid injury to the frontal branch of the facial nerve, which courses over the zygomatic arch in a superficial plane of loose areolar tissue anterior to the temporal hairline. Knowledge of the scalp layers in this region is essential to avoid injury to the facial nerve. The course of the frontal branch of the facial nerve and layers of the scalp are shown in Figures 102-4 and 102-5, respectively.

The temporoparietal fascia, considered a continuum of the superficial muscular aponeurosis of the midface, fuses with the superficial layer of the deep temporal fascia approximately 1 cm above the zygoma. The facial nerve, which starts deep to the temporoparietal fascia in the midface, pierces through this fused

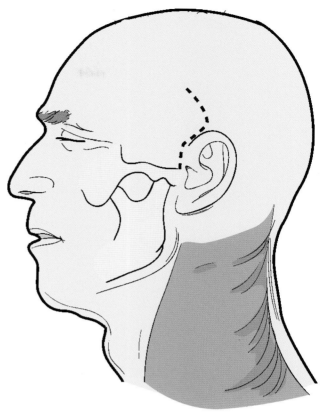

Figure 102-2. Standard skin incision used for the middle fossa approach to the internal auditory canal.

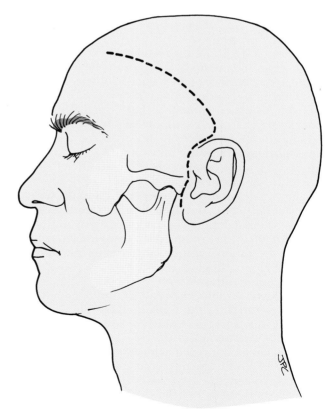

Figure 102-3. Modification of the temporal incision used for exposure of a petrous carotid artery or for petrous apicectomy.

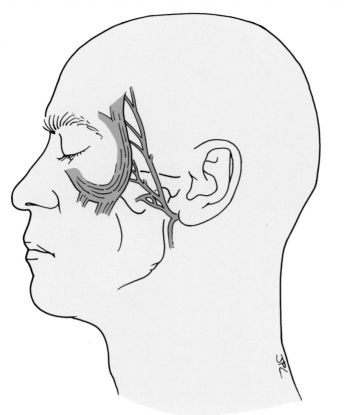

Figure 102-4. Anatomy of the frontal branch of the facial nerve.

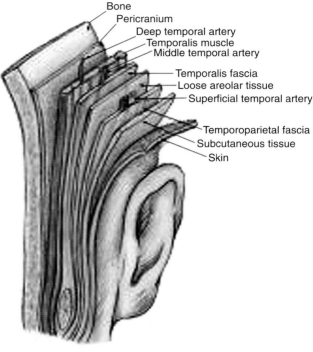

Figure 102-5. Layers of the scalp.

fascial layer 1 cm above the zygoma and runs superficial to the superficial temporal fascia until its termination on the medial surface of the frontalis muscle. To protect the facial nerve during anterior elevation of the skin flap, the dissection should be performed deep to the superficial layer of the temporal fascia. At the level of the superior brow line, 2 cm above the zygomatic arch, the deep temporal fascia splits into a deep layer and superficial layer to envelop the zygomatic arch, between which the superficial temporal fat pad can be found. At this level the superficial temporal fascia is typically incised (Fig. 102-6), and dissection is extended deep to the superficial temporal fat pad, anteriorly and inferiorly along the surface of the deep temporal fascia to the zygoma, to preserve the facial nerve in the skin flap (Fig. 102-7).

The zygomatic arch, with or without the roof of the glenoid fossa, is then removed via surgical osteotomies to allow elevation of the remaining temporalis muscle inferiorly out of the field of dissection. This lowers the level of the craniotomy to the floor of the middle fossa and provides an improved angle of exposure under the temporal lobe with less retraction of the temporal lobe. The junction of the zygomatic arch and malar eminence is divided via a chevron-shaped osteotomy with an oscillating saw (Fig. 102-8). The glenoid fossa osteotomies are then performed medial to the glenoid fossa

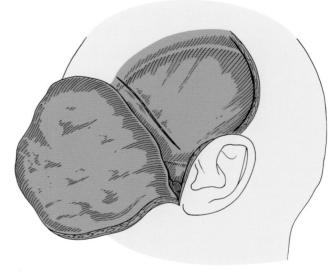

Figure 102-6. Dissection of the superficial layer of the deep temporal fascia to preserve the frontal branch of the facial nerve.

to allow removal of the zygomatic arch over the roof of the glenoid fossa.

An inferiorly based temporalis muscle flap is then created by incising the muscle along the linea temporalis while taking care to leave a superior cuff of muscle attached to its insertion to facilitate subsequent muscle reapproximation. Dissection of the temporalis muscle is carried as inferiorly as possible to permit a low subtemporal approach and placement

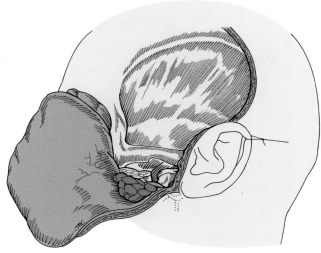

Figure 102-7. The frontal branch of the facial nerve is preserved within the anterior skin flap.

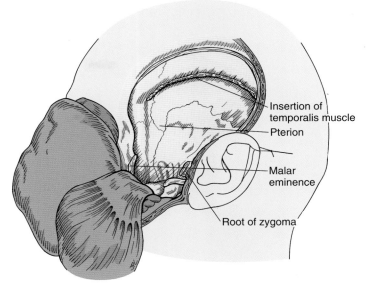

Insertion of
temporalis muscle
Pterion

Malar
eminence

Root of zygoma

Figure 102-9. Surface anatomy of the lateral skull base.

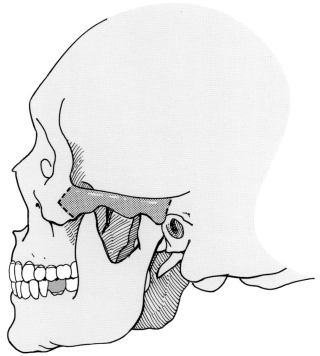

Figure 102-8. Osteotomies used for removal of the zygomatic arch and medial aspect of the glenoid fossa.

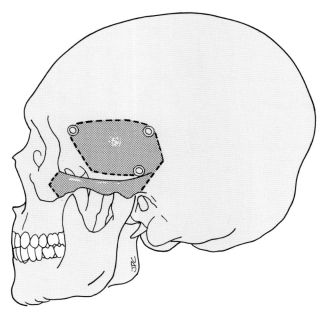

Figure 102-10. Location of the temporal craniotomy and removal of the zygomatic arch.

of self-retaining retractors or stay sutures. In this manner the lateral surface of the skull is exposed (Fig. 102-9). Posteriorly, the root of the zygoma, the glenoid fossa, and the external auditory canal are identified. Anterior dissection has exposed the confluence of the frontal, sphenoidal, and temporal bones in an area known as the pterion. Superiorly, the temporalis muscle has been released from its insertion. The malar eminence and the lateral and superior orbital rim are also exposed.

A low temporal craniotomy is then performed with a cutting burr or craniotome along the floor of the middle fossa from the external auditory canal to the orbital wall, which is possible only after removal of the zygomatic arch. The superior aspect of the craniotomy often extends posterior to the external auditory canal, and burr holes are often made for drilling access when the craniotome is used (Fig. 102-10). Using a dural elevator, the bone flap is carefully elevated off the dura and soaked in saline until completion of the procedure. The completed craniotomy is shown in Figure 102-11. Next, a cutting burr or rongeur is used to lower

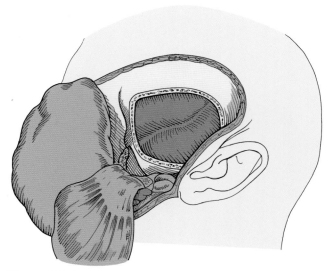

Figure 102-11. Completed craniotomy for petrous carotid dissection and petrous apicectomy.

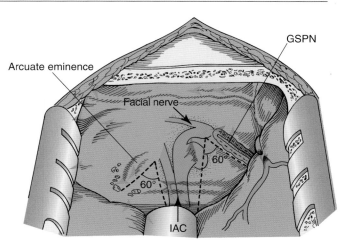

Figure 102-12. Surface anatomy of the middle cranial fossa. GSPN, greater superficial petrosal nerve; IAC, internal auditory canal.

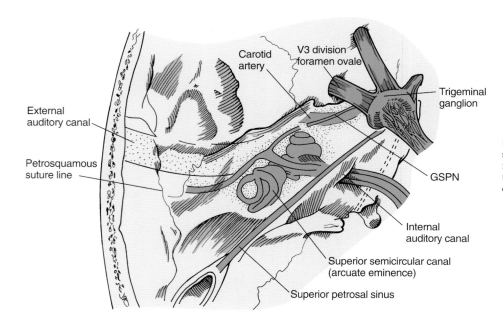

Figure 102-13. Anatomic relationships of the internal auditory canal, labyrinth, carotid artery, facial nerve, and trigeminal nerve. GSPN, greater superficial petrosal nerve.

the inferior border of the craniotomy to the level of the floor of the middle fossa.

The temporal lobe is then elevated extradurally from the floor of the middle fossa in a posterior-to-anterior direction. Familiarity with the surface anatomy of the floor of the middle fossa is essential (Fig. 102-12). The arcuate eminence, a round elevation of bone overlying the superior semicircular canal (the arcuate eminence may be absent in 15% of patients[8]), is first identified posteriorly. The sulcus of the superior petrosal sinus forms the medial boundary of the floor of the middle fossa and dural exposure for this approach. Knowledge of the relative locations of the vestibular labyrinth, cochlea, facial nerve, and internal and external auditory canal within the temporal bone is essential

for safe bony dissection (Fig. 102-13). As dural elevation is continued anteriorly, the greater superficial petrosal nerve (GSPN) is identified coursing within the spheno-petrosal groove. Posteriorly, the sphenopetrosal groove forms the facial hiatus where the GSPN exits from the geniculate ganglion. This portion of the facial nerve is dehiscent in up to 15% of normal individuals, so gentle dissection and minimal traction on the overlying dura will avoid trauma to the facial nerve. The first landmark in the area overlying the horizontal segment of the petrous carotid artery is the middle meningeal artery as it emerges from the foramen spinosum anterior and medial to the petrosquamous suture (Fig. 102-14). After cauterizing and transecting this artery (Fig. 102-15), the lesser superficial petrosal nerve, foramen ovale, and

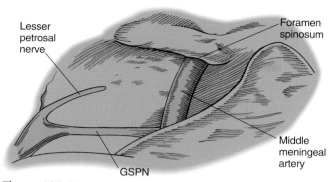

Figure 102-14. Anatomic relationship of the middle meningeal artery to the lesser and greater superficial petrosal nerves. GSPN, greater superficial petrosal nerve.

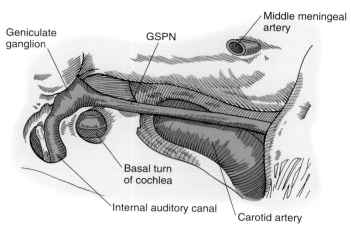

Figure 102-16. Anatomic relationships of the petrous carotid artery. GSPN, greater superficial petrosal nerve.

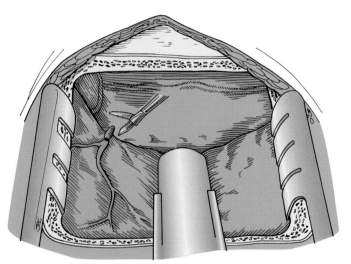

Figure 102-15. The middle meningeal artery is coagulated and divided.

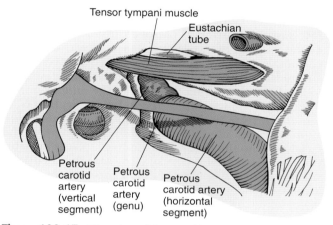

Figure 102-17. Dissection of the carotid artery to the level of the eustachian tube and tensor tympani muscle.

third division of the trigeminal nerve are identified. To expose the horizontal petrous carotid artery, bone must be removed medial to the middle meningeal artery and inferomedial to the GSPN, from the facial hiatus to the sphenopetrosal groove. Attempts should be made to preserve the GSPN whenever possible to avoid postoperative "dry eye" secondary to impaired lacrimation. In rare cases the GSPN may be sacrificed to prevent traction injury to the geniculate ganglion.

The horizontal segment of the petrous carotid artery lies under the GSPN and runs along an axis approximately 15 degrees medially to the course of the GSPN (Fig. 102-16). A natural bony dehiscence of the carotid canal can often be found immediately posterior to the V3 division of the trigeminal ganglion, and the internal carotid artery may easily be injured in this location. If this natural bony dehiscence is absent, a window of bone over the petrous carotid artery can be drilled down to eggshell thickness and then carefully elevated off the carotid artery. A blunt elevator is then used to free the carotid artery and its surrounding periosteum from the bony canal. A 2-mm rongeur can be used to

complete bone removal around the carotid artery in piecemeal fashion. A 180-degree circumference of the bone of the carotid canal should be removed to provide adequate access for reliable vascular control at the time of tumor removal. Bony dissection can then proceed in a posterolateral direction along the horizontal course of the petrous carotid canal to expose the genu and vertical segments of the carotid artery.

At the genu of the petrous carotid artery, the eustachian tube and tensor tympani muscle course superolateral to the vertical segment of the carotid artery (Fig. 102-17). When pursuit of a lesion involves exposure of the genu and vertical segment of the petrous carotid artery, the eustachian tube and tensor tympani must be transected, thus compromising middle ear function and increasing the risk for postoperative CSF rhinorrhea. In such cases, the eustachian tube must be clearly identified and oversewn at the conclusion of the procedure.

Wound closure is accomplished in layered fashion, beginning with a watertight dural closure. The craniotomy bone plate is replaced and secured with a microplating system. The temporalis muscle is reapproximated and the overlying soft tissues are closed in two layers. A mastoid dressing is then left in place for 72 hours and the patient is observed in the hospital for 4 to 5 days.

Petrous Apicectomy

The middle fossa approach can be extended to allow further exposure of the petrous apex. This approach may be useful in the management of neoplastic and inflammatory lesions of the petrous apex, including petrous apicitis. The petrous apex is a pyramidal region, also referred to as Kawase's rhomboid, in the antero-medial aspect of the temporal bone with variable degrees of pneumatization. It is bordered superomedi-ally and inferomedially by the superior and inferior petrosal sinuses, respectively[9]; the trigeminal nerve and ganglion anterosuperiorly; the IAC, cochlea, and genic-ulate ganglion posteriorly; the GSPN laterally; and the petrous carotid anteriorly and inferolaterally (Fig. 102-18).

The key landmarks for the petrous apex are the IAC and the horizontal petrous carotid artery, which define the field of dissection to ensure exposure of the petrous apex and preservation of the cochleovestibular and facial nerves. Several methods have been described to locate the IAC along the floor of the middle cranial fossa. Early approaches describe following the GSPN posteriorly from the facial hiatus to the geniculate gan-glion and then along the labyrinthine segment of the facial nerve to the IAC.[10] This approach places the laby-rinthine segment of the facial nerve and the cochlea at risk for injury. A second method proposes using the arcuate eminence (superior semicircular canal) as the major landmark to localize the IAC because the IAC lies along a 60-degree plane from the ampulla of the supe-rior semicircular canal. However, this approach, which involves skeletonizing the superior semicircular canal to view the ampulla, increases the risk of sensorineural hearing loss secondary to violation of the vestibular

labyrinth. Our group uses the technique described by Garcia-Ibanez.[11-14] The IAC is located medially by drill-ing along the medial border of the petrous temporal bone along a line bisecting the 120-degree angle formed by the arcuate eminence and the GSPN (Fig. 102-19). Bony dissection may be accomplished with a 2- to 3-mm diamond burr until the porus acusticus is identified. Drilling is then continued laterally toward the fundus to unroof the entire length of the IAC. At the fundus, bone resection is limited anteriorly by the basal turn of the cochlea and posteriorly by the ampulla of the supe-rior semicircular canal and the vestibule. The petrous carotid artery is then identified as described earlier.

With the IAC and petrous carotid artery skeleton-ized, the petrous apex can be drilled out to provide exposure of the posterior fossa all the way anterior to the precavernous portion of the ICA and medially to the inferior and superior petrosal sinuses (Fig. 102-20). The final limits of this extended middle fossa exposure are the inferior petrosal sinus inferiorly, the horizontal petrous carotid artery laterally, the gasserian ganglion anteriorly, and the IAC posteriorly. After complete petrous apicectomy, the superior petrosal sinus is ligated to allow opening of the tentorium to the incisura, thereby exposing the contents of the middle and pos-terior cranial fossae (Fig. 102-21).

Wound closure and postoperative care are as described for the middle fossa approach.

Posterior Petrosal Approaches

Depending on the patient's preoperative hearing status and the need for additional surgical exposure, a retro-labyrinthine, partial labyrinthine, translabyrinthine, transcochlear, or complete petrosectomy approach is chosen. The patient is positioned supine with the head turned to the opposite side and the ipsilateral shoulder raised slightly. Intraoperative facial nerve monitoring is established at the beginning of the procedure. Paralytic agents are not used after induction of general anesthe-sia. Brain stem auditory evoked responses are also mon-itored routinely because hearing preservation is desired.

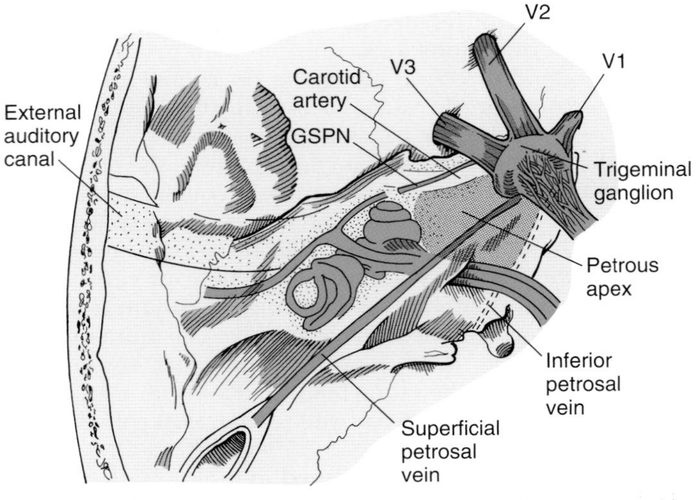

Figure 102-18. Anatomy of the petrous apex. GSPN, greater super-ficial petrosal nerve.

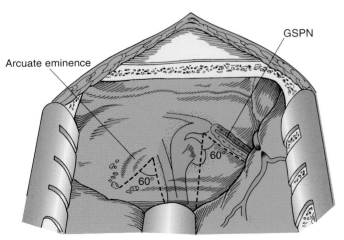

Figure 102-19. Landmarks for the internal auditory canal. GSPN, greater superficial petrosal nerve.

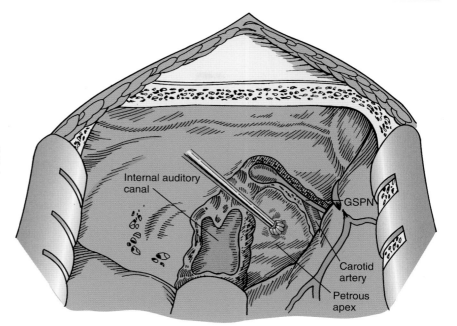

Figure 102-20. Removal of the petrous apex after exposure of the petrous carotid artery and the internal auditory canal. GSPN, greater superficial petrosal nerve.

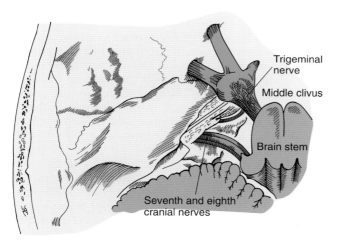

Figure 102-21. Intracranial exposure via a transpetrous apex approach.

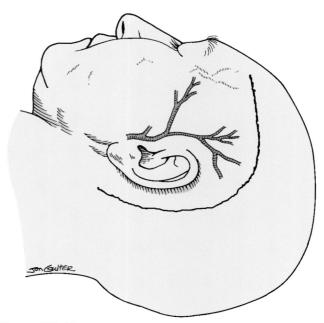

Figure 102-22. Skin incision for a combined anterior and posterior petrosal approach.

Perioperative medications administered include broad-spectrum antibiotics with good CSF penetration (Ceftriaxone, 2 g); furosemide (Lasix, 20 mg); mannitol, 0.5 mg/kg; and dexamethasone, 10 mg. Bacitracin (50,000 U/L of saline solution) is used in the irrigation fluid. Lumbar drainage is not routinely performed.

The planned incision is injected with a solution of 1% lidocaine with 1 : 100,000 epinephrine. A large C-shaped postauricular skin incision is made and extended superiorly above the pinna to provide surgical exposure for the temporalis muscle and inferiorly to expose the mastoid tip, as shown in Figure 102-22. This incision may be modified according to the bony exposure required. If hearing is absent, the external auditory canal is transected and oversewn. Anterior and posterior skin flaps are elevated over the temporalis fascia

and mastoid periosteum. The frontal branch of the facial nerve is preserved as described earlier. The temporalis muscle is incised along its attachment along linea temporalis. Posteroinferiorly, this incision is extended through the mastoid periosteum to the mastoid tip to develop a large anteroinferiorly based musculoperiosteal flap (Fig. 102-23). Exposure of the lateral surface of the skull is demonstrated in Figure 102-24. Inferiorly, the external auditory canal and glenoid fossa are identified. Anteriorly, the frontal,

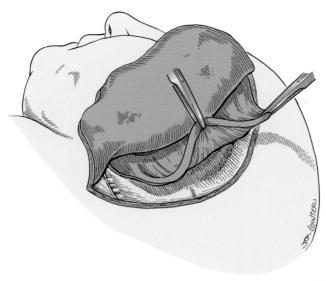

Figure 102-23. Musculoperiosteal flap. *(Redrawn from Cass SP, Sekhar LN, Pomeranz S, et al: Excision of petroclival tumors by a total petrosectomy approach. Am J Otol 15:474-484, 1994.)*

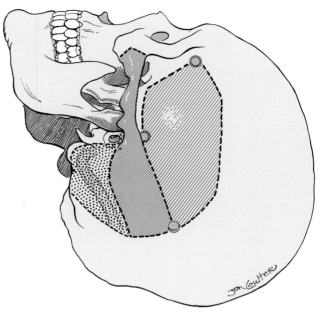

Figure 102-25. Cranial, zygomatic, and mastoid bone work separated into three components.

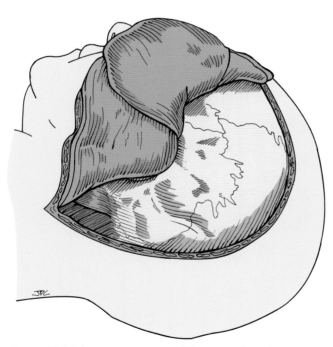

Figure 102-24. Surface anatomy of the exposed cranium.

sphenoid, and temporal bones are exposed at the pterion.

Osteotomies of the zygoma, a temporal craniotomy, and a mastoidectomy are performed. The size of the temporal craniotomy and the extent of petrosal exposure through the mastoid are determined by the size and location of the tumor. The zygomatic arch and glenoid fossa are removed to improve inferior exposure, and a complete mastoidectomy is performed with variable amounts of additional petrosal bone removal.

We prefer to perform the temporal craniotomy, removal of the zygomatic arch, and mastoidectomy in separate segments (Fig. 102-25). The temporal craniotomy plate and zygomatic arch can then be reattached at closing with a microplating system. It is also possible to perform the bone work in such a manner that the temporal craniotomy and mastoid cortex are removed en bloc with or without the zygomatic arch and glenoid fossa (Fig. 102-26).

To create a bone flap that includes a temporal craniotomy and a large portion of the mastoid cortex, the sigmoid sinus is exposed from the level of the jugular bulb to the confluence of the sigmoid sinus, superior petrosal sinus, and transverse sinus (Fig. 102-27). Approximately 2 cm of bone is removed posteriorly over the transverse sinus. Once the sigmoid and transverse sinuses are exposed, the mastoid cortex is cut with a small cutting burr along the external auditory canal forward into the glenoid fossa. Burr holes are made anteriorly in the temporal fossa, posteriorly above the transverse sinus, and superiorly near the insertion of the temporalis muscle (Fig. 102-28). A footed attachment on a craniotome is used to cut a temporal craniotomy, and the mastoid cortex is freed from the underlying air cells and middle fossa plate with a small cutting burr and chisel.

The zygomatic arch is removed along with the roof of the glenoid fossa by dividing the junction of the zygomatic arch and malar eminence via a chevron-shaped osteotomy with an oscillating saw. The glenoid fossa osteotomies are then performed medial to the glenoid fossa to allow removal of the zygomatic arch along with the roof of the glenoid fossa. Exposure of the middle and posterior fossa dura after completion of the initial bone work is shown in Figure 102-29.

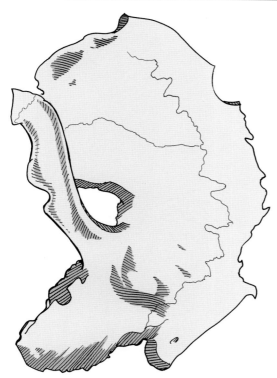

Figure 102-26. Combined temporal craniotomy, osteotomy of the zygoma, and preservation of the mastoid cortex.

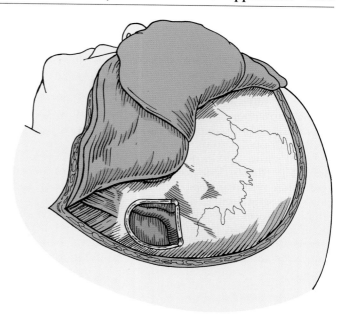

Figure 102-27. Exposure of the sigmoid and transverse sinuses.

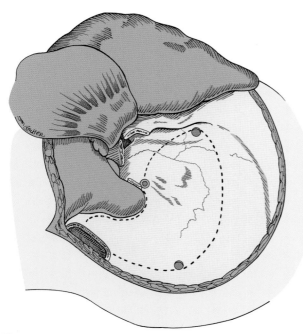

Figure 102-28. Outline of osteotomies within the mastoid and temporal squama.

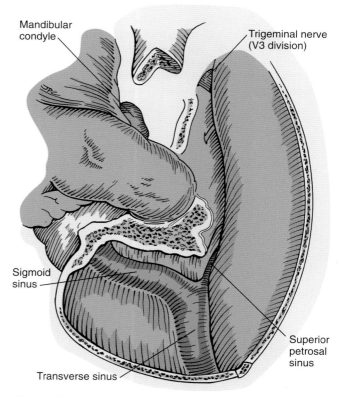

Figure 102-29. Surgical exposure after craniotomy and before transmastoid petrosal bone work.

The dura is opened along the floor of the temporal fossa and in the presigmoid region. Care is taken to locate and protect the vein of Labbé. The superior petrosal sinus is coagulated and ligated. The tentorium is divided parallel to the petrous ridge along the inci-sura. The fourth cranial nerve should first be isolated and protected. With the posterior temporal lobe elevated superiorly and the sigmoid sinus retracted posteriorly, wide field access to the supratentorial and infratentorial regions of the posterior cranial fossa is obtained.

Retrolabyrinthine Approach

The patient is placed supine with the ipsilateral shoulder elevated and the head turned to the opposite side so that the mastoid process is at the highest point in the field. A complete mastoidectomy is performed with an operating microscope, suction irrigation, and high-speed cutting burr, as described in Chapter 115. Special attention is paid to exposing the sigmoid sinus, jugular bulb, fallopian canal, vestibular labyrinth, superior petrosal sinus, middle fossa dura, and posterior fossa dura (Fig. 102-30). The porus of the IAC is then exposed by further removing bone medial to the superior and posterior semicircular canals. The endolymphatic sac, which lies over the posterior fossa dura between the sigmoid sinus and posterior semicircular canal, is preserved along with the endolymphatic duct. The endolymphatic duct and sac are useful landmarks to help preserve the vestibular labyrinth, but violation of the sac or duct increases the risk for sensorineural hearing loss. The dura over the middle and posterior fossae is then incised to expose the infratentorial portion of the tumor (Fig. 102-31). Once the superior petrosal sinus and tentorium are divided, both the supratentorial and infratentorial portions of the tumor are exposed (Fig. 102-32).

This approach alone provides exposure of the cerebellopontine angle but does not offer the surgeon adequate visualization of the anterior brain stem or petroclival region. Adequate exposure of the medial portion of the IAC is possible in most cases, but a high-

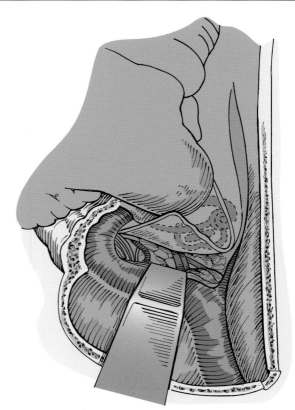

Figure 102-31. The infratentorial portion of the tumor is exposed through the retrolabyrinthine petrosal approach.

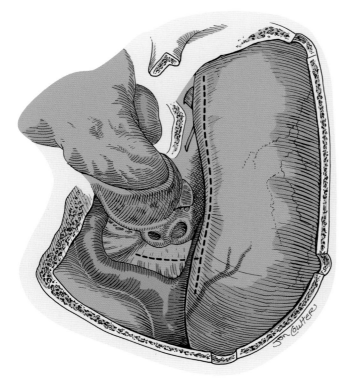

Figure 102-30. Dural exposure after an anterior and retrolabyrinthine petrosal approach and dural incisions.

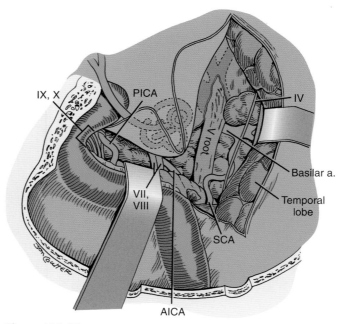

Figure 102-32. Both the supratentorial and the infratentorial portions of the tumor are exposed through the combined anterior and posterior petrosal exposure. AICA, anterior inferior cerebellar artery; PICA, posterior inferior cerebellar artery; SCA, superior cerebellar artery.

riding jugular bulb, anteriorly displaced sigmoid sinus, or dominant sigmoid sinus may prevent adequate visualization.

At the completion of the procedure, the dura is reapproximated in watertight fashion. The mastoid cavity is loosely packed with an abdominal fat graft, and the postauricular wound is closed in layers. A firm mastoid dressing is then left over the ear for 72 hours and the patient is observed in the hospital for 4 to 5 days.

Partial Labyrinthectomy Approach

This approach is an extension of the retrolabyrinthine approach. The decision to proceed with a partial labyrinthectomy approach is often an intraoperative decision made when the anatomy of the temporal bone is limited by variations that result in a small presigmoid dural window, such as a high-riding jugular bulb, unfavorable sigmoid sinus location, or contracted mastoid. Partial removal of the posterior and superior semicircular canals will provide additional access to the lateral portion of the IAC, cerebellopontine angle, and petrous apex. After completion of a retrolabyrinthine approach as described earlier, the posterior and superior semicircular canals are carefully skeletonized. The ampullated and nonampullated ends of the posterior and superior semicircular canals are then isolated from the vestibule to allow safe removal of the intervening segments of the semicircular canals.

The technique for fenestration of the semicircular canals is similar to that described for occlusion of the posterior semicircular canal in Chapter 131. A small diamond burr is used to create a small bony window at the common crus and ampullated ends of both canals (Fig. 102-33). The membranous canal must be preserved to maintain hearing. The membranous canal is then compressed by packing a mixture of bone wax and bone dust into the bony labyrinth (Fig. 102-34). After adequate packing of the semicircular canals in these four locations, the isolated segments of the superior

and posterior semicircular canals can be safely drilled away to expose the jugular bulb region, posterior fossa, and IAC (Fig. 102-35). Further anterior and medial dissection of bone above the IAC will lead to the petrous apex. After tumor removal, wound closure and postoperative care are as described for the retrolabyrinthine approach.

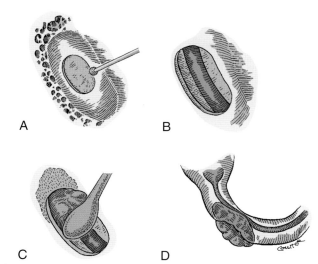

Figure 102-34. Technique for semicircular canal occlusion. **A,** Skeletonization of the semicircular canal with a small diamond burr. **B,** Semicircular canal fenestrated without violating the membranous labyrinth. **C,** Bone wax, bone paste, or soft tissue is applied to the fenestrated portion of the semicircular canal with a duckbill elevator. **D,** The membranous labyrinth is compressed and occluded.

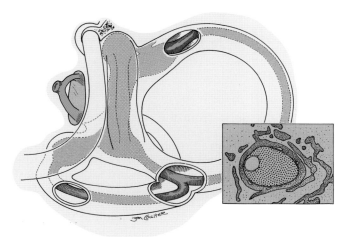

Figure 102-33. Location of the semicircular canal fenestra for partial labyrinthectomy. The *inset* shows the eccentric location of the membranous canal within the bony semicircular canal.

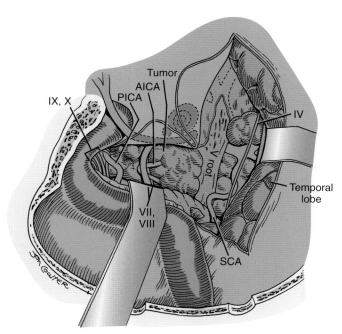

Figure 102-35. Exposure of tumor via a combined partial labyrinthectomy and posterior petrosal approach. AICA, anterior inferior cerebellar artery; PICA, posterior inferior cerebellar artery; SCA, superior cerebellar artery.

Translabyrinthine Approach

When hearing is absent and greater petrosal exposure is required, a translabyrinthine approach can be combined with an anterior petrosal approach. This approach is described in detail in Chapter 124.

Transcochlear Approach and Total Petrosectomy

The transcochlear approach is an anterior extension of the translabyrinthine approach that is used to gain additional exposure to the petrous apex and petroclival region. This approach requires posterior transposition of the facial nerve from the meatal segment to the stylomastoid foramen. The facial nerve remains in the posterior aspect of the surgical field as tumor dissection proceeds anteriorly and medially over the clival region.

In addition to the exposure provided by the translabyrinthine approach, the external auditory canal is transected at the bony-cartilaginous canal and oversewn in two layers to achieve a watertight seal. The facial recess is opened and the facial nerve is skeletonized along the tympanic and mastoid segments, down to the stylomastoid foramen. The incus is removed through the mastoid antrum. The skin of the ear canal is then removed in continuity with the tympanic membrane and malleus, and the canal wall is lowered to the level of the facial nerve in the mastoid segment. Both the chorda tympani and GSPN are sectioned at their origins from the facial nerve to allow posterior transposition of the facial nerve out of the fallopian canal.

Next, the cochlea is drilled out and bone between the basal turn of the cochlea and the horizontal segment of the petrous ICA is removed, including the carotid ridge, to completely expose the jugular bulb and pars nervosa. Cranial nerves IX, X, and XI will be within the field of dissection as they exit the jugular foramen and are at risk for injury.

To access lesions of the clivus, anteromedial brain stem, infratemporal fossa, and posterior nasopharynx, this approach is combined with a middle fossa approach. The surgical steps are modified accordingly. After transecting and oversewing the external auditory canal, the subtemporal sphenoid bone is removed up to the foramen ovale with a rongeur to completely expose the mandibular nerve (V3) (Fig. 102-36). The petrous carotid is completely unroofed from the precavernous segment to the upper cervical segment while leaving the artery sheathed in periosteum (Fig. 102-37). As mentioned earlier, the middle meningeal artery and GSPN are transected, and the cartilaginous eustachian tube is cauterized, packed with fat, and sutured closed. At this point the cochlea and medial petrous bone are removed through the posterior approach to expose the jugular bulb deep to the facial nerve, including the pars nervosa. Skeletonization of the facial nerve is then completed anteriorly via the middle fossa approach. The facial nerve is completely decompressed and mobilized posteriorly and inferiorly to provide wide surgical exposure for tumor removal. When the facial nerve is mobilized in this manner, the proximal and distal blood

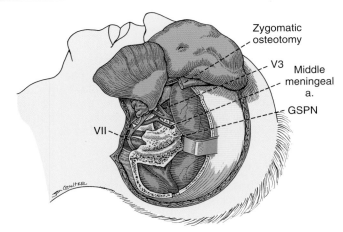

Figure 102-36. Total petrosectomy: radical mastoidectomy with removal of the subtemporal bone to expose V3. The middle meningeal artery is divided. GSPN, greater superficial petrosal nerve. *(Redrawn from Cass SP, Sekhar LN, Pomeranz S, et al: Excision of petroclival tumors by a total petrosectomy approach. Am J Otol 15:474-484, 1994.)*

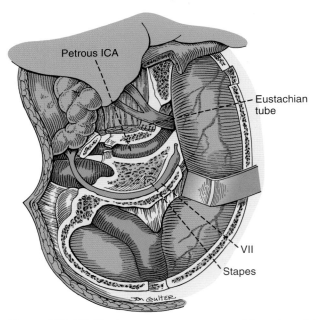

Figure 102-37. Total petrosectomy: exposure of the petrous internal carotid artery (ICA). *(Redrawn from Cass SP, Sekhar LN, Pomeranz S, et al: Excision of petroclival tumors by a total petrosectomy approach. Am J Otol 15:474-484, 1994.)*

supply to the nerve from the intracranial vessels and stylomastoid artery, respectively, is preserved.

Once the inferior fibrocartilaginous ring surrounding the upper cervical carotid artery is divided, the carotid artery can be mobilized forward without tension and held in place with a suture along the periosteum of the carotid canal. The medial petrous apex clival bone can then be removed to the midline to provide wide exposure with direct views of the midclivus, anterior brain stem, and basilar artery (Fig. 102-38).

A rarely used variant of the transcochlear approach is the transotic approach, in which the facial nerve is

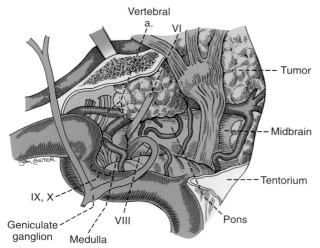

Figure 102-38. Total petrosectomy: exposure of the clivus and tumor after mobilization of the facial nerve and carotid artery. ICA, internal carotid artery; JB, jugular bulb. *(Redrawn from Cass SP, Sekhar LN, Pomeranz S, et al: Excision of petroclival tumors by a total petrosectomy approach. Am J Otol 15:474-484, 1994.)*

not transposed and tumor resection is performed in front of and behind the facial nerve within the fallopian canal.

Wound closure for the posterior petrosal approaches involves meticulous inspection and obliteration of potential CSF fistulas. Bone wax is used to seal off any remaining air cells within the temporal bone. The middle ear and mastoid cavity are packed with autologous muscle or fat grafts. The wound is closed in layers, including reapposition of the temporalis flap to its superior cuff and application of a pressure dressing and a subgaleal drain. In addition, when the facial nerve is fully exposed, as in a transcochlear or total petrosectomy approach, covering the nerve with Silastic at the time of closure helps aid in identification of the nerve if future surgery is warranted. The extensive operative time needed for the combined approaches and total petrosectomy often necessitates staged surgery 1 week apart.

Expanded Endoscopic Nasal Approach

Kassam and coauthors at the University of Pittsburgh have published landmark papers on the use of endoscopic expanded endonasal approaches for skull base surgery.[5,15] All patients for endoscopic skull base surgery undergo preoperative imaging, including high-resolution CT angiography and sometimes additional contrast-enhanced MRI of the brain, depending on the tumor type and location. Patients are positioned supine with the head in neutral position and secured with three-point fixation in a Mayfield head frame. Intraoperative frameless stereotactic image guidance is used in every case. When lesions involve or abut critical neurovascular structures, we recommend monitoring the patient intraoperatively with somatosensory evoked potentials, brain stem evoked responses, and electromyography as indicated. The nasal cavities are packed with

oxymetazoline-soaked pledgets, and a third- or fourth-generation cephalosporin is administered perioperatively for prophylaxis. We recommend a team surgery approach that includes an otolaryngologist and neurosurgeon, with both nares used simultaneously for surgery. The use of an endoscope holder by an independent surgeon prohibits dynamic intraoperative examination and adaptation.

Surgery begins with the development of a transnasal corridor, which involves rigid nasal endoscopy with a 0-degree endoscope, oftentimes with an irrigating sheath. The right middle turbinate is lateralized. Frequently, the inferior aspect of the right middle turbinate is resected with curved scissors to accommodate the instruments and the endoscope in the right nasal cavity. Suction electrocautery is then used to obtain hemostasis. At this time, if the surgical defect is anticipated to be large or extend intracranially, a posterolaterally pedicled vascularized septonasal mucosa flap based on the posterior nasal branch of the sphenopalatine artery is raised via electrocautery.[16] The anterior extent of the flap should come to the caudal septum. The width of the flap should be maximized by careful dissection of the superior limit and the inferior extension along the floor of the nasal cavity. The flap is then displaced into the maxillary sinus if an antrostomy is indicated or rotated into the nasopharynx to protect it from trauma during the remainder of the procedure.

A 1- to 2-cm posterior septectomy is performed just anterior to the rostrum of the sphenoid to allow bilateral dissection without contamination of the endoscope. After cauterization of the underlying mucosa, large pituitary forceps are used to remove the rostrum and thereby enter the sphenoid sinus. Wide bilateral sphenoidotomies are created with a Kerrison rongeur and extended laterally and inferiorly to the level of the medial pterygoid plates (pterygoid wedge, where the vidian canal is located). If a septal flap is not used, the posterior septal artery is coagulated and transected as it crosses the inferior aspect of the rostrum to facilitate removal of this portion of the rostrum and the floor of the sphenoid sinus.[5,15] Within the wide sphenoidotomies, the optic nerve canals, carotid arteries, lateral optic-carotid recesses, planum sphenoidale, and clival indentation or recess are identified. Often the sphenoid sinus is asymmetrically pneumatized and as a result one or both of the intersinus septa lead directly back to the carotid artery. Therefore, these septa should be removed with biting instruments and not pulled off. Occasionally, the optic nerve and carotid artery may be dehiscent within the sphenoid sinus. Finally, the large sphenoidotomy provides room for surgical access and maneuverability.

After the transnasal corridor is established, various approaches can be taken to the skull base. To approach the medial petrous apex, the basopharyngeal fascia is stripped away from the superior nasopharynx, and the sphenoid floor is then drilled until it is flush with the clival recess. As mentioned earlier, if not elevated in a flap, the sphenopalatine and posterior nasal arteries are isolated and ligated. A posterior maxillary antrostomy is performed to identify the key surgical landmark, the medial pterygoid plate. This plate is drilled for about 1 cm along the vidian artery, perpendicular to the clivus, to the anterior genu of the internal carotid artery. The bone is drilled eggshell thin with a coarse 3-mm diamond burr, and the internal carotid artery is exposed. The bone lateral to the internal carotid artery is removed to allow lateral translocation of the vessel without compressing it. Once the internal carotid artery is moved laterally, the underlying petrous apex can be directly accessed and the approach can be extended to the medial anterior margin of the IAC. This approach is ideal for extradural lesions such as cholesterol granulomas and cholesteatomas.

The expanded endonasal approach can also be used for direct access to the medial aspect of the petroclival junction, previously only accessed by conventional lateral skull base approaches, which require a significant degree of petrous bone resection.[15] The vidian canal is identified at the level of the medial pterygoid plate and followed to its origin from the anterior genu of the internal carotid artery. The bone over the horizontal segment, genu, and parasellar carotid protuberance can be removed with a combination of high-speed drills with extended burr shafts and fine 1-mm Kerrison rongeurs. The medial portion of the clivus at the petroclival junction is drilled to expose the dura and venous plexus. Dorello's canal can be followed superolaterally to the cavernous sinus. The cavernous sinus represents the superior boundary of this exposure and the middle fossa represents the lateral boundary. Venous bleeding from the cavernous sinus and basilar venous plexus is controlled with Avitene microfibrillar collagen packing (Davol, Inc., Cranston, RI). The dura medial to the posterior margin of the cavernous sinus can be opened to provide access to the pontine cistern. This approach has been used for chondrosarcomas, chordomas, and sinonasal lesions of the petroclival space, such as meningiomas, to provide a direct route to the tumor without significant neurovascular manipulation.[5]

Expanded endoscopic nasal surgery can be further extended to the quadrangular space.[15] The borders of the quadrangular space include the middle fossa laterally, the horizontal petrous internal carotid artery inferiorly, and the abducens nerve superiorly.[5] The approach to the quadrangular space involves isolating the maxillary division of the trigeminal nerve, V2, through a wide maxillary antrostomy. After the vidian canal is followed to the anterior genu of the internal carotid artery, V2 is isolated and followed superiorly to the foramen rotundum. Care should be taken during bone removal because the space between V2 and the vidian canal narrows posteriorly. The bone over the horizontal portion of the internal carotid artery is removed, and dissection continues superiorly to the lateral portion of the cavernous sinus, where V2 disappears into the dura mater. The dura is opened in a medial-to-lateral direction from the genu of the internal carotid artery toward V2. This approach allows access into Meckel's cave, the petrous bone, and the posterior fossa for tumor resec-

tion. The use of angled telescopes enhances the surgical view around corners and in tight areas. By remaining below the abducens nerve and lateral to the internal carotid artery throughout the procedure, the superior portion of the cavernous sinus, where cranial nerves III, IV, V1, and VI are located, can be avoided, thus reducing the risk for postoperative cranial nerve palsy.

Finally, when tumors invade and thrombose the superior aspect of the cavernous sinus, this region can be accessed via a dural opening above the quadrangular space in a medial-to-lateral direction over the superior lateral portion of the cavernous sinus.[15] Initially, bleeding is reduced secondary to tumor-induced thrombosis. The medial margin of the internal carotid artery is identified by opening the sella. With the internal carotid artery protected with a dissector, the tumor can be safely stripped away from the cranial nerves. The incidence of cranial neuropathy is significantly increased when the tumor is adherent to the cranial nerves and when aggressive packing of postresection venous bleeding from the inferior petrosal sinus is necessary. Therefore, this approach should be reserved for tumors that are refractory to medical or radiosurgical management or for tumors with preexisting cranial nerve deficits. Another advantage of the endonasal route is the ability to follow tumor into the pterygopalatine and infratemporal fossae with angled telescopes. Endonasal approaches have been successful in removing tumor as far lateral as the masticator space and pterygoid musculature.

Reconstruction

For open lateral approaches, reconstruction begins with primary dural repair or a dural graft of fascia lata or temporalis fascia, or both repair and a graft, for residual defects or extra support. Abdominal fat is typically used to obliterate the surgically created mastoid or petrous cavities. The bone graft removed at the start of the procedure is reapplied with miniplates and screws. The temporalis muscle is reattached to the superior cuff on the skull so that it reassumes its anatomic position. The skin is closed in dermal and epidermal layers, and a pressure dressing is applied. Depending on the field of dissection, a suction drain may be applied between the musculature and dermal layers.

For the expanded endonasal approach, reconstruction varies from simple packing of the sphenoid defect with duricel or autologous fat grafts for extradural lesions to more involved layered packing with AlloDerm (LifeCell Corporation, Branchburg, NJ) inlay or onlay grafts for repair of the resulting dural defect and subsequent packing of the bony defect with autologous fat, DuraGen (Integra Life Sciences Corporation, Plainsboro, NJ), and a vascularized septal mucosa flap.[5,15] A temporary balloon catheter positioned in the nasopharynx is filled with saline to reinforce the packing and prevent migration of the grafts. When the cavernous sinus is involved, packing with Avitene for hemostasis plus placement of autograft composed of abdominal or thigh fat is required to protect the exposed internal carotid artery.

POSTOPERATIVE CARE AND COMPLICATIONS

Petrosal approaches expose larger portions of the skull base and thus place the patient at risk for significant complications, including CSF leak, wound infection, meningitis, cranial neuropathy, cerebral edema, pneumocephalus, seizures, temporal lobe hemorrhage, stroke, and pulmonary embolism.

Cerebrospinal Fluid Leak

The key to avoiding postoperative CSF leak is prevention intraoperatively the time of surgery through meticulous repair of dural defects, dural grafting, and restrictions in postoperative activities, such as straining with bowel movements, nose blowing, and weight bearing. CSF usually leaks through the eustachian tube or though the incision. Because primary repair of the surgical wound is not always possible with the more extensive petrosal approaches, closure of the dural defects with free or vascularized grafts and packing of the dead space and the eustachian tube with fat and connective tissue, respectively, are essential. For hearing-preserving posterior petrosal approaches, such as the retrolabyrinthine and partial labyrinthine approaches, the eustachian tube and middle ear are not packed. Instead, only the mastoid antrum and cavity are loosely packed with an abdominal fat graft to minimize the risk of postoperative conductive hearing loss from adhesions involving the ossicular chain. Some postoperative conductive hearing loss is expected for 4 to 6 weeks as a result of hemotympanum. The transcochlear and total petrosectomy approaches require transection and blind sac closure of the external auditory canal and eustachian tube.

As mentioned, the surgical cavities are packed with fat and muscle grafts to limit the risk of CSF leaking through the incision. Additional measures to minimize this risk include oversewing the incision with nonabsorbable suture material, applying a compressive mastoid dressing for up to 72 hours, bed rest with the head elevated 30 to 45 degrees, and occasionally, lumbar drainage. Planning the incisions and dissection preoperatively also helps reduce the risk of leaks. The skin and muscle incisions should be stair-stepped. For larger defects, temporalis muscle flaps can be used to line the defects. When all the aforementioned measures have been attempted and CSF leakage persists, surgical re-exploration should be considered in an otherwise stable patient.

The risk of CSF leakage is increased in expanded endonasal approaches because of limitations with dural closure. The size of the defect, location of the defect, and experience of the surgeon are the most important factors in preventing postoperative leaks. Endoscopic repairs depend on the ability of the brain to settle over the repair and hold the tissues in place over the defect. Thus, excessive lumbar drainage will actually increase the likelihood of repair failure. A multilayered closure is the best way to seal endoscopic approaches. Typically,

AlloDerm inlay or onlay grafts (or both) are used to cover the dural defect and are fixed in place with tissue adhesives such as Dura Seal (Confluent Surgical, Inc., Waltham, MA) and Tisseel VH (Baxter, Deerfield, IL). Abdominal fat grafts are used to fill the extradural surgical defect, and frequently a vascularized nasal septal flap with tissue adhesive is used to cover the surface. To minimize postoperative leaks, a Foley balloon catheter can be left in place for 5 to 7 days. Alternatively, the nasal cavity may be packed with Merocel sponges to secure the flaps in place, with removal after 3 to 5 days. Systemic antibiotics should be administered for the duration that the packing remains in place. If a CSF leak occurs despite these measures, passive lumbar drainage and bed rest are often effective in controlling the leak, and in refractory cases, the defect can typically be repaired endoscopically.

Infections

The majority of infectious complications can be prevented with appropriate perioperative antibiotics, sterile surgical technique, and meticulous wound closure. Localized wound infections, pneumonia, and urinary tract infections are risks associated with any major surgical procedure, and standard postoperative care should be undertaken to prevent these problems, including postoperative incentive spirometry for pulmonary toilet, prompt removal of indwelling lines and catheters, and early ambulation. Specifically for petrosal approaches, the risk of meningitis and epidural abscess is real, and they can be catastrophic. Perioperative antibiotics should be administered for at least 24 hours after surgery and longer if nasal packing was placed. Postoperative fevers or elevated white blood cell counts should be investigated by blood culture, complete blood count, urinalysis, sputum culture, chest radiography, head CT, and lumbar puncture if clinically warranted. Empirical antibiotics with good CSF penetration should be initiated according to Gram stain results or evidence of clinical deterioration.

Cranial Neuropathies and Temporal Lobe Injury

Cranial neuropathies and temporal lobe injuries, including seizure, hemorrhage, stroke, and functional atrophy, are the result of traction injury to the brain during attempts to increase exposure during surgery. Using a combination of anterior and posterior petrosal approaches for larger and anteriorly located tumors within the skull base and lowering the level of the craniotomy to the floor of the middle cranial fossa in anterior petrosal approaches help limit such injuries. With more midline lesions in the petroclival region, endoscopic nasal approaches offer the advantage of direct access to the tumor with less risk for postoperative cranial neuropathy.

If the lower cranial nerves are at risk because of the size or location of the tumor, preoperative or early postoperative assessment of speech and swallowing is essential to limit aspiration and expedite recovery and rehabilitation. If the lower cranial nerves are compromised at the time of surgery, the patient should be treated promptly by tracheostomy, and safe enteral access should be obtained via a nasogastric or gastrostomy tube. If injury is anticipated preoperatively, concurrent medialization thyroplasty may be performed to prevent postoperative voice and swallowing difficulties. When the GSPN is sacrificed, postoperative dry eye syndrome should be anticipated and managed with aggressive eye protection and lubrication. If injury occurs to the main trunk of the facial nerve, eye protection with a moisture chamber, lubrication, and early surgical rehabilitation with an upper eyelid gold weight or palpebral spring should be considered.

Postoperative seizure activity should be controlled with neuroleptic medications, and neurology should be promptly consulted for management. For all anterior petrosal approaches in which the temporal lobe is retracted for prolonged periods, prophylactic anticonvulsants such as phenytoin are indicated.

Pneumocephalus and Cerebral Edema

Pneumocephalus and cerebral edema tend to be early complications that result in focal neurologic deficits and progressive deterioration in mental status, although pneumocephalus can also occur as a late complication secondary to violation of the dural closure with Valsalva maneuvers.

Mild asymptomatic pneumocephalus is commonly seen on early postoperative imaging and is a result of the surgical exposure. It usually resolves within 1 to 2 weeks. However, large or increasing pneumocephalus (tension pneumocephalus), particularly in the setting of mental status changes, should be managed by prompt surgical decompression because the expanding air will result in brain compression and potentially brain herniation. Sources of pneumocephalus are identical to those for CSF leaks and include the nasal cavity, the eustachian tube, and the surgical incision. Imaging studies can be used to localize the defect. Although prevention with meticulous wound closure is essential, avoiding disruption of the repair in the postoperative period is also paramount in preventing pneumocephalus. Excessive lumbar spinal drainage may draw air into the cranial cavity through the nasal cavity, and excessive positive pressure ventilation may displace grafts used to repair nasal defects resulting from endoscopic surgery. Care should therefore be exercised when managing lumbar drains and tracheostomy tubes after surgery.

Cerebral edema can also lead to brain herniation and mortality if not recognized and treated promptly. We routinely perform CT or MRI of the head within 24 hours after surgery to assess for the presence and degree of edema. In the event that clinically significant edema occurs, treatment includes osmotic diuresis with mannitol, systemic steroids, and hyperventilation to reduce Pco_2. An extraventricular drain may be placed at the bedside to decompress the brain and monitor intracranial pressure. If the cerebral edema is refractory to these measures, the inferior temporal gyrus may have to be partially resected.

Deep Venous Thrombosis and Pulmonary Embolism

Deep venous thrombosis and pulmonary embolism are postoperative complications with high morbidity and mortality that are typically preventable. Prolonged surgery and postoperative immobility drastically increase the risk for thrombotic events. The use of pneumatic compression stockings in the postoperative period dramatically reduces the incidence of such events. Early postoperative ambulation and physical therapy are also helpful. The risk for thromboembolic events is increased in patients with meningiomas and paragangliomas.

Tachycardia and tachypnea are often the first indicators of pulmonary embolism and thus should be thoroughly evaluated in a postoperative patient. Once hypoxia, shortness of breath, chest pain, hypotension, or syncope develop, the prognosis is much poorer because they signify a larger, more hemodynamically compromising clot. Immediate evaluation with a contrast-enhanced spiral CT scan of the chest and intervention are warranted, including thrombectomy, Greenfield filter placement in the inferior vena cava, and in some cases, thrombolytic therapy. Anticoagulation is not routinely used in intracranial surgery because of the risk for intracranial hemorrhage.

PEARLS

- Open petrosal approaches are useful for petroclival lesions within the middle and posterior cranial fossae above the lower third of the clivus. Lower clival tumor extension will require a transcondylar approach.
- Exposure of the central clival depression requires a transcochlear, total petrosectomy, or endonasal approach.
- The petrous carotid artery is the central landmark for anterior petrosal approaches; exposure and isolation of this artery are essential for vascular control.
- In the expanded endonasal approach, the vidian canal is used as a landmark to locate the petrous carotid artery.
- The asymmetrical intrasinus septum in the sphenoid sinus often leads to the vertical petrous carotid artery, and careful removal is necessary to prevent injury to the carotid artery.

PITFALLS

- Surgical dissection should proceed with caution because the carotid artery and optic nerve may be dehiscent on the lateral wall of the sphenoid sinus.
- Tumor extending into the posterior fossa is not accessible through an anterior petrosal approach alone and often necessitates combined anterior and posterior petrosal exposure.

- Surgical exposure through a retrolabyrinthine craniotomy is limited when the sigmoid sinus is located anteriorly and the jugular bulb is high.
- Scalp flap elevation in a plane superficial to the superficial layer of the temporalis fascia places the frontal branch of the facial nerve at risk for injury.
- Excessive spinal fluid drainage through a lumbar drain may produce a counterproductive siphon effect leading to graft displacement and pneumocephalus.

References

1. Abdel Aziz KM, Sanan A, van Loveren HR, et al: Petroclival meningiomas: Predictive parameters for transpetrosal approaches. Neurosurgery 47:139-150, discussion 150-152, 2000.
2. Al-Mefty O, Fox JL, Smith RR: Petrosal approach for petroclival meningiomas. Neurosurgery 22:510-517, 1988.
3. Cass SP, Hirsch BE, Stechison MT: Evolution and advances of the lateral surgical approaches to cranial base neoplasms. J Neurooncol 20:337-361, 1994.
4. Erkmen K, Pravdenkova S, Al-Mefty O: Surgical management of petroclival meningiomas: Factors determining the choice of approach. Neurosurg Focus 19(2):E7, 2005.
5. Kassam AB, Gardner P, Snyderman CH, et al: Expanded endonasal approach: Fully endoscopic, completely transnasal approach to the middle third of the clivus, petrous bone, middle cranial fossa, and infratemporal fossa. Neurosurg Focus 19(1):E6, 2005.
6. Tummala RP, Coscarella E, Morcos JJ: Transpetrosal approaches to the posterior fossa. Neurosurg Focus 19(2) E6, 2005.
7. Solares CA, Fakhri S, Batra PS, et al: Transnasal endoscopic resection of lesions of the clivus: A preliminary report. Laryngoscope 115:1917-1922, 2005.
8. Kartush JM, Kemink JL, Graham MD: The arcuate eminence. Topographic orientation in middle cranial fossa surgery. Ann Otol Rhinol Laryngol 94:25-28, 1985.
9. Kawase T, Shiobara R, Toya S: Anterior transpetrosal-transtentorial approach for sphenopetroclival meningiomas: Surgical method and results in 10 patients. Neurosurgery 28:869-875, discussion 875-866, 1991.
10. House WF, Hitselberger WE: The transcochlear approach to the skull base. Arch Otolaryngol 102:334-342, 1976.
11. Fisch U, Mattox DE: Microsurgery of Skull Base. New York, Thieme, 1988.
12. Garcia-Ibanez E, Garcia-Ibanez JL: Middle fossa vestibular neurectomy: A report of 373 cases. Otolaryngol Head Neck Surg 88:486-490, 1980.
13. Lawton MT, Daspit CP, Spetzler RF: Transpetrosal and combination approaches to skull base lesions. Clin Neurosurg 43:91-112, 1996.
14. Rhoton AL Jr: The temporal bone and transtemporal approaches. Neurosurgery 47(Suppl):S211-S265, 2000.
15. Kassam A, Thomas AJ, Snyderman C, et al: Fully endoscopic expanded endonasal approach treating skull base lesions in pediatric patients. J Neurosurg 106:75-86, 2007.
16. Hadad G, Bassagasteguy L, Carrau RL, et al: A novel reconstructive technique after endoscopic expanded endonasal approaches: Vascular pedicle nasoseptal flap. Laryngoscope 116:1882-1886, 2006.

Endonasal Approach to the Sella and Parasellar Areas

Carl H. Snyderman, Ricardo L. Carrau, and Amin B. Kassam

The evolution of cranial base surgery over the last 2 decades is best exemplified by the evolution of surgical approaches for pituitary tumors. There has been a transition from an open microscopic approach to a "minimally invasive" endoscopic approach. For many years, a sublabial, transseptal microscopic approach was the standard of care. It entailed a sublabial mucosal incision with dissection of the nasal septum in a submucoperichondrial/subperiosteal plane. The septal cartilage was displaced to the side and the vomer was removed. After removal of the sphenoid rostrum, a self-retaining retractor was placed. The main limitations of this approach were the narrow nasal corridor and poor visualization. Postoperative discomfort was significant.

The next stage in pituitary surgery was a transnasal, transseptal approach. The transseptal approach avoided the morbidity of the sublabial incision but provided a smaller surgical corridor. It entailed a hemitransfixion incision in the septal mucosa with disarticulation of the cartilaginous septum and creation of a submucoperichondrial/subperiosteal tunnel. The remainder of the dissection was the same as for the sublabial approach, with placement of a self-retaining retractor in one nostril. The major deficiency of this approach was a narrow surgical corridor with limited visualization and room for instrumentation.

After introduction of the nasal endoscope in the 1980s, a completely endonasal endoscopic approach to the sphenoid sinus and sella was developed.[1] Refinements included the binarial approach, the development of new instrumentation for endonasal skull base surgery, the concept of a modular approach to the skull base with extensions from the sella in the sagittal and coronal planes, and the introduction of septal mucosal flaps for dural reconstruction.[2-4] Advantages of the endonasal

endoscopic approach include less soft tissue morbidity and postoperative pain than with the sublabial approach, improved visualization, and increased access.

The endonasal approach to the sella is the starting point for many endonasal surgeries on the ventral skull base. A midline approach to the sphenoid can also be used for other sphenoid sinus pathology such as chronic sinusitis, mucoceles, and meningoceles, especially when normal sinus anatomy is obscured by pathology or previous surgery. A midline approach provides a reliable means of accessing the sphenoid contents and minimizes the risk of inadvertent injury to lateral structures (optic nerve, internal carotid artery [ICA]).

ANATOMY

The sphenoid sinus is geometrically shaped like a cube. The rostrum of the anterior wall is shaped like the prow of a ship and articulates with the vomer bone of the septum in the midline (Fig. 103-1). The sphenoid ostium is located at the superolateral corner of the sinus behind the attachment of the superior turbinate. The roof of the sphenoid sinus is the planum sphenoidale and is bounded by the cribriform plates and the fovea ethmoidalis anteriorly. The posterior wall of the sphenoid sinus is characterized by the bulge of the sella superiorly and the depression of the clival recess inferiorly (Fig. 103-2). The brain stem and vertebrobasilar arteries are situated deep to this bone. The tubercular strut is a thick ridge of bone overlying the superior intercavernous sinus at the junction of the sella and planum sphenoidale. The degree of pneumatization of the sphenoid sinus is variable and can be categorized as presellar, sellar, or postsellar pneumatization patterns.

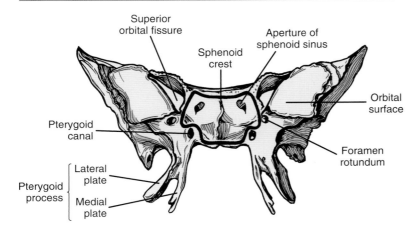

Figure 103-1. Anterior view of the sphenoid bone with bony landmarks identified. The extent of the sphenoidotomy is outlined; it extends between the foramen rotundum and pterygoid canal and includes the lateral recess.

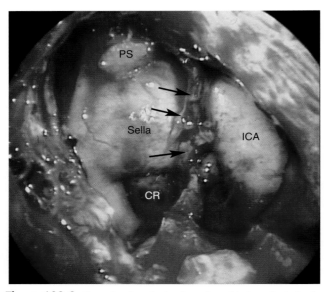

Figure 103-2. Bony landmarks in the sphenoid sinus include the planum sphenoidale (PS), the sella, the clival recess (CR), and the internal carotid artery (ICA) canal. Sphenoid septations *(arrows)* that deviate laterally attach to the carotid canal.

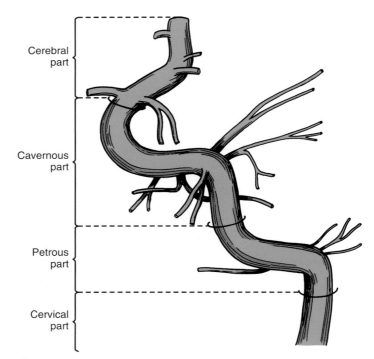

Figure 103-3. Segments of the internal carotid artery.

The most important anatomic structures for the surgeon are situated laterally. The ICA courses along the lateral wall from the petrous carotid artery to the ophthalmic artery (Fig. 103-3). The paraclival segment is located at the level of the clival recess; the cavernous segment forms an S-shaped siphon lateral to the sella. The ICA then courses lateral to the optic nerve to become the supraclinoid segment and contributes to the circle of Willis. Deep to the paraclival ICA at the level of the floor of the sella, the sixth cranial nerve courses superolaterally in Dorello's canal. The optic nerves are superomedial to the carotid arteries and converge at the level of the tubercular strut. Laterally, the junction of the ICA and the optic nerve is bounded by the lateral optic-carotid recess (Fig. 103-4). This recess is formed by pneumatization of the anterior clinoid process. The medial optic-carotid junction is less apparent but represents a "danger zone" where the ICA courses medially toward the sella. The pneumatization of the sphenoid sinus may extend laterally into the base of the pterygoid plates. When this occurs, the pneumatized sinus extends between the pterygoid canal (vidian artery and nerve) inferiorly and the foramen rotundum (second division of the trigeminal nerve) superiorly.

Anatomic variations of the sphenoid are common and may increase the risk for inadvertent injury to structures bordering the sphenoid sinus. The sphenoid sinus often contains multiple septations. Lateral septations always attach to the carotid canal (see Fig. 103-2). The prominence of the carotid canal is quite variable and it may be dehiscent in approximately 10% of patients (Fig. 103-5). Tortuosity of the carotid arteries is pro-

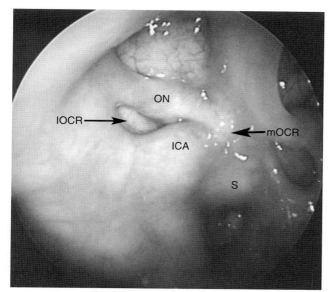

Figure 103-4. Cadaveric dissection with a view of the right optic nerve (ON) and internal carotid artery (ICA). The pneumatization of the anterior clinoid forms the lateral optic-carotid recess (lOCR). The medial junction of the ON and ICA is the medial optic-carotid recess (mOCR).

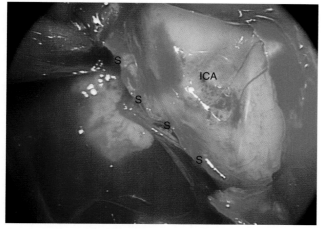

Figure 103-5. The left cavernous segment of the internal carotid artery (ICA) is dehiscent and susceptible to injury. A lateral sphenoid septation (S) attaches to the carotid canal.

nounced in patients with acromegaly. The prominence of the optic canals depends on the degree of pneumatization of the sinus; the optic nerves may be at risk in patients with posterior extension of the ethmoidal air cells (Onodi cell). An Onodi cell may be recognized on preoperative radiographs by horizontal septations within the sphenoid sinus on a coronal view or by an oblique anterior sphenoid wall on an axial view.

PATIENT SELECTION

Indications for an endonasal approach to the sphenoid sinus include inflammatory disease, benign and malignant neoplasms, congenital malformations, and trauma.

Inflammatory conditions include acute and chronic sinusitis, invasive fungal sinusitis, mucocele/mucopyocele, nasal polyposis, and cholesterol granulomas of the petrous apex. Neoplasms may arise from the mucosal lining of the sinus or the underlying bone or may extend into the sinus from the nasal cavity or cranial cavity. Pituitary tumors are among the most common neoplasms and may be confined to the sella or extend superiorly to the suprasellar region, laterally to the cavernous sinus, or anteriorly to the sphenoid sinus. Tumors arising from bone encountered in this region include fibrous dysplasia, chordoma, and chondrosarcoma. Meningiomas frequently involve the planum sphenoidale and petroclival regions. Sinonasal neoplasms that can involve the sphenoid include inverting papilloma, squamous cell carcinoma, adenocarcinoma, adenoid cystic carcinoma, and sinonasal undifferentiated carcinoma. Congenital malformations include meningoceles of the lateral sphenoid recess. Rarely, traumatic injuries may result in a cerebrospinal fluid (CSF) leak within the sphenoid sinus or compression of the optic nerve.

PREOPERATIVE EVALUATION

Symptoms of sphenoid disease are often nonspecific and patients may remain asymptomatic or attribute their minor symptoms to "sinus disease." When headaches occur, they are poorly localized and may be experienced in a frontal or occipital location. Neoplastic disease may be associated with mild epistaxis or nasal obstruction. Patients should be queried about associated symptoms from involvement of adjacent structures, such as visual loss, diplopia, and facial hypoesthesia. Neoplastic invasion of the sella may result in symptoms of hypopituitarism.

Physical examination of a patient with suspected sphenoid sinus pathology should include nasal endoscopy to look for intranasal pathology and assess the patency of the sphenoid ostia. Assessment of cranial nerve function includes visual acuity, motility of the extraocular muscles (cranial nerves III, IV, and VI), and midfacial sensation (V2). A complete ophthalmic evaluation by a neuro-ophthalmologist is indicated if there is evidence of orbital involvement.

A computed tomography (CT) scan of the sinuses is essential to establish a differential diagnosis and determine the extent of disease. Magnetic resonance imaging (MRI) provides complementary information and is helpful in narrowing the diagnostic possibilities. It is especially helpful for visualizing tumor involving the dura and perineural extension and in differentiating soft tissue from obstructed secretions.

PREOPERATIVE PLANNING

Preoperative consultation with specialists in other disciplines may include ophthalmology, endocrinology, and neurosurgery, depending on the initial symptoms and findings. Complete evaluation of visual function may establish the urgency of surgery in patients with visual loss and their potential for recovery. Testing of pituitary function determines the need for hormonal replacement, especially perioperative coverage with stress steroids. Collaboration with a neurosurgeon is recommended for surgeries that involve the cranial base.

Radiologic imaging with CT of the sinuses or skull base is used to plan the best approach (laterality) and to look for variations in normal anatomy (pneumatization, lateral sphenoid septations, Onodi cell, course of the ICA) that may create technical problems during surgery. Intraoperative image guidance is very helpful in surgical approaches to the sella and is used routinely with an image guidance protocol consisting of detailed scanning of the skull base. A CT angiogram provides bony detail with visualization of the ICA. When normal anatomy is obscured, image guidance can help direct the trajectory to the sella and avoid one that is too high and risks a CSF leak. It is also helpful in identifying anatomic structures beneath the bone surface, such as the ICA and optic nerves, and delineating the margins of pathology. Tumors that have a significant soft tissue interface (intracranial, orbital, or infratemporal skull base extension) are also imaged with MRI, and a fusion image is created for intraoperative guidance.

SURGICAL APPROACHES

The sella and surrounding areas may be approached unilaterally when disease is very limited. A bilateral or binarial approach is preferred in most cases because of improved visualization and increased room for instrumentation. The basic approach to the sella may be expanded in any direction, depending on the pathology, and may include a transplanum approach for suprasellar lesions,[2] a transclival/transodontoid approach for lower clival lesions, and a transpterygoid approach for access to the lateral recess of the sphenoid and middle fossa.[5]

Techniques

The patient is positioned in a supine position and registration with an image guidance system is instituted. If immobility of the head is desired, the head is fixed in position with a Mayfield clamp, and the image guidance registration is transferred to the head holder; otherwise, a mask or tracker secured to the skull is used to track the position of the head. The nasal cavity is decongested with pledgets soaked in oxymetazoline, and the anterior nares are prepared with povidone-iodine solution.

The potential need for a reconstructive flap must be considered at the beginning of the surgery.[4] If exposure of the ICA or dura is anticipated, a septal mucosal flap is elevated at the beginning of surgery. It is elevated opposite the side that requires greater exposure. The inferior aspect of the middle turbinate on one side (right side for a right-handed surgeon) is resected to provide additional room for the endoscope during the later stages of surgery (see Video 103-1). The inferior turbinate is lateralized and the sphenoid ostium is visu-

alized (see Video 103-2). A needle-tip electrocautery is used to incise the mucosa and perichondrium/periosteum of the nasal septum while leaving a 5-mm margin at the skull base and nasal vestibule (see Video 103-3). The incision extends along the junction of the nasal septum and nasal floor to the inferior surface of the sphenoid sinus. A vascular pedicle containing the posterior nasal artery and extending from the sphenoid os to the inferior sphenoid surface is preserved. The flap is elevated deep to the perichondrium/periosteum and displaced into the oropharynx for later reconstruction (see Video 103-4).

The posterior septum is incised with a Cottle elevator at its attachment to the sphenoid rostrum, and mucosa is elevated from the contralateral sphenoid surface and resected (see Video 103-5). If bleeding from the contralateral posterior nasal artery is encountered, it is controlled with monopolar or bipolar electrocautery. The bone of the rostrum is removed in the midline with bone rongeurs to create an opening into both sphenoid sinus air cells. The posterior 1 to 2 cm of the transected septum is resected with back-biting rongeur to enhance binarial exposure (see Fig. 103-2) (see Video 103-6). The anterior face of the sphenoid sinus is then resected with Kerrison rongeurs to maximize the sphenoidotomy (see Fig. 103-1). Laterally, bone is removed to the edge of the pterygoid (vidian) canal, which is located inferolateral to the lateral recess of the sphenoid sinus. Superiorly, bone is removed to the planum sphenoidale. This may require opening the posterior ethmoid air cells for visualization. Resection of soft tissue and bone anterior to the planum sphenoidale in the midline is minimized to avoid injury to olfactory nerves and possible CSF leak. Additional room for instrumentation can be gained by removing thick bone along the floor of the sphenoid sinus with a drill (4-mm diamond hybrid bit).

Both nasal passages can now be used for instrumentation. The sphenoid sinus is inspected to confirm the location of the sella, carotid arteries, and optic nerves (Fig. 103-6). The relationship of sphenoid septations to these structures is determined, and the septations are carefully removed with rongeurs or a drill (see Video 103-7). Aggressive removal of lateral septations that attach to the carotid canal can result in vascular injury. Although sinus mucosa can be preserved when removing small pituitary tumors, it is usually stripped from the sinus to improve visualization of bony landmarks and to prepare the surgical bed for reconstruction with the septal mucosal flap or fat grafts.

In patients undergoing pituitary surgery, the bone over the sella is thinned with the drill and fractured with an elevator. The bone fragments are elevated from the dura of the sella and removed. Removal of bone continues to the margin of the cavernous sinus with a 1-mm angled Kerrison rongeur (Fig. 103-7) (see Video 103-8). The tip of the rongeur should be directed parallel to the cavernous ICA to avoid perforating the vessel. The ICA is especially prone to injury at the medial optic-carotid recess, where the ICA deviates medially before passing lateral to the optic nerve. Opening of

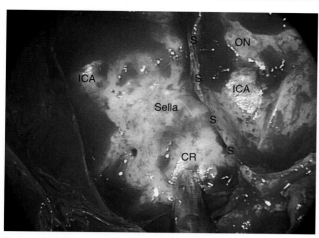

Figure 103-6. Endoscopic view of the sphenoid sinus and bony landmarks after bilateral sphenoidotomy and resection of the posterior nasal septum. CR, clival recess; ICA, internal carotid artery; ON, optic nerve; S, lateral sphenoid septation.

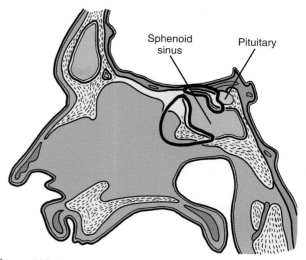

Figure 103-8. The planum sphenoidale and sella may be removed in continuity to provide access to tumors with suprasellar extension.

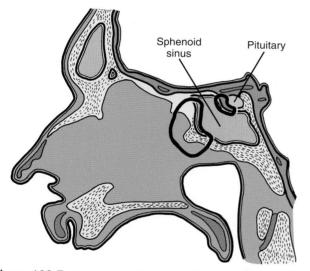

Figure 103-7. The extent of resection of the anterior face of the sphenoid sinus, posterior nasal septum, and sella is outlined.

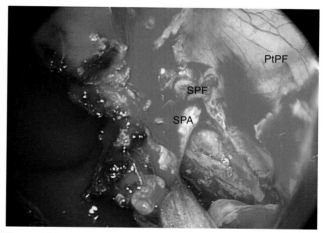

Figure 103-9. A left antrostomy has been performed and the sphenopalatine artery (SPA) exposed at the sphenopalatine foramen (SPF). Overlying bone is removed to expose the pterygopalatine space (PtPF).

the dura and removal of pituitary pathology are then performed in conjunction with a neurosurgeon. The otolaryngologist maintains visualization with the endoscope while the neurosurgeon uses two hands to dissect the tumor. For tumors that have suprasellar extension, a transplanum approach is combined with a transsellar approach (Fig. 103-8). The bone of the planum sphenoidale over the dura is thinned with a drill (3- to 4-mm hybrid diamond bit) until it is thin enough to fracture and elevate from the dura. Drilling should be limited to the midline initially until the course of the optic nerves is well visualized. Continuous irrigation when drilling is essential to prevent thermal injury to the optic nerves. Once the bone of the sella and posterior planum is removed, the remaining strut of bone along the tuberculum sellae is thinned laterally adjacent to the middle clinoid (medial optic-carotid recess). The

strut of bone can then be fractured and elevated from the superior intercavernous sinus. Bleeding from the sinus is controlled by gentle application of hemostatic material. The dura can now be opened in the midline to avoid injury to the optic nerves, and the superior intercavernous sinus is transected to provide maximal visualization.

Pathology that extends into the lateral recess of the sphenoid sinus requires a transpterygoid approach if the sinus is well pneumatized.[5,6] A middle meatal antrostomy is performed on the side of the pathology, and the sphenopalatine foramen is identified (see Video 103-9). The overlying bone is removed with a 1-mm angled Kerrison rongeur to expose the contents of the pterygopalatine space (Fig. 103-9) (see Video 103-10). The vessel is cauterized with bipolar electrocautery and transected. The soft tissues of the pterygopalatine space are elevated from the underlying pterygoid bone medi-

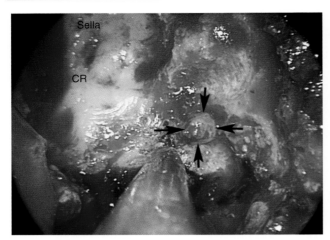

Figure 103-10. The contents of the left pterygoid canal *(arrows)* have been exposed and the surrounding bone has been drilled. CR, clival recess.

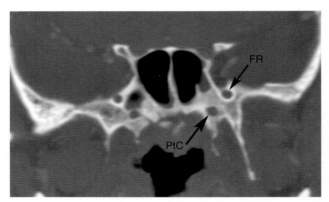

Figure 103-11. The lateral recess of the sphenoid sinus is bounded laterally by the pterygoid canal (PtC) inferiorly and the foramen rotundum (FR) superiorly.

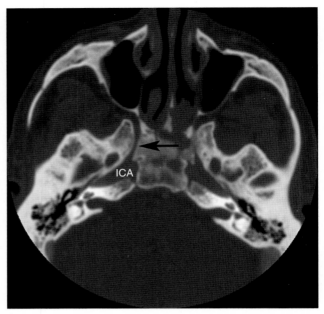

Figure 103-12. The pterygoid canal *(arrow)* is a reliable landmark for locating the petrous internal carotid artery (ICA) at the second genu.

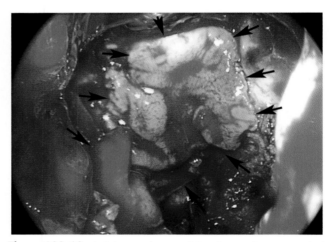

Figure 103-13. A right septal mucosal flap *(arrows* denote margins) has been transposed to cover the defect in the skull base.

ally and displaced laterally. The vidian artery and nerve are identified at the point where they exit the pterygoid canal, and additional bone superolateral to the pterygoid canal is removed to open the lateral recess (Fig. 103-10). The lateral recess is bounded superolaterally by the foramen rotundum (second division of the trigeminal nerve) and the floor of the middle cranial fossa (Fig. 103-11). Wide exposure requires sacrifice of the vidian artery and nerve. The vidian artery courses superolateral to the ICA and is a key landmark for identification of the second genu of the ICA (Fig. 103-12).[7] The surrounding bone is drilled to the plane of the petrous ICA, starting with removal of bone inferiorly from the 3-o'clock to the 9-o'clock position (see Video 103-11). This avoids injury to the ICA until the depth of the artery can be ascertained. Identification of the course of the petrous ICA is a prerequisite for additional dissection of the petrous apex and parasellar region.[8]

Any dural defects are repaired with inlay and onlay fascial grafts; a synthetic dural substitute may be used. The septal mucosal flap is then retrieved from the oropharynx and rotated to cover the grafts and exposed bone (Fig. 103-13). If there is a deep space that is not suitable for contouring of the flap, the space is first obliterated with an abdominal fat graft to create a planar surface for the flap. The flap is covered with a layer of oxycellulose (Surgicel) followed by a synthetic glue (DuraSeal). This is supported by nasal tampons or a Foley urinary catheter inflated with saline to counteract intracranial CSF pressure. The nasal septum is protected with Silastic splints.

POSTOPERATIVE CARE

In the absence of a CSF leak, any nasal packing is removed in 1 to 2 days. If dural repair has been performed, packing is maintained for 5 to 7 days. Prophylaxis with oral antibiotics is maintained as long as the nasal packing is in place. Patients are instructed to use a saline nasal spray after the packing is removed and to avoid strenuous activities that may increase intracranial pressure, such as nose blowing, bending, and lifting. Silastic nasal splints are maintained for 1 week if a septal mucosal flap is not harvested and for 3 weeks if it has. Protection of the exposed cartilage with Silastic splints prevents desiccation and promotes mucosalization. After the splints are removed, saline irrigation is instituted to prevent the accumulation of crust. Gentle endoscopic débridement of crust is performed periodically during the first month while taking care to not disrupt the dural repair. Healing is usually complete within 3 months, and the nasal crusting diminishes.

Patients are monitored for evidence of a CSF leak in the first few weeks postoperatively. Most CSF leaks are apparent once the nasal packing is removed and are characterized by clear rhinorrhea that is often unilateral, a reservoir sign, and occasionally, low-pressure headaches. When the diagnosis is questionable, the leak is confirmed by testing of a rhinorrhea sample for β_2-transferrin. Most leaks are managed by early surgical intervention consisting of endoscopic repair and placement of a lumbar spinal drain for 3 to 5 days.

COMPLICATIONS

Complications associated with the endonasal approach to the sella and parasellar areas can be categorized as nasal, vascular, and neural. Most otolaryngologic complications are minor but have a significant impact on quality of life: sinusitis, chronic rhinitis with nasal crusting, loss of olfactory function, nasal synechiae and obstruction, septal perforation, minor epistaxis, decreased tearing, and palatal or facial hypoesthesia. Patients require significant postoperative care with endoscopic removal of nasal crusts for approximately 3 months after surgery. A subset of patients will continue to have problems, however, especially after radiation therapy. Although a binarial approach increases the potential for nasal crusting, it appears that use of a septal flap greatly decreases the amount of crusting in the sphenoid region. Loss of olfactory function (and decreased taste) is observed for several months after surgery and probably reflects a combination of factors: mucosal edema, nasal obstruction from crusting, and some loss of olfactory mucosa. A transpterygoid approach often results in loss of vidian nerve function. Most patients will not notice an appreciable change in tearing except in situations in which tearing is normally increased: emotional tearing, windy conditions, and cold weather. Dissection posterior to the sphenopalatine artery can injure the descending palatine nerve and result in palatal hypoesthesia. The infraorbital nerve may be injured along the roof of the maxillary sinus or at the foramen rotundum and result in numbness of the cheek.

Dreaded complications of endonasal surgery include injury to the ICA and optic nerves. These injuries can be avoided with a good understanding of endo-scopic anatomy and its variations and by careful surgical technique. Most injuries to the ICA occur at the medial optic-carotid recess, where the ICA deviates medially. The vidian artery is a reliable landmark for locating the petrous ICA at the second genu (see Fig. 103-8). Injury to the optic nerve may occur as a result of direct trauma or thermal injury from electrocautery or drilling. The presence of an Onodi cell should be determined preoperatively to avoid injury during opening of air cells.

CSF leaks are a common sequela of endonasal skull base surgery and should be anticipated. A trajectory to the sphenoid sinus that is too high risks violation of the skull base through the posterior ethmoid air cells or planum sphenoidale and can be avoided by visualizing the inferior attachment of the nasal septum to the rostrum and using image guidance intraoperatively.

SUMMARY

The sphenoid sinus is the starting point for endonasal approaches to the sella and ventral skull base. A binarial approach maximizes visualization and allows bimanual dissection. The parasellar areas can be visualized by extending the sphenoidotomy superiorly or laterally. Reliable anatomic landmarks within the sphenoid sinus are used to avoid injury to the ICA and optic nerves.

PEARLS

- The need for a septal mucosal flap for reconstruction should be considered before performing a sphenoidotomy.
- The safest area to open the sphenoid sinus is in the midline at the sphenoid rostrum.
- The lateral recess of the sphenoid sinus extends between the pterygoid canal and the foramen rotundum.
- Lateral septations of the sphenoid sinus attach to the carotid canal.
- The lateral optic-carotid recess is a useful landmark for visualizing the course of the optic nerve and the ICA; it is formed by pneumatization of the anterior clinoid.

PITFALLS

- A high trajectory to the sphenoid sinus may result in violation of the planum sphenoidale and a CSF leak.
- Monopolar electrocautery should not be used within the sphenoid sinus because of the risk of injury to the ICA or optic nerve.
- The ICA deviates medially at the medial optic-carotid recess and may be injured when opening the sella.
- An unrecognized Onodi cell can result in injury to the optic nerve.
- The increased tortuosity of the carotid arteries in acromegalic individuals results in a narrowed surgical field.

References

1. Carrau RL, Kassam AB, Snyderman CH: Pituitary surgery. Otolaryngol Clin North Am 34:1143-1155, ix, 2001.
2. Kassam A, Snyderman CH, Mintz A, et al: Expanded endonasal approach: The rostrocaudal axis. Part I. Crista galli to the sella turcica. Neurosurg Focus 19(1):E3, 2005.
3. Kassam AB, Mintz AH, Snyderman CH, et al: Expanded endonasal approach to the sella and anterior skull base. In Badie B (ed): Neurosurgical Operative Atlas. New York, Thieme, 2007, pp 21-30.
4. Hadad G, Bassagasteguy L, Carrau RL, et al: A novel reconstructive technique after endoscopic expanded endonasal approaches: Vascular pedicle nasoseptal flap. Laryngoscope 116:1882-1886, 2006.
5. Alnashar IS, Carrau RL, Herrera A, Snyderman CH: Endoscopic transnasal transpterygopalatine fossa approach to the lateral recess of the sphenoid sinus. Laryngoscope 114:528-532, 2004.
6. Tosun F, Carrau RL Snyderman CH, et al: Endonasal endoscopic repair of cerebrospinal fluid leaks of the sphenoid sinus. Arch Otolaryngol Head Neck Surg 129:576-580, 2003.
7. Vescan AD, Snyderman CH, Carrau RL, et al: Vidian canal: Analysis and relationship to the internal carotid artery. Laryngoscope 117:1338-1342.
8. Snyderman CH, Kassam AB, Carrau R, Mintz A: Endoscopic approaches to the petrous apex. Op Tech Otolaryngol 17:168-173, 2006.

Chapter **104**

Endoscopic Management of Cerebrospinal Fluid Leaks

Ricardo L. Carrau, Allan D. Vescan, Carl H. Snyderman, and Amin B. Kassam

A cerebrospinal fluid (CSF) leak implies a fistula between the subarachnoid space and the sinonasal tract. Patients with CSF leaks have symptoms such as clear nasal discharge and headache or complications such as pneumocephalus, meningitis, or a brain abscess. Immediate identification plus repair of a CSF fistula avoid the development of life-threatening complications.[1,2]

CSF leaks can be classified in a number of ways. Etiology, anatomic site, age of the patient, and underlying intracranial pressure are the most common classification systems used. Etiologic classification can be subdivided into traumatic and nontraumatic in origin. In the traumatic category, leaks can be either accidental or iatrogenic. Most CSF leaks are caused by trauma-induced fractures of the cranial base or by injuries produced during endoscopic sinus surgery or cranial base surgery. CSF leaks are diagnosed in 3% of patients suffering closed head injuries and in up to 30% of patients with a fracture of the skull base.[3] Similarly, iatrogenic trauma such as that caused by traditional cranial base surgery and endoscopic sinus surgery is associated with CSF leaks. Endoscopic sinus surgery remains one of the most common causes of CSF rhinorrhea despite an overall incidence of 1% in patients undergoing such surgery.[4-21] Nontraumatic CSF leaks may occur secondary to tumors of the skull base, congenital malformations, or high-pressure hydrocephalus (HPH). The etiology of HPH includes tumors, trauma, infections, and hemorrhagic cerebrovascular accidents (CVAs). Occasionally, no cause is identified for the HPH and it is therefore deemed "idiopathic."

Multiple techniques have been reported for the repair of a CSF fistula. In 1952, Hirsch described the first endonasal repair of CSF rhinorrhea with a septal flap.[22] Subsequently, Montgomery described his experience with septal flaps through an external nasal approach to treat CSF rhinorrhea.[23] In 1976, McCabe reported his experience with the use of osteomucoperiosteal flaps from the septum or middle turbinate through an external ethmoidectomy approach.[24] In 1989, a publication of McCabe's updated experience reported a 100% closure rate with follow-ups of 1.6 to 22 years.[25] The use of these and other local flaps to treat CSF fistulas via an endoscopic approach was subsequently reported.[13,26]

In 1985, Calcaterra[27] described the use of free muscle or fascia grafts to treat CSF fistulas via an external ethmoidectomy approach, and in 1989, Papay and colleagues[28] described an endoscopic technique. Multiple publications followed with reports of the use of free grafts or local flaps, or both, for the repair of CSF fistulas. Recently, a vascularized nasoseptal flap has been devised to reconstruct skull base defects of various causes, and early follow-up data have revealed a remarkable improvement in CSF fistula rates after expanded endonasal approaches to the skull base.[29]

The availability of biologic material and the experience and familiarity of the operating surgeon with various techniques are the most important factors influencing the choice of which technique is used during endoscopic endonasal closure of CSF fistulas. Most techniques yield similar results in experienced hands, as confirmed by a meta-analysis of the literature by Hegazy and coworkers.[1] After analyzing all reports in the English literature, these authors found no significant differences in outcome regardless of which surgical technique or which homologous material was used for the repair.

PATIENT SELECTION

Diagnosis plus management of a CSF leak involve three critical steps: distinguishing a CSF leak from other sources of rhinorrhea, locating the fistula, and ruling out high intracranial pressure secondary to altered CSF dynamics.

Clinical diagnosis of a CSF leak is based on a history of clear, watery nasal drainage that is generally unilateral and commonly associated with headache. Increased rhinorrhea when the patient leans over, tilts the head forward, or performs a Valsalva maneuver further suggests the presence of a CSF leak. A history of tumor, trauma, or previous surgery involving the paranasal sinuses or cranial base heightens the level of suspicion. Occasionally, a life-threatening complication arising from the CSF leak, such as pneumocephalus, brain abscess, or ascending bacterial meningitis, may be the initial manifestation.

Conditions such as vasomotor rhinitis and sympathetic denervation can cause profuse rhinorrhea that may be confused with a CSF leak. Nasal irrigation fluid used during endoscopic sinus surgery or as part of postoperative care may accumulate in the paranasal sinuses and later manifest as postoperative rhinorrhea. Thus, biochemical testing is indicated to confirm the true nature of the nasal drainage. CSF will be high in glucose and low in protein. However, normal nasal discharge has been shown to be falsely positive for glucose in 45% to 75% of cases.[30] β_2-Transferrin is a protein found in CSF, aqueous humor, and perilymph, but not in blood or nasal secretions; therefore, β_2-transferrin is a reliable chemical marker of CSF leakage.[31-35] In addition to β_2-transferrin, a new chemical marker called β-trace protein is being explored for the diagnosis of CSF fistula.[36]

PREOPERATIVE PLANNING

When CSF rhinorrhea develops after sinus surgery, the endoscopic surgeon typically has an impression about the possible site of injury to the cranial base (i.e., site of the CSF fistula).

Therefore, a thorough endoscopic office examination of the nasal cavity may identify the site of leakage. Fistulas with low-pressure leaks are difficult to identify, especially in the presence of postoperative tissue edema and blood clots.

Intrathecal injection of contrast material and radioactive tracers has been advocated to confirm a CSF leak and identify the site of origin. Intrathecal fluorescein may be used to aid in the diagnosis and localization of a CSF leak. During this test, 0.5 mL of fluorescein at a concentration not greater than 5% is diluted with 10 mL of CSF obtained through lumbar puncture and then injected intrathecally. Fluorescein is neurotoxic, so a low-concentration, low-volume injection is mandatory to avoid the neurologic complications associated with higher concentrations. After intrathecal injection of the fluorescein solution, the CSF leak may be visualized with a nasal endoscope.[31-35,37] Under Wood's lamp (i.e., black light), fluorescein will appear as bright yellow-green. The yellowish color of fluorescein may also be identified without the need for special lighting.

The logistics of performing a lumbar puncture in an outpatient setting and medicolegal considerations (the fluorescein drug package insert includes an advisory warning against intrathecal use) have discouraged us from using this technique. Intrathecal injections are rarely critical to identification of a CSF fistula. Exceptional patients are those with multiple fistulas, such as those patients who have suffered skull base fractures, and the rare patient with repeated episodes of meningitis in the absence of an apparent cranial base defect or other predisposing factors such as rhinosinusitis or otitis media.

Others have advocated intrathecal injection of air, which can "bubble" out at the fistula site and therefore aid in identification.[37] Air, however, is an irritant to the brain and may induce seizures. Normal saline solution may be injected into the intrathecal space to increase the pressure within the subarachnoid space and thus aid in identification of the leak.

Scintigraphy with indium-111 has been advocated for the identification of a CSF leak. Radiotracing is a very sensitive test; however, it is associated with a high false-positive rate[31] and has a poor resolution that precludes establishing the specific point of leakage. In general, we do not advocate scintigraphy. In our practice, the presence of a CSF leak is ascertained with β_2-transferrin electrophoresis, and its site of origin is identified by computed tomography (CT) scanning, magnetic resonance imaging (MRI), or CT cisternography, with or without endoscopy (Fig. 104-1).

An important consideration in a patient with spontaneous rhinorrhea or rhinorrhea after skull base trauma is to distinguish whether the CSF rhinorrhea is arising from the sinonasal tract or from other sites such as the middle ear or mastoid (Fig. 104-2). A CSF fistula in the temporal bone may drain into the nose through the eustachian tube. Imaging is critical to locate the site of the fistula. Radiographically, high-resolution computed tomography (HRCT) can be used to identify a cranial base defect. HRCT is our preferred initial imaging study to aid in identification of the site of injury and its extent (Fig. 104-3). HRCT with contrast enhancement also provides information about the possibility of intracranial complications that occur in the setting of acute trauma (iatrogenic or accidental), such as hematoma or brain contusion. HRCT with views taken at a plane perpendicular to the suspected site of injury better evaluates the integrity of the bony wall in question. Coronal CT views are best to evaluate defects of the cribriform plate, fovea ethmoidalis, or planum sphenoidale, whereas axial views are superior for evaluation of the posterior wall of the frontal or sphenoid sinuses. We use MRI to ascertain the contents of a meningocele or meningoencephalocele (Fig. 104-4).

HRCT, however, may not identify small areas of surgical trauma or linear nondisplaced fractures. In this

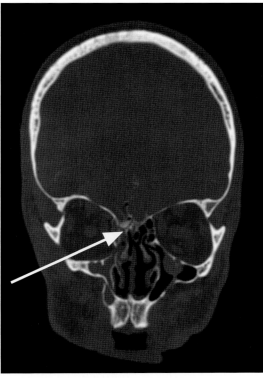

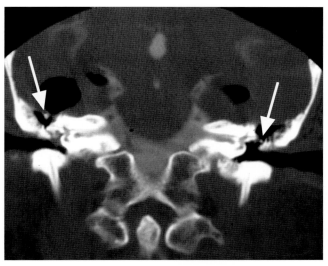

Figure 104-2. Coronal CT cisternogram demonstrating bilateral tegmen defects with contrast material penetrating through existing defects *(arrows)*.

Figure 104-1. Coronal CT cisternogram demonstrating a right cribriform defect leading to a post-traumatic cerebrospinal fluid fistula *(arrow)*.

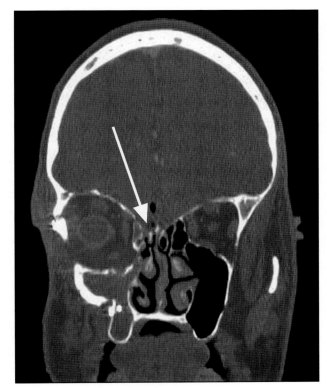

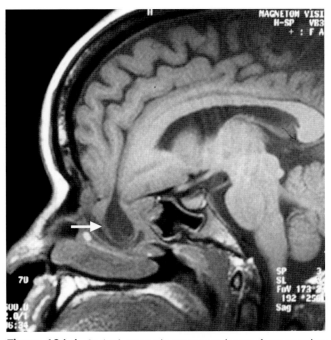

Figure 104-4. Sagittal magnetic resonance image demonstrating large meningoencephaloceles of the anterior cranial base *(arrow)*.

Figure 104-3. Coronal CT scan demonstrating a defect in the right cribriform plate after trauma as the cause of the cerebrospinal fluid fistula *(arrow)*.

case, HRCT can be used in conjunction with intrathecal injection of contrast material to identify the fistula. CT cisternography has been documented to be both sensitive and reliable. Water-soluble nonionic contrast agents with less associated toxicity, headache, nausea, and arachnoiditis have replaced metrizamide. Identification of the fistula with contrast-enhanced studies, however, requires the presence of an active leak. Intermittent leaks that are temporarily sealed by swelling, inflammation, or brain herniation may yield a false-negative result. Intrathecal injection of saline solution to increase the CSF pressure, "a saline challenge," enhances the sensitivity of the test.

Others have suggested MR cisternography to complement the information offered by HRCT without the need for an intrathecal contrast agent.[38] In our experience, however, this technique has yielded inconsistent results.

SURGICAL TECHNIQUE

Ethmoid Sinus Roof and Cribriform Plate

If a CSF leak is suspected during endoscopic sinus surgery, the overlying mucosa should be reflected away to closely examine the area and determine the extent of injury. An inlay or onlay free tissue graft may be used to patch the site of injury.

Fascia lata, temporalis muscle, abdominal fat, septal or middle turbinate mucosa or composite grafts, periosteum, and perichondrium are all suitable grafting materials. Whenever possible, the dural edges are undermined with a small elevator and the edges of the graft are tucked between the dura and bone (i.e., epidural inlay graft). Alternatively, the dura may be separated from the brain, and the inlay graft may be placed in the subdural space. When an inlay graft is not possible because of technical difficulties, because the fistula involves a linear fracture that does not expose the dural defect, or because dissection of the dura may place neurovascular structures at risk, the graft is placed as an onlay over the defect (outside the cranial cavity). Free muscle or fat grafts can also be used as a dumbbell–type plug. Fibrin glue, platelet-rich serum, or other biologic glue may be used to increase the adhesiveness of the muscle or fascia graft.

The graft is supported in place with layers of Gelfoam or Gelfilm (Upjohn Co., Kalamazoo, MI), followed by packing of bacitracin-impregnated gauze or sponge packing. The use of Gelfoam or Gelfilm (or both) prevents adherence of the packing material to the graft, thereby preventing accidental avulsion when the packing is removed 3 to 7 days after surgery.

Alternatively, a vascularized tissue flap may be fashioned with mucoperichondrium from the middle turbinate or septum and harvested transnasally. If the fistula involves the cribriform plate, the mucosa and bone of the lateral aspect of the middle turbinate are removed and the remaining mucoperiosteal flap is rotated to cover the defect or cover a muscle or fascia free graft.

Similarly, the mucosa and bone of the lateral aspect of the middle turbinate may be removed to cover a defect of the fovea ethmoidalis. An additional option includes removal of mucosa from a portion of the ipsilateral septum, removal of the corresponding septal cartilage or perpendicular plate of the ethmoid, and rotation of the contralateral mucoperichondrial flap to cover the defect. The flap is then supported by Gelfoam or Gelfilm (or both) and bacitracin-impregnated gauze. This type of septal flap is the preferred flap for defects of the planum sphenoidale that may not be reached by middle turbinate flaps (i.e., defects that are posterior to the posterior attachment of the middle turbinate). Recently, we have been using the Hadad-Bassasteguy flap, which consists of a septal mucoperichondrial/mucoperiosteal flap based on the posterior septal artery. The entire mucoperichondrium/mucoperiosteum may be harvested on one side to cover very large defects of the skull base.

Exposure of the entire defect is essential. In fact, exposure of the defect may be a more important factor in determining success of the repair than its size or site.[39]

Sphenoid Sinus

The sphenoid sinus can be approached transseptally or, preferably, through a direct endoscopic approach such as the one described for pituitary surgery. CSF leaks involving the sphenoid sinus are amenable to a repair that includes obliteration of the sinus. After proper identification of surgical landmarks such as the carotid canal, optic nerve canal, and optic carotid recesses and establishing the extent of the defect identifying the leak, the sinus mucosa is thoroughly removed. Onlay or inlay free tissue grafts are placed and the sinus is then obliterated with abdominal free fat. Anteriorly, the exposed fat is covered with a layer of Surgicel followed by Gelfilm, and the nose is packed with a ½-inch nasal strip that has been impregnated with antibiotic ointment.

An intraoperative CSF leak arising from the sella turcica during pituitary surgery can most often be repaired by obliterating the sella with free fat and reconstructing the floor of the sella with a free bone or cartilage graft harvested during the endoscopic approach.[41] Thus, it does not require postoperative packing or removal of the entire mucoperiosteum of the sinus. The previously described Hadad flap has been very effective in repairing these defects.

The risk of accidental injury to adjacent neurovascular structures is a critical consideration when dealing with defects at the lateral wall of the sphenoid sinus. Adequate visualization of this area is mandatory. Leaks that arise in the lateral recess present technical difficulties as a result of poor visualization after a traditional sphenoidotomy (Fig. 104-5). Repair often requires ligation of the sphenopalatine artery and extension of the sphenoidotomy toward the pterygopalatine fossa.[42] The transpterygoid approach can be combined with endoscopic medial maxillectomy as necessary to allow ade-

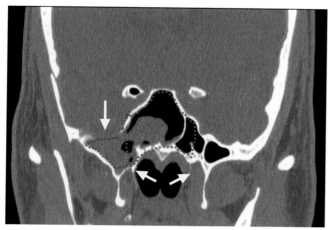

Figure 104-5. Coronal CT scan of the sphenoid sinus depicting the limit of visualization of a traditional sphenoidotomy *(green dots)*. The lateral recess of the sphenoid sinus can be visualized with a transpterygoid approach *(red dots)*. The *diagonal arrows* point to the medial pterygoid plates. The *vertical arrow* points to a bone defect of the right middle cranial fossa.

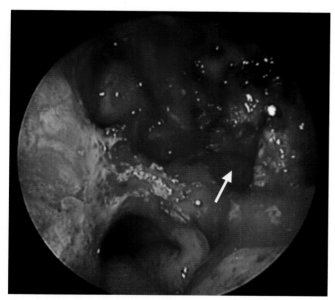

Figure 104-6. Endoscopic view using a zero-degree scope of the left lateral recess of the sphenoid sinus via a transpterygoid approach *(arrow)*.

quate range of motion and visualization of even the most lateral of sphenoid defects. Through this extended lateral approach to the sphenoid sinus the endoscopic surgeon is now able to use a zero-degree scope and straight instruments to replace angled scopes and working around corners (Fig. 104-6).

Frontal Sinus

CSF leaks involving the frontal sinus are usually repaired via a transfrontal sinus approach. The Draf III approach,[43] which involves medial widening of the frontal recesses and removal of the superior nasal

septum and inferior frontal sinus septum, may provide exposure of leaks around the frontonasal recess, thus allowing endoscopic repair.

POSTOPERATIVE MANAGEMENT

As previously mentioned, the general principles of managing a CSF fistula include adjunctive measures that may facilitate healing of the repair, including avoidance of activities that raise intracranial pressure, such as straining, leaning forward, or lifting weights greater than 15 pounds. Other measures include bed rest, stool softeners, 30- to 45-degree elevation of the head of the bed, sneezing with an open mouth, and absolute avoidance of nose blowing. "Deep extubation" to prevent straining and coughing is used, and positive pressure mask ventilation is contraindicated.

The use of prophylactic antibiotics for the prevention of meningitis in patients with CSF fistulas continues to be controversial. However, antibiotics are warranted when the patient has an active sinus infection. In patients with indwelling lumbar catheters, prophylactic antibiotics are routinely administered, and although the concept is not universally accepted, antibiotics are believed to decrease the incidence of catheter-related infections.[44] The routine use of antibiotics for traumatic CSF leaks is not of proven efficacy, however, and may select resistant bacteria.[45] Nonetheless, we do favor the use of perioperative prophylactic antibiotics during repair of the CSF leak. Antibiotics are continued until the nasal packing is removed.

A postoperative CT scan without contrast enhancement in the first 24 hours after surgery is important to rule out evidence of intracranial bleeding, parenchymal injury, or tension pneumocephalus. We favor a routine CT scan of the brain, even in the absence of any neurologic deficit.

In our practice, we work in conjunction with a neurosurgical team during the repairs; although we do not consider it necessary in all cases, neurosurgical consultation provides an important perspective on intraoperative and postoperative management, especially on the need for a CSF drain or a shunt. A lumbar drain with a designated amount of CSF removed daily based on CSF production is helpful to control intracranial pressure, but it is used only for patients suspected of having HPH. Overdrainage should be avoided because it creates negative intracranial pressure (i.e., suction effect) that may result in pneumocephalus and promote bacterial contamination of the CSF with resultant meningitis.

High-Pressure Hydrocephalus

Normal intracranial pressure ranges from 5 to 15 cm H_2O when the patient is in the supine position. However, intracranial pressure increases with positional changes, with the Valsalva maneuver, and during rapid eye movement (REM) sleep. Increased intracranial pressure, or HPH, is defined as sustained or intermittent pressure of 20 to 30 cm H_2O.[48] Post-traumatic, postsurgical, and

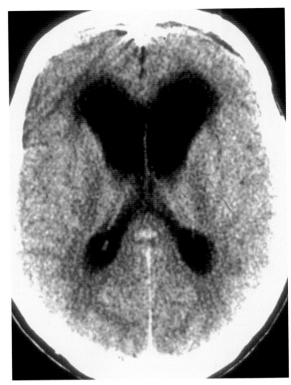

Figure 104-7. Axial CT scan of the head in a patient with high-pressure hydrocephalus and ventriculomegaly of the temporal horns.

High-risk patient:
"Spontaneous" CSF fistula
Recurrent CSF fistula
Hx of:
Head trauma
SBS
Subarachnoid hemorrhage

↙ ↘

Sphenoid sinus obliteration and nasal packing   Intraoperative lumbar spinal drain

↓   ↓

3-5 days post-op measure CSF opening pressure

↓   ↓

Normal CSF pressure   Elevated CSF pressure

↓   ↓

Discharge home   VP shunt

↓

CT 6 weeks post-op

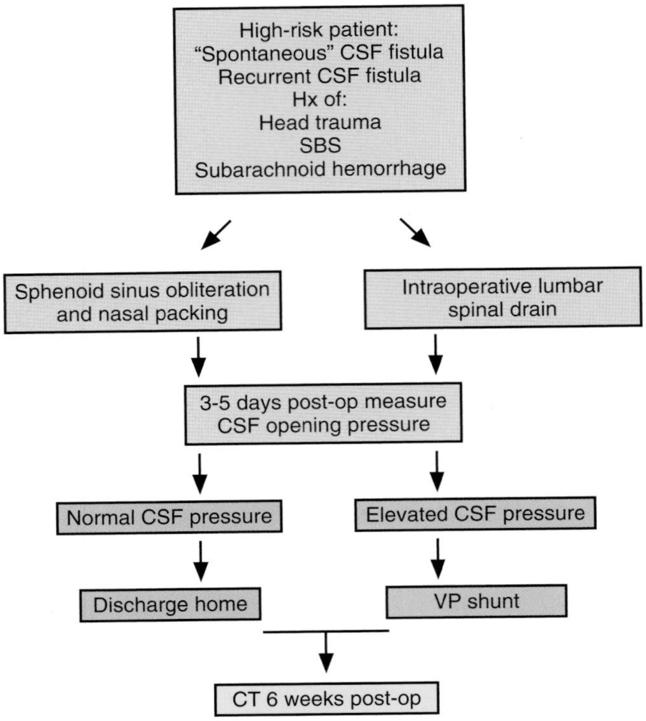

Figure 104-8. Management algorithm for patients at high risk for high-pressure hydrocephalus and failure of repair of a cerebrospinal fluid (CSF) fistula. CT, computed tomography; Hx, history; SBS, skull base surgery; VP, ventriculoperitoneal.

postinfectious hydrocephalus can result from obstruction of the arachnoid villi, thus preventing adequate CSF reabsorption with subsequent increased intraventricular pressure. In post-CVA, post-traumatic and postsurgical hydrocephalus, the obstruction arises from subarachnoid hemorrhage, whereas in the case of infection, inflammatory changes are responsible for obstructing the arachnoid villi (Fig. 104-7).[46-51]

Radiation therapy causes vascular changes in the brain and elevation of CSF protein, scarring, and adhesions, all of which may contribute to impairment of CSF reabsorption. Likewise, meningitis causes scarring of the CSF cisterns and absorptive sites, thus leading to chronic hydrocephalus.[46-48]

Patients with recurrent CSF leaks, a past history of head or cranial base trauma (or both), and a history of cranial base surgery and those with "spontaneous" CSF leaks are considered at high risk for HPH and are enrolled in the following protocol (Fig. 104-8).[52] The CSF leak is repaired via an endonasal endoscopic approach by following surgical principles such as adequate exposure, hemostasis, preparation of the fistula for grafting, and stabilization of the graft. A lumbar spinal drain is inserted intraoperatively or immediately after surgery. Three to 5 days postoperatively, the lumbar spinal drain is clamped, and if no CSF leak is identified for 24 hours, the drain is removed. Twenty-four to 48 hours later, a lumbar puncture is performed to measure CSF opening pressure. A ventriculoperitoneal (VP) shunt is recommended if CSF opening pressure is elevated. IF CSF opening pressure is normal, the patient is discharged home and monitored in our outpatient offices.

Patients with CSF leaks in the sphenoid sinus are treated by obliteration of the sinus with abdominal fat, which is then stabilized with nasal packing. A postoperative lumbar spinal drain is not required. A lumbar puncture is performed 3 to 5 days postoperatively to measure opening pressure and establish the need for a VP shunt.

In patients with normal CSF opening pressure, a CT scan of the brain is performed 6 weeks after surgical closure. Ventriculomegaly of the temporal horns or transependymal edema will identify patients with HPH who may have escaped identification (false negative).

CSF leaks in patients who did not have any of the previously mentioned high-risk factors are repaired endoscopically and without the use of a spinal drain.

Nasal irrigation with nasal saline solution plus gentle débridement of crusting is started 1 week postoperatively.

PEARLS

- Early identification plus repair of CSF fistulas avoids the development of life-threatening complications.
- Most traumatic CSF leaks will heal with conservative management.
- Endoscopic repair is as successful as open repair given localization of the leak.
- β_2-Transferrin is an extremely reliable marker for CSF leak because it is found only in CSF, perilymph, and vitreous humor.
- A CT cisternogram with water-soluble contrast material is a very useful localizing study in cases in which intrathecal fluorescein is not used.

PITFALLS

- Traumatic CSF fistulas after skull base fracture are often multifocal in nature.
- Failure of CSF fistula repair is frequently a result of inadequate exposure versus inadequate repair.
- High-pressure hydrocephalus is a factor in failure of CSF fistula repair.
- Intrathecal administration of an inappropriate concentration of fluorescein can lead to neurologic sequelae.
- Positive pressure ventilation should be avoided in the immediate postoperative period to prevent pneumocephalus.

References

1. Hegazy HM, Carrau RL, Snyderman CH, et al: Transnasal-endoscopic repair of cerebrospinal fluid rhinorrhea: A meta-analysis. Laryngoscope 110:1166-1172, 2000.
2. Bernal-Sprekelsen M, Bleda-Vazquez C, Carrau RL: Ascending meningitis secondary to traumatic cerebrospinal fluid leaks. Am J Rhinol 14:257-259, 2000.
3. Dagi FT, George ED: Management of cerebrospinal fluid leaks. In Schmidek HH, Sweet WH (eds): Operative Neurosurgical Techniques: Indications, Methods and Results. Orlando, FL, Grune & Stratton, 1988, pp 49-69.
4. Wigand ME: Transnasal ethmoidectomy under endoscopic control. Rhinology 19:7-15, 1981.
5. Hoffman DF, May M: Endoscopic sinus surgery—experience with the initial 100 patients. Trans Pa Acad Ophthalmol Otolaryngol 41:847-850, 1989.
6. Kainz J, Stammberger H: The roof of the anterior ethmoid: A place of least resistance in the skull base. Am J Rhinol 3:191-199, 1989.
7. Benninger MS, Mickelson SA, Yaremchuk K: Functional endoscopic sinus surgery: Morbidity and early results. Henry Ford Hosp Med J 38:5-8, 1990.
8. Levine HL: Functional endoscopic sinus surgery: Evaluation, surgery, and follow-up. Laryngoscope 100:79-84, 1990.
9. Sterman BM, DeVore RA, Lavertu P, Levine HL: Endoscopic sinus surgery in a residency training program. Am J Rhinol 4:207-210, 1990.
10. Duplechain JK, White JA, Miller RH: Pediatric sinusitis. The role of endoscopic sinus surgery in cystic fibrosis and other forms of sinonasal disease. Arch Otolaryngol Head Neck Surg 117:422-426, 1991.
11. Salman SD: Complications of endoscopic sinus surgery. Am J Otolaryngol 12:326-328, 1991.
12. Wigand ME, Hosemann WG: Results of endoscopic surgery of the paranasal sinuses and anterior skull base. J Otolaryngol 20:385-390, 1991.
13. Stankiewicz JA: Cerebrospinal fluid fistula and endoscopic sinus surgery. Laryngoscope 101:250-256, 1991.
14. Vleming M, Middelweerd RJ, de Vries N: Complications of endoscopic sinus surgery. Arch Otolaryngol Head Neck Surg 118:617-623, 1992.
15. Freedman HM, Kern EB: Complications of intranasal ethmoidectomy: A review of 1,000 consecutive operations. Laryngoscope 89:421-434, 1979.
16. Eichel BS: The intranasal ethmoidectomy: A 12-year perspective. Otolaryngol Head Neck Surg 90:540-543, 1982.
17. Stevens HE, Blair NJ: Intranasal sphenoethmoidectomy: 10-year experience and literature review. J Otolaryngol 17:254-259, 1988.
18. MacKay IS: Endoscopic sinus surgery—complications and how to avoid them. Rhinology 14(Suppl):151-155, 1992.
19. Friedman WH, Katsantonis GP: Intranasal and transantral ethmoidectomy: A 20-year experience. Laryngoscope 100:343-348, 1990.
20. Cumberworth VL, Sudderick RM, Mackay IS: Major complications of functional endoscopic sinus surgery. Clin Otolaryngol 19:248-253, 1994.
21. Kennedy DW, Shaman P, Han W, et al: Complications of ethmoidectomy: A survey of fellows of the American Academy of Otolaryngology–Head and Neck Surgery. Otolaryngol Head Neck Surg 111:589-599, 1994.
22. Hirsch O: Successful closure of cerebrospinal fluid rhinorrhea by endonasal surgery. Arch Otolaryngol 56:1-13, 1952.
23. Montgomery WW: Cerebrospinal rhinorrhea. Otolaryngol Clin North Am 6:757-771, 1973.
24. McCabe BF: The osteo-muco-periosteal flap in repair of cerebrospinal fluid rhinorrhea. Laryngoscope 86:537-539, 1976.
25. Yessenow RS, McCabe BF: The osteo-mucoperiosteal flap in repair of cerebrospinal fluid rhinorrhea: A 20-year experience. Otolaryngol Head Neck Surg 101:555-558, 1989.
26. Mattox DE, Kennedy DW: Endoscopic management of cerebrospinal fluid leaks and cephaloceles. Laryngoscope 100:857-862, 1990.
27. Calcaterra TC: Diagnosis and management of ethmoid cerebrospinal rhinorrhea. Otolaryngol Clin North Am 18:99-105, 1985.
28. Papay FA, Maggiano H, Dominquez S, et al: Rigid endoscopic repair of paranasal sinus cerebrospinal fluid fistulas. Laryngoscope 99:1195-1201, 1989.
29. Hadad G, Bassagasteguy L, Carrau RL, et al: A novel reconstructive technique after endoscopic expanded endonasal approaches: Vascular pedicle nasoseptal flap. Laryngoscope 116:1882-1886, 2006.
30. Yamamoto Y, Kunishio K, Sunami N, et al: Identification of CSF fistulas by radionuclide counting. AJNR Am J Neuroradiol 11:823-826, 1990.
31. Oberascher G, Arrer E: Efficiency of various methods of identifying cerebrospinal fluid in oto- and rhinorrhea. ORL J Otorhinolaryngol Relat Spec 48:320-325, 1986.
32. Fransen P, Sindic CSM, Thavroy C, et al: Highly sensitive detection of beta-2 transferrin in rhinorrhea and otorrhea as a marker for cerebrospinal fluid (C.S.F.) leakage. Acta Neurochir (Wein) 109:98-101, 1991.
33. Oberascher G: Cerebrospinal fluid otorrhea—new trends in diagnosis. Am J Otol 9:102-108, 1988.
34. Oberascher G: A modern concept of cerebrospinal fluid diagnosis in oto- and rhinorrhea. Rhinology 26:89-103, 1988.
35. Skedros DG, Cass SP, Hirsch BE, Kelly RH: Sources of error in use of beta-2 transferrin analysis for diagnosing perilymphatic and cerebral spinal fluid leaks. Otolaryngol Head Neck Surg 109:861-864, 1993.
36. Meco C, Oberascher G, Arrer E, et al: Beta-trace protein test: New guidelines for the reliable diagnosis of cerebrospinal fluid fistula. Otolaryngol Head Neck Surg 129:508-517, 2003.

37. Kelly TF, Stankiewicz JA, Chow JM, et al: Endoscopic closure of postsurgical anterior cranial fossa cerebrospinal fluid leaks. Neurosurgery 39:743-746, 1996.

38. Sillers MJ, Morgan CE, Gammal TE: Magnetic resonance cisternography and thin coronal computerized tomography in the evaluation of cerebrospinal fluid rhinorrhea. Am J Rhinol 11:387-392, 1997.

39. Weber R, Keerl R, Draf W, et al: Management of dural lesions occurring during endonasal sinus surgery. Arch Otolaryngol Head Neck Surg 122:732-736, 1996.

40. Carrau RL, Jho HD, Ko Y: How I do it: Transnasal-transsphenoidal endoscopic surgery of the pituitary gland. Laryngoscope 106:914-918, 1996.

41. Gjuric M, Goede U, Keimer H, Wigant ME: Endonasal endoscopic closure of cerebrospinal fluid fistulas at the anterior cranial base. Ann Otol Rhinol 105:620-623, 1996.

42. Al-Nashar IS, Carrau RL, Herrera A, Snyderman CH: Endoscopic transnasal transpterygopalatine fossa approach to the lateral recess of the sphenoid sinus. Laryngoscope 114:528-532, 2004.

43. Weber R, Draf W, Kratzsch B, et al: Modern concepts of frontal sinus surgery. Laryngoscope 111:137-146, 2001.

44. Janecka IP, Sen C, Sekhar LN, et al: Cranial base surgery: Results in 183 patients. Otolaryngol Head Neck Surg 110:539-546, 1994.

45. Sen C, Snyderman CH, Sekhar LN: Complications of skull base operations. In Sekhar LN, Janecka IP (eds): Surgery of Cranial Base Tumors. New York, Raven Press, 1993, pp 831-839.

46. Fuhrmeister U, Ruether P, Dommatsch D: Alterations of CSF hydrodynamics following meningitis and subarachnoid hemorrhage. In Shulman K, Marmarou A, Miller JK (eds): Intracranial Pressure IV. Berlin, Springer Verlag, 1980, pp 241-244.

47. Bagley C Jr: Blood in the cerebrospinal fluid: Resultant functional and organic alterations in the central nervous system. Part B: Clinical data. Arch Surg 17:39-81, 1928.

48. Brown JK: Mechanisms of production of raised intracranial pressure. In Minns RA (ed): Problems of Intracranial Pressure in Childhood. London, MacKeith Press, 1991, pp 13-35.

49. Vale FL, Bradley EL, Fisher WS III: The relationship of subarachnoid hemorrhage and the need for postoperative shunting. J Neurosurg 86:462-466, 1997.

50. Noren G, Greitz D, Hirsch A, Lax I: Gamma knife radiosurgery in acoustic neuromas. In Tos M, Thomsen J (eds): Acoustic Neuroma. Amsterdam, Kugler, 1992, pp 289-292.

51. Duong D, O'Malley S, Sekhar L, Wright D: Postoperative hydrocephalus in cranial base surgery. Skull Base Surg 10:197-200, 2000.

52. Carrau RL, Snyderman CH, Kassam AB: The management of CSF leaks in patients at risk for high-pressure hydrocephalus. Laryngoscope 115:205-212, 2005.

Chapter **105**

Reconstruction after Skull Base Surgery

Ricardo L. Carrau, Allan D. Vescan, Carl H. Snyderman, and Amin B. Kassam

The goals of reconstruction after any oncologic resection are preservation and rehabilitation of function, restoration of cosmesis, and avoidance of morbidity. Any reconstruction after anterior craniofacial resection should strive to separate the cranial cavity from the upper aerodigestive tract, obliterate the dead space, preserve neurovascular and ocular function, and restore cosmesis (Table 105-1). Multiple free tissue grafts, vascularized local flaps, free microvascular flaps, and allografts are available for these purposes (Table 105-2).

PATIENT SELECTION

Any patient who requires a skull base resection that produces a pathway of communication between the cranial cavity and the upper aerodigestive tract will need some form of reconstruction. Before embarking on reconstruction of the surgical defect, key patient factors must be considered, including underlying medical comorbid conditions such as diabetes mellitus and peripheral vascular disease and, most importantly, the size and site of the defect. It is often the complexity of the resection that dictates the option most suitable for reconstruction. Defects may involve a significant volume of soft tissue and facial or cranial bones, and there may be functional concerns such as resection of walls of the orbit or communication with the oral cavity. An important point to consider with respect to patient selection is what additional treatments may be required. Postoperative radiation therapy is often necessary after oncologic resection of malignant tumors of the skull base. Vascularized tissue is superior to any other source to avoid the complications of radiation therapy.

PREOPERATIVE PLANNING

Estimation of the extent of resection by thorough analysis of the preoperative imaging studies, including computed tomography (CT) and magnetic resonance imaging, is fundamental in planning the reconstruction and obtaining informed consent. In addition, angiography may be necessary to assess for peripheral vascular disease if a free microvascular flap is necessary. Doppler ultrasonography is another technique available to assess flow through vessels that supply the possible regional or free flaps.

It is important to communicate with other team members regarding the types of reconstruction being considered. Frequently, the members of the skull base team who perform the ablation may be different from the ones who perform the reconstruction.

SURGICAL TECHNIQUES

Pericranial Flap/Galeopericranial Flap

The majority of defects after anterior craniofacial resection involve the area of the anterior skull base located between the orbits and extending from the crista galli anteriorly to the planum sphenoidale posteriorly (Fig. 105-1). This area is amenable to reconstruction with a pericranial or galeopericranial flap.[1-3] Both pericranial and galeopericranial flaps are vascular pedicled flaps supplied by the supraorbital and supratrochlear vessels (Fig. 105-2). Thus, sacrifice of the supraorbital and supratrochlear vessels would render the pericranial flap nonviable. Harvesting of the pericranial flap does not impair the blood or sensory supply to the remaining

Table 105-1	GOALS OF RECONSTRUCTION
Separation of cranial cavity from upper aerodigestive tract	
Obliteration of dead space	

Function
  neurovascular
  ocular	

Cosmesis	

Table 105-2	MATERIALS FOR RECONSTRUCTION
Free tissue grafts	
Vascularized flaps Pericranial/galeal Temporalis muscle Forehead Scalp Facial	
Free microvascular flaps Rectus abdominis Radial forearm Latissimus dorsi	
Allografts Plates/mesh Bone cement	

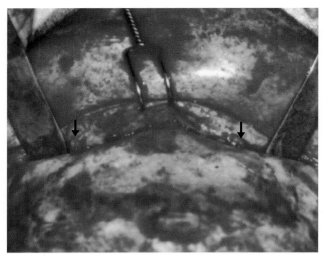

Figure 105-2. The vascular supply of both pericranial and galeo-pericranial flaps includes the supratrochlear and supraorbital vessels (*arrows*).

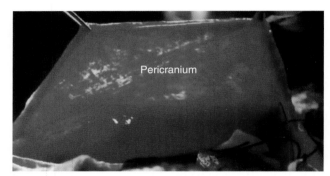

Figure 105-3. Intraoperative photograph demonstrating a pericranial flap.

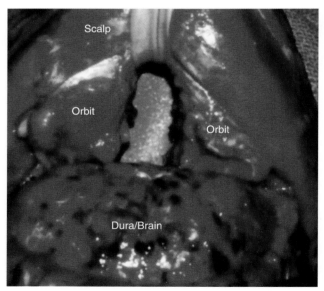

Figure 105-1. Intraoperative photograph demonstrating the defect after anterior craniofacial resection.

scalp. Both flaps can be designed to reach the clival region or be divided longitudinally to reconstruct two different defects (i.e., anterior skull base and nose or orbit).

The pericranium comprises the periosteum and the areolar tissue that separates the periosteum from the galea. Both tissue layers are raised as a single unit with a combination of sharp and blunt dissection extending from the bicoronal incision to the supraorbital neurovascular bundles. Additional length could be gained by planning harvesting of the flap distal to the bicoronal incision. We prefer to harvest the pericranial flap at the end of surgery (Fig. 105-3) to prevent desiccation and avoid inadvertent injury to the flap during the extirpative part of the operation. The flap is inserted under the supraorbital and craniotomy bone grafts to cover the anterior skull base defect (Fig. 105-4). Compression of the flap by the supraorbital bone graft should be avoided.

Temporalis Muscle Flap

Defects of the anterolateral and infratemporal skull base, as well as defects of the orbit, oral cavity, oropharynx, and nasopharynx, may be reconstructed with a temporalis muscle flap.[4-6] This muscle flap may be divided vertically to reconstruct two separate defects (i.e., subtemporal skull base and orbit), or most commonly, the anterior half of the muscle is used for reconstruction and the posterior half is transposed anteriorly

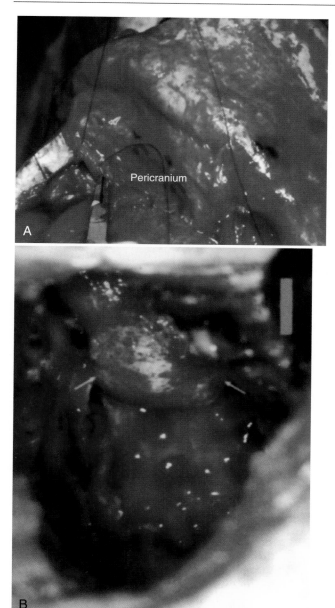

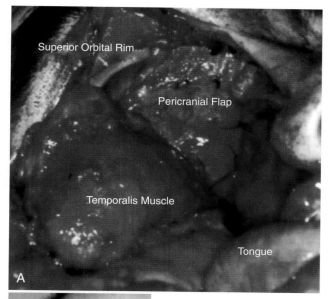

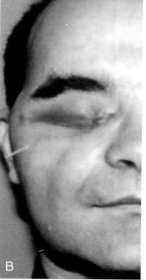

Figure 105-4. A, Intraoperative photograph of a pericranial flap inset between the dura and skull base. **B,** Pericranial flap seen from the nasal side (*arrows*).

Figure 105-5. A, Intraoperative photograph of reconstruction of the skull base and orbit with the temporalis muscle. **B,** Postoperative appearance.

to fill the anterior temporal fossa. In our practice, the temporalis muscle flap is most commonly used to provide soft tissue cover for the bone grafts or titanium mesh used for reconstruction of the orbital walls, to reconstruct the infratemporal fossa or skull base, or to obliterate the orbital cavity after exenteration. A temporalis muscle flap may be used as an adjunct to a pericranial flap when resection of the skull base has been extended laterally (Fig. 105-5).

The temporalis muscle flap is harvested by dissecting the temporalis muscle from the temporal fossa with a combination of electrocautery and blunt dissection. Its insertion to the zygoma (superficial and deep layers

of the deep temporal fascia) should be transected to gain adequate mobilization. To protect the frontal branches of the facial nerve, the superficial layer of the deep temporal fascia is incised along an imaginary line that extends from the superior orbital rim to the root of the zygoma. The plane of dissection proceeds deep to this fascial layer, which corresponds to a subperiosteal plane over the zygomatic arch and malar process. Its reach or arc of rotation may be increased by dividing the insertion of the temporalis muscle to the coronoid process of the mandible.

The muscle is then rotated and sutured into place. If the posterior half was not used, it is transposed anteriorly and sutured to the lateral orbital rim and to a curvilinear plate screwed at the level of the temporal line. The temporalis muscle flap is supplied by the deep temporal artery, a terminal branch of the internal maxillary artery. Dissection of the flap in its medial aspect or oncologic resection or preoperative embolization of the muscular branches of the internal maxillary artery will render the flap nonviable.

Temporoparietal Fascia Flap

The temporoparietal (superficial temporal fascia) fascia flap is supple and offers an extended reach that allows it to be used for reconstruction of anterior, lateral, and posterior skull base defects, as well as maxillofacial defects.[7-13] It can be harvested bilaterally as two separate flaps or as a bipedicle flap, which may provide enough tissue to reconstruct the entire anterior skull base.

The temporoparietal fascia flap includes the superficial temporal fascia and galea, which is supplied by the superficial temporal artery. Its vascular supply encompasses an area that extends from the ipsilateral temporal artery to the midline and covers up to 15 cm in width (Fig. 105-6). It is critical to plan harvesting of this flap in advance. To preserve its integrity and blood supply, the flap should be harvested at the time of the bicoro-

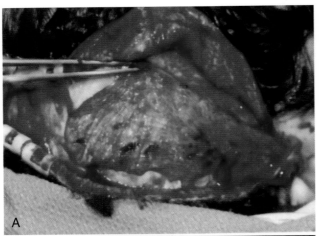

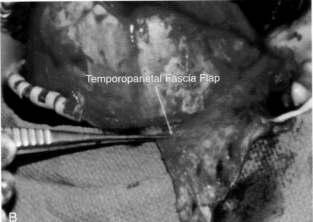

Temporoparietal Fascia Flap

Figure 105-6. **A,** Intraoperative photograph demonstrating dissection of a temporoparietal fascia flap. **B,** Temporoparietal fascia flap.

nal incision. Because a customary hemicoronal or bicoronal incision would divide the flap and sacrifice its blood supply, anterior harvesting of the flap should be limited to the hairline since the frontal branch of the facial nerve may be injured if the dissection is extended anterior to this point. To harvest the temporoparietal fascia, the coronal incision is extended to but not through the galea, and the flap is then harvested by sharp dissection. The dissection is somewhat cumbersome and tedious because of the rich blood supply of the scalp. Hemostasis is achieved with bipolar cautery.

Microvascular Free Flaps

Microvascular free flaps lengthen the time of surgery and increase its cost and morbidity, so these flaps are recommended only in certain situations, such as the need to reconstruct a defect left by an extended resection that includes all the soft tissues from the skin to the brain, to support the brain, after extended maxillectomies that produce defects that will not retain a prosthesis, or when local or regional flaps are not available.[3,11,12,14-17] Contraindications to the use of free flaps include severe peripheral vascular disease, lack of availability of adequate host vessels, medical instability, and the need for vasopressors. Commonly used microvascular free flaps include the radial forearm flap, the rectus abdominis flap, and the latissimus dorsi flap (Fig. 105-7). A thorough discussion of these flaps is included in Chapter 81.

Reconstruction of the Craniofacial Skeleton

Wires, stitches, titanium alloy plates, or mesh may be used to fix free bone grafts such as the craniotomy bone, the supraorbital block, and other parts of the maxillofacial skeleton[18-21] (Fig. 105-8). We prefer the use of plates or mesh because they yield stable fixation and a more predictable long-term result. Titanium plates and mesh osseointegrate very well; in addition, they produce minimal imaging artifact and radiation scattering. Titanium mesh can also be used to replace parts of the bony framework that had to be resected, such as frontal bone, orbital bone, or anterior maxilla (Fig. 105-9). We cover the mesh with acellular dermis to prevent subsequent indentation of the skin over the mesh pattern.

Reconstruction of the Orbit

Reconstruction of the orbital walls is recommended when more than a third of the circumference of the orbit is sacrificed (i.e., more than the lamina papyracea) or when the periorbita had to be removed with the adjacent bony wall.[18-21] This latter defect produces significant enophthalmos and may also lead to hypoophthalmia in the case of resection of the orbital floor.

The orbital walls are better reconstructed with rigid materials that resist contraction and provide an immediate and predictable outcome. This can be achieved with bone grafts, titanium mesh, porous polyethylene, or other alloplastic material. We generally use titanium

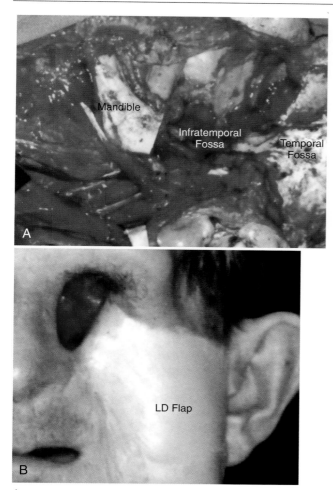

Figure 105-7. A, Extensive anterior and lateral skull base and intraoral defect. **B**, Postoperative photograph demonstrating a nasocutaneous fistula and retraction of the left oral commissure. A latissimus dorsi (LD) free microvascular flap has a tendency to sag because of its bulk and weight.

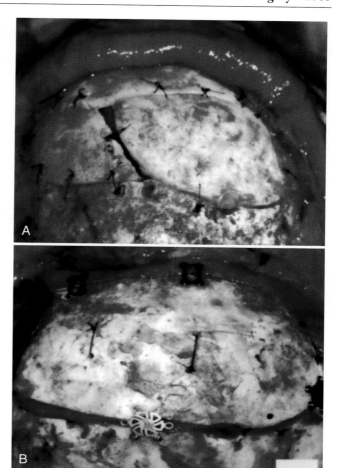

Figure 105-8. A, Fixation of bone grafts with sutures. **B**, Fixation of bone grafts with titanium plates.

mesh because of its availability and ease of conforming to the orbital walls (Fig. 105-10). Another consideration when choosing the reconstructive material is that these patients usually require postoperative radiation therapy, which raises the possibility of osteoradionecrosis of bone grafts. Titanium mesh, however, needs to be covered with an acellular dermis graft over the orbital side or the soft tissues of the orbit will "grow" into the mesh holes and lead to tethering of the extraocular muscles and severe contraction of the lower eyelid (i.e., ectropion). The medial canthus is repositioned with a titanium plate that is screwed to the remaining nasal bones (Fig. 105-10). The lateral canthus should also be repositioned and sutured to the lateral orbital rim to avoid lower eyelid ectropion.

POSTOPERATIVE CARE

Postoperatively, the patient is transferred to an intensive care unit for continuous cardiovascular and neurologic monitoring. Postoperative anemia, hypovolemia, and electrolyte imbalances are corrected when present.

A CT scan of the brain is performed on the first or second postoperative day to identify intracranial complications such as cerebral contusion, edema or hemorrhage, fluid collections, or pneumocephalus.

The scalp drains are kept on bulb suction only. High-pressure suction can produce rapid shifting of the brain or brain stem (or both), with life-threatening effects. Drains are removed when the drainage is less than 30 mL/day. If the dura was opened or resected during the ablation, the drain puncture site should be closed with an encircling stitch on removal of the drain to prevent infection.

COMPLICATIONS[22-25]

Scalp Wound

Necrosis of the scalp is rare and most often the result of poorly designed incisions or prolonged use of hemostatic clamps. The latter may result in areas of ischemia, particularly around the auricle, that can make the tissue susceptible to secondary infection. Scalp necrosis may

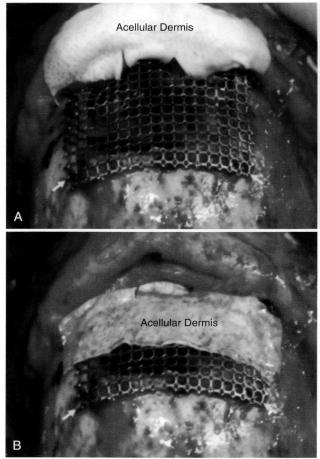

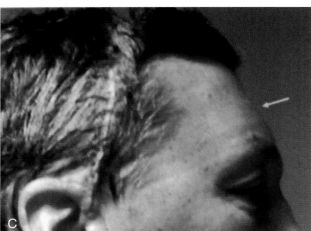

Figure 105-9. A, Intraoperative photograph. The frontal and glabellar area is reconstructed with titanium mesh *(arrows)*. **B,** Acellular dermis is layered over the titanium mesh (*arrows*). **C,** Postoperative appearance of frontal contour (*arrow*).

also be the result of previous irradiation, which when combined with harvesting of the galeopericranial flap, may render the scalp ischemic.

Postoperative intracranial infection usually results from inadequate separation between the cranial cavity or grafts and the sinonasal tract, from a large dead space, or from noncompliance and blowing the nose in the immediate postoperative period. Partial necrosis of the scalp flap may lead to a wound infection, as well as contamination of the grafts. Restoration of the separation between the cranial cavity and the sinonasal tract, débridement (removal of the free bone grafts), and prolonged antibiotic therapy (45 days, guided by culture and sensitivity testing) are the recommended treatment.

Postoperative Sinonasal Bleeding

Significant postoperative nasal bleeding most commonly arises from a branch of the internal maxillary or anterior ethmoidal artery and is amenable to endoscopic control. Angiography with embolization is reserved for patients in whom the bleeding site is not readily apparent, such as those who underwent reconstruction with a microvascular free flap. Intracranial postoperative bleeding or bleeding from the vascular

anastomosis of a free microvascular flap requires surgical intervention.

Cerebrospinal Fluid Leak

In a patient with postoperative rhinorrhea, testing of the fluid for β_2-transferrin is prudent to confirm a cerebrospinal fluid (CSF) leak. Accumulation of irrigation fluid in the sinonasal tract, with subsequent drainage, can mimic a CSF leak in the immediate postoperative period.

A postoperative CSF leak is managed conservatively with bed rest, stool softeners, and a lumbar drain (50 mL every 6 to 8 hours). Persistence of the leak beyond 3 to 5 days, unabated by conservative measures, indicates the need for surgical repair. Surgical exploration, however, may be indicated as initial therapy if loss of the reconstructive flap or dehiscence of the dural repair is suspected.

Tension Pneumocephalus

Trapped intracranial air can act as a space-occupying lesion that compresses the brain parenchyma and gives rise to lethargy, disorientation, slow mentation, or hemiparesis. A CT scan without contrast enhancement

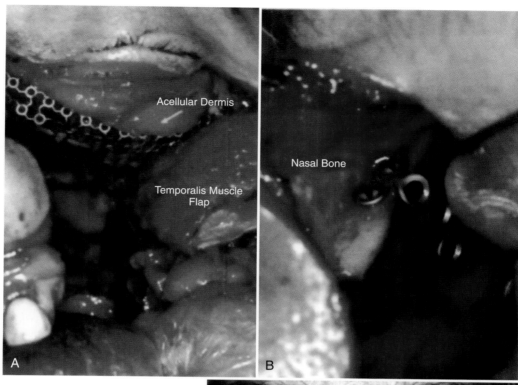

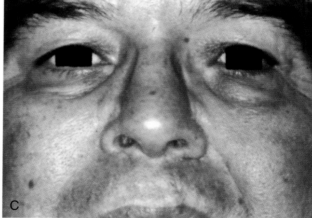

Figure 105-10. A, Intraoperative view of a titanium mesh plate used for reconstruction of the orbital floor. A temporalis muscle flap will cover the mesh on its inferior area. The soft tissues of the orbit are separated from the mesh with acellular dermis to avoid ingrowth of the tissues and a frozen globe. **B,** Intraoperative view of a titanium plate used for medial canthopexy. **C,** Postoperative photograph demonstrating less lagophthalmos and enophthalmos than with traditional techniques.

confirms the diagnosis and may be used to guide aspiration of the air with a needle placed through a burr hole or osteotomy gap. Recurrent tension pneumocephalus is usually associated with loss of the pericranial flap or may be due to nose blowing by a noncompliant patient despite instructions otherwise. Recurrent pneumocephalus requires bypassing the sinonasal tract airway with a tracheostomy or endotracheal tube or surgical closure of any cranionasal communication, or both.

Limitation of Extraocular Muscle Movement

Some degree of postoperative diplopia is present in most patients and is caused by dissection of the trochlea, postoperative edema, or removal of the orbital walls. It is usually self-limited and typically lasts less than 4 weeks. Reconstructive grafts may entrap the medial, lateral, or inferior rectus muscles and result in restriction of range of motion and permanent diplopia. Intraorbital dissection, such as that required when the periorbita is resected, or surgery on the cavernous sinus may injure the motor innervation of these muscles. A forced duction test helps differentiate between muscle entrapment and loss of muscle innervation.

Enophthalmos

Enophthalmos is caused by expansion of the volume of the orbital cavity as a result of resection of the orbital walls and is more pronounced when the periorbita is resected. It is best to prevent this complication by reconstructing the orbital walls with autogenous bone or titanium mesh (i.e., rigid reconstruction).

PEARLS

- Vascularized tissue is preferred over nonvascularized tissue such as free tissue grafts.
- Local and locoregional flaps are associated with less morbidity, less operative time, and less cost than microvascular free flaps are.
- Microvascular free flaps provide better coverage or support (or both) for defects that include the skin or lateral skull base.
- Trauma to the skull base tends to produce multiple defects.
- High ventricular pressure should be suspected in patients with recurrent CSF leaks.

PITFALLS

- Patients who undergo preoperative radiation or chemoradiation therapy are at a higher risk for devascularization of the scalp from harvesting of a pericranial or galeopericranial flap.
- Patients who have undergone radiation therapy are at higher risk for delayed healing or nonhealing of the defect.
- No reconstruction provides immediate protection against high CSF pressure.
- Patients who have skull base defects are at higher risk for meningitis, even after reconstruction.
- Oncologic resection may destroy the blood supply to local or regional flaps.

References

1. Snyderman CH, Janecka IP, Sekhar LN, et al: Anterior cranial base reconstruction: Role of galeal and pericranial flaps. Laryngoscope 100:607-614, 1990.
2. Potparic Z, Fukuta K, Colen LB, Jackson IT: Galeo-pericranial flaps in the forehead: A study of blood supply and volumes. Br J Plast Surg 49:519-528, 1996.
3. Neligan PC, Mulholland S, Irish J, et al: Flap selection in cranial base reconstruction. Plast Reconstr Surg 98:1159-1166, 1996.
4. Kiyokawa K, Tai Y, Inoue Y, et al: Efficacy of temporal musculopericranial flap for reconstruction of the anterior base of the skull. Scand J Plast Reconstr Surg Hand 34:43-53, 2000.
5. Hanasono MM, Utley DS, Goode RL: The temporalis muscle flap for reconstruction after head and neck oncologic surgery. Laryngoscope 111:1719-1725, 2001.
6. Burggasser G, Happak W, Gruber H, Freilinger G: The temporalis: Blood supply and innervation. Plast Reconstr Surg 109:1862-1869, 2002.
7. Har-Shai Y, Fukuta K, Collares MV, Stefanovic PD: The vascular anatomy of the galeal flap in the interparietal and midline regions. Plast Reconstr Surg 89:64-69, 1992.
8. David SK, Cheney ML: An anatomic study of the temporoparietal fascial flap. Arch Otolaryngol Head Neck Surg 121:1153-1156, 1995.
9. Pinar YA, Govsa F: Anatomy of the superficial temporal artery and its branches: Its importance for surgery. Surg Radiol Anat 28:248-253, 2006.
10. Pollice PA, Fondel JL Jr: Secondary reconstruction of upper midface and orbit after total maxillectomy. Arch Otolaryngol Head Neck Surg 124:802-808, 1998.
11. Telliouglu AT, Tekdemir I, Erdemli EA, et al: Temporoparietal fascia: An anatomic and histologic reinvestigation with new potential clinical applications. Plast Reconstr Surg 105:40-45, 2000.
12. Lai A, Cheney ML: Temporoparietal fascial flap in orbital reconstruction. Arch Facial Plast Surg 2:196-201, 2000.
13. Olson KL, Manolidis S: The pedicled superficial temporalis fascial flap: A new method for reconstruction in otologic surgery. Otolaryngol Head Neck Surg 126:538-547, 2002.
14. Yamada A, Harii K, Ueda K, Asato H: Free rectus abdominis muscle reconstruction of the anterior skull base. Br J Plast Surg 45:302-306, 1992.
15. Bridger GP, Baldwin M: Anterior craniofacial resection for ethmoid and nasal cancer with free flap reconstruction. Arch Otolaryngol Head Neck Surg 115:308-312, 1989.
16. Schwartz MS, Cohen JI, Meltzer T, et al: Use of radial forearm microvascular free-flap graft for cranial base reconstruction. J Neurosurg 90:651-655, 1999.
17. Valentini V, Fabiani F, Nicolai G, et al: Use of microvascular free flaps in the reconstruction of the anterior and middle skull base. J Craniofac Surg 17:790-796, 2006.
18. Janecka IP: New reconstructive technologies in skull base surgery: Role of titanium mesh and porous polyethylene. Arch Otolaryngol Head Neck Surg 126:396-401, 2000.
19. Badie B, Preston JK, Hartig GK: Use of titanium mesh for reconstruction of large anterior cranial base defects. J Neurosurg 93:711-714, 2000.
20. Rapidis AD, Day TA: The use of temporal polyethylene implant after temporalis myofascial flap transposition: Clinical and radiographic results from its use in 21 patients. J Oral Maxillofac Surg 64:12-22, 2006.
21. Ruiz RL, Turvey TA, Costello BJ, Tejera TJ: Cranial bone grafts: Craniomaxillofacial applications and harvesting techniques. Atlas Oral Maxillofac Surg Clin North Am 13:127-137, 2005.
22. Kraus DH, Shah JP, Arbit E, et al: Complications of craniofacial resection for tumors involving the anterior skull base. Head Neck 16:307-312, 1994.
23. Haughey BH, Gates GA, Skerhut HE, Brown WE: Cerebral shift after lateral craniofacial resection and flap reconstruction. Otolaryngol Head Neck Surg 101:79-86, 1989.
24. Clayman GL, DeMonte F, Jaffe DM, et al: Outcome and complications of extended cranial-base resection requiring microvascular free-tissue transfer. Arch Otolaryngol Head Neck Surg 121:1253-1257, 1995.
25. Newman J, O'Malley BW Jr, Chalian A, Brown MT: Microvascular reconstruction of cranial base defects: An evaluation of complication and survival rates to justify the use of this repair. Arch Otolaryngol Head Neck Surg 132:381-384, 2006.

Chapter **106**

Transnasal and Transoral Approaches to the Cervical Spine

Carl H. Snyderman, Ricardo L. Carrau, Amin B. Kassam, and Paul A. Gardner

The superior aspects of the cervical spine (C1 and C2) are not easily reached from a transcervical route and have traditionally been accessed through a transoral/transpalatal approach. Innovations in recent years include the introduction of endoscopes for assistance with the transoral approach and the development of a completely endoscopic transnasal approach. Although not widely used yet, we believe that the transnasal approach has distinct advantages that will make it the preferred technique. The otolaryngologist does not typically perform cervical spine surgery in isolation but cooperates with other specialties (neurosurgery, orthopedic surgery) to provide access to the upper cervical spine. With the transnasal endoscopic approach, the otolaryngologist maintains an endoscopic view for the neurosurgeon after the initial exposure is achieved.

Resection of the odontoid process is sometimes necessary for the treatment of basilar invagination with brain stem compression. This may be the result of rheumatoid degeneration with pannus formation or traumatic fracture and dislocation of the odontoid. With the advent of transnasal endoscopic approaches to the ventral skull base, resection of the odontoid may also be performed to provide access to tumors of the foramen magnum and adjacent areas.

ANATOMY

The transoral and transnasal approaches to C1 and C2 are midline approaches. C1 and C2 articulate with the skull at the inferior edge of the clivus (foramen magnum). The dens or odontoid process is covered anteriorly by the arch of C1. The vertebral bodies are covered by the paraspinal muscles anteriorly (longus colli and longus capitis). The body of C2 is typically at the level of the soft palate. The posterior pharyngeal wall covers the bodies of C3 and C4. Laterally, the vertebral artery is exposed between C1 and C2, where it exits the vertebral canal and loops superficially. The parapharyngeal segment of the internal carotid artery is situated laterally and is not in the surgical field, but an ectatic artery may occasionally deviate medially into the retropharyngeal region.

The palatal mucosa receives its blood supply from the greater palatine vessels, which exit the greater palatine foramina medial to the second molars. The arteries course anteriorly to supply the mucosa over the hard palate. Passavant's ridge is a muscular ridge that is physiologically but not anatomically distinct and provides contact with the soft palate during nasopharyngeal closure.

The clivus is the anterior portion of the occipital bone and extends from the floor of the sphenoid sinus to the foramen magnum. The bone of the clivus thins as it approaches the foramen. Laterally, the clivus is bounded by the medial pterygoid plates and the base of the pterygoids. The pterygoid canal and vidian artery lead to the second genu of the petrous carotid artery, which is situated superolaterally. The lateral limit of the surgical field is the eustachian tube.

PATIENT SELECTION

Indications for surgery on C1 and C2 include infectious, inflammatory, traumatic, and neoplastic conditions. Infectious problems are rare but could include a localized retropharyngeal abscess, which is best accessed directly, and osteomyelitis. Traumatic injuries of C1 and C2 that compress the spinal cord cannot be repaired directly but may require decompression of displaced bone fragments. Stabilization of the spine with posterior fusion is usually necessary.

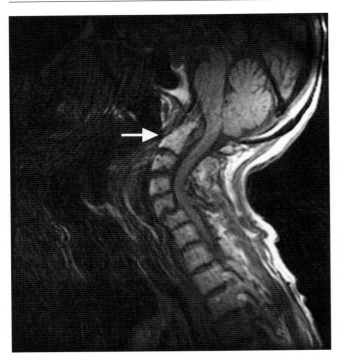

Figure 106-1. Basilar invagination with brain stem compression secondary to rheumatoid pannus *(arrow)*.

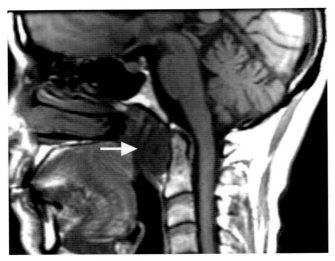

Figure 106-2. Neoplasms at the level of the foramen magnum *(arrow)* are most commonly chordomas, chondrosarcomas, or meningiomas.

The most common indication for surgical approaches to C1 and C2 is rheumatoid degeneration of the ligaments with resultant destruction of the odontoid and creation of an inflammatory pannus (Fig. 106-1). Symptoms are a consequence of cervical instability, as well as basilar invagination and compression of the brain stem.

Resection of the lower clivus and odontoid provides a surgical corridor to tumors at the foramen magnum (Fig. 106-2). These tumors are a heterogeneous group consisting of chondrosarcomas, meningiomas, chordomas, and other types. This approach may be combined with other modules of the expanded endonasal approach to the ventral skull base to obtain optimal exposure.[1]

PREOPERATIVE EVALUATION

Patients with basilar invagination are typically elderly patients and often have severe pharyngeal dysfunction at the time of surgery. A complete neurologic examination with assessment of evidence of long-tract compression should be performed. The larynx is examined to evaluate laryngeal function, swallowing, and risk of aspiration.

Computed tomography (CT) is best suited to assess changes in bone anatomy, the relationship of C1 to the lower clivus, and the position of the odontoid. Magnetic resonance imaging (MRI) is superior for visualization of the pannus and the amount of brain stem compression. If an intraoperative navigational system is used, a CT angiogram is obtained preoperatively for image guidance. It is necessary to modify the standard scanning protocol to include the upper cervical spine to the C3 level.

Consultation with an anesthesiologist should be obtained for evaluation of the airway and consideration of airway options. Increased difficulty of intubation because of cervical instability may be encountered. There is also a risk of accidental extubation with repositioning of the patient for posterior cervical fusion if performed during the same operative setting.

PREOPERATIVE PLANNING

After endotracheal intubation and induction of general anesthesia, the patient undergoes baseline somatosensory evoked potential (SSEP) monitoring before positioning. Brain stem evoked responses to monitor brain stem function may also be indicated. Cervical instability during repositioning requires continued monitoring, especially with movement of the patient. The patient is then placed in Mayfield pins in a neutral position, and postpositioning SSEPs are used to confirm the safety of the positioning. Image guidance registration, including the cervicomedullary junction, is undertaken.

Adequate preparation of the nares or pharynx is carried out, and the patient is given a third-generation cephalosporin for perioperative antibiotic prophylaxis. Topical antibiotics may also be used in this situation because the entire dissection is usually extradural.

SURGICAL APPROACHES

Although the transoral/transpalatal approach is still the standard of care at most institutions, we prefer the transnasal route for decompression of the brain stem. The transnasal route is limited inferiorly and can reliably reach only the body of C2. If more inferior resection is needed, a transnasal route can be combined with a transoral route. A transoral route is contraindicated in patients with severe trismus and is difficult in patients with a full set of restored teeth.

Transoral/Transpalatal Approach

Surgery may be performed with nasal or oral endotracheal intubation. If the patient is nasally intubated, the tube can be displaced to one side in the pharynx. Alternatively, an oral RAE tube can be held between the retractor and the tongue. Various retractors (Dingman, Crockard) are available and allow self-retained retraction of the mandible and tongue, as well as the lateral oral commissure (Fig. 106-3). One of the biggest challenges is finding a proper fit of the tongue blade so that the base of tongue does not bulge into the field. During lengthy cases, the retractor should be released for several minutes intermittently to prevent excessive tongue pressure and the potential for ischemic necrosis or edema.

If the superior extent of the resection is the odontoid, incision of the palate is not necessary. A red rubber catheter is passed transnasally and sutured to the soft palate adjacent to the uvula. It is then retracted to pull the soft palate into the nasopharynx and secured to the drapes. If the exposure needs to extend to the rostrum of the sphenoid, incision of the palate is generally necessary. A paramedian incision is made adjacent to the uvula and curves in a lazy "S" fashion behind the maxillary alveolus so that the majority of the palatal flap is based on one greater palatine artery. The mucoperiosteal flaps are elevated laterally to the edge of the greater palatine foramen with preservation of the blood supply. The posterior edge of the hard palate may be resected to provide additional exposure superiorly.

Electrocautery is used to make a vertical midline incision in the posterior pharyngeal wall from the level of C3 to the nasopharynx. The incision continues through the soft tissues in the midline between the longus capitis and longus colli muscles. The paraspinal muscles are elevated from the vertebral bodies and ring of C1. Excessive lateral dissection is avoided because of

the risk of injuring the vertebral artery. A self-retaining retractor is placed and the bone work is then performed with a drill and Kerrison rongeurs. Visualization is enhanced with use of the operating microscope or even endoscopes.

After completion of the decompression, the pharyngeal incision is closed in two layers: a deep layer of interrupted 3-0 polyglycolic acid suture and a superficial layer of 3-0 polyglycolic acid suture placed with a vertical mattress technique. Obtaining watertight closure can be difficult at the superior and inferior limits of the incision. If a palatal incision has been made, the soft palate incision is closed in two layers: a deep intramuscular layer of interrupted 4-0 polyglycolic acid suture and a superficial layer of interrupted 4-0 polyglycolic acid suture. The mucoperiosteal flap over the hard palate is thin and closed in a single layer with a vertical mattress technique. A paraffin nasal splint can be molded to the contour of the hard palate and secured with sutures around the teeth. This protects the palatal mucosa during mastication.

Transnasal Approach

The technique has been described elsewhere[2,3] and is performed by a surgical team consisting of an otolaryngologist and neurosurgeon operating simultaneously. The first step is bilateral sphenoidotomy with resection of the posterior attachment of the nasal septum to the rostrum of the sphenoid (see Video 106-1). The mucosa of the posterior nasopharynx is then cauterized and elevated to expose the underlying paraspinal muscles (longus capitis and longus colli). The soft tissues and muscles are then resected to expose the underlying pharyngobasilar fascia (see Video 106-2). Resection of this dense fascia is facilitated by using a drill with a 3-mm coarse diamond bit to remove the cortical bone of the clivus starting at the sphenoidotomy and progressing inferiorly (see Video 106-3). The limits of exposure include the eustachian tubes laterally, the floor of the sphenoid sinus superiorly, and the level of the soft palate inferiorly.

An image guidance system is used to identify the level of the ring of C1, and the bone is then exposed (Fig. 106-4). The lower edge of the clivus is thinned with a drill and resected with a Kerrison rongeur. The central portion of C1 is then removed with the drill and the defect is widened laterally with a bone rongeur (Fig. 106-5) (see Video 106-4). The location of the underlying dens is confirmed with image guidance and the central portion of the dens is drilled (see Video 106-5). When only a shell of outer cortical bone remains, the base of the dens is detached from the body of C2. Blunt and sharp dissection of the attachments of the dens to the surrounding pannus allows mobilization and removal of the remaining bone (Fig. 106-6) (see Video 106-6).

Although resection of the pannus may not be necessary, we prefer to partially resect the pannus with an ultrasonic aspirator until pulsations transmitted from the brain stem are observed (see Video 106-7). No

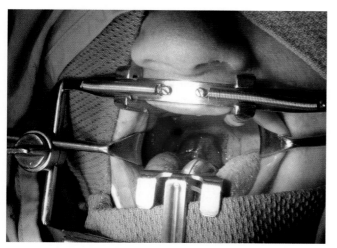

Figure 106-3. A Dingman retractor distracts the mandible and maxilla and displaces the endotracheal tube, tongue, and cheeks.

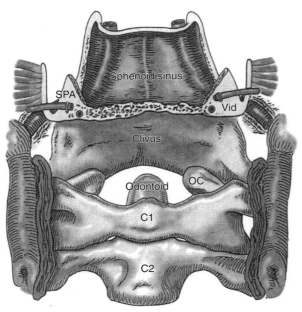

Figure 106-4. The nasopharyngeal soft tissues are resected to expose the lower clivus and ring of C1. OC, occipital condyle; SPA, sphenopalatine artery; Vid, vidian artery. (*Reprinted with permission from Kassam AB, Snyderman C, Gardner P, et al: The expanded endonasal approach: A fully endoscopic transnasal approach and resection of the odontoid process: Technical case report. Neurosurgery 57[1 Suppl]:E213, discussion E213, 2005.*)

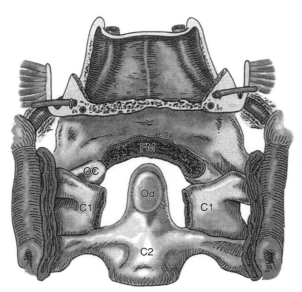

Figure 106-5. The central ring of C1 is removed with a drill and the gap is widened with a Kerrison rongeur. FM, foramen magnum; OC, occipital condyle; Od, odontoid. (*Reprinted with permission from Kassam AB, Snyderman C, Gardner P, et al: The expanded endonasal approach: A fully endoscopic transnasal approach and resection of the odontoid process: Technical case report. Neurosurgery 57[1 Suppl]:E213, discussion E213, 2005.*)

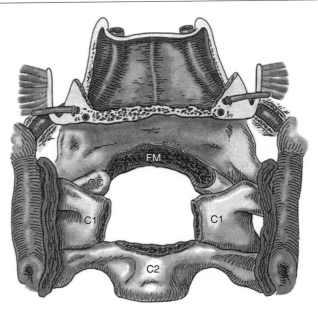

Figure 106-6. The odontoid is removed with a drill and dissection of the ligamentous attachments. FM, foramen magnum; OC, occipital condyle. (*Reprinted with permission from Kassam AB, Snyderman C, Gardner P, et al: The expanded endonasal approach: A fully endoscopic transnasal approach and resection of the odontoid process: Technical case report. Neurosurgery 57[1 Suppl]:E213, discussion E213, 2005.*)

reconstruction is necessary if the dura has not been violated. The defect is covered with fibrin glue (see Video 106-8).

Because of inherent instability of the cranioverte-bral junction in these patients, posterior fusion of the cervical spine to the occiput is usually performed during the same operative event.

POSTOPERATIVE MANAGEMENT

These patients are at increased risk for aspiration post-operatively, and reintubation can be difficult because of posterior neck fusion. Consideration should be given to leaving the patient intubated postoperatively until a safe airway can be ensured, or a temporary tracheos-tomy should be performed. With the transnasal approach, we have found tracheostomy to be necessary only in patients with significant preoperative pharyn-geal dysfunction.

Patients may start a full liquid diet and progress to a soft diet as soon as they are able to swallow without aspiration. Formal evaluation with a modified barium swallow may be helpful in determining swallowing capa-bility. With the transnasal approach, patients can resume an oral diet immediately. Return of swallowing function is often delayed for several days with a transoral route.

If used, nasal septal or palatal splints are removed 1 week postoperatively.

COMPLICATIONS

The transoral/transpalatal approach to the upper cervi-cal spine and foramen magnum provides limited exposure, especially in patients with impaired jaw opening or enlarged oropharyngeal tissues. Although C2 and C3 can be exposed with retraction of the soft palate, exposure plus removal of bone of C1 and the lower clivus are difficult, even with a palatal incision. Resection of the posterior edge of the hard palate provides additional exposure but increases the risk for a palatal fistula postoperatively. Other potential risks include dental injury, edema or necrosis of the tongue, upper airway obstruction secondary to edema, dysphagia, pain with swallowing, nasal regurgitation/hypernasal speech as a result of palatal incompetence, retropharyngeal hematoma or abscess, and temporomandibular joint syndrome secondary to excessive opening of the jaw. Because of concerns about the airway postoperatively, patients may remain intubated or require a tracheostomy. The angle of approach to the tip of the odontoid is less than 90 degrees and may hinder visualization with a microscope and increase the difficulty of dissection. Although the introduction of endoscopes through the oral cavity has the potential of decreasing the extent of exposure and improving visualization, it does not solve all these issues.

Palatal dysfunction is a significant problem with transoral/transpalatal procedures. Palatal incisions result in some degree of retraction, and partial dehiscence of the closure can create a gap at the palatal edge. Additionally, resection of vertebral bone and retropharyngeal soft tissues increases the distance between the palate and the posterior pharyngeal wall and prevents good contact during nasopharyngeal closure. This results in hypernasal speech and nasal reflux of liquids. There is less risk of palatal dysfunction with a transnasal approach. Because the posterior pharyngeal defect is above the level of the contact point for the soft palate and posterior pharyngeal wall (Passavant's ridge), there is no risk of hypernasal speech or nasal regurgitation.

Closure of the pharyngeal incision is difficult after a transoral approach, and ongoing contamination of the wound by saliva with heavy bacterial flora can occur. In contrast, the defect created by a transnasal approach is above the level of the soft palate and should not be exposed to the same degree of bacterial contamination. The wound is protected with a layer of fibrin glue at the end of the procedure.

The extracranial parapharyngeal segment of the internal carotid artery is lateral to the fossa of Rosenmüller and deep to the eustachian tube. On occasion, a tortuous internal carotid artery may course medially in the retropharyngeal area. This a relative contraindication to a transoral approach but would not preclude a transnasal approach.

Far lateral dissection at the level of C1 and C2 may injure the vertebral artery and should be performed only under image guidance.

If a cerebrospinal fluid (CSF) leak should occur with a transoral approach, obtaining a watertight closure can be difficult, depending on the length and accessibility of the superior extent of the incision. With the transnasal approach, there is a greater risk of a dural opening and CSF leak if dissection is performed in the region of the occipital condyle superolaterally. A CSF leak in this area can be effectively sealed with a fat graft or septal mucosal flap.

SUMMARY

The transnasal endoscopic approach to the odontoid is direct and provides access to the lower clivus, C1, and body of C2. Visualization with the endoscope is superior to that with the microscope and facilitates more complete removal of pannus if indicated. The only limitation is the ability to dissect below the body of C2 because of the level of the hard palate. Avoidance of pharyngeal and palatal incisions circumvents the potential airway and swallowing morbidity associated with the transoral approach. Because the surgical opening is above the level of the soft palate, palatal dysfunction is avoided and there is no need to close the mucosal defect. No infections have been observed. There is also minimal pain, and patients are able to resume an oral diet immediately if there were no swallowing problems preoperatively. A more rapid return to normal function and avoidance of operative morbidity should result in shorter hospitalization with decreased cost of care.

PEARLS

- A palatal incision can usually be avoided by retraction of the soft palate into the nasopharynx with a catheter sutured to the base of the uvula.
- With a transnasal route, resection of the posterior nasal septum to the nasal floor is necessary to provide adequate lateral access.
- Resection of the nasopharyngeal mucosa and underlying muscle and fascia improves exposure of C1 and C2.
- Removal of a thickened pannus should be performed until transmitted pulsations are evident; complete removal risks a CSF leak.
- The inferior extent of the transnasal approach is limited by the posterior edge of the hard palate.

PITFALLS

- Patients with preoperative pharyngeal dysfunction are at increased risk for airway problems and should have a tracheostomy performed at the same time.
- Patients with cervical instability should undergo neurophysiologic monitoring during positioning and throughout surgery to avoid neural injury.
- Excessive pressure from an oral retractor can result in ischemic necrosis of the tongue.
- Loss of retropharyngeal soft tissue and bone increases the risk for postoperative palatal insufficiency.
- Retropharyngeal dissection lateral to the eustachian tube should be avoided because of the risk of injury to the internal carotid artery.

References

1. Kassam AB, Snyderman CH, Mintz A, et al: Expanded endonasal approach: The rostrocaudal axis. Part II. Posterior clinoids to the foramen magnum. Neurosurg Focus 19(1):E4, 2005. Available at http://www.aans.org/education/journal/neurosurgical/July05/19-1-4.pdf.
2. Kassam AB, Snyderman CH, Gardner PA, et al: The expanded endonasal approach: A fully endoscopic transnasal approach and resection of the odontoid process: Technical case report. Neurosurgery 57(1 Suppl):E213, discussion E213, 2005.
3. Kassam AB, Mintz AH, Gardner PA, et al: The expanded endonasal approach for an endoscopic transnasal clipping and aneurysmorrhaphy of a large vertebral artery aneurysm: Technical case report. Neurosurgery 59(1 Suppl 1):ONSE162-ONSE165, 2006.

OTOLOGY

Chapter **107**

Office-Based Procedures in Otology

Alyssa Hackett and Yael Raz

In otolaryngology, as in other surgical disciplines, minimally invasive procedures are increasingly being performed in the office setting. Some even envision a day when certain otosclerosis patients will routinely undergo office-based stapedectomy.[1]

There are many advantages to an office-based surgical approach.[2] The procedures are carried out under local anesthesia, and patients do not need to abstain from oral intake. The cost of both the facility and the anesthesia is significantly lower, and a family member or friend may be present throughout the procedure. However, an office-based approach is not appropriate for every patient. Patients who are poor candidates for office surgery include those with narrow ear canals or those whose anatomy makes the procedure too complex; highly anxious patients; most children, particularly those who are 3 to 6 years of age; and patients with neurocognitive deficits.[2]

As with any procedure, the key to patient satisfaction is fostering trust between the patient and physician. Before selecting an office approach to any procedure, it is imperative that the patient/parent know what to expect during the procedure. The duration, noise, pain, and possibility of vertigo are all components that may have an impact on overall patient satisfaction with the experience. Attaching a video camera to the microscope and allowing the patient to watch the procedure on a monitor can sometimes reduce anxiety.

This chapter presents various techniques for anesthetizing the ear, as well as commonly performed office procedures. For foreign bodies involving the external auditory canal (EAC) or myringoplasty, readers are referred to Chapters 108 and 113, respectively.

ANESTHESIA

Giving proper care and consideration to anesthetic options before starting the procedure will minimize patient discomfort and the propensity to move during the procedure. Options include topical anesthesia (often used for myringotomy), local anesthesia (often used for biopsy of a mass in the ear canal), and regional blocks (useful for repairing lacerations or draining a hematoma of the auricle).

Topical Anesthesia of the Tympanic Membrane

Phenol, lidocaine, and tetracaine are all commonly used to topically anesthetize the tympanic membrane (TM). Before initiating anesthesia, an otoscopic examination should be performed to remove debris from the ear canal and completely visualize the TM for perforations, desquamated skin, and retraction pockets. The anesthetic agent is less effective if it must diffuse through debris to reach the TM. Perforations may allow anesthetic agents to reach the middle ear space and thereby result in temporary facial nerve palsy or vertigo.[3]

Phenol

Phenol creates a small chemical burn at the point where it is directly applied to the TM. Therefore, when used in large uncontrolled quantities, phenol can cause significant chemical otitis externa. When used in small controlled quantities and directly applied to the eardrum, however, phenol can produce safe, effective, and rapid anesthesia. It is our preferred anesthetic for topical application to the TM.

An appropriately sized aural speculum is first used to visualize the TM. Moisture and debris, if present, are suctioned from its lateral surface. It is particularly important to ensure a dry TM when using phenol; otherwise, it will spread and cauterize the entire moist region. The tip of a phenol applicator is dipped in phenol such that a small drop is collected between the prongs (Fig. 107-1). The applicator is gently touched to the inside of the bottle to remove excess liquid. The phenol is applied to the area or areas of the TM to be manipulated (e.g., small dots for intratympanic injections or linear streaks for myringotomy). Immediate blanching will occur and indicates that the TM has been anesthetized. The phenol can also be applied with cotton over a metal applicator or via a phenol kit with a prepackaged sponge applicator (see Fig. 107-1). Patients should be warned that they will experience a transient burning sensation on application of the phenol. Used in these small amounts, phenol does not cause any permanent damage to the TM.

Tetracaine or Lidocaine

The literature does not support a standard concentration of lidocaine or tetracaine. Solutions of 4% to 10% lidocaine (amide) or 8% to 16% tetracaine (ester) dissolved in isopropyl alcohol are some of the more commonly described anesthetics used for TM anesthesia.

The patient is positioned supine with the head tilted to the side. The anesthetic should be room to body temperature before use to avoid a caloric effect. The solution is dropped into an ear canal with an intact TM until it is filled one third to one half full. The solution must remain in contact with the TM for at least 15 to 20 minutes for lidocaine and 60 minutes for tetracaine. A piece of cotton or a wick may be placed in the ear canal to allow the patient to ambulate during this time. The wick should be inserted slowly until it makes contact with the TM to ensure adequate exposure of the anesthetic to the TM. Before initiating the procedure, the wick is removed and a pick or the tip of the suction device (disconnected) is used to touch the TM to assess the effectiveness of the anesthesia. If the patient experiences pain distinct from noise produced by touching the TM, the anesthetic should be given more

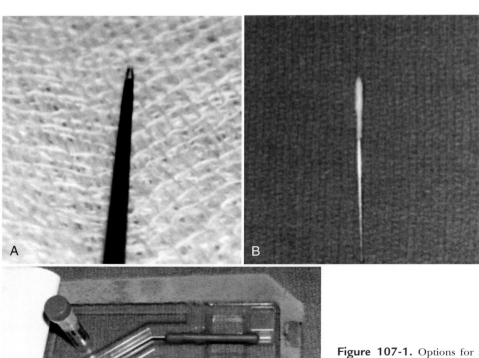

Figure 107-1. Options for application of phenol to the tympanic membrane. **A,** Phenol applicator. **B,** Cotton on a metal applicator. **C,** Prepackaged kit with sponge tip.

time to work. Once adequate anesthesia is achieved, the residual anesthetic is aspirated from the canal.

EMLA Cream

EMLA (eutectic mixture of local anesthetics) cream has been used for anesthesia of the eardrum by some authors. The cream is easy to apply directly to the eardrum with minimal risk of entry into the middle ear, but it does not always provide adequate anesthesia.[4] This may in large part be attributed to the long latency period for EMLA's full potency to be realized. One hour or more is generally accepted as the appropriate waiting period after application of EMLA, thus making it suboptimal for use in a busy office setting.

External Ear and Canal Anesthesia

Biopsy or repair of the external ear can be done in the office under local anesthesia. It is usually accomplished with local or regional injection of lidocaine or with a variety of topically applied anesthetics.

Topical Anesthetics

Topical anesthesia is often a good choice for children who cannot tolerate injectable anesthetic. EMLA or LET (lidocaine-epinephrine-tetracaine) is frequently used on both intact and broken skin.

EMLA or LET is applied directly to the surgical field while taking care to completely cover the area to be worked on. A temporary occlusive dressing can be placed over the medication for a minimum of 30 minutes for LET and 60 minutes for EMLA. Alternatively, LET can be mixed from its components (1% to 4% lidocaine, 1:1000 to 1:2000 epinephrine, 0.5% to 2% tetracaine) and applied with a cotton ball soaked in the mixture. Finally, a wide variety of commercially available patches, usually impregnated with lidocaine, are available for local procedures. Regardless of the local anesthetic used, it is prudent to test the sensation of the site with a needle prick or pinprick.

Local Injection of Lidocaine with Epinephrine

Traditionally, epinephrine has not been used for local anesthesia in regions of the body such as the outer ear, tip of the nose, fingers, toes, and penis because of the risk of skin necrosis from decreased blood flow. However, several recent studies have shown that epinephrine can be safe for local injection in the ear.[5-7]

The injection site is sterilized with an alcohol swab or a surgical preparation of choice. A 1-mL syringe is filled with a solution of 1% lidocaine with 1:200,000 epinephrine. A 1:10 bicarbonate-to-lidocaine dilution can be formulated to buffer the acidity of lidocaine and reduce burning at the injection site. This solution must be used within 1 week of mixing. A 25-gauge or smaller needle is used to inject the deep dermis. The needle is inserted under the skin at a 10- to 15-degree angle as the anesthetic is simultaneously slowly injected until the entire region to be operated on has been infiltrated. A bleb of fluid can be both visualized and palpated as the anesthetic is injected. Pain during injection can be reduced by injecting slowly and minimizing the total

number of skin punctures. A single needle puncture may be sufficient to cover small areas. If the skin is broken, injection can be performed through the open skin edges. The amount of anesthetic necessary depends on the size of the field but should be enough to completely cover the operative field. Despite being used locally, some of the lidocaine will reach the systemic circulation. The maximum dose of 1% lidocaine with epinephrine is 7 mg/kg up to 500 mg or 50 mL. The maximum dose of lidocaine without epinephrine is 4.5 mg/kg. Lidocaine provides adequate anesthesia within 2 minutes of injection, and the effect should last for several hours.

Regional Anesthesia

Regional anesthesia can be used for procedures involving the auricle, as well as the TM. Four nerves supply sensation to the ear (Fig. 107-2). The auriculotemporal nerve, a branch of the mandibular portion of the trigeminal nerve, supplies the superior portion of the outer ear. The great auricular nerve, which originates from the cervical plexus, supplies the inferior auricle. The middle section of the outer ear is supplied by the lesser occipital nerve, another branch of the cervical plexus. Finally, the auditory branch of the vagus nerve supplies the concha and the EAC. The EAC also has some innervation from the auriculotemporal nerve and branches from the tympanic plexus of the facial nerve.

Sound knowledge of this anatomy is necessary to choose an effective regional anesthetic modality. Two are discussed here: an outer ear block and a four-quadrant canal block. An outer ear block does not supply anesthesia to the EAC or the TM. Conversely, a four-quadrant canal block does not supply anesthesia to the outer ear but does provide good anesthesia to the EAC and TM.

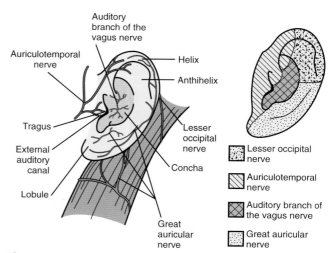

Figure 107-2. Innervation of the auricle. (*Adapted from Roberts R, Hedges JR [eds]: Clinical Procedures in Emergency Medicine, 4th ed. Philadelphia, WB Saunders, 2004.*)

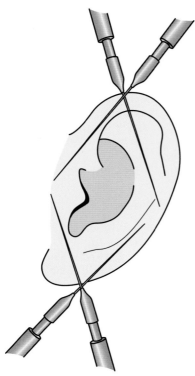

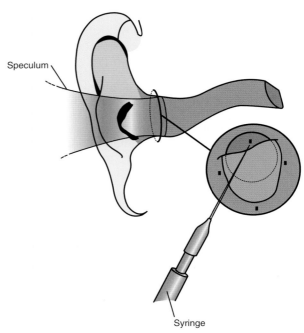

Figure 107-4. Four-quadrant canal block. *(Adapted from Roberts R, Hedges JR [eds]: Clinical Procedures in Emergency Medicine, 4th ed. Philadelphia, WB Saunders, 2004.)*

Figure 107-3. Outer ear block. *(Adapted from Roberts R, Hedges JR [eds]: Clinical Procedures in Emergency Medicine, 4th ed. Philadelphia, WB Saunders, 2004.)*

Outer Ear Block

Injections for an ear block are made at the junction of the most superior and inferior portions of the auricle with the head. The injection sites are disinfected with an alcohol swab, and a 10-mL syringe is filled with 1% lidocaine with epinephrine. A 25-gauge or smaller-bore needle is positioned at the superior pole. It is inserted at a 10- to 15-degree angle to the surface of the skin and directed toward the tragus (Fig. 107-3). The needle is inserted along the subcuticular plane while drawing back on the syringe. If no blood is returned as it is inserted, it can safely be assumed that the anesthetic can be injected as the needle is withdrawn without danger of intravenous injection. A total of 2 to 3 mL is injected. The needle is not completely removed from its initial puncture site as it is being repositioned to anesthetize along the posterior aspect of the pinna. A total of 2 to 3 mL of lidocaine is injected in the same manner as discussed earlier. The inferior pole is then injected. Anesthesia is obtained within a few minutes and lasts for more than one hour.

Four-Quadrant Canal Block

Again, 1% lidocaine with epinephrine is used for anesthesia. This technique involves injection at the bony cartilaginous junction of the EAC. The most medial aspect of the hair-bearing portion of the EAC can approximate this junction. A 25- or 27-gauge needle is used on a small syringe (1 or 3 mL with a Luer-Lok). The EAC is injected anteriorly, inferiorly, superiorly,

and posteriorly (Fig. 107-4). Slight pressure is applied with the speculum just lateral to the injection site to drive the anesthetic medially until blanching of the bony canal skin is noted. A moderate amount of resistance should be felt when the correct plane is infiltrated. If the injection is too superficial, a bleb may occur and hinder view of the canal for the procedure to be performed. Visualizing the more medial bony canal during the injection is helpful because blebs can be recognized early and the injection site may be adjusted.

DISIMPACTION OF CERUMEN

Disimpaction of cerumen is the most common procedure performed in the office. The ear is normally self cleaning; it expels cerumen, dust, dirt, and skin cells through gradual outward migration of the epithelium of the auditory canal. However, several conditions can interrupt this process and necessitate cleaning by a physician. Individuals with a narrow canal who wear hearing aids or ear plugs, those who have undergone surgery involving the ear canal, and chronic cotton swab users are among those most at risk for impaction of cerumen.

The task of cleaning an ear canal frequently falls on primary care physicians, with the removal technique of choice being irrigation of the ear canal. Not every ear can be completely disimpacted in this manner, and in the otolaryngologist's office, direct microscopic visualization is available to manually remove the cerumen. It is the preferred method when available and has the added benefit of providing an opportunity for trainees to reinforce the skills required for otologic surgery—working through a speculum, holding instruments in a manner that does not block view of the canal/TM, and maintaining fine control of the tip of the instrument. In nearly every situation, cerumen can be removed without causing discomfort or bleeding.

TECHNIQUE

An appropriately sized aural speculum is inserted into the ear canal and held in place with the nondominant hand. Under microscopic vision, cerumen is removed with suction, wax curettes, or various picks. Loop curettes can be sharp and should be used with caution. Ridged spatula-type curettes are less traumatic and handy when there is a small to moderate amount of cerumen that does not completely occlude the canal. If the cerumen forms a complete plug, it should be manipulated by working at the interface between the plug and the skin. This allows the physician to follow the contours of the canal and anticipate variations in anatomy (i.e., a prominent anterior bulge from the temporomandibular joint) and enables visualization of the TM. Depending on the consistency of the wax, curettes, picks, or suction may be used. A small right-angled pick is particularly handy in establishing the plane between firm wax and the canal skin. This pick is also ideal for removing cerumen that is impacted against the TM. When aspiration is used, a 5F suction device is generally sufficient but should be changed to 3F when close to the TM. A 7F suction device should be used only when absolutely necessary because the noise generated can be uncomfortable and it is harder to avoid inadvertently injuring the skin of the ear canal.

The same principles apply to cleaning a mastoid cavity. Ideally, one should be familiar with the previous operative reports and the status of the TM and middle ear anatomy. The ease of cleaning a cavity depends greatly on whether proper attention was given to critical issues at the time of surgery, particularly lowering the facial ridge sufficiently, sizing the meatoplasty adequately, and drilling the roof and floor of the ear canal so that they are flush with the superior and inferior aspects of the mastoid bowl. It is important to clear all pockets of desquamation and cerumen. Frequently, suctioning the bowl results in dizziness, so cleaning should rely on picks or curettes when possible. If the debris is moist, small suction devices should be used in patients prone to vertigo.

DRAINAGE OF A HEMATOMA OF THE AURICLE

Hematoma of the auricle is commonly seen in patients engaged in contact sports such as rugby, boxing, and wrestling because of the high potential for shearing the skin and perichondrium off the underlying cartilage. Wrestling has traditionally accounted for such a large proportion of auricular hematomas that the term "wrestler's ear" is sometimes used to describe the resul-

tant "cauliflower ear" deformity from an untreated injury. The requirement for head or ear protection during wrestling matches has greatly reduced but not eliminated the incidence of auricular hematoma in this population.

Cartilage receives its blood supply from the overlying perichondrium. Shearing injuries cause disruption of the normal anatomic relationship of the perichondrium to the cartilage, with resultant cartilage necrosis. The characteristic appearance of a cauliflower ear is the consequence of subsequent fibrosis, contracture, and neocartilage formation. To reduce this risk, it is important that the position of the perichondrium over the cartilage be restored as soon as possible after the formation of a hematoma.

Most auricular hematomas are believed to develop in the potential space between the perichondrium and cartilage; however, it has recently been shown that hematomas, particularly those that are recurrent, are often located *intra*cartilaginously.[8] Intracartilaginous hematomas can be multiloculated and, when incompletely evacuated, have a high potential to cause a cauliflower ear deformity.

PREOPERATIVE PLANNING

A careful history is important to determine the mechanism of injury and the time course of formation of the hematoma. A complete otoscopic examination should also be performed to assess for additional external or middle ear trauma. It is likewise important to determine the likelihood that the ear may be reinjured before it has healed. Athletes, in particular, may be likely to reinjure the ear because they are often unwilling to miss practice or a competition while the ear is healing. Bulky compression dressings and needle drainage should be avoided in this patient population. Recurrent hematomas may require open exploration.

SURGICAL TECHNIQUE
Incision and Drainage

Incision plus drainage is the preferred method for evacuation of a hematoma because the risk of recurrence is lower than with needle aspiration. All hematomas, even those that are multiloculated and intracartilaginous, can be successfully managed with this technique. The ear is appropriately prepared on both its medial and lateral surfaces. The periaural area should also be draped in such a fashion that hair is kept out of the surgical field. Anesthesia of the ear is obtained with a regional nerve block. An incision is made in the helical or antihelical fold to conceal the incisional scar (Fig. 107-5). It should be a minimum of 4 to 5 mm or larger if complete exploration is necessary. Blood or fluid is manually expressed from the incision by digital compression. A hemostat may be needed to explore the cavity and completely evacuate any loculations present. Once the fluid has been totally removed, a small rubber band or Penrose drain may be used to prevent

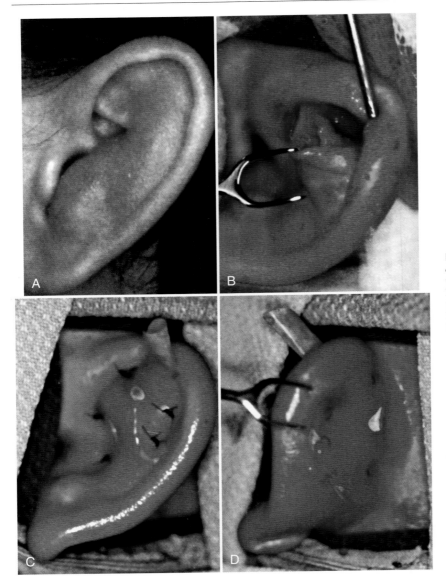

Figure 107-5. Hematoma of the auricle. **A,** The contours of the pinna are distorted by a hematoma. **B,** The auricle is incised parallel to the helical rim. **C,** A Penrose drain is placed, and trimmed Silastic sheeting is secured to both the lateral and medial (**D**) surface of the auricle with bolster stitches. *(Courtesy of Barry E. Hirsch, MD.)*

reaccumulation of fluid (Fig. 107-5). Regardless of whether a drain is placed, success of the procedure relies on an adequate compression-type dressing. A bolster-type dressing sutured to the ear has been shown to be effective against recurrence while allowing return to normal activity, including contact sports.[9] A dental roll is cut to the size of the hematoma. For large hematomas involving both the helical and antihelical rims, a bolster may be necessary at both sites. Size 3-0 silk or nylon suture is inserted through the dental roll and the lateral side of the auricle. On the medial side of the auricle, the suture is passed through another smaller piece of dental roll and back through the medial roll, the ear, and the lateral roll to complete the stitch (Fig. 107-5). The dental rolls and suture are then coated in antibiotic ointment.

Needle Aspiration

Hematoma of the auricle can be managed by needle aspiration followed by a period of compressive dressing. Alhough less invasive, this technique does carry a significantly higher risk of recurrence. Hematomas that are very firm on palpation are probably composed of clot and are unlikely to be drained successfully by needle aspiration. The ear is appropriately prepared on both its medial and lateral surfaces. Anesthesia of the ear is obtained with a regional nerve block as detailed earlier in this chapter. An 18-gauge needle is inserted into the hematoma and then a syringe is used to evacuate the hematoma. When the needle is withdrawn, the ear is digitally manipulated to ensure complete evacuation. A bolster is then fashioned and sutured in place as described earlier. Alternately, some practitioners prefer to use thermal splints or a whole-ear compressive dressing.

POSTOPERATIVE MANAGEMENT

After drainage, the patient should be monitored closely for signs of recurrence or infection. Antibiotics are used while the bolster is in place. The bolster is removed within approximately 5 days and patients are observed closely for recurrence of the hematoma.

INCISION AND DRAINAGE OF EAR ABSCESS

The external ear is a common site of local infections that require incision and drainage of a fluctuant collection of purulent exudate and necrotic tissue. These collections can be as small as a furuncle in the canal or as extensive as a subperiosteal abscess. Draining such collections not only contributes to their resolution but also helps alleviate some of the patient's pain and discomfort by releasing pressure and tension on the involved tissue. As with most infections, there is an increased incidence of these types of infections in immunocompromised hosts and diabetics.

Obstruction and infection of hair follicles resulting in a painful collection of purulent exudate give rise to furuncles and carbuncles. The most common location for them to develop on the ear is in the cartilaginous canal, with *Staphylococcus aureus* being the most frequent causative pathogen. These infections will sometimes drain spontaneously or after treatment with warm compresses and manual manipulation. Furuncles that are persistent require incision and drainage for resolution. Antibiotics are seldom necessary but should be considered in cases with significant concomitant cellulitis.

Although furuncles and carbuncles often develop without a history of trauma, allowing the organism to gain access to the skin, perichondritis and chondritis of the auricle are frequently associated with trauma or cosmetic cartilage piercing. Perichondritis, or inflammation of the perichondrium, and chondritis, or inflammation of the cartilage, may lead to frank abscess formation and require incision and drainage. Débridement may be necessary to contain or resolve the infection.

The auricular cartilage is relatively avascular, with a consequent diminished capacity to both clear an infection and deliver systemic antibiotics at adequate minimal inhibitory concentrations. Antibiotics are of use for intralesional therapy during prolonged drainage,[10] but evidence is inconclusive concerning the efficacy of systemic antibiotics.[11-13] In complicated infections requiring hospital admission, transdermal iontophoretic antibiotics should be considered because they have been found to be superior to diffusion of antibiotics through the skin or through the eschar of a burn.[14] Samples should be taken for culture at the time of drainage/débridement and broad-spectrum antibiotics

started. Although *S. aureus* is the pathogen most frequently isolated, *Pseudomonas aeruginosa* is common in both burn and piercing injuries.

A postauricular abscess develops when mastoiditis extends to invade the subperiosteal space. Mastoidectomy is required; however, performing incision and drainage in the office can diminish the pain and inflammation while arrangements are made for intravenous antibiotics and surgery.

PATIENT SELECTION

All patients with the acute formation of a painful fluctuant mass in the ear require drainage. Although some furuncles can be managed with warm compresses and manual expression, other types of infection must be incised to be drained. In the very early stages of infection of the ear there may not yet be a frank abscess. High-dose systemic antibiotics can sometimes prevent this early infection from developing into an abscess with corresponding cartilage damage. These patients need to be monitored daily for the infection to either resolve or develop into an abscess to be drained.

PREOPERATIVE PLANNING

A complete history and focused examination that includes otoscopy should be done before surgery. Individuals with a history of valvular heart disease should receive appropriate endocarditis prophylaxis. Antibiotic prophylaxis for bacteremia should also be given to immunocompromised patients, including those with human immunodeficiency virus infection or acquired immunodeficiency syndrome, patients with diabetes mellitus, those receiving chemotherapy or steroids, transplant patients, and alcoholics.

The size and cause of the furuncle/abscess will dictate whether or what type of drainage procedure to incorporate. Small abscesses that are complications of ear piercing may require only a small drain or wick, which can be removed in a few days. Larger abscesses, usually those resulting from trauma to an extended portion of the ear, will require a more elaborate drainage scheme.

For infections likely to cause cartilaginous destruction, the incision site should be planned so that it does not hinder future reconstructive procedures. Generally, reconstruction of the helical rim is accomplished through an incision in either the helical or antihelical fold in an attempt to conceal the scar.

SURGICAL TECHNIQUE

Furuncles

Injection of local anesthetic at several points lateral to the abscess generally suffices for incision and drainage of furuncles. Needle localization of the pocket before incision is useful to confirm the presence of pus. Abscesses situated quite laterally may be incised with a no. 15 blade. More medially situated abscesses may be accessed more readily with a myringotomy blade.

Auricular Abscesses

The patient is positioned supine with the affected ear up. The ear is prepared and draped. A regional ear block is the preferred method. For smaller abscesses, local injection of anesthetic can also be effective, although a very cooperative patient is required because manipulating the abscess is intensely painful. If sufficient anesthesia is not achieved with a regional block, local injection can be a useful adjunct. Injecting the skin centrally overlying the abscess allows the anesthetic to gradually diffuse through the skin/subcutaneous tissue plane and provides excellent anesthesia to the most sensitive portion of the abscess. An injection angle parallel to the skin helps prevent injection into the abscess cavity instead of subcutaneous tissue.

Once anesthesia has been obtained, the abscess is incised with a no. 15 blade along the natural contour of either the helical or antihelical fold. The pus is collected and sent for culture. The abscess cavity must be completely evacuated with all loculations eliminated. A hemostat or other blunt-tipped instrument may be used to probe the cavity and eliminate loculations. The cartilage is examined and any necrotic cartilage is débrided. This should be done conservatively to minimize the cartilage defect. It is possible that the cartilage will need to be débrided again, but staged débridement helps manage the size of the rim deformity. If extensive cartilage necrosis is noted, performing the procedure in the operating room may be good judgment. Once the cavity is adequately débrided, it is flushed with saline to remove residual debris. The incision is not closed. Depending on the size of the cavity, a drain or a small catheter may be used for infusion of antibiotics.

Subperiosteal Abscesses

One percent lidocaine with epinephrine is injected in curvilinear fashion approximately 1 cm posterior to the postauricular sulcus. The incision used for drainage should overlie the planned incision for mastoidectomy (Fig. 107-6). A hemostat is then used to enter the abscess cavity. Once the purulent exudate has been aspirated, the wound is irrigated with saline. Definitive surgical treatment should be scheduled to take place shortly after incision and drainage of a subperiosteal abscess.

POSTOPERATIVE MANAGEMENT

Furuncles do not generally require follow-up, but the patient should return if the pain or swelling worsens or the condition is not healing within 1 week. Postoperative management of other types of drained infections is dependent on the extent of the infection. Patients with significant chondritis or a subperiosteal abscess should be admitted for careful follow-up, administration of antibiotics, and possible surgical management.

Patients with an auricular abscess should be instructed that it may take several weeks for the infection to clear completely and that they are at risk for recurrence during this time. If the infection recurs, it should again be drained immediately with débridement

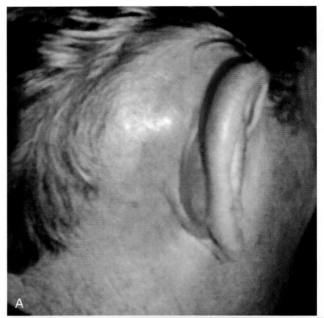

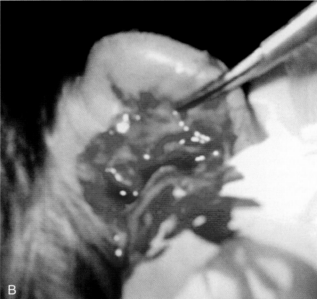

Figure 107-6. Postauricular abscess. **A,** The postauricular region was erythematous and fluctuant. **B,** Copious pus was cleared via a small postauricular incision performed in the office. A mastoidectomy was done the following morning.

of necrotic tissue. If an auricular rim defect develops, the patient should be referred for rim reconstruction. Reconstruction will generally take place 6 to 9 months after the infection has cleared to ensure that it has been completely eliminated.

BIOPSY OF A MASS IN THE EXTERNAL AUDITORY CANAL

Masses in the EAC are often asymptomatic and recognized on routine screening otoscopic examination.

Table 107-1	MASSES IN THE EXTERNAL EAR CANAL

Benign
Cholesteatoma
Eosinophilic granuloma
Exostosis
Fibrous dysplasia
Keratosis obturans
Neurofibroma
Osteoma
Paraganglioma/schwannoma
Stenosis
Temporomandibular joint herniation
Vascular lesions

Malignant
Adenocystic carcinoma
Basal cell carcinoma
Cerumen gland tumor
Malignant melanoma
Metastatic cancer
Soft tissue sarcoma
Squamous cell carcinoma

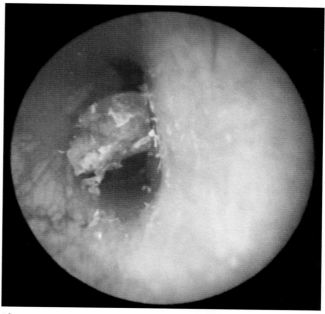

Figure 107-7. Pink, fleshy mass in the right external auditory canal. The mass was pulsating and noted to be protruding from the middle ear, which was also filled with tumor. Further evaluation confirmed the diagnosis of a large glomus tympanicum tumor.

However, they may be accompanied by hearing loss, aural fullness, otalgia, or otorrhea. Masses in the EAC can be benign or malignant (Table 107-1). The most commonly encountered malignant masses in the EAC are squamous cell, basal cell, and adenocystic carcinoma. The first step in planning the appropriate intervention for treatment or removal of the growth is to have an accurate diagnosis, which is often accomplished by biopsy of the lesion. Some benign masses in the EAC (i.e., osteomas, exostoses) can be diagnosed by their classic appearance and location and do not require intervention unless they are associated with conductive hearing loss or interfere with the ability to clear the ear of cerumen and squamous debris. Canal cholesteatomas can be addressed in the office setting by careful cleaning (see Chapter 110). Masses associated with a recent onset of pain and otorrhea may represent inflammatory polyps associated with otitis externa. Topical drops containing both a steroid and an antibiotic component may resolve these masses without need for biopsy. When a mass is suspected to be inflammatory in nature and topical therapy is used, close monitoring for resolution of the mass is critical, with subsequent biopsy of masses that fail to resolve.

More medially situated masses, such as polyps associated with blockage of an attic retraction pocket, may also be encountered. Removal of the bulk of these polyps followed by steroid/antibiotic drops can resolve the mass. Once the polyp has resolved, the attic may be cleaned of cerumen and squamous debris, and if the attic pocket is sufficiently wide to allow complete visualization and cleaning, it may be managed conservatively. Even when a large cholesteatoma necessitating surgical treatment is noted, addressing the polyp in the office setting may reduce inflammation and allow a smoother surgical procedure. In these situations the polyp can be removed with cup forceps. Care should be taken to avoid pulling on the lesion because it may be associated with the ossicular chain.

It is also important to recognize the appearance of malignant otitis externa, particularly in a patient with diabetes. This severe infection is typically manifested by granulation tissue at the bony-cartilaginous junction and requires aggressive management with antibiotics. Malignancies may masquerade as otitis externa, thereby resulting in delays in diagnosis and treatment. Although a diagnosis may be suggested by the physical appearance of many of the remaining lesions, biopsy should still be performed to confirm the diagnosis. Finally, one should be familiar with the pulsatile, fleshy appearance of glomus tumors. Large glomus tumors (Fig. 107-7) may protrude into the ear canal, and biopsy of these lesions in the office is not wise because excessive bleeding may result.

PREOPERATIVE PLANNING

Biopsy of any lesion can be a more anxiety-filled procedure than other types of office procedures because of the fear associated with the diagnosis. If at all possible, the biopsy should be done at the initial evaluation to expedite a tissue diagnosis. It is important to communicate with the patient regarding the types of expected diagnoses and the lag time until the pathology report is available. Time should be taken to carefully answer all the patient's questions without painting an overly dismal or overly optimistic picture.

SURGICAL TECHNIQUE

The patient is positioned supine with the affected ear up. A four-quadrant canal block is the anesthetic method of choice for this procedure. Once adequate anesthesia has been achieved, microscopic cup forceps can be used to remove the lesion. Pedunculated lesions may easily be removed with Bellucci scissors. It is advisable to have vials of epinephrine available in the office. In the event that extensive bleeding is encountered, small cotton balls soaked in epinephrine may be applied to the biopsy site. Silver nitrate sticks may be broken into small pieces and applied to the site with alligator forceps, or a small amount of liquid silver nitrate may be used on a small cotton-tipped swab.

POSTOPERATIVE MANAGEMENT

The patient should be seen in 1 week for evaluation of the biopsy site, as well as to discuss the results of the biopsy.

INTRATYMPANIC INJECTIONS

Intratympanic aminoglycoside or corticosteroid injection is an increasingly popular procedure performed in the office for the treatment of conditions such as Meniere's disease (MD) and sudden sensorineural hearing loss (SSNHL). Intratympanic injections are generally well tolerated with few side effects from the procedure itself. The puncture sites are typically closed within several weeks, and infections and persistent perforations are rare.[15]

It is well established that the main mode for chemicals to gain access to the inner ear is through absorption at the round window. Obstruction at the round window reduces absorption of the medication.[16] Intratympanic injection is the delivery technique preferred by the authors. Other techniques for the delivery of medications to the inner ear include injection of medication onto material such as Gelfoam placed directly on the round window niche, insertion of pressure equalization tubes with the self-administration of drops, wick placement in the round window through a tympanostomy tube, and microcatheter devices. Detailed information on alternative techniques is discussed by Jackson and Silverstein in their article, "Chemical Perfusion of the Inner Ear."[17]

Intratympanic Gentamicin

MD-associated vertigo can be incapacitating for the patient, and a significant number of patients do not achieve control of vertigo with conservative measures such as diuretic therapy and salt restriction. The use of intratympanic aminoglycosides is a minimally invasive approach to partial or total vestibular ablation. This chemical vestibular ablation may obviate the need for surgical management.

Gentamicin is the most commonly used aminoglycoside for injection because it is associated with vestibular toxicity more than cochlear toxicity. Streptomycin is similar to gentamicin in its predilection for the vestibular system but is less commonly used today because it has been shown that intratympanic gentamicin (IT-

GENT) has a higher success rate in the control of vertigo with a lower incidence of hearing loss.[18] The ototoxic effect of aminoglycosides is well established, with the risk of permanent mild to profound hearing loss increasing with increased use of the drug. Some individuals have reportedly lost hearing with the first IT-GENT injection, whereas other individuals, surprisingly enough, had improvement of their hearing loss once their vestibular symptoms were controlled.[4,19,20] A review of the literature on intratympanic aminoglycosides for MD reported control of vertigo in around 90% of patients, but hearing loss also occurred in approximately 30%.[21] Some hearing loss can be attributed to the natural course of MD, which is characterized by fluctuations in hearing. Nonetheless, there is a significant risk of profound hearing loss directly associated with the use of IT-GENT that increases with higher dosing. This risk is quoted to be as low as 3% when a conservative dosing scheme is used and as high as 15% in a more aggressive scheme. The current trend is toward titrating treatment to control vertigo rather than using a defined number of injections or total ablation as an end point of treatment. This method is believed by some to minimize the risk for hearing loss.[4,19,22] Before committing to IT-GENT, patients need to be well informed of the risks of injection and take into account how serviceable their current hearing is and the impact that losing hearing would have on their lives. Regardless of the risks to hearing, physicians and patients now often favor a trial of IT-GENT for medically uncontrolled vertigo in an attempt to avoid invasive surgery.

Intratympanic Dexamethasone

Various steroids are also injected into the ear, particularly for the treatment of SSNHL. Classically, steroids have been believed to exert an effect in both MD and SSNHL through their anti-inflammatory properties, the assumption being that a viral or autoimmune-type process is affecting the cochlea. However, this may not actually be the case. It has recently been shown that mice with autoimmune hearing dysfunction respond equally well to aldosterone as they do to prednisolone, thus suggesting that the mechanism behind the drug effect may be through stimulation of a mineralocorticoid receptor.[23]

Regardless of the mechanism of action, the goal of steroid therapy is to create the maximal effect through achieving the highest possible concentration of steroid in the perilymph while minimizing systemic side effects. Studies of steroid concentrations in the perilymph of guinea pigs have shown that it is possible to produce much higher concentrations with intratympanic injection than via systemic routes.[24,25] Although most studies refer to intratympanic injection of steroids as a salvage technique for the treatment of SSNHL and sudden hearing loss associated with MD, some practitioners are now considering it first-line treatment because of the relative ease of the procedure and avoidance of systemic side effects.[26]

PATIENT SELECTION

Intratympanic Gentamicin

IT-GENT is appropriate to consider in patients with MD that is unresponsive to conservative measures. Such measures include diuretics and salt and caffeine restriction, which can adequately control symptoms in the majority of patients. Conservative treatments should be tried for at least 3 months before considering IT-GENT. Use of IT-GENT has increased greatly over the past decade but remains controversial, with some centers relying more heavily on surgical procedures or including a trial of histamine injections or the Meniett device (Medtronic) before proceeding with an ablative procedure. Although the procedure is relatively quick and easy to perform, it carries a significant risk of permanent sensorineural hearing loss, as well as chronic disequilibrium. Because MD is diagnosed by history, careful discussion of the nature of the patient's dizzy spells must take place before any treatment. Migraine-associated dizziness, benign paroxysmal positional vertigo, superior semicircular canal dehiscence, and other causes of episodic vertigo must be ruled out by history, physical examination, or imaging. The vertigo spells must occur with sufficient frequency to be truly disabling, and nonablative alternatives, both clinical and surgical, must be extensively discussed. IT-GENT is also sometimes useful in the setting of vestibular hypofunction when a small amount of residual balance function in the affected ear impairs vestibular compensation. Patients should be instructed to expect a period of significant disequilibrium, usually for several days after the injection. All patients are enrolled in vestibular rehabilitation to optimize vestibular compensation. Ideally, the first session takes place before the injection is performed.

Usually, the affected ear is readily identified on the basis of unilateral aural symptoms, including fullness, tinnitus, and hearing loss. If it is not clear which ear is affected or if there are symptoms of bilateral MD, ablative procedures much be approached with great caution and only after nonablative treatments have been fully explored. Patients with poor vision or impaired proprioception (e.g., peripheral neuropathy) and older patients may have an impaired capacity to compensate for the resultant unilateral vestibular loss. The risk of MD developing in the unaffected ear with possible oscillopsia must be discussed with the patient. Gentamicin is contraindicated in patients when the only hearing ear is affected.

Intratympanic Dexamethasone

Currently, there is no well established set of criteria to select patients who will benefit most from intratympanic dexamethasone (IT-DEX). A multicenter trial is under way to help clarify questions concerning indications, timing, frequency, type of steroid used, and concentration. The authors' approach is to use oral steroids only for mild SSNHL. For moderate or severe SSNHL, IT-DEX is administered in conjunction with oral steroids.

Patients who cannot tolerate oral steroids (e.g., severe diabetics) are considered for IT-DEX even with mild SSNHL.

PREOPERATIVE PLANNING

For both IT-GENT and IT-DEX, pure-tone audiometry should be performed before each injection. Vestibular testing should be performed before proceeding with IT-GENT. Significant hypofunction in the unaffected ear would represent a contraindication to ablation. Some clinicians include electrocochleography because an elevated summating potential to action potential (SP/AP) may suggest hydrops; however, MD may be present with a normal SP/AP ratio and a high ratio may be present in the absence of symptoms.[27] In MD, the affected ear often has elevated thresholds on vestibular evoked myogenic potential recordings.[28] Patients with SSNHL should undergo magnetic resonance imaging with gadolinium enhancement to rule out a retrocochlear process because a fraction of acoustic neuromas may be manifested in this manner. However, because there is a benefit to delivering the steroid early, the first injection is usually performed immediately on detecting the sudden loss, with imaging studies scheduled to coincide with the 1-week follow-up visit.

SURGICAL APPROACH

The patient is positioned supine with the head at a 45-degree angle, an appropriately sized aural speculum is introduced into the ear canal, and an otoscopic examination is performed with removal of any obstructing cerumen or debris from the canal and TM. Anesthesia of the eardrum is then induced. If using phenol, the applicator is touched to the anterosuperior and posteroinferior TM (Fig. 107-8). A 25-gauge needle on a tuberculin syringe loaded with the appropriate medication is used. The syringe is filled to 0.6 mL. Loading more than this amount into the syringe can make it awkward for the thumb of the injecting hand to reach the plunger comfortably. The needle is bent to a 25-degree angle at the hub and inserted via microscopic visualization through an aural speculum. Bending the needle helps prevent obstruction of the view of the TM during the injection. The needle should be angled so that the bevel will face superiorly as the middle ear is entered. Because the drum is positioned with its inferior aspect located more medially than its superior aspect, it is easier to insert the bevel fully into the middle ear and avoid spillage into the ear canal during the injection. Spillage into the ear canal not only makes it more difficult to determine whether an appropriate volume has been injected but also makes it difficult to visualize the rising air-fluid level during the injection. A puncture is made in the anterosuperior quadrant within the area anesthetized by the phenol. This allows air to exit the middle ear space and tends to ease the aural fullness and discomfort associated with the injection. The needle is then inserted through a separate puncture site in the posteroinferior TM and the

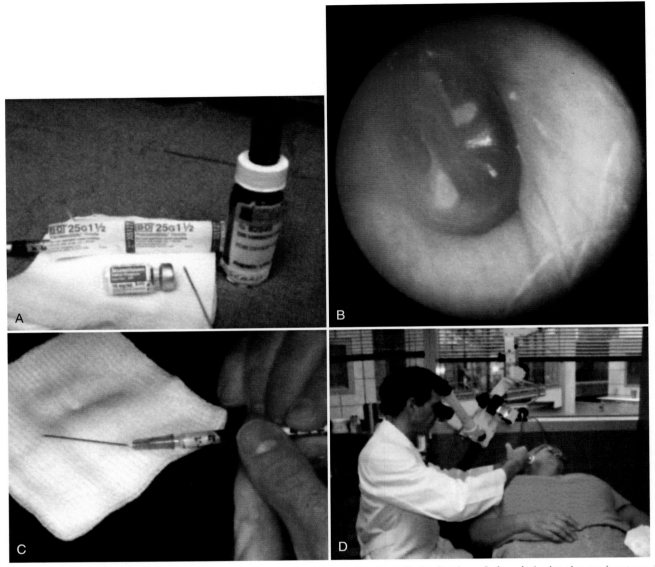

Figure 107-8. Intratympanic injection. **A,** Phenol, applicator, and loaded syringe. **B,** Application of phenol. A pinpoint myringotomy is established anterosuperiorly to allow air to escape the middle ear during the injection. The medication is injected via a posteroinferior myringotomy. **C,** Bending the needle slightly allows better visualization during the injection. **D,** The injection is performed with the patient's head tilted 45 degrees away from the affected ear. Once the injection has been completed, the patient is asked to turn so that the injected ear faces straight up. The patient maintains this position for 25 minutes.

medication is injected. Typically, 0.4 mL can be injected into the middle ear space. The authors use gentamicin buffered with sodium bicarbonate at a final concentration of 30 mg/mL and dexamethasone at a concentration of 10 mg/mL. However, it should be noted that different concentrations and other types of steroids have been used successfully. If it is difficult to stabilize the needle as the TM is approached, steadying the syringe with the thumb of the nondominant hand can be helpful. The thumb of the injecting hand should be in position on the plunger so that no adjustments are required once the needle has been placed through the TM. This prevents tearing at the myringotomy and

maintains a seal around the puncture site as the middle ear is filled. The medication is slowly injected into the middle ear space and the resultant air-fluid level is observed as it rises up to the anterosuperior puncture site. Once the middle ear has been filled and efflux of medication into the ear canal is noted, the needle is withdrawn and the patient remains supine with the injected ear up for 25 to 30 minutes. The patient is given tissues and a basin and is instructed to spit secretions instead of swallowing them to minimize clearance of the middle ear by the eustachian tube. The risk of persistent perforation or infection has been very low with this technique.

POSTOPERATIVE MANAGEMENT

Intratympanic Gentamicin

The patient is instructed to maintain dry ear precautions until the follow-up visit at 3 weeks. Typically, by this time the injection site will have healed and these restrictions can be lifted. Some practitioners report that more than 50% of patients experienced at least 2 years of control of episodic vertigo with a single injection.[20] Vestibular physical therapy is initiated and the patient is seen in follow-up 3 weeks after the injection. An audiogram is performed. If the patient reports persistent severe attacks at the follow-up visit, a second injection is considered. Repeat injections may be performed, separated by at least 3 to 4 weeks, in patients with persistent symptoms. Treatment is discontinued when the vertigo is controlled. This may occur despite persistent vestibular function in the treated ear. Audiometry is repeated before each injection and 2 months after the last injection. Gentamicin may be associated with an initial decline in hearing for up to 1 month after treatment, but patients may subsequently regain some or all of the hearing lost as a result of treatment.[4] Diuretic therapy and salt restriction are both maintained during the course of treatment. Of the patients who achieve control of vertigo, approximately 70% to 80% will continue to have their vertigo controlled at 2 years, and of those who relapse, a second course of IT-GENT can often achieve a sustained remission.[19,20]

Intratympanic Dexamethasone

The patient is instructed to maintain dry ear precautions and is seen in follow-up within 1 week for a repeat hearing test. If there has been an improvement but the hearing has not returned to baseline, a second injection is performed. Injections proceed on a weekly basis until hearing returns to baseline or a plateau is reached.

MYRINGOTOMY AND INSERTION OF TUBES

Myringotomy, with or without insertion of pressure equalization tubes, has become a mainstay in the management of recurrent otitis media, chronic otitis media with effusion, complicated acute otitis media, or chronic eustachian tube dysfunction. On occasion, tubes are also used to provide access to the middle ear for delivery of medications, to provide ventilation of the middle ear during hyperbaric oxygen therapy, or to enable use of the Meniett device. Although children are most often taken to the operating room for placement of tubes, most adults can easily tolerate performance of the procedure in the office under local anesthesia. Various tubes should be available in the office. Small tubes (i.e., tiny titans) are often useful for short-term aeration. They may become clogged more easily, particularly with viscous effusions. Midsize tubes (i.e., beveled Armstrong tubes) typically remain in place for 6 to 9 months. Patients with mucoid otitis media may benefit from short tubes with a wide internal diameter (i.e., Paparella II tubes). In a cooperative patient with an adequately sized ear canal, even the longer-lasting Goode T tubes may be inserted in the office setting, although they are more commonly placed in the operating room. Myringotomy and tympanostomy tubes are both discussed extensively in Chapter 112. This section focuses on modifications of the procedure when performed in the office setting.

PATIENT SELECTION

All patients are examined carefully with an otologic microscope. Pneumatic otoscopy should always be included in the examination, because on occasion a serous effusion may not be readily apparent even with careful otomicroscopy. Tuning fork testing should also be used to confirm a conductive hearing loss. Even when the history and physical examination clearly indicate a chronic effusion, it is wise to formally test the hearing before manipulating the TM for both medicolegal and diagnostic purposes. Occasionally, chronic effusions are associated with normal hearing, thus leaving less reason to proceed with drainage. When conductive loss is present, determining the degree of loss can be helpful in ruling out additional pathology involving the conductive apparatus.

As for all office procedures, the surgeon must determine whether the patient will be able to tolerate the potential noise and discomfort without excess motion. Unilateral effusion in adults merits careful examination of the nasopharynx for adenoid hypertrophy or a mass lesion obstructing the orifice of the eustachian tube. The patient is instructed regarding the need for maintenance of a dry ear and the potential risk of TM perforation. Patients who are avid swimmers and disinclined to practice dry ear precautions may prefer to live with an effusion or undergo fitting with custom plugs before the procedure. Insertion of pressure equalization tubes may be difficult in patients with severe middle ear atelectasis. However, a small titanium tube can usually be inserted into the anteroinferior quadrant and often provides significant relief of aural fullness. The decision regarding whether to perform myringotomy alone versus proceeding with placement of pressure equalization tubes hinges on the desired duration of middle ear ventilation. A myringotomy may close within days and is therefore used when very short-term ventilation is needed. Serous effusions that occur acutely in the setting of an upper respiratory infection or after a flight will often resolve spontaneously, particularly if the patient is able to perform autoinsufflation or a Valsalva maneuver with successful ventilation of the middle ear space. A 3-day course of a nasal decongestant such as oxymetazoline (Afrin), as well as a nasal steroid spray, should be considered before myringotomy in these situations. Myringotomy should not be used as first-line therapy for uncomplicated acute otitis media. However, when significant otalgia is present, myringotomy does provide symptomatic relief. Myringotomy with tube insertion is indicated when acute otitis media persists despite antibiotics or is complicated by sensorineural hearing loss, vertigo, facial nerve paresis, mastoiditis or intracranial extension, meningitis, or a brain abscess. Vascular anomalies (aberrant carotid, dehiscent jugular bulb), as well as glomus tumors, may be mistaken for otitis media with effusion. When this possibility cannot be ruled out, imaging should be obtained before proceeding with a myringotomy because extensive bleeding and neurovascular complications may occur.

PREOPERATIVE PLANNING

Myringotomy "kits" containing the various instruments to be used may be prepared in advance. Otherwise, the surgeon should have ready access to speculums of various size, wax curettes, phenol, a phenol applicator, a myringotomy knife, 3F and 5F suction devices, fine alligator forceps, and a fine right-angled or gently curved pick. Although most often the procedure can be performed without bleeding, on occasion an inflamed TM will bleed despite adequate application of phenol. It is helpful to have access to epinephrine in these instances.

SURGICAL TECHNIQUE

Depending on the anatomy of the ear canal and the degree of prominence of the anterior bulge from the temporomandibular joint, myringotomies may be performed in the anteroinferior to posteroinferior aspects of the TM. The posterosuperior quadrant must be avoided given the location of the ossicles. Phenol is applied at the planned myringotomy site, typically in radial fashion (Fig. 107-9). The area to be anesthetized depends on the procedure. If the procedure is a planned myringotomy only and the effusion is serous, a small area is anesthetized and a small linear incision is performed that is adequate to allow aspiration of the middle ear space with a 3-mm suction device. When pressure equalization tubes are to be inserted, the size of the myringotomy depends on the size of the tube to be inserted. A myringotomy that is significantly longer than the diameter of the tube should be avoided because it is unnecessary and carries a greater potential for loss of the tube in the middle ear space. An angled myringotomy blade facilitates visualization of the TM during the incision. Particularly because the patient is not under sedation or general anesthesia, it is important to avoid the discomfort and bleeding associated with trauma to the EAC during the myringotomy and tube insertion. Excess magnification should be avoided. The resulting loss of depth of the field makes it difficult to protect the canal because it is not in focus while the drum is manipulated. Many different tubes are available, and over time, each clinician will develop a preference. Tubes may be grasped at their lateral lip, which often has a small tab. Although the tube may be inserted in one fluid motion with alligator forceps, it is often more comfortable for the patient if the inferior aspect of the medial flange of the tube is placed through the

myringotomy and then a fine pick is used to gently insert the upper aspect of the flange through the TM. Bleeding during the procedure may cause blockage of the tube and should be controlled. In most instances the bleeding resolves within minutes and can be suctioned. However, on occasion, epinephrine-soaked cotton may be necessary to control persistent bleeding.

POSTOPERATIVE MANAGEMENT

Follow-up intervals depend on the indication for the procedure, with complicated otitis media requiring very close monitoring as opposed to other conditions (i.e., chronic serous otitis media), which may not require follow-up for 6 months. When a myringotomy has been performed, the patient is asked to return within several weeks. If the effusion has recurred at the follow-up visit, the procedure is repeated, but with insertion of a tube. The patient is maintained on dry ear precautions while the myringotomy remains patent or a tube remains in place. If there is active infection at the time of the procedure, topical antibiotics are prescribed. Serous effusions do not require treatment with antibiotic drops. Steroid-containing drops are helpful when there is significant middle ear mucosal inflammation or a mucoid effusion. Drops are also used when there has been bleeding during the procedure in an attempt to prevent crusting and blockage of the tube.

MIDDLE EAR ENDOSCOPY

Middle ear endoscopy can be used to clarify the diagnosis of some causes of conductive hearing loss, including interruption of the ossicular chain, otosclerosis, and chronic otitis media with or without cholesteatoma. Endoscopy has been found by some groups to change treatment in as many as 17% of patients on whom it is used.[29] Other physicians seldom or never perform middle ear endoscopy and instead opt to confirm the suspected diagnosis at the time of surgery.

PATIENT SELECTION

Most patients with conductive hearing loss will have a cause defined by traditional methods of evaluation (i.e., history, otoscopy, tympanometry, stapedial reflex evaluation, in conjunction with audiometry). Good candidates for middle ear endoscopy are those who have a conductive or mixed hearing loss in which the cause is unclear and an exact diagnosis may affect the need for or approach to surgery. Two situations in which this is likely to occur are questionable cholesteatoma and suspected otosclerosis or other ossicular chain problems.[29]

Children and other patient populations unlikely to tolerate the procedure should be taken to the operating room and have endoscopy performed under general anesthesia. The endoscope may be used to palpate the ossicles, but any sudden movement may cause them to be damaged or dislocated.

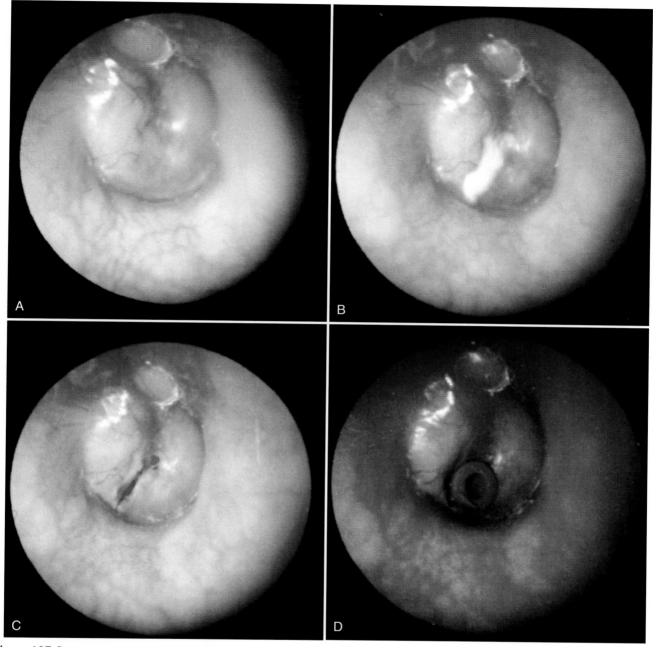

Figure 107-9. Insertion of a pressure equalization tube. **A,** A thick mucoid effusion is noted in the right middle ear. **B,** Phenol is applied in radial fashion in the posteroinferior quadrant. **C,** The myringotomy has been performed. **D,** A Paparella II tube has been inserted.

PREOPERATIVE PLANNING

A complete otoscopic examination and an audiogram showing evidence of conductive hearing loss should be done before endoscopy. A computed tomography scan may also be useful to evaluate the presence and extent of cholesteatoma, as well as to attempt to evaluate the integrity of the ossicular chain. If the TM is already perforated, the perforation should be used for the endoscopy; if not, a myringotomy "kit" is used. A full

set of endoscopes should be available because the optimal angle required to evaluate middle ear structures will change, depending on placement of the tympanostomy window. Currently 0-, 30-, and 90-degree Olympus endoscopes are available with an outer diameter of 1.7 mm. Storz 30- and 70-degree endoscopes with an outer diameter of 1.9 mm are also available.

The success of endoscopy in the office hinges on good communication with the patient before and during the procedure. The patient should be aware that it is imperative for the head to remain still when the endoscope is in use. Patients also need to be informed that they may experience discomfort from palpation of middle ear structures and that heat from the endoscope light can induce vertigo. Patients should be informed that at any point during the procedure they can ask to stop or pause it and the endoscope will be removed immediately; otherwise, the patient may be more likely to move while the endoscope is in place, thereby causing more damage.

SURGICAL TECHNIQUE

The patient is placed supine with the head tilted toward the unaffected side and positioned at a height at which the physician is comfortable and able to steadily maneuver the endoscope. The ear is examined, and any obstructing cerumen or debris is cleared. No anesthesia of the eardrum is required if there is a concomitant TM perforation of 2 mm or greater, thereby allowing easy passage of the endoscopes. Otherwise, for both very small perforations and intact TMs, appropriate local anesthesia of the eardrum should be obtained in the posterosuperior quadrant. An arc incision is then made between the oval and round windows. The incision should be large enough to allow passage of the endoscopes. Alternatively, a laser myringotomy may be made in this location.

The endoscope is inserted into the ear canal and advanced slowly toward the myringotomy. It is held at the edge of the myringotomy, and when necessary, the scope is advanced through the opening. The endoscopy is begun with a 0- or 30-degree scope to obtain a feel for proper positioning of the endoscope through the opening. It is difficult to visualize straight ahead with a 70- or 90-degree scope, thus making it difficult to accurately advance the scope to the opening. The choice of scope is dependent on the position of the myringotomy, as well as the patient's anatomy. Through the standard posterosuperior myringotomy, a 0- or 30-degree scope should be able to visualize the stapes and part of the incus, but a larger angle is generally needed to evaluate the remainder of the chain (Fig. 107-10).

The status of the middle ear mucosa is evaluated with particular attention paid to signs of cholesteatoma. The integrity of the ossicular chain is then closely examined for signs of otosclerosis, dislocation, deformation, or other abnormality. In a very cooperative patient, the ossicles may be palpated by passing a pick through the myringotomy under endoscopic visualization. The endoscope is held in place with the nondominant hand and is used to guide the pick to the myringotomy by sliding the tip of the pick down the barrel of the endoscope until it can be visualized. This technique will help reduce the risk of accidentally touching or perforating an unanesthetized part of the TM. The pick is slowly advanced into the middle ear cavity, and the stapes and long process of the incus are then touched to assess their movement. The myringotomy window may be closed with a paper patch.

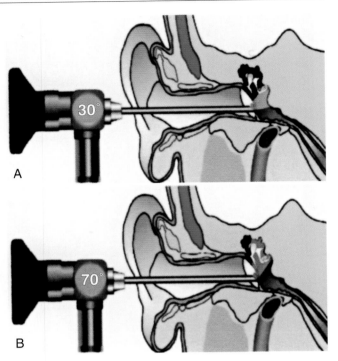

Figure 107-10. The visual field of 30- and 70-degree endoscopes. *(Reprinted with permission from Kakehata S, Futai K, Kuroda R, et al: Office-based endoscopic procedure for diagnosis in conductive hearing loss cases using OtoScan laser-assisted myringotomy. Laryngoscope 114:1285-1289, 2004.)*

POSTOPERATIVE MANAGEMENT

Dry ear precautions should be in place until the myringotomy has healed. The patient should be seen at follow-up in 3 weeks to ensure closure of the myringotomy.

PEARLS

- In any office procedure, communicating with the patient to maximize comfort is the key to success.
- Anxiety surrounding office procedures can be reduced through installation of a video monitoring system so that the patient can watch the procedure in progress.
- Any solution introduced into either the ear canal or the middle ear should first be warmed to body temperature to avoid inducing vertigo.
- When a mass in the EAC is suspected to be inflammatory in nature and topical therapy is instituted, close monitoring for resolution of the mass is critical, with biopsy of persistent lesions.

PITFALLS

- Patients with deep retraction pockets, TM perforations, or a mastoid bowl are particularly susceptible to transient facial paralysis from local anesthetics.
- If the temporal artery is punctured with an outer ear block, pressure should be maintained for 20 to 30 minutes to avoid the formation of a hematoma.
- Biopsy of pulsatile, highly vascular lesions should not be performed in the office.
- Although relatively easy to perform, intratympanic injection of gentamicin is associated with significant potential morbidity; therefore, nonablative options should be exhausted and the patient must be fully informed of the risks.

References

1. Krouse JH, Mirante JP, Christmas DA: Office-Based Surgery in Otolaryngology. Philadelphia, WB Saunders, 1999, p 273.
2. Siegel GJ, Chandra RK: Laser office ventilation of ears with insertion of tubes. Otolaryngol Head Neck Surg 127:60-66, 2002.
3. Hoffman RA, Li CL: Tetracaine topical anesthesia for myringotomy. Laryngoscope 111:1636-1638, 2001.
4. Smith WK, Sandooram D, Prinsley PR: Intratympanic gentamicin treatment in Meniere's disease: Patients' experiences and outcomes. J Laryngol Otol 120:730-735, 2006.
5. Hafner HM, Rocken M, Breuninger H: Epinephrine-supplemented local anesthetics for ear and nose surgery: Clinical use without complications in more than 10,000 surgical procedures. J Dtsch Dermatol Ges 3:195-199, 2005.
6. Gessler EM, Hart AK, Dunlevy TM, et al: Optimal concentration of epinephrine for vasoconstriction in ear surgery. Laryngoscope 111:1687-1690, 2001.
7. Watson D: Torn earlobe repair. Otolaryngol Clin North Am 35:187-205, vii-viii, 2002.
8. Ghanem T, Rasamny JK, Park SS: Rethinking auricular trauma. Laryngoscope 115:1251-1255, 2005.
9. Schuller DE, Dankle SD, Strauss RH: A technique to treat wrestlers' auricular hematoma without interrupting training or competition. Arch Otolaryngol Head Neck Surg 115:202-206, 1989.
10. Bassiouny A: Perichondritis of the auricle. Laryngoscope 91:422-431, 1981.
11. Llera JL, Levy RC: Treatment of cutaneous abscess: A double-blind clinical study. Ann Emerg Med 14:15-19, 1985.
12. Noel SB, Scallan P, Meadors MC, et al: Treatment of *Pseudomonas aeruginosa* auricular perichondritis with oral ciprofloxacin. J Dermatol Surg Oncol 15:633-637, 1989.
13. Margulis A, Bauer BS, Alizadeh K: Ear reconstruction after auricular chondritis secondary to ear piercing. Plast Reconstr Surg 111:891-897, discussion 898, 2003.
14. Kaweski S, Baldwin RC, Wong RK, et al: Diffusion versus iontophoresis in the transport of gentamicin in the burned rabbit ear model. Plast Reconstr Surg 92:1342-1349, discussion 1350-1351, 1993.
15. Doyle KJ, Bauch C, Battista R, et al: Intratympanic steroid treatment: A review. Otol Neurotol 25:1034-1039, 2004.
16. Silverstein H, Rowan PT, Olds MJ, et al: Inner ear perfusion and the role of round window patency. Am J Otol 18:586-589, 1997.
17. Jackson LE, Silverstein H: Chemical perfusion of the inner ear. Otolaryngol Clin North Am 35:639-653, 2002.
18. Blakley BW: Clinical forum: A review of intratympanic therapy. Am J Otol 18:520-526, discussion 527-531, 1997.
19. Horii A, Saika T, Uno A, et al: Factors relating to the vertigo control and hearing changes following intratympanic gentamicin for intractable Meniere's disease. Otol Neurotol 27:896-900, 2006.
20. Wu IC, Minor LB: Long-term hearing outcome in patients receiving intratympanic gentamicin for Meniere's disease. Laryngoscope 113:815-820, 2003.
21. Blakley BW: Update on intratympanic gentamicin for Meniere's disease. Laryngoscope 110:236-240, 2000.
22. Pender DJ: Gentamicin tympanoclysis: Effects on the labyrinthine sensory cells. Laryngoscope 113:343-348, 2003.
23. Trune DR, Kempton JB, Gross ND: Mineralocorticoid receptor mediates glucocorticoid treatment effects in the autoimmune mouse ear. Hear Res 212:22-32, 2006.
24. Parnes LS, Sun AH, Freeman DJ: Corticosteroid pharmacokinetics in the inner ear fluids: An animal study followed by clinical application. Laryngoscope 109:1-17, 1999.
25. Chandrasekhar SS: Intratympanic dexamethasone for sudden sensorineural hearing loss: Clinical and laboratory evaluation. Otol Neurotol 22:18-23, 2001.
26. Kakehata S, Sasaki A, Oji K, et al: Comparison of intratympanic and intravenous dexamethasone treatment on sudden sensorineural hearing loss with diabetes. Otol Neurotol 27:604-608, 2006.
27. Ferraro JA, Durrant JD: Electrocochleography in the evaluation of patients with Meniere's disease/endolymphatic hydrops. J Am Acad Audiol 17:45-68, 2006.
28. Timmer FC, Zhou G, Guinan JJ, et al: Vestibular evoked myogenic potential (VEMP) in patients with Meniere's disease with drop attacks. Laryngoscope 116:776-779, 2006.
29. Kakehata S, Futai K, Kuroda R, et al: Office-based endoscopic procedure for diagnosis in conductive hearing loss cases using OtoScan laser-assisted myringotomy. Laryngoscope 114:1285-1289, 2004.

Chapter 108

Foreign Bodies of the External Auditory Canal

Barry E. Hirsch

A foreign body of the external auditory canal can pose a real challenge to otolaryngologists. Foreign bodies are more commonly seen in the pediatric population but they do occur in adults. Insects, vegetable matter, and inorganic material are the objects seen most frequently. Removal of the material is important not only for relieving acute symptoms of pain, pressure, and hearing loss but also to avoid potential sequelae of infection, canal stenosis, and further hearing loss.

PATIENT SELECTION

The acute event resulting from entrapment of a foreign body in the ear canal will bring most patients to the attention of a physician. Such patients also include adults, who become immediately aware that an object that they were using to clean or manipulate the ear becomes dislodged and is left in the external auditory canal. The most common inorganic object creating this problem is the end of a cotton-tipped applicator. After ear cleaning, people may realize that the cotton tip is no longer attached to the end of the applicator. Similarly, other materials, such as facial tissue and paper, can be rolled in an elongated fashion and used to probe the ear. Institutionalized adults and children may also use these materials for ear cleaning or packing. In this population, if drainage, infection, or odor has not developed, such material may be found only on routine physical examination.

Along with using instrumentation to clean their ears, adults also place objects in the ear canal for protection, including devices to minimize water exposure because of recurrent otitis externa or perforation of the tympanic membrane. Material used for hearing protection can become lodged or break off and remain in the external canal. Examples of such products include sili-cone putty used for sound or water protection and Silastic occlusive plugs or foam inserts for sound protection. Again, patients become acutely aware of broken off material remaining in the ear canal.

The list of objects that children can put in their ears is endless. Unless a witness observes a child placing a foreign body in the canal, its presence may not be discovered until routine physical examination detects the object or problems arise because of its presence. Objects that occlude the ear canal could produce hearing loss. This is a common chief complaint in an aware child or adult. Inflammation caused by the foreign object may result in infection and drainage. Localized aural discharge, cellulitis of the concha and external meatus, or serosanguineous otorrhea would prompt further evaluation. Certain materials pose more of a challenge to extract from the canal. Once water enters the external canal, vegetable materials such as beans and peas can swell and cause obstruction, pain, and maceration. Other materials that have been found in the ear canal include small toys, beads, erasers, crayons, pits from fruit, disc batteries, nuts, and stones. Disc batteries should be removed as soon as possible to avoid the liquefaction necrosis that results when moisture and secretions permit flow of electrons.[1] Irrigation of the ear canal should be avoided to minimize the risk of generating an electric current. Similarly, unsuccessful attempts at removal of the battery that result in trauma and bleeding in the ear canal would also allow flow of current and therefore further tissue destruction.

Insects occasionally find their way into the ear canals of children and adults alike. These are usually flying insects, but crawling insects may also enter the canal, especially when people are asleep. Patients become acutely aware of their presence because of the insect's noise and the induced pain. Management in this situation becomes more urgent than that needed for inanimate objects.

PREOPERATIVE PLANNING

In most situations, removal of a foreign body is an elective event. This permits planning in terms of the appropriate instrumentation, lighting, the need for and type of anesthesia, and the method of extraction. Adult or pediatric patients with otorrhea, hearing loss, and obstruction or occlusion of the ear canal who fail to respond to topical and systemic therapy may have pathology of the middle ear and mastoid or foreign bodies causing their symptoms and findings. If medical therapy fails to reduce the inflammation that limits visualization of the medial canal and tympanic membrane, computed tomography is appropriate to assess the status of the external canal, middle ear, and mastoid.

Management of insects in the ear canal requires additional material. A live insect can be difficult and painful to extract. Various solutions, including ether, isopropyl alcohol, and mineral oil, are effective in drowning and killing the insect before flushing or extraction. Topical tetracaine (Pontocaine) or lidocaine (Xylocaine) solution can also be used to submerge and paralyze the insect in the ear canal.[2] This is readily available in all emergency room settings.

Foreign bodies can be categorized not only by their chemical composition but also by their shape and consistency. Understanding the physical properties of a foreign body facilitates the choice of method for removal. Soft and wet objects similar to cerumen can be suctioned or flushed from the canal. Firm or hard foreign bodies require specific instruments for extraction. Round objects may get wedged at the bony isthmus or the cartilaginous-bony junction. Small foreign bodies may shift to the medial canal and get caught in the anteroinferior sulcus between the tympanic membrane and the bony canal.

Another classification system categorizes the foreign bodies into two groups: objects with smooth surfaces and not easily grasped (nongraspable) and objects with irregularly shaped surfaces and easily grasped. In a study of pediatric patients treated in emergency departments for foreign bodies in the ear canal, it was noted that beads were the most common objects. When the foreign bodies were group by nongraspable and graspable, the success rate for removal of a graspable object was 64% with a 14% complication rate. In contrast, successful removal of a nongraspable object occurred in only 45% of cases with a 70% complication rate. It was concluded that skilled emergency department personnel could handle pediatric patients with graspable foreign bodies in the ear canal with low complication rates. Nongraspable foreign objects should be referred to an otolaryngologist early in the course of their management.[3]

A variety of instruments need to be available before extracting a foreign body in the ear canal. Otologic examination of the external auditory meatus (or mastoid cavity) identifies the presence of the foreign object. Its shape and consistency are noted. Small objects can readily be removed with a hand-held otoscope and operating head.

In a series of 698 pediatric patients with foreign bodies in the external auditory canal, Schulze and colleagues proposed indications for referral for otomicroscopy-guided removal. These indications were categorized by the type of foreign body (spherical or sharp-edged shape, disc batteries, and vegetable matter), location of the foreign body (adjacent to the tympanic membrane), time in the ear (>24 hours), patient description (<4 years of age with difficulty visualizing the foreign object, agitation, or both), and a history of previous attempts at removal.[4]

Objects with an unusual shape that are wedged in the ear canal often require maximal lighting and more dexterous manipulation. An operating microscope provides the necessary light and the means for bimanual removal. Some of the instruments that should be available include various-sized ear specula; a water irrigation kit; small, medium, and large suction devices; ring and wire loop curettes; right-angled hooks; and picks. If necessary, the use of progressively larger specula facilitates exposure and dilatation of the canal. Injectable local anesthetics such as lidocaine with epinephrine should be available when manipulation and extraction are potentially painful.

It is important to determine whether the foreign object has penetrated the tympanic membrane or middle ear. Patients with acute hearing loss and dizziness should be suspected of injury transmitted to the inner ear. If available, an audiogram should be obtained to determine the nature and degree of the hearing loss. Exploration of the ear under intravenous sedation or general anesthesia should be considered for patients in whom damage to the ossicular chain or inner ear is suspected. General anesthesia will probably be necessary for most children and anxious, uncooperative adults.

SURGICAL TECHNIQUES

Removal of Insects

Flying or crawling insects that enter the external canal typically need to be removed urgently. Live insects can cause pain and ongoing irritation because of their movement and potential trauma to the tympanic membrane. The noise and disturbing sensation created by live insects drive patients to seek urgent medical attention. The ear canal and tympanic membrane are inspected to identify the species of insect and the trauma it may have caused. The presence of loose appendages such as wings or legs should be noted. The patient is placed supine with the involved ear facing up. The ear canal is filled with one of the previously mentioned solutions (ether, isopropyl alcohol, mineral oil, tetracaine, or lidocaine). This may incur a flurry of activity as the insect drowns. Should the patient have severe pain, the skin of the external canal can be infiltrated with local anesthetic. The insect is extracted from the canal with suction, which also removes the excess solution. Ideally, the insect is removed with the suction tip as well. It may be necessary to remove the insect with alligator forceps. Once the insect is removed, the canal is carefully inspected for residual body parts, which are carefully removed with forceps or a fine, cotton-tipped applicator. The integrity of the ear canal skin and tympanic membrane is verified.

Removal of Vegetable Material

Foreign bodies such as peas, beans, nuts, and corn have the potential to swell as a result of oil secretions from the canal, water from swimming or showering, or attempts at flushing the ear. If the object is relatively dry and intact, extraction with suctioning may simply remove the material. It may be necessary to place a small, right-angled hook behind the object to manipulate it into the lateral canal. Flushing these objects out is not recommended to avoid swelling, maceration, and disruption of the integrity of the object. However, if the object is soft, crumbling, and friable and cannot be extracted with suction, irrigation may be necessary. Warm tap water typically suffices for such irrigation. Mixing hydrogen peroxide with an equal volume of water mechanically facilitates aural flushing. An irrigating system such as that shown in Figure 108-1 is most effective. Other systems would include a large-gauge angiocatheter attached to a syringe. Large metal ear syringes are also available for this purpose. Care is taken to avoid directing excessive pressure at the tympanic membrane.

Management of foreign bodies in children is particularly challenging. One must assess the nature of the foreign body and the anticipated degree of technical difficulty that will be necessary to extract it. If the object is relatively intact and can be removed with suction or just a few passes of a right-angled instrument, effort should be made to extract it without general anesthesia, which may require that the child be restrained by the parents or an assistant or be wrapped in a sheet like a papoose. If the foreign body is impacted, it is usually necessary to take the child to the operating room and, under masked general anesthesia, extract the object.

Objects that are wedged in the ear canal medial to the cartilaginous-bony junction pose a significant challenge. By using sequentially larger ear specula, attempts are made to dilate the lateral external auditory meatus to facilitate extraction. A large-gauge suction placed on the object may remove it from the canal. Care must be taken to avoid further impaction and medialization with this technique (Fig. 108-2). If this method is unsuccessful, a right-angled hook (Fig. 108-3) is passed beyond the object and withdrawn laterally. Passing the instrument in the anterior inferior canal should be avoided because of the thin skin and sensitivity of the canal. The superior and posterior quadrants have thicker skin that is more readily compressed. If manipulation of the ear is uncomfortable, a local anesthetic can be injected into the canal skin. A small volume should be used to minimize further edema from the injected solution. After adequate anesthesia has been achieved, extraction can proceed in a more relaxed setting.

A novel idea for removing an object that is difficult to extract is to attach an anchor to the foreign body. Isaacson described applying a quick-setting epoxy adhesive to a foreign body that is spherical in shape with a smooth surface and impacted medially in the canal. This was done in a two-step procedure by applying the first layer of glue to the foreign body in the clinic 1 to 2 days in advance. After 10 minutes, a second layer was applied to a small metal anchor (a no. 8 machine screw with a fashioned concave surface), which was then attached to the foreign object. The child was taken to

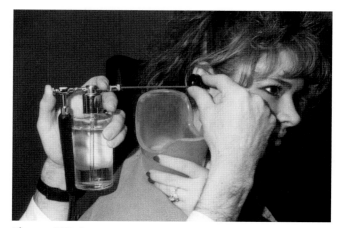

Figure 108-1. A DeVilbiss irrigating system (syringe and bottle DV177) connected to a positive pressure air source is used to flush soft material from the external auditory canal.

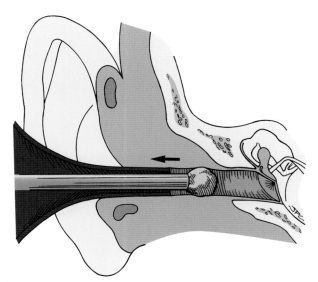

Figure 108-2. A large-gauge suction is usually successful in removing most objects from the external auditory canal. Care must be taken to not push the foreign body more medially.

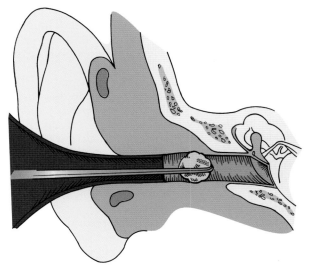

Figure 108-3. A right-angled hook is passed beyond the object, which is then extracted laterally.

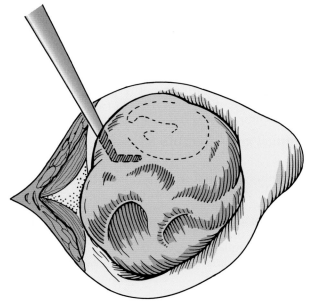

Figure 108-4. An incision is made in the incisura (12-o'clock position) of the external auditory meatus to widen the meatus and permit an instrument to be passed medial to the foreign body.

the operating room 2 days later, at which time a firm grasp on the anchor permitted extraction through the ear canal.[5]

On rare occasions, larger objects cannot be extracted despite the techniques previously described. This usually occurs when the foreign body has been wedged medially beyond the cartilaginous meatus. Children and rarely adults may require general anesthesia for more complete foreign body removal. The ear canal and postauricular area are prepared and draped in sterile manner. The largest ear speculum that fits into the external auditory meatus is placed into the meatus. If a hook cannot be advanced beyond the object, it may be necessary to open the incisura with an incision made at the 12-o'clock position down to the bony canal. This permits further dilatation of the external canal and facilitates advancement of an instrument (Fig. 108-4).

Perforation of the tympanic membrane with possible disruption of the ossicular chain may occur as a result of a foreign object placed in the ear. The penetrating object, such as a cotton-tipped applicator, pencil, bobby pin, stick, or knitting needle, is usually long and narrow. It is often removed or readily extracted at the time of injury.

Intravenous sedation or general anesthesia is preferred for patients in whom perforation of the tympanic membrane is suspected. After removal of the foreign body, the tympanic membrane is carefully inspected. Small central perforations or lacerations are repaired with Gelfoam placed in the middle ear medial to the tympanic membrane defect or with a paper patch applied to the lateral surface of the tympanic membrane (see Chapter 113). Patients with significant conductive or sensorineural hearing loss should undergo exploratory tympanotomy for evaluation of the integrity of the ossicular chain and the round and oval windows. Details regarding repair of the ossicular chain and oval

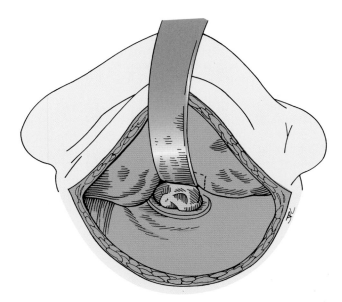

Figure 108-5. The ear has been reflected anteriorly to expose the lodged foreign object medially.

window can be found in Chapters 114 and 117, respectively.

Occasionally, it may be necessary to undertake a postauricular approach. In such cases, a postauricular incision is made down to the posterior wall of the bony external auditory canal, similar to the postauricular approach for exostoses of the external auditory canal (see Chapter 109). A lateral conchal flap is incised through the ear canal. A postauricular incision is made and connected with the conchal flap, and tracheostomy tape and a self-retaining retractor are positioned to reflect the auricle anteriorly for postauricular exposure of the meatus lateral to the foreign body (Fig. 108-5). A right-angled hook can be passed anterosuperiorly beyond the object and extracted laterally. If excessive trauma and laceration of canal skin are anticipated with extraction of the object, a flap of canal skin pedicled inferiorly is raised. The foreign body is removed, and the canal skin and auricle are returned to their original positions. The ear canal should be stented to immobilize any skin flaps and avoid stenosis. Care is taken to avoid trapping of epithelium by unrolling folded edges and reapproximating skin flaps to the best fit. Methods for packing the ear canal include the use of Gelfoam, a Merocel ear pack, or a rosebud packing made of silk strips and cotton balls (see Chapter 113).

POSTOPERATIVE MANAGEMENT

Patients having foreign bodies extracted from the ear canal who incur minimal trauma and have no associated inflammation require no further treatment. Should maceration or cellulitis preexist or laceration and inflammation occur during extraction, topical eardrops are advised. Ototopical antibiotics, usually containing steroids, are instilled twice daily, depending on the severity of inflammation. The patient is instructed to avoid further water contamination by keeping the ear free of swimming pool or shower water. Vaseline applied to a cotton ball is usually effective in keeping the ear canal dry.

If significant cellulitis has developed or the patient is diabetic, the use of systemic antibiotics may be necessary. *Staphylococcus aureus* and *Pseudomonas aeruginosa* are the organisms most likely to be involved. Oral ciprofloxacin should be effective in treating external canal cellulitis.

Patients who require external canal stenting or packing are also treated with topical antibiotic drops. The Gelfoam, canal pack, or rosebud pack serves as a wick for delivering the topical drops. Wicks meant to be placed for a short time, such as a Pope otowick, are generally removed after 3 days unless there is severe inflammation or laceration of the canal skin. The wick then remains for 1 week. The patient removes the wick and continues applying topical drops. Patients in whom a Merocel ear pack or rosebud pack is placed are seen in approximately 1 week. The packing is removed and the canal inspected. Topical drops are continued for a few more days. The patient continues to keep the ear free of water exposure for a few weeks, at which time examination of the ear canal is performed to confirm complete healing.

PEARLS

- Aural irrigation to remove foreign bodies (other than insects) in the external auditory canal should be avoided because the object is rarely flushed out and skin maceration often results.
- Live insects can be drowned with alcohol, mineral oil, or topical anesthetics (Pontocaine, Xylocaine).
- A large nasal suction (9F) device may make sufficient contact with the object to remove it from the canal.
- Passing a right-angled hook parallel to the object and then beyond it allows optimal placement of instruments for extraction.
- Injection of a local anesthetic followed by canal dilatation with progressively larger specula may facilitate removal of the foreign body.

PITFALLS

- Instrumental removal of a live insect without drowning it can intensify the pain and stimulation experienced by the patient.
- Instrumentation directed medially along the posterior ear canal may contact and traumatize the tympanic membrane.
- Aggressive manipulation may result in more medial impaction and possible injury to the tympanic membrane and ossicular chain.
- Failure to recognize and properly reapproximate lacerated canal skin may lead to trapped epithelium and the development of canal cholesteatoma.
- Repeated unsuccessful attempts at foreign body removal will result in canal trauma, further obstruction, and an uncooperative patient.

References

1. Capo JM, Lucente FE: Alkaline battery foreign bodies of the ear and nose. Arch Otolaryngol Head Neck Surg 112:562-563, 1986.
2. Bressler K, Shelton C: Ear foreign-body removal: A review of 98 consecutive cases. Laryngoscope 103:367-370, 1993.
3. DiMuzio J Jr, Deschler DG: Emergency department management of foreign bodies of the external ear canal in children. Otol Neurotol 23:473-475, 2002.
4. Schulze SL, Kerschner J, Beste D: Pediatric external auditory canal foreign bodies: A review of 698 cases. Otolaryngol Head Neck Surg 127:73-78, 2002.
5. Isaacson G: Two-stage removal of an impacted foreign body with an epoxied anchor. Ann Otol Rhinol Laryngol 112:777-779, 2003.

Chapter **109**

External Canal Osteomas and Exostoses

Barry E. Hirsch

The contour of the cartilaginous and bony external auditory canal is S shaped. Direct inspection of the tympanic membrane may be obscured by a prominent anterior canal wall forming an acute angle with the tympanic membrane. Normal aural hygiene is facilitated by epithelial migration from the tympanic membrane to the external auditory meatus. Irregular bony overgrowth may impede this process and predispose the ear to epithelial entrapment and recurrent otitis externa.

Exostoses of the external auditory canal represent hyperplasia of the periosteum and underlying bone. When exostoses are present, they are typically seen in men, and a history of cold-water swimming can frequently be obtained. Examination of 307 surfers at a California surfing competition revealed a 73.5% prevalence of exostoses.[1] In a recent study of 202 avid surfers on the east coast of the United States, the prevalence and degree of canal obstruction were assessed. Their surfing habits (location/water temperature) and duration of practicing the sport were recorded, along with the patency of their ear canals. Most of the surfers (84%) were categorized as warm-water surfers (>60° F). There was a 38% overall prevalence of external canal exostoses, with 69% graded as mild and 31% as moderate to severe. Those participating in the sport for a longer time and exposed to cold water had a much greater incidence of exostoses. In addition, surfers with moderate to severe obstruction were significantly more willing to surf in cold water than those who had mild exostoses.[2]

Occasionally, patients will deny any water exposure yet will still manifest these bony overgrowths. Exostoses are usually multiple in number and have a smooth contour. They are broad-based, convex, epithelium-covered nodules located in the medial aspect of the external auditory canal (Fig. 109-1). These lesions are typically found bilaterally. Dense lamellae of bone are evident histologically.[3]

Osteomas are benign bony lesions of unknown origin that have an outer cortex of bone with inner cancellous trabeculations. Osteomas are singular, pedunculated, unilateral lesions generally located at the tympanomastoid or tympanosquamous suture lines. Osteomas may vary in size from a few millimeters to larger than 2 cm (Fig. 109-2).[4]

Exostoses are relatively common and are seen in 6.36 of every 1000 patients treated by ear, nose, and throat departments, in contrast to the rare incidence of osteomas. Osteomas are to be considered true bone tumors, and exostoses are believed to be reactions to irritation from cold-water immersion or chronic otitis externa. However, in a histopathologic review by Fenton and coworkers, many of the features of trabeculated bone, such as lamellar deposition of bone and fibrovascular channels, were seen in specimens clinically diagnosed as osteoma and exostoses.[5]

Osteomas and exostoses are usually asymptomatic. They are often identified by an internist or family practitioner, who subsequently requests otologic consultation. Significant canal obstruction or chronic skin changes initiate recurrent ear symptoms. Osteomas or exostoses that significantly encroach on the canal lumen may impede migration of desquamated epithelium, thereby predisposing the patient to recurrent episodes of otitis externa. Both lesions, when extensive, may produce hearing loss by either occlusion of the canal or impacted epithelial debris inhibiting vibration of the tympanic membrane. Exostoses usually encroach on the external auditory canal in an anteroposterior direction. Superiorly based lesions located near the pars flaccida may grow inferiorly and restrict movement of the malleus. It is estimated that approximately 80% of the ear canal needs to be obstructed to cause symptoms of recurrent otitis externa and conductive hearing loss. Occlusion less than this degree rarely necessitates operative intervention.[6]

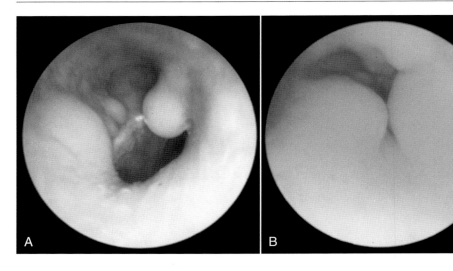

Figure 109-1. A, View of the right external auditory canal revealing multiple broad-based exostoses located medially near the tympanic membrane. **B,** Left external auditory canal with multiple obstructing exostoses obscuring the tympanic membrane.

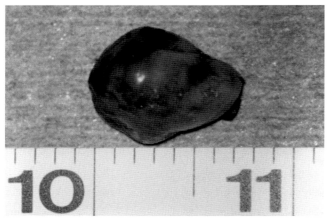

Figure 109-2. Excised osteoma of the external auditory canal with its narrow pedicle located on the right side of the bony tumor.

Recurrent otitis externa occurs when epithelial debris is trapped between the tympanic membrane and osteoma and becomes macerated and colonized with bacteria. Débridement of the external auditory canal and the use of topical otic preparations are necessary for each acute infectious episode. These recurrent infections frequently result in chronic dermatitis and further canal obstruction.

PATIENT SELECTION

Surgical intervention is not usually necessary when exostoses or osteomas are identified. Periodic cleaning of cerumen and epithelial debris medial to the lesions may be necessary. The prophylactic use of eardrops is recommended for patients who are continually exposed to water. Swimming without ear protection may have to be curtailed if it is the predisposing event for recurrent infections. Surgical intervention is indicated when patients experience chronic or recurrent otitis externa

or when reaccumulation of epithelial debris and cerumen impaction cause conductive hearing loss.

Surgical treatment of external auditory canal exostoses may be associated with complications and the need for revision surgery. Initial symptoms include hearing loss, recurrent otitis externa, and cerumen impaction. In a series of 136 patients undergoing surgery for exostoses, it was found that 21% had no symptoms and were advised to have surgery based on their clinical examination. The author of this review emphasized that surgery should be reserved for patients with ear symptoms because, even in experienced hands, surgery is associated with a potential risk for complications.[7]

Patients with a perforated tympanic membrane or conductive hearing loss from ossicular chain problems, in addition to exostoses, may have to undergo a staged procedure. The obstruction of the external auditory canal and recurrent infection may need to be addressed initially, and after subsequent healing, the second procedure may be performed.

PREOPERATIVE PLANNING

Patients undergoing surgery for recurrent otitis externa should have optimal preoperative medical care, including cleaning of the external auditory canal and minimizing inflammation with topical otic preparations. An audiogram is necessary to determine the presence and degree of conductive or sensorineural hearing loss. If symptoms are present bilaterally, surgical intervention is directed at the more involved ear. In the event of significant bilateral disease, the procedure should be staged to ensure unilateral healing and avoid the handicap of bilateral ear packing.

On occasion, lesions may totally obstruct the ear canal and thus prohibit examination of the tympanic membrane. In this situation, computed tomography is necessary to define the origin and extent of the bony lesions, particularly with osteomas located laterally in the canal (Fig. 109-3). Coronal and axial bone window images assist the surgeon in identifying the lesion and the appropriate approach (Fig. 109-4). The radiologic characteristics differentiating osteomas from exostoses have been described. An osteoma arises from the tympanosquamous or tympanomastoid suture line, and its density is slightly lower than that of normal bone, which suggests that it consists of mainly cancellous bone.[8] An isolated osteoma, as demonstrated, may easily be removed with the patient under local anesthesia. Obstructive exostoses that require drilling are performed with the patient under general anesthesia. Removal of multiple large irregular exostoses may result in trauma to the canal epithelium. If the canal skin is not suitable for replacement or is inadequate at the time of surgery, it may be necessary to harvest a split-thickness skin graft (Thiersch graft). Along with informed consent for the canal procedure, patients should be told of the possible need for a skin graft.

SURGICAL TECHNIQUE

The pedunculated attachment of osteomas to suture lines in the external auditory canal can be removed through a transmeatal approach. A four-quadrant block consisting of an anesthetic solution of 2% lidocaine (Xylocaine) with 1:100,000 epinephrine is injected into the external auditory meatus. After adequate local anesthesia has been achieved, a middle ear curette or right-angled hook is passed beyond the osteoma. If exposure is inadequate for visualization or instrumentation, the soft tissue at the incisura at the 12-o'clock position may be compressed or incised to permit passage of an instrument beyond the osteoma (Fig. 109-5). An overlying skin flap can be incised and preserved if the osteoma is attached by a broad base (Fig. 109-6A and B). If the osteoma is on a narrow pedicle, the osteoma can usually be fractured with a curette and removed. Occasionally, it may be necessary to use a small osteotome or drill to weaken the base. Once the osteoma is removed, the bony base is further drilled to the level of the bony external canal. A small strip of silk or a piece of Gelfoam impregnated with antibiotic ointment is used as a topical dressing (see Fig. 109-6C).

Exostoses are generally multiple and broad based. Greater surgical exposure routinely requires a postauricular approach, usually performed with the patient under general anesthesia. The postauricular hair is shaved and the ear is prepared and draped in the usual sterile fashion. A solution of 2% lidocaine with 1:100,000 epinephrine is injected in a four-quadrant block into the external auditory meatus and the postauricular crease. The exposure and approach are similar to those used for postauricular tympanoplasty techniques (see Chapter 113). Endaural incisions in the 12- and 6-o'clock positions are made in the lateral meatus and

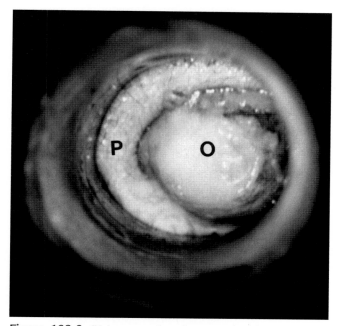

Figure 109-3. Right external auditory canal with a posteriorly based osteoma (O) obstructing complete examination of the medial canal and tympanic membrane. P, posterior.

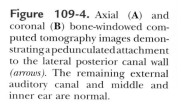

Figure 109-4. Axial (**A**) and coronal (**B**) bone-windowed computed tomography images demonstrating a pedunculated attachment to the lateral posterior canal wall (*arrows*). The remaining external auditory canal and middle and inner ear are normal.

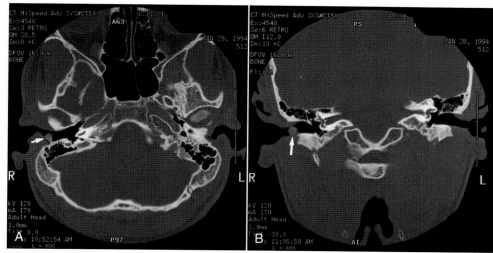

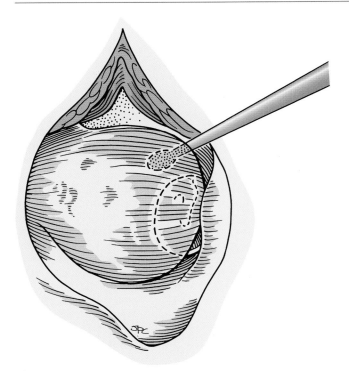

Figure 109-5. An incision made in the incisura widens the aperture to the external auditory meatus. A curette is positioned medial to the osteoma in preparation for removal. The tympanic membrane is ghosted in.

connected vertically to create a conchal flap. The medial extent of the skin flap extends approximately 3 to 4 mm beyond the hair-bearing canal (Fig. 109-7). A postauricular incision is made, the conchal flap is elevated from the lateral posterior canal wall, and the two incisions are connected. A tracheostomy tape is used to reflect the conchal flap with the external auditory meatus anteriorly (Fig. 109-8). A self-retaining retractor holds the auricle and posterior conchal skin flap anteriorly to provide direct exposure to the more medial canal.

Skin flaps based medially are carefully dissected from the anterior and posterior canal walls. A medium-sized cutting burr is used to remove the bony exostoses while leaving a thin shell of bone attached to the canal skin. Dissection is performed in a lateral-to-medial direction toward the tympanic membrane. The suction tip is used to protect the canal skin flap from the shaft and burr of the drill. If space permits, thin Silastic sheeting or a section of foil from a suture pack is positioned to provide additional protection to the canal wall skin (Fig. 109-9). As the bony overgrowth is removed, direct examination of the tympanic membrane becomes feasible. Once exposure is gained, the flap is returned to its newly contoured canal and the opposite wall is treated in a similar fashion. A thick, crescent-shaped section of bone often remains at the medial aspect of the dissection. Care is taken to further elevate the medially based skin flap distal to this shelf of bone as it approaches the tympanic membrane. The remainder of

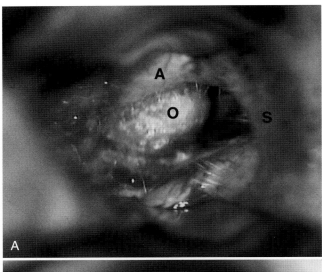

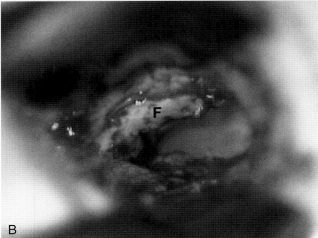

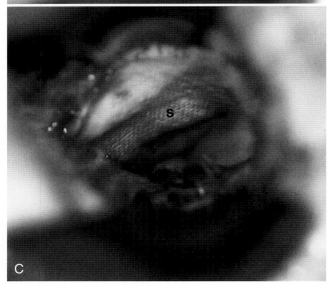

Figure 109-6. A, Broad-based osteoma (O) of the left ear located on the anterior external auditory canal wall. A, anterior; S, superior. **B,** A skin flap (F) based medially was created and returned to cover the exposed bone. **C,** A strip of silk (S) is positioned on the anterior canal wall to secure the skin flap.

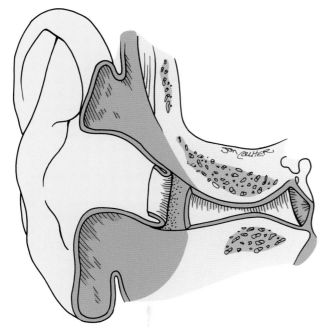

Figure 109-7. Through the external auditory meatus, a conchal flap is incised and back-elevated. Note the narrowed bony canal medially.

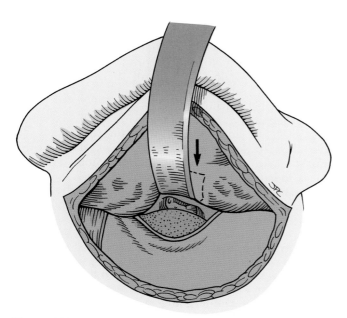

Figure 109-8. A postauricular incision has been made and a tracheostomy tape is placed to evert the conchal flap within the canal (*arrow*). A self-retaining retractor (not shown) provides the necessary exposure.

the bone is removed to create a smoothly contoured canal. More aggressive bone removal can be undertaken anteriorly. Because such bone removal encroaches on the posterior aspect of the temporomandibular joint, care must be taken to avoid trauma to the periosteum surrounding the joint capsule. Medium and small diamond burrs are used to further smooth the walls of

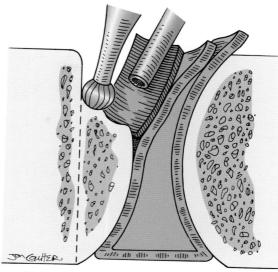

Figure 109-9. Beginning laterally, the posterior canal wall skin is elevated and protected with a sheet of suture pack foil or Silastic. The suction tip is used to retract the skin and maintain a clean surgical field. The bony exostosis is drilled to contour the canal.

the bony canal. Care is taken to avoid drilling into the tympanic membrane, the bony lateral process of the malleus, and the tympanic annulus. Aggressive drilling of the posterior canal wall can lead to injury to the mastoid air cells and should be avoided.

It may be difficult to leave the anterior or posterior skin pedicled medially. Should additional bone work be necessary in an area obstructed by the skin flap, rather than tearing it with the drill burr or shaft, the skin can be removed in a large rectangular section to provide the exposure needed. The skin can subsequently be replaced when the bony canalplasty is completed.

Once drilling is completed, the skin is repositioned, although it is not necessary to completely cover all areas of denuded bone. If the skin flaps have been preserved, they are adequate for epithelial coverage. However, large areas of exposed bone should be grafted to facilitate more rapid and uncomplicated healing. Freehand split-thickness skin sections (Thiersch grafts) measuring approximately 1.0 by 1.5 cm are harvested with a no. 10 blade from the postauricular skin overlying the mastoid (Fig. 109-10). The feathered edges of the skin graft are trimmed sharply. The grafts are placed over areas of raw bone while avoiding overlapping the edges of the surrounding skin. It is necessary to secure the skin flaps (and grafts) by packing the medial and lateral canal. If the original canal skin was pedicled and preserved, the canal can be packed with a single Merocel stent (Fig. 109-11). When the original skin or graft is replaced in sections, firm reapproximation and immobilization are achieved with rosebud packing, which consists of multiple strips of silk placed in the ear canal. Cotton or Merocel balls impregnated with antibiotic ointment are placed in the depth of the packing and brought out to the level of the midcanal. The ear is returned to its anatomic position, the conchal flap is

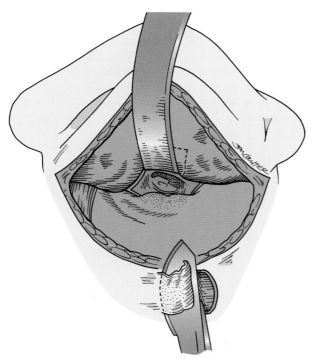

Figure 109-10. Excessive loss of canal skin should be replaced. A freehand split-thickness Thiersch graft is harvested from the postauricular skin overlying the mastoid.

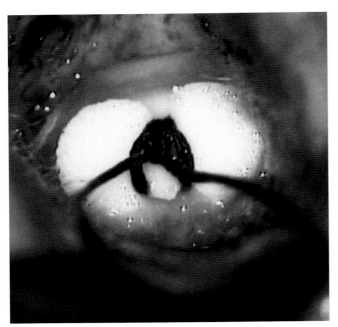

Figure 109-11. A Merocel ear pack secures the canal wall skin flaps.

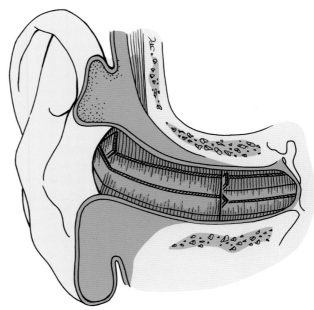

Figure 109-12. Double-rosebud packing is used to secure skin that was replaced in sections.

The routine method for removing these bony lesions is to use a high-speed otologic drill. Some surgeons advocate the use of a mallet and a thin 1- to 3-mm chisel or osteotome. It has been proposed that the bony mass can be serially shaved with these instruments. This technique may also minimize noise and vibration trauma from the drill.[6,9]

Rather than completely removing all the exostoses from both the anterior and posterior canal walls, an alternative strategy is to address only exostoses of the anterior wall of the external auditory canal. This still places the temporomandibular joint at risk but minimizes complications related to disruption of the ossicular chain and injury to the chorda tympani and facial nerve.[10]

POSTOPERATIVE MANAGEMENT

Systemic antibiotics are not administered unless there is concern for ongoing low-grade chronic infection and cellulitis. Patients undergoing a postauricular approach have the mastoid dressing removed the following morning. Oral narcotic analgesics are prescribed when necessary. The cotton ball in the conchal meatus may need to be changed frequently in the first few postoperative days, depending on the amount of serosanguineous drainage. Antibiotic-steroid eardrops are administered twice daily. After 7 to 10 days, patients are seen for follow-up. Sutures and the lateral rosebud packing are removed from those who have undergone postauricular canalplasty. Antibiotic-steroid eardrops are continued twice a day, and the patient is seen the following week, at which time the medial rosebud packing is removed.

repositioned, and a second rosebud packing is placed (Fig. 109-12) (see Chapter 113). The postauricular wound is closed with 5-0 fast-absorbing suture and Steri-Strips. A cotton ball is placed in the external meatus, and a Glasscock or sterile mastoid dressing is applied.

The donor site for the split-thickness skin graft is treated with topical antibiotic ointment twice a day. Patients are asked to wash their hair in a sink to avoid potential water contamination or maceration.

Patients who have isolated lesions (osteomas) removed by the endomeatal approach are seen 10 days postoperatively, at which time the silk sleeve or Gelfoam packing is removed. Flat de-epithelialized areas are allowed to heal further by secondary intention. Topical eardrops are continued for a few weeks until complete healing has occurred.

Despite attempts to meticulously approximate epithelial flaps within the external auditory canal, there may be areas of exposed bone medially and de-epithelialized subcutaneous tissue laterally. Careful cleaning and débridement of the ear are performed when the second packing is removed. Areas of hypertrophied granulation tissue are cauterized with silver nitrate, and antibiotic-steroid drops are continued. Frequent, diligent, and meticulous care should be given to canal hygiene to avoid postoperative stenosis. Should encroachment of the canal lumen develop, a stent consisting of multiple Pope otowicks or strips of Merocel microporous sponge is placed in the canal and remains for an additional week. The canal is reevaluated and appropriate local care is given. Patients demonstrating irregular epithelization and midcanal stenosis or medial canal soft tissue blunting may need to be returned to the operating room. In this situation, hypertrophied soft tissue is débrided and a single firm stent consisting of long rosebud silk packing is inserted. Topical eardrops are administered, and the stent is removed in 10 days. Silver nitrate is usually effective for control of excessive granulation tissue. 5-Fluorouracil cream may also be applied if silver nitrate alone is unsuccessful.

The first few postoperative weeks are critical to the healing process. It may be necessary to see patients weekly to monitor and control wound healing. Despite the appearance of appropriate epithelialization, patients are restricted from water exposure for at least 2 months. A cotton ball with Vaseline is used while showering. Swimming is prohibited until complete healing has taken place.

COMPLICATIONS

Patients undergoing removal of exostoses usually have a history of chronic otitis externa. They are prone to wound-healing problems and thus require close observation. Exuberant granulation tissue may heal with a midcanal stenosis or medial blunting at the level of the tympanic membrane.

The structures surrounding the external auditory canal are subject to potential injury during the operative procedure. Aggressive drilling of bony lesions on the posterior wall may result in injury to the mastoid air cell system. Migration of epithelium into these cells would potentially lead to fistulization or cholesteatoma formation. Similarly, drilling the anterior canal wall may lead to entry into the capsule of the temporomandibular joint. Small areas of bony dehiscence are tolerated if the periosteum is not violated. However, large areas of bone removal lead to prolapse of the soft tissues of the temporomandibular joint into the external auditory canal. This not only retards wound healing in the immediate postoperative period but may also produce subsequent aural hygiene problems. Clicking or other auditory sounds may occur with mandibular movement.

Structures potentially at risk when drilling the canal medially are the chorda tympani nerve, the tympanic membrane, and the malleus. The chorda tympani may be drilled in the area just medial to the posterior annulus. The tympanic membrane may be torn by the drill or other instruments used during dissection of the canal skin. The lateral process of the malleus may also be hit by the drill and result in conductive or sensorineural hearing loss.

Inadequate bone removal may give rise to persistent symptoms. This typically occurs at the interface of the tympanic membrane and the anteromedial canal wall. An acutely angled anterior sulcus may continue to trap epithelial debris and promote the persistence of symptoms.

When the skin of both the anterior and posterior canals is violated, postoperative canal stenosis can occur. Caution is needed during the procedure, and heightened awareness is necessary during the immediate postoperative period to avoid and recognize this problem. Débridement of exuberant granulation tissue and repacking of the canal should be undertaken once this process is recognized.

Patients experiencing persistent inflammation or chronic otitis externa should be suspected of having allergic dermatitis secondary to topical otic drops. Preparations containing aminoglycosides should be discontinued in favor of other topical agents. Steroid cream preparations may be necessary if an allergic reaction develops.

Facial nerve injury is a devastating complication after surgery for exostoses. The facial nerve is relatively close to the posteroinferior annulus. A facial nerve with an aberrant course that is lateral and more anterior to its normal position may potentially be damaged and result in inadvertent facial paresis. The surgeon should anticipate this problem while drilling the bony posteroinferior canal. Facial nerve monitoring during the procedure should help minimize the likelihood of this untoward event.

PEARLS

- Surgical intervention is not usually necessary when exostoses and osteomas are asymptomatic.
- Computed tomography scans of the temporal bone should be obtained when the ear canal and tympanic membrane cannot be examined.
- A single osteoma located laterally in the ear canal and attached by a narrow pedicle can be removed with a curette under local anesthesia.

- Caution is needed when drilling the posterior and inferior bony canal walls because of the proximity of the facial nerve.
- Facial nerve monitoring is advisable during surgical removal of exostoses.

PITFALLS

- Surgical intervention in patients with limited symptoms may result in greater problems postoperatively than before surgery.
- Aggressive drilling of the posterior inferior external auditory canal may result in injury to the facial nerve.
- Contact between the surgical drill and the ossicular chain may cause sensorineural hearing loss.
- External canal stenosis can occur when excessive skin is sacrificed or traumatized.
- Failure to recognize and intervene when significant narrowing of the canal is seen in the early postoperative period will result in inflammatory stenosis and conductive hearing loss.

References

1. Wong BJ, Cervantes W, Doyle KJ, et al: Prevalence of external auditory canal exostoses in surfers. Arch Otolaryngol Head Neck Surg 125:969-972, 1999.
2. Kroon DF, Lawson ML, Derkay CS, et al: Surfer's ear: External auditory exostoses are more prevalent in cold water surfers. Otolaryngol Head Neck Surg 126:499-504, 2002.
3. Nager GT, Hyams VJ: Pathology of the Ear and Temporal Bone. Baltimore, Williams & Wilkins, 1993, p 1341.
4. Senturia BH, Marcus MD, Lucente FE: Diseases of the External Ear: An Otologic-Dermatologic Manual, 2nd ed. New York, Grune & Stratton. 1980, p 204.
5. Fenton JE, Turner J, Fagan PA: A histopathologic review of temporal bone exostoses and osteomata. Laryngoscope 106:624-628, 1996.
6. Whitaker SR, Cordier A, Kosjakov S, Charbonneau R: Treatment of external auditory canal exostoses. Laryngoscope 108:195-199, 1998.
7. Vasama JP: Surgery for external auditory canal exostoses: A report of 182 operations. ORL J Otorhinolaryngol Relat Spec 65:189-192, 2003.
8. Hsiao SH, Liu TC: Osteoma of the external ear canal. Otol Neurotol 24:960, 2003.
9. Hetzler D, Longridge NS: Exocytosis of the external auditory canal. Otol Neurotol 24:523, author reply 523, 2003.
10. Longridge NS: Exostosis of the external auditory canal: A technical note. Otol Neurotol 23:260-261, 2002.

Chapter 110

Keratosis Obturans and Canal Cholesteatoma

Yael Raz

Keratosis obturans and canal cholesteatoma were initially attributed to the same pathologic process, and the two terms were used interchangeably.[1] Both conditions are associated with disruption in the normal outward migration of external auditory canal epithelium, a process critical for extrusion of desquamated skin.[2] Piepergerdes and colleagues are credited with defining these two entities as unique processes requiring distinct management algorithms.[3] Nevertheless, partial overlap between these two conditions has led to continued debate in the recent literature over appropriate nomenclature.[4,5]

In keratosis obturans, the defect in lateral epithelial migration is circumferential and results in the formation of a laminar keratin plug that can frequently be removed intact as a cast of the external canal (Figs. 110-1 and 110-2). The keratin plug may extend medially to the tympanic membrane. Conductive hearing loss is common secondary to an occlusive effect. The condition is typically bilateral and may be accompanied by otalgia. Widening of the external auditory canal can occur as a result of circumferential bony resorption, presumably secondary to constant pressure induced by the keratin plug. The canal epithelium typically remains intact and can become thickened or inflamed. Early reports suggested an association with bronchiectasis and sinusitis, particularly in children.[6,7] Otorrhea is rare.

Canal cholesteatoma, in contrast, appears most commonly as a keratin "pearl," usually situated on the floor of the external canal (Fig. 110-3). Canal cholesteatomas are generally unilateral and characterized by ulceration of the canal skin and focal bony erosion (Fig. 110-4). Hearing is not usually affected because the canal is not completely occluded and the middle ear is spared.

After removal of the cholesteatomatous matrix, the bony canal is exposed and often eroded. Epithelium surrounding the bony defect will generally show sharply demarcated edges, although bleeding and granulation tissue are occasionally present. Whereas the appearance of keratosis obturans is difficult to confuse with other entities, the same cannot be said for canal cholesteatoma. Suspicion of carcinoma must be entertained and biopsy of the margins of the crater in the canal should be performed routinely. Bone exposure within the external auditory canal and the presence of granulation tissue may also be confused with acute necrotizing otitis (malignant external otitis). However, the latter condition is accompanied by significant pain and a greatly elevated erythrocyte sedimentation rate and is almost universally seen in diabetic patients. Furthermore, identification of *Pseudomonas* in culture would be expected in acute necrotizing disease, whereas normal canal flora is generally cultured from canal cholesteatoma.

The chief distinction between keratosis obturans and canal cholesteatoma lies in circumferential widening of the bony canal in the former as opposed to focal bony erosion in the latter and visual determination of whether the canal epithelium remains intact or whether bone has become exposed. As yet, there is no clear understanding of the cause of the abnormalities in epithelial migration that characterize keratosis obturans and canal cholesteatoma. However, recent work on factors involved in the regulation of cell-cell adhesion and epithelial proliferation has begun to shed light on the molecular processes that may be involved.[8,9] Although this discussion is limited to idiopathic canal cholesteatomas, entrapment of squamous epithelium may occur in the setting of congenital or acquired canal atresia or after temporal bone trauma or surgery.

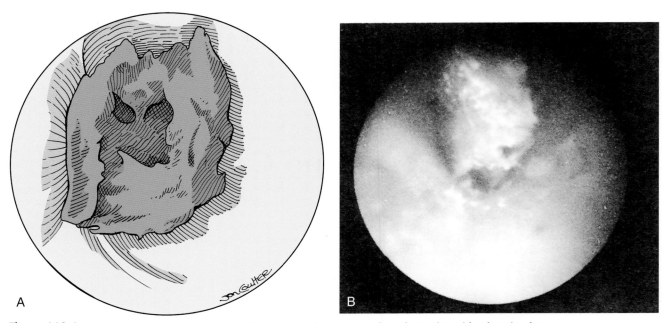

Figure 110-1. **A** and **B,** Views of the external auditory meatus showing complete obstruction with a keratin plug.

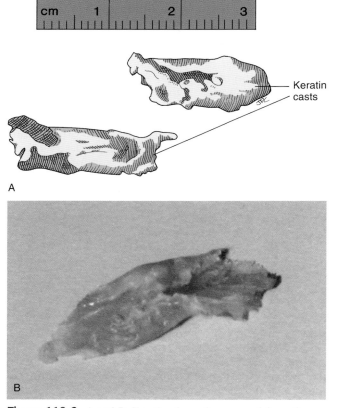

Keratin casts

Figure 110-2. **A** and **B,** Keratin plugs after removal from the ear canals.

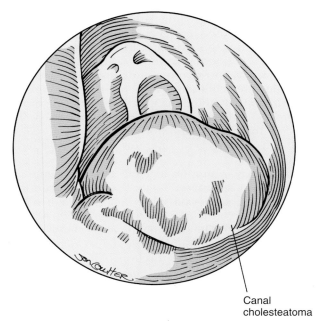

Canal cholesteatoma

Figure 110-3. Otoscopic view of a canal cholesteatoma forming in the inferior canal wall.

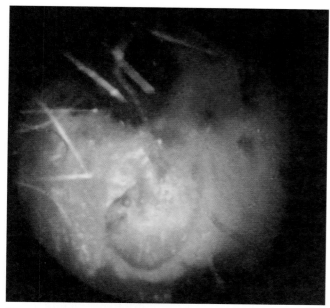

Figure 110-4. Otoscopic view of exposed and eroded bone after removal of a cholesteatoma matrix.

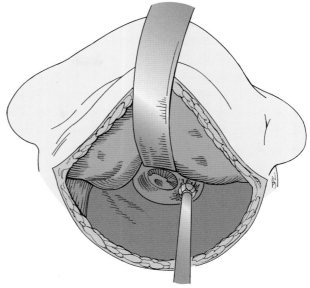

Figure 110-5. Postauricular approach for resculpting and grafting of a canal wall defect.

PATIENT SELECTION

Canalplasty has been described on rare occasions for intractable keratosis obturans[10]; however, conservative management suffices in most cases. Emollients and lubricants will aid in the removal of keratotic plugs, but no drugs have been found to successfully eliminate the problem. Steroid and exfoliative agents have been tried with limited success, but simple lubrication of the keratin plug before removal remains the most effective treatment. Over time, each patient will determine the correct interval necessary for serial canal cleaning to prevent hearing loss, obstruction, and secondary infection.

Small canal cholesteatomas can also be managed conservatively, provided that the patient is free of otalgia and the entire extent of the affected area can be visualized and accessed for cleaning. Even extensive canal erosion with bone exposure can be managed conservatively in elderly patients for long periods without resorting to surgical intervention. Significant otalgia is rare and permits consideration of surgery in patients with the following criteria: (1) those living at a great distance or who have difficulty traveling regularly for cleaning of the ear; (2) individuals with repeated bleeding from ulcerated skin margins and those in whom repeated secondary canal infections develop; (3) patients who electively wish a more permanent alternative to repeated cleaning of the ear canal; and (4) large lesions with involvement of the middle ear, facial canal, or mastoid air cells. Reassurance, as well as biopsy in cases of canal erosion, will suffice in the great majority of cases to satisfy patients that ongoing conservative treatment is the method of choice.

PREOPERATIVE EVALUATION

In large canal cholesteatomas, preoperative imaging with temporal bone computed tomography can be helpful in determining the extent of involvement of mastoid air cells or the facial nerve canal and assist in deciding whether facial nerve monitoring will be necessary.

SURGICAL APPROACHES

Local anesthesia is the method of choice in patients who elect to undergo surgery. The purpose of surgery is to remove infected or unhealthy skin, eliminate devitalized bone, smooth the contours of the bony canal, and finally, reline the denuded area of the canal.

A postauricular approach provides the best exposure of the affected canal. The postauricular incision is combined with a short conchal flap extending to the level of the defect in the canal. The auricle is then reflected anteriorly in the standard tympanoplasty-mastoidectomy fashion (Fig. 110-5). After exposing the area of canal erosion, unhealthy tissue is débrided from the epithelial border, and the skin adjacent to the defect is reflected medially for optimal exposure. Appropriately sized cutting and diamond burrs are then used to removed devitalized bone and smooth the contours of the canal defect. Bone is removed until healthy bleeding osseous tissue is encountered (Fig. 110-6). Lesions of the posteroinferior canal may extend into the mastoid air cells. When the cells are of sufficient size, they should be obliterated with fat or fascia before applying the skin graft. At this point, the area of denuded bone is determined. If minimal coverage is required, the bony canal can be lined with temporalis fascia. Extensive areas of bone exposure can be resurfaced with a split-thickness skin graft approximately

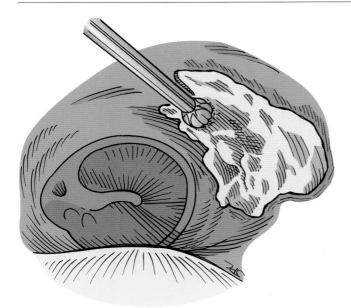

Figure 110-6. Use of cutting and diamond burrs to remove sequestrum and expose fresh, viable bone.

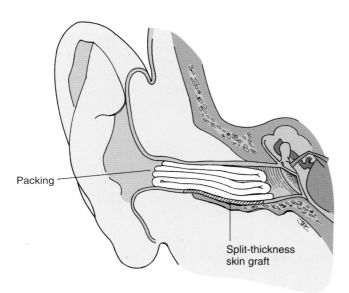

Packing

Split-thickness
skin graft

Figure 110-7. Packing is placed in the canal to stabilize the split-thickness skin graft.

0.012-inch thick. The authors prefer the upper inner aspect of the arm as a donor site, but other convenient areas may be used as well. It is seldom necessary to take more than about 1 square inch of skin for repair of canal defects of this type. Previously elevated skin flaps in the canal are replaced, and the conchal flap is returned to its original position. After the skin graft is placed over the defect, a strip of silk or rayon mesh is laid over the graft to protect and prevent movement of it. Finally, continuous packing soaked in antibiotic ointment is gently layered into the canal (Fig. 110-7). The postauricular incision is then closed and dressed in the usual manner.

Larger canal cholesteatomas involving significant exposure of the mastoid air cells may require reconstruction of the canal wall (i.e., with hydroxyapatite) or a modified radical mastoidectomy. Facial nerve monitoring should be considered for these lesions because the cholesteatoma can erode into the facial canal.

POSTOPERATIVE MANAGEMENT

The packing is removed in 10 to 14 days, and simple débridement of the skin edges is carried out until healing is complete. It is rare for canal cholesteatomas to recur, but desquamation from the skin graft site may continue for a period of several months. During this time, the application of mineral oil in small amounts will prevent desquamated epithelium from accumulating. Healing is usually complete within 6 to 10 weeks.

COMPLICATIONS

Complications include facial nerve injury, recurrence of cholesteatoma, injury to the tympanic membrane or malleus, and persistent exposed bone. The facial nerve is particularly at risk when drilling in the medial, postero-inferior aspect of the canal and caution is required in this region. If the mastoid air cell system is entered, skin may grow through the defect resulting in a fistula or recurrent cholesteatoma. This can be prevented by using fat, fascia or cartilage to obliterate the exposed cells. If the pathology is located medially, the tympanic membrane or malleus may be injured during drilling of the bony canal. The surgeon must be mindful of the deep aspect of the rotating burr and downsize appropriately to avoid iatrogenic hearing loss or a perforation. Assuring the removal of all devitalized bone, as well as careful positioning of an adequately sized graft, can help prevent incomplete epithelialization.

PEARLS

- It is important to remove all devitalized bone because failure to do so will lead to loss of the overlying skin graft. Bleeding must be seen from all newly freshened bone surfaces to ensure an adequate nutritional bed for the graft.
- Histologic examination of skin edges must be performed to rule out malignancy.
- Desquamation from the skin graft may continue for several months postoperatively and requires frequent débridement until healing is complete.

PITFALLS

- Extensive drilling of the posteroinferior canal wall may expose the vertical portion of the facial nerve, and thus caution must be exercised in this region.
- Otorrhea or recurrence of canal cholesteatoma may result if the mastoid air cells are not obliterated with fat or fascia before skin grafting.

- Preoperative consent for harvesting of a split-thickness skin graft should be obtained lest the operating room staff be caught unprepared in the event that an extensive area of bony exposure is encountered.

References

1. Paparella M, Shumrick D: Otolaryngology, vol 2. Philadelphia, WB Saunders, 1973, p 37.
2. Naiberg J, Berger G, Hawke M: The pathologic features of keratosis obturans and cholesteatoma of the external auditory canal. Arch Otolaryngol 110:690-693, 1984.
3. Piepergerdes MC, Kramer BM, Behnke EE: Keratosis obturans and external auditory canal cholesteatoma. Laryngoscope 90:383-391, 1980.
4. Persaud RA, Hajioff D, Thevasagayam MS, et al: Keratosis obturans and external ear canal cholesteatoma: How and why we should distinguish between these conditions. Clin Otolaryngol 29:577-581, 2004.
5. Kuczkowski J, Mikaszewski B, Narozny W: Immunohistochemical and histopathological features of keratosis obturans and cholesteatoma of the external auditory canal. Atypical keratosis obturans. J Laryngol Otol 118:249-250, author reply 250-251, 2004.
6. Black JIM, Clayton RG: Wax keratosis in children's ears. BMJ 2:673-675, 1958.
7. Morrison AW: Keratosis obturans. J Laryngol Otol 70:317-321, 1956.
8. Naim R, Riedel F, Bran G, Hormann K: Expression of beta-catenin in external auditory canal cholesteatoma (EACC). Biofactors 19:189-195, 2003.
9. Adamczyk M, Sudhoff H, Jahnke K: Immunohistochemical investigations on external auditory canal cholesteatomas. Otol Neurotol 24:705-708, 2003.
10. Paparella MM, Goycoolea MV: Canalplasty for chronic intractable external otitis and keratosis obturans. Otolaryngol Head Neck Surg 89:440-443, 1981.

Chapter 111

Congenital and Acquired Atresia of the External Auditory Canal

Elizabeth H. Toh and Barry E. Hirsch

Atresia of the external auditory canal may be congenital or acquired (Figs. 111-1 and 111-2). Congenital atresia is much more common, with a reported incidence of 1 in 10,000 to 20,000 births, and is often associated with deformities of the auricle and middle ear. Congenital atresia results from developmental abnormalities in the first and second branchial arches during the first trimester of fetal life. Although the vast majority of these defects are sporadic, 10% occur as part of a syndromic abnormality. Acquired atresia of the external auditory canal is unusual and may occur secondary to trauma, chronic inflammation, radiation therapy, or iatrogenic injury after surgery. Other terminology used to describe this acquired condition includes postinflammatory acquired atresia of the external auditory canal, postinflammatory medial canal fibrosis, and chronic stenosing external otitis.[1-3]

Congenital atresia occurs more commonly in males than females and is most often unilateral, with the right ear affected more often than the left. The atresia is more frequently bony than membranous. Associated anomalies of the inner ear occur in less than 20% of patients, so most atresia cases are amenable to surgical correction. The pinna is rarely completely normal or totally absent (anotia). At minimum, there are usually cartilaginous or soft tissue remnants from faulty embryologic development. Mild deformity or microtia is common (Fig. 111-3). In general, the appearance of the external ear correlates well with development of the middle ear.[4]

Because of anomalous development of the first and second branchial arches, anatomic anomalies of the facial nerve are generally present. Middle ear abnormalities such as fixation of the malleus, fusion of the malleus-incus complex, fixation of the stapes footplate, anomalous position of the chorda tympani, and a per-sistent stapedial artery have also been described. Inner ear dysplasia may involve the cochlea, the vestibule, the semicircular canals, and the internal auditory canal.

Congenital atresia of the external auditory canal has been seen in association with hydrocephalus, posterior cranial hypoplasia, hemifacial microsomia, cleft palate, and genitourinary anomalies. Syndromes in which congenital atresia has been described include Treacher Collins, Goldenhar, trisomy 22, Klippel-Feil, cleidocranial dysplasia, Fanconi, Crouzon's, DiGeorge, and thalidomide toxicity.

PATIENT SELECTION

Congenital Atresia

The goals of reconstruction of atresia of the ear include provision of functional hearing and creation of a dry and patent external auditory canal. In 1992, Jahrsdoerfer and associates devised a grading scale using preoperative computed tomography (CT) scans to evaluate a child's candidacy for correction of atresia.[5] These authors assigned one point for each of eight factors detected on CT imaging (Table 111-1), plus two points if the stapes was normal. A perfect score of 10 yields an excellent prognosis for hearing improvement to within a 15 to 20 dB speech reception threshold, and the converse would hold true for a diminishing number of normal structures identified on CT imaging. The prognosis for hearing improvement is expressed as a percentage relative to the assigned CT score. A zero added to each score indicates the percent chance of achieving closure within 15 to 20 dB. Surgery is not usually recommended when the score is 5 or less. When applying the results of this evaluation, surgeons must also consider their own experience, as well as other potential prob-

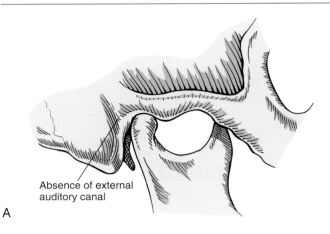

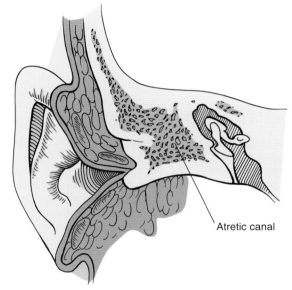

Figure 111-1. Lateral (**A**) and coronal (**B**) views of the temporal bone in a patient with congenital aural atresia.

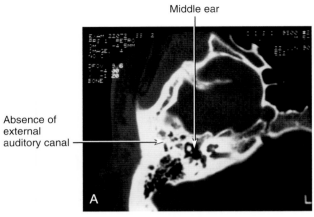

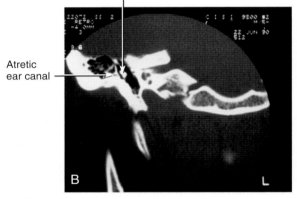

Figure 111-2. Computed tomography scans of aural atresia in the axial (**A**) and coronal (**B**) planes.

Table 111-1	GRADING SYSTEM TO DETERMINE CANDIDACY FOR SURGICAL CORRECTION OF CONGENITAL AURAL ATRESIA	
Parameter		**Points**
Stapes present		2
Oval window open		1
Middle ear space		1
Facial nerve		1
Malleus-incus complex		1
Mastoid pneumatized		1
Incus-stapes connection		1
Round window		1
Appearance of the external ear		1
Total available points		10

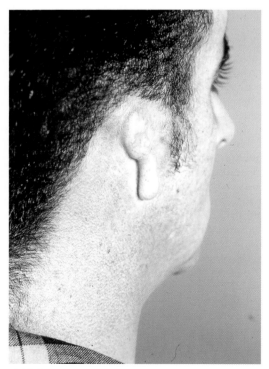

Figure 111-3. Typical appearance of microtia associated with aural atresia.

lems with the child's general health and otologic status.

In the great majority of patients with congenital atresia, reconstruction of the pinna must also be planned and timed appropriately along with the atresia repair. Surgical reconstruction of the pinna should be completed or at least initiated before atresia repair to take advantage of the uncompromised blood supply in the temporal area. Reconstruction of the pinna is a complex and often multistage procedure that may be performed with rib cartilage or synthetic material. The use of rib and rib cartilage for reconstruction of the pinna results in an external ear that is more resistant to trauma, infection, and extrusion. However, synthetic Silastic or porous polyethylene material may result in a cosmetically superior pinna. Regardless of the method of reconstruction, the otologist must ensure that the atresia surgery does not jeopardize the circulation of the auricular reconstruction.

Correction of the atresia at or after the age of 5 years allows optimal development of the mastoid process, adequate time for initiating repair of the microtia, and maturity of the child to participate in postoperative care. When corrective surgery for unilateral atresia is delayed past early childhood, cosmetic correction of the microtia can and should be accomplished in the usual manner. A 4- to 6-month interval between microtia and atresia repair is generally recommended. The presence of cholesteatoma in the atretic canal may be identified by bone erosion on preoperative CT and may dictate the need for earlier surgery.

Acquired Atresia

The most common form of acquired canal atresia involves soft tissue obliteration of the external auditory canal only. The intervening segment between the patent canal laterally and the tympanic membrane usually consists of fibrous tissue. Chronic otitis externa and chronic suppurative otitis media are the most common inciting causes. Acquired atresia may develop after severe trauma to the temporal bone with fracture of the anterior or posterior canal walls. Inflammation, such as severe seborrheic dermatitis and other dermatologic conditions, may result in severe scarring and obliteration of the soft tissues of the external canal over time. Acquired atresia may also occur after burns and may represent the mid-canal or medial canal type of fibrosis after tympanomastoid surgery. The final common pathway in the development of an atretic canal is an exuberant fibroproliferative inflammatory response, which typically occurs over the course of years.

In the early inflammatory phase of the disease, conservative medical management with aggressive aural toilet and the application of steroid-containing ototopical antibiotics plays some role in controlling any underlying infection and minimizing the development of granulation tissue. Once mature fibrosis of the canal has developed, the ear is generally dry and hearing loss remains the only functional concern. Because the goal of surgery is hearing improvement when the acquired atresia is unilateral, as is usually the case, the option for amplification should be offered to the patient. Dermatologic disease processes must be made quiescent before surgical repair is attempted. Active seborrheic dermatitis with scaling and exudation does not provide a good environment for surgical repair and reconstruction. When thickened skin obstructs the external meatus and there is no evidence of further active disease after the formation of pachyderma, reconstruction is a plausible approach for hearing improvement. Aural rehabilitation with a bone-anchored hearing aid (BAHA) may be offered to select patients who do not elect to undergo atresia repair and are unable to use a conventional hearing aid in the affected ear because of auditory feedback or fitting problems. Candidates for BAHA use must have an underlying cochlear reserve of at least 40 dB in the better-hearing ear.

PREOPERATIVE EVALUATION

Congenital Atresia

When first evaluating a child with congenital atresia of the external auditory canal, the physician must obtain a comprehensive history and perform a physical examination to determine whether the atresia is an isolated finding or part of a syndromic or hereditary problem. When the latter appears to be the case, genetic counseling may be indicated for future family planning.

The educational needs and philosophy of atresia repair must be considered. Because the great majority of affected children have unilateral atresia, it must be determined whether hearing is normal in the opposite ear. Sensorineural hearing loss is occasionally identified in the nonatretic ear and must be investigated further. When hearing in the nonatretic ear is normal, the option for conservative management should be weighed against the risks associated with surgery. Speech and language acquisition can be ensured in these children, even if surgery is delayed until they reach their teens or if a decision is made to not proceed with surgery. The presence of atresia at birth will almost certainly ensure that audiometric testing is performed early in childhood. In very young children, auditory brain stem response (ABR) measurements can easily approximate auditory threshold levels. By the age of 4 or 5 years, behavioral audiometric testing can be performed. Reliable responses typically demonstrate maximal conductive hearing loss with normal cochlear reserve. It used to be recommended that surgery for unilateral atresia be postponed until a child had reached the age of self determination. With advances in CT, intraoperative facial nerve monitoring, and greater surgical experience, these guidelines are less rigid. Elective surgery is now performed on unilateral atresia when the parents have been carefully counseled and strongly desire it.

A child with bilateral atresia will undergo the same audiologic evaluation as previously described but requires careful and expert evaluation with bone conduction ABR testing. In these cases, the "near-field" effect of the generator site ensures a larger wave I on the ipsilateral side. Immediate amplification with bone conduction hearing aids is well accepted by small children and will ensure normal speech acquisition and language development until the child is old enough for surgery. It is generally agreed that children with bilateral atresia should undergo surgical repair in one ear by the age of 5 years for the reasons indicated earlier. The higher-graded ear is generally operated on first.

Evaluation of a patient with aural atresia must include high-resolution, thin-cut CT in both the axial and coronal planes. Newer spiral CT machines offer the ability to generate high-quality reconstructed coronal images from the axial sequences obtained, thus reducing the overall dose of radiation delivered. These views permit thorough evaluation of the degree of mastoid and middle ear pneumatization, inner ear morphology, facial nerve anatomy, and ossicular abnormalities. Inner ear dysplasia, such as Mondini's malformation or a large vestibular aqueduct, increases the risk for sensorineural hearing impairment with surgery, which must be discussed with the parents. Review of the CT scans will also inform the surgeon of the presence of canal cholesteatoma, as suggested by an expansile soft tissue density with adjacent bony erosion.

A word is necessary regarding BAHAs in the treatment of congenital atresia. They are not generally advised if repair of microtia is being considered because the surgery necessary for their implantation jeopardizes the blood supply necessary for cosmetic reconstruction of the pinna. In addition, children with favorable results on the CT rating scale have an excellent chance of achieving reasonable hearing. Even when children attain speech reception thresholds that are slightly worse than normal, they will benefit from using in-canal hearing aids once atresia surgery has been performed. BAHAs remain a rehabilitative recommendation for children in whom imaging suggests a poor prognosis for successful hearing improvement and in those who elect to not undergo surgery. The recommended lower age limit for implantation of a BAHA device is currently 5 years.

Acquired Atresia

Because the primary goal of surgery for acquired atresia is improvement in hearing, preoperative audiologic testing will help confirm the nature and extent of loss in the affected ear. The fibrous plug alone will often result in a 25- to 30-dB conductive hearing loss. The patient should be counseled that any additional underlying sensorineural hearing loss would probably necessitate the use of a conventional hearing aid in the operated ear once the ear canal has healed.

Preoperative high-resolution CT imaging of the temporal bone in the axial and coronal planes is helpful in differentiating bony from soft tissue atresia, detecting the presence of underlying cholesteatoma, and assessing the status of the middle ear and ossicular chain.

SURGICAL APPROACHES

Congenital Atresia

Surgical correction should not be attempted before the pinna has been reconstructed and correctly placed in relation to the anticipated location of the external canal. This can easily be determined by palpating the mastoid tip and temporomandibular joint to ensure that the proposed meatus will be properly located just behind the condyle of the mandible. The preoperative CT scan is reviewed again and particular attention is paid to the intratemporal course of the facial nerve, level of the tegmen, and depth of the middle ear cavity from the surface of the skull. Intraoperative facial nerve monitoring should be performed in all cases.

A standard postauricular C-shaped incision is made after infiltration with a solution of 1% lidocaine with 1:100,000 epinephrine. Every attempt is made to preserve all circulation to the auricle originating from the anterior, inferior, and superior aspects (Fig. 111-4), which may occasionally require placement of the incision further posteriorly than would ordinarily be done for routine mastoid surgery. The mastoid periosteum is incised and the soft tissue overlying the mastoid is then elevated anteriorly until the glenoid fossa is well identified (Fig. 111-5). A temporalis fascial graft is harvested, thinned, and dried for construction of a new tympanic membrane. The external canal should be created just behind the glenoid fossa and just inferior to the temporal line (Fig. 111-6). The temporal bone sometimes has a small depression or cribriform area that marks the location of the undeveloped external auditory canal. In other cases, a soft tissue plug is present that may be followed directly into the atretic plate or the tympanic membrane. When external canal landmarks are absent, drilling should begin as close to the glenoid fossa and

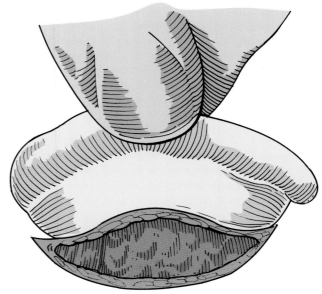

Figure 111-4. Postauricular incision with an attempt to maintain the blood supply to the pinna.

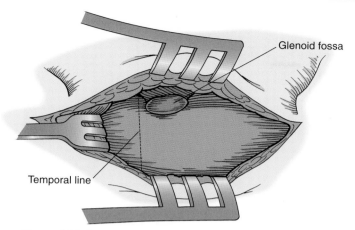

Figure 111-5. Identification of the glenoid fossa (right ear).

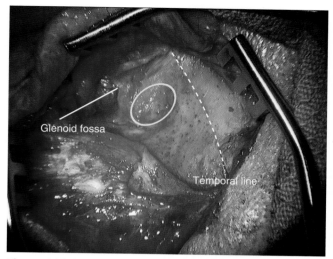

Figure 111-6. Creation of an external meatus just inferior to the tegmen and just posterior to the glenoid fossa (left ear).

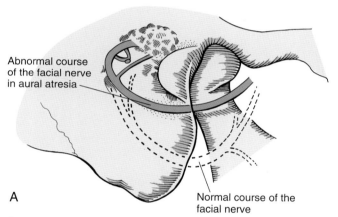

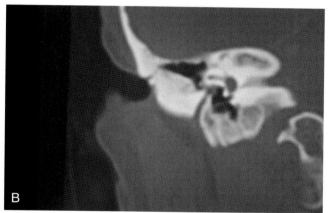

Figure 111-7. A, Normal course of the facial nerve and the course usually seen in atresia. **B,** Coronal computed tomography scan showing anterior displacement of the mastoid segment of the facial nerve.

middle fossa dural plate as possible. In doing so, bone must be preserved between the glenoid fossa and what is to become the anterior canal wall. By following the middle fossa dural plate medially, the atretic plate will generally be encountered at a depth of approximately 1.5 cm. Unlike routine mastoid surgery, drilling should be confined to a relatively small circumference to avoid the creation of a mastoid cavity. Mastoid air cells may be encountered, but they should be minimally exposed if the drilling is confined to the location of the atretic canal. The diameter of the external auditory canal that is being created should be only 1.5 times larger than normal (about 1.3 cm in diameter).

Although intraoperative monitoring helps the surgeon minimize trauma to the facial nerve, the general location of this structure should be carefully reviewed on the CT scan preoperatively. In the great majority of cases, the horizontal portion and the second genu of the facial nerve will be in relatively normal posi-

tions. The most common anomaly is an anterior and sometimes lateral deviation of the vertical trunk of the facial nerve (Fig. 111-7), which occurs in up to 25% of cases. The nerve may traverse the promontory, round window, or hypotympanum, or it may be inferior to the tympanic annulus, if present. In this situation the surgeon will generally encounter the atretic plate without exposing the nerve, assuming that drilling has been confined to the area described earlier. When soft tissue is initially encountered, drilling should be performed with diamond burrs from that point on. The atretic plate is then thinned until the bone is paper-thin and can be gently lifted away from the fibrous remnants of the tympanic membrane and ossicular chain with angled picks or elevators (Fig. 111-8). Trauma to the ossicular chain must be avoided during drilling to prevent sensorineural hearing loss. The most common ossicular abnormality is a fused malleus-incus complex. Incudostapedial connection by means of a fibrous

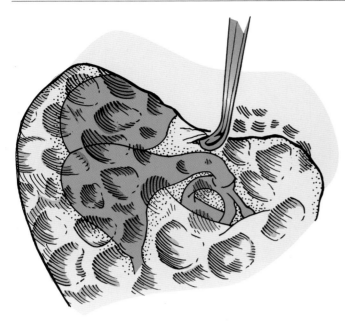

Figure 111-8. Curetting away the remnants of the bony atresia plate overlying the lateral ossicular chain.

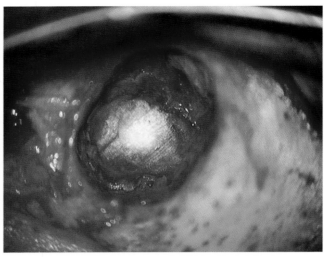

Figure 111-9. The fascial graft is placed over the ossicular mass and placed into the bony annulus and canal.

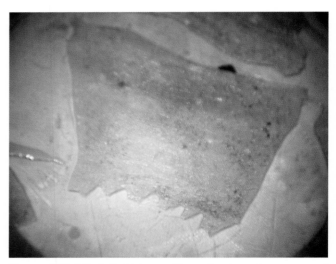

Figure 111-10. Split-thickness skin graft trimmed to measured dimensions and contoured along its medial border to allow placement over the fascial graft.

strand or stapedial arch discontinuity is sometimes found. Footplate fixation occasionally occurs as well. When necessary, ossiculoplasty is performed as it would be during tympanoplasty with bony or cartilaginous autografts or various PORPs (partial ossicular replacement prostheses) and TORPs (total ossicular replacement prostheses). Separation of the incudomalleal complex is generally unnecessary because it is usually mobile. Occasionally, the malleus neck is fixed to the atretic plate by means of a bony spur, in which case it must be separated and mobilized. In rare cases, the ossicular chain may be fixed at more than one location, and complete mobilization of the chain is necessary to ensure optimal postoperative hearing results. The use of an argon laser for lysis of soft tissue adhesions and bony attachments during this portion of the procedure will help minimize the risk of sensorineural hearing loss from excessive manipulation of the ossicular chain.[6]

After ossiculoplasty, a 1.5-mm diamond burr is used to create a bony annulus and sulcus on which to place the fascial graft used for creating the new tympanic membrane. Anteriorly, this minimizes blunting of the anterior meatal angle. Thorough irrigation of the newly created ear canal and middle ear space is critical at this point to prevent postoperative bony refixation of the ossicular chain. If a PORP or TORP has been used for ossiculoplasty, irrigation should be performed before placement of the prosthesis. The fascial graft is then centered over the ossicular mass to optimize hearing results (Fig. 111-9). The fascia is extended for 1 to 2 mm onto the newly developed bony annulus, and when possible, a small extension of the fascial graft may be placed into the hypotympanum or protympanum to prevent lateralization of the new tympanic membrane. Any air cells uncovered in the process of drilling the new canal are obliterated with connective tissue plugs to prevent iatrogenic cholesteatoma resulting from ingrowth of skin into the mastoid cavity.

A split-thickness skin graft 0.008- to 0.010-inch thick and approximately 2 × 3 inches in dimension is harvested from one of several donor sites, including the medial surface of the upper part of the arm, the superior lateral quadrant of the buttocks, or lower part of the abdomen. A thinner graft is less likely to curl at the edges and will reduce the rate of postoperative canal stenosis. The circumference of the tympanic membrane, the length of the canal, and the circumference of the external meatus are measured with a length of suture material. The skin graft is then cut to the appropriate size with these measurements (Fig. 111-10). The external meatus must be created by excising conchal skin and any underlying rib graft or prosthesis when

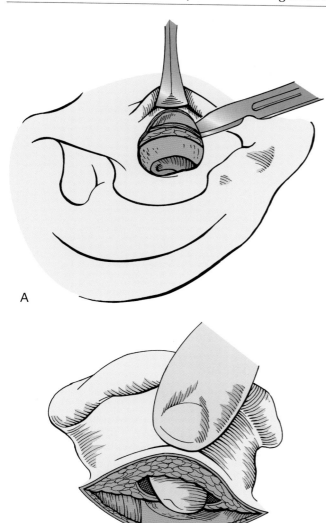

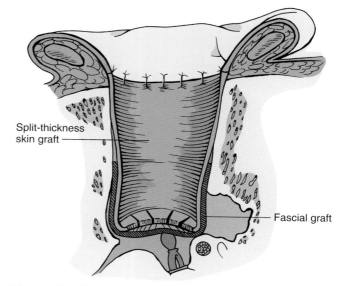

Figure 111-12. The split-thickness skin graft is placed with its medial border overlapping the fascial graft by 1 mm.

Figure 111-11. A, Creation of the meatus in the pinna. **B,** Ensuring adequate diameter of the meatus to make allowance for shrinkage.

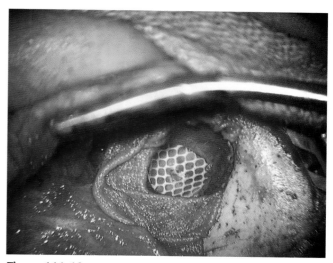

Figure 111-13. A reinforced Silastic disc is placed over the fascial graft after the split-thickness skin graft has been placed.

they are present in this area. The meatal opening should overlie the newly created canal and should admit the surgeon's thumb to compensate for postoperative contracture (Fig. 111-11).

The previously measured skin graft is then placed epithelial side down onto a Silastic sheeting template that is 0.04 inch thick. Bacitracin ointment is spread onto the Silastic sheeting to enhance adherence of the skin graft. The Silastic template is cut to the same size as the overlying skin. The Silastic is curled and placed in the canal, where it then unfurls and holds the graft against the canal wall. The medial edges of the skin graft are extended 1 mm over the fascial graft (Fig. 111-12). An additional disc of Silastic marginally smaller than the diameter of the newly created canal may be placed against the tympanic membrane to discourage blunting of the new tympanic membrane (Fig. 111-13). The lateral edges of the skin graft are sutured to the meatus with 4-0 chromic suture (Fig. 111-14). Packing is then

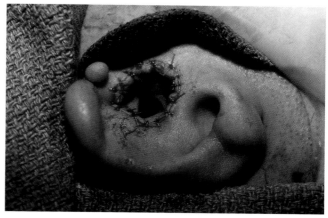

Figure 111-14. The lateral border of the split-thickness skin graft is sutured to the external meatus.

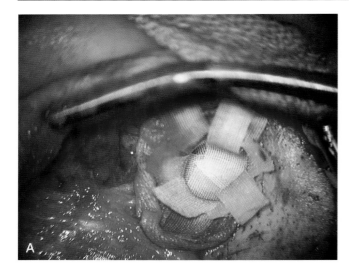

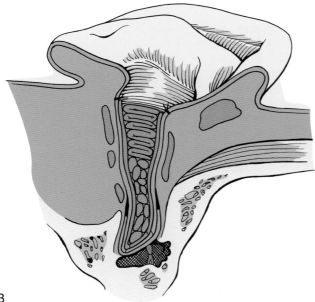

Figure 111-15. **A,** Silk strips are layered in the ear canal. **B,** Packing is placed within the silk lining to maintain the skin graft in place.

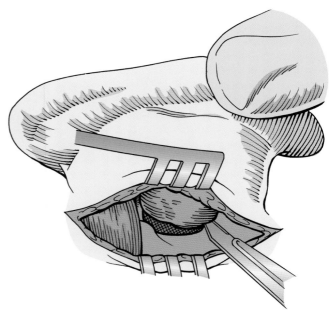

Figure 111-16. Postauricular approach for acquired atresia.

Acquired Atresia

Most of these patients will have soft tissue atresia as a result of previous surgery or a chronic inflammatory process. The goals of surgery are to remove the fibrous plug, expose the tympanic membrane, and re-epithelialize the ear canal with normal healthy skin. Preoperative CT scanning will confirm the presence of any bony atresia. If drilling will be necessary for bony atresia, intraoperative facial nerve monitoring should be performed. A postauricular approach is generally recommended for wide surgical access. Repair via endaural approaches has been uniformly unsuccessful.[7]

After infiltrating the postauricular region and ear canal with a solution of 1% lidocaine with 1:100,000 epinephrine, a circumferential canal incision is initially made at the junction of the normal medial conchal skin margin and the lateral aspect of the canal stenosis/atresia. A standard postauricular incision is then made down to the level of the temporalis fascia superiorly and the mastoid periosteum inferiorly. The mastoid periosteum is incised in along the linea temporalis and then down to the mastoid tip. Surgical dissection is continued under the periosteum anteriorly to the level of the cartilaginous ear canal. Ear canal skin and soft tissue are then gently elevated off the bony external auditory canal (Fig. 111-16). This dissection proceeds medially until the tympanic membrane is identified (Fig. 111-17). There is usually an identifiable plane between the fibrous external canal plug and the fibrous layer of the tympanic membrane. In cases of bony atresia, a combination of small cutting and diamond drill burrs is used to carefully enlarge the bony canal. Care should be exercised to not expose mastoid air cells posteriorly when doing so. The goal of canalplasty should be to provide a direct unobstructed view of the entire tympanic membrane through the external auditory meatus.

placed in the canal and consists of a single large Merocel wick, which once positioned in the newly created canal is hydrated with an ototopical solution to hold the skin graft in place. Alternatively, silk strips may be layered in the canal and the canal packed with Merocel sponges soaked with an ototopical solution (Fig. 111-15). The postauricular incision is then closed in the usual fashion with 4-0 Vicryl or Dexon, and a soft mastoid dressing is applied.

Some surgeons used to prefer a mastoidectomy technique wherein a "canal wall–down" type of cavity is created to correct congenital atresia. Although this technique may be successful in restoring hearing, it introduces the added problem of a mastoid cavity. We do not advocate this technique.

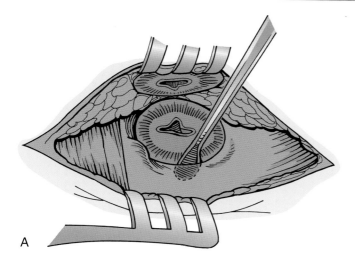

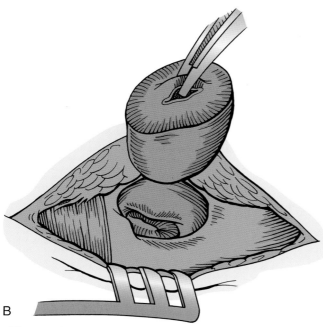

Figure 111-17. **A** and **B,** Elevation and elimination of the canal stenosis.

Once this has been completed satisfactorily, the ear is thoroughly irrigated to remove all bone dust. Middle ear exploration is advised if preoperative audiometric testing indicates a conductive hearing loss greater than the 20 to 30 dB expected for canal atresia alone.

Generally, little skin can be salvaged from the canal in such cases because the soft tissue is composed almost entirely of scar tissue. For this reason, a skin graft is used in the manner previously described for reconstructing a congenital atretic canal. Once again, it is not prudent to remove and replace skin from the external auditory canal that is actively inflamed, such as in chronic external otitis, because the same problem will usually recur. Resolution of acute and chronic inflammation should be ensured before proceeding in this manner.

POSTOPERATIVE MANAGEMENT

Self-absorbing suture material is used for both the skin graft and the postauricular incision. The mastoid dressing is removed 24 hours after surgery and the ear is kept dry. The canal wick is continually hydrated with antibiotic eardrops. Patients are seen 7 days postoperatively to remove Steri-Strips from the postauricular incision and inspect the canal wick. After removal of the canal wick at day 10 to 14, the patient is seen every 2 weeks until the skin graft is completely healed. Desquamation during this period is common, and frequent cleaning of the ear canal may be necessary. Small layers of granulation tissue may also develop in the seams between the edges of the skin graft, but frequent examination allows débridement and cauterization of this tissue before it becomes bothersome or obstructive. The use of steroid-containing ototopicals may be of benefit in this situation. The initial postoperative audiogram is obtained 6 to 8 weeks after surgery, when healing is mostly complete. Thereafter, the patient is seen at 6- to 12-month intervals for routine cleaning of the ear.

Hearing is generally improved immediately postoperatively but may deteriorate over time. The best hearing results have been reported by Jahrsdoerfer and coworkers, with 67% of patients attaining speech reception thresholds of 30 dB or better.[5] These results are similar to those achieved by Tuefert and De La Cruz,[6] although the number of patients who maintained an air-bone gap of 30 dB or less fell from 63.1% to 50% over time. Our experience supports the fact that roughly two thirds of patients achieve these thresholds. The risk for severe sensorineural hearing loss related to atresia surgery is 2% to 7.5%.[5,6]

When hearing improvement does not exceed a 30-dB speech reception threshold, some patients may wish to use an in-canal type of hearing aid once healing within the canal is complete. Typically, only a small amount of amplification is necessary to restore hearing to acceptable levels, which is why the creation of a canal alone has sometimes been helpful.

COMPLICATIONS

Canal restenosis and lateralization of the tympanic membrane are by far the most common complications after atresia surgery. Other complications include blunting of the tympanic membrane, sensorineural hearing loss, and facial nerve injury. For an inexperienced surgeon, the facial nerve is at its greatest risk in the inferoposterior portion of atretic bone just lateral to the middle ear.[8] Facial nerve problems occur much less frequently because intraoperative facial nerve monitoring is now routine.

Stenosis in the midcanal area seems to take place only in unepithelialized areas in which bare bone persists. If early signs of canal stenosis are evident on postoperative follow-up, gentle stenting and dilatation of the canal will usually limit the extent of stenosis. Any areas of granulation within the canal should be aggressively cauterized with silver nitrate and treated with steroid-containing ototopicals.

In the case of midcanal or medial canal stenosis after a previous attempt at tympanoplasty or mastoidectomy, special precautions may be taken to prevent recurrence. A steroid solution may be placed in the packing at the time of surgery and a short course of oral steroids given in the immediate postoperative period. If despite these measures medial fibrosis begins again in the postoperative period, triamcinolone acetonide (Kenalog), 10 mg/mL, is injected with a 27-gauge needle into the medial canal stenotic area. This will usually prevent restenosis.

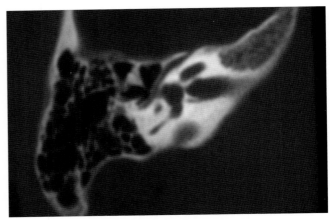

Figure 111-18. Axial computed tomography scan showing the facial nerve coursing over the oval window.

PEARLS

- In the absence of any identifiable ear canal in an atretic ear, drilling should always begin at the level of the linea temporalis, just posterior to the glenoid fossa.
- Lateralization of the tympanic membrane graft in atresia surgery is best prevented by tucking a small flap of fascia anteromedial to the bony annulus or under the malleus handle.
- Blunting in the anterior sulcus is minimized by creating a good bony annulus to seat the fascial graft, minimizing the amount of skin-fascia overlap medially, and tightly packing the anterior sulcus with a Silastic disc over the tympanic membrane.
- Meatal stenosis is prevented by creating a large meatus 1.5 times the normal size and careful suturing of the lateral margins of the skin graft to the newly created meatus to facilitate early healing in this area.
- Patients who are poor surgical candidates for atresia repair may be rehabilitated with a BAHA, provided that their underlying cochlear reserve is 40 dB or less in the better-hearing ear, and microtia repair is not planned in the future.

- The most common causes of sensorineural hearing loss after atresia are drilling on the ossicular chain and overzealous manipulation of the ossicular chain.
- The presence of any active dermatologic condition involving the meatus and canal at the time of atresia repair will compromise healing and result in restenosis of the canal.
- Soft tissue stenosis of the ear canal often results from nonepithelialized bone within the ear canal.

References

1. Becker BC, Tos M: Postinflammatory acquired atresia of the external auditory canal: Treatment and results of surgery over 27 years. Laryngoscope 108:903-907, 1998.
2. Slattery WH, Saadat P: Postinflammatory medial canal fibrosis. Am J Otol 18:294-297, 1997.
3. Birman CS, Fagan PA: Medial canal stenosis—chronic stenosing external otitis. Am J Otol 17:2-6, 1996.
4. Kountakis SE, Helidonis E, Jahrsdoerfer RA: Microtia grade as an indicator of middle ear development in aural atresia. Arch Otolaryngol 121:885-886, 1995.
5. Jahrsdoerfer RA, Yeakley JW, Aguilar EA, et al: Grading system for the selection of patients with congenital aural atresia. Am J Otol 13:6-12, 1992.
6. Teufert KB, De La Cruz A: Advances in congenital aural atresia surgery: Effects on outcome. Otolaryngol Head Neck Surg 131:263-270, 2004.
7. Jacobsen N, Mills R: Management of stenosis and acquired atresia of the external auditory meatus. J Laryngol Otol 120:266-271, 2006.
8. Jahrsdoerfer RA, Lambert PR: Facial nerve injury in congenital aural atresia surgery. Am J Otol 19:283-287, 1998.

PITFALLS

- An aberrant facial nerve that crosses the oval window will increase the risk of trauma to the nerve at the time of ossiculoplasty (Fig. 111-18).
- Failure to mobilize the entire ossicular chain before tympanic membrane grafting will result in residual postoperative conductive hearing loss.

TYMPANIC MEMBRANE, MIDDLE EAR, AND MASTOID

Chapter 112

Otitis Media, Myringotomy, and Tympanostomy Tubes

Barry E. Hirsch

The middle ear is an air-containing space in which the pressure is equalized to that of the outside atmosphere via the eustachian tube. Most of the pathology occurring in the middle ear and mastoid results from eustachian tube dysfunction. Some of the acute and chronic middle ear disorders can be reversed or prevented by temporary or permanent ventilation via myringotomy, with or without a tube.

Return of normal middle ear aeration is most frequently needed in the pediatric population. Children are predisposed to middle ear problems because of eustachian tube dysfunction with subsequent otitis media with effusion and recurrent acute otitis media. Indications for placement of tympanostomy tubes in children remain highly controversial. Some physicians advocate that pediatric patients with otitis media with effusion be managed with prophylactic or multiple courses of antibiotics or simple observation. Such management is controversial because of the threat of delayed language development during these formative years.

Over a decade ago, guidelines were proposed to provide a management algorithm for otitis media with effusion. Until recently, the indications for myringot-omy with or without tube placement for otitis media with effusion were not critically defined. Clinical practice guidelines were developed by a subcommittee of experts from the American Academy of Pediatrics, American Academy of Family Physicians, and American Academy of Otolaryngology–Head and Neck Surgery. They stated that identification of serous otitis media does not require antibiotics or removal of the fluid. Effort needs to be made to distinguish children who are at risk for speech, language, or learning problems and provide appropriate intervention. Those who are not at risk can be observed for 3 months from the date of onset or diagnosis. If hearing loss, language delay, or learning problems are suspected, hearing testing should be conducted. If sequelae are not identified, the children can be re-examined at 3- to 6-month intervals. Once surgery becomes indicated, insertion of a tympanostomy tube is the preferred initial treatment. Adenoidectomy is reserved for patients who require repeat surgery. It was also concluded that antihistamines and decongestants are ineffective for otitis media with effusion. Furthermore, antimicrobials and corticosteroids do not have long-term efficacy and should not be used for routine management.[1]

LASER MYRINGOTOMY

The use of lasers in the practice of medicine has had direct application in otology. Laser myringotomy was proposed as a safe method to ventilate the middle ear. It is not clear whether laser myringotomy is an effective alternative to ventilation tubes. Koopman and associates conducted a randomized trial comparing laser myringotomy with ventilation tubes in children who had otitis media with effusion.[2] The mean time until closure of the laser perforation was 2.4 weeks, as opposed to a mean of 4 months with tubes. The success rate was 40% for the laser and 78% for tubes. We have not found laser myringotomy to be of clinical benefit in the treatment of eustachian tube dysfunction, and we have continued the use of myringotomy knives for opening the middle ear to provide ventilation.

Other clinical situations warrant removing fluid from the middle ear space or providing aeration. Factors that influence such treatment include the age of the patient, the nature of the pathology, the likelihood of persistent eustachian tube dysfunction, and the appearance of the tympanic membrane. Whether myringotomy alone or with tube placement is performed is also dictated by the clinical situation. In this chapter some of the more common indications for middle ear aeration or drainage are reviewed.

VACCINATION

The potential role of enhanced immunologic surveillance against the bacteria associated with otitis media raises the question of whether immunizations would decrease the need for myringotomy and tubes. Prevnar is a pneumococcal heptavalent conjugate vaccine that has been approved for use in children younger than 24 months. The prevalence of resistance to oral antibiotics emphasized the need to seek other methods of preventing acute otitis media. A study by Caspary and colleagues revealed that children vaccinated with Prevnar were two times less likely to have non–*Streptococcus pneumoniae* isolated from the middle ear. Children who were vaccinated were three times as likely to be infected with *Haemophilus influenzae,* but these strains produced β-lactamase less often.[3]

The most common organisms isolated from effusions in the middle ear are *S. pneumoniae* and *Moraxella catarrhalis.* The yield for identification through routine culture techniques is approximately 25%. There is further evidence that otitis media with effusion is associated with persistent bacterial infection in the absence of positive culture.

The development of biofilms is hypothesized to be the reason that otitis media with effusion is recalcitrant to antibiotic treatment. Biofilms are described as a collection of bacteria coated by an extracellular matrix, which may effectively protect the bacteria from penetration by the antibiotic. A recent study investigated whether chronic otitis media is related to biofilms. Biopsy of ear mucosa was performed and fluid aspirated from 26 children undergoing placement of tympanos-

tomy tubes. Using polymerase chain reaction–based diagnostics, at least one otitis media pathogen was positively identified in 24 of 24 effusions. Confocal laser scanning microscope images were obtained from middle ear mucosa biopsy specimens. By using organism-specific probes for the three most common bacteria, mucosal biofilms were visualized on 46 of 50 (92%) of the specimens. This information may change the philosophy on how best to medically manage chronic otitis media.[4]

PATIENT SELECTION

The indications for tympanocentesis, myringotomy, or myringotomy with tube placement are individualized for specific manifestations of eustachian tube dysfunction and middle ear pathology. The choice of procedure and the design of the myringotomy tube are based on the anticipated needs of the patient's middle ear problems. Hearing loss is the primary symptom for which ventilation of the middle ear is needed. Clinical situations can be characterized under the headings of otitis media with effusion (children and adults), acute otitis media, craniofacial abnormalities, barotrauma, otitis media and sepsis, and chronic eustachian tube dysfunction.

Otitis Media with Effusion

Children

Otitis media with effusion is probably the most common and most controversial pathologic condition for which tympanostomy tubes are placed. The immature development of the eustachian tube and the frequency at which children are exposed to pathologic organisms account for the higher incidence of middle ear effusion in this age group.

Parents may notice children pulling at their ear or, if old enough, complaining of ear discomfort. Audiometric and tympanometric screening tests performed in daycare centers and elementary schools have identified young children with hearing impairment and abnormal mobility of the tympanic membrane, respectively. Appropriate referral to a pediatrician or otolaryngologist will determine whether significant tympanic membrane, middle ear, or inner ear disease is present. Examination of the ear frequently reveals a dull, retracted tympanic membrane that is opaque or amber. Pneumatic otoscopy is often the most helpful technique for confirming lack of tympanic membrane mobility. A flat tympanogram also supports the diagnosis. However, we rely primarily on physical examination and rarely find this adjunctive diagnostic test to be necessary. An audiogram is obtained to determine the type and degree of hearing loss (conductive, sensorineural, or mixed).

Otitis media occurs in 40% to 70% of preschool children. However, otitis media with effusion frequently resolves within 3 months with or without the use of systemic antibiotics.[5] There are a few algorithms that are used in the management of otitis media with effusion. An option for medical therapy consists of three courses of antimicrobial therapy given for 10 days at a time, separated by one month. Another method of treatment is long-term, low-dose antibiotic prophylaxis. Children who have bilateral ear disease with significant hearing impairment and in whom medical treatment has failed are candidates for tympanostomy tubes. In a child younger than 6 months, it may be difficult to accurately assess hearing thresholds. Other methods for determining hearing loss include parents' observation of behavioral manifestations of hearing loss, such as sitting close to a television set, requesting higher listening volumes, poor school performance, inattentiveness, or failure to meet milestones for language development. If it is determined that one ear is involved and the contralateral ear is normal and if the hearing loss appears to be minimal, continued observation may be prudent in children younger than 3 years.

Adults

Otitis media with effusion occurs in adults as well as children. Adults with a history of recurrent childhood infections may have borderline eustachian tube dysfunction throughout their adult years. These people may have difficulty achieving middle ear aeration after an airplane flight or, more commonly, after an upper respiratory tract infection. Patients will complain of unilateral or bilateral ear "stuffiness," occasional popping sensations in the ear, and hearing loss. Examination of the ear reveals a retracted tympanic membrane that may be dull or amber. Pneumatic otoscopy, especially when used with the operating microscope, facilitates identification of fluid in the middle ear. Tuning fork testing may confirm a conductive hearing loss. If a patient complains of new-onset hearing loss that appears to be conductive and one is uncertain whether the middle ear contains fluid, diagnostic myringotomy will provide a diagnosis.

Patients with new-onset unilateral or bilateral serous effusions must undergo a complete examination of the head and neck. To provide comprehensive care, one must determine the cause of the effusion. New-onset unilateral or bilateral serous effusion of the middle ear may be a manifestation of eustachian tube dysfunction resulting from pathology in the nasopharynx. Marked adenoid hypertrophy or a neoplasm in the nasopharynx, such as nasopharyngeal carcinoma or lymphoma, can obstruct the eustachian tube orifice and cause serous effusion. Tumors of the infratemporal fossa and petrous apex may compress the eustachian tube. Fluid in the middle ear may also result from sinonasal allergic rhinitis. In particular, attention is directed to the nasopharynx. If examination with a mirror is inadequate, flexible fiberoptic or rigid nasopharyngoscopy is necessary.

If examination of the tympanic membrane reveals air bubbles within the middle ear space or air-fluid levels, aeration with a Valsalva maneuver or politzerization is attempted. These tests may also be facilitated by vasoconstriction of the nasal mucosa with topical oxymetazoline (Afrin). If the middle ear can readily be ventilated by either of these maneuvers, observation is warranted. Additional medical treatment with oral decongestants, short-term vasoconstrictive nasal sprays, or intranasal steroid sprays should be provided. However, if the patient is unable to ventilate the ear, myringotomy alone is performed. A tube is not necessary for patients seen for the first time with otitis media with effusion. Patients known to have a longstanding history of chronic eustachian tube dysfunction will probably require a tympanostomy tube.

Acute Otitis Media

Acute otitis media is also a disease most common to pediatric patients, although adolescent and adult patients may experience this painful infection as well. Symptoms of hearing loss, unilateral ear pain, and fever are typical of this acute infection. Systemic antibiotics are usually effective in reversing the infectious and inflammatory process. However, symptomatic relief may require 24 to 72 hours. Myringotomy alone provides immediate relief from distention of the tympanic membrane secondary to an abscess in the middle ear space. A tympanostomy tube is not necessary in this clinical situation.

Another manifestation of eustachian tube dysfunction in children is recurrent acute otitis media. This condition generally responds to oral antibiotics with clearing of the subsequent serous effusion. Prophylaxis with daily doses of antibiotics is an alternative strategy for medical management. Tympanostomy tube placement should be considered in patients who experience multiple recurrent infections despite appropriate medical therapy. In addition, if the infections become burdensome to the patient and parents or if the child's academic performance, school attendance, and physical health are repeatedly being compromised, tympanostomy tubes should be advocated.

Acute Otitis Media with Complications

Despite the relatively common occurrence of acute otitis media, complications associated with this infection are rare. Such complications include mastoiditis, meningitis, brain abscess, and facial paralysis. Along with systemic antibiotics, wide myringotomy with tube placement is warranted in this acute setting. This provides middle ear ventilation to facilitate decompression of the pressure and drainage of toxins affecting the facial nerve.

Craniofacial Abnormalities

The eustachian tube is rendered dysfunctional in numerous craniofacial abnormalities. A flattened cranium maintains the orientation of the eustachian tube in a horizontal plane, which may impede normal eustachian tube function. Patients with trisomy 21 abnormalities characteristically have poor tubal function and require myringotomy tubes. Similarly, patients with compromised soft palate function secondary to a cleft palate or tumor resection have a dysfunctional eustachian tube opening that predisposes them to middle ear fluid and disease. Patients with such abnormalities should be screened early in life for compromised eustachian tube function.

Barotrauma

Patients requiring hyperbaric oxygen therapy for disorders other than carbon monoxide intoxication may experience eustachian tube dysfunction. Consultation with an otologist may be requested for patients with pain or hearing loss during hyperbaric oxygen therapy. Typically, these patients have wound-healing problems that require 2 to 3 weeks of treatment. Medical management of their "middle ear squeeze" usually consists of oral and topical decongestants, along with slowing the rate of rise in pressure in the chamber. If pain or hearing loss still persists, tympanostomy tube placement is warranted.

Sepsis and Otitis Media

The ears and sinuses of hospitalized patients who are systemically ill with no obvious cause for their fever are often evaluated as a potential source. Consultation is frequently requested for patients with fluid signal from the middle ear as seen on magnetic resonance imaging (MRI) or computed tomography (CT) of the head and temporal bones. Should an effusion or obvious infection be identified, myringotomy with culture or tympanocentesis may be warranted.

Chronic Eustachian Tube Dysfunction

In patients with a longstanding history of eustachian tube dysfunction, an atrophic, retracted, flaccid tympanic membrane that is hypermobile may develop. Retraction may predispose to the formation of pockets extending posteriorly toward the sinus tympani or superiorly toward the epitympanum. The tympanic membrane may drape over the ossicular chain and create a natural type II or III tympanoplasty (Fig. 112-1).

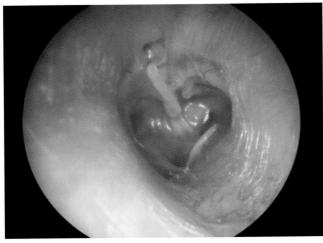

Figure 112-1. Severe atelectasis with a natural type II/III tympanoplasty. Ventilation of the middle ear aims to lateralize the tympanic membrane off the promontory and ossicles.

Further progression of these retraction pockets may promote the formation of cholesteatoma. Placement of a tympanostomy tube will eliminate the negative middle ear pressure and minimize the likelihood of further progression.

PREOPERATIVE PLANNING

Otitis Media with Effusion

The parents of children who are candidates for placement of tympanostomy tubes should be given the chance to review the indications, operative procedure, and postoperative management of tube placement. Unless it is an older, mature child, the procedure is typically performed under general oral anesthesia. Ideally, an audiogram should be obtained before tube placement, but this may not be feasible in a very young child. Patients with recurrent acute otitis media requiring tube placement are managed similarly.

Patients with extremely small external auditory canals may require myringotomy tubes that are not normally stocked. Stenotic canals may permit only a straight tympanostomy tube with a very small inner flange. Should it be anticipated that a smaller tube is necessary, a call to check on the operating room tube inventory is warranted. Placement of myringotomy tubes in adults is typically performed in the clinic under topical anesthesia. The instruments and technique are described later in this chapter.

Acute Otitis Media

Both pediatric and adult patients will benefit from myringotomy when they experience severe pain from acute otitis media. Topical anesthesia applied to an inflamed tympanic membrane may not be effective. An adult, however, is better able than a child to cope with myringotomy. Nursing assistance may be necessary to restrain or wrap the child in a sheet.

Myringotomy is also performed for diagnostic evaluation of otitis media. The predominant indications are a child with persistent acute otitis media in whom antibiotic therapy fails or any person who may be immunocompromised when identification of the organism is important for appropriate management. Myringotomy provides prompt relief of fullness, pressure, pain, and hearing loss in persons with acute otitis media unresponsive to antibiotics. When identification of the organism is critical, a Senturia trap is used for diagnostic tympanocentesis. In clinical situations in which the bacteriology of the middle ear effusion must be known, appropriate planning is necessary. Communication with the patient's physician and microbiology laboratory will expedite handling of the aspirated specimen.

Patients with acute otitis media who experience complications such as facial paralysis, mastoiditis, or meningitis require imaging to detect any other intracranial complications. Along with CT or MRI, neurosurgical consultation is warranted should an intracranial abscess be identified. Administration of intravenous antibiotics with close monitoring in a hospital is necessary. If coalescent mastoiditis is present, mastoidectomy along with a wide myringotomy and tube insertion should be performed.

Choice of Tubes

The tympanostomy tube is placed through an incision in the tympanic membrane to aerate the middle ear. Depending on the nature of the middle ear pathology, short- or long-term ventilation may be needed. Given the patient's findings and previous otologic history, along with the anticipated need, one may then decide how long ventilation will be necessary. The variety of tube designs and material available allows ventilation of the middle ear from a few weeks to indefinitely. Adult patients with new-onset otitis media with effusion who require ventilation should undergo placement of a tube that would remain in place from a few weeks to 3 months. Patients who meet this criterion are those who have persistent serous otitis media despite myringotomy drainage. In addition, patients who have recently undergone otologic surgery and are having problems with aeration may need short-term ventilation while the middle ear and eustachian tube recover. Such ventilation consists of a straight polyethylene tube for which the medial flange has been removed (Fig. 112-2). The tip of the tube is beveled to facilitate insertion.

Tubes with an inner flange remain in the tympanic membrane and middle ear space for a longer time. A Tytan tube provides middle ear ventilation for 4 to 6 months. If more time is needed for additional ventilation, a grommet tube is used. The long-term results of using Armstrong beveled grommet tubes in children were reported by Lindstrom and coauthors. The median and mean times to extrusion were 16.5 and 15.5 months, respectively. The incidence of perforations that did not resolve was 1.32%. Tubes were retained longer than 2 years in 12.2% of the patients.[6] We prefer the design of the Armstrong beveled grommet tube (Fig. 112-2).

Should ventilation of the middle ear be required indefinitely, other tubes are available. A Per-Lee tube has a soft Silastic shaft attached to a large flexible middle ear flange. When placed through the tympanic membrane, this tube will last for many years. The Goode T tube also provides long-term ventilation. Figure 112-3 demonstrates the Per-Lee and Goode T tubes. The physician and patient must be aware that extrusion of the tube may lead to a residual perforation in the tympanic membrane. In the first edition of this text we described the use of a tube composed of hydroxyapatite, which we no longer use.[7]

SURGICAL TECHNIQUE

Tympanocentesis

Tympanocentesis is performed when an infectious agent is believed to be the cause of otitis media. The external auditory meatus is carefully cleaned of cerumen or keratin debris. Concomitant otitis externa with a serous discharge requires further cleaning with a small suction device or a cotton-tipped applicator, or both. If bacterial or fungal colonization in the external meatus is suspected, the canal is flushed with 95% alcohol. Once the canal is suctioned free of this solution and it has dried, tympanocentesis is performed. In a cooperative adult, a small (2 to 3 mm) dot of phenol is applied to the tympanic membrane to provide local anesthesia. Either the posteroinferior or the anterior quadrants are readily accessible for this procedure (Fig. 112-4).

Children

Children warranting ventilation with tubes routinely require general anesthesia for insertion of the tube. Once general oral anesthesia has been induced, the operating microscope is positioned and the ear examined. With an ear loop, small cotton-tipped applicator, suction device, or alligator forceps, the ear is cleaned of cerumen. We prefer to place the myringotomy tube in the anterior or anterosuperior quadrant (Fig. 112-5). These areas retain a tube longer because of the migration pattern of the epithelium of the tympanic membrane. After the myringotomy, a 5F suction device is used to evacuate fluid from the middle ear. Thicker

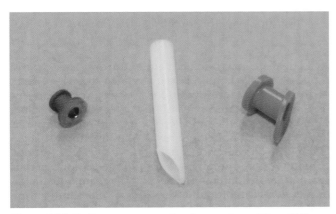

Figure 112-2. Tympanostomy tubes frequently used for middle ear ventilation: *left,* Tytan tube with a 0.76-mm inner diameter (ID) (Medtronics, Inc.); *center,* straight-shank tube (Micromedics); *right,* Armstrong modified beveled grommet, 1.14-mm ID (Medtronics, Inc.).

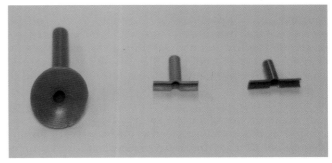

Figure 112-3. Long-term ventilation tubes: *left,* Per-Lee 600 flange angled vent tube, 1.5-mm inner diameter (ID) (Medtronics, Inc.); *center,* Goode T tube, 1.14-mm ID, 6-mm length; *right,* Goode T tube modified, 1.27-mm ID, 4.5-mm length (Medtronics, Inc.).

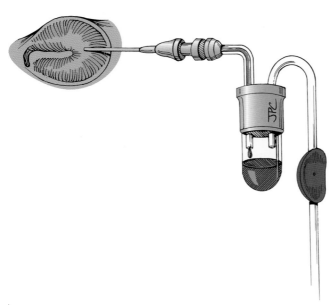

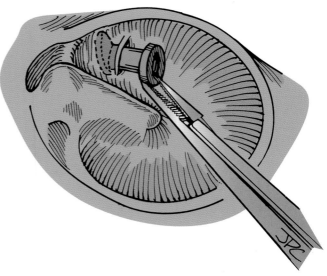

Figure 112-6. An Armstrong beveled grommet tube is placed after aspiration of fluid in the middle ear. *(From Bluestone CD: Otologic surgical procedures. In Bluestone CD, Stool SE [eds]: Atlas of Pediatric Otolaryngology. Philadelphia, WB Saunders, 1995, p 35.)*

Figure 112-4. Tympanocentesis of the inferior tympanic membrane with a Senturia trap. *(From Bluestone CD: Otologic surgical procedures. In Bluestone CD, Stool SE [eds]: Atlas of Pediatric Otolaryngology. Philadelphia, WB Saunders, 1995, p 31.)*

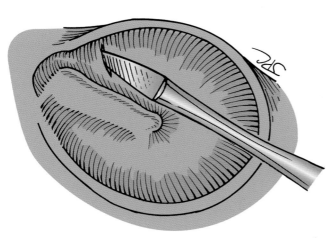

Figure 112-5. Myringotomy is performed in the anterosuperior quadrant. *(From Bluestone CD: Otologic surgical procedures. In Bluestone CD, Stool SE [eds]: Atlas of Pediatric Otolaryngology. Philadelphia, WB Saunders, 1995, p 33.)*

secretions may require suctioning with a 7F suction device. If fluid removal proves difficult, a second myringotomy is performed in the posteroinferior quadrant to better ventilate the ear. Once the fluid is evacuated, the size of the myringotomy is noted. If the myringotomy site is inadequate, it can be enlarged with the myringotomy knife. Alligator forceps may also be opened in the myringotomy site to dilate the incision. A grommet tube is typically inserted in children requiring such ventilation (Fig. 112-6). Once a grommet tube is placed, its proper location and orientation are verified. One should avoid placing the myringotomy tube right at the annulus or immediately adjacent to the

malleus. The former may result in marginal perforation and the latter in pulsatile tinnitus.

An antibiotic-steroid drop is instilled into the ear if the middle ear had mucoid fluid, excessive serous fluid, or a purulent collection. In addition, unwarranted bleeding merits the use of drops to minimize the likelihood of tubal obstruction.

Adults

Most teenagers and adults tolerate myringotomy and tube placement under local anesthesia in an office setting. The patient is informed about the indications for tube placement, and the potential risks of inserting and having a myringotomy tube in place are discussed. Operative consent is obtained. The instruments needed for the procedure are prepared. Instruments that should be available include an applicator wrapped with a wisp of cotton, topical phenol, a myringotomy knife, a suction tip, alligator forceps, and a fine micropick to facilitate myringotomy tube positioning should it be necessary (Fig. 112-7).

The ear canal is cleaned under the operating microscope. Ideally, the tube is placed in the anterior aspect of the tympanic membrane. On occasion, because of the prominent convexity of the anterior bony canal wall, access to the anterior tympanic membrane is limited. In this situation a myringotomy tube is placed in the posteroinferior quadrant. Topical anesthetic (phenol applied to a fine cotton-tipped applicator) is placed on the lateral surface of the tympanic membrane. A myringotomy is performed, and fluid is aspirated from the middle ear. The ventilation tube is inserted and optimally positioned.

Topical anesthesia is occasionally insufficient, possibly because of the patient's intolerance to manipulation of the ear or narrowness of the ear canal. After

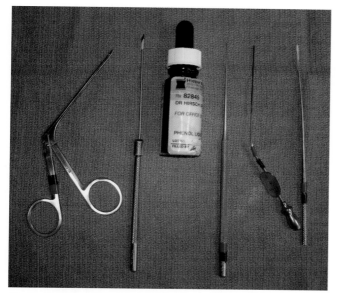

Figure 112-7. Instruments needed for placement of a myringotomy tube in the office (from left to right): fine alligator forceps, myringotomy knife, phenol, fine micropick, suction tip, and applicator wound with a wisp of cotton.

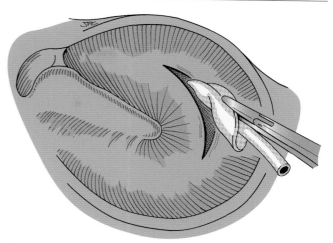

Figure 112-8. The flange of a Per-Lee tube has been trimmed, folded on itself, and grasped with alligator forceps in preparation for insertion. A wide myringotomy has been incised to fit the larger tube.

POSTOPERATIVE MANAGEMENT

Myringotomy and placement of tympanostomy tubes are usually done in the office in adults with serous otitis media. Patients are advised that some drainage may occur. A cotton ball is placed in the external meatus. Once drainage has ceased, patients are instructed to leave the ear open to air.

All patients, including children and adults, are instructed to keep their ears dry. Patients are particularly advised to minimize water exposure while showering or swimming. During showering, a cotton ball with petrolatum (Vaseline) placed on its medial surface is recommended for water protection. We permit swimming with tympanostomy tubes in place. Again, however, precautions are still given to minimize water exposure. We advocate the use of ear plugs for swimming (e.g., silicone putty, a molded ear plug, Doc's Proplugs). The latter has been most effective for protecting the ear during showering and swimming.

Patients undergoing myringotomy tube placement for purulent otitis media, mucoid effusion, or blood coming through the tube from the middle ear are instructed to use topical antibiotic eardrops to minimize the likelihood of tube obstruction from inspissated secretions or dried blood. Parents or patients are advised to use 4 to 5 drops of a quinolone ear preparation twice a day. Children receiving myringotomy tubes are usually checked within a few weeks of placement. The position and patency of the tube are verified. Patients are seen every 4 to 6 months, depending on the ear pathology.

Postoperative tympanostomy tube otorrhea occurs in approximately 20% of untreated children. In a study comparing topical ciprofloxacin/hydrocortisone and neomycin/polymyxin B/hydrocortisone with no treatment, it was noted that there was less otorrhea in the treated ears than in the untreated ears. Given the prophylactic efficacy of drops, it was recommended that the quinolone preparation be used because of its lack

informing the patient, a local anesthetic consisting of 1% lidocaine (Xylocaine) with 1:100,000 epinephrine is infiltrated into the external canal. Topical phenol is also placed to cauterize the drum and minimize bleeding. Patients are advised that the tongue may feel temporarily numb on the side of the injection.

Patients requiring ventilation for an indefinite period are usually taken to the operating room for tube placement under the operating microscope. Our first choice is a T tube, given its relative ease of insertion and lower incidence of tympanic membrane perforation after extrusion. The Per-Lee tube provides indefinite middle ear ventilation. The large flange of a Per-Lee tube is trimmed. Myringotomy is performed in the anterior aspect of the tympanic membrane. The flanges of the Per-Lee tube are folded on themselves with alligator forceps, and the tube is advanced into the middle ear (Fig. 112-8). It is often necessary to use middle ear hooks or picks to facilitate tucking the flanges of the tube medial to the tympanic membrane. In the first edition of this text we mentioned using the Jahn hydroxyapatite tube for long-term ventilation. This tube requires a lengthier procedure for proper placement. It was necessary to elevate an inferior tympanomeatal flap to drill a trough in the bony tympanic ring for placement of the tube in the middle ear. Problems encountered with this tube included the development of organized occlusion of the lumen of the tube that defied achieving patent communication from the ear canal to the middle ear. In addition, the shaft of the tube became incorporated into the bony tympanic ring, and a surgical drill was required to remove the tube.

of ototoxicity.[8] As a result of the broad spectrum of coverage provided by quinolones, they are the medication of choice when tube otorrhea develops. Other factors that may contribute to otitis media and otorrhea include exposure to other children in daycare and to second-hand smoke.

Persistent drainage despite the use of topical eardrops warrants microscopic evaluation of the ear. Purulent material draining through the myringotomy tube should be cultured for identification of the organism and antibiotic sensitivity. The presence of polypoid tissue implies a foreign body reaction to the tube or keratin debris in or around the tube. Ototopical drops containing steroids are often effective in reversing the pathology, but persistent granulation tissue or polyp formation will probably necessitate biopsy and removal of the tube. CT may be appropriate to evaluate the middle ear for cholesteatoma.

On occasion, granulation tissue may develop around the outer flange of a myringotomy tube and manifest as aural bleeding and localized infection. Management consists of removing the polyp with either a suction device or cup forceps. Liquid silver nitrate is applied with a fine cotton-tipped applicator to cauterize the granulation tissue base. Topical eardrops are prescribed for 1 week.

COMPLICATIONS

Myringotomy or placement of a myringotomy tube is usually straightforward and without complications. However, as with any surgical procedure, problems can occur. One must determine that the observed pathology merits myringotomy or a tube, or both. The indications mentioned include ventilation for retraction pockets, middle ear effusion, aeration for barotrauma, and conductive hearing loss in which the status of the middle ear space is in question. If the tympanic membrane is opaque or does not readily move, diagnostic myringotomy is performed. However, caution must be exercised to not confuse congenital or aberrant blood vessels in the middle ear space with fluid. In particular, a dehiscent high-riding jugular bulb or aberrant carotid artery may look like a blue or salmon effusion. Careful inspection of the tympanic membrane should allow recognition of these unusual findings. Similarly, a glomus tumor may also be confused with acute otitis media with effusion.

During myringotomy and tube insertion, caution must be taken to not traumatize the canal wall. In particular, the anterior bony canal is covered with thin skin that bleeds easily when abraded or lacerated. Should this occur, a cotton wick impregnated with adrenaline is placed in the ear canal for 5 minutes, and topical eardrops are provided for 5 days.

Creating too large a myringotomy may also be a problem. A tube placed in a large perforation may readily fall into the middle ear. If the tube can be removed through the myringotomy site, this effort should be undertaken. Identifying a tube in the middle ear behind an intact tympanic membrane does not

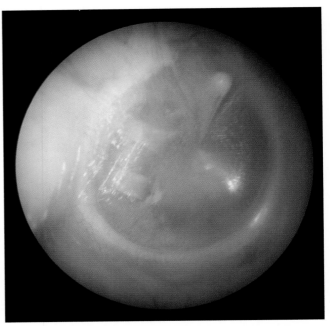

Figure 112-9. Right ear demonstrating a retained myringotomy tube in the middle ear.

mandate removal of the tube (Fig. 112-9). Occasionally, the tube may fall into the hypotympanum and make access difficult unless a large tympanomeatal flap is elevated. If the tube drops out of sight, it is best to not blindly try to retrieve it. The patient or family should be told of the complication and apprised of the rare but potential problems, including chronic otitis media or a sense of the object shifting with head movement. This is unusual and surgical intervention is warranted if patients are symptomatic. Preoperative imaging may be useful in planning the procedure.

A large tympanic membrane defect may also occur when a large suction device for aspiration is applied to a severely atrophic tympanic membrane. There are two options for management. One is to place Gelfoam medial to the perforation and paper-patch the defect. A second myringotomy and tube are then placed in the posterior or posteroinferior quadrant. Another method is to place the tube at a margin of the large perforation and apply a paper patch to the remaining portion of the defect.

In some patients the ear canal is exceedingly small. This often occurs in children with trisomy 21 abnormalities. If the stenotic canal is small, a smaller tube is often necessary. If a beveled grommet tube is preferred, one is available in a smaller size. This smaller tube is preferentially used in children younger than 3 months or, again, in patients with very small ear canals. On rare occasion the canal is so stenotic that only a straight tube can be placed.

Myringotomy tubes should not be placed in the posterosuperior quadrant. Concern for the ossicular chain in this area demands that this quadrant not be violated. A tube with short depth, such as a Tytan tube, may be placed carefully if the ear canal is so narrow that this is the only quadrant visible.

Myringotomy tubes can become plugged. Diligent care is required for patients who are prone to this problem. In particular, patients with hydroxyapatite tubes require meticulous attention. It is for this reason that we no longer use this type of tube design. The diameter of a 3F suction device is sufficiently comparable with that of the tube lumen to permit placement within its lumen. A desiccated mucous plug may often be removed in this fashion. Otherwise, a straight or curved pick can be used to mobilize the plug to facilitate suctioning and extraction. On occasion, the plug can also be pushed into the middle ear space. Patients with mucoid effusions are susceptible to plugging the lumen of their tube, which may be prevented with the use of topical eardrops containing steroids.

Patients with poor eustachian tube function and a retracted tympanic membrane may undergo myringotomy tube placement to improve ventilation. Sometimes, there is a fibrous union between the incus and stapes. Before myringotomy tube placement, a natural type III tympanoplasty may exist (see Chapter 114), which describes a tympanic membrane directly adherent to the stapes. After placement of the tube, the tympanic membrane may lateralize, thereby causing partial ossicular disarticulation and increasing the air-bone gap. Careful inspection of the incudostapedial area may identify this potential problem. Although rare, patients are advised that hearing may actually deteriorate after tube placement.

Despite the presence of fluid in the middle ear and mild conductive hearing loss, patients may not acknowledge improved hearing after tube placement. Immediately after tube placement, patients may complain of a hollow sound or describe their hearing as though they "are in a barrel." They are reassured that this is a short-lived problem and that hearing will sound more normal by the next day.

After myringotomy tube extrusion, a perforation in the tympanic membrane may persist. If additional time for middle ear ventilation is necessary, the perforation functions like a myringotomy tube. However, a persistent perforation may need to be repaired with either a paper patch or formal tympanoplasty (see Chapter 113).

Post-tympanostomy tube otorrhea (PTTO) occurring within 2 weeks of placement is considered an early complication. Its reported incidence is between 5% and 49%. Late PTTO occurs greater than 2 weeks postoperatively and is caused by the same mechanism as for acute otitis media and by external contamination. It has been noted to develop in 26% of patients. Chronic PTTO refers to otorrhea lasting longer than 8 weeks and has an incidence of 4%.[1] Some of the factors that may predispose to PTTO include children in an urban setting, lower socioeconomic status, repeated exposure to unrelated children (daycare), and the presence of mucoid or purulent effusions at the time of placement of the tympanostomy tubes. In children older than 3 years, the bacteriology of the drainage mirrors the organisms of acute otitis media: *S. pneumoniae, H. influenza, M. catarrhalis,* and *Streptococcus pyogenes.* The incidence of *Pseudomonas aeruginosa* and *Staphylococcus aureus* is higher in children older than 3 years, and it occurs with even greater frequency in the summer months.[9]

PEARLS

- Myringotomy without a tube may be more appropriate if the compromise in middle ear aeration is only short lived.
- Do not place a myringotomy tube in the posterior superior quadrant to avoid the possibility of injury to the ossicular chain.
- Use a wider-diameter tube and topical steroid eardrops if mucoid fluid is encountered in the middle ear.
- When placing a myringotomy tube in the office setting, have a fine 1-mm right-angled pick available to facilitate positioning of the tube.
- Persistent otorrhea, especially when granulation tissue is present around the tube, may require removal of the myringotomy tube.

PITFALLS

- Application of phenol or placement of a myringotomy tube in an atrophic flaccid portion of the tympanic membrane is more likely to result in residual tympanic membrane perforation.
- Placing a myringotomy tube at the annulus or juxtaposed to the malleus handle may lead to marginal perforation or pulsatile tinnitus, respectively.
- Aggressive aspiration of an atrophic tympanic membrane through the myringotomy site with a large-diameter suction device may result in perforation at another area of the tympanic membrane.
- Re-establishing aeration in an ear with severe retraction, possible erosion of the incus, and a natural type III tympanoplasty may cause greater conductive hearing loss if the tympanic membrane lateralizes away from the stapes.
- Hitting the promontory while placing a myringotomy tube in a severely retracted tympanic membrane can be avoided by placement in the anterior superior quadrant, over the air space of the eustachian tube opening.

References

1. Rosenfeld RM, Culpepper L, Doyle KJ, et al: Clinical practice guideline: Otitis media with effusion. Otolaryngol Head Neck Surg 130(5 Suppl):S95-S118, 2004.

2. Koopman JP, Reuchlin AG, Kummer EE, et al: Laser myringotomy versus ventilation tubes in children with otitis media with effusion: A randomized trial. Laryngoscope 114:844-849, 2004.

3. Caspary H, Welch JC, Lawson L, et al: Impact of pneumococcal polysaccharide vaccine (Prevnar) on middle ear fluid in children undergoing tympanostomy tube insertion. Laryngoscope 114:975-980, 2004.

4. Hall-Stoodley L, Hu FZ, Gieseke A, et al: Direct detection of bacterial biofilms on the middle-ear mucosa of children with chronic otitis media. JAMA 296:202-211, 2006.

5. Bluestone CD: Eustachian Tube: Structure, Function, Role in Otitis Media. Ontario, BC Decker, 2005.

6. Lindstrom DR, Reuben B, Jacobson K, et al: Long-term results of Armstrong beveled grommet tympanostomy tubes in children. Laryngoscope 114:490-494, 2004.

7. Hirsch BE: Otitis media, myringotomy, and tympanostomy tubes. In Myers EN (ed): Operative Otolaryngology: Head and Neck Surgery. Philadelphia, WB Saunders, 1997, pp 1236-1245.

8. Morpeth JA, Bent JP, Watson T: A comparison of Cortisporin and ciprofloxacin otic drops as prophylaxis against post-tympanostomy otorrhea. Int J Pediatr Otorhinolaryngol 61:99-104, 2001.

9. Oberman JP, Derkay CS: Posttympanostomy tube otorrhea. Am J Otolaryngol 25:110-117, 2004.

Chapter **113**

Myringoplasty and Tympanoplasty

Barry E. Hirsch

Myringoplasty and *tympanoplasty* are descriptive terms defining surgical procedures that address pathology of the tympanic membrane and the middle ear, respectively. Myringoplasty is an operative procedure used to restore the integrity of a perforated tympanic membrane. This assumes that the middle ear space, its mucosa, and the ossicular chain are free of active disease. Inspection of the middle ear is undertaken through the tympanic membrane. A tympanomeatal flap is not raised and the middle ear is not directly exposed. The only procedure performed is directed at reconstruction of the tympanic membrane. In contrast, tympanoplasty also implies reconstruction of the tympanic membrane but in addition deals with pathology in the middle ear cleft, such as chronic infection, cholesteatoma, or problems with the ossicular chain. Zollner[1] and Wullstein[2] provided a classification of tympanoplasty that focuses on the type of ossicular chain reconstruction needed. This classification is of historical interest because reconstruction of the ossicular chain was not undertaken at that time. It does provide a standardized method for analyzing pathology of the ossicular chain and for reporting outcomes of middle ear reconstruction. The five types of tympanoplasty that these authors described define the status of the ossicular chain as a result of pathologic changes from eustachian tube dysfunction and middle ear disease. Progression from type I to type V describes the status of the remaining ossicular chain. Type I has all ossicles intact and requires reconstruction of only the tympanic membrane. Type V consists of no ossicles and connection to the inner ear through a fenestrated horizontal semicircular canal or the vestibule at the oval window.

A variety of symptoms and signs indicate the need for either myringoplasty or tympanoplasty. Acute tympanic membrane perforation or lacerations may occur as a result of local trauma, such as a hand slap to the ear, from a misdirected cotton-tipped applicator inserted in the external canal, or from barotrauma.

Another source of perforation of the tympanic membrane is water compression, which can occur while diving or falling onto a body of water with the ear making direct contact with its surface. It can also occur as a result of a wave hitting the ear while swimming or as a consequence of forceful irrigation of the ear canal during removal of cerumen. Patients with trauma to the tympanic membrane typically complain of a sudden onset of pain with associated hearing loss and occasional bloody otorrhea. The tympanic membrane in such cases may heal spontaneously or might require myringoplasty only. In contrast, patients requiring tympanoplasty more often have a longstanding history of hearing loss, perforation of the tympanic membrane, and chronic otitis media with intermittent otorrhea. Frequent otorrhea often implies chronic mastoid disease, and mastoidectomy may be required.

This chapter focuses on repair of the tympanic membrane. The indications and techniques of ossicular chain reconstruction are covered in Chapter 114. Pathologic processes requiring mastoidectomy, such as chronic otitis media with or without cholesteatoma, are addressed in Chapter 115.

PATIENT SELECTION

Indications for reconstruction of the middle ear and tympanic membrane are to eliminate recurrent disease, provide a dry ear canal and middle ear space with an intact tympanic membrane, and maintain or improve hearing. Achieving an intact tympanic membrane eliminates the precautions that patients must take to avoid potential contamination of the middle ear with water and subsequent otorrhea.

Otologic management is dictated by the patient's symptoms and findings. The status of the tympanic membrane and eustachian tube function greatly influences the alternatives for otologic care. Patients with conductive hearing loss and an intact tympanic membrane who have an aerated middle ear or a clean dry perforation have three options: (1) periodic observation and monitoring of hearing status, (2) surgical reconstruction of the tympanic membrane, and (3) amplification with a hearing aid. Electing no further treatment with a dry tympanic membrane perforation incurs the risk of recurrent otorrhea after an upper respiratory tract infection or contamination with water. Patients should not swim or be exposed to water. If the conductive hearing loss is greater than 30 to 35 dB, the patient is often functionally compromised. Along with reduced hearing in the ipsilateral ear, it may be difficult to localize sound. Patients reluctant to undergo surgery may opt for aural amplification. Although the risks associated with anesthesia and a surgical procedure are avoided, problems inherent with hearing aid use must be accepted, including the need to frequently replace batteries, instrument malfunction, amplification of unwanted background noise, reduced hearing while the hearing aid is out (such as during sleep), and occasionally noisy feedback.

Perforation of the tympanic membrane does not necessarily have to be accompanied by conductive hearing loss. Small perforations, such as those seen after extrusion of a myringotomy tube, may be associated with normal hearing, whereas a patient with a nearly total perforation may have conductive hearing loss of 35 to 40 dB. A similar loss in the setting of a small perforation raises concern that the ossicular chain may not be intact or may be fixed. The surgeon must anticipate the potential need for reconstruction of the ossicular chain and have appropriate surgical instruments and prostheses available at the time of surgery.

The presence of a mixed loss of hearing may alter the advice given by the surgeon. Although surgical correction of conductive loss may close the air-bone gap, a sensorineural component may still require amplification. In this situation, surgery may not be in the patient's best interest. However, if severe mixed loss precludes adequate gain and comfort from an ear-level aid, surgical correction of the conductive component would better facilitate aural rehabilitation. The diagnosis of otosclerosis must be considered when there is a history of slowly progressive hearing loss, bilateral disease is present, and the family history is positive. Surgical management of fixation of the stapes footplate is addressed in Chapter 117.

Examination of patients with a perforated tympanic membrane via the microscope is helpful in revealing the nature of the pathology. Inspection of the canal and middle ear space may provide evidence of recurrent or chronic otorrhea. The location of the defect in the tympanic membrane may raise the surgeon's suspicion of cholesteatoma. Marginal perforations with thin keratin migrating laterally from the edge ("trail sign") suggests squamous epithelium or cholesteatoma in the middle ear. These findings, along with hypertrophied mucosa or extensive granulation tissue, suggest the need for tympanoplasty with mastoidectomy. Tympanoplasty without mastoidectomy would be considered if recurrent drainage is infrequent.

The role of mastoidectomy in improving the success rate of tympanic membrane grafting is controversial. This issue was examined in a recent study. Similar success was achieved in two groups of patients undergoing tympanoplasty in which the only variable was whether mastoidectomy was performed at the time of tympanoplasty. Neither group had (1) active infection (active otorrhea, abnormal middle ear mucosa, or granulation tissue), (2) ossicular abnormalities (ossicular fixation, ossicular discontinuity, ossicular malformation, or absence of an ossicle), (3) cholesteatoma, or (4) previous attempt at tympanic membrane repair (previous tympanoplasty or mastoidectomy). The authors noted that the need for subsequent revision surgery was diminished in those undergoing mastoidectomy at the initial procedure.[3] It is our opinion that tympanoplasty alone, without mastoidectomy, is indicated in patients with normal-appearing mucosa in the middle ear. Despite a well-organized preoperative plan, the surgeon must be prepared to modify the surgical approach and technique based on the intraoperative findings.

Other issues can influence whether surgical intervention is offered. The nature of the patient's disease and desire for intervention typically dictate the type of rehabilitation recommended. An audiogram is always obtained and typically repeated if the patient has not been seen in the office within 6 months. Along with the physical examination, the hearing status of the contralateral ear also influences the method of aural rehabilitation. A patient with mixed or conductive hearing loss and a contralateral anacoustic ear is offered a hearing aid unless the hearing ear has significant active disease unresponsive to medical management.

Collecting additional information and identifying other findings on physical examination may influence the decision for or against surgical intervention. The issue of timing of tympanoplasty, especially in children, remains controversial. The status of the contralateral ear may provide caution or reassurance that the eustachian tube is functioning normally in the involved ear. A recent study in children noted that a dry perforation or the presence of a myringotomy tube in the contralateral ear did not negatively affect successful tympanic membrane repair in the ipsilateral ear. Poor prognostic findings included more objective evidence of ongoing contralateral eustachian tube dysfunction, as evidenced by otitis media with effusion or negative middle ear pressure (atelectasis). Surgery in these children less often resulted in an intact tympanic membrane and a normal middle ear space.[4]

Operative reports of previous otologic procedures performed on either ear should be reviewed. This may provide insight into the status of eustachian tube function, because patients with tympanic membrane perforation who have undergone repeated tympanoplasty procedures usually have poor tubal function. In addition, evaluating the status of contralateral middle ear aeration and tubal function may predict the probable success of yet another tympanoplasty.

Other physical findings and symptoms may affect the decision to surgically address the tympanic membrane and middle ear. Patients with cleft palate deformities are prone to recurrent and chronic middle ear infection. Symptoms such as vertigo should be investigated to avoid operating on an ear that may have ongoing vestibulopathy. If a patient has an actively draining ear, every effort should be made to dry the ear with topical drops or possibly systemic antibiotics, or both. A dry ear before surgery increases the likelihood of success. It is also important for the physician to know whether the patient will be compliant and return for follow-up care.

The risks and benefits of the planned operative procedure must be explained. Potential complications, although rare, include worsening of hearing or complete hearing loss, vertigo, change in taste on the ipsilateral side of the tongue, and failure of the graft to heal. Taste disturbance results when the chorda tympani nerve is stretched, desiccated, or divided. Patients may remain symptomatic for 4 to 6 months. In some cases this results in permanent dysfunction. Patients undergoing a postauricular approach should be told that the top of the pinna often feels numb or there may be a sense of "pins and needles" along the midhelix. Sensation usually returns in approximately 3 months.

PREOPERATIVE PLANNING

Imaging studies are not generally obtained before routine myringoplasty or tympanoplasty procedures. If readily available, the operative notes should be reviewed if previous procedures were performed on the involved ear. However, previous operative reports may not reflect the current situation in the middle ear and mastoid. After numerous otologic procedures, local tissue for grafting may not be readily available. If this is the case, alternative sources such as perichondrium, periosteum, or even areolar tissue or fascia from the contralateral side should be considered. The integrity of the skin and patency of the canal should be assessed. A split-thickness skin graft may be necessary if canal atresia or stenosis is present after previous procedures. Before surgical intervention, informed consent must be obtained.

ANESTHESIA

Tympanoplasty for reconstruction of the tympanic membrane and correction of conductive hearing loss is typically performed through a postauricular approach, especially in patients with large or anterior perforations and revision operations. Most of the procedures that we perform entail lateral grafting techniques, usually performed under general endotracheal anesthesia. Adult patients who are reluctant to undergo general anesthesia may be given a local anesthetic and regional block supplemented with monitored intravenous sedation. In cases of conductive hearing loss with an intact tympanic membrane or a small perforation in which a medial graft is anticipated, a transcanal approach is used. In this case either local or general anesthesia may be considered. However, intravenous sedation with local anes-

thesia is preferred and typically well tolerated by the patient. A sedated but awake patient with additional local anesthesia presents distinct advantages during ossicular reconstruction procedures. The surgeon can assess the patient's hearing result during the procedure and detect any untoward symptoms, such as dizziness. Antibiotic prophylaxis is not given for routine myringoplasty and tympanoplasty procedures.

SURGICAL TECHNIQUES

Medial and lateral grafting are probably equally successful in the hands of experienced surgeons. Nevertheless, we typically choose lateral grafting because of our consistent results, which are in part due to the greater exposure provided by this approach. A graft is placed medially when the patient has an infrequent history of otorrhea; when the perforation in the tympanic membrane is small, not marginal, and located in the posterior half of the tympanic membrane, or when there is minimal evidence of middle ear disease. Myringoplasty by definition addresses only the tympanic membrane in patients in whom the ossicular chain is assumed to be intact. Tympanoplasty techniques incorporate inspection of the middle ear and reconstruction of the ossicular chain when necessary.

An operative approach recently described for difficult or failed tympanoplasty procedures involves the use of a palisading technique of cartilage and perichondrium. It may be indicated in patients with severe atelectasis, in those with high-risk perforations and an intact ossicular chain, and in association with ossiculoplasty when the malleus is present. High-risk perforation is defined as a tympanic membrane perforation that persists after unsuccessful attempts at surgical repair, a perforation anterior to the malleus, a perforation larger than 50%, or a bilateral perforation.[5] Our preference is not to use cartilage because inspection of the middle ear to monitor for the recurrence or development of cholesteatomas may be compromised. Cartilage is necessary when the scutum is eroded or removed to access the epitympanum for mucosal disease and cholesteatoma. Cartilage harvested from the tragus, including an island of perichondrium, can help secure the graft in its desired position.

Myringoplasty

Myringoplasty is performed for small or acute traumatic perforations of the tympanic membrane. Acute traumatic tympanic membrane lacerations or perforations require that the edges of the drum be unfolded to remove squamous epithelium from the medial surface of the tympanic membrane. Analgesia is often necessary and is provided by a four-quadrant external canal block applied just lateral to the cartilaginous-bony junction with 2% lidocaine (Xylocaine) with 1:100,000 epinephrine through a 27-gauge dental needle (Fig. 113-1) (see Video 113-1). The edges of the tympanic membrane perforation are unfolded so that not all squamous epithelium is removed from the middle ear (Fig. 113-2). Often, approximation is not precise, and small

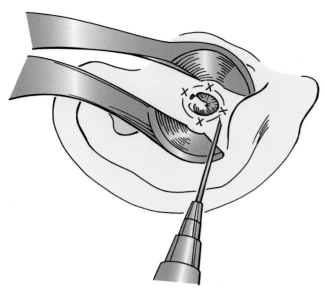

Figure 113-1. With a Lempert speculum, local anesthetic is injected in a four-quadrant fashion into the external auditory meatus. The needle tip is placed just lateral to the bone-cartilage junction, and the solution is infiltrated until the skin blanches. *(Redrawn from Bluestone CD, Stool S: Atlas of Pediatric Otolaryngology, 3rd ed. Philadelphia, WB Saunders, 1996.)*

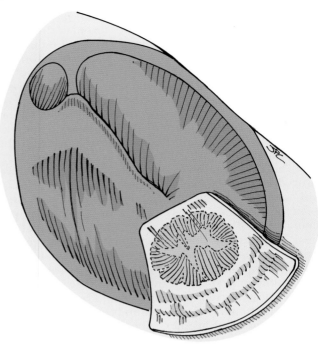

Figure 113-3. The edges of the stellate perforation are approximated and supported with a cigarette paper patch or a Steri-Strip.

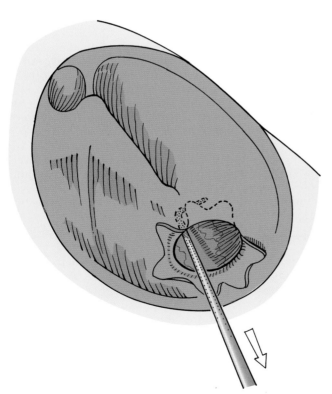

Figure 113-2. The edges of a fresh stellate perforation are everted from the medial surface of the tympanic membrane. When squamous epithelium is no longer present in the middle ear, the edges are reapproximated. *(Redrawn from Naumann HH: Head and Neck Surgery, vol 3: Ear. Stuttgart, Germany, Georg Thieme, 1982.)*

pieces of Gelfoam impregnated with a suspension of ciprofloxacin and hydrocortisone (Ciprodex) or plain ciprofloxacin solution (Floxin) is placed medial to the laceration or perforation. A cigarette paper patch, Steri-Strip, or silk patch is applied to the lateral surface of the tympanic membrane (Fig. 113-3).

Small chronic perforations may also be treated by lateral patching techniques. In this situation, topical phenol or trichloroacetic acid is applied to the edges of the perforation with a wisp of cotton on an applicator. A sharp pick is then used to freshen the margins of the tympanic membrane perforation to allow removal of the edges of the perforation. This technique removes any squamous epithelium that may have migrated under the medial surface of the tympanic membrane at the edge of the perforation and stimulates bleeding and healing from the local vascular supply (Fig. 113-4). If the perforation is small and the edges are well defined, Gelfoam is not needed in the middle ear. A paper patch is applied to the lateral surface of the tympanic membrane.

Small central perforations may be reconstructed with an autogenous tissue graft if paper patching is unsuccessful. This technique requires similar preparation of the tympanic membrane while ensuring that no squamous epithelium has migrated to the medial surface of the edges of the perforation. Depending on the age of the patient, myringoplasty with placement of the graft medially can be performed in the operating room under local anesthesia. Fat from the earlobe or areolar tissue from the postauricular area is harvested, compressed, and allowed to dry. After the edges of the tympanic membrane perforation are freshened,

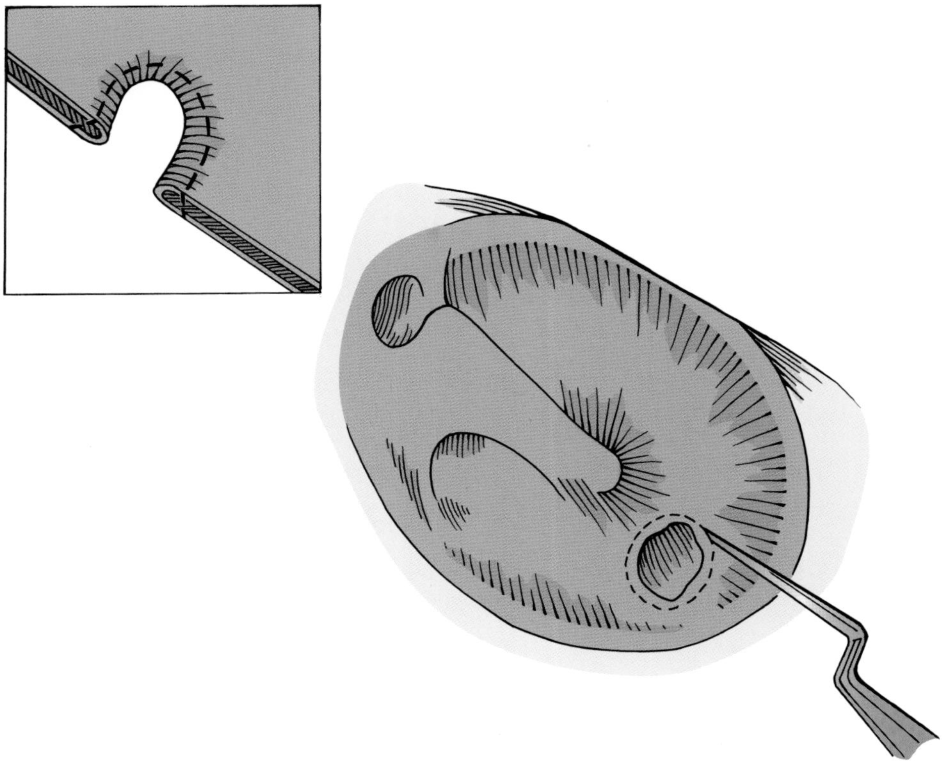

Figure 113-4. The edge of the perforation is circumferentially freshened to remove epithelium from the medial margin and promote local bleeding. The *inset* emphasizes that the medial edge of the perforation must be removed to eliminate squamous epithelium from the middle ear. *(Redrawn from Naumann HH: Head and Neck Surgery, vol 3: Ear. Stuttgart, Germany, Georg Thieme, 1982.)*

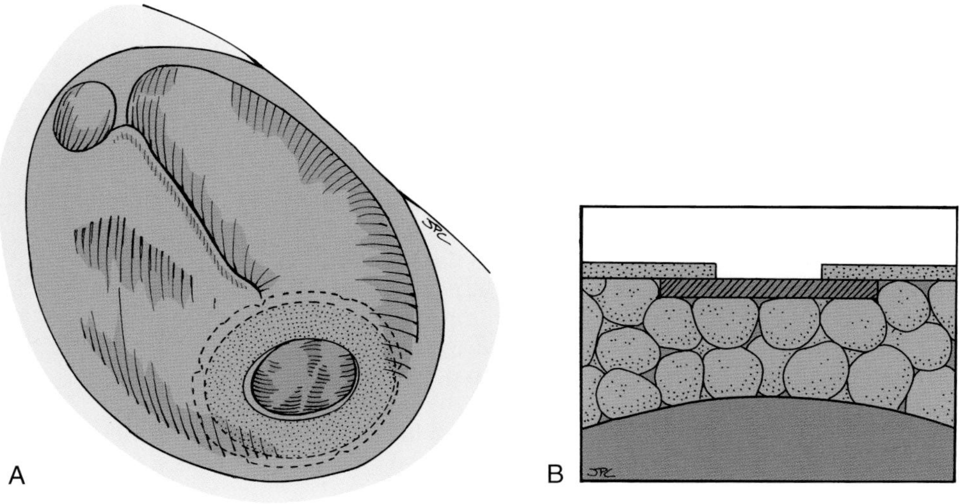

Figure 113-5. A, Myringoplasty of the right tympanic membrane with a posteroinferior perforation. The edges of the perforation are freshened, Gelfoam is placed in the middle ear, and an areolar or compressed fat graft *(stippled area)* is placed through the perforation, positioned medial to the tympanic membrane, and supported by the Gelfoam. **B,** Gelfoam supports the graft on the medial surface of the tympanic membrane.

A

B

Gelfoam is placed through the perforation into the middle ear space. A properly sized tissue graft is placed through the perforation and sandwiched between the medial surface of the tympanic membrane and the Gelfoam (Fig. 113-5). In the absence of significant conductive hearing loss, this technique can be used to reconstruct such small defects without elevating a tympanomeatal flap. A small piece of Surgicel placed lateral to the grafted perforation may be used to further secure the graft. Gelfoam soaked in antibiotic solution is placed lateral to the tympanic membrane to fill the medial external canal.

Tympanoplasty

Lateral Grafting Technique

The patient's head is turned toward the contralateral side, and the hair is shaved superior and posterior to the pinna to provide approximately 1 to 2 cm of hairless skin. After adequate general anesthesia has been obtained and the operative field has been prepared and draped, 2% lidocaine with 1:100,000 epinephrine is injected into the external canal with a dental syringe and a 27-gauge needle. This is done in at least four quadrants by placing the needle just at the medial

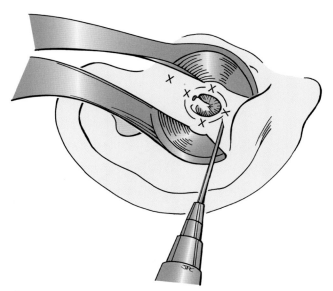

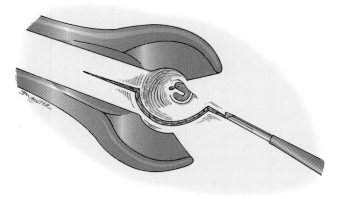

Figure 113-7. With a Lempert speculum and a no. 64 Beaver blade, 12- and 6-o'clock incisions are connected with a posterior canal wall incision, just medial to the conchal cartilage.

Figure 113-6. Local anesthetic is injected in a four-quadrant fashion into the external auditory meatus and incisura.

margin of the cartilaginous canal and injecting approximately 1 mL. Additional infiltration is placed at the 12-o'clock position at the incisura down to the root of the zygoma (Fig. 113-6) (see Video 113-1). The same anesthetic is also injected into the post-auricular area a few millimeters posterior to the post-auricular crease.

Using the operating microscope, incisions are made in the skin of the external meatus at 12 o'clock and 6 o'clock with a no. 64 Beaver blade. An endaural Lempert speculum is used to facilitate exposure of these incisions. The 12-o'clock incision begins approximately 1 cm lateral to the lateral process of the malleus and extends to the tragal incisura. The 6-o'clock incision is a short incision in the bony canal down to the junction of the bone and cartilage (see Video 113-2). These two incisions are then connected vertically along the posterior bony canal wall, about 3 mm medial to the bony-cartilaginous junction, to create a conchal flap (Fig. 113-7). Through this endaural approach the conchal flap dissection is initiated by back-elevating the canal skin (Fig. 113-8) (see Video 113-3). The 12-o'clock corner of the flap must be completely dissected and mobilized to facilitate elevation of the skin from the postauricular approach.

Hatch marks are placed in the postauricular area over the planned postauricular incision and the skin is incised a few millimeters posterior to the sulcus. The skin is initially incised with a no. 15 blade. The incision can be continued through subcutaneous tissue and the postauricular muscle with a knife or electrocautery (Fig. 113-9). Subcutaneous dissection is performed along the posterior aspect of the conchal cartilage to define the posteriorly based conchal flap. The skin of the external auditory canal is elevated from the postauricular approach and dissected toward the previously made endaural incisions (see Video 113-4). A prominent

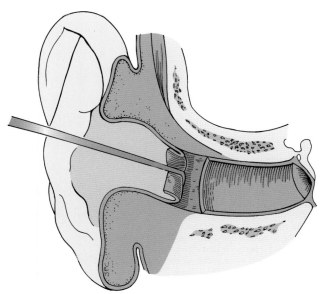

Figure 113-8. A large duckbill dissector is used to back-elevate the conchal flap to facilitate subsequent mobilization.

spine of Henle may be encountered and requires more vigorous soft tissue dissection. The endaural 12-o'clock incision is connected with the postauricular incision by placing a no. 15 blade through the subcutaneous tissue at the zygomatic root. From the postauricular approach, the knife is beveled toward the bony canal wall, and the conchal cartilage flap is further defined (Fig. 113-10). The flap is then elevated off the posterior canal wall via the original vertical conchal flap incision made endaurally. When the two incisions are connected, the conchal flap is retracted with either a tracheostomy tape and a self-retaining retractor or a Perkins retractor alone (Fig. 113-11) (see Video 113-5). Incision into and exposure of the cartilage of the external canal may result in pain and possibly chondritis. This complication is more likely if the 6-o'clock incision is carried too far laterally or with extension of the post-

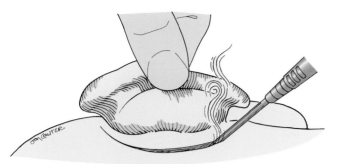

Figure 113-9. An incision with a no. 15 blade is made posterior to the postauricular sulcus. Electrocautery is used to continue the incision and maintain hemostasis.

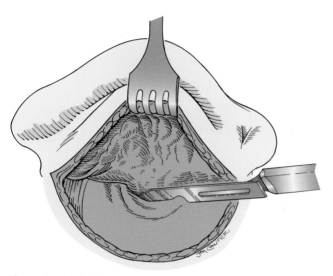

Figure 113-10. Through the postauricular incision, a knife is used to dissect the skin from the bony wall of the posterior canal. The blade is directed toward the bony canal wall to avoid laceration of the skin of the canal.

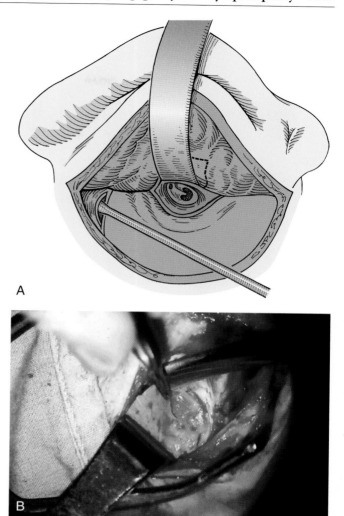

A

B

Figure 113-11. A, The conchal flap has been dissected and inverted toward the external auditory meatus *(dotted lines).* A tracheostomy tape maintains retraction on the soft tissue of the canal. This is then secured with a self-retaining retractor. A Freer dissector is used to harvest areolar tissue or temporalis fascia. **B,** The skin is retracted with an Army-Navy retractor. Temporalis fascia is removed from the temporalis muscle.

auricular dissection toward the posterior inferior aspect of the conchal cartilage.

If the areolar tissue (fool's fascia) obtained from the lateral surface of the fascia covering the temporalis muscle is hearty and well defined, this tissue layer is chosen for grafting. The area over the temporalis muscle is exposed and a self-retaining retractor is placed. An Army-Navy retractor may be needed to lift the temporal skin to facilitate better exposure. A no. 15 Bard-Parker blade is used to superficially incise the areolar tissue layer, and a plane is developed between this layer and underlying fascia with a Freer dissector (Fig. 113-11A). Scissors are used to remove a 2 by 2-cm section. If this proves to be too thin or is deemed to be inadequate, true temporalis fascia is harvested in a similar manner (see Fig. 113-11B). Hemostasis may be necessary for regional vessels. The graft is spread on a cutting block, cleaned of attached muscle fibers or adipose tissue with the side of the knife blade, and allowed to dry.

The medial aspect of the canal skin is then removed by circumferentially incising the anterior canal wall at the bulge (see Video 113-6). The skin remaining in the canal medial to the incision is then sequentially elevated toward the fibrous tympanic annulus with duckbill elevators or an oval knife (Fig. 113-12) (see Video 113-7). Dissection extends medially to remove the canal skin and epithelium over the tympanic membrane as an intact sleeve. The easiest area to obtain a clean dissection plane is at the posterior inferior medial canal and annulus, which is at the 8-o'clock position in the demonstrated right ear (Fig. 113-12) (see Video 113-8). Care is taken to elevate all the squamous epithelium off the remaining tympanic membrane. This dissection is facilitated superiorly, where the pars flaccida can be stripped off the lateral process of the malleus in a down-

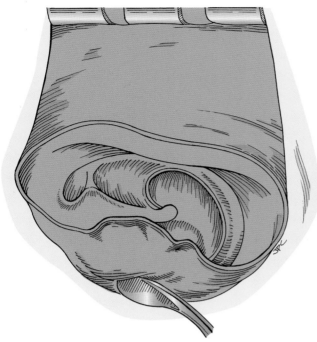

Figure 113-12. With a duckbill elevator, the skin of the bony external meatus is elevated in a medial direction until the bony annulus is encountered. Dissection follows the circumference of the collagenous fibrous layer of the tympanic membrane.

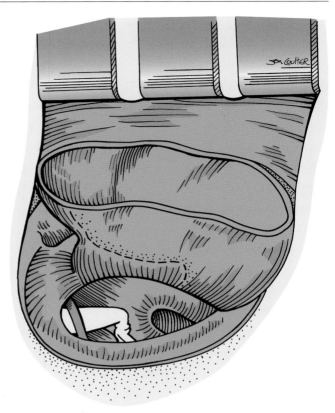

Figure 113-13. Most of the epithelial layer of the tympanic membrane has been elevated off the anterior and posterior canal walls and fibrous tympanic membrane. It remains pedicled along the handle of the malleus and can be stripped off readily with cup forceps.

ward fashion with cup forceps, and posteriorly at the inferior fibrous annulus, where anterior dissection can be easily performed parallel to the plane of the fibrous annulus (Fig. 113-13) (see Video 113-9). Often, a small perforation of the tympanic membrane is made larger by removing this epithelial layer because of the underlying fibrous layer defect.

A prominent anterior canal wall may obstruct the view of the anterior annulus. The anterior canal wall skin is back-elevated in a medial-to-lateral direction to provide access to the bony anterior canal wall (see Video 113-10). This area of bone of the anterior canal may have to be removed with a drill to provide unobstructed exposure of the anterior canal. This reduces the incidence of blunting of the angle between the anterior canal wall and tympanic membrane and facilitates postoperative examination and cleaning (see Video 113-11). If the bony overhang prohibited visualization of the anterior sulcus, the improved exposure facilitates performance of this step in the procedure (see Video 113-12). Epithelial remnants may remain in the anterior and inferior sulcus. Retention of this skin would result in the development of a middle ear or intratympanic cholesteatoma. If there is concern that all the skin was not removed, an angled curette is used to further dissect the anterior and inferior sulcus just lateral to the annulus (see Video 113-13).

Tympanoplasty requires inspection of the middle ear space and reconstruction of the ossicles, when necessary. A sickle knife or curved pick (Rosen needle) is used to elevate the posterior fibrous annulus while taking care to preserve the chorda tympani nerve. The ossicular chain must be completely inspected and palpated (Fig. 113-14). If visualization of the incudostapedial joint and stapes footplate is not adequate, bone of the posterior superior bony canal wall may be removed with a curette or drill (Fig. 113-15). The status of the ossicular chain is assessed by palpation. Limited mobility of the lateral chain (malleus-incus) and fixation of the incus-stapes complex will require separation of the incudostapedial joint. If a cholesteatoma is present in the middle ear, the incus may need to be removed to evaluate the integrity of the stapes (see Videos 113-14 and 113-15). Repair of the ossicular chain is reviewed in Chapter 114.

Middle Ear Disease

Common pathologic processes found in the middle ear include granulation tissue, hyperplastic mucosa, cholesteatoma, and tympanosclerosis. Each is managed in a different way.

Granulation tissue and mucosal hyperplasia require reconstruction of an aerated middle ear space. Early assessment of eustachian tube patency directs one's decision regarding reconstruction. Failure of tympanoplasty is likely if irreversible mucosal disease or eustachian tube obliteration is present. Deciding that a eustachian tube will never function normally is difficult

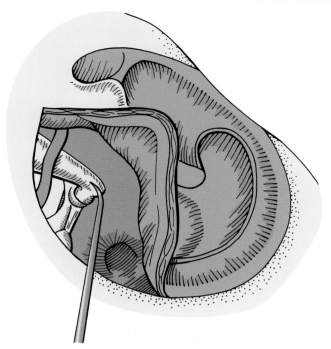

Figure 113-14. The posterior fibrous annulus has been elevated to inspect the middle ear space and the integrity of the ossicular chain. *(Redrawn from Naumann HH: Head and Neck Surgery, vol 3: Ear. Stuttgart, Germany, Georg Thieme, 1982.)*

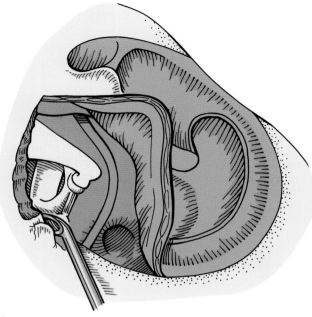

Figure 113-15. A curette or small cutting burr is used to remove bone from the posterosuperior tympanic annulus to provide additional exposure of the incudostapedial joint and the footplate of the stapes. *(Redrawn from Naumann HH: Head and Neck Surgery, vol 3: Ear. Stuttgart, Germany, Georg Thieme, 1982.)*

because judgment depends largely on one's surgical experience. If the lining of the middle ear and eustachian tube is hyperplastic and the eustachian tube is patent, removal of the thickened mucosa usually warrants an intervention that would avoid the development of adhesions from the denuded promontory to the tympanic membrane graft and malleus umbo. A thin Silastic disc (0.005 to 0.01 inch) is placed on the promontory in the mesotympanum and can remain indefinitely. More extensive disease extending into the epitympanum may require mastoidectomy. Thicker Silastic sheeting (0.02 to 0.04 inch) is used if it is believed that ossicular reconstruction will be more likely to succeed once the middle ear space is aerated. The decision to stage the procedure and return in 4 to 9 months for subsequent reconstruction is generally made at the time of surgery.

Staging is undertaken if there is concern for incomplete removal or residual cholesteatoma. The incus is usually removed to facilitate elimination of middle ear disease, regardless of whether it is cholesteatoma, granulation tissue, or hyperplastic mucosa. Extensive cholesteatoma around the stapes footplate may be easier to remove after the inflammatory response has subsided. Cholesteatoma may become more focally organized into a ball or "pearl" and thus facilitate complete removal during a subsequent procedure. Silastic sheeting can maintain a middle ear space between the promontory and tympanic membrane graft. The Silastic sheet is contoured to have a pointed end extend toward the meatus of the eustachian tube and the superior end lay

over the facial nerve into the epitympanum. Nearly complete closure of the conductive component of the hearing loss may result if Silastic is placed over an intact stapes superstructure.

Cholesteatoma must be totally eradicated. Cholesteatoma pearls or a localized matrix is easily removed. Layered epithelium covering the stapes superstructure or footplate or extending into the sinus tympani must be meticulously removed. Extension of disease into the epitympanum generally requires access and inspection of the attic through a transcortical mastoidectomy approach (see Chapter 115). Recently, the use of endoscopes has proved to be most helpful in closely inspecting the epitympanum.[6]

Tympanosclerosis is a unique reparative response believed to be secondary to middle ear inflammation. Tympanosclerosis consists of brittle chalk-like plaque that is typically found within the tympanic membrane, affecting the ossicles, and on the medial wall of the middle ear. Reversing the inflammatory process is believed to eliminate the future development of tympanosclerosis. Both fixation and erosion of the ossicles from tympanosclerosis may be seen. The stapes footplate is occasionally found to be fixed. Reconstruction of the tympanic membrane is facilitated by removing the myringosclerotic plaque if it is restricting the mobile portion of the drum to either the annulus or the malleus handle. Stapedioplasty is not performed when the tympanic membrane is perforated. If the stapes is fixed because of tympanosclerosis, manipulation may result in fracture of the footplate or dislodgement of the footplate from the annular ligament. Repair of stapes fixation should be staged and performed only after the tympanic membrane is intact.

The ossicular chain must be adequately visualized and palpated to determine its mobility. Ossicular reconstruction is undertaken when indicated. Specific details regarding these techniques are discussed in Chapter 114.

After inspection and treatment of the middle ear and ossicular chain, the posterior fibrous tympanic membrane and cartilaginous annulus are returned to their original positions. The areolar tissue or fascia is harvested and cut to the proper size, typically an 11- by 13-mm oval disc, although smaller grafts can be used if the perforation is not large. If the posterior annulus is deficient or a large amount of bone from the posterior canal wall has been removed, a longer, more oblong graft is tailored. The longer portion of the graft is laid on the posterior canal wall. The graft is positioned on the annular margin, lateral to the handle of the malleus (Fig. 113-16).

When the perforation is nearly total and the malleus is not supported by any remaining fibrous tympanic membrane, the graft can still be positioned lateral to the malleus. However, when the malleus is directed medially, approximating the promontory, the graft should be positioned medial to the umbo of the malleus to prevent lateralization. The graft is then cut radially for a few millimeters from the 12-o'clock position and placed medial to the umbo and distal handle of the malleus, with the superior edges of the graft overlapping in the pars flaccida area (Fig. 113-17) (see Video 113-16). The graft must be positioned so that it lies on the cartilaginous annulus and does not extend onto the anterior or inferior bony canal walls. A graft that is too thick, placed beyond the fibrous annulus, and extended onto the anterior inferior canal wall may result in blunting of the angle between the tympanic membrane and

the bony canal wall. This problem is avoided by trimming the graft to the appropriate size and shape. When the graft must be wrapped around the medial surface of the malleus, the superior margins of the incised graft are overlapped over each other (see Video 113-17).

The skin that had been harvested from the external canal is then inspected under the microscope. Scissors are used to open up the sleeve of skin that was obtained from the medial external canal. It is thinned and subcutaneous tissue is removed if necessary (see Video 113-18). The separate pieces are placed on a plastic cutting block with the epithelial side up and cut into rectangular shapes. It is necessary to remove extremely thin or irregular edges of the skin to ensure that all of the epithelial surfaces face the ear canal lumen. Preparation and trimming of the skin should be done with use of the microscope to eliminate unfurled edges. An accurately sized graft should be placed so that it is just overlapping the anterior annulus to avoid blunting (see Video 113-19).

Each piece of skin is then carefully placed lateral to the areolar (or fascial) graft with the epithelial surface toward the auricle. Attention is directed to the anterior sulcus, where skin is placed on the anterior canal with the thinner edge positioned lateral to the areolar or fascial graft. The skin overlying the graft should be thin. The first piece of skin is placed in this area, and subsequent grafts are placed over the pars flaccida area and, when available, posteriorly onto the bony canal wall (Fig. 113-18) (see Video 113-20). If there is insufficient skin to provide coverage of the bony canal, a thin split-thickness skin graft (Thiersch graft) is harvested from the non–hair-bearing postauricular skin with a no. 10 blade.

Packing of the external ear canal is necessary. Packing keeps canal flaps and epithelial grafts in their

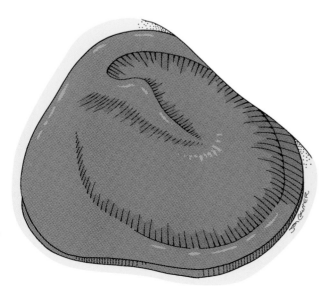

Figure 113-16. The areolar graft is routinely placed lateral to the annulus, and the remaining fibrous tympanic membrane is draped over the malleus.

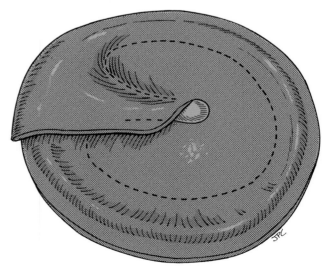

Figure 113-17. If the handle of the malleus is directed medially within the middle ear, the areolar graft is cut vertically at the 12-o'clock position and positioned medial to the malleus handle and lateral to the fibrous tympanic membrane and annulus. The edges of the areolar graft overlap superiorly, lateral to the proximal handle and the short process of the malleus and pars flaccida area.

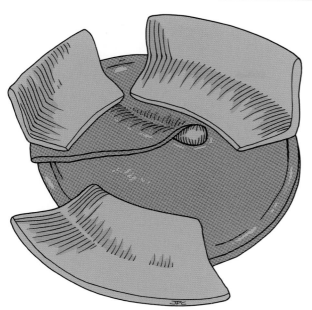

Figure 113-18. The skin of the medial bony canal wall and lateral tympanic membrane was thinned and cut into rectangular pieces. The thicker part of the skin graft is initially placed on the anterior bony canal wall. The thinner edges overlie the areolar graft. Depending on the availability of skin, multiple pieces are placed.

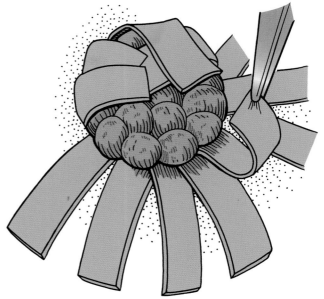

Figure 113-20. Small cotton or Merocel balls are packed within the rosebud dressing, and the edges are folded over one another.

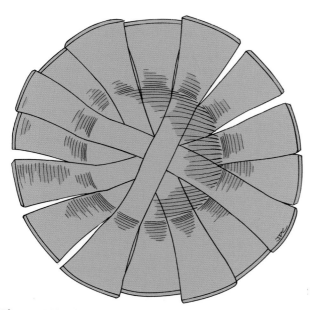

Figure 113-19. Medial rosebud packing consists of strips of silk that are placed radially to completely cover the areolar graft.

proper positions, which greatly aids in the healing process. The cylindrical channel of the ear canal is maintained to preclude narrowing from blood products and granulation tissue. The contour and patency are preserved until the packing is removed or dissolves. It is important to prevent blunting of the anterior sulcus with one of the following techniques: Gelfoam, ointment, Merocel sponges, or a silk rosebud pack. We use two methods of packing, depending on the preference

of the surgeon. The first consists of Gelfoam soaked in antibiotic suspension. The initial piece is approximately 5 to 7 mm in length and 4 mm in width, compressed, and folded on itself. While firmly holding the anterior canal wall skin graft, the Gelfoam is secured anteriorly to define the anterior tympanomeatal sulcus. The remainder of the ear canal is filled with small to progressively larger pieces of Gelfoam.

The other packing technique that we use is precise but tedious. It consists of using strips of silk, 4×25 mm, placed in rosebud fashion into the medial canal (Fig. 113-19) (see Video 113-21). Merocel balls impregnated with bacitracin ointment are then placed within the rosebud, and the lateral leaves are folded over one another to create a mold or cast of the medial canal. This accurately defines the anterior sulcus, which will minimize the risk of anterior blunting and lateralization (Fig. 113-20) (see Video 113-22).

The tracheostomy tape and self-retaining retractors are then released and the ear is returned to its anatomic position. The conchal flap is thinned if there is too much subcutaneous tissue and returned into the external canal. Lateral rosebud packing consisting of silk strips 7 to 10 mm $\times$ 30 to 35 mm is then placed in a similar rosebud fashion and secured with larger Merocel balls (Fig. 113-21) (see Video 113-23). Another method for stenting the lateral canal is with a small-pore Merocel sponge (Schindler ear pack) impregnated with antibiotic otic suspension. The postauricular wound is closed with interrupted 4-0 Monocryl suture and running 5-0 fast-absorbing chromic suture and Steri-Strips. A cotton ball is placed at the external meatus, and a sterile mastoid or Glasscock dressing is applied. Most patients undergo surgery as an outpatient and are discharged the day of the procedure. The mastoid or Glasscock dressing is maintained overnight and removed by the

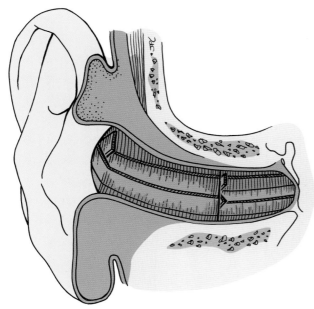

Figure 113-21. The medial rosebud pack secures the grafted tympanic membrane. The lateral pack stents the lateral canal and conchal flap.

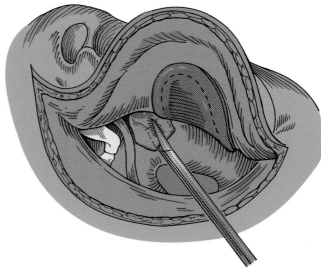

Figure 113-22. Medial grafting technique. After the edges of the tympanic membrane perforation are freshened, a tympanomeatal flap is elevated. A tissue graft *(shaded area)* is positioned medial to the perforation and supported by packing Gelfoam into the middle ear. *(Redrawn from Naumann HH: Head and Neck Surgery, vol 3: Ear. Stuttgart, Germany, Georg Thieme, 1982.)*

patient or family after 24 hours. The cotton ball placed in the external meatus is removed and replaced every few hours as needed.

✣ *Medial Grafting Technique*

The external canal is injected as described earlier. Once anesthesia is adequate, the edges of the perforation are trimmed with a perforating pick or sickle knife (see Fig. 113-4). A graft is then harvested. Small perforations can be repaired with compressed adipose tissue harvested from the earlobe or with areolar tissue from the post-auricular area. For larger defects, an incision posterior to the superior aspect of the helix is made over the temporalis area, where areolar tissue or fascia is obtained. (This is incorporated into the postauricular approach if greater exposure of the tympanic membrane is necessary.) A tympanomeatal flap is elevated by incising the medial canal skin over the scutum superior to the lateral process of the malleus. It is extended posteriorly while keeping a distance of 4 to 5 mm from the annulus. The incision is then curved inferiorly, running parallel to the annulus, and is directed toward the 6-o'clock position. The tympanomeatal flap is then elevated along with the annulus. The ossicular chain is next inspected and palpated as mentioned earlier. The graft is then brought into the middle ear, placed up against the medial aspect of the tympanic membrane perforation, and supported with Gelfoam placed within the middle ear space (Fig. 113-22). The flap is then returned to its anatomic position. Packing consists of a strip of silk supported with cotton balls impregnated with bacitracin ointment or Gelfoam to fill the external canal.

POSTOPERATIVE MANAGEMENT

After myringoplasty for repair of tympanic membrane perforation or lacerations, the packing is removed 7 to 10 days after the procedure. Patients in whom a paper patch has been applied to the lateral surface of the repair are monitored until the paper patch migrates onto the skin of the bony canal wall. This process may take 6 to 12 weeks, during which time the patient is instructed to avoid getting water into the ear.

With the lateral grafting technique, the Glasscock or mastoid dressing is removed on the first postoperative day. Patients are instructed to keep the incision dry for 1 week; they are permitted to shower but should avoid getting the incision and Steri-Strips soaking wet. Topical eardrops are used twice daily for repairs packed with Gelfoam. Lateral packing involving the rosebud technique can remain dry. Topical eardrops are not needed during the first postoperative week. The ointment around the Merocel balls keeps the lateral packing moist. Drainage normally occurs through the external canal, and the cotton ball is changed frequently. Analgesics are provided. The patient is seen 7 to 10 days after surgery, and the postauricular Steri-Strips and the lateral rosebud packing are removed. Antibiotic-steroid drops are prescribed for use twice a day.

One week later, the medial rosebud pack is removed. The canal is cleaned with a thin wisp of cotton on an applicator. The cotton applicator is used to gently wipe or absorb any residual blood that may collect or pool in the inferior or anterior sulcus. Cleaning the medial canal will help avoid the development of granulation tissue, scarring, and blunting. A 3F suction device or cotton on an applicator can be used to remove excessive blood or serum, but caution is needed to avoid accidental removal of the replaced skin. The ear canal may attempt to heal with cicatricial midcanal soft tissue stenosis. If not recognized, it can progress to complete stenosis and give the appearance of a lateralized tympanic membrane. In the immediate postoperative period, most patients have a relatively insensate ear canal that permits office débridement and stenting. Occasionally, the patient must be returned to the operating room for aggressive débridement and repacking. Granulation tissue, if present, is cauterized with silver nitrate. Excessive granulation tissue can be removed with a curette. Topical 5-fluorouracil can also be used. It may be necessary to place a wick with antibiotic drops for another week to ensure smooth healing of the ear canal.

The tympanic membrane should be intact and mobile. Tuning fork testing is performed and the results compared with those obtained preoperatively. If the middle ear space is incompletely aerated, positive nasal pressure (Valsalva maneuver) is occasionally used to aerate the middle ear space. No additional drops are used if the canal and tympanic membrane are well epithelialized. Otherwise, drops are continued for approximately 2 to 3 weeks. The patient is instructed to continue avoiding getting water in the ear when showering until healing is complete (usually 1 month). Patients are instructed to use Vaseline on a cotton ball for protection from water.

Postoperative care of medial grafts is similar to that for myringoplasty. The lateral packing is removed 7 to 10 days later. Drops are used twice a day, and the patient is instructed to keep the ear dry. For all techniques, the patient returns in approximately 3 to 4 weeks or at a total of 5 to 6 weeks after surgery. If healing is adequate, audiometric testing is performed at that time.

PEARLS

- Anticipate and inform patients who may not achieve successful tympanoplasty repair, including those who have failed multiple previous procedures; patients with severe contralateral atelectasis, middle ear effusion, or otorrhea; and those with obvious sources of eustachian tube dysfunction, such as abnormalities of the soft palate.
- Preparation and trimming of the skin should be done under the microscope to ensure that no unfurled edges are present.

- If there is insufficient skin to provide coverage of the bony canal, a thin split-thickness skin graft (Thiersch graft) from the non–hair-bearing postauricular skin is used.
- Place an accurately sized graft that just overlaps the anterior annulus to avoid blunting.
- Once the medial packing is removed from the ear canal, diligent local care of the external canal is necessary to avoid midcanal stenosis.

PITFALLS

- Incision into and exposure of the cartilage of the external canal may result in pain and possibly chondritis.
- Leaving remnants of epithelium from the tympanic membrane or on the anterior inferior sulcus when elevating the external canal skin from the medial canal can result in residual drum or canal cholesteatoma.
- Injury to the chorda tympani nerve results in sensation disturbances of the tongue, especially taste.
- The ear canal may attempt to heal with cicatricial midcanal soft tissue stenosis.
- Failure to recognized significant mucosal disease or compromised eustachian tube function will probably result in graft failure.

References

1. Zollner F: The principles of plastic surgery of the sound-conducting apparatus. J Laryngol Otol 69:637-652, 1955.
2. Wullstein H: Theory and practice of tympanoplasty. Laryngoscope 66:1076-1093, 1956.
3. McGrew BM, Jackson CG, Glasscock ME 3rd: Impact of mastoidectomy on simple tympanic membrane perforation repair. Laryngoscope 114:506-511, 2004.
4. Collins WO, Telischi FF, Balkany TJ, Buchman CA: Pediatric tympanoplasty: Effect of contralateral ear status on outcomes. Arch Otolaryngol Head Neck Surg 129:646-651, 2003.
5. Dornhoffer J: Cartilage tympanoplasty: Indications, techniques, and outcomes in a 1,000-patient series. Laryngoscope 113:1844-1856, 2003.
6. Tarabichi M: Endoscopic management of limited attic cholesteatoma. Laryngoscope 114:1157-1162, 2004.

Chapter 114

Ossicular Chain Reconstruction

Barry E. Hirsch

Conductive hearing loss results from restriction of sound wave energy in displacing the basilar membrane of the organ of Corti. Conductive hearing loss not of middle ear or tympanic membrane origin can result from obstruction in the external auditory canal and possibly from fluid distention within the inner ear, such as that seen in early Meniere's disease. Inner ear conductive hearing loss also occurs when a "third window" exists in the otic capsule. Dehiscence of the superior semicircular canal provides a site for expansion of inner ear fluid, which prevents the fluid wave from providing full stimulation to the basilar membrane of the cochlea. This may result in conductive hearing loss even though acoustic reflexes will still be present.

Conductive hearing loss of middle ear origin may be congenital or acquired and results from ossicular chain fixation, erosion, dislocation, or fracture. Ossicular chain reconstruction (OCR) re-establishes the sound-transforming mechanism to provide a mobile connection from the tympanic membrane through an aerated middle ear space to the perilymph. This chapter focuses on the surgical techniques for OCR. Tympanic membrane grafting, surgery for stapes fixation secondary to otosclerosis, and chronic otitis media with cholesteatoma are addressed in other chapters.

The term *tympanoplasty* describes procedures that address the status of the middle ear from the tympanic membrane to the vestibule. OCR is frequently performed in conjunction with tympanic membrane grafting for eliminating middle ear and mastoid disease. Zollner and Wullstein were early pioneers in the concepts of middle ear reconstructive surgery.[1,2] Wullstein provided a classification system consisting of five types (I to V) of tympanoplasty that focus on reconstruction with the remaining ossicular chain. Each type refers to the most lateral intact structure that remains connected to the inner ear on which the tympanic membrane is grafted or the ossicular chain reconstructed. Type I tympanoplasty indicates that all three ossicles are present and mobile. Thus, OCR is not needed. In type II tympanoplasty, the tympanic membrane is grafted to an intact incus and stapes. In practice, the need for type II tympanoplasty is rarely encountered. According to Wullstein, a type III tympanoplasty exists when an intact mobile stapes superstructure is present and the tympanic membrane or graft remains directly on the stapes superstructure. Type IV tympanoplasty describes an absent or eroded superstructure with the graft or tympanic membrane overlying a mobile stapes footplate. Type V tympanoplasty refers to a fenestration created in the horizontal semicircular canal (Fig. 114-1).

Use of this classification system was subsequently encouraged by Farrior,[3] who clarified the terminology by basing the type of OCR on the pathologic anatomy at the completion of surgery rather than the method of reconstruction used. According to Farrior, type III tympanoplasty refers to establishing continuity of the stapes to the more lateral tympanic membrane or malleus by interposing a sculpted ossicle, bone, or other alloplastic material. A type IV tympanoplasty denotes reconstruction of the ossicular chain from a mobile stapes footplate to the malleus, tympanic membrane, graft, or rarely, the incus. Type V tympanoplasty has been subdivided into types Va and Vb. Type Va designates a true fenestration procedure into the horizontal canal, whereas type Vb implies that the footplate is fixed or absent. After the vestibule is sealed with a tissue graft, continuity is restored from the oval window to the incus, malleus, tympanic membrane, or graft. Technically, stapedectomy would be characterized as a type Vb tympanoplasty, but this terminology is not proposed for otosclerosis surgery.

This classification system is supplemented by describing the method of reconstruction used for each case. This is applied particularly to type III tympanoplasty. The most common type III tympanoplasty performed is an incus interposition with the patient's own incus (autograft). We had used homograft (cadaver)

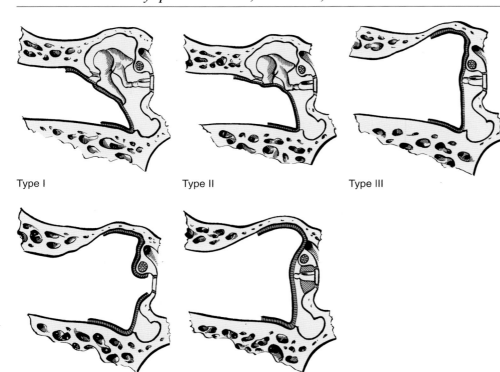

Type I   Type II   Type III

Type IV   Type V

Figure 114-1. The Wullstein classification of types of tympanoplasty. *(From Kley W: Surgical treatment of chronic otitis media and its immediate consequences. In Naumann HH [ed]: Head and Neck Surgery, vol 3: Ear. Stuttgart, Germany, Georg Thieme, 1982, p 221.)*

ossicles in the past, but concern regarding possible infection or contamination with viral or prion particles has eliminated their use. A type III tympanoplasty with stapes augmentation entails increasing the height of the stapes above the fallopian canal when a canal wall–down mastoidectomy is performed and the malleus is absent. This technique frequently uses the body of the incus, the head of the malleus, or a cortical bone graft. We use the term *partial ossicular replacement prosthesis* (PORP) when a synthetic biocompatible prosthesis is positioned from the stapes superstructure to the tympanic membrane, graft, or malleus. Types IV and Vb tympanoplasty are performed with either a *total ossicular replacement prosthesis* (TORP) or the patient's own incus from the footplate or grafted oval window to the malleus, tympanic membrane, or graft.

PATIENT SELECTION

OCR is performed for conductive hearing loss or when the ossicular chain must be disarticulated for access to other middle ear pathology. A chief complaint of hearing loss may result from trauma, chronic eustachian tube dysfunction, congenital anomalies, chronic otitis media, tumors of the middle ear space, or ossicular chain fixation resulting from tympanosclerosis. Physical examination may demonstrate an intact or perforated tympanic membrane. It is important to examine the contralateral ear, which provides a means of predicting the likelihood of successful tympanoplasty and OCR when eustachian tube function is compromised.

Patients sustaining head trauma with fractures involving the temporal bone may present with a conductive, sensorineural, or mixed hearing loss. Hemotympanum often occurs but is usually resorbed in 4 to 6 weeks. This time frame is necessary to determine the type and degree of residual hearing loss after return of middle ear aeration. The anatomy of the external canal should be examined along with the integrity of the tympanic membrane. Pneumatic otoscopy is useful for confirming a small tympanic membrane perforation by demonstrating lack of mobility. Myringosclerosis can also restrict movement of the tympanic membrane. In contrast, hypermobility suggests a flaccid membrane or possible fracture of the malleus handle. Tuning forks are used to both confirm the presence and estimate the magnitude of a conductive hearing loss.

Pure-tone audiometry is performed to determine the degree of conductive hearing loss and the quality of cochlear function. A persistent conductive hearing loss typically indicates ossicular chain disruption. This may be repaired electively or rehabilitated by aural amplification. Patients demonstrating a large mixed hearing loss should be considered surgical candidates for OCR (Fig. 114-2). In patients with significant mixed hearing loss, bone-windowed thin-cut computed tomography (CT) helps define the status of the cochlea, ossicles, and middle ear space. Disruption of the ossicular chain can be demonstrated in these scans (Fig. 114-3). Patients with severe to profound mixed hearing loss may have hearing aid tolerance problems. Closing the air-bone gap restores hearing thresholds to levels at which routine hearing aid amplification is more feasi-

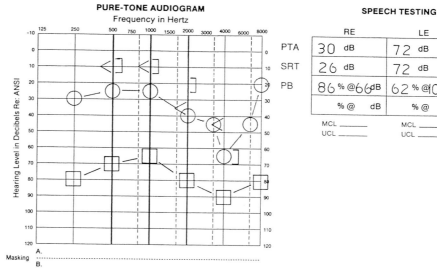

PURE-TONE AUDIOGRAM
Frequency in Hertz

SPEECH TESTING

	RE	LE	MASK
PTA	30 dB	72 dB	
SRT	26 dB	72 dB	
PB	86 % @66dB	62 % @102dB	
	% @ dB	% @ dB	

MCL _____   MCL _____
UCL _____   UCL _____

Figure 114-2. The audiogram shows a left moderate to severe mixed hearing loss with fair word recognition. Options for rehabilitation include amplification or ossicular chain reconstruction. ANSI, American National Standards Institute; LE, left ear; MCL, most comfortable loudness level; PB, phonetic balance; PTA, pure-tone average; RE, right ear; SRT, speech reception threshold; UCL, uncomfortable loudness level.

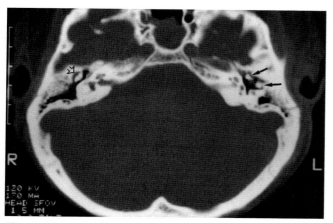

Figure 114-3. Computed tomography scan demonstrating temporal bone trauma with disruption of the ossicular chain. The normal incudomalleus complex is indicated with the *open arrow*. The *solid arrows* identify the separated malleus and incus.

ble. OCR may not be warranted in patients with cochlear concussion and poor speech discrimination.

Patients undergoing tympanoplasty with or without mastoidectomy and are found to have significant middle ear mucosal disease may not be ideal candidates for immediate reconstruction. On occasion, the procedure is staged in anticipation of achieving an aerated middle ear space with healthier mucosa. Our philosophy on staging the procedure has evolved over the past 2 decades. It was our routine approach to remove pathologic disease, reconstruct the ossicular chain, and graft the tympanic membrane in one procedure. We believed that recurrent or persistent disease would become evident by the findings of subsequent progressive conductive hearing loss, recurrent otorrhea, or evidence of cholesteatoma in an ear with cholesteatoma as the original pathology. Our approach has been modified slightly based on the findings in the middle ear and the age of

the patient. In initial procedures or operations performed on young people in whom taking the canal wall down would minimize the likelihood of persistent disease, we would attempt total removal of the disease and keep the canal wall intact but plan to re-explore the ear in 6 to 12 months.

A staged procedure is performed when cholesteatoma is mixed within granulation tissue around the stapes footplate and superstructure and cannot be completely removed. Another situation follows removal of thickened hyperplastic inflamed mucosa from the promontory and eustachian tube orifice when a large graft to the tympanic membrane is necessary. If the incus or head of the malleus is available and free of disease (cholesteatoma), it is removed and banked for planned subsequent reconstruction. A piece of sculpted Silastic sheeting (0.02 to 0.04 inch) with a rounded tip extending into epitympanum is place over the promontory. The video shows a disc of reinforced Silastic sheeting being placed on the promontory and medial to the malleus (see Video 114-1). A fascia graft is positioned lateral to the Silastic and rests on the bony annulus (see Video 114-2). Placement of the Silastic block over a mobile stapes superstructure occasionally provides an effective columellar connection between the stapes and the tympanic membrane and results in near closure of the air-bone gap. If good hearing has been achieved with the initial procedure, re-exploration is not mandatory unless concern exists about residual or recurrent disease.

On rare occasion, reconstruction at a subsequent staged procedure may not require access through the external auditory canal and tympanic membrane. If the original tympanomastoidectomy procedure entailed opening the facial recess, it is possible to reconstruct the ossicular chain from the postauricular approach. Endoscopes may be necessary to fully evaluate the attic and mesotympanum. This technique allows improvement in hearing and avoids canal incisions, middle ear packing, and restrictions from water exposure.[4]

In keeping with otologic principles, the surgeon is cautioned about operating on the better-hearing ear. As with all rules, there are exceptions. Surgical intervention could be considered in a better-hearing ear if other pathologic findings are present, such as cholesteatoma in the involved ear. However, the status of the contralateral ear is most important to consider.

Age does not impose a limitation for tympanoplasty and OCR. In children who do not have a recent history of recurrent episodes of otitis media and demonstrate a dry ipsilateral perforation and normal contralateral ear on physical examination, it can be assumed that eustachian tube function is competent and they are candidates for tympanoplasty. Similarly, elderly patients in good health have the option of amplification or middle ear reconstruction.

The decision regarding elective reconstruction for conductive hearing loss remains with the patient. If there is no evidence of active infection, potential tumor, or cholesteatoma, the option of hearing aid amplification should be discussed. If a patient has chronic otitis media with perforation and it is believed that a hearing aid would exacerbate the underlying disease and promote drainage, appropriate counseling should be given.

Patients with a large conductive loss in the involved ear and normal hearing in the contralateral ear require further counseling. Despite a technically successful operation, complete closure of the air-bone gap is frequently not achieved in some type III and more complicated reconstructive procedures. Although hearing can be improved substantially, a residual difference between the two ears may be perceived by the patient as being an unsuccessful result. Realistic expectations must be conveyed when discussing anticipated goals of the procedure.

It may be difficult to decide what to recommend to patients with residual conductive hearing loss who have undergone previous attempts at OCR. Although previous operative dictations are occasionally unreliable, in this situation it is often helpful to review them. Nearly complete closure of the air-bone gap should be anticipated with a type I tympanoplasty. Patients with a type III or IV tympanoplasty and residual conductive hearing loss of 15 to 20 dB with normal hearing on the contralateral side may desire further improvement. Surgeons must have an appreciation of the hearing results before contemplating revision surgery.

PREOPERATIVE PLANNING

Physical examination of the external auditory canal and tympanic membrane is important in determining the status of the ear. Primary inflammation of the skin of the external canal or inflammation secondary to disease from the middle ear requires medical management to optimize postoperative healing. A few weeks of topical and systemic antibiotics may be necessary. The integrity of the tympanic membrane and middle ear space is noted. Tuning fork testing with 256-, 512-, and 1024-Hz forks is performed to determine whether a conductive

hearing loss is present and to estimate the degree of loss. The most commonly used frequency is 512 Hz. Obtaining an audiogram is mandatory to establish the nature and degree of the conductive hearing loss and cochlear function. Patients with an intact tympanic membrane, no history of chronic ear disease, and progressive conductive hearing loss most likely have otosclerosis. Fixation of the lateral ossicular chain is relatively uncommon. An astute clinician may detect decreased mobility of the malleus during pneumatic otoscopy. It is typically diagnosed at the time of exploratory tympanotomy. The cause may be congenital. Delayed lateral chain fixation is probably due to tympanosclerosis secondary to chronic inflammation of the middle ear. Acoustic reflexes should be absent in the setting of conductive hearing loss caused by pathology within the middle ear. Dehiscence of the superior semicircular canal may give findings of conductive hearing loss of inner ear origin. Acoustic reflexes are characteristically present in this form of conductive hearing loss. We now request acoustic reflex testing of patients with conductive hearing loss and an intact tympanic membrane.

CT is not routinely performed unless symptoms or signs of complications of chronic otitis media and cholesteatoma are present, including asymmetrical cochlear function, dizziness, severe headaches, facial paresis, or cerebrospinal fluid otorrhea. Repair of congenital atresia also requires CT scanning to define the otic capsule, middle ear space, ossicular chain, bony plate, and course of the facial nerve. This topic is covered more thoroughly in Chapter 111.

The method for providing anesthesia is dictated by the status of the tympanic membrane, the presumed status of the ossicular chain, the presence or absence of inflammatory middle ear disease, the anticipated approach, the patient's tolerance for a procedure under sedation, and the experience of the surgeon. Patients with an intact tympanic membrane and conductive hearing loss can undergo an endaural approach under local anesthesia and intravenous sedation. General anesthesia is recommended for children and patients with a tympanic membrane perforation who require a postauricular approach. Facial nerve monitoring is not used for routine tympanoplasty procedures; however, monitoring is indicated for patients with evidence of facial nerve signs of weakness, fasciculations, or spasm and during procedures for repair of congenital aural atresia. Antibiotics are not given perioperatively. As with all procedures, the patient is informed of the risks, benefits, and alternative treatments.

PROSTHESIS OPTIONS AND ADJUNCTIVE TECHNIQUES

Over the past 60 years there have been significant advances in the development and application of new materials available for reconstruction of the ossicular chain. In a poll of members of the American Otologic Society published in 2001, hydroxyapatite was the preferred alloplastic material because it provided biocompatibility, rigidity for sound transmission, durability, longevity, ease of use, and good hearing results.[5] Plastipore prostheses, which had been widely used in the latter part of the past century, were reported to have the lowest satisfaction rate, of all prostheses.

The newest material currently available is titanium, which is lightweight, has great tensile strength, and is rigid yet slightly malleable. It requires a cartilage interface between the prosthesis and the tympanic membrane. The design for partial prostheses incorporated a bell-shaped configuration that fits over the stapes superstructure (Fig. 114-4). Jackson and colleagues compared titanium with synthetic non–titanium-based prostheses and showed improved hearing outcomes with titanium prostheses but thought that there was a minimal learning curve needed to successfully achieve closure of the air-bone gap.[6] A consortium of otologists from different regions of the United States were similarly in favor of titanium prostheses given their good hearing results and low rate of extrusion.[7] Our only reservation with using this material is the requirement for a cartilage graft under the tympanic membrane. This inhibits visual monitoring of the middle ear for recurrent cholesteatoma after surgery for that pathology.

The use of bone cement in skull base surgery and cranioplasty has led to applications in otology and reconstruction of the ossicular chain. The chemical composition of these products includes hydroxyapatite, cyanoacrylates, polymethyl methacrylates, and glass ionomers. Great care must be taken with the latter product to avoid contact with any neural tissue because of the severe neurologic complications that can occur from aluminum being leached from the product. A study using SerenoCem (Corinthian Laboratory, Nottingham, UK) for repair of an eroded incus confirmed that the product was not exothermic when reconsti-tuted but required at least 20 minutes to harden in a dry operative field.[8]

Hydroxyapatite bone cement is available from numerous manufacturers. It too is minimally exothermic, is malleable for a few minutes, sets in 4 to 6 minutes, and undergoes osteointegration over time. It can provide an adjunct or alternative to ossiculoplasty with preformed prostheses. Goebel and Jacob reported successful use of hydroxyapatite bone cement in challenging cases with difficult ossicular reconstruction.[9] The products currently available include Mimix (Walter Lorenz Surgical, Jacksonville, FL), BoneSource (Stryker Leibinger, Portage, MI), and Norian (Synthes USA, Paoli, PA).

SURGICAL TECHNIQUES

The approaches to and methods for tympanic membrane grafting are reviewed in Chapter 113. Frequently, the preoperative status of the ossicular chain is unknown when correction of conductive hearing loss is attempted. The surgeon must be prepared to have access to the entire ossicular chain. When elevating a tympanomeatal flap, the superior limb of the incision should be superior to the pars flaccida and approximately 4 to 5 mm from the posterosuperior annulus (Fig. 114-5). This longer flap permits removal of bone from this area to provide exposure of the malleus neck and the entire stapes footplate and to gain access for removal of the body of the incus, if necessary.

Reconstruction of the tympanic membrane and ossicular chain demands a precise and stable connection between the drum and the stapes or footplate. The reconstructed ossicle or prosthesis should not make direct contact with the surrounding tympanic ring, which would restrict transmission of sound to the cochlea. A prosthesis that is too short will have a tendency to fall or become displaced. On the other hand, excessive length and poor eustachian tube dysfunction

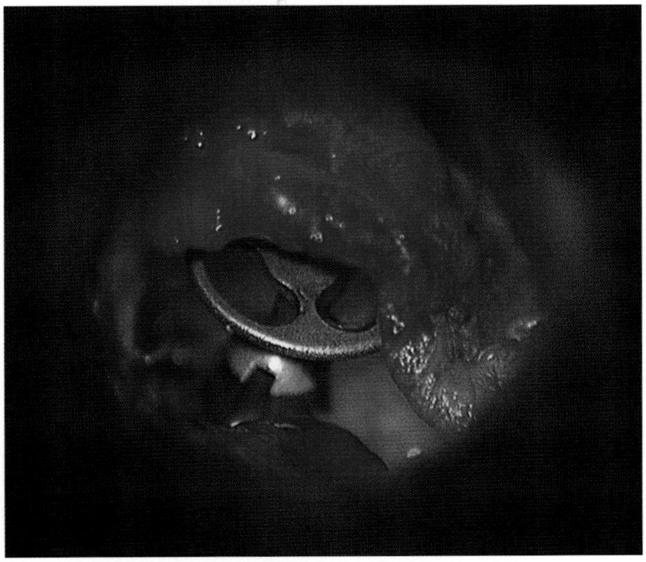

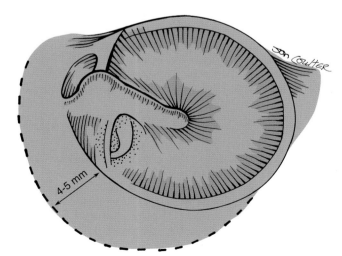

Figure 114-4. Titanium partial ossicular replacement prosthesis with a cage or bell that fits over the stapes superstructure.

Figure 114-5. The tympanomeatal incision for exploratory tympanotomy should be 4 to 5 mm away from the posterosuperior annulus.

4-5 mm

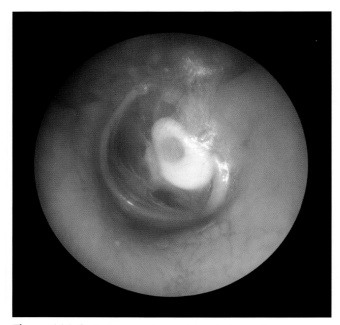

Figure 114-6. Hydroxyapatite partial ossicular replacement prosthesis making direct contact with the tympanic membrane. Note the very slight tenting over the prosthesis.

set the stage for extrusion of the prosthesis. The prosthesis should not only touch the tympanic membrane but should also be under slight tension to create minimal tenting of the tympanic membrane over the prosthesis (Fig. 114-6). The following text focuses on isolated problems encountered in OCR and the methods and techniques for reconstruction.

Problems with the Incus

The most commonly encountered abnormality in the ossicular chain involves the incus. Rarely, it is manifested as incudomalleal fusion or fixation. More commonly, the long process and lenticular process of the incus are eroded or connected by a fibrous union (Fig. 114-7). In patients with an intact mobile malleus and stapes, incus interposition is the most commonly used method for OCR. This technique has been used for the past 50 years. A variety of techniques are available for modification of the incus to provide a mobile yet firm connection from the stapes superstructure to the malleus. The surgeon should note the status of the middle ear mucosa and the relationship of the malleus to the stapes.

The stapes may be located directly medial to the handle of the malleus. The other anatomic variation occurs when the malleus is located anterior to the vertical plane of the stapes. This relationship is important in determining how the incus will be sculpted so that it can be interposed between the stapes and the malleus (Fig. 114-8). In addition, the height of the stapes relative to the promontory and facial nerve is noted. This is more of an issue when disease in the middle ear and mastoid requires a canal wall–down mastoidectomy. The patient's incus (autograft) is usually available for

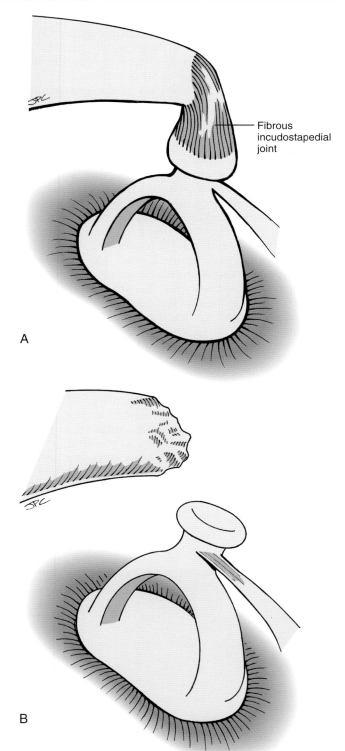

Fibrous incudostapedial joint

A

B

Figure 114-7. A, Erosion of the lenticular process with a residual fibrous joint. **B,** Erosion of the long process of the incus.

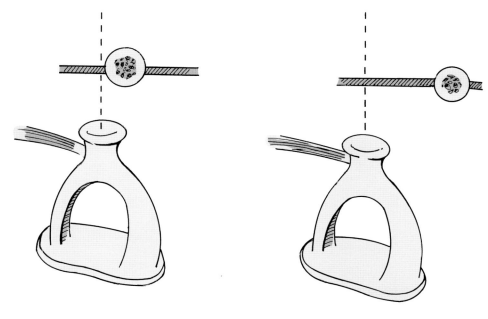

Figure 114-8. The position of the malleus relative to the stapes determines how the incus will be sculpted to perform an interposition. **Left,** The malleus is located lateral to the stapes. **Right,** Reconstruction requires augmenting the vertical height of the stapes and its anterior span to the malleus.

reconstruction, but it may be necessary to remove additional bone from the posterosuperior canal to extract the incus. A right-angled hook or curved needle is used to disarticulate any remaining attachments of the incus body to the malleus head. Cup forceps are used to grasp the proximal long process of the incus. With a rotating downward maneuver the surgeon extracts the incus from the epitympanum entering into the middle ear (Fig. 114-9) (see Video 114-3). Care is taken to avoid displacement of the stapes superstructure and injury to the chorda tympani nerve.

Various designs for sculpting an incus for interpositioning between the stapes and the malleus are demonstrated in Figure 114-10. The incus should be held with an instrument such as a fine hemostat or forceps designed for holding ossicles (Fig. 114-11). Should the incus be inadequate because of significant erosion or infiltration by cholesteatoma, we had used a homograft incus in the past but now use a synthetic PORP prosthesis. If a mastoidectomy had been performed, the same variable high-speed drill is used for incus sculpting. Otherwise, a battery-powered microdrill is used (see Video 114-4).

When the stapes and malleus are in a nearly vertical plane, height is needed to connect the two ossicles. The acetabulum for the stapes head is drilled into the short process of the incus. A groove for the malleus handle is created in the articulating surface of the incus body. This is initially positioned underneath the malleus handle, and the malleus-incus complex is lifted and rolled onto the stapes (Fig. 114-12). A very common configuration is one used to gain some height and horizontal span. The acetabulum for the stapes is created in the body of the incus near its junction with the long process (Fig. 114-13A). A more oval aperture is drilled to accommodate the shoulder of the crura (see Fig. 114-13B). Care must be taken to ensure that the undersurface of the short process of the incus is not resting

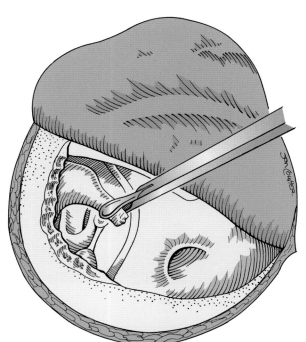

Figure 114-9. The incus body is disarticulated from the malleus head and extracted with cup forceps.

on the promontory of the cochlea. With all interpositioning techniques, placement of the incus superior or inferior to the chorda tympani nerve can provide further support to the sculpted ossicle (see Fig. 114-13C). When considerable height is needed to be bridged, the incus is configured as shown in Figure 114-14A. This relationship can be appreciated when the tympanic membrane is atrophic and translucent (see Fig. 114-14B).

Occasionally, the incus is eroded just at the incudostapedial joint (see Fig. 114-7). Rather than removing

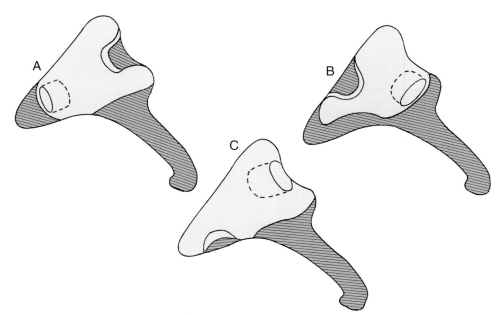

Figure 114-10. The incus body can be sculpted in a variety of forms to accommodate each particular relationship between the malleus and stapes. **A,** Gains vertical height. **B,** Gains some vertical height and mostly horizontal span. **C,** Gains mostly vertical height and some horizontal span.

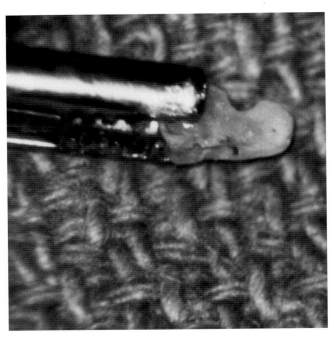

Figure 114-11. Ossicle holder firmly grasping a sculpted incus.

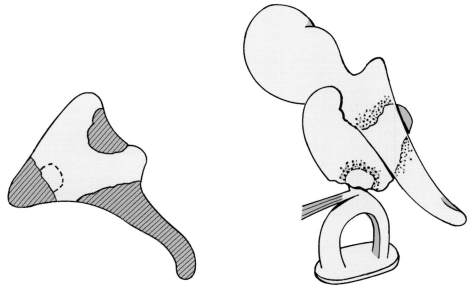

Figure 114-12. Incus interposition to gain height from the stapes to the malleus.

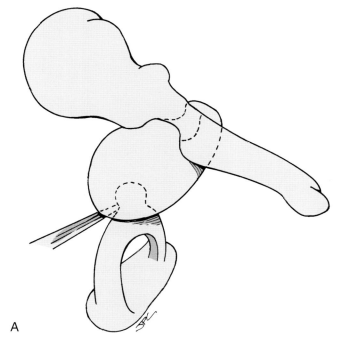

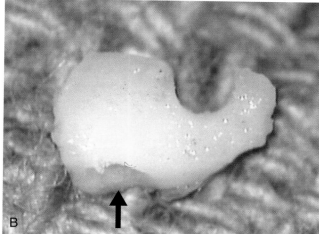

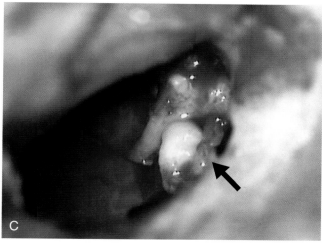

Figure 114-13. A, Incus interpositioning to gain some height and mostly horizontal span. **B,** The sculpted incus has an oval aperture that fits snugly on the stapes *(arrow).* **C,** In a left ear, the incus has been positioned superior to the stapes and medial to the malleus handle. The chorda tympani nerve provides additional support *(arrow).*

the incus, an alternative method for reconstructing this joint is to use an Applebaum hydroxyapatite prosthesis. This prosthesis fits on the stapes superstructure and supports the remaining long process of the incus (Fig. 114-15) (see Video 114-5).

Type III tympanoplasty is also performed with synthetic prostheses. Products containing hydroxyapatite are well tolerated. A cartilage interface between the dense hydroxyapatite prosthetic head and the tympanic membrane or graft is not needed. The shafts are made of a combination of hydroxyapatite and polyethylene or fluoroplastic. In a technique similar to that used for incus interpositioning, a PORP can be positioned from the stapes to the mobile membrane (Fig. 114-16). It can easily be shortened to provide the appropriate distance from the stapes to the malleus handle and tympanic membrane (see Video 114-6). We do not strictly apply

the terms *PORP* and *TORP* to indicate ossicular reconstruction directly to the tympanic membrane or its graft. We use the terms *PORP* and *TORP* synonymously with *incus replacement prosthesis* and *incus-stapes replacement prosthesis,* respectively. The malleus may be present and can provide further support for the prosthesis.

Reconstruction of the ossicular chain in patients undergoing a canal wall–down mastoidectomy may also require a type III tympanoplasty. After the head of the malleus is removed, a connection from the stapes to the malleus handle is necessary. This can be accomplished with incus interposition techniques or with a synthetic prosthesis. When the level of the tympanic membrane is displaced medially because of an absent malleus, minimal height is needed for the stapes to reach the tympanic membrane. The membrane could be grafted directly onto the stapes superstructure as described by

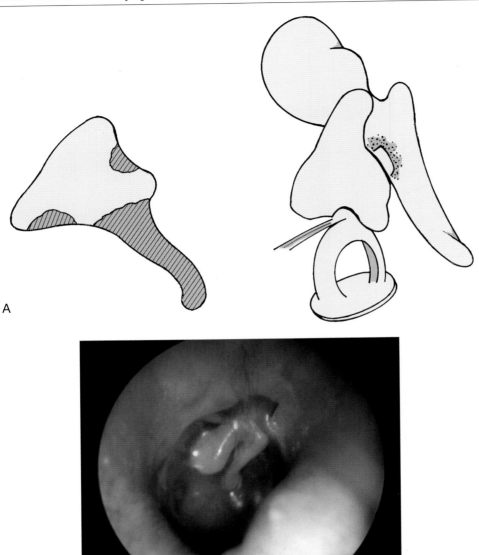

A

Figure 114-14. A, Incus interposition to gain mostly vertical height and some horizontal span. **B,** Postoperative photograph of a right ear with a translucent tympanic membrane. A groove was drilled into the short process of the incus so that it can rest against the neck of the malleus.

B

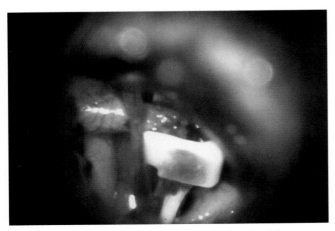

Figure 114-15. Intraoperative photograph of an Applebaum prosthesis placed between the stapes and an eroded long process of the incus.

Wullstein. However, greater surface contact is achieved when an ossicular graft is placed on the stapes. The body of the incus, the head of the malleus, or a small cortical bone graft harvested from the root of the zygoma or the outer table of the squamosa portion of the temporal bone can be drilled to form a dome for the stapes superstructure (Fig. 114-17).

Under high magnification, the relationship of the facial nerve and horizontal semicircular canal to the height of the stapes can be appreciated. When the tympanic membrane or graft is returned to cover the middle ear, it is supported laterally by the horizontal semicircular canal and the facial ridge. The height of the stapes must be augmented to make better contact with the tympanic membrane (Fig. 114-18). The vertical height of a PORP is too great in this situation. It cannot be trimmed sufficiently to provide the necessary height of 2 to 3 mm.

On rare occasion, the malleus can be directly attached to the stapes superstructure. This situation occurs in a canal wall–down procedure when the incus is absent and the stapes superstructure is intact. If the malleus remains attached to the tympanic membrane along the distal handle and umbo, its attachment to the tensor tympani tendon can be divided and the malleus rotated posteriorly and placed on top of the stapes.

Problems with the Stapes

If the stapes superstructure is partially eroded, interposing an ossicle or prosthesis from the stapes arch or one of its crura will probably fail. Reconstruction from the undersurface of the malleus to the mobile stapes footplate provides a more secure connection of the ossicular chain.

An autograft incus occasionally provides adequate length to meet these requirements. The distance should be measured before sculpting the incus. The size of the incus from the short process to its articulating surface often satisfies the length needed from the footplate to the undersurface of the malleus.

The incus is sculpted by flattening the short process to rest on the stapes footplate. A groove in the articulating surface of the incus is further defined to secure the incus to the medial surface of the malleus (Fig. 114-19A). Additional length is available when the long process of the incus remains. The lenticular process is removed, and the groove for the malleus is drilled on the superior surface of the incus (see Fig. 114-19B) (see Video 114-7). The sculpted ossicle is placed on the footplate between the remaining crura. While the malleus handle is lifted, the incus is rotated into position (Fig. 114-20). The chorda tympani nerve can be positioned to further secure the ossicular assembly.

When the oval window niche is narrow and deep, a wide incus body may have to be thinned to fit between the promontory and the facial nerve. More often, a synthetic prosthesis is necessary. The principle for reconstruction is connection of the malleus to the footplate. Any columella-type prosthesis can be used. In the past, a stainless steel wire incus replacement prosthesis was fashioned from the neck of the malleus to the footplate. However, placement of this prosthesis was technically difficult and occasionally resulted in extrusion.

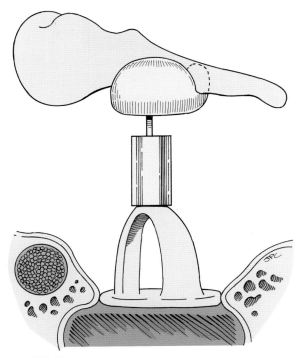

Figure 114-16. A partial ossicular replacement prosthesis is positioned between the stapes and the malleus handle. It can be placed directly onto the medial surface of the tympanic membrane or graft without intervening cartilage when the dome of the prosthesis is made of hydroxyapatite.

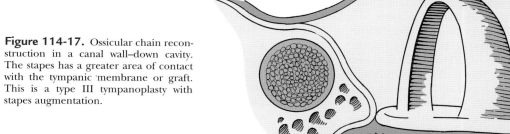
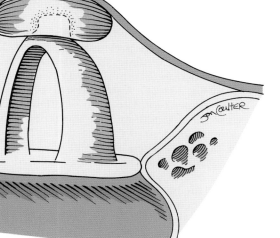

Figure 114-17. Ossicular chain reconstruction in a canal wall–down cavity. The stapes has a greater area of contact with the tympanic membrane or graft. This is a type III tympanoplasty with stapes augmentation.

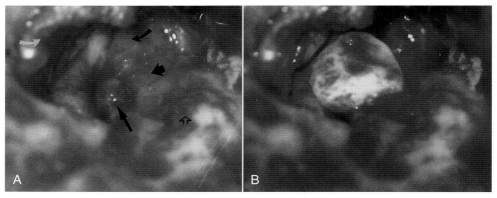

Figure 114-18. A, Left ear, canal wall–down mastoidectomy in preparation for ossicular chain reconstruction. Note that the stapes head *(long arrow)* is at the level of the tympanic segment of the facial nerve *(short arrow).* The tympanic membrane *(curved white arrow)* will rest on the facial ridge and the horizontal semicircular canal *(open arrow).* The cochleariform process is identified *(curved black arrow).* **B,** A sculpted cortical bone graft is placed as a dome over the stapes. This augments the height of the stapes and provides greater surface contact with the tympanic membrane.

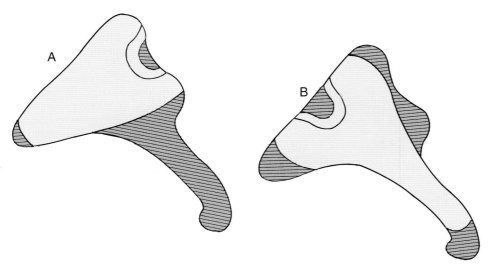

Figure 114-19. Techniques for sculpting the incus for a type IV tympanoplasty. **A,** The short process of the incus is flattened. The long process is removed and a groove drilled for the malleus handle. **B,** The long process is flattened, and the notch for the malleus handle is on the superior surface of the incus.

Materials such as polytetrafluoroethylene, titanium, Polycel with wire, and prefabricated prostheses of hydroxyapatite are currently available.

We currently use either a titanium prosthesis or one with a dense hydroxyapatite dome attached to a shaft that can be trimmed easily. This is the same composition as the PORPs previously described. The TORP is secured from the stapes footplate to the malleus in a manner similar to that for a type IV tympanoplasty with an incus (Fig. 114-21). A straight strut of hydroxyapatite from the stapes footplate to the malleus neck has also been used. The length must be shortened appropriately to permit placement of this prosthesis. We have experienced problems when the shaft was made of dense hydroxyapatite. This ceramic material had a tendency to shatter or crack when the length was shortened. This problem can be remedied by holding the prosthesis firmly between one's thumb and forefinger. The shaft can then be shortened with a fine diamond burr drill and drip irrigation. The shaft of the prostheses that we currently use is a combination of hydroxyapatite and polytetrafluoroethylene (Teflon). It is readily trimmable and does not osteointegrate when there is direct contact with the promontory.

Titanium prostheses are available in fixed lengths or with a trimmable shaft. A sizing set is used to determine the proper length needed. The video demonstrates use of a 5-mm sizing prosthesis to verify the appropriate length needed for the prosthesis implanted (see Video 114-8).

Type IV tympanoplasty often requires temporary support of the prosthesis. Wet Gelfoam is placed around the shaft base up to the level of the facial nerve if the malleus handle is present. When the prosthesis is in direct contact with the tympanic membrane, as will be described, Gelfoam is positioned around the entire prosthesis to the level of the tympanic membrane (see Video 114-9).

Problems with the Malleus

A relatively uncommon source of conductive hearing loss is fixation of the malleus and incus, also known as

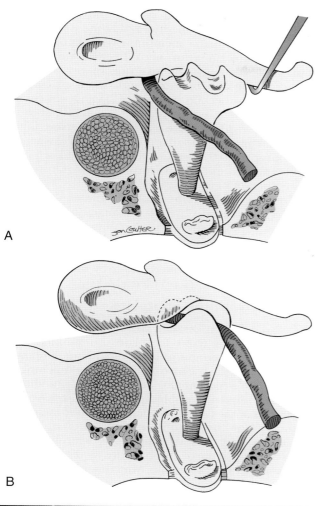

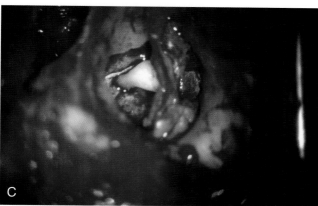

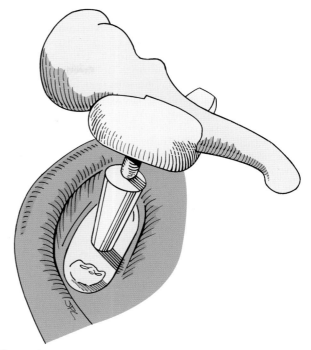

Figure 114-21. Type IV tympanoplasty from the footplate to the malleus with an incus-stapes replacement prosthesis (total ossicular replacement prosthesis).

Figure 114-20. Type IV tympanoplasty with incus. **A,** The sculpted short process of the incus is placed on the stapes footplate. Note the small groove created for the chorda tympani nerve (shown in red). The malleus is lifted laterally to permit the incus to be rotated into position. **B,** The incus is secured between the footplate and the proximal malleus handle. The chorda tympani nerve provides additional support. **C,** Intraoperative photograph of a type IV tympanoplasty using the incus.

lateral chain fixation. This may entail ankylosis of the head of the malleus and body of the incus to the scutum, immobility of the incudomalleal joint, or calcification of the anterior malleus ligament restricting its movement.

A recently described technique for liberating the lateral ossicular chain addressed both the head of the malleus and the body of the incus in the epitympanum. A tympanomeatal flap is elevated beginning anterior to the malleus and extended more superiorly to provide access to the scutum. A laser was used to release the areas of bony fixation anterior to the malleus head and the superior body of the incus. A small drill provided greater space between the ossicles and surrounding bone, and a small piece of thin Silastic sheeting was placed to prevent refixation.[10] A problem with this technique is the possibility of contacting the ossicular chain with the drill and causing sensorineural hearing loss. Exposure of the epitympanum by removal of the scutum may also result in retraction of the pars flaccida and acquired cholesteatoma.

Our method for handling lateral chain fixation does not require as much exposure of the epitympanum, but the tympanomeatal flap must be designed to be superior to the pars flaccida. The flap is elevated anterior to the neck of the malleus. Palpation of the malleus confirms immobility of the lateral chain. It is necessary to separate the incudostapedial joint to ensure that limitation of movement is not being caused by otosclerosis. The joint between the malleus and incus is disarticulated with a curved pick to allow the entire incus to be removed (see Video 114-10).

Typically, fixation of the malleus persists. A 1-mm microdrill is used to divide the head of the malleus from its handle at the neck of the malleus. Care must be taken to avoid injury to the chorda tympani nerve, which runs just medial to the neck of the malleus. This technique creates a malleus handle that is mobile and supported by its attachment to the tympanic membrane and tensor tympani tendon. At this point the incus is sculpted and interposed between the head of the stapes and the handle of the malleus.

On rare occasion, the malleus handle alone may be absent or deficient. Difficulty arises in situations in which the malleus handle is shortened and the surgeon must decide whether its length is adequate to use for reconstruction. As a general rule, shortening beyond a third of its length will probably preclude satisfactory closure of the air-bone gap. This is a more difficult decision and a problem for reconstruction. Again, an incus interposition can be performed. However, the incus should be sculpted to maintain sufficient height for connecting the stapes superstructure to the grafted tympanic membrane. Improved transmission of tympanic membrane vibration is achieved by directing the position of the short process of the incus toward the center of the membrane.

When the malleus handle is absent, we more frequently use a synthetic prosthesis. In canal wall–up procedures, the remaining malleus head can be ignored. If the stapes superstructure is present, a PORP is used (Fig. 114-22). If the stapes superstructure is absent but the footplate is present and mobile, a TORP is placed (Fig. 114-23).

A unique situation arises when there is a total or near-total perforation of the tympanic membrane and all the ossicles are gone except for a mobile footplate. The options for reconstruction are grafting the tympanic membrane and placing a TORP from the footplate to the graft or placing a thick piece of Silastic sheeting (0.04 inch) in the middle ear, grafting the

tympanic membrane, and staging the procedure. A problem with the first method is that the final position of the grafted tympanic membrane is not known. It may heal in a more lateral or, more likely, a more medial position. This creates potential uncertainty about how to choose the appropriate length when placing the prosthesis. The second method of staging will circumvent this problem, but the patient is committed to two procedures. Unless there is minimal disease in the middle ear and the ossicular reconstruction can achieve the appropriate connection to the grafted tympanic membrane, we opt for performing the grafting and reconstruction in two stages.

On rare occasion, the malleus handle may be fractured. Preoperative physical examination with pneumatic otoscopy can show hypermobility of the tympanic membrane and malleus. If exploration and palpation of the malleus can verify this pathologic condition, reconstruction is performed either by incus interposition or with a PORP (see Video 114-11).

Problems with the Footplate

The most common cause of stapes footplate fixation is otosclerosis. If a fixed footplate is identified while repairing a perforation of the tympanic membrane, it is best to stage the reconstruction to avoid opening the vestibule to a potentially contaminated middle ear space. The same philosophy applies to extensive tympanosclerosis of the footplate when a tympanic membrane perforation or chronic otitis media is present. Tympanosclerosis describes deposition of sclerotic plaque after recurrent acute or chronic otitis media. This brittle calcification can restrict the tympanic membrane and ossicular chain. Movement of the stapes footplate can also be restricted by tympanosclerosis, which can be confirmed by gentle palpation of the stapes while observing for a round window reflex. If the tympanic membrane is perforated, it should be repaired and the operation staged for a subsequent procedure. Healing is typically complete within 4 to 6 months, at which time

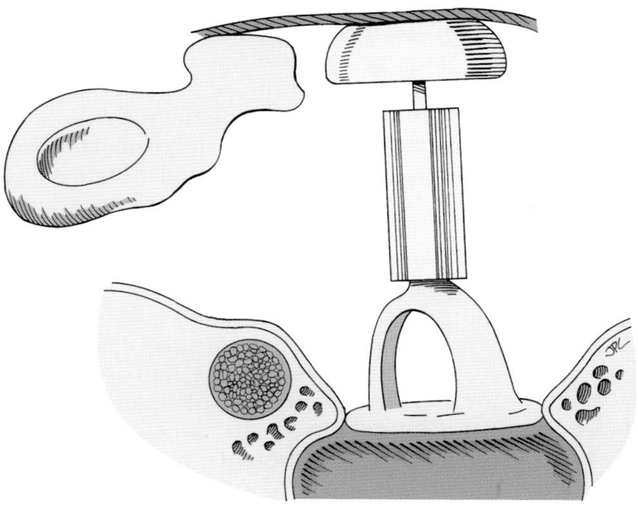

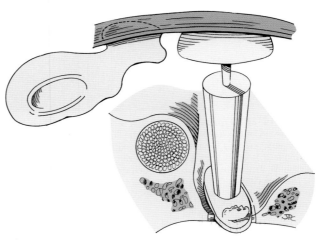

Figure 114-22. Type III tympanoplasty with a partial ossicular replacement prosthesis when the malleus is absent (stapes to the tympanic membrane or graft).

Figure 114-23. Type IV tympanoplasty with a total ossicular replacement prosthesis when the malleus handle is absent (stapes footplate to the tympanic membrane or graft).

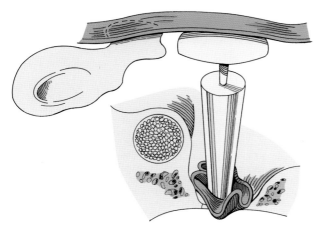

Figure 114-24. Type Vb tympanoplasty with a total ossicular replacement prosthesis. A graft covers the vestibule on which the shaft of the prosthesis is embedded. The dome of the prosthesis tents the grafted tympanic membrane. The malleus handle is absent.

the footplate can be safely addressed. There is controversy about how to best manage the stapes when it becomes fixed by this process. Options include not intervening surgically and providing amplification, performing stapes mobilization, or removing the footplate (stapedectomy) and placing a prosthesis. The concern for mobilization is based on the possibility of refixation of the stapes by new plaque formation. If the status of the ear disease is stable, both short- and long-term hearing results are similar, thus indicating that refixation is unlikely to occur after mobilization. It has also been shown when tympanosclerosis affects the footplate, stapedectomy in a sterile middle ear is a safe and effective procedure.[11]

In cases of chronic otitis media with cholesteatoma, the stapes footplate may be eroded. If the vestibule is opened inadvertently or by disease, OCR is warranted at that time. It is rare to have such extensive disease yet still have an intact incus. Therefore, reconstruction is frequently done from the vestibule to the malleus, tympanic membrane, or graft (type Vb tympanoplasty). The vestibule is covered with a thin but strong graft that will support a prosthesis. The grafted tympanic membrane may heal in a more medial position when exposed to the negative pressure of the middle ear space. This puts further demand on the support needed from the oval window graft. If there is concern that the prosthesis may sublux into the vestibule, a perichondrial graft is harvested from the posterior conchal cartilage or the tragus. Otherwise, true fascia is obtained from the temporalis muscle. The graft is air-dried, cut to approximately 3 × 4 mm, and placed over the vestibule. The shaft of the prosthesis is placed in the center of the graft and the cap or dome is positioned under the malleus handle or directly to the grafted tympanic membrane (Fig. 114-24).

POSTOPERATIVE MANAGEMENT

The principles of care and instructions given to patients postoperatively are similar to those after tympanoplasty.

Patients are instructed to keep the ear free of water and avoid blowing the nose or other forms of Valsalva maneuvers. It is also recommended that significant changes in barometric pressure, such as during an air flight, be avoided for several weeks postoperatively. Although difficult to enforce, attempts are made to minimize vigorous head movement in the postoperative period. Parents are encouraged to restrict pediatric patients from engaging in gymnastic or other excessive physical activities.

Less caution is needed for patients undergoing OCR with an intact tympanic membrane. In this situation, significantly compromised eustachian tube dysfunction is less likely to be present, so middle ear aeration is more predictable. Patients with tympanic membrane perforations more likely have compromised eustachian tube function or middle ear disease that must also be taken into consideration.

Patients with an intact tympanic membrane who are undergoing OCR have silk packing placed supported by small cotton balls or Gelfoam. The packing is removed 7 to 10 days postoperatively. If inflammation exists, topical ear drops are used for 1 week. The patient is seen again in 4 weeks for examination of the ear and audiometry testing. Patients requiring lateral graft tympanoplasty (tympanic membrane reconstruction) usually have double–silk rosebud packing in place. The outer pack is removed in 1 week and topical eardrops are prescribed. Postauricular Steri-Strips are removed from the tympanic membrane graft donor site. The second medial pack is removed 1 week later. Topical drops are continued twice daily for 2 weeks. Patients are seen a few weeks later to assess healing of the canal and tympanic membrane. When the tympanic membrane inflammation has resolved and the membrane is thin and mobile, audiometric testing is performed (see Chapter 113).

PEARLS

- The surgeon should be prepared to manage all reconstructive problems within the middle ear by being familiar with the various techniques for OCR should unanticipated problems arise.
- Careful palpation plus inspection of the tympanic membrane and all ossicles is critical to decide whether myringosclerosis and tympanosclerosis, separately or in combination, have caused the conductive hearing loss.
- To avoid restriction of movement, an interposed ossicle or prosthesis should not be placed so that it makes direct contact with the surrounding tympanic ring or rests on the cochlear promontory.
- Reconstruction of the tympanic membrane and ossicular chain demands a precise connection between the drum and the stapes or footplate.
- In the postoperative period, should significant retraction of a tympanic membrane cause to it drape over a prosthesis, placement of a myringotomy tube may prevent extrusion.

PITFALLS

- Normal mobility must be confirmed by palpation of the malleus and incus because lateral ossicular chain fixation may be missed by an inexperienced surgeon.
- Reconstruction with a partially eroded stapes (type III tympanoplasty) may not provide adequate support of a partial ossicular replacement prosthesis, and the reconstruction may need to be taken medially to the footplate.
- Excessive manipulation of the stapes when tympanosclerosis is present on the footplate may result in fracture or unanticipated removal of the stapes.
- A prosthesis will become displaced unless there is adequate tension between its medial site of contact (footplate or stapes) and the tympanic membrane or intervening cartilage.
- Excessive removal of the scutum without the support of a block of cartilage may result in retraction of the attic and cholesteatoma.

References

1. Zollner F: The principles of plastic surgery of the sound-conducting apparatus. J Laryngol Otol 69:637-652, 1955.
2. Wullstein H: Theory and practice of tympanoplasty. Laryngoscope 66:1076-1093, 1956.
3. Farrior JB: Classification of tympanoplasty. Arch Otolaryngol 93:548-550, 1971.
4. Blevins NH: Transfacial recess ossicular reconstruction: Technique and early results. Otol Neurotol 25:236-241, 2004.
5. Goldenberg RA, Emmet JR: Current use of implants in middle ear surgery. Otol Neurotol 22:145-152, 2001.
6. Gardner EK, Jackson CG, Kaylie DM: Results with titanium ossicular reconstruction prostheses. Laryngoscope 114:65-70, 2004.
7. Krueger WW, Feghali JG, Shelton C, et al: Preliminary ossiculoplasty results using the Kurz titanium prostheses. Otol Neurotol 23:836-839, 2002.
8. Chen DA, Arriaga MA: Technical refinements and precautions during ionomeric cement reconstruction of incus erosion during revision stapedectomy. Laryngoscope 113:848-852, 2003.
9. Goebel JA, Jacob A: Use of Mimix hydroxyapatite bone cement for difficult ossicular reconstruction. Otolaryngol Head Neck Surg 132:727-734, 2005.
10. Seidman MD, Babu S: A new approach for malleus/incus fixation: No prosthesis necessary. Otol Neurotol 25:669-673, 2004.
11. Teufert KB, De La Cruz A: Tympanosclerosis: Long-term hearing results after ossicular reconstruction. Otolaryngol Head Neck Surg 126:264-272, 2002.

Chapter 115

Mastoid Surgery

Michele St. Martin and Yael Raz

Mastoidectomy is one of the most common otologic operations performed today. Indications for mastoidectomy range from eradication of chronic infection or cholesteatoma to approaches for various neurotologic procedures. Mastoidectomy was first described by Louis Petit in the 1700s, although the concept did not gain wider acceptance until espoused by von Troltsch and Schwartze.[1,2] Modifications of the original radical procedure followed. Bondy described a technique in 1910 in which mastoidectomy was performed and the posterior canal wall removed while leaving the pars tensa and ossicular chain intact.[3] This procedure represents the origin of today's modified radical mastoidectomy.

Although the terms canal wall down (CWD) mastoidectomy and modified radical mastoidectomy are sometimes used interchangeably, there are in fact distinctions between these various procedures. In modified radical mastoidectomy, usually reserved for attic cholesteatomas, the mesotympanum is not entered.[4] Removal of the canal wall externalizes the cholesteatoma, and there is no need to elevate a tympanomeatal flap to address disease in the mesotympanum or explore the ossicular chain. When the middle ear is entered, the procedure is referred to as tympanoplasty with CWD mastoidectomy.

In 1958, the canal wall up (CWU) mastoidectomy was popularized by William House.[5] This procedure attempted to avoid the common problems with radical mastoidectomy, such as the lifelong requirement for cleaning, a propensity toward caloric stimulation by cold water or air, and restrictions on water exposure while bathing or swimming. In addition, hearing results improved with this procedure when compared with the standard modified radical mastoidectomy. CWU mastoidectomy has the advantage of preserving the normal anatomy of the ear. Generally, there is no need for maintenance of dry ear precautions. However, the exposure granted by this approach is more restricted, and it is technically more difficult to fully eradicate cholesteatomas. Frequently, a second-look procedure is required to rule out recurrent or residual disease, and recurrent disease is more likely.

Removal of the posterior ear canal affords better exposure that usually allows the cholesteatoma to be addressed at a single stage. It is technically easier to fully eradicate a cholesteatoma and the recurrence rate is lower. Disadvantages of CWD procedures include a more protracted postoperative healing period, the need for indefinite mastoid bowl care, a higher possibility of recurrent otorrhea, poorer hearing results, and a need for restricting water exposure.

The technique of removing and reconstructing the posterior bony canal wall has been espoused by numerous authors over the years.[6-8] This technique theoretically provides the advantage of improved surgical exposure with recurrence rates similar to those with CWD procedures yet avoiding the disadvantages of an open mastoid cavity. McElveen and Chung[8] described en bloc removal of the posterior bony canal wall with an oscillating microsaw. In certain cases this technique allows the surgeon to leave the ossicular chain intact, thereby improving hearing results in comparison with the use of partial or total ossicular reconstruction prostheses. The canal wall is then replaced and secured with bone cement. Dornhoffer[7] advocates removal of the upper one third of the canal wall and reconstructs the defect with cymba cartilage. Gantz and colleagues[6] have further modified the technique to involve obliteration of the mastoid with bone pâté and creation of an attic block with bone chips to isolate the mesotympanum from the attic and mastoid. This is done to reduce the amount of nitrogen-absorbing epithelium to discour-

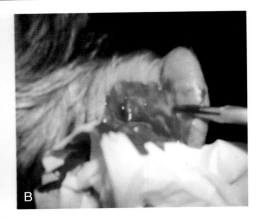

Figure 115-1. A, Erythema and fluctuance overlying the right mastoid secondary to a subperiosteal abscess. The patient had a history of having undergone mastoidectomy for chronic otitis media. **B,** Incision and drainage revealed extensive purulent debris. Treatment included antibiotics and revision mastoidectomy.

age the formation of a retraction pocket. Both authors advocate second-look procedures when the canal wall is reconstructed.

PATIENT SELECTION

Cortical mastoidectomy may be used for the treatment of complicated acute otitis media, chronic otitis media unresponsive to medical management, cholesteatoma, neoplasm of the temporal bone, repair of cerebrospinal fluid (CSF) leaks, and decompression of the facial nerve, as well as for exposure of deeper structures in the temporal bone or posterior fossa (Fig. 115-1). The decision to perform a CWU or CWD procedure must be individualized to each patient. Important factors include the location and extent of cholesteatoma, the presence of defects in the bone of the posterior canal wall, patient compliance, the presence of complications of otitis media or cholesteatoma, the presence of malignancy, the patient's hearing status, and the general medical condition of the patient.

Removal of the canal wall is indicated when it has already been destroyed to a significant degree by disease. Although small dehiscences can be repaired, a large erosion of the posterior canal wall by cholesteatoma is often best dealt with by removing the remaining canal wall. A fistula in the horizontal semicircular canal (HSC) (Fig. 115-2) is often best managed by leaving the skin in situ and externalizing the matrix into a CWD mastoid cavity. However, successful preservation of hearing has been reported with complete removal of the matrix overlying the dehiscence via a CWU technique.[9] Sclerotic mastoids may necessitate the use of a CWD approach (Fig. 115-3). When there is extensive cholesteatoma that would require a second stage in a patient with significant comorbid disease, removal of the canal wall can allow single-stage eradication of the disease. Recurrent cholesteatoma despite multiple attempts at CWU procedures is another indication for CWD mastoidectomy. Some authors would argue that cholesteatoma in an only-hearing ear constitutes an indication for a CWD procedure; however, this depends on the extent of the cholesteatoma and the surgeon's experience. Finally, poor compliance has frequently been cited as an indication for CWD surgery.

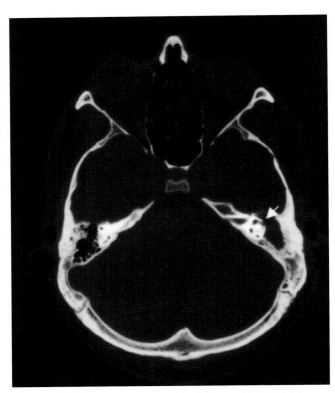

Figure 115-2. Cholesteatoma in the left mastoid with dehiscence of the horizontal semicircular canal *(arrow)*. Matrix was left over the dehiscent area and exteriorized with a canal wall down mastoidectomy.

PREOPERATIVE EVALUATION

Before surgery, patients should undergo routine audiometry, in addition to imaging studies as indicated. It is never advisable to operate on an ear in which hearing status is unknown. Preoperative audiometry will also allow the surgeon to determine whether the better- or worse-hearing ear is being operated on, which can affect the operative strategy. Additionally, the surgeon should note the presence and degree of any conductive hearing loss, whose source should be sought at the time of surgery.

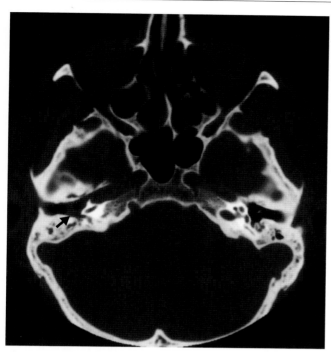

Figure 115-3. Cholesteatoma *(arrow)* in a right contracted mastoid cavity. A canal wall down mastoidectomy was planned from the outset.

Imaging studies are not mandatory before simple mastoidectomy, but high-resolution computed tomography (CT) allows assessment of the size and degree of pneumatization of the mastoid cavity, as well as the position of the tegmen mastoideum and sigmoid sinus. In addition, one should evaluate for dehiscence of the tegmen, facial nerve, or HSC. CT of the temporal bone is usually performed before cochlear implantation to assess the cochlea for congenital abnormality or ossification.

Barring extenuating circumstances such as severe comorbid conditions, mastoidectomy is performed under general anesthesia. Long-acting muscle relaxants should be avoided to allow monitoring or electrical stimulation of the facial nerve. Nerve monitoring is not essential for initial mastoidectomy, and disposable nerve stimulator units can be used if an unanticipated need arises. Formal nerve monitoring should be available for patients undergoing mastoidectomy in the setting of congenital ear anomalies, cochlear implantation, and revision mastoid surgery. Although electrophysiologic nerve monitoring is not a substitute for solid understanding of the course of the facial nerve through the temporal bone, it is a useful tool, particularly when an unanticipated anomaly is encountered. It is our practice to monitor the facial nerve for all mastoidectomies. Even though this may not represent the current standard of care, regular use of the nerve monitoring unit ensures familiarity with the equipment when the need arises and makes sense from a medicolegal standpoint as well.

Although evidence supporting the perioperative administration of antibiotics to patients undergoing mastoidectomy is limited, we routinely administer one dose preoperatively (generally 2 g of cefazolin). This may serve to reduce the incidence of postoperative wound infection in a contaminated ear inasmuch as most chronically draining ears harbor polymicrobial infections. A special note should also be made regarding preparation for revision mastoidectomy. Regardless of whether the patient has previously been operated on by the same or another surgeon, the operative report should be reviewed to allow the surgeon to anticipate potential pitfalls such as a dehiscent tegmen or facial nerve. It is generally advisable to use facial nerve monitoring in all revision surgery because the potential for dehiscence is greater in this group of patients. A preoperative CT scan is also recommended to delineate changes related to the previous surgery. The revision ear must be approached with caution because of the obliteration of normal landmarks.

SURGICAL APPROACH

The patient is positioned supine on the operating table, usually with the head at the foot of the bed to allow the surgeon's knees to fit under the table. The head is turned toward the side away from the operated ear, while taking care to ensure that the contralateral auricle is not being compressed. A small amount of hair in the postauricular region is shaved to keep the operating field free of hair. The patient's remaining hair is then secured with tape to keep it out of the field. The postauricular crease is cleaned with alcohol and injected with lidocaine with epinephrine. If a facial nerve monitor is to be used, the electrodes are placed at this time. The patient should be secured to the table with straps because rotating the bed will be necessary during the procedure. Bed controls may be retained by the anesthesiologist or may be wrapped in sterile plastic and placed on the bed for the surgeon to control. The operating table is turned either 90 or 180 degrees, depending on the surgeon's preference.

The operative field is then prepared with povidone-iodine (Betadine) and the ear canal is flooded with preparative solution. Drapes are applied as the individual surgeon prefers; it is common to use a drape with a plastic bag attached to collect irrigation fluid and prevent it from running onto the floor or the surgeon's lap. Suction and irrigation tubing is set up, the drill is connected to the motor and foot pedal, and the instrument table and operating microscope are brought into position. Before the start of the procedure, the surgeon should ensure that the microscope is properly balanced and that the correct lens (usually 225 to 300 mm) is attached.

The external auditory canal (EAC) and tympanic membrane (TM) are examined under the operating microscope. Cerumen or debris in the EAC is removed while taking care to not cause bleeding.

Four-Quadrant Injection

If a tympanomeatal flap is to be elevated in conjunction with the mastoidectomy, injection of lidocaine with epinephrine is performed at the bony-cartilaginous junction. The location of this junction can be estimated by the medial-most aspect of the hair-bearing canal skin. A 1.5-inch, 25-gauge needle with the bevel aimed toward the bone is used to inject the four quadrants of the canal. Light pressure is applied with the speculum to create a cushion into which the local anesthetic is injected and to direct the anesthetic medially. The correct plane for injection offers a moderate amount of resistance. The bony canal should be monitored to ensure that the skin of the EAC has blanched down to the TM without blebs.

Establishing a Vascular Strip

If a tympanomeatal flap is to be elevated in conjunction with the mastoidectomy, a vascular strip is established via an endaural approach at this point. The canal incision can be fashioned in an H shape (Fig. 115-4). Alternatively, the vascular strip (the lateral aspect of the "H") can be defined at this point and the tympanomeatal flap (medial aspect of the "H") deferred until exposure of the canal is established via the postauricular incision. The superior (12 o'clock) incision is placed in line with the lateral process of the malleus. The superior and inferior incisions are established with a flap knife or Beaver blade. They are connected approximately halfway between the annulus and the bony-cartilaginous junction with an angled Beaver blade or a round knife. A cotton ball soaked in topical adrenaline may be inserted into the EAC for additional hemostasis if necessary. Alternatively, the canal incisions can be fash-

ioned via the postauricular incision. In this case it is useful to have cotton or Gelfoam in the medial ear canal to provide resistance and protect the anterior canal. A no. 11 blade is useful for this approach.

Planning the Postauricular Incision

The microscope is moved aside and a postauricular incision is made with a no. 15 blade. The incision extends from just superior and posterior to the root of the helix down to the mastoid tip (Fig. 115-5). The incision should be placed several millimeters behind the postauricular sulcus. When the mastoidectomy is performed for access to deeper structures, a more posterior incision is made to provide better exposure of the sigmoid sinus and posterior fossa (Fig. 115-6). In young children without a well-developed mastoid tip, the inferior aspect of the incision is more posterior and is not carried down as far to avoid injuring the facial nerve (Fig. 115-7). The incision is carried down to the level of the loose areolar tissue overlying the temporalis fascia (Fig. 115-8). Identification of this plane is facilitated by pulling laterally on the auricle as the incision is made. Once the correct plane has been entered, the knife blade is turned flat and dissection is carried anteriorly toward the posterior EAC while taking care to not

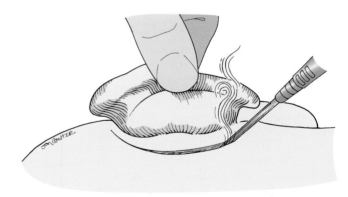

Figure 115-5. Postauricular skin incision used in adults.

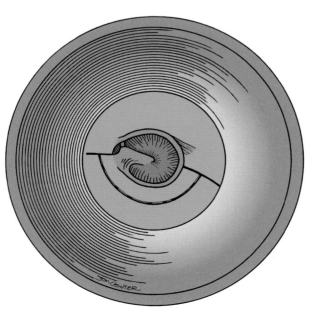

Figure 115-4. Skin flaps within the external auditory canal. An H-shaped skin incision creates a laterally based vascular strip-type flap and a medially based tympanomeatal flap.

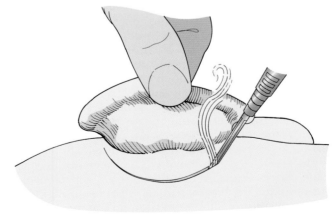

Figure 115-6. Skin incision used for transmastoid neurotologic surgery.

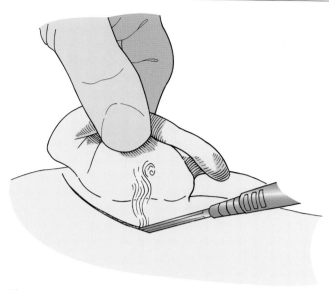

Figure 115-7. Postauricular skin incision used in children.

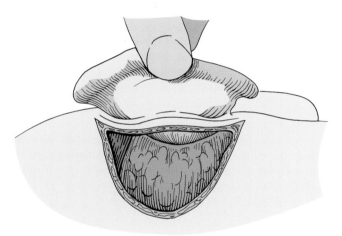

Figure 115-8. Dissection of subcutaneous tissue to expose the temporalis fascia and musculoperiosteal tissue overlying the mastoid cortex.

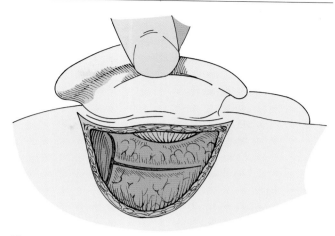

Figure 115-9. Incisions used to expose the mastoid cortex.

brought out through the postauricular incision to retract the ear anteriorly. Self-retaining retractors are positioned and the surface landmarks of the mastoid are identified, including the spine of Henle, the cribriform area, and the linea temporalis (Fig. 115-10). MacEwen's (suprameatal) triangle provides an approximation of the location of the antrum (Fig. 115-11).

Intact Canal Wall Mastoidectomy

During the course of training in otologic surgery it is imperative that the surgeon first gain exposure to temporal bone drilling in the laboratory. This invaluable experience will allow familiarity with the anatomy and equipment and facilitate safe and speedy mastoidectomy in the operating room. Adequate irrigation is essential for safe drilling. Constant flow prevents accumulation of bone dust and thereby allows underlying structures such as the tegmen to be identified through intact bone. Irrigation also prevents thermal injury to underlying structures, such as the facial nerve. Either suction irrigators or a self-irrigating drill can be used. Generally, the drill is used in the forward direction and drilling performed in a clockwise direction. Counterclockwise drilling in the "forward" setting can result in "skipping" of the burr and potentially damage underlying structures. The use of long smooth strokes parallel to the underlying structures is safer and more effective and provides better visualization. Larger burrs are safer because they are less likely to plunge into critical structures, and the general rule is to use the largest burr that can safely be used in that particular region. Drilling typically starts with a large (6 mm) cutting burr that is downsized to a 4-mm cutting burr more medially, after entry into the antrum. A diamond burr should be used for the final thinning of bone overlying structures such as the middle fossa tegmen or sigmoid sinus or when drilling near the facial nerve. Drilling with a diamond burr in the "reverse" direction can also control small bleeders in the bone. The drilling trajectory should parallel the underlying structure to be identified to reduce the chance of unintentional injury. During the procedure it is important to "saucerize" the edges

enter the EAC at this point. Temporalis fascia may now be harvested if TM grafting is anticipated. The inferiormost aspect of the fascia harvest site should be placed at least one centimeter above the linea temporalis. Preserving the fascia at the linea temporalis allows more solid closure of the superior periosteal incision.

The mastoid cortex is exposed by incising the periosteum along the linea temporalis. A vertical limb is extended from the posterior aspect of the periosteal incision toward the mastoid tip. This can be performed in a T fashion (Fig. 115-9) or in a "7" shape with the apex positioned posterosuperiorly. A heavy Lempert or Fisch periosteal elevator is used to free the cortex of soft tissue. A large duckbill or Joseph elevator is used to expose the posterior aspect of the EAC. If a vascular strip was fashioned, it can now be elevated from bone with a round knife. Tracheostomy tape or a $\frac{1}{4}$-inch Penrose drain can be placed through the canal and

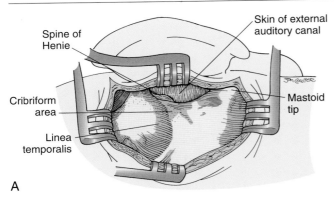

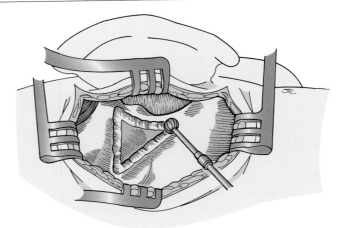

Figure 115-12. Location and direction of the initial bone cuts on the mastoid cortex.

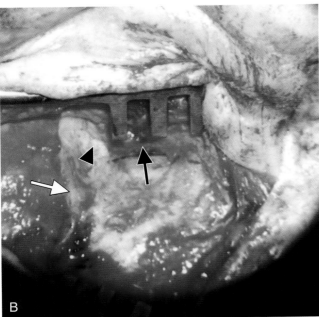

Figure 115-10. A, Surgical landmarks on the lateral surface of the temporal bone. **B,** Intraoperative view. The mastoid periosteum has been incised and reflected anteriorly to expose the linea temporalis *(white arrow),* spine of Henle *(arrowhead),* and posterior aspect of the external auditory canal *(arrow).*

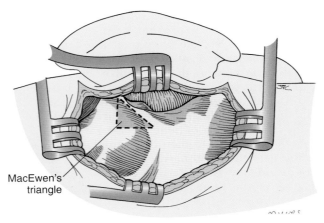

Figure 115-11. MacEwen's triangle (suprameatal triangle).

of the mastoid cavity to provide excellent visualization of structures as they are identified and help prevent inadvertent injury. The exception to such saucerization occurs in cochlear implant surgery, where a ledge of bone laterally may help retain the coiled wire within the mastoid cavity. In general, injury is best avoided by clearly identifying vital structures such as the tegmen, facial nerve, sigmoid sinus, horizontal canal, and incus. In this manner, structures may be followed throughout their course in the mastoid rather than risking injury by haphazard identification.

The initial drilling is often performed more readily without use of the operating microscope. If the surgeon prefers to use the microscope, a low-power view should be used so that the entire mastoid cortex is in view. A large cutting burr is used to begin drilling. The first cuts are made parallel to the linea temporalis and then posterior to the EAC to create a 90-degree angle. The third side of the triangle roughly approximates the course of the sigmoid sinus posteriorly (Fig. 115-12). The mastoid cortex is removed and the air cell system is exposed (Fig. 115-13). Drilling proceeds with identification of the tegmen mastoideum through bone. The tegmen will be visible as a pink color change in the bone superiorly in the mastoid cavity; small vessels signal that dissection is close to the dura. The sound of the drill may become higher pitched as the bone becomes thin. The tegmen should remain covered with a thin layer of bone to avoid injury to the dura or the future development of an encephalocele. The posterior canal wall is thinned while taking care to not enter the canal. Drilling proceeds along a wide plane to avoid drilling in a hole, and the edges are saucerized so that one does not have to drill unseen under a ledge. The deepest point of the dissection should always be centered over the antrum, approximated by MacEwen's triangle. This will ensure that the antrum with its critical landmarks will be entered before reaching the plane of the facial nerve. The sigmoid sinus will come into view posteriorly in the mastoid cavity as the air cells are removed. Care must be taken to remove disease present in the sinodural

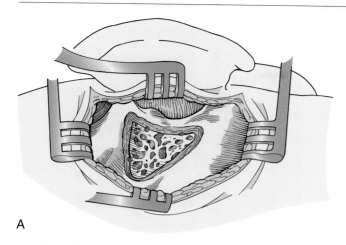

A

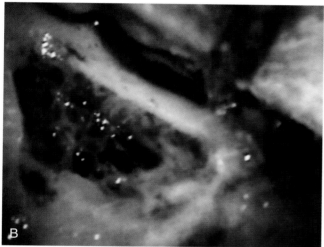

B

Figure 115-13. A, Removal of the mastoid cortex exposes the mastoid air cell system. **B,** Intraoperative view.

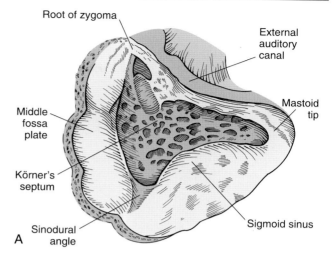

A

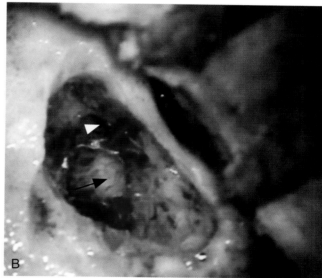

B

Figure 115-14. A, Körner's septum. The lateral semicircular canal and mastoid antrum lie under Körner's septum. **B,** Exposure of the mastoid air cells will vary depending on the nature of the surgery. For this right-sided cochlear implantation, the posterior and superior margins of the mastoidectomy have not been saucerized. The dome of the horizontal semicircular canal (arrow) is identified, and the short process of the incus (arrowhead) is just visible in the fossa incudis.

angle, as well as in the mastoid tip. The digastric ridge can be identified posteroinferiorly; the cephalic edge of this ridge provides an important landmark for the course of the vertical portion of the facial nerve.

Körner's septum will be present to a varying degree just lateral to the mastoid antrum. Using the tegmen as the superior landmark and the posterior canal wall as the anterior landmark, Koerner's septum is removed and the antrum is entered (Fig. 115-14). This step highlights the importance of identifying the tegmen and following it toward the antrum. Failure to identify the tegmen may result in entering the antrum too low and risking injury to the HSC and facial nerve. Drilling through the septum will allow visualization of the HSC. Once the antrum has been entered, cholesteatoma matrix or mucosal disease should be removed so that the HSC may be identified. Once the HSC and tegmen are clearly visible, the short process of the incus may be identified. The burr is downsized at this time and drilling continues toward the root of the zygoma until the incus is seen in the fossa incudis. It is helpful to tilt the bed away from the surgeon to visualize the incus. Frequently, the incus is visible through the irrigation fluid

filling the antral air cell before being visible through air because of the refractive properties of water. Care must be taken to not touch the incus with the drill or high-frequency sensorineural hearing loss may result. The completed intact canal wall mastoidectomy should be bounded by a thin but intact middle fossa plate, the sigmoid sinus should be visible through intact bone, the posterior wall of the EAC should be thinned yet intact, the short process of the incus should be visible via the aditus ad antrum, and the horizontal SCC should be clearly identifiable (Fig. 115-15). Additional work may be undertaken to clean Trautmann's triangle, the mastoid tip, and the retrofacial air cell tracts as necessary. If cholesteatoma is present in the aditus ad antrum, it may be necessary to disarticulate the incudostapedial

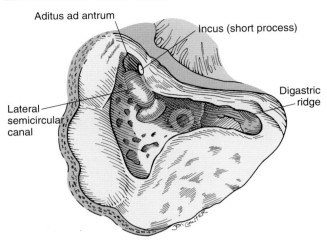

Figure 115-15. Completed intact canal wall mastoidectomy.

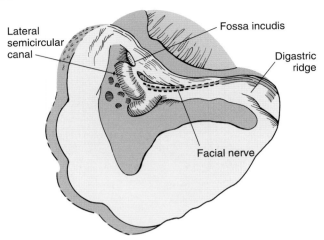

Figure 115-16. Landmarks for identification of the facial nerve.

joint and remove the incus to facilitate more complete resection of cholesteatoma medial to the canal wall by working from both the mastoid cavity and the middle ear. Umbilical tape may then be used in a "flossing" technique to further remove squamous epithelium from the antrum. This is done by passing the tape from the mastoid cavity through the antrum to the middle ear and out of the ear canal and then moving it back and forth over the medial surface of the canal wall (see Video 115-1). For certain procedures such as endolymphatic sac decompression or labyrinthectomy, it may be desirable to identify the posterior semicircular canal by removing the retrolabyrinthine air cells.

Drilling the Facial Recess

The facial recess is a triangle defined by the incus buttress, the facial nerve, and the chorda tympani. Opening the facial recess allows access to the posterior mesotympanum, through which inflammatory tissue or cholesteatoma may be removed. This technique is also referred to as a posterior tympanotomy and is used to create access to the round window niche for drilling of the cochleostomy during cochlear implantation. Safely entering the recess relies on identification of landmarks for the facial nerve, including the incus, HSC, posterior EAC, and digastric ridge (Fig 115-16). The posterior EAC should be thinned laterally to medially to improve visualization of the chorda tympani and facial recess; air cells lateral to the plane of the incus should be removed. The short process of the incus points to the second genu of the facial nerve. Because it lies in the same plane, the incus provides a very useful landmark for identification of the facial nerve. The HSC is another critical landmark, and the second genu of the facial nerve is just anterior and medial to the HSC. The digastric ridge may also be useful; the cephalic edge of the digastric ridge leads to the stylomastoid foramen and is a good inferior landmark for the vertical portion of the facial nerve.

A 2- or 3-mm diamond burr should be used for drilling medial to the plane of the incus. Drilling should

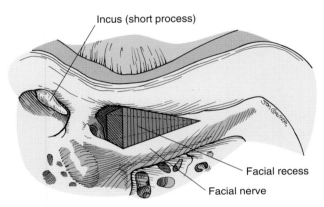

Figure 115-17. Anatomy of the facial recess.

commence just inferior to the short process of the incus. The bridge of bone between the incus and the recess is termed the incus buttress. Removal of bone between the chorda tympani nerve and the vertical facial nerve proceeds just below the incus buttress by drilling parallel to the course of the facial nerve. Copious irrigation prevents thermal injury and enhances visualization through bone. Because the facial recess is larger superiorly than inferiorly, it is safest to enter the recess at its superior aspect (Fig. 115-17). Once the recess has been entered, drilling can proceed medial to the chorda tympani with caution to expand the view toward the round window niche. Bone is thinned over the facial nerve as necessary to provide a sufficient view of the middle ear (Fig. 115-18). A thin shell of bone is maintained over the nerve. Care must be taken to not allow the shaft of the burr to contact the facial nerve because such contact may cause thermal injury to the nerve. After the middle ear has been entered, the recess can be expanded to allow visualization of the incudostapedial joint, round window niche, promontory, and other middle ear structures (Fig. 115-19).

Once drilling has been completed, the mastoid and middle ear are irrigated thoroughly to remove bone dust and debris. To close the postauricular wound in a

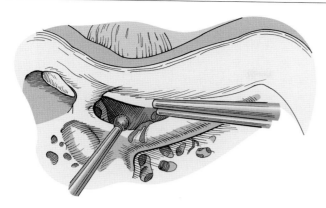

Figure 115-18. Removal of air cells to open the facial recess.

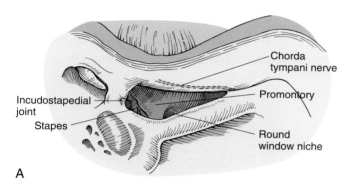

Incudostapedial joint
Stapes
Chorda tympani nerve
Promontory
Round window niche

A

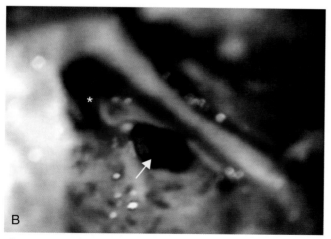

B

Figure 115-19. A, Exposure of middle ear structures through the completed facial recess. **B,** Using the short process of the incus *(asterisk),* horizontal semicircular canal, and thinned posterior wall of the external auditory canal as landmarks, the facial recess has been entered. The cochlear promontory and the round window niche *(arrow)* are visible.

CWU procedure, the mastoid periosteum should be reapproximated to avoid unsightly retraction of postauricular skin into the bony defect. We use 3-0 Vicryl interrupted sutures for closure of periosteum. The deep layer of skin is then closed with interrupted 3-0 or 4-0 Vicryl, depending on skin thickness. If a vascular strip was elevated, a rolled Telfa strip coated with bacitracin

ointment is used to stent the meatus. The superficial layer of skin is then closed with running 5-0 fast-absorbing plain gut suture. The incision is then dressed with bacitracin ointment, Xeroform, Telfa, and a Glasscock cup. The dressing may be removed 24 hours postoperatively; the patient is instructed to keep the operated ear dry.

Again, special care must be taken in the case of revision surgery. When making periosteal incisions and entering the previously drilled mastoid cavity, bony dehiscences may be encountered over the tegmen, sigmoid sinus, or facial nerve. The surgeon must use caution to prevent inadvertent injury to these structures. Often, cortical bone has regrown to some extent in a previously drilled cavity. This must be removed to provide adequate identification of landmarks via the same principles as described earlier.

Canal Wall Down Mastoidectomy

A problem-free mastoid bowl begins with a complete cortical mastoidectomy to identify the tegmen mastoideum, the short process of the incus if present, and the HSC. Successful CWD mastoidectomy entails more than simply drilling down the posterior wall of the EAC. It is especially critical to saucerize the bony edges of the mastoidectomy superiorly and posteriorly to allow the surrounding soft tissue to collapse into the mastoidectomy defect and ultimately create a smaller cavity. Trouble spots that can result in a wet cavity include the sinodural angle and the mastoid tip. Removal of the mastoid tip is accomplished by identifying the digastric ridge posteroinferiorly and following its cephalic edge toward the stylomastoid foramen. Once this has been completed, the bone lateral to the ridge can be removed safely with the drill.

The posterior wall of the EAC is thinned and maintained as a useful landmark until the facial recess has been opened. Sequentially smaller diamond burrs are used to remove the bone between the chorda tympani and the facial nerve. It is important to establish the location of the facial nerve and maintain a thin layer of bone over it. Identification of the facial nerve is critical for two reasons. First, the best way to protect the nerve is to positively establish its location. Second, attempts at protecting the nerve by leaving excess bone over it result in a bony ledge, referred to as a "high facial ridge," which makes subsequent mastoid bowl care challenging and may ultimately require revision surgery (Fig. 115-20).

Once the level of the nerve is identified, the EAC wall can be removed. The area to be drilled can be conceived of as an anterior buttress (involving the tympanosquamous suture and lateral wall of the epitympanum or scutum), a posterior buttress (involving the facial ridge), and the intervening bridge of bone (Fig. 115-21). Removal can be accomplished with a 4-mm cutting burr (Fig 115-22). Frequently, disease that necessitates CWD surgery also requires removal of the incus, in which case it is preferable to proceed with separation of the incudostapedial joint and removal of

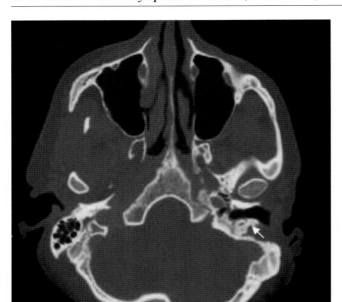

Figure 115-20. High facial ridge. Excess bone has been left in place lateral to the fallopian canal *(arrow).* This results in excess buildup of cerumen and squamous debris, which is difficult to clear in the office.

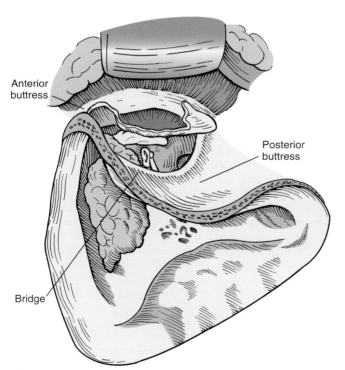

Figure 115-21. Buttresses and bridge of the posterior canal wall.

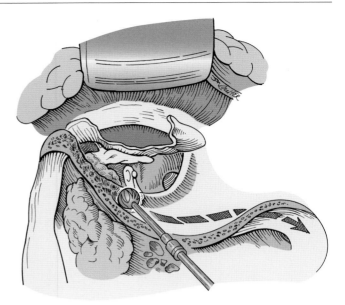

Figure 115-22. Technique of removing the canal wall.

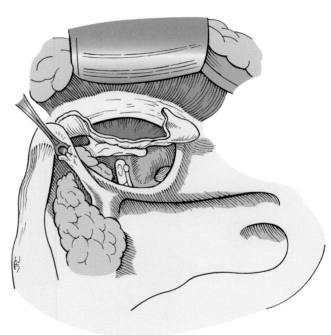

Figure 115-23. The last bridge of the posterior canal wall is removed while using a curette to protect the ossicles and facial nerve.

the incus before removing the canal wall. However, if the ossicular chain is mobile and the ear pathology is such that the incus can be kept in situ, a small bridge of bone thinned to an eggshell thickness can be maintained over the short process of the incus. The remain-ing bone overlying the short process of the incus can then removed with a pick or curette (Fig 115-23). Once the canal wall has been removed, a smooth transition must be established between the roof of the EAC and the tegmen mastoideum at the anterior buttress. Similarly, inferiorly the floor of the ear canal must be con-toured such that there is a smooth transition to the facial ridge at the posterior buttress. With an anteriorly positioned sigmoid or low tegmen in the setting of a contracted mastoid cavity, the canal wall must some-

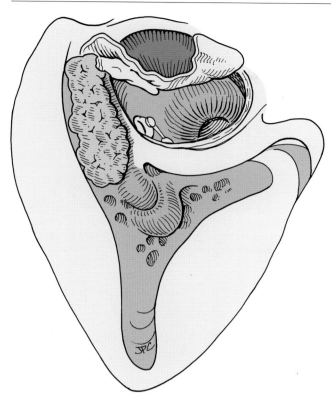

Figure 115-24. Completed canal wall down mastoidectomy with tympanoplasty.

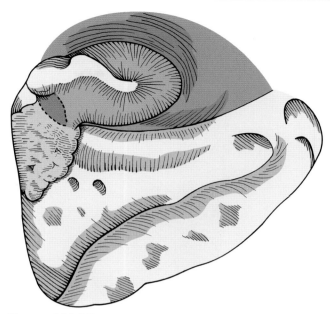

Figure 115-25. Completed Bondy-modified radical mastoidectomy.

times be removed to permit safe identification of deeper structures. The mastoid cavity should then be inspected to ensure that all diseased cells have been exenterated with a smoothly contoured appearance (Fig 115-24). Once the middle ear disease, if present, has been addressed, the middle ear is packed with Gelfoam. The previously harvested, pressed, and dried fascia can then be used in an underlay fashion by draping the graft onto the horizontal facial nerve superiorly and onto the facial ridge posteriorly, followed by further packing lateral to the drum and graft.

Bondy-Modified Radical Mastoidectomy

A Bondy mastoidectomy refers to removal of the posterior canal wall for attic disease without entering the middle ear space. This technique may be used for attic cholesteatoma in the setting of an intact ossicular chain and normal or nearly normal hearing. The pars tensa is not disrupted and the mesotympanum is not entered. The epitympanic cholesteatoma is exteriorized through an endaural approach. The anterior buttress is removed and the canal wall is lowered to the level of the incus. In this instance, the cholesteatoma matrix is left in situ as the epithelial lining to the now exteriorized epitympanum (Fig. 115-25). A meatoplasty is necessary to facilitate cleaning of the Bondy mastoid cavity.

Radical Mastoidectomy

When middle ear disease cannot be fully or safely addressed during a CWD procedure, the surgeon may elect to proceed with grafting of the TM with plans to return for a second look. For example, when significant squamous debris is present in the oval window and the surgeon believes that it cannot be removed adequately, sometimes a second look 6 to 9 months later allows the epithelium to form a pearl, which is more readily dissected. However, in some instances when it is believed that the middle ear disease is irreversible, radical mastoidectomy is performed. Drilling proceeds as for a CWD mastoidectomy. The malleus, incus, and TM are removed and hearing restoration is not attempted. The middle ear mucosa is removed, including the lining of the eustachian tube orifice. The eustachian tube is then obliterated with muscle and bone. The epitympanum, mesotympanum, and hypotympanum are thus all exteriorized into the EAC (Fig 115-26). A meatoplasty is then performed.

Meatoplasty

A meatoplasty should always be performed when the canal wall has been removed. This step is critical in allowing access for mastoid bowl care in the office. An inadequate meatoplasty results in accumulation of squamous debris or cerumen and contributes to chronic otorrhea. To enlarge the meatus, the skin of the external auditory meatus must be incised and cartilage removed. On the other hand, excessive enlargement of the meatus results in an unsightly cosmetic defect. The meatoplasty should be sized so that it matches the cavity and allows access to the most superior, posterior, and inferior aspects of the mastoid bowl for cleaning. Some contraction will occur in the postoperative period.

The meatoplasty begins with removal of a crescent of conchal cartilage. A Senn retractor or double-pronged skin hook is used to retract the auricle. The

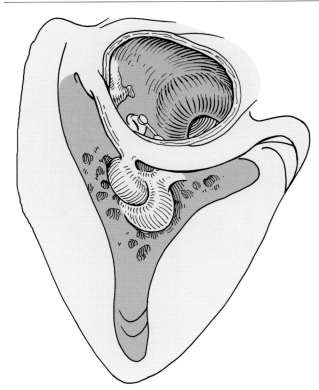

Figure 115-26. Completed radical mastoidectomy.

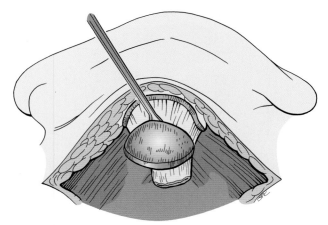

Figure 115-28. A Freer elevator is used to elevate the conchal cartilage from the overlying skin.

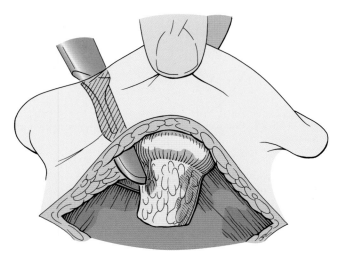

Figure 115-29. A superior canal incision is made and connected to the postauricular exposure to create a long Koerner flap.

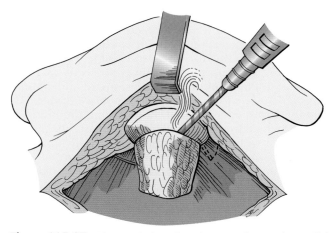

Figure 115-27. The conchal cartilage is exposed up to the medial edge of the cartilage at the bone-cartilage junction of the external auditory canal.

middle or ring finger of the retracting hand, when placed within the concha laterally, can provide resistance as the subcutaneous tissue overlying the concha is incised via the postauricular approach. The underlying cartilage is exposed to its medial rim (Fig 115-27). The conchal cartilage is then incised with a no. 15 blade. A round knife or Freer elevator can be used to elevate the cartilage from the conchal skin, and this segment of cartilage is removed (Fig. 115-28). A no. 15 blade is then placed in the auditory canal, and 12- and 6-o'clock incisions are made through the canal skin and

subcutaneous tissue (Fig. 115-29). Two or three 3-0 Vicryl sutures are placed in the subdermal tissue and used to anchor the posterior meatal skin to the deep periosteal tissue posterior to the mastoidectomy. When tied, these sutures should establish an open meatus that matches the size of the mastoid cavity (Fig 115-30). The attached vascular strip is pulled posteriorly by the stay sutures to line the lateral and posterior aspects of the mastoid cavity. The meatoplasty is stented for 10 to 14 days with a roll of bacitracin-coated Telfa. The mastoid periosteum is not reapproximated. Closure of the postauricular skin incision then proceeds as for intact canal wall procedures.

Postoperative Management

The patient is instructed to wear a Glasscock ear dressing for 2 days postoperatively. After removal of the dressing, the patient may shower but is instructed to keep the ear dry. Bacitracin is applied to the postauricular incision twice a day for 1 week. The first postopera-

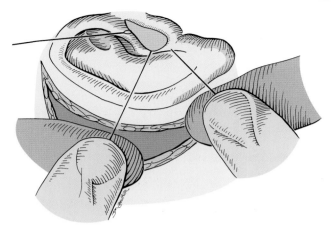

Figure 115-30. Stay sutures are used to properly match the size of the meatus to the size of the mastoid cavity.

tive visit occurs in 7 to 10 days, at which time the incision is checked and any packing in the EAC is removed. If a meatoplasty has been performed, the stent is left in place for 10 to 14 days. The second follow-up visit takes place 3 to 4 weeks later. Frequently, the TM will be healed sufficiently to allow an early postoperative audiogram at this time. Thereafter, the patient may be monitored routinely per the surgeon's usual practice. CWD mastoidectomies require more frequent follow-up for the first few months after surgery until the bowl is lined with healthy epithelium. During this healing period, silver nitrate cautery may be necessary to address granulation tissue.

COMPLICATIONS

Potential complications of tympanomastoidectomy include TM perforation, altered taste, vertigo, sensorineural hearing loss, facial paralysis, injury to the tegmen or underlying dura, iatrogenic injury to the ossicular chain, hemorrhage from injury to the sigmoid sinus, and inadvertent entry into the EAC. An intact TM may be perforated during elevation of the tympanomeatal flap in a tympanomastoidectomy, particularly if the TM is atrophic or tethered to middle ear structures. If perforation should occur, the torn TM should be grafted at the end of the procedure. Stretching or cutting the chorda tympani nerve can lead to dysgeusia; symptoms of altered taste often resolve within several months if it does occur.

Vertigo or sensorineural hearing loss (or both) may result from inadvertently dislocating the stapes or from entering the HSC. Touching the incus with the drill during the mastoidectomy may also result in high-frequency sensorineural loss. If the patient shows evidence of severe vertigo on awakening, inpatient admission may be required for control of nausea and vomiting and supportive care. Consideration should be given to high-dose corticosteroids if sensorineural hearing loss has occurred. Tuning fork testing performed in the postoperative care unit will help diagnose

sensorineural loss, and an urgent audiogram may be obtained in cases with significant concern.

The facial nerve may be injured by direct trauma, either from the burr or from instrumentation of a dehiscent nerve, or by thermal injury if the rotating shaft of the burr comes in contact with a thin layer of bone overlying the nerve. The patient's facial nerve function should always be evaluated in the postoperative care unit. If facial weakness is discovered that did not exist preoperatively, the surgeon should observe the patient until any local anesthesia has worn off to ensure that the palsy is not due to infiltration of the nerve by local injection. In addition, if a compressive dressing or ear packing has been used, it should be loosened immediately. If the weakness persists, the surgeon should note whether it is partial or complete paralysis. If partial, the patient should be treated with high-dose corticosteroids and monitored closely for the development of complete paralysis. In the case of immediate complete paralysis, the appropriate response depends on whether the surgeon is confident that the nerve has been visualized during surgery and left intact. If so, the patient should be treated with steroids and observed. If the nerve was not visualized, the patient should undergo electroneuronography and temporal bone CT. If indicated by CT or electrical testing, re-exploration of the ear should be undertaken for decompression or anastomosis. Strong consideration should be given to consultation with another surgeon because anxiety can run high when faced with this significant complication and affect one's ability to best deal with the situation.

Bony defects in the tegmen result from overly aggressive drilling along the roof of the mastoid cavity; on occasion, the dura is violated and a CSF leak results. If the bony defect is small (<1 cm) and the surgeon is certain that the dura has not been injured, the defect need not be repaired because the risk of encephalocele is low. Alternatively, larger bony defects or injury to dura necessitate repair, which may be accomplished at the time of surgery by using fascia or muscle to graft over the defect from below. Temporalis muscle may also be rotated into the cavity to cover the defect.

Any of the ossicles may be dislocated during surgery on the attic or mesotympanum, although the incus and stapes are more at risk. When dissecting cholesteatoma or inflammatory tissue off the ossicles, care must be taken to not use undue force. Dissection on the stapes should proceed in a posterior-to-anterior direction to take advantage of the countertraction provided by the stapedius tendon.

If significant bleeding is encountered because of a large emissary vein or injury to the sigmoid sinus, hemostasis can often be achieved by applying pressure over the bleeding site with Gelfoam soaked in epinephrine. Alternatively, Surgicel may be placed over the injury and held in place until the bleeding is controlled.

Finally, during a CWU mastoidectomy, the EAC may inadvertently be violated as the posterior canal wall is thinned. To prevent retraction of skin into the mastoid cavity and subsequent EAC cholesteatoma, the surrounding skin should be elevated and the defect covered with fascia in an underlay technique. Larger bony defects should be repaired with conchal or tragal cartilage as well to reinforce the skin.

PEARLS

- The use of long drilling strokes in a direction parallel to important structures such as the facial nerve, tegmen, and sigmoid sinus facilitates identification and minimizes injury to these structures.
- Constant irrigation prevents bone dust from obscuring underlying structures and prevents thermal injury, particularly to the facial nerve.
- Important structures should always be positively identified rather than relying on avoidance to prevent injury.
- Removal of the mastoid tip, lowering of the facial ridge, removal of air cells at the sinodural angle, and an adequate meatoplasty can prevent the need for revision surgery in CWD mastoidectomy.
- When performing CWD procedures, the canal wall should be left intact until all the landmarks have been identified—the thinned canal wall serves as an additional landmark that can be followed medially to identify the chorda tympani nerve and enter the facial recess.

PITFALLS

- Touching the ossicles with the high-speed drill may result in sensorineural hearing loss.

- Facial nerve injury may occur through failure to positively identify the nerve or as a result of bony dehiscence.
- Inadvertent injury to the tegmen and underlying dura may result in CSF leak or encephalocele, or both.
- Breaches of the posterior EAC wall during CWU procedures should be repaired by elevating the canal skin and covering the defect with fascia; cartilage may be added for larger defects.
- Inadequate meatoplasty is probably the most common reason for difficulties in CWD surgery—a large meatoplasty should be created and stented for at least 10 days postoperatively.

References

1. Von Troltsch AF: Lehrbuch der Ohrenheilkunde mit Einschluss der Anatomie des Ohres. Leipzig, Germany, Foegel, 1873.
2. Milstein S: The history of mastoid surgery. Am J Otol 1:174-178, 1980.
3. Bondy G: Totalaufmeisselung mit Erhaltung von Trommelfell und Gehorknockelchen. Monatsschr Ohrenheilk 44:15, 1910.
4. Sheehy JL: Surgery for chronic otitis media. In English GL (ed): Otolaryngology. Philadelphia, JB Lippincott, 1989.
5. Sheehy JL, Patterson ME: Intact canal wall tympanoplasty with mastoidectomy. A review of eight years' experience. Laryngoscope 77:1502-1542, 1967.
6. Gantz BJ, Wilkinson EP, Hansen MR: Canal wall reconstruction tympanomastoidectomy with mastoid obliteration. Laryngoscope 115:1734-1740, 2005.
7. Dornhoffer JL: Retrograde mastoidectomy with canal wall reconstruction: A follow-up report. Otol Neurotol 25:653-660, 2004.
8. McElveen JT Jr, Chung AT: Reversible canal wall down mastoidectomy for acquired cholesteatomas: Preliminary results. Laryngoscope 113:1027-1033, 2003.
9. Copeland BJ, Buchman CA: Management of labyrinthine fistulae in chronic ear surgery. Am J Otolaryngol 24:51-60, 2003.

Chapter 116

Congenital Malformations of the Middle Ear

Arpita I. Mehta and Yael Raz

The various manifestations of middle ear malformations provide an interesting clinical challenge for physicians. In the adult population undergoing exploratory tympanotomy for presumed otosclerosis, such anomalies may be unexpected. The otologic surgeon must be prepared to deal with unanticipated findings such as partial or complete absence of components of the ossicular chain, lateral chain fixation, a persistent stapedial artery, abnormal course of the facial nerve, or absence of the oval window. Knowledge of the embryologic origins of middle ear structures is useful in understanding the various anomalies that arise and anticipating associated defects. For example, branchial arch anomalies may accompany defects of the ossicular chain, which is derived in part from the first two arches. Additionally, the stapes and facial nerve develop simultaneously.[1] An inferiorly displaced facial nerve may prevent contact between the developing stapes and the inner ear, thereby inhibiting further development of the stapes and preventing proper induction of the oval window.[2] Thus, an abnormal course of the facial nerve should be suspected when anomalies of the stapes or oval window are encountered.

Middle ear malformations should always be considered in the differential diagnosis for children with conductive hearing loss. Congenital ear deformities are estimated to occur in 1 in 11,000 to 15,000 individuals.[3,4] Isolated anomalies of the middle ear with a normal auricle and external auditory canal account for only a small percentage of these deformities.[5] Approximately one quarter of congenital middle ear anomalies occur in the setting of a disorder such as Treacher Collins, Klippel-Feil, or branchio-oto-renal syndrome.[6] In an adult patient, congenital middle ear anomalies should be suspected when hearing loss has been present since childhood, thus making otosclerosis unlikely, and the history is negative for otitis media.

This chapter focuses on the operative management of isolated middle ear malformations. Management of aural atresia is addressed in Chapter 111, and microtia repair is discussed in Chapter 85.

PATIENT SELECTION

Depending on the nature of the middle ear anomaly, the resultant hearing loss can be purely conductive or mixed, unilateral or bilateral, and range from mild to profound. Whereas bilateral middle ear anomalies are often recognized in early childhood, in the past, unilateral middle ear abnormalities were frequently not identified until a school-aged child received a screening hearing test. However, with the recent adoption of universal newborn hearing screening tests by most states, the age at identification of children with developmental middle ear abnormalities can be expected to decrease significantly. Non–otitis-related unilateral conductive hearing loss should be managed conservatively until the child is at least 5 to 7 years of age. The age at which surgery is appropriate must be tailored to each patient and depends on eustachian tube function and the reliability of the results of behavioral audiometric testing. In the setting of significant bilateral hearing loss, amplification should be pursued as soon as possible. Given the significant possibility that stapedial fixation will be encountered, it is not advisable to proceed with surgery while there is a significant risk of otitis media. Stapes surgery at an early age presents an unnecessary risk of perioperative labyrinthitis with resultant sensorineural hearing loss. Surgery is not warranted unless the hearing loss is in the moderate to severe range, with a speech reception threshold greater than 35 and a pure-tone average greater than 30 dB.[7] Once the child reaches an age when hearing can be reliably tested and is beyond the time period of increased vulnerability to otitis media, stapes surgery can be performed quite safely.[8,9]

Conductive hearing loss should always be confirmed with tuning fork testing before proceeding with surgical intervention. Children who are unable to respond reliably to tuning fork testing will probably not prove reliable for behavioral air and bone conduction testing. It is safer to provide amplification until the audiometric test results are reliable. Surgery for conductive hearing loss in the setting of a normally formed ear canal is an elective procedure. The hearing loss can be effectively managed with hearing aids, and it is imperative that parents understand the alternatives to surgery before proceeding with exploration in a pediatric patient, particularly for anomalies that are associated with significant risk to the facial nerve or inner ear (i.e., congenital stapedial fixation or absence of the oval window). Some authors argue that it is not appropriate to proceed with surgical management of unilateral conductive hearing loss not attributable to otitis media until the child can participate in the informed consent process.

When stable conductive hearing loss has been documented in children, the possibility of congenital fixation of the stapes must be entertained. This disorder is caused by failure of differentiation of the lamina stapedialis into the annular ligament, which results in ankylosis of the stapes footplate. The chief risk associated with fenestration of the footplate in such cases is the occurrence of a perilymphatic gusher. Although the true incidence of a perilymphatic gusher is unknown, it has been reported to be significantly higher than the incidence seen in otosclerosis (<1%).[10] Congenital stapedial footplate fixation can occur in the setting of an X-linked familial disorder characterized by progressive mixed hearing loss associated with inner ear anomalies, including Mondini's malformations and dilatation of the internal auditory canal (Fig. 116-1). The excessive flow of perilymph that follows opening of the footplate in these children is believed to be due to either a patent cochlear aqueduct or a defect in the lateral end of a dilated internal auditory canal. Mutations in the gene encoding the POU3f4 transcription factor have been implicated in at least one form of X-linked progressive mixed hearing loss.[11,12] The presence of mixed loss, particularly in males, should alert the surgeon to a potential gusher. Although some surgeons have obtained successful hearing results, it is generally conceded that computed tomography (CT) evidence of a widened cochlear aqueduct or internal auditory canal should be considered a relative contraindication to surgery.

Superior canal dehiscence syndrome, in which the bone overlying the superior semicircular canal is absent, can be manifested as conductive hearing loss and probably accounts for a fraction of the patients whose air-bone gap fails to close after stapes surgery.[13] The conductive hearing loss persists postoperatively because it is not secondary to stapes fixation. Rather, the con-

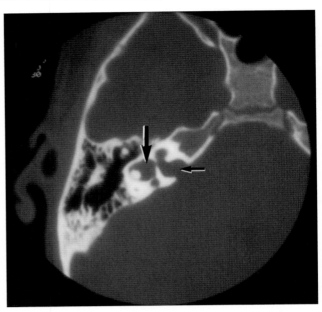

Figure 116-1. Computed tomography scan of a dysplastic inner ear showing a dilated and tortuous internal auditory canal (*small arrow*, internal auditory canal; *large arrow*, Mondini's deformity).

ductive loss is due to bony deficiency in the otic capsule and the resultant "mobile third window." This problem can be avoided by confirming the absence of a middle ear reflex before proceeding with middle ear exploration. Ossicular fixation should result in an elevated or absent stapedial reflex, whereas in superior canal dehiscence syndrome, this reflex will be preserved. Another situation in which caution is advised is an adult patient with conductive hearing loss and a history suggestive of Meniere's disease. Stapes surgery in the setting of endolymphatic hydrops is associated with a higher risk of sensorineural hearing loss and dizziness, which may be related to the proximity of the distended saccular epithelium to the stapes footplate.

PREOPERATIVE EVALUATION

History and Physical Examination

A thorough history should be elicited from the patient or caregivers, or both. In children it is important to note the onset of symptoms to help differentiate a congenital disorder from the juvenile onset of an acquired disorder. Prenatal history, school performance, social interactions, and language development should be assessed. Previous otologic history, particularly the frequency of otitis media and requirement for pressure equalization tubes, should be assessed. The history will often be limited in a pediatric patient, but when possible, it should address otologic symptoms such as otalgia, otorrhea, tinnitus, or vertigo. A careful review of symptoms may reveal associated cardiac, renal, or other medical problems suggestive of a syndromic diagnosis. A family history of hearing loss is important to address.

Physical examination should include inspection for other developmental anomalies, particularly those originating in the first and second branchial arches. Children with disorders affecting the mandibular arch (i.e., Treacher Collins syndrome) are at risk for airway compromise, so appropriate precautions must be taken in the operating room. Identification of even minor flaws in the pinna or surrounding area, such as preauricular tags and pits, should alert the surgeon to a higher probability of an anomaly. Conductive hearing loss in a normal-appearing ear in a patient with contralateral atresia or microtia should be assumed to represent an abnormality of the middle ear. Occasionally, ossicular anomalies, especially those involving the malleus, may be visible on otomicroscopy. However, most often the otoscopic examination is unremarkable. Weber and Rinne tests must always be included and the results should be consistent with the audiometric findings.

Audiologic Testing

Identification and treatment of significant hearing loss in the pediatric population are critical for appropriate development of speech and language. Assessment of hearing loss can be challenging in this population because of the limitations inherent in patient histories and the questionable reliability of audiologic testing. Because conductive hearing loss is so commonly associated with otitis media, hearing loss caused by an ossicular malformation is occasionally inappropriately attributed to recurrent infection and eustachian tube dysfunction. It is important to confirm closure of the air-bone gap once a child's middle ear has been ventilated to avoid overlooking a congenital anomaly.[7] Audiologic testing is performed in an age-appropriate fashion. Children as young as 2 years old can be trained, with repeated testing, to respond reliably to masked air and bone conduction tests.[7] Tympanometry should be included as well because even the most astute clinician can sometimes miss a middle ear effusion, particularly in a poorly cooperative child. When appropriate, acoustic reflexes should be determined as well.

Progressive versus Stable Hearing Loss

An important determination in children is the distinction between progressive and stable hearing loss. Progressive conductive loss in the absence of significant otoscopic findings is most often compatible with a diagnosis of childhood otosclerosis. Although unusual, especially before the age of 12 years, this condition may be handled with the same surgical techniques as those used to perform stapes surgery in adults (see Chapter 117). Several authors have attested to the safety of stapes surgery in children.[14] Congenital fixation of the stapes, in contrast, carries some increased risk for sensorineural deafness and requires additional preparation. Otosclerosis may be diagnosed by documentation of progressive impairment in hearing, whereas congenital stapedial fixation is stable. The family history may provide an important clue in establishing this diagnosis,

and CT may identify characteristic radiolucency of the otic capsule.

Imaging

Developments in radiologic evaluation of the temporal bone have facilitated the management of middle ear malformations. Careful evaluation of radiographic information will allow the surgeon to assess the chance of successful hearing restoration and provide specific details for informed patient consent. Dilatation of the internal auditory canal or enlargement of the cochlear aqueduct can be identified preoperatively and may lead the surgeon to recommend conservative management (Fig. 116-1). All pediatric patients with conductive hearing loss not attributable to otitis media merit high-resolution temporal bone CT. Radiologic imaging is not indicated in an adult patient undergoing exploration for conductive hearing loss unless there is strong suspicion of a congenital middle ear malformation or neoplasm.

SURGICAL APPROACH

Most of the operative techniques used to correct middle ear malformations are similar to or modifications of tympanoplasty methods. Procedures that are successful in middle ear reconstruction after eradication of chronic disease are highly adaptable in dealing with a great variety of congenital ossicular problems. Various approaches to reconstruction of the conductive apparatus can be used, with technical details varying according to surgeon preference and the individual patient's anatomy. Thus, a "cookbook" approach to surgical correction of middle ear abnormalities can be difficult, and surgeons will ultimately develop their individual preferences for materials and reconstructive approaches. Materials must be available in the operating room to adequately replace or reconstruct any ossicular abnormality. Incus sculpting is often a viable option in these cases. An assortment of partial and total ossicular replacements, as well as stapes prostheses, should also be kept on hand. The Skeeter drill should be available for incus sculpting, as well as possible drill outs for thickened stapes footplates. Depending on surgeon preference for stapes procedures, CO_2, argon, or other otologic lasers can provide less traumatic access to the vestibule.

Regardless of the material chosen for reconstruction, the basic principles for reconstructing the middle ear conductive apparatus include the use of appropriately sized material in an adequately aerated middle ear and a stable, columnar mechanism for conduction of sound from the most lateral mobile structure (capitulum or footplate) to the malleus or tympanic membrane. Appropriate sizing of the reconstruction requires patience and experience—short prostheses are prone to slippage, whereas prostheses that are excessive in length may sublux into the vestibule. The more angled the reconstruction, the higher the chance for slippage. Some prosthetic materials (i.e., titanium) require placement of a small cartilage graft between the prosthesis and the tympanic membrane to prevent extrusion. Cartilage can be harvested from the tragus or concha via a small incision. With a postauricular incision, often a necessity in a pediatric patient, conchal cartilage is preferred because it can be harvested without a second incision.

Anesthesia

In an adult it is preferable to perform exploratory surgery under local anesthesia with intravenous sedation whenever possible. Local anesthesia results in the advantages of less bleeding, cost-effectiveness, postoperative analgesia, quicker patient mobilization, reduced risk for aspiration, the ability to test hearing during surgery, and immediate feedback regarding potential vestibular injury.[15] Young children require general anesthesia. The surgeon must balance the increased latitude provided by deeper anesthesia with the loss of feedback information from the patient. If the course of the facial nerve is found to be significantly aberrant on preoperative CT, general anesthesia with the use of a facial nerve monitor may prove safer than local anesthesia with sedation.

Elevation of a Tympanomeatal Flap and Exploration of the Middle Ear

Regardless of the mode of anesthesia, four-quadrant injection of a local anesthetic in combination with epinephrine is useful in minimizing bleeding during elevation of the tympanomeatal flap. When planning the tympanomeatal flap, one must always ensure that the superior limb of the tympanomeatal flap extends far enough superiorly to allow considerable removal of the scutum in the case of a lateral ossicular chain procedure (Fig. 116-2). In adults a transcanal approach typically provides adequate exposure. Younger children may require a postauricular approach. Once the middle ear is entered, each component of the ossicular chain

is palpated independently. It is important to recognize that multiple defects may coexist—as highlighted by the increased incidence of lateral ossicular chain fixation identified on re-exploration after unsuccessful stapes surgery.[14]

Anticipating an Aberrant Facial Nerve

In approaching a malformed ear, identification of the facial nerve is critical. The preoperative CT scan should be reviewed carefully and the course of the nerve delineated. The surgeon must be familiar not only with the usual landmarks for the tympanic segment of the facial nerve but also with the most common aberrant courses. Dehiscence of the horizontal portion of the facial nerve is such a common finding that it may be considered a normal variant. Usually, the surgeon need only recognize the condition and avoid trauma to the nerve. Overhanging of the nerve may, on the other hand, present some difficulty in accessing the oval window (Fig. 116-3). The facial overhang can be managed by gentle retraction of the nerve while working in the oval window area. A stapes prosthesis may be placed in close contact with the nerve and may occasionally even cause a small indentation in the epineurium. When this abnormality is combined with shortening of the long process of the incus, the situation is more difficult. It can usually be solved by bending a crimp-on prosthesis to fit around the facial nerve (Fig. 116-4).

The facial nerve may subdivide into several branches and in some cases may not traverse the bony fallopian canal. Occasionally, its course across the oval window prevents surgical access to the vestibule; to avoid injury to the facial nerve, these cases should be abandoned in favor of amplification. Anterior deviation of the vertical portion of the facial nerve is usually associated with congenital aural atresia, but it may exist alone; it is identified as it courses across the hypotympanum. In a

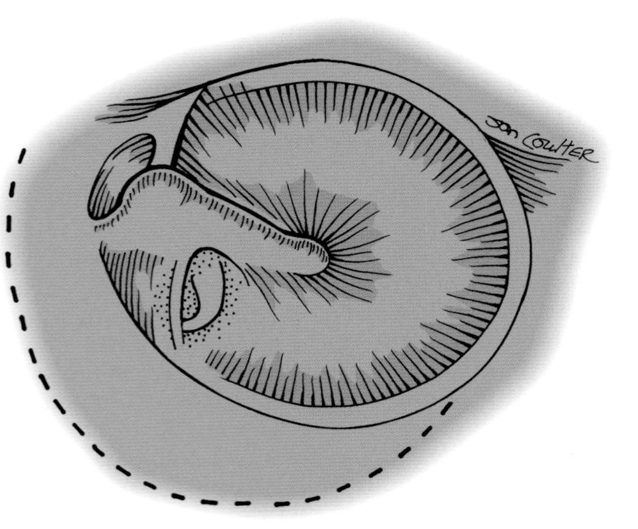

Figure 116-2. Correct incision for middle ear exploration to evaluate for conductive hearing loss.

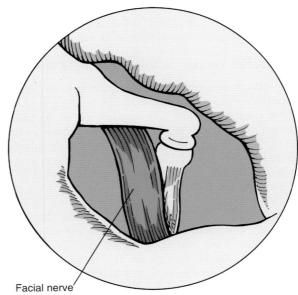

Facial nerve

Figure 116-3. Dehiscent and overhanging facial nerve.

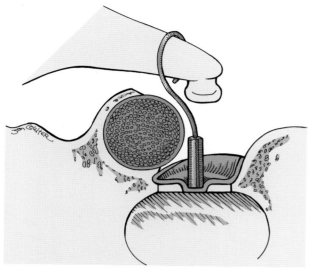

Figure 116-4. Use of a fashioned crimp-on piston prosthesis to circumvent an overhanging facial nerve.

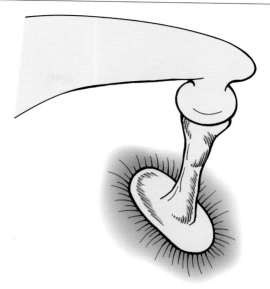

Figure 116-5. Monopedal stapes superstructure.

series of 94 patients with congenital malformations of the ear (50 of whom had anomalies confined to the middle ear), Jahrsdoerfer reported an aberrant course of the facial nerve in 12 cases.[16] Most commonly, the tympanic segment of the nerve was displaced inferiorly and obscured the oval window. The nerve was often dehiscent in the middle ear. The free-floating facial nerve was mistaken for fibrous tissue in two cases previously operated on elsewhere and resulted in injury to the nerve.

Modifications in the anatomy of the chorda tympani nerve are common. This nerve may be larger or smaller in diameter than normal and may be displaced inferiorly or superiorly relative to the posterosuperior canal wall. On occasion, the chorda tympani may enter the middle ear from a position lateral to the annulus of the tympanic membrane. In this situation, the nerve travels beneath the skin of the posterior canal wall for a short distance and may be injured on elevation of the tympanomeatal flap.

In cases in which a middle ear malformation is suspected, intraoperative facial nerve monitoring provides a definite advantage. Unfortunately, these defects are often not suspected preoperatively. When unexpected questions arise regarding the location of the facial nerve, disposable stimulators can be used. If the intraoperative findings suggest that facial function may be jeopardized, the procedure should be terminated, appropriate imaging studies obtained, and formal nerve monitoring used in a subsequent procedure.

The following discussion reviews middle ear anomalies in accordance with the likelihood of their appearance. Congenital anomalies of the incus or malleus in the setting of a mobile stapes (i.e., epitympanic fixation or ossicular discontinuity) are quite amenable to reconstruction, as is congenital fixation of the stapes footplate in the setting of a normal incudomalleolar complex. However, when stapedial fixation occurs in the context of an abnormal lateral chain, the chance for closure of the air-bone gap drops significantly.[14,17,18] Aplasia or severe dysplasia of the oval or round window carries an even worse prognosis for restoration of hearing, and controversy exists regarding whether reconstruction should be attempted at all in this situation. However, some authors have reported successful reconstruction of even these severe malformations.[16]

Defects of the Stapes

Although abnormalities of the stapes are the most frequently encountered of all ossicular defects, the variations seen are most often minor and inconsequential. Differences in the tilt and shape of the superstructure of the stapes are common. Hough has comprehensively reviewed these many variations.[19] The size of the obturator foramen and the shape of the crura often vary. Even defects as significant as a monopedal stapes are clinically unimportant unless hearing loss is present (Fig. 116-5).

Abnormalities requiring surgical correction are related to stapes fixation and incomplete articulation of the stapes with the incus. Bony bridges may connect the superstructure to the promontory (Fig. 116-6) or the facial nerve, or the stapes tendon may be ossified. These bony bridges probably represent failure of detachment of the developing stapes from Reichert's cartilage (second branchial arch).[20] These bridges may be separated by fracturing them or dividing them with a CO_2 laser. Occasionally, the superstructure of the stapes is separated from the footplate (Fig. 116-7). The defective arch should be removed and replaced with a prosthesis. Reconstruction can proceed with a total ossicular prosthesis or a stapes prosthesis, depending on the mobility of the footplate.

Footplate thickness varies but is important only relative to fixation. Congenital fixation is recognized as

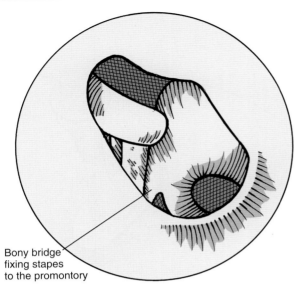

Figure 116-6. Bony attachment fixing the stapes to the promontory.

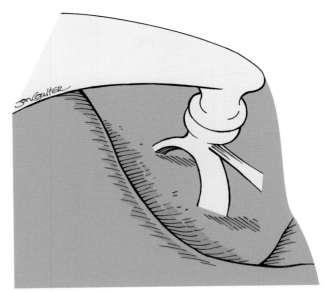

Figure 116-8. Congenital footplate fixation with absence of the annular ligament.

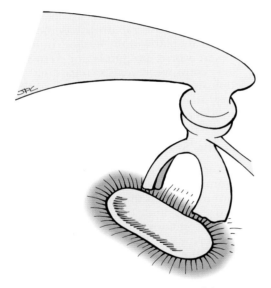

Figure 116-7. Congenital failure of the stapedial superstructure to articulate with the footplate.

a blending of the bone of the footplate with the surrounding otic capsule and the absence of a visible annular ligament (Fig. 116-8). Congenital fixation of the stapes may occur as a sporadic abnormality or in the setting of various syndromes. The fixed stapes is often deformed. In one series, one half the cases of stapedial footplate fixation were accompanied by associated anomalies of the incudomalleolar complex.[18] Although the reported results of stapes surgery in the setting of isolated stapedial fixation are quite good, the presence of associated abnormalities of the lateral ossicular chain suggests a less favorable chance for a satisfactory hearing result. In a series from De la Cruz and associates, the air-bone gap was closed to within 10 dB in 71% of patients with normal incudomalleolar com-

plexes as opposed to only 12.5% of those with anomalies involving the lateral chain.[14] The drop in hearing results can be attributed to the decreased stability of the reconstruction when the prosthesis must extend from the footplate to the malleus or tympanic membrane. The thickness of the footplate may necessitate a drill-out procedure. This is performed in much the same manner as for obliterative otosclerosis. The oval window is gradually saucerized with a microdrill until the footplate is "blue-lined." At this point, fenestration is carried out in the usual manner, followed by stapes replacement with an appropriate prosthesis. Total absence of the stapes is rare, as is true of the other ossicles.

Handling a Perilymphatic Gusher

Excessive flow of perilymph on accessing the vestibule is more common in the setting of congenital stapedial fixation than otosclerosis.[10] Perilymph flow may be terminated by elevating the head of the table and packing the oval window with connective tissue. This situation must be handled with extreme patience. It is critical to avoid suctioning the vestibule. On occasion, a lumbar drain is necessary for controlling the flow of fluid at the oval window; however, it should be performed only if conservative measures fail. The patient may experience a spinal headache postoperatively. The preoperative CT scan should be reviewed carefully for the presence of a dilated internal auditory canal with inadequate definition of the habenula perforata, enlargement of the cochlear aqueduct, or the presence of a Mondini malformation, all of which suggest a risk for a perilymphatic gusher and may warrant management with amplification in lieu of surgical reconstruction.

Defects of the Incus

Hypoplasia or fibrous replacement of the long or lenticular process is the most common defect of the incus

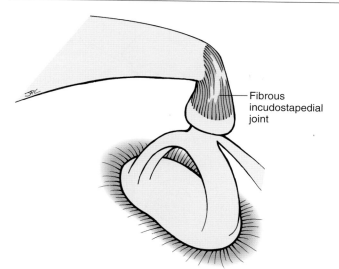

Figure 116-9. Fibrous incudostapedial joint.

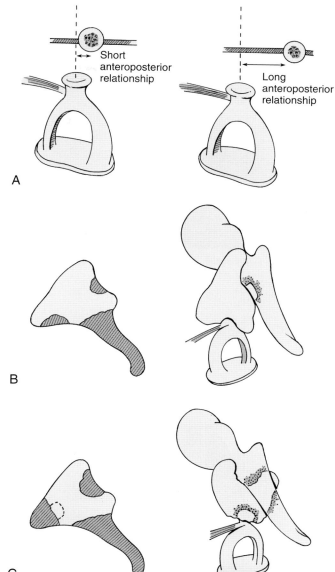

Figure 116-10. A, Variation in the anteroposterior (AP) dimensions between the malleus and the stapes head. **B,** Method of interpositioning the incus when the AP distance is long. **C,** Method of interpositioning the incus when the AP distance is short.

(Fig. 116-9). The appearance is much the same as with incus erosion after chronic otitis media with drum retraction. Complete lack of an incudostapedial joint is rare. These defects are most easily remedied by incus interposition, provided that mobility of the malleus and stapes is normal. This time-tested technique is associated with little risk of extrusion or absorption. There are many variations in modeling the incus for use, and surgeons have their own preferences. Figure 116-10 illustrates two options for fashioning and positioning the incus, depending on the anteroposterior distance between the malleus and stapes. Another option in dealing with this problem is a partial ossicular reconstructive/replacement prosthesis (PORP).

Fixation of the incus may occur secondary to bony attachments within the attic or from the horizontal semicircular canal. Failure of complete development of the incudomalleal joint (fusion) is common in aural atresia, but it may also occur as an isolated finding (Fig. 116-11). Minor spurs or projections sometimes emanate from the long process of the incus, and rarely, a bony bridge may connect the long process to the malleus handle. The latter problem is easily solved by separation of the bony ridge from the malleus with a malleus nipper. Fixation occurring in the epitympanum, however, should be corrected by separation of the incudostapedial joint, removal of the incus, and interposition of the incus between the stapes and the handle of the malleus. In this instance, mobilization procedures are associated with a significant risk of refixation.

Variations in angulation and size of the distal portion of the long process are common in the setting of a congenital malformation. These aberrations may affect the use of certain stapedial prostheses, particularly the bucket-handle variety. A prosthesis with a large well may be necessary, and failure to engage the bucket handle may result.

Defects of the Malleus

Developmental anomalies of the malleus are the most uncommon of the ossicular defects. Complete absence of this structure is extremely rare and has been described only in the presence of multiple abnormalities. Separation of the manubrium from the neck and head of the malleus has occasionally been reported,[21] and the manubrium is also sometimes twisted or rotated anteriorly or posteriorly from its normal position. Absence or discontinuity of the malleus handle (Fig. 116-12) constitutes a major conductive hearing loss that is most easily handled by removing the incus and placing a PORP from the stapes to the tympanic membrane. Preservation of the incus in these cases makes reconstruc-

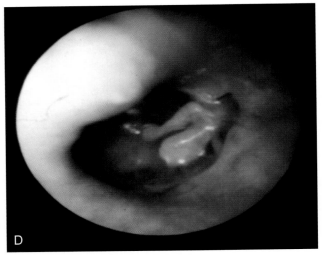

Figure 116-10, cont'd. D, Postoperative photograph of a left tympanic membrane after incus interposition.

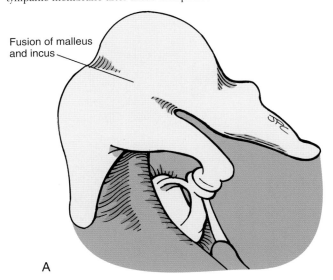

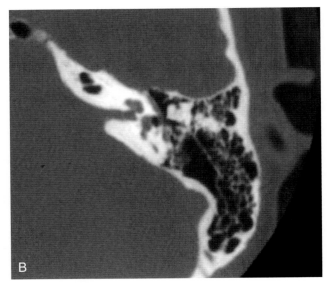

Figure 116-11. A, Fusion of the malleus and the incus. **B,** Radiographic appearance of malleoincudal fusion.

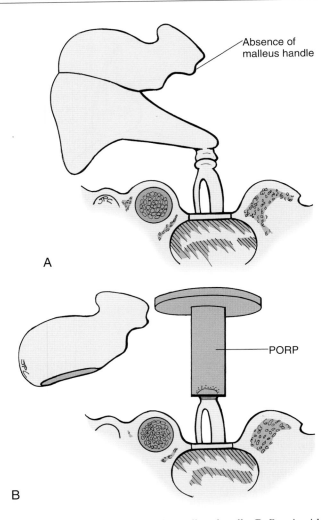

Figure 116-12. A, Absence of the malleus handle. **B,** Repair with a partial ossicular replacement prosthesis (PORP).

tion difficult. Use of a PORP ensures that the center of the tympanic membrane is used to provide the maximal driving force to the ossicular chain. The authors' choice of prosthesis is a hydroxyapatite PORP with a flexible shaft. Another rare defect is absence of contact between the malleus handle and the tympanic membrane (Fig. 116-13). This defect can be addressed by a lateral tympanoplasty with placement of the graft medial to the malleus handle. Alternatively, the incus can be removed and a PORP used to bridge between the stapes and the tympanic membrane.

Fixation of the head of the malleus occurs in about 1 in every 100 ears explored for conductive hearing loss (Fig. 116-14).[21] Bony attachments to the scutum may be present superiorly or laterally; fusion to the incus was described earlier. Early attempts at correction by merely fracturing these attachments were met with a relatively high incidence of refixation. For this reason, the head should be separated from the malleus with malleus nippers or a microdrill after separation of the incudostapedial joint. The incus is then removed, sculpted,

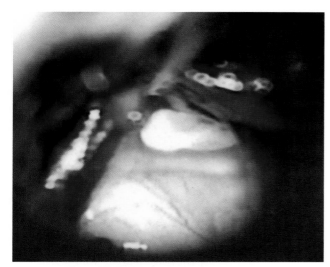

Figure 116-13. The long process of the malleus has failed to attach to the tympanic membrane.

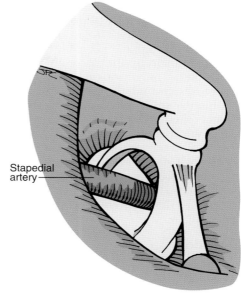

Figure 116-15. Stapedial artery remnant coursing through the obturator foramen of the stapes.

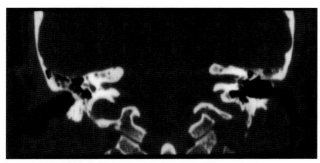

Figure 116-14. Computed tomography scan revealing fixation of the left malleus head.

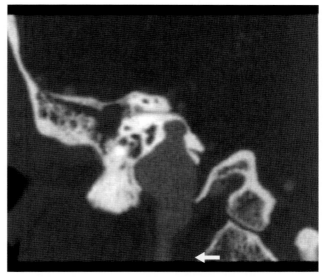

Figure 116-16. Contrast-enhanced coronally reconstructed computed tomography scan demonstrating a high-riding jugular bulb with a small diverticulum arising from the superior surface *(arrow).*

and interposed between the stapes and malleus. Thus, lateral fixation of the ossicular chain is actually managed in the same fashion regardless of whether the malleus or the incus is involved.

Vascular Abnormalities

Small remnants of the stapedial artery are frequently noticed in the course of middle ear exploration. These tiny vessels usually present no problem, and the small amount of bleeding that they engender will cease spontaneously. Large remnants of the stapedial artery require more careful attention (Fig. 116-15). Access to the footplate and even its removal can usually be accomplished by working anterior or posterior to these vessels. Ligation of large vessels with clips or laser hemostasis should be avoided because of potential injury to the facial nerve. The persistent stapedial artery substitutes for the middle meningeal artery, and the foramen spinosum is congenitally absent.[22]

The presence of a high jugular bulb is relatively common and may be associated with dehiscence into the middle ear. The jugular bulb is most often defined as high riding when the most cephalad portion of the bulb reaches beyond the level of the floor of the inter-

nal auditory canal.[23] Occasionally, a high-riding bulb may contain a diverticulum, which projects even further cephalad (Fig. 116-16). This anomaly is usually asymptomatic and does not require intervention. If the high-riding bulb is symptomatic (pulsatile tinnitus, conductive hearing loss), it may be skeletonized and held inferior to the round window by a graft of tragal cartilage or cortical bone.

The rarest of vascular abnormalities is an aberrant carotid artery. The normal petrous carotid turns from its vertical course to a horizontal and medial trajectory.

This genu is normally anteromedial to the cochlea. An aberrant carotid artery results from inadequate development of the cervical internal carotid artery. Blood flow is redirected through the normally very small inferior tympanic branch of the ascending pharyngeal artery and to the caroticotympanic artery.[24] The aberrant vessel courses through the middle ear and appears on CT as a tubular soft tissue mass along the promontory that enters the horizontal carotid canal through a dehiscence in the lateral carotid plate (Fig. 116-17). An aberrant carotid artery is not amenable to surgical therapy. The chief danger with this entity is failing to recognize its true identity or mistaking it for a glomus tumor. Misdiagnosis with puncture or biopsy of the vessel can result in significant hemorrhage and possibly neurologic sequelae.[25]

Round Window

Complete absence of the round window is perhaps the rarest of middle ear defects. As the otic capsule ossifies during development, a cartilaginous ring prevents bony deposition at the site of the nascent round window membrane.[26] Absence of the round window is presumed to be secondary to improper formation of this cartilaginous ring. Jahrdoerfer reported successful hearing outcomes in three patients with congenital oval window aplasia who had no apparent round window, so this finding does not necessarily represent a contraindication to ossicular reconstruction.[16] Fenestration of the promontory to create a round window is not advisable because of a significant risk of sensorineural hearing loss.

Other Lesions

Congenital cholesteatomas are discussed in Chapter 126. These lesions are usually seen transtympanically or occasionally discovered at the time of myringotomy, but they are rarely encountered unexpectedly in the course of middle ear exploration. Choristomas are unusual lesions consisting of heterotopic tissue and may be found in the middle ear as well. In both instances, treatment requires complete surgical ablation followed by reconstructive measures common with tympanoplasty. Other soft tissue lesions, such as hemangiomas and adenomas, are rare.

POSTOPERATIVE MANAGEMENT

Postoperative management of patients undergoing surgery for congenital middle ear abnormalities is generally the same as that after tympanoplasty with reconstruction. The exception is a perilymph gusher. In these cases the head is maintained at an elevation of at least 30 degrees for 48 hours. When perilymphatic drainage continues postoperatively, a lumbar subarachnoid catheter is inserted, and 50 mL of cerebrospinal fluid is removed every 8 hours in adults and older children. Correspondingly, younger children require withdrawal of lesser amounts. Minimal hydration is maintained, and the catheter can usually be removed within 48 to

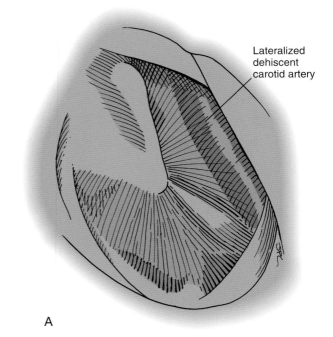

Lateralized dehiscent carotid artery

A

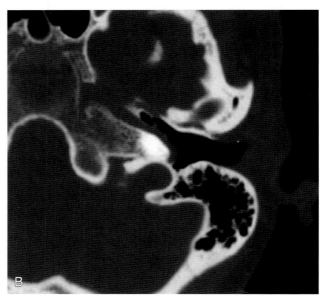

B

Figure 116-17. A, Aberrant carotid artery as seen through the tympanic membrane. **B,** Computed tomography scan demonstrating an aberrant internal carotid artery.

72 hours. Strenuous activity is forbidden for 2 to 3 weeks. The usual precautions against blowing the nose and avoidance of water in the ear are given.

Packing in the external canal consists of a small silk sleeve held in place over the tympanomeatal flap and supported with several small cotton balls or Merocel spheres moistened with antibiotic ointment. This material is removed 1 week after surgery, but water is avoided until the canal is completely healed. Audiometry is performed when it can be determined that the flap is completely healed and there is no longer fluid or blood within the middle ear, typically within 3 to 4 weeks postoperatively. Antibiotics are not routinely administered after middle ear surgery, and analgesics are necessary for several days only.

COMPLICATIONS

Complications after surgical correction of middle ear anomalies include hearing loss, vertigo, perilymphatic drainage, and facial paralysis. Treatment of perilymphatic drainage has been addressed.

In the early postoperative period, hearing loss may usually be assessed with a tuning fork. Conductive loss is common because of packing in the canal and middle ear effusion, but sensorineural loss may follow a drill-out procedure or one associated with a perilymph gusher. Stopping the fluid leakage is the most effective way to prevent permanent hearing loss. Steroids have no proven value in these cases but are often administered in divided doses of 60 to 80 mg of prednisone daily in adults.

Mild to moderate vertigo can follow any middle ear procedure but is most common after opening of the oval window. Severe vertigo, especially when not present intraoperatively under local anesthesia, is unexpected and may signal a serious problem. The surgeon should consider a fistula, subluxation of the footplate, or a prosthesis that extends too far into the vestibule. Sensorineural hearing loss often accompanies this complication. If one of the listed causes is believed to be possible, surgical exploration should be carried out immediately to correct the problem.

Temporary facial paralysis may result from diffusion of local anesthetic toward the stylomastoid foramen or, less commonly, from the use of topical anesthesia in the middle ear in the presence of dehiscence in the fallopian canal. An appropriate period of observation will soon delineate these cases. When facial weakness persists, the surgeon must question whether the nerve was exposed and injury may have occurred. This situation is unusual after middle ear surgery but is more common after mastoidectomy or procedures for aural atresia. When paralysis is unexpected and without explanation, re-exploration is mandatory to rule out disruption of the nerve.

Acknowledgments

The authors would like to acknowledge Dr. Donald B. Kamerer for his major contribution to the first edition of this chapter and Dr. Barton Branstetter for generously sharing radiologic images of congenital temporal bone malformations.

PEARLS

- A chance encounter with a middle ear abnormality is a probability for every otologic surgeon.
- Middle ear malformations should always be considered in the differential diagnosis of children with conductive or mixed hearing loss.

- Preoperative CT should be obtained in all pediatric patients with conductive hearing loss not attributable to otitis media to fully assess the middle ear for an aberrant course of the facial nerve and abnormalities of the ossicular chain.
- A variety of materials should be available so that the otologic surgeon is equipped to deal with any unexpected finding in the course of middle ear exploration for conductive hearing loss.
- If a perilymph gusher is encountered, avoid suctioning at the fenestra, elevate the head of the bed until the flow stops, and pack the oval window with connective tissue.

PITFALLS

- Middle ear anomalies are accompanied by a higher risk of an aberrant facial nerve and require vigilance.
- Stapes surgery should not be performed when there is radiologic evidence of a widened internal auditory or cochlear aqueduct.
- Failure to recognize vascular anomalies such as an aberrant carotid and attempted myringotomy or biopsy may result in significant complications—temporal bone CT allows this entity to be recognized readily.
- Inappropriate exploratory tympanotomy can be avoided by confirmation of the absence of stapedial reflex before surgery.
- Unexpected postoperative vertigo should raise concern for a possible fistula, subluxation of the footplate, or a prosthesis that extends too far into the vestibule.

References

1. Gulya AJ, Schuknecht HF: Phylogeny and Embryology. In Anatomy of the Temporal Bone with Surgical Implications. New York, Parthenon, 1994, pp 235-273.
2. Lambert PR: Congenital absence of the oval window. Laryngoscope 100:37-40, 1990.
3. Farrior JB: Surgical management of congenital conductive deafness. South Med J 80:450-453, 1987.
4. Nager GT, Levin LS: Congenital aural atresia: Embryology, pathology, classification, genetics, and surgical management. In Paparella M, Shumrick D (eds); Otolaryngology. Philadelphia, WB Saunders, 1980, pp 1303-1344.
5. Stewart JM, Downs MP: Congenital conductive hearing loss: The need for early identification and intervention. Pediatrics 91:355-359, 1993.
6. Cremers CW, Teunissen E: The impact of a syndromal diagnosis on surgery for congenital minor ear anomalies. Int J Pediatr Otorhinolaryngol 22:59-74, 1991.
7. Briggs RJ, Luxford WM: Correction of conductive hearing loss in children. Otolaryngol Clin North Am 27:607-620, 1994.
8. House JW, Sheehy JL, Antunez JC: Stapedectomy in children. Laryngoscope 90:1804-1809, 1980.
9. Cole JM: Surgery for otosclerosis in children. Laryngoscope 92:859-862, 1982.

10. Dornhoffer JL, Helms J, Hoehmann DH: Stapedectomy for congenital fixation of the stapes. Am J Otol 16:382-386, 1995.

11. Vore AP, Chang EH, Hoppe JE, et al: Deletion of and novel missense mutation in POU3F4 in 2 families segregating X-linked nonsyndromic deafness. Arch Otolaryngol Head Neck Surg 131:1057-1063, 2005.

12. de Kok YJ, van der Maarel SM, Bitner-Glindzicz M, et al: Association between X-linked mixed deafness and mutations in the POU domain gene POU3F4. Science 267:685-688, 1995.

13. Minor LB, Carey JP, Cremer PD, et al: Dehiscence of bone overlying the superior canal as a cause of apparent conductive hearing loss. Otol Neurotol 24:270-278, 2003.

14. De la Cruz A, Angeli S, Slattery WH: Stapedectomy in children. Otolaryngol Head Neck Surg 120:487-492, 1999.

15. Caner G, Olgun L, Gultekin G, et al: Local anesthesia for middle ear surgery. Otolaryngol Head Neck Surg 133:295-297, 2005.

16. Jahrsdoerfer R: Congenital malformations of the ear. Analysis of 94 operations. Ann Otol Rhinol Laryngol 89:348-352, 1980.

17. Teunissen B, Cremers CW: Surgery for congenital stapes ankylosis with an associated congenital ossicular chain anomaly. Int J Pediatr Otorhinolaryngol 21:217-226, 1991.

18. Teunissen EB, Cremers WR: Classification of congenital middle ear anomalies. Report on 144 ears. Ann Otol Rhinol Laryngol 102:606-612, 1993.

19. Hough J: Malformations and anatomical variations seen in the middle ear during the operation for mobilization of the stapes. Laryngoscope 68:1337-1338, 1958.

20. Tos M: Embryology of Stapes Ankylosis. Surgical Solutions for Conductive Hearing Loss. Stuttgart, Germany, Thieme, 2000, pp 240-246.

21. Bergstrom L: Anomalies of the ear. Otolaryngology 1:24-28, 1994.

22. Silbergleit R, Quint DJ, Mehta BA, et al: The persistent stapedial artery. AJNR Am J Neuroradiol 21:572-577, 2000.

23. Swartz JH, Harnsberger HR: Temporal Bone Vascular Anatomy, Anomalies, and Diseases, Emphasizing the Clinical-Radiological Problem of Pulsatile Tinnitus. In Imaging of the Temporal Bone. New York, Thieme, 1998, pp 170-239.

24. Fisher NA, Curtin HD: Radiology of congenital hearing loss. Otolaryngol Clin North Am 27:511-531, 1994.

25. Sauvaget E, Paris J, Kici S, et al: Aberrant internal carotid artery in the temporal bone: Imaging findings and management. Arch Otolaryngol Head Neck Surg 132:86-91, 2006.

26. Martin C, Tringali S, Bertholon P, et al: Isolated congenital round window absence. Ann Otol Rhinol Laryngol 111:799-801, 2002.

Chapter 117

Otosclerosis

Barry E. Hirsch

Otosclerosis is a two-stage, metabolic bone-remodeling process of the otic capsule characterized by bone resorption (otospongiosis) and recalcification (otosclerosis). The term *otosclerosis* was ascribed to Politzer in 1894.[1] The etiology is believed to be familial, with inheritance occurring by autosomal dominant transmission with varying penetrance. Konigsmark and Gorlin[2] reported the incidence of clinical otosclerosis to be 3 per 1000 in whites and much less in blacks, although histologic evidence of disease has been reported in as many as 8% of temporal bones.

Investigations over the past few years have focused on other causes of stapes fixation, including viral infections. It is postulated that a systemic viral infection may cause an inflammatory vascular reaction with the subsequent development of otosclerosis. Reverse transcriptase–polymerase chain reaction (RT-PCR) has provided evidence suggesting that a paramyxovirus responsible for measles may be the cause of otosclerosis. An excellent summary of the association of viruses as the cause of otosclerosis was published by Ferlito and colleagues.[3]

Among adults, otosclerosis is the chief cause of conductive hearing loss, which occurs in several well-known patterns. It most frequently begins in young adulthood but may occur from adolescence to old age. Otosclerosis is more common in females by a ratio of 2:1 or 3:1, and the family history is positive in 50% of patients, which implies that the disease develops spontaneously in the remaining 50% of people affected by otosclerosis.

Although conductive hearing loss secondary to stapedial fixation is the classic manifestation, mixed hearing loss and even pure sensorineural hearing impairment can result from disease in the otic capsule. In addition, it is not uncommon for hearing loss to change in type over time. A sensorineural component may develop in people with conductive loss, and those who start with sensorineural hearing loss can acquire conductive loss as well.

Surgeons have recognized the mechanical impediment to sound transmission caused by otosclerosis since the late 19th century. Since then, surgical procedures for correction of otosclerosis have been modified, abandoned, and then re-established to provide one of otolaryngology's most fascinating stories. Today, a properly selected patient in the hands of an experienced otologic surgeon has a better than 95% chance of hearing restoration, with a low incidence of complications by closure of the air-bone gap. Certainly, these expectations rival those of any surgical procedure and have resulted in stapes surgery for otosclerosis being an extremely successful method of restoring hearing.

PATIENT EVALUATION AND SELECTION

Patients typically have a complaint of slowly progressive hearing loss in one or both ears identified by themselves or others such as coworkers, friends, and family. Associated complaints may include tinnitus that is occasionally described as "hearing one's heartbeat" in one or both ears. This form of pulsatile tinnitus can occur with otosclerosis, especially when otospongiosis is active. Patients with active disease may describe mild dizziness or motion intolerance. This complaint can be troubling because stapes surgery should be avoided if there are other sources of vestibular dysfunction. Dehiscence of the superior semicircular canal can be manifested as pressure-induced dizziness and conductive hearing loss. This is discussed later in this chapter. If the disequilibrium, lightheadedness, or motion intolerance can be ascribed to otosclerosis, surgery will probably resolve the problem. Patients may have a varied degree of hearing loss once confirmed on audiometric testing. Some people are acutely aware of 10 to 15 dB of hearing difference between the two ears. Others may need to incur greater loss to bring the impairment to their attention. Individual tolerance to hearing impairment varies greatly. For this reason it is not unusual for hearing loss to progress to moderate levels, especially when the patient's hearing needs have not been complex. The patient's subjective assessment of the hearing loss does not always match the physician's objective evaluation.

Physical examination of the ears should identify a healthy ear canal and tympanic membrane with no evidence of middle ear pathology. Tuning fork testing remains an essential factor in helping determine the type and degree of hearing loss. Positive results on the Rinne test (air conduction greater than bone conduction) with 256- and 512-Hz tuning forks suggest that if an air-bone gap is identified on audiometric testing, it is probably less than 15 dB. Such patients are not usually considered candidates for surgical intervention at that time. They are apprised of their hearing levels and advised to be seen again in 6 months to monitor their audiometric and tuning fork results. An audiogram is mandatory in evaluating candidacy for otosclerosis surgery. There should be evidence of a 25-dB air-bone gap in the involved ear to consider offering surgery for correction of the hearing loss. Conductive hearing loss on audiometric testing should always be confirmed by the tuning fork examination. Mixed hearing loss should prompt the surgeon to consider the phenomenon of Carhart's notch (Fig. 117-1). This will allow as much as 15 dB of "overclosure" at 2000 Hz, 10 dB at 1000 and 3000 Hz, and 5 dB at 500 Hz.

Ideally, successful surgery will restore hearing to normal levels, but many patients are happy with modest improvement that lessens their dependency on amplification. Each patient requires a thoughtful discussion of the realistic expectations for hearing improvement, in addition to counseling about alternative methods. For persons who are not certain about their treatment preference, a trial of amplification should be suggested.

Some clinical situations can present a significant challenge to obtaining accurate audiometric data. First is the presence of a large air-bone gap, particularly when asymmetrical. Correct use of adequate masking in this case is mandatory to avoid errors related to crossover to the other ear. Likewise, unilateral sensorineural impairment can create a "shadow curve" that mimics conductive loss. Tuning fork confirmation of audiometric data will save the physician from being misled.

Profound mixed hearing loss will challenge audiologists and otolaryngologists alike. In this situation, the bone conduction thresholds may exceed the maximum output of the audiometer, and the amount of air-bone gap is difficult to ascertain. Several clues, however, will help make the diagnosis of otosclerosis, including a positive family history of otosclerosis, documentation of progressive loss of hearing, evidence of conductive loss on previous audiograms, and success with amplification beyond that expected from examination of the audiometric thresholds. Reasonable word recognition scores in association with severe to profound sensorineural hearing loss should also heighten the clinician's suspicion of a conductive component. In these patients, surgical restoration of even 20 dB produces a grateful patient. They are in a much better position to successfully use a hearing aid at lower levels of amplification and avoid problems with acoustic feedback.

There are only two relatively hard-and-fast rules in surgery for otosclerosis: the first is never to operate on an only-hearing ear, and the second is always to operate on the poorer-hearing ear. These simple principles have been proved to serve the best interest of the patient. As with any rules, there are rare exceptions. If a person has profound mixed hearing loss in one ear, is anacoustic in the other, and is unable to successfully use a hearing aid, the option of attempting partial hearing restoration is reasonable. The only remaining option would be a cochlear implant. In a similar approach, if a patient who successfully underwent stapes surgery should lose hearing in the contralateral ear and serious complications develop in the operated ear, such as a perilymphatic fistula, surgical intervention is warranted.

Differential Diagnosis and Concomitant Otologic Disease

Conductive hearing loss does not always guarantee the diagnosis of otosclerosis, especially when only one ear is involved. This is an important principle to be remembered when counseling patients for surgery. The surgeon must always look for and be prepared to manage problems other than stapes fixation when exploring the impaired ear. Congenital middle ear anomalies, tympanosclerosis, and lateral fixation of the ossicular chain are among the other causes of conductive loss.

A new clinical entity has recently been described that provides an explanation for "inner ear conductive hearing loss." Minor noted that patients with dehiscence of the superior semicircular canal present with

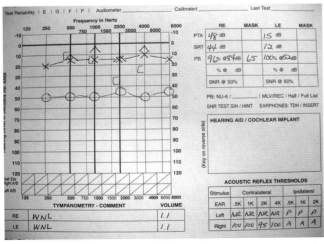

Figure 117-1. Audiogram showing right mixed hearing loss and a sensorineural dip at 2000 Hz indicative of Carhart's notch.

signs and symptoms indicative of having a third window in the otic capsule, including a positive Tullio phenomenon (sound-induced vertigo); dizziness with a Valsalva maneuver, coughing, belching, or sneezing; pulsatile or thumping tinnitus; and occasionally, conductive hearing loss. Tuning fork testing can still show a negative Rinne test (bone conduction greater than air conduction). Conductive hearing loss coming from the middle ear routinely exhibits absence of elicited acoustic reflexes. In contrast, acoustic reflexes are typically present when the conductive hearing loss is due to dehiscence of the superior semicircular canal.[4] Patients suspected of having otosclerosis should undergo testing for acoustic reflexes preoperatively to help avoid performing middle ear surgery when an alternative source of conductive hearing loss may exist.

Concomitant disease must be considered in several instances. Meniere's disease in the involved ear is generally considered to be a contraindication to surgery because of a higher incidence of postoperative cochlear impairment. Active Meniere's disease in the contralateral ear is also a relative contraindication because the final hearing status of that ear is unknown. Tympanic perforations should be repaired before stapes surgery because of the risk of contamination of the middle ear and vestibule by organisms from the external auditory canal. The same strategy is maintained when a ventilation tube is in place. The tube needs to be removed and the tympanic membrane repaired. If needed, a ventilation tube can be placed later in the postoperative period. Osteogenesis imperfecta (van der Hoeve's syndrome) is often associated with conductive hearing loss, but more often it is secondary to erosion of the incus or crura of the stapes. Likewise, patients with Paget's disease may have fixation of the stapes, but long-term results are unfavorable because of the development of sensorineural loss.

Otosclerosis in the Pediatric Age Group

Children with conductive hearing loss are less likely to have otosclerosis than other problems with the ossicular chain. Fixation of the stapes can be present from birth as a result of congenital fixation or can be acquired from tympanosclerosis or otosclerosis. The outcome after surgery can vary for each condition and may differ from surgeon to surgeon. Welling and coauthors reviewed the literature and reported their experience with pediatric stapes surgery. In general, similar results should be expected after stapes surgery for otosclerosis in children and adults. This implies hearing loss that develops late in the first decade or early teen years and is not associated with a history of recurrent otitis media. Surgical treatment of stapes fixation secondary to tympanosclerosis does not achieve as good or lasting results as treatment of fixation secondary to otosclerosis.[5] Computed tomography scanning must be performed in all pediatric patients with conductive hearing loss when surgical exploration is planned. The ear is examined for anomalies of the otic capsule such as a large vestibular aqueduct, cochlear dysplasia such as Mondini's deformity, or a wide internal auditory canal. These findings can be associated with a perilymphatic gusher, which may have disastrous effects on postoperative hearing. We would also recommend directing attention to the course of the facial nerve within the temporal bone to ensure that no anatomic anomalies are present. Such anomalies should temper the surgeon's judgment in favor of the use of amplification.

Selection of the correct ear for surgery is usually straightforward because the ear with the worse hearing is chosen. Word recognition scores are seldom a consideration in otosclerosis, but rarely these and other deficits in cochlear reserve must be factored in when presenting the options and risks to the patient. When hearing thresholds are similar in each ear, it is helpful to ask patients which side is most impaired in their judgment. Again, the worse ear is chosen for initial exploration. If the candidate cannot make a choice, it is useful to consider the side on which the telephone is usually held. Finally, if there is neither sufficient information nor patient preference to pick which side should be done first, the surgeon then has the option. It is easier for a right-handed surgeon to operate on a patient's left ear, especially if the patient has a large chest and short neck. The opposite holds for a left-handed surgeon.

In the past, some physicians have maintained that after successful surgery, the second ear should not undergo surgery. Today, most experienced surgeons believe that elective surgery in the second ear is desirable and carries the same risks as surgery on the first side. The advantages of binaural hearing in eliminating noise and providing sound localization are believed to outweigh the small risk of sensorineural loss. There is no correct period before which the second ear may undergo surgery, but most surgeons prefer to wait at least 6 months. Certainly, during that period hearing in the operated ear should improve with no signs of complications.

Counseling of a patient considering surgery must always be based on the tenet that these procedures are elective. Some patients will choose no treatment despite what the surgeon and family believe is an obvious need for amelioration. Each individual has the right to make an informed choice, whether seemingly wise or not. No surgeon wishes to be in the position of defending an unfavorable result in a patient who was reluctant to undergo surgery in the first place. This is why unhurried and careful preoperative counseling is so important. A frank discussion of the results expected and potential risks necessarily includes the experience of the surgeon and not merely statistics quoted from the literature.

Although every potential complication cannot be anticipated, it is imperative to discuss those that present the greatest dangers and those that occur with the greatest frequency. Among the specific risks to be addressed are worsening or total hearing loss, possible infection, vertigo, disturbances in taste, perforation of the tympanic membrane, and facial weakness. It is also important to address postoperative restrictions so that patients can properly plan the few weeks after their surgery, including avoiding heavy strenuous work or exercise and keeping the ear dry from water.

PREOPERATIVE PLANNING

A complete medical and drug history is important in each case. Pain in the back or neck or restriction of motion of the head or neck may limit the surgeon's ability to operate, particularly under local anesthesia. Advance knowledge of these potential problems will save a great deal of intraoperative delay. When lateral cervical rotation is restricted, the patient can be carefully strapped to an electric tilting operating table, which should provide adequate access to the ear, although patients with extreme immobility may technically be unable to undergo surgery. Patients who cannot lie flat or require special positioning may do better under general anesthesia. All medications that affect platelet function and coagulation should be discontinued 10 days before the procedure. Maintenance doses of warfarin (Coumadin) require consultation with the patient's primary care physician to discuss possible strategies for discontinuing the medication temporarily. As with any patient, a detailed history of drug allergies and sensitivities is necessary not only for the surgeon but also for the anesthesiologist.

The initial examination should recognize special problems related to the individual's anatomy, including the presence of a narrow external cartilaginous or bony meatus. Admission of a 4.5-mm speculum is generally sufficient for surgery, depending on the configuration of the canal. Constriction of the meatus can easily be alleviated by a 12-o'clock incision in the lateral canal between the helix and tragus. Unusual inclination or overhang of a canal wall should be noted preoperatively. Rarely, limited canal diameter or anterior displacement relative to the middle ear requires a postauricular approach. The presence of a very thin atrophic tympanic membrane, especially in its posterior portion, may alert the surgeon to the potential for a torn tympanic membrane and the need for supplemental tissue grafting of the tympanic membrane.

In the past our method for anesthesia was preoperative sedation and a local infiltration block. Exceptions were children, adults with special pain or positioning problems, and patients who request general anesthesia because of anxiety. We acknowledge the advantage of local anesthesia so that the surgeon can verify whether the patient's hearing is improved while on the operating table. The surgeon can also monitor for the development of vertigo in an awake patient. Complaints of vertigo should alter the surgeon's procedure or technique being taken at that time. Our approach then switched to the use of narcoleptic anesthesia administered intravenously by an anesthesiologist. This form of conscious sedation too often provided varying levels of sedation. The anesthesia would be "too light" or even "too deep," and patients would suddenly startle. They also experienced occasional paradoxical agitation and inability to hold still. Over the past few

years we have used general anesthesia. It is our thinking that a motionless patient is less likely to have complications. We are confident in our technical abilities to execute the procedure in the same manner as though the patient were awake or sedated. The ear canal is still infiltrated by local injection via dental carpules containing 2% lidocaine (Xylocaine) with a 1:100,000 solution of epinephrine through a 27-gauge needle.

Imaging

Imaging is rarely necessary in the routine evaluation of otosclerosis if only conductive hearing loss is present. During the active phase of otospongiosis, demineralization may be evident in the anterior aspect of the footplate at the fissula ante fenestram. Patients with sensorineural hearing loss may demonstrate demineralization of the otic capsule by the presence of a doublering or halo sign. Visualization of the otic capsule with magnetic resonance imaging (MRI) typically reveals a signal void characteristic of bone. Scanning after gadolinium enhancement may demonstrate active foci of otospongiosis. In advanced cases of cochlear otosclerosis, high-resolution, T2-weighted MRI sequences give useful information about the patency of the basal turn of the cochlea when a cochlear implant procedure is being considered.[6]

PROSTHESES AND SURGICAL TECHNIQUES

The intended technique for implantation of stapes prostheses dictates the design and material composition of the device. Small fenestra stapedotomy calls for a narrow piston with a wire extension that is crimped over the distal long process of the incus. It should be relatively firm and lightweight to avoid undue tension on the incus. The hooked portion can be secured over the incus by using crimping forceps to close the loop around the incus. A prosthesis that is too tight around the incus will probably lead to necrosis of the ossicle given the tenuous blood supply along the long process of the incus. A prosthesis that is too loose will also cause traumatic erosion because of the "sawing" action that occurs with reciprocating vibration of the incus against the wire loop. Efforts to avoid this complication of stapes surgery have been made through changes in design and materials. The original round configuration of the wire that is crimped over the incus was modified from the shape of a cylinder to a flat ribbon, which disperses the surface area of contact. The earlier material used in crimp-on prostheses was stainless steel. The ribbon design incorporates platinum, which is softer and more malleable.

The process of crimping the hooked portion around the incus entails a scissors-like action of the fingers to close an instrument with its operating end consisting of slotted jaws that do not close completely. This maneuver may be fraught with minute arcs of hand rotation that make it slightly difficult to remain in the same plane of closure. The mechanical effort of closing

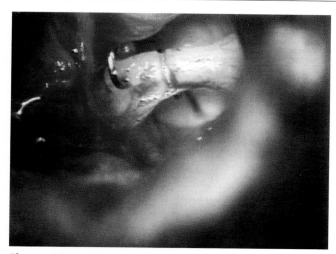

Figure 117-2. Left ear showing a crimp-on prosthesis that had eroded the long process of the incus.

the jaws can be delivered with excessive force, thereby crimping the hooked portion too tightly. Similarly, insufficient closure will probably result in the patient complaining of sound distortion and a sense of vibration. If the prosthesis is too loose, erosion of the incus will eventually occur, with return of the conductive hearing loss (Fig. 117-2).

Numerous investigators have researched outcomes based on the material used for stapes piston prostheses. Massey and coworkers conducted a study to compare the effectiveness of titanium and Teflon wire prostheses for hearing improvement in patients undergoing stapes surgery for otosclerosis. Closure of the air-bone gap to less than 10 dB was achieved in 86% of patients with a Teflon prosthesis versus 71% of those receiving titanium prostheses.[7] A smaller number of patients received the titanium prosthesis, which at the time was used when the diameter of the incus was smaller. The design of the prosthesis allows a more circumferential crimp around the incus. A similar study comparing gold and titanium prostheses was reported by Tange and coauthors.[8] They found that the heavier gold piston gave more overclosure (gain) than the lighter titanium prosthesis did; however, they thought that the lighter but stiffer titanium piston provided a higher air-bone gap closure within 10 dB.[8]

Developments in metallurgy over the past few decades have brought new alloys into medicine with applications in otology. Nitinol is a shaped memory alloy composed of nickel and titanium. To remove the forceps from the crimping process, Nitinol is now available in stapes prostheses. The application of heat activates a phase transformation in the metal that causes it to revert to its closed position around the incus. Heat is typically delivered with a laser on low energy settings. The use of this material and technique precludes overcrimping at the attachment to the incus. The piston portion of the device is made of Teflon (Gyrus Corp., Jacksonville, FL). Knox and Reitan published an excel-

lent review of the history, chemical and mechanical properties, and in vitro and in vivo testing of Nitinol stapes prostheses.[9]

There have been minimal changes in the surgical method of treating otosclerosis. In the early years, stapes mobilization was initially successful but routinely succumbed to refixation. Over the past 50 years, postoperative results have consistently demonstrated that removal of a portion or the entire stapes footplate (stapedectomy) or bypass of the obstruction with a fenestration piston (stapedotomy) successfully resolves the source of conductive impairment. Silverstein introduced a novel technique for overcoming otosclerosis limited to the anterior portion of the footplate (fissula ante fenestram) when the remainder of the footplate is blue, thin, and without fixation. He described a minimally invasive stapes procedure termed stapedotomy minus prosthesis (STAMP). The anterior crus is vaporized with a handheld argon laser. The anterior footplate is then vaporized linearly in a superior-to-inferior direction to allow the posterior footplate to be mobile and still be attached by the stapes tendon. The decision whether this procedure could be performed was made during exploration of the middle ear. The preoperative audiogram was not predictive of the degree and location of otosclerosis. Statistical analysis suggested that there was improvement in high-frequency hearing results as compared with conventional laser stapedotomy procedures. The rate of refixation was 9%, but revision surgery was not precluded.[10]

Positioning of the Patient

Positioning of the patient on the operating table must be optimal to facilitate proper exposure for the surgeon. The patient should be as close to the surgeon as the table comfortably permits. Elevation of the head should be minimized; in persons with a short neck or a large chest, it may even be helpful to slightly lower the head of the table relative to the horizontal plane of the body. Comfort should be achieved by padding the arms, elevating the knees, or placing support under the lumbar area as necessary. It is not necessary to remove any hair, but it must be secured to allow easy and unobstructed access to the ear canal. The arm opposite the ear undergoing surgery is positioned on an arm board, and an appropriate vein on the dorsum of the hand is identified for use as a tissue graft in the oval window. Preparation is carried out with either alcohol or povidone-iodine (Betadine) solution as the surgeon chooses. After conventional draping for a transcanal procedure, the solution is gently suctioned from the ear canal, and cerumen is removed as necessary.

Anesthesia

Anesthetic block is achieved with a 27-gauge needle and dental carpules containing 2% lidocaine with a 1:100,000 solution of epinephrine. Injection is begun at the 6-o'clock position in the canal and carried out slowly because of resistance of the skin, which is adherent to cartilage or bone. Gradual blanching of the canal skin signals successful injection. Too rapid an injection may also cause ballooning of the canal skin with a subcutaneous collection of fluid. When this occurs, the ballooned area should be punctured immediately with a needle tip. Gradual progression of the injections then proceeds from the 6-o'clock position in both directions until circumferential anesthesia is complete. Slow injection in this manner usually results in patients feeling only the first injection if they are awake. Care must be taken to inject only a minimum of solution because overzealous injection results in reduction of the size of the meatus and canal. When general anesthesia is administered, the same local agents are injected to provide a bloodless field because of the vasoconstrictive effect of the epinephrine.

Exposure

Creation of an incision to maximize exposure is important in every operation. When exploring an ear with conductive hearing loss, however, it is wise to anticipate other situations. Discovery of lateral ossicular chain fixation, for example, may necessitate greater removal of bone from the scutum and potentially cause a defect impossible to close with a short tympanomeatal flap. Correct canal incisions are three dimensional and extend from the posteroinferior annulus to a point well superior to Shrapnell's area (Fig. 117-3). The length of the canal flap is 5 to 7 mm, and it is dissected gently to avoid tearing the edges. The flap is elevated until the fibrous annulus is well exposed inferiorly and the notch of Rivinus is seen superiorly (Fig. 117-4). The tympanic membrane is then elevated anteriorly by sharp dissection. Sectioning of the posterior plica (mallear fold) will allow complete reflection of the tympanic membrane. When this does not suffice, the superior incision has generally not been developed far enough anteriorly.

The amount of bone that must be removed from the posterior canal wall for adequate visualization varies

considerably. When bone must be removed, curettage should begin at the notch of Rivinus and proceed inferiorly as care is taken to preserve the chorda tympani nerve (Fig. 117-5). When exploring the middle ear for otosclerosis or any conductive hearing impairment, the following landmarks should be visible to the surgeon to ensure adequate exposure (Fig. 117-6):

- Anteriorly—the neck and handle of the malleus
- Inferiorly—the round window
- Posteriorly—the pyramidal process
- Superiorly—the horizontal portion of the facial nerve

Good visualization of these structures will allow surgical correction of any conductive pathology encountered. Bone removal is generally performed with microcurettes but may also be achieved with a small cutting burr. The latter method usually presents a greater risk to the chorda tympani.

The chorda tympani can be preserved in more than 90% of cases. In the event of partial sectioning, the fibers should be reapproximated because good function will typically be restored. Some authors advise complete sectioning of the nerve when partial damage has occurred, but this is not justified in our experience. Even when complete sectioning is necessary, patients rarely complain of taste disturbance for more than a few months.

Determining Pathology

After adequate exposure, the entire ossicular chain and middle ear should be examined. Foci of otosclerosis may be immediately recognized as chalky white. There may be increased vascularity on the promontory, but recognition of the disease can sometimes be difficult. The ossicular chain is palpated gently with a slightly angled pick. Palpation should begin with the handle of the malleus and proceed medially to the long process of the incus and finally to the superstructure of the stapes. Extreme fixation sometimes precludes determination of the location of pathology. In this situation, the incudostapedial joint should be separated with a right-angled hook or a joint knife. This maneuver will allow separate palpation of the lateral chain and stapes. The site of fixation can then be determined.

In addition to confirming the pathology to be located at the footplate of the stapes, the degree of otosclerotic involvement must be observed. The surgeon must determine whether the footplate is thin enough for easy penetration or whether obliteration is present. Anatomic difficulties such as a dehiscent or overhanging facial nerve should also be noted at this time. It is always better to recognize potential difficulties before beginning disassembly of the ossicular chain. Failure to see any "blue area" within the central footplate may signal partial or complete obliterative disease. In this situation, the surgeon must judge whether adequate management of all problems that may ensue is possible, such as a floating footplate or the necessity for a drill-out procedure.

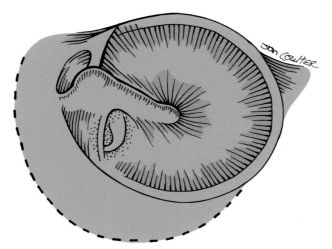

Figure 117-3. Correct incision in the canal allows adequate removal of bone and exposure of the ossicular chain.

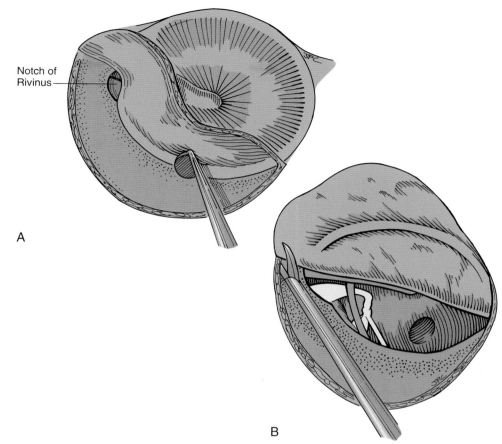

Figure 117-4. A, Elevation of the tympanomeatal flap. **B,** Exposure of the middle ear is enhanced by ensuring adequate anterior development of the flap.

A

B

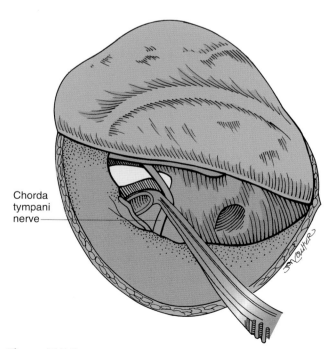

Figure 117-5. Curetting the posterosuperior bony canal wall with preservation of the chorda tympani nerve.

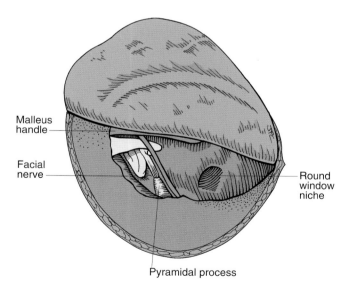

Figure 117-6. Demonstrating adequate middle ear exposure for management of any conductive problem encountered.

Philosophy of Footplate Removal

Beginning with the revival of stapes surgery by Dr. John Shea, Jr., in the 1950s, complete removal of the stapes footplate was considered the norm and resulted in satisfactory hearing results in a high percentage of cases. In recent years, the "small fenestra" technique has had a number of proponents because of the perception of improved results, particularly in the higher frequencies of 4 kHz and above. Careful review of the many articles' pros and cons reveals significant flaws in case study conclusions. In almost all the studies, the cases of more than one surgeon or more than one prosthesis were combined to arrive at conclusions regarding hearing results. A significant article on methodology was authored by Rizer and Lippy,[11] who compared results in three groups of patients, all of whom underwent surgery by Lippy. The three groups consisted of total removal of the footplate, partial removal of the footplate, and small fenestra stapedotomy. The Robinson prosthesis and identical tissue grafts were used in all cases. Although not statistically significant, the best hearing results in all frequencies actually occurred in the group with total removal of the footplate. Accordingly, it is safe to conclude that the amount of footplate removal is insignificant in comparison with the skill of the surgeon. With these facts in mind, two techniques for stapes surgery will be described. The first is the standard procedure without use of the laser, and the second embraces the newer laser technology available for otologic surgeons. Both techniques are used by our group, and hearing results have been equivalent.

Several general comments can be made. Conventional stapes surgery avoids the risk of high-energy lasers within the middle and inner ear. Laser techniques, on the other hand, better handle bleeding and avoid the potential complication of a floating footplate. Laser surgery is not applicable to obliterative disease.

Conventional Stapedectomy

After careful assessment of the degree and location of the otosclerosis, the incudostapedial joint is separated (Fig. 117-7). At this time, connective tissue is harvested for use in the oval window. When harvesting tissue, the surgeon may use the tragal perichondrium, areolar tissue, or temporalis fascia because of their proximity to the operative field. An alternative strategy is for an assistant to harvest a vein graft from the dorsum of the hand opposite the ear undergoing surgery (Fig. 117-8) while the otologic surgeon proceeds uninterrupted with the middle ear surgery. The type of connective tissue used for sealing the oval window is unimportant, provided that it is thin. When using vein, either the adventitial or the intimal surface may seal the oval window. Brief drying of the vein graft, as would be done for temporalis fascia, will make the graft easier to handle, thereby facilitating introduction and placement in the oval window. As the tissue graft comes in contact with perilymphatic fluid, it becomes soft and pliable

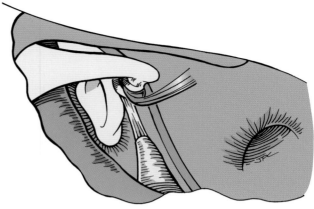

Figure 117-7. Separation of the incudostapedial joint while being careful to preserve the lenticular process of the incus.

once again. Preparation of the tissue graft should precede opening of the footplate so that the period of exposure of the vestibule is shortened.

Next, the footplate is fenestrated with a fine, sharp needle (Fig. 117-9). Although fenestration should ideally be performed in the center of the footplate, it may be done wherever the blue color indicates the bone to be thinnest. The stapedius tendon should be kept intact through this step to supply resistance against which to push during the fenestration. If gentle pressure does not perforate the bone, slow to-and-fro rotation of the needle point will generally complete the procedure. Successful fenestration is recognized when the needle point gives way slightly. Perilymph will be seen at the point of entry. Successful creation of the fenestra accomplishes two important purposes. First, the vestibule is already decompressed in the unlikely event of total footplate avulsion on fracture of the superstructure. Second, an area of purchase is now available for instrumentation in the case of footplate flotation. The stapedial tendon is sectioned (Fig. 117-10), and fracture of the stapedial superstructure is next accomplished by quick downward pressure toward the promontory (Fig. 117-11) (see Video 117-1). Occasionally, fixation of the superstructure to the promontory necessitates careful superior fracturing toward the horizontal facial nerve. In either case, the entire stapedial arch is then removed.

Small angled footplate hooks are next used to remove a sufficient amount of the central area of the footplate for placement of the graft and insertion of the prosthesis (Fig. 117-12). The amount of footplate removed is the portion that can easily be taken out, which usually amounts to approximately one fourth of the surface area of the footplate. Occasionally, larger portions of the footplate become elevated when enlarging the fenestra; in such cases, they may be removed with no fear of complications.

The appropriate length for the prosthesis is measured, although 4 mm is almost always the correct size for a bucket-handle prosthesis of the Robinson type

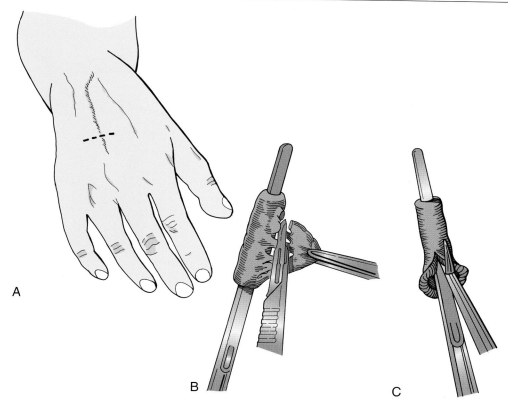

Figure 117-8. **A,** A 2-cm transverse incision is made on the dorsum of the hand for harvesting the vein graft. **B,** Removal of connective tissue from the vein graft. **C,** Opening the vein graft.

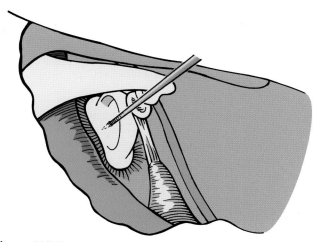

Figure 117-9. Fenestration of the central area of the stapes foot-plate with a fine needle.

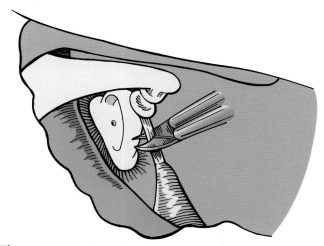

Figure 117-10. Sectioning of the stapedial tendon.

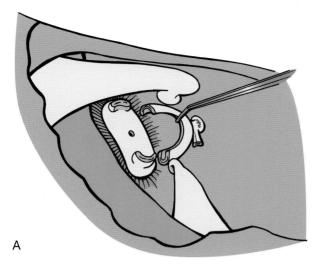

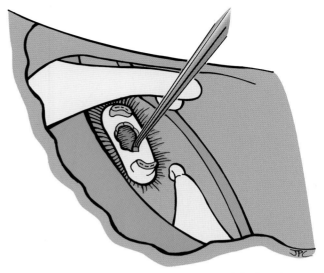

Figure 117-12. Removal of the central area of the footplate.

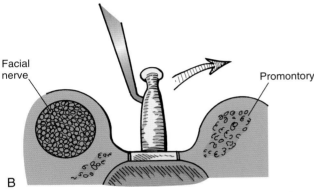

Figure 117-11. A and **B,** Down-fracturing of the stapes superstructure toward the promontory.

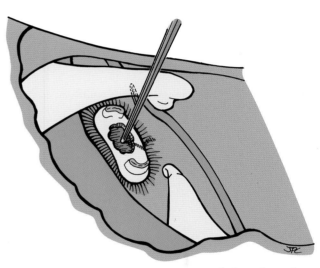

Figure 117-13. Measurement from the vestibule to the undersurface of the incus for the Robinson prosthesis.

(Fig. 117-13). The Robinson prosthesis is favored for several reasons:

1. It is self-centering within the fenestration.
2. Its weight favors good hearing results.
3. Because it is not a "crimped-on" prosthesis, the chance of ischemic pressure necrosis of the incus is negligible.
4. It can be used with minimal footplate removal.

The vein graft is placed over the oval window and gently depressed into the fenestra to identify the location of placement for the medial end of the prosthesis (Fig. 117-14) (see Video 117-2). Next, the prosthesis is placed by inserting the device into the fenestra and leaning it against the posterior surface of the incus, where it will remain standing by capillary attraction (see Video 117-3). A right-angled pick is then used in one hand to lift the long process of the incus while a second pick slides the bucket forward and under the lenticular process (Fig. 117-15). The entire shaft is rotated until the bale or bucket handle becomes aligned with the axis of the incus. The bucket handle is then lifted over the incus and into place (Fig. 117-16). Routine positioning

of the prosthesis and swinging the bucket handle over the incus are demonstrated in Video 117-4. A few minor maneuvers may be necessary to place the well of the prosthesis beneath the lenticular process of the incus (see Video 117-5). If the lenticular process is missing from the incus, a Bailey modification of the Robinson prosthesis is used. This modification consists of an elliptical notch in the bucket, which allows one to slide the prosthesis along with its handle superiorly onto the long process until it is well stabilized. If the bucket handle is deemed to be too loose as it rests over the incus, a small piece of tissue graft (residual vein) can be placed to cover it and the distal incus. This provides a "band-aid" to secure the handle in position (see Video 117-6).

Next, the ossicular chain is palpated at the malleus handle to ensure continuity of the chain; gentle pres-

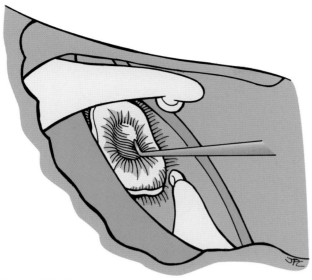

Figure 117-14. Placement of the vein graft over the fenestrated footplate.

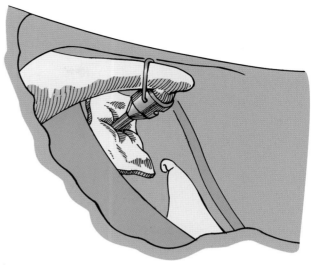

Figure 117-16. The prosthesis in place with the handle over the incus.

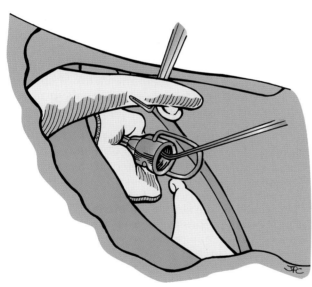

Figure 117-15. Placement of the Robinson prosthesis via a two-handed technique.

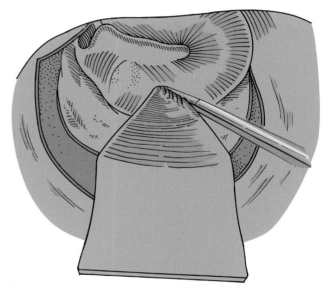

Figure 117-17. Packing of the tympanomeatal flap with a silk sleeve to maintain its position.

sure is placed on the incus to ensure good "bounce" of the prosthesis. This maneuver helps center the prosthesis. If this bounce is absent, the medial portion of the strut may not be within the fenestra. Finally, the tympanomeatal flap is reflected to its original position, and the flap is packed with a single silk strip and several small cotton balls impregnated with antibiotic ointment (Fig. 117-17).

Surgeons should have more than one technique at their disposal when performing stapes surgery because of occasional unanticipated findings. Shortening or absence of the long process of the incus may require a wire-piston device or even the use of a malleus-to–oval window prosthesis. Likewise, lateral chain fixation may necessitate incus interpositioning or the use of a partial ossicular reconstructive/replacement prosthesis.

CO₂ Laser–Assisted Stapedotomy

The laser should be set up with safe energy parameters and test-fired to confirm accuracy of the aiming beam. The HeNe aiming beam can be set on auto-HeNe so that when the foot pedal is depressed, the aiming beam remains off, thereby allowing an undistorted view of the last laser strike. Alcohol should not be used as a preparative solution when the laser is used.

With the CO_2 laser set at a continuous-mode 200-μm spot size, 0.1-second duration, and 1.25 W, a fenestration is made in the superior central area of the

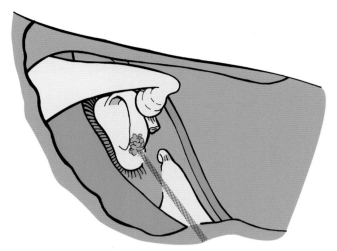

Figure 117-18. CO_2 laser vaporization of the posterior crus.

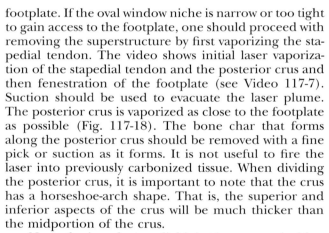

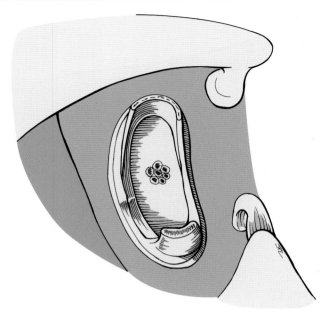

Figure 117-19. Rosette pattern of laser strikes on the central footplate.

footplate. If the oval window niche is narrow or too tight to gain access to the footplate, one should proceed with removing the superstructure by first vaporizing the stapedial tendon. The video shows initial laser vaporization of the stapedial tendon and the posterior crus and then fenestration of the footplate (see Video 117-7). Suction should be used to evacuate the laser plume. The posterior crus is vaporized as close to the footplate as possible (Fig. 117-18). The bone char that forms along the posterior crus should be removed with a fine pick or suction as it forms. It is not useful to fire the laser into previously carbonized tissue. When dividing the posterior crus, it is important to note that the crus has a horseshoe-arch shape. That is, the superior and inferior aspects of the crus will be much thicker than the midportion of the crus.

Next, the incudostapedial joint is separated with a joint knife, and the stapes superstructure is down-fractured. It has not been necessary to directly divide the anterior crus with the laser because the anterior crus is normally thinner than the posterior crus and otosclerosis usually firmly fixes the anterior footplate. The laser is then focused on the footplate. It is useful to confirm proper depth of focus by using high-power magnification (25 ×) temporarily to focus on the footplate and then return to a comfortable working magnification. Laser strikes are made on the footplate in a rosette pattern (Fig. 117-19) (see Video 117-8). Six to eight laser strikes are usually required to form a fenestra about 0.8 mm in diameter. The proper size of the fenestra may be confirmed by using a no. 26 suction device that has a 0.6-mm diameter at its tip or estimated by the 200-μm size of the laser strikes. It is easier to form a fenestra that is slightly on the larger side than to increase the size of the fenestra once the vestibule is open. If the stapedotomy is not adequate, it can be enlarged with the laser and footplate instruments (see Video 117-9). It is important to not fire the laser into an open vesti-

bule. Next, a Farrior stapes rasp or a fine 45-degree pick is used to remove the char. The rasp has the shape of a disc (per style) so that small fragments of char may be removed in any direction, which avoids turning or twisting of the instrument as must be done when using angled picks. This instrument comes in two sizes, 0.5 and 0.6 mm, and is manufactured by Gyrus ENT. (Memphis, TN). Once the char is removed, a small fenestra stapedotomy is completed. If the opening in the footplate is irregular, a 6-mm drill set on low speed can be used to optimize the stapedotomy.

Alternatively, the author still prefers using a Robinson bucket-handle prosthesis over a vein graft for all routine stapedectomy procedures as described earlier. If the surgeon prefers a wire-piston prosthesis, it is placed in the oval window and carefully crimped to the incus (Figs. 117-20 and 117-21). The newer prosthesis does not have to be manually crimped around the incus (Smart; Gyrus ENT). After placing the wire-Teflon prosthesis, the laser is used to heat the hook portion of the prosthesis to secure it around the incus (see Videos 117-10 and 117-11).

An alternative to using multiple 200-μm laser strikes to form the fenestra is to use one 0.6-mm laser strike in the middle of the footplate. The oval window may be sealed with clotted blood or tissue. The tympanic membrane is then returned to its normal position and secured as described earlier. As mentioned, the laser is not only useful when there is a narrow oval window niche but can also help avoid a floating footplate.

Revision Stapes Surgery

Revision surgery after stapedectomy or stapedotomy is performed for two reasons. The first indication is for

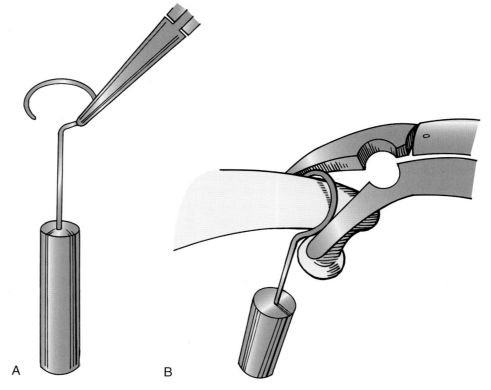

Figure 117-20. A, Method of grasping the piston with alligator forceps for insertion onto the incus. **B,** Tightening of the piston onto the long process of the incus.

A

B

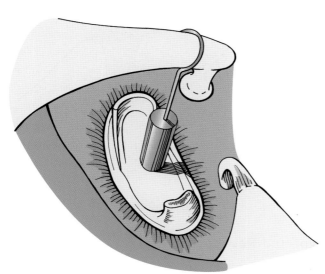

Figure 117-21. Piston in place with insertion into the fenestrated footplate.

correction of postoperative complications. Such problems typically occur during the first few weeks after the initial procedure. Patients complain of decreased hearing or dizziness, or both. Other complaints may include increased tinnitus, distortion of sound, motion intolerance, and vertigo associated with coughing, straining, sneezing, acute alteration in barometric or middle ear pressure, or change in body position. In the immediate postoperative period this could occur as a result of the formation of a granuloma. In the past,

development of a granuloma was ascribed to a complication related to the use of Gelfoam as sealant for the oval window. Synthetic materials are no longer used to cover the vestibule when a stapedectomy is performed. Various autogenous tissues, such as vein, fascia, areolar tissue, perichondrium, periosteum, fat, and blood, are used to seal the opening to the vestibule. Other possible sources include inflammatory tissue formed as a result of reaction to talcum powder on the surgeon's operating room gloves. On rare occasion, people may be allergic to an element included in the metal composition of the prosthesis.

The other urgent indication for surgical intervention is the possibility of a perilymphatic fistula. Similar to the signs and symptoms mentioned earlier, patients can have complaints related to hearing or balance (or both). Hearing loss may be sudden or rapidly progressive and is characteristically sensorineural. Fistula testing (pneumatic otoscopy with recording or observation of eye movements) is not reliable because it can be falsely positive in patients undergoing stapedectomy.

The second indication for revision surgery occurs when conductive hearing loss persists or develops over time. It must be emphasized, similar to the discussion regarding the initial procedure, that this is an elective procedure to restore hearing. The other alternative is amplification with a hearing aid. The hearing status of the contralateral ear must be defined to determine how best to advise a patient. Given the small but real risk of total hearing loss after revision stapes surgery, absent hearing in the contralateral ear is a contraindication to an elective revision procedure. Possible exceptions to operating on an only-hearing ear are severe complications from the first procedure (progressive hearing loss and dizziness) or a severe to profound mixed hearing loss in which amplification is insufficient and cannot provide adequate gain.

Revisions of this type should be reserved for surgeons with considerable experience because hearing results, even in the best of hands, do not approach those of primary cases. Lesinksi reviewed his series of 279 cases of revision stapes surgery performed with a laser. Sources of failure included unrecognized fixation of the lateral ossicular chain, erosion of the incus, displacement of the prosthesis from the oval window, and regrowth of otosclerosis. The most common finding was a displaced or malfunctioning prosthesis (81%), followed by erosion of the incus (30%). It was believed that erosion of the incus was caused by continued vibration of the incus bone against a prosthesis that was immobile at the interface with the otic capsule. Residual fixed stapes footplate was found in the center of the oval window in 14% of patients, and 4% had complete fixation of the malleus.[12]

Correction of prosthetic slippage and problems with the incus is statistically more successful than reopening of a bony window closure. The laser has a definite advantage in the presence of middle ear fibrosis or scarring and is invaluable in minimizing trauma to the inner ear associated with removing soft tissue in the oval window niche. The benefits of using the laser for revision stapes procedures were emphasized by Lippy and colleagues. The success rate increased to 80% for closure of the air-bone gap within 10 dB with the use of an argon laser. Hearing results were least successful when the incus could not be used for reconstruction.[13]

Obliterative Disease

Replacement of normal footplate anatomy by obliterative otosclerosis presents a greater, but not insurmountable challenge to the surgeon. Forewarning may occur in the form of a positive Schwartze sign, a pinkish blush behind the tympanic membrane indicative of enhanced vascularity. Unfortunately, no typical audiometric pattern suggests this occurrence. Experience in using a microdrill is mandatory for this procedure, and lack thereof requires abandonment of the operation (Fig. 117-22). Visible superstructure is fractured and removed without fear of footplate flotation. A small microdrill with an angled handpiece is used to saucerize the oval window area (Fig. 117-23). Cutting burrs are used initially, and then small diamond burrs are used to remove the remaining focus of bone until the blue line of perilymph is visualized through the thinned footplate area (see Video 117-12). It is important to keep the saucerization at the same depth throughout the circumference of the drilled-out area. When the site has been sufficiently thinned, fenestration is performed in the usual manner, and surgery proceeds as described earlier. Although drill-out procedures have been associated with a greater risk of sensorineural hearing loss,

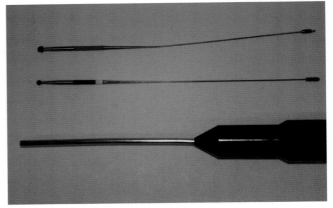

Figure 117-22. Micro–ear drills can fit through the ear speculum and still provide good visualization.

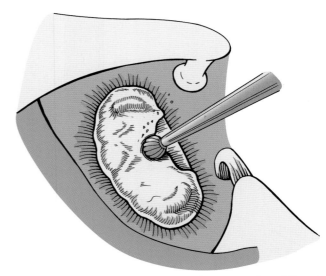

Figure 117-23. Use of a microdrill to saucerize obliterative disease.

the risk is small in the hands of an experienced operator.

Expected Results

There is no otologic procedure (save perhaps myringotomy) in which hearing improvement will exceed that of stapes surgery. Conservative estimates of at least 90% success in restoration of conductive loss to air-bone gaps of less than 10 dB are realistic and seen in nearly all series reported. Results that differ significantly from these bear investigation for faulty patient selection or surgical technique. Occasional reduction or catastrophic loss of hearing is known to even the most experienced surgeons, but the incidence should be 1% or less. These statistics make surgery an acceptable risk for most patients seeking improvement in hearing. Although otolaryngologists must decide about their own qualifications as stapes surgeons, experience clearly leads to superior hearing results.

POSTOPERATIVE MANAGEMENT

The demands of third-party insurers over the past decade have greatly reduced the length of hospital stay. Today, surgery for otosclerosis is performed as an outpatient procedure regardless of the type of anesthesia provided. Fortunately, most surgeons have discovered that reduction of stay has not altered the outcome in otosclerosis surgery. Nevertheless, each physician must maintain the ability to determine which patients require overnight observation for any of numerous reasons, including age, general health, complicating medical problems, and distance from the hospital. Complications encountered during surgery or symptoms suffered postoperatively should also be sufficient reason for extension of hospital stay.

Patients are allowed to ambulate soon after surgery, but they are advised to not lie on the ear that has undergone surgery for 24 hours. Precautions are given about sudden head movements to avoid dizziness, and prohibitions are also outlined against nose blowing, straining or lifting, or getting water into the ear that has been repaired. Clean cotton is kept in the external meatus as necessary until the packing is removed in approximately 1 week. Patients are encouraged to report any occurrence of worsening of vertigo, as well as any diminution in hearing. Sedentary work is permitted within 48 hours, but more strenuous occupations are banned for at least 3 weeks. Air travel is discouraged until the middle ear is seen to be well aerated, although this restriction may be impractical for some patients living at great distances. Antibiotics are not prescribed routinely. Analgesics with codeine are given when necessary.

COMPLICATIONS

Complications encountered during surgery range from the insignificant to those that may require abandonment of the procedure. Even when completion of surgery is not possible, it is of primary importance to preserve auditory nerve function whenever possible. Reliance on a hearing aid as a fall-back position is infinitely preferable to severe loss of cochlear reserve. Complications are considered individually in the following sections.

Tympanic Membrane Perforations

A tear in the tympanic membrane is most often due to failure to elevate the flap throughout its entire width before separation of the fibrous annulus from its sulcus (Fig. 117-24). A small tear may easily be repaired with tiny pledgets of Gelfoam inserted through the perforation. Larger defects should be reinforced with any remaining harvested tissue as an underlay graft. Occasionally, an extremely atrophic and thinned tympanic membrane is recognized preoperatively, and myringoplasty should be anticipated at the time of surgery. Tympanic membrane problems rarely have an impact on the outcome of surgery.

Injuries to the Chorda Tympani Nerve

Careful removal of bone from the posterior canal wall allows preservation of the chorda tympani nerve in approximately 90% of cases. Stretching of the nerve or partial sectioning of less than one half its diameter should prompt preservation with reapproximation of

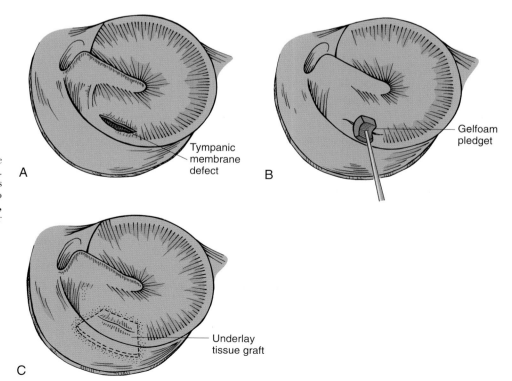

Figure 117-24. A, Postoperative defect in the tympanic membrane. **B,** A moist Gelfoam pledget is inserted through the defect to support it from the medial side. **C,** Use of an underlay tissue graft for repair of the defect.

the fibers as well as possible. Complete or nearly complete sectioning of the nerve is inevitable in a small percentage of cases. Even complete sectioning of the nerve most often results in only temporary dysgeusia. Most patients seem to compensate for taste disturbances within 6 months, although a small number may complain indefinitely. When taste is of utmost importance to the patient and when taste disturbance has resulted from surgery in the opposite ear, amplification for the second ear should be advised.

Ossicular Dislocation

This unusual complication involves incudomalleal dislocation. It results from inadvertent lateral displacement of the long process of the incus. Careful placement of the incus in its original position will usually give a good hearing result despite somewhat greater difficulty in placing the prosthesis because of instability of the incus.

Floating Stapedial Footplate

A floating footplate occurs when the superstructure is down-fractured and the entire footplate becomes loosened from the surrounding annular attachment at the oval window. This event is relatively rare and occurs in less than 1% of cases. It is best avoided by awareness of the factors that lead to it. Fracture of the stapedial superstructure before gaining a fenestration or control hole in the footplate may lead to this problem. Excessive pressure exerted on a thickened footplate may also result in circumferential dislodgement of it. It is necessary to get a purchase of the footplate when it is mobilized and floating. If a fenestration was initially performed, a footplate hook can be used to engage the footplate and extract it laterally. When this is not possible, the undersurface of the footplate is best accessed by drilling or curetting a small opening in the promontory side of the footplate until a fine right-angled pick can be inserted under the footplate and turned to complete extraction of it (Fig. 117-25). Another method for removing a large floating fragment is to place a few drops of blood over the window and remove the coapted fragments once a clot has formed. If the footplate becomes subluxated too far medially within the vestibule, attempts at retrieval should not be undertaken to avoid traumatic injury to the inner ear. A wire or bucket-handle prosthesis should be placed over a tissue graft.[14] Slight displacement of small fragments should be left alone because they rarely cause hearing loss. Larger fragments may induce persistent postural vertigo.

Perilymph Gushers

Preoperative computed tomography should be performed in children to identify anomalies of the otic capsule and potential gushers. On occasion, perilymph gushers are encountered in adults. The problem consists of excessive perilymphatic flow into the middle ear because of enlargement of the cochlear aqueduct or communication between the medial internal auditory

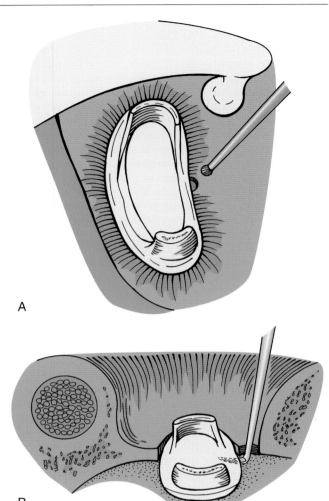

Figure 117-25. **A,** Creation of a small "rescue hole" in the vestibule for removal of a floating footplate. **B,** Insertion of a fine right-angled pick through the rescue hole for retrieval of the footplate.

canal (fundus) and the inner ear (Fig. 117-26). Control is best achieved by elevating the head of the table and continuing to suction the perilymph until the reservoir of the cerebellar pontine cistern is exhausted. Fat is harvested from the ear lobule and placed snugly in the oval window after removal of the footplate. The fat is held in place with the stapes prosthesis. Elevation of the head is continued postoperatively and may be supplemented by insertion of a spinal drain. This condition increases the incidence of sensorineural hearing loss.

Round Window Otosclerosis

Complete obliteration of the round window niche as a result of otosclerosis is rare, although partial narrowing occurs occasionally. The procedure should be abandoned in the case of complete obliteration because drill-out of the round window has been associated with a high rate of sensorineural loss. Surgery may proceed as usual with partial closure.

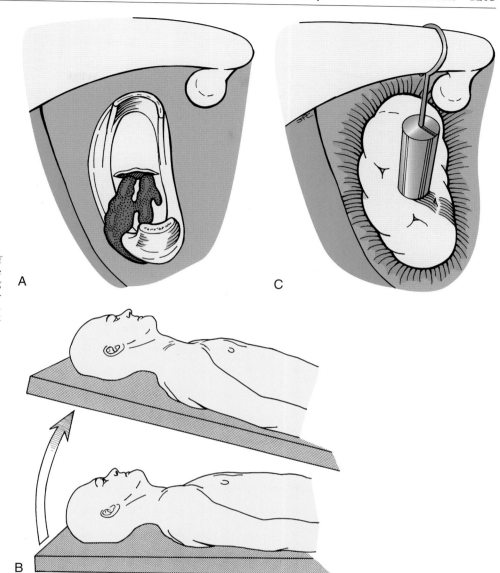

Figure 117-26. A, A gusher of perilymph through the footplate fenestra. **B,** Reverse Trendelenburg position for relief of the perilymphatic gusher. **C,** Use of a piston prosthesis with an adipose tissue graft to seal the perilymphatic gusher.

Persistent Stapedial Artery

Small remnants of this second branchial arch vessel often course across the stapedial footplate (Fig. 117-27). In a few cases, the artery may be large enough to create potential bleeding problems when disrupted. Even the larger arteries can most often be worked around by fenestration of the footplate and placement of the prosthesis anterior or posterior to the intact vessel. If the obturator foramen is obliterated by the artery, wise judgment may dictate termination of the procedure and the use of amplification with a hearing aid.

Dehiscence and Displacement of the Facial Nerve

Partial or total dehiscence of the horizontal portion of the facial nerve is a fairly common finding during middle ear surgery. Recognition of this anomaly is usually only important in that it encourages one to avoid instrumentation that could damage the nerve. Much less commonly, the facial nerve may overhang the oval window and, in rare cases, even travel directly across its surface (Fig. 117-28). Stapes surgery can usually be successfully completed in the presence of moderate overhang of the facial nerve, although visualization of the oval window is somewhat more difficult. Gentle retraction of the nerve with the side of a suction tip will ordinarily allow fenestration of the footplate and placement of the prosthesis. When the overhang is more pronounced, a crimp-on prosthesis of tantalum or platinum may be bent to curve around the dehiscence. Nitinol prostheses are also available, but great caution must be taken to ensure that tightening of the metal alloy with the laser does not injure the exposed nerve. The oval window may also be compromised by

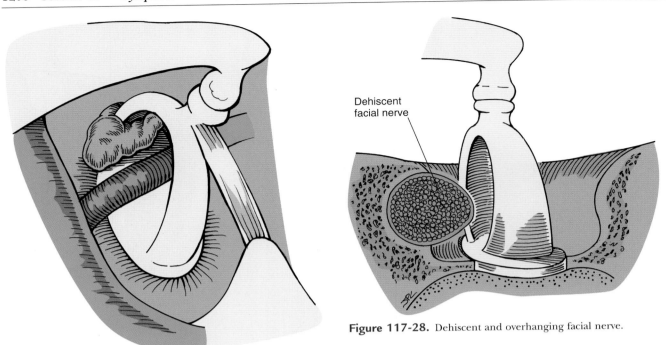

Figure 117-28. Dehiscent and overhanging facial nerve.

Figure 117-27. Persistent stapedial artery.

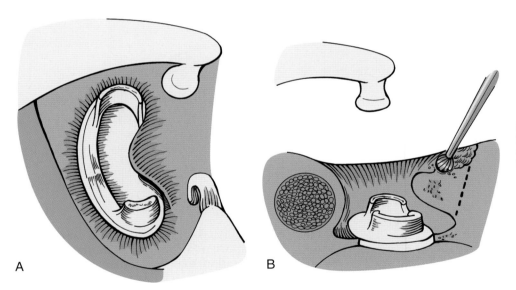

Figure 117-29. A, Promontory focus of otosclerosis. **B,** Use of a microdrill to remove the promontory overhang.

A   B

an overhang of bone from the promontory. This situation may be corrected with a microdrill until visualization is adequate (Fig. 117-29). Extreme situations of nerve displacement with coverage of the footplate dictate abandonment of the surgery.

Intraoperative Vertigo

The onset of vertigo during surgery is related to stimulation of the labyrinthine receptors, which may occur because of excessive manipulation of the stapes or emp-

tying of the fluid compartment of the vestibule. Local anesthesia permits the surgeon to rely on this symptom as a sign of impending damage to the inner ear. General anesthesia obviates this important signal. Vertigo is often transient or mild, but when it persists, it may imperil the completion of surgery because of associated nausea and vomiting. In this situation, rapid measures must be instituted to relieve symptoms and permit completion of the procedure. Droperidol is the most expeditious drug in this emergency; 1.25 mg is given slowly as a direct intravenous push, and larger doses can be used if necessary. Relief of symptoms is rapid and permits completion of the operation with patient comfort. Intraoperative monitoring is necessary when using this drug because of potential cardiac complications and hypotension. Intravenous ondansetron (4 mg) is also effective in this regard.

The use of general anesthesia does not permit the surgeon to monitor inner ear complications. However, under general anesthesia the patient will not move or become intolerant of minor middle ear stimulation. It is our preference to use general anesthesia rather than local or intravenous sedation for stapes surgery.

Reparative Granuloma

The formation of reactive granulation tissue in and around the oval window is a catastrophic complication of stapes surgery that is seen less and less commonly today. Some have attributed it to particulate foreign matter from the prosthesis or possibly from the surgeon's gloves, but this hypothesis remains unproved. Possibly, washing of powder from surgical gloves, use of powderless gloves, and rinsing of prosthetics before introduction have reduced the incidence of granuloma. A granuloma typically develops approximately 1 week after surgery. Patients complain of diminished hearing and dizziness after initially exhibiting no significant problems. Examination reveals a violaceous fullness in the posterosuperior quadrant of the tympanic membrane. Audiometric testing confirms sensorineural impairment, which is usually accompanied by reduction in word recognition.

Although some authors have advocated systemic therapy with high-dose steroids, the generally accepted treatment is immediate surgical intervention with removal of the granuloma. This entails removal of the prosthesis and tissue graft and insertion of new material. Rapid recognition of the condition and surgical correction may reverse the hearing loss, but a permanent sensorineural deficit is more likely. In extreme cases or when recognition is delayed, granulomatous tissue has been shown to invade the oval window and fill the vestibule.

Perilymphatic Fistula

In addition to reparative granuloma, postoperative perilymphatic fistula is the other chief cause of poor hearing results. Although each patient has a temporary fistula after footplate fenestration, the usual manner of healing seals the fluid leak within a short time. Persistence or redevelopment of the fistula after healing may be the result of imperfect tissue graft placement, dislodgment of the prosthesis, or sudden expulsion of fluid because of coughing or sneezing. Symptoms related to perilymphatic leakage are typically fluctuant hearing loss and dizziness. Although physical examination of the ear is unremarkable, audiograms confirm

deterioration of cochlear function. When this complication is suspected, immediate exploration is indicated if hearing is to be salvaged. If a fistula is confirmed, tissue grafting and prosthetic placement are repeated.

Preoperative Problems with the Tympanic Membrane

When the tympanic membrane is extremely thin or atrophic, plans for grafting should be included in the preoperative counseling. Even if such grafting is unnecessary during surgery, it is better to have forewarned the patient. A larger piece of fascia, vein, or perichondrium can be harvested if a tissue graft is used for closure of the oval window. Severe atrophy and atelectasis can be supported with cartilage harvested from the tragus (see Video 117-13).

Magnetic Resonance Imaging

With few exceptions, almost all middle ear prosthetics in use today are nonferromagnetic. The Robinson prosthesis is included in the group of devices that can be safely subjected to MRI. Patients are instructed in this regard to arm them for future questions about their eligibility for scanning. It is anticipated that magnet strength will increase in the future. The Robinson prosthesis is available in titanium, as well as the original stainless steel configuration. Titanium is a safe metal in a magnetic field. Prostheses made of nitinol are also safe during MRI.

PEARLS

- An appropriate candidate for middle ear exploration to diagnosis otosclerosis is a patient with a normal ear examination, negative Rinne test, conductive hearing loss of 25 dB, absent acoustic reflexes, and an understanding of the risks and benefits of the procedure.
- Offer surgery to the worse-hearing ear and do not undertake elective surgery on an only-hearing ear unless maximum amplification has been tried and deemed unsuccessful.
- Ensure that adequate surgical exposure has been achieved before addressing the status of the stapes.
- Palpate the lateral ossicular chain after the incudostapedial joint has been separated, confirm that the lateral chain is not fixed, and then check the mobility of the stapes.
- Do not apply suction directly to the stapedotomy and vestibule.
- If a floating footplate develops and it sinks into the vestibule, place a tissue graft over the oval window and reconstruct with a wire or bucket-handle prosthesis.

PITFALLS

- Proceeding with footplate work before optimizing exposure of the oval window niche may result in prolongation of the procedure and untoward results.
- Attempts at recovering segments of the footplate that fall into the vestibule may result in iatrogenic sensorineural hearing loss.
- Failure to close the air-bone gap after surgery for presumed otosclerosis may be due to fixation of the lateral ossicular chain or dehiscence of the superior semicircular canal.
- Despite closure of the air-bone gap, residual sensorineural hearing greater than a 35-dB speech reception threshold may still require hearing aid amplification.
- In unilateral otosclerosis, the patient's perception of complete success is having the operated ear improve to air conduction scores within 15 dB of the better ear.

References

1. Politzer A: Über primäre Erkrankung der knöcheren Labyrinthkapsel. J Ohrenheilk 25:309-327, 1894.
2. Konigsmark BW, Gorlin RJ: Genetic and Metabolic Deafness. Philadelphia, WB Saunders, 1976.
3. Ferlito A, Arnold W, Rinaldo A, et al: Viruses and otosclerosis: Chance association or true causal link? Acta Otolaryngol 123:741-746, 2003.
4. Minor LB: Clinical manifestations of superior semicircular canal dehiscence. Laryngoscope 115:1717-1727, 2005.
5. Welling DB, Merrell JA, Merz M, Dodson EE: Predictive factors in pediatric stapedectomy. Laryngoscope 113:1515-1519, 2003.
6. Sakai O, Curtin HD, Fujita A, et al: Otosclerosis: Computed tomography and magnetic resonance findings. Am J Otolaryngol 21:116-118, 2000.
7. Massey BL, Kennedy RJ, Shelton C: Stapedectomy outcomes: Titanium versus Teflon wire prosthesis. Laryngoscope 115:249-252, 2005.
8. Tange RA, Grolman W, Dreschler WA: Gold and titanium in the oval window: A comparison of two metal stapes prostheses. Otol Neurotol 25:102-105, 2004.
9. Knox GW, Reitan H: Shape-memory stapes prosthesis for otosclerosis surgery. Laryngoscope 115:1340-1346, 2005.
10. Silverstein H, Hoffmann KK, Thompson JH Jr, et al: Hearing outcome of laser stapedotomy minus prosthesis (STAMP) versus conventional laser stapedotomy. Otol Neurotol 25:106-111, 2004.
11. Rizer FM, Lippy WH: Evolution of techniques of stapedectomy from the total stapedectomy to the small fenestra stapedectomy. Otolaryngol Clin North Am 26:443-451, 1993.
12. Lesinski SG: Revision stapedectomy. Curr Opin Otolaryngol Head Neck Surg 11:347-354, 2003.
13. Lippy WH, Battista RA, Berenholz L, et al: Twenty-year review of revision stapedectomy. Otol Neurotol 24:560-566, 2003.
14. Jaisinghani VJ, Schachern PA, Paparella MM: Stapes mobilization in otosclerosis. Ear Nose Throat J 80:586-590, 2001.

Chapter **118**

Bone-Anchored Hearing Devices

Yael Raz

Conductive and mixed hearing loss can often be treated surgically or with conventional hearing aids. However, certain patients are not candidates for standard surgical approaches or traditional amplification—for example, those whose external auditory meatus has been closed off during lateral temporal bone resection, mastoid cavities that continue to drain despite surgical treatment, or congenital aural atresia not favorable for repair. Bone-anchored hearing devices conduct sound via bone vibration, thereby effectively bypassing the middle ear conductive apparatus, and represent a viable alternative for this subset of patients. Although conventional bone-conducting hearing aids can also provide amplification in such cases, these devices can cause discomfort and possible skin erosion as a result of pressure from the headband. Bone-anchored devices are osseointegrated and thus do not place pressure on the surrounding skin. Bone-anchored hearing devices are also an appealing alternative to the CROS (contralateral routing of offside signal) aid in the treatment of single-sided deafness. Sound from the deafened side is transmitted to the intact contralateral cochlea with little attenuation. Multiple studies suggest that the Baha is better accepted than amplification with the CROS aid.[1,2]

Coupling of a bone vibrator to an osseointegrated implant was initiated in Sweden in the early 1970s.[3] Several companies have marketed bone-anchored hearing aids in the past; however, at present there is one dominant device in the marketplace, the Baha (manufactured by Cochlear Corporation, which recently acquired Entific Corporation). The Baha consists of three parts: an implanted titanium flange fixture, a sound processor, and an external abutment that couples the titanium fixture to the sound processor (Fig. 118-1).

Successful placement of the Baha depends on the creation of a healthy, permanent percutaneous connection. Osseointegration of the flange fixture is a critical factor. The implant is made of titanium, a metal that is highly biocompatible and corrosion free. The microstructure of the implant has been designed with a rough surface containing micropits that enhance interaction between osteocytes and the implant, thus maximizing osseointegration.[4] The fixture is threaded to maximize contact with the surrounding bone and enhance stability. The implant is inserted with a high-torque drill at slow speed to avoid thermal damage to the surrounding osteocytes. Disposable drill bits ensure a sharp bit for each step, and irrigation prevents thermal damage. Another critical factor in ensuring the health of the percutaneous connection is avoidance of infection or inflammation. Modeled after the natural interface between fingernails, talons, or teeth and the surrounding skin or gingival bed, the skin at the fixture penetration site must be free of hair and immobile.[5] Movement of skin at the implant-skin interface or the presence of hair follicles can provide an entry point for bacterial infection or inflammation. Meticulous attention to technique in the soft tissue work is critical for stabilization of the surrounding skin. Insertion of the titanium device requires a specialized handpiece that is fitted with multiple adaptors to elevate the skin graft, establish a guide hole, and countersink and insert the fixture. Attention to detail such as handling the titanium components with titanium forceps, using appropriate drill speeds, and irrigation can be critical in ensuring osseointegration of the device and a healthy percutaneous connection. Complications with the Baha consist primarily of adverse soft tissue reaction surrounding the fixture and failure of osseointegration.[6,7]

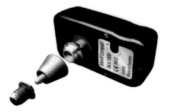
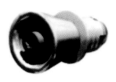

Figure 118-1. The Baha system includes a flange fixture, an external abutment, and a sound processor that snaps on to the external abutment. In adults undergoing a single-stage procedure, the flange fixture is preattached to the external abutment, and both pieces are inserted as a unit. *(Permission granted from Cochlear Corporation.)*

PATIENT SELECTION

When the Baha is being considered for mixed or conductive hearing loss, the bone line should be better than 45-dB pure-tone average (PTA; 0.5, 1, 2, 3 kHz) in the affected ear, and word recognition should be greater than 60%. When bone conduction is worse than 45 dB, a body-level sound processor is more suitable. For single-sided deafness, the contralateral ear should have a PTA air conduction threshold better than 20 dB. Insertion of the titanium flange fixture is a relatively safe and quick procedure that can be performed under local anesthesia, and there are relatively few contraindications. The patient must be comfortable with the concept of having a device protruding from the scalp. Certain patients actually prefer the aesthetic appearance of the Baha as opposed to a conventional hearing aid because it can be hidden with certain hairstyles. It is important to communicate to patients that it is necessary to permanently remove the hair follicles surrounding the abutment and that the scalp will be concave at the site of the implant to immobilize the surrounding skin. Extensive preoperative counseling with photographs enhances patient satisfaction. A test band coupled to the sound processor can provide a simulation of the sound input achieved with the Baha; however, sound fidelity is not as high as with the actual implanted device because of soft tissue attenuation.

The patient's ability to care for the implant site must be taken into consideration in selection for this procedure. Patients with certain psychiatric or other disorders that impair the ability to maintain proper hygiene may not be able to perform the appropriate local skin care required to keep the implant site healthy. Patients with a history of external beam irradiation to the scalp, diabetes, or dermatologic conditions such as psoriasis may be more prone to adverse skin reactions and need to be monitored closely, but these conditions have not been found to increase the risk of implant loss.[8] Before surgery, the patient meets with an audiologist to select the sound processor.

PREOPERATIVE EVALUATION

In children, a computed tomography (CT) scan of the temporal bone can be helpful, particularly in the presence of developmental abnormalities that affect the thickness of the skull. In adults, there is no indication for imaging studies. One potentially frustrating aspect of the preoperative evaluation is the preauthorization process. The Baha device falls in the gray zone between cochlear implants, which are routinely covered by insurance, and hearing aids, which are not generally covered. Insurance policies regarding the Baha seem to vary from state to state and among various companies. It is critical to address this issue before surgery and to clarify whether the insurance company will cover the cost of the sound processor in addition to placement of the flange fixture. On occasion, coverage can be obtained with physician advocacy on the patient's behalf in the form of a letter indicating that the patient is not a candidate for conventional amplification and explaining how the device differs from a conventional hearing aid.

SURGICAL APPROACH

We prefer to insert the titanium flange fixture under general anesthesia. However, when there are concerns regarding a patient's ability to withstand general anesthesia, the procedure can be performed under intravenous sedation with local anesthesia or even with local anesthesia alone. In adults, insertion of the device is performed in a single-stage procedure in which the flange fixture is inserted with the abutment preattached. Once the site has healed and osseointegration has occurred, the sound processor is attached to the abutment. In children or in adults with irradiated skin or poor bone quality, the flange fixture is inserted at the first stage and the abutment is placed at a second stage once osseointegration has occurred.

Planning the Flap

We typically use an inferiorly based skin flap. A mock device is useful in outlining the size of the skin flap. However, We have found that the fixture is ideally placed at the center of the skin flap and not at its superior aspect, as marked in the present generation of mock devices. If the fixture site is marked too superiorly within the outline of the mock device, gravity often results in a superior overhang of tissue that makes contact with the sound processor. The implant site should be 5 to 5.5 cm away from the ear canal to prevent the sound processor from contacting the pinna (Fig. 118-2). Placing the fixture in the region of the temporal line will make it most likely that adequately thick cortical bone will be encountered. It is our preference to use the dermatome because it is rapid and consistently results in an even, thin skin flap (0.6-mm thickness, 24-mm width). However, equally thin flaps can also be achieved manually. When two-stage surgery is performed, if the cover screw projects from the skin surface, the dermatome can tear at this site and therefore manual elevation plus thinning of the flap is recommended.

The postauricular region is shaved and topical anesthetic is infiltrated at the planned flap site. If using the dermatome, the local anesthetic should be massaged into the skin so that the skin surface is smooth before harvesting the graft. A superficial skin incision at the superior aspect of the planned flap is helpful in allowing the dermatome to engage the skin. Use of mineral oil and application of pressure with a tongue depressor in advance of the dermatome is helpful in developing the skin graft. Steady downward pressure and slow, even progress ensure an intact graft that remains attached to the scalp inferiorly. If constant downward pressure is not maintained until the dermatome has been stopped, the skin graft may be severed at the base. The graft can still be used; it should be maintained in moist gauze and sutured as a free graft over the implant site. Once the flap has been elevated, its undersurface is freed of hair follicles with a horizontal sweeping motion of the scalpel (Fig. 118-2). Even for thin flaps elevated with the dermatome, this step is helpful in keeping the percutaneous connection clean and infection free. The skin graft is then reflected inferiorly and covered with moist gauze.

Drilling the Fixture Site

The soft tissue is incised superiorly, anteriorly, and posteriorly; elevated off the underlying periosteum; and reflected inferiorly. The inferior attachment is not divided until adequate cortical thickness has been established by drilling the guide hole. Thus, if the drill site needs to be altered significantly, the soft tissue can be replaced while avoiding unnecessarily large and unsightly defects. This area of the mastoid cortex is denuded of periosteum in an amount sufficient to

accept the countersink. Once the initial drilling steps (guide hole and countersinking) establish adequate cortical depth, more extensive removal of soft tissue can be performed.

Drilling of the guide hole is performed at high speed with irrigation and use of the guide drill and a plastic spacer to ensure that depth of drilling is not greater than 3 mm (Fig. 118-3). It is critical that this step and all subsequent drilling steps be carried out precisely perpendicular to the mastoid cortex. Acute angles during the early drilling steps will result in angling of the flange fixture, which will lead to contact between the sound processor and the surrounding tissue and may result in discomfort or acoustic feedback. A drill indicator attachment is available to facilitate visualization of the drill's trajectory (see Fig. 118-3). The guide hole is examined to ensure that the sigmoid sinus, dura, and mastoid air cells have not been violated. The plastic spacer is then removed and drilling continues to a depth of 4 mm, again using copious irrigation. Some authors have recommended proceeding with implantation in the event of violation of the dura or sigmoid sinus because the flange fixture effectively stops leakage of cerebrospinal fluid or bleeding. However, a cerebral abscess has been reported with the Baha system.[9] Additionally, osseointegration may be impaired by the absence of bone at the deep surface of the fixture. If multiple attempts do not reveal bone

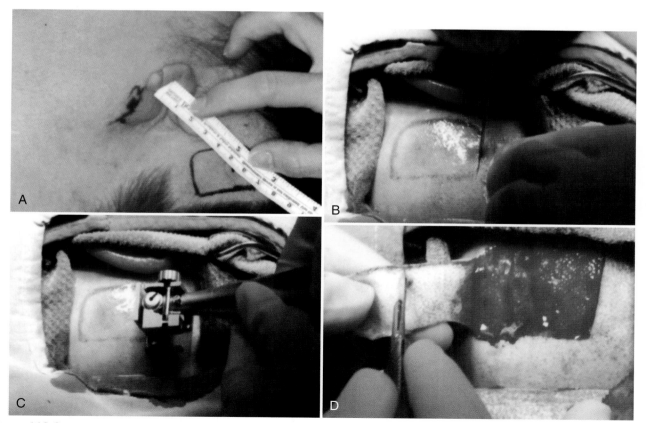

Figure 118-2. A, A mock device is used to plan the size of the skin flap. The implant should be placed 5.0 to 5.5 cm from the ear canal to ensure that the sound processor will not contact the auricle. **B,** The skin is incised superficially to allow the dermatome to engage the skin. **C,** The Baha dermatome is used to elevate an inferiorly based skin flap. **D,** Hair follicles are removed from the undersurface of the skin flap.

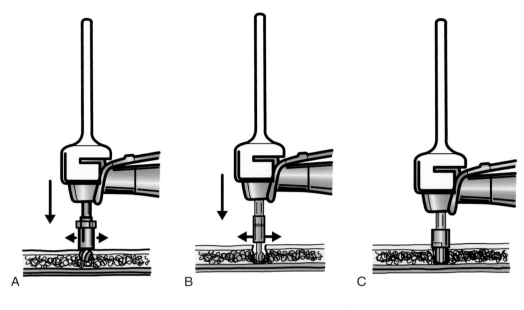

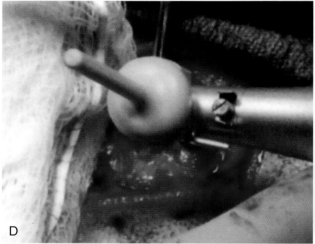

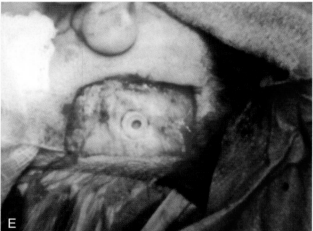

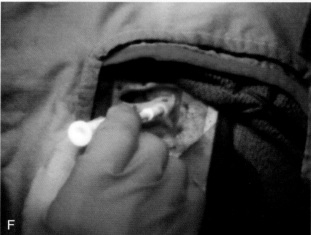

Figure 118-3. A, Drilling commences with use of the guide drill and a plastic spacer to ensure a depth no greater than 3 mm. **B,** The spacer is then removed and the guide hole is drilled to a depth of 4 mm if cortical bone thickness is sufficient. **C,** The appropriately sized countersink is then used. Drilling of the guide hole and countersink is performed under high speed (≈2000 rpm) with copious irrigation. **D,** The drill indicator facilitates visualization of the drill's trajectory. **E,** If the countersink has been drilled precisely perpendicular to the cortex, a concentric ring should be visible surrounding the guide hole. **F,** A 4-mm biopsy punch is used to remove skin directly overlying the drill site.

depth sufficient to handle a 4-mm fixture, the surgeon may elect to proceed with a 3-mm fixture, although it is somewhat more prone to failure of osseointegration.[10] In a young child with a thin skull, exposure of the dura is often unavoidable, thus frequently necessitating use of the 3-mm fixture.[11]

Once the guide hole has been established, the appropriately sized countersink drill bit is attached to the handpiece (3 or 4 mm, depending on the depth of the guide hole). The drilling motion for making the countersink and the guide hole should be up and down rather than plunging the drill in a single downward trajectory. This allows irrigation fluid to enter the drilled area and protects against thermal damage. The countersink drill widens the guide hole to an appropriate diameter and creates an even surface for the flange, thereby enhancing contact between the fixture and the surrounding bone. Care should be taken to remove bone from the threads of the drill. If drilling has been

performed directly perpendicular to the cortex, a concentric countersink should be visible surrounding the drill hole. A cruciate incision is then made in the skin graft overlying the drill site. Alternatively, a 4-mm biopsy punch can be used (see Fig. 118-3).

Soft Tissue Removal

After drilling of the guide hole and countersink, the inferior attachment of the soft tissue underlying the skin flap is divided. The periosteum is left intact except for the area of the countersink. Absence of soft tissue between the skin graft and the periosteum is essential to ensure fixation of the skin surrounding the flange fixture and prevent infection and inflammation. The margins surrounding the graft site are then retracted with double skin hooks, and the soft tissue surrounding the graft site is removed anteriorly, posteriorly, and superiorly (Fig. 118-4). The result is a beveled, gentle

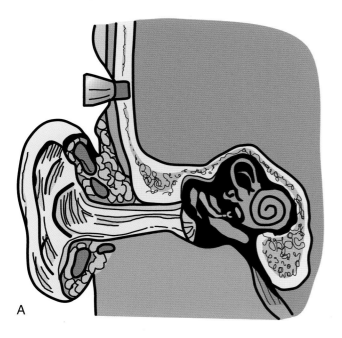

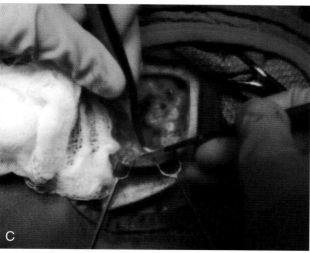

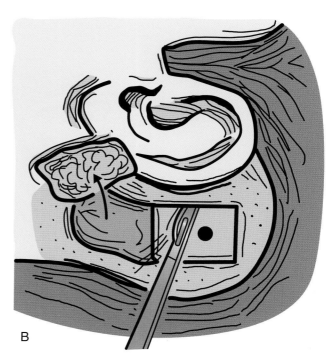

Figure 118-4. **A,** The bone underneath the skin graft site is covered only by periosteum. Note the absence of soft tissue. **B** and **C,** The tissue surrounding the graft site is also thinned aggressively to allow the skin margins surrounding the graft to slope gently toward the graft site.

slope onto the skin flap and implant site. Individuals who are obese or have a particularly thick scalp are more prone to the development of this superior soft tissue overhang. Beveling of the margins is particularly important in this population to avoid contact between this superior shelf of skin and the sound processor.

Insertion of the Device

For adults undergoing a planned single-stage insertion, the abutment is packaged preattached to the titanium fixture (Fig. 118-5). An abutment inserter attachment is used to pick up the implant, which is inserted at low speed. The fixture is self tapping. Irrigation should be avoided until the first threads have engaged so that fluid is not trapped between the screw and bone. No pressure is necessary at this stage, and the fixture should be allowed to find its own way. The final turns can be performed manually to ensure a tight fit; however, care must be taken to not tighten the screw excessively and damage the surrounding bone. The implant must be

stable once inserted or connective tissue will form at the bone-screw interface and prevent osseointegration of the fixture. If a biopsy punch was used previously, a small incision may be necessary to enlarge the opening sufficiently to accept the abutment. Alternatively, a small cruciate incision can be made in the skin overlying the abutment and the abutment delivered through the skin.

Shrinkage of the skin graft, as well as the added surface area created by beveling of the margins, sometimes makes the closure tight. Tension can be diminished by tacking the margins surrounding the skin flap to the periosteum, particularly at the corners. It is better to leave some of the beveled margin to granulate than to approximate the graft under tension. The incision is closed with interrupted chromic suture. Alternate sutures incorporate the underlying periosteum (Fig. 118-6). Tacking sutures, particularly at the base of the flap, and small incisions in the center of the graft prevent hematoma formation and subsequent separa-

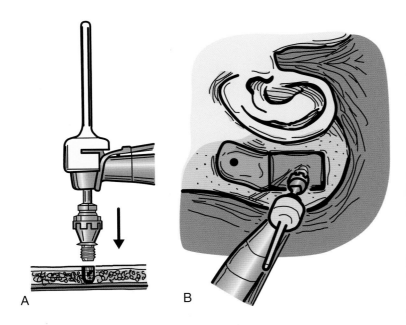

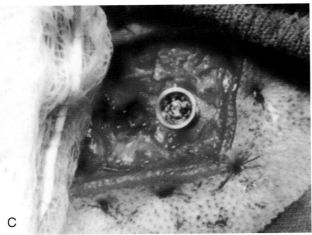

Figure 118-5. **A,** The abutment adaptor is placed on the drill and used to pick up the flange fixture with the preattached abutment. **B,** The fixture is inserted at slow speed. **C,** The flange fixture is self tapping, and the drill stops automatically once complete insertion has been achieved.

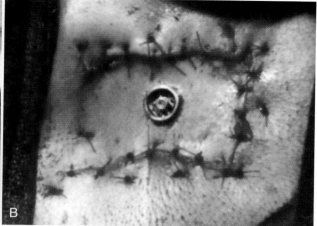

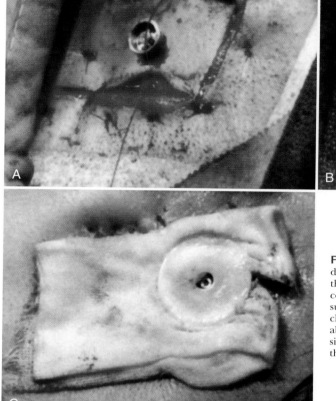

Figure 118-6. A, The abutment is delivered through the skin flap and draped over the underlying periosteum. The skin margins surrounding the graft site have been tacked to the periosteum at the two superior corners and inferiorly. For closure, simple sutures are alternated with sutures incorporating the underlying periosteum. **B,** The completed closure is free of tension. **C,** A healing cap is snapped onto the external abutment, and a large sheet of folded Xeroform with an inverted Y incision at one edge is tucked under the healing cap. The Xeroform keeps the skin graft secure against the underlying periosteum.

tion of the skin graft from the periosteum. A healing cap is snapped onto the abutment. An inverted Y-shaped incision is made at one edge of a folded Xeroform sheet, which is placed under the healing cap. A mastoid dressing is applied and left in place for 1 to 2 days.

Special Considerations in the Pediatric Population

The Baha has been approved by the U.S. Food and Drug Administration for children 5 years of age and older, although reports from outside the United States suggest that the first stage can be performed successfully in younger children.[12] The optimal age for Baha insertion depends on the thickness of the skull, which correlates with height more than with age. The procedure should be staged in young children, particularly if the calvaria is less than 3 mm thick. A longer period—between 6 and 12 months—should be allotted for osseointegration. The procedure can be performed in a single stage between 9 and 12 years of age. If a staged procedure is planned, a cover screw is threaded into the inner threads of the fixture to maintain its patency for later attachment of the abutment. At the second stage this screw is removed and the abutment is attached and externalized. The sound processor may be coupled to

the abutment 4 weeks after the second stage. In children, the thickness of the skull may limit the fixture to 3 mm instead of the 4-mm implant typically used in adults.

Children with craniofacial anomalies, such as Treacher Collins syndrome or microcephaly, are more likely to have thin cortical bone or a low-hanging middle fossa tegmen. In this population, preoperative CT scanning can be useful for assessing the thickness of the skull and determining the position of the middle fossa relative to the mastoid. Techniques have been described for building up the bone surrounding the fixture with the use of a Gore-Tex membrane.[13]

Children who are too young for insertion of the Baha may be fitted with a Baha soft band, which maintains the sound processor over the mastoid with light pressure. Infants with unilateral hearing loss often do not allow the band to remain in place for long; however, children with bilateral conductive hearing loss enjoy the sound and thus tolerate the soft band quite well. When the hearing loss is due to microtia or anotia, insertion of the Baha must be coordinated with reconstructive efforts. Special planning and perhaps more posterior placement of the device might be required to keep the device from contacting the anticipated helical rim of the reconstructed auricle and avoid disruption

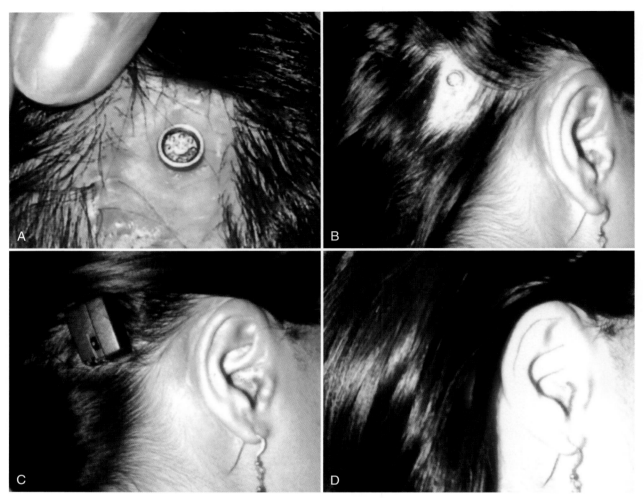

Figure 118-7. A, The graft site with external abutment 3 months postoperatively. Note the absence of hair follicles, a key factor in preventing infection at the percutaneous connection. **B,** The graft site 1 year postoperatively. **C,** The sound processor has been coupled to the external abutment. **D,** With certain hairstyles, the BAHA can be quite inconspicuous.

of the vascular supply to the temporoparietal skin flap used for its coverage. Alternatively, osseointegrated flange fixtures can be used to affix a prosthetic auricle. The location of these fixtures must be coordinated with an experienced prosthetist. In children, consideration should be given to the insertion of a "sleeper" fixture. This additional fixture is maintained under the skin flap with an internal cover screw and serves as a backup in case of failure of osseointegration or secondary trauma with loss of the initial fixture.

POSTOPERATIVE MANAGEMENT

One week postoperatively, the folded Xeroform is replaced. Two weeks after surgery, if the site has healed satisfactorily, the healing cap can be removed. The patient is instructed to clean the site with soap and water. The sound processor is coupled to the abutment after allowing 3 months for osseointegration to take place (Fig. 118-7). Premature loading of the abutment can result in failure of osseointegration. The patient is then monitored at 6-month intervals to ensure stability of the abutment.

PEARLS

- The planned fixture site should be marked at the center of the skin flap rather than superiorly, as indicated by the marker hole in the present generation of mock devices.
- Successful osseointegration depends on copious irrigation and maintenance of the appropriate drill speed when establishing the guide hole and countersink, as well as insertion of the flange fixture.
- Removal of surrounding hair follicles, a thin skin graft, and excision of soft tissue underlying the skin graft will ensure a reaction-free penetration site.
- The mastoid cortex is thickest at the temporal line, thus making it an optimal site for the flange fixture.
- Extra care must be taken to ensure that all drilling steps are performed perpendicular to the mastoid cortex.
- Maintenance of the periosteum surrounding the drill site is vital for ensuring a satisfactory blood supply to the skin flap.

PITFALLS

- A skin graft that has inadvertently been severed at the base can still be used; it should be maintained in moist gauze and sutured as a free graft over the implant site.
- Inadequate removal of tissue at the margins of the skin graft, particularly superiorly, can result in a soft tissue overhang that makes contact with the sound processor.
- Skin growth over the external abutment can usually be managed by excision of the skin in the office, followed by silver nitrate cautery, injection of triamcinolone (Kenalog), and application of the healing cap.
- When the Baha is selected for patients with microtia, the fixture must not violate the blood supply to the skin flaps used for construction of the auricle.
- Tension on the suture line can be diminished by tacking the margins surrounding the skin flap to the underlying periosteum.
- In children with thin skin undergoing a second-stage procedure, consideration should be given to raising the skin flap manually because the internal hexagonal screw may catch on the dermatome and cause a tear in the flap.

References

1. Wazen JJ, Spitzer JB, Ghossaini SN, et al: Transcranial contralateral cochlear stimulation in unilateral deafness. Otolaryngol Head Neck Surg 129:248-254, 2003.
2. Niparko JK, Co KM, Lustig LR: Comparison of the bone anchored hearing aid implantable hearing device with contralateral routing of offside signal amplification in the rehabilitation of unilateral deafness. Otol Neurotol 24:73-78, 2003.
3. Tjellstrom A, Lindstrom J, Hallen O, et al: Osseointegrated titanium implants in the temporal bone. A clinical study on bone-anchored hearing aids. Am J Otol 2:304-410, 1981.
4. Eriksson E, Branemark PI: Osseointegration from the perspective of the plastic surgeon. Plast Reconstr Surg 93:626-637, 1994.
5. Branemark PI, Albrektsson T: Titanium implants permanently penetrating human skin. Scand J Plast Reconstr Surg 16:17-21, 1982.
6. Tjellstrom A, Hakansson B: The bone-anchored hearing aid. Design principles, indications, and long-term clinical results. Otolaryngol Clin North Am 28:53-72, 1995.
7. Lustig LR, Arts HA, Brackmann DE, et al: Hearing rehabilitation using the BAHA bone-anchored hearing aid: Results in 40 patients. Otol Neurotol 22:328-334, 2001.
8. Tjellstrom A, Hakansson B, Granstrom G: Bone-anchored hearing aids: Current status in adults and children. Otolaryngol Clin North Am 34:337-364, 2001.
9. Scholz M, Eufinger H, Anders A, et al: Intracerebral abscess after abutment change of a bone anchored hearing aid (BAHA). Otol Neurotol 24:896-899, 2003.
10. Tjellstrom A, Granstrom G: One-stage procedure to establish osseointegration: A zero to five years follow-up report. J Laryngol Otol 109:593-598, 1995.
11. Papsin BC, Sirimanna TK, Albert DM, et al: Surgical experience with bone-anchored hearing aids in children. Laryngoscope 107:801-806, 1997.
12. Seemann R, Liu R, Di Toppa J: Results of pediatric bone-anchored hearing aid implantation. J Otolaryngol 33:71-74, 2004.
13. Granstrom G, Tjellstrom A: Guided tissue generation in the temporal bone. Ann Otol Rhinol Laryngol 108:349-354, 1999.

Chapter 119

Perilymphatic Fistulas

Barry E. Hirsch

Perilymphatic fistulas (PLFs) define a communication from the inner ear to the middle ear that occurs as a result of disruption of the natural bony or soft tissue barrier between the perilymphatic and middle ear spaces. It can be through the round or oval windows, fractures, neoplastic erosion, microfissures of the otic capsule, or disruption of the endosteal membrane after a fenestration procedure. Despite this clear definition, the existence of PLF as a spontaneous event remains a controversial issue in otology.

The clinical features of PLF became evident as experienced otolaryngologists correlated patients' symptoms with operative findings during middle ear surgery. Three different types of otologic findings have brought PLF into the differential diagnosis when acute auditory or vestibular dysfunction occurs. One form of PLF became recognized in the early era of otosclerosis surgery. On rare occasion, sudden onset of rapidly progressive hearing loss and dizziness would develop after stapedectomy. Middle ear exploration in these patients often revealed an opening in the oval window. A greater incidence of oval window PLFs was observed when a wire-Gelfoam prosthesis had been used. Likewise, polyethylene prostheses were found to erode through the oval window membrane and create a PLF. After repair of the PLF, the symptoms were frequently controlled. A second clinical entity described was erosion of the otic capsule by tumors of the middle ear or cholesteatoma and creation of a PLF, also eliciting symptoms of hearing loss or vertigo. A third clinical situation in which PLF was identified occurred with implosive or explosive injury to the inner and middle ear. Fee proposed this concept in 1968.[1] Patients subjected to significant barotrauma followed by hearing loss or dizziness were found to have a tear in the round window membrane or disruption of the stapes footplate.

PLFs may be categorized as *spontaneous* (idiopathic) or *post-traumatic*. A spontaneous PLF, by definition, has no predisposing events or factors that would induce a leak. It is often associated with congenital anomalies of the inner ear.[2] The incidence of spontaneous PLFs without an inner ear anomaly is apparently quite low. Post-traumatic PLFs include those that occur as a result of erosive tumors or cholesteatomas, secondary to iatrogenic leaks after otologic surgery, or subsequent to head trauma, barotrauma, or acoustic injuries.

The differential diagnosis should include a PLF when patients have hearing loss and vertigo, as well as a recent history of otologic surgery, head trauma, or barotrauma or evidence of middle ear pathology. Skepticism regarding the incidence of spontaneous PLF abounds because of isolated reports of large series of patients undergoing middle ear exploration for this diagnosis. We do not believe that spontaneous PLF is a cause of constant disequilibrium, tinnitus, aural fullness, and cognitive defects. Thus, PLFs in most adult patients can typically be categorized as post-traumatic in origin. In contrast, children and adolescents would be more likely to have spontaneous PLFs. It was shown that pediatric patients evaluated for hearing loss or vertigo had a higher incidence of congenital inner and middle ear anomalies. This group of patients had a significantly higher incidence of β_2-transferrin present in fluid samples collected at the time of exploratory tympanotomy.[2] Symptoms related to congenital anomalies of the temporal bone should become apparent in the earlier years rather than after the third decade of life.

An astute physician must have a high index of suspicion in rendering a diagnosis of PLF. The patient's immediate history is critical in linking the onset and activities with the symptoms of hearing loss, tinnitus, and vertigo. It is also imperative to know the patient's past history of otologic diseases and surgery, any congenital malformations that may be present, previous ear or head trauma or barotrauma, or a history of recurrent meningitis.

Trauma is the leading cause of PLF. It may be in the form of barotrauma, head trauma, or a penetrating injury. The latter is often associated with vertigo and routinely requires surgical repair. We have had clinical experiences with unusual forms of ear trauma. One involved a metal choker necklace and the other a branch of a tree entering the middle ear and extracting and subluxating the stapes, respectively. A similar report described a patient with severe itching; penetration of the ear with a paint brush resulted in perforation of the tympanic membrane, anacusis, and severe vertigo. The vestibular symptoms are often relieved once the fistula is sealed.[3]

It may be difficult to differentiate the symptom complex of Meniere's disease (fluctuating hearing loss, vertigo, tinnitus, and aural fullness) from those of a PLF. Loss of perilymph may result in a relative increase in endolymph with resultant secondary endolymphatic hydrops. Fitzgerald proposed a diagnostic strategy to manage surgical intervention. Simultaneous repair of a PLF and performance of an endolymphatic sac procedure may incur an unnecessary operation. A positive fistula test or immediate onset of Meniere's disease symptom complex after head or ear trauma points toward the pathology being a PLF, and surgery should be directed to the middle ear alone.[4]

There are other rare causes of PLF. An unusual form of trauma is from a lightning strike. Perforation of tympanic membrane is a known complication in this setting. If otorrhea should occur, the discharge, especially if watery and clear, should be assayed for β_2-transferrin. Exploration for a PLF should be considered when mixed hearing loss is identified.[5]

A formidable problem inherent in making the diagnosis of PLF is that there are no specific tests diagnostic of PLF, including both preoperative assessment and intraoperative determination. The current "gold standard" method of diagnosing a PLF is based on subjective interpretation of the surgeon's observations at the time of exploratory tympanotomy. The surgeon looks for reaccumulation of clear fluid in the round or oval window niche, especially after suction aspiration, or for a microfissure of the otic capsule. Identification of clear fluid can be falsely interpreted as perilymph in that a serous transudate or injected lidocaine may also pool in niches in the middle ear. Unless a unique marker for perilymph is identified, PLF at the time of exploration may be overdiagnosed.

In summary, based on our experience with exploration of the middle ear, we do acknowledge that PLFs exist but the incidence is low. It is important to consider a PLF in the differential diagnosis of sudden or rapidly progressive hearing loss or disequilibrium. However, one's criteria for exploring an ear must be defined and understood.

PATIENT SELECTION

Given that most cases of presumed PLF in adults can be categorized as post-traumatic, a critical feature necessary to entertain a diagnosis of PLF is the history given by the patient. In contrast, progressive hearing loss in children cannot be assumed to be hereditary in origin. The physician must extract and synthesize a complete otologic history. Complaints of aural fullness, hearing loss or dizziness, vertigo, or disequilibrium suggest the need for further information. The present history must clarify the onset of symptoms along with predisposing factors or associated physical activities. The duration and frequency of symptoms are the most important to ascertain. A history of episodic hearing loss with aural fullness, tinnitus, and vertigo lasting a few hours is more suggestive of Meniere's disease than PLF. Sudden hearing loss after an upper respiratory infection is probably a postviral loss unless violent sneezing or coughing preceded the acute event. Consideration of the diagnosis of PLF requires that if hearing loss is present, its onset be sudden, fluctuating, or rapidly progressive. Vestibular complaints may range from symptoms as vague as episodic lightheadedness or mild disequilibrium to unsteadiness, vertigo with nausea and vomiting, or ataxia.

Sudden auditory or vestibular symptoms may develop after abrupt changes in middle ear or subarachnoid space pressure. Injury to membranes of the scala tympani, media, or vestibuli (intracochlear fistula) or to the round or oval windows may occur as a result of severe barotrauma, acoustic trauma, or extreme physical exertion. Patients would be considered at risk for having a PLF if symptoms developed within a day or two after barotrauma from a poorly pressurized air flight; swimming pool or scuba diving; closed compressive ear trauma (hand slap to the ear); violent sneezing; forceful straining from constipation, labor and delivery, or weightlifting; or a blast injury.

Patients are questioned about whether they have recently or previously undergone any otologic surgery. Attempts are made to extract information regarding the precise nature of any procedure and whether any untoward complications occurred. In particular, it is helpful to determine whether the surgery was for otosclerosis, cholesteatoma, or other tumor of the middle ear and mastoid. The differential diagnosis for patients describing episodic dizziness or fluctuating progressive hearing loss after stapedectomy includes serous labyrinthitis, reparative granuloma (in the early postoperative period), or PLF (see Chapter 117).

Patients complaining of unrelenting vertigo should be examined for nystagmus. A spontaneous vestibular (horizontal) nystagmus may be identified. It can be observed on gross eye examination or by limiting visual fixation by having the patient wear Frenzel's lenses or infrared video goggles with display on a monitor. Another method for identifying nystagmus is via ophthalmoscopy. One looks for rhythmic retinal movement when examining the fundus. Assessment of hearing status is essential. Interpretation of tuning fork testing in the immediate postoperative period after otologic surgery may be difficult, depending on the hearing status of the contralateral ear. Complete closure of the air-bone gap may not be evident because of canal packing or middle ear fluid. Tuning fork lateralization to the operative ear confirms that cochlear function is preserved. Lateralization to the contralateral ear may indicate contralateral conductive hearing loss (bilateral otosclerosis) or significant ipsilateral sensorineural loss. The packing should be removed from the ear canal, and the tympanic membrane should be carefully inspected. The integrity of the tympanic membrane and the presence of middle ear fluid should be confirmed.

A fistula test with a pneumatic otoscope is performed to look for pneumatic-induced nystagmus (Hennebert's sign) or pneumatic-induced vertigo (Hennebert's symptom). Gentle pneumatic otoscopy may elicit horizontal nystagmus with positive or negative pressure. However, these findings must be interpreted cautiously in the immediate postoperative setting. The presence or absence of nystagmus does not confirm that a fistula does or does not exist. An audiogram will provide helpful information by identifying the type and degree of hearing loss present. Erythema of the tympanic membrane with a mild conductive hearing loss may be treated medically with antibiotics, steroids, and close observation. Another possibility is that this manifestation of hearing loss or disequilibrium may be a result of serous labyrinthitis. Significant progressive change in sensorineural hearing levels or speech discrimination scores in the face of new-onset dizziness is strongly suggestive of a PLF or possible reparative granuloma. Despite the surgeon's reluctance to re-explore a recently operated ear, the history and findings warrant intervention.

Indirect injuries to the tympanic membrane by an open hand slap to the ear often result in rupture of the tympanic membrane. A similar injury could occur with significant acoustic trauma, such as a blast injury. Blunt trauma to the tympanic membrane may also result in direct damage to the ossicular chain. In all three types of injuries, the compressive energy could be transmitted through the ossicular chain with subluxation of the stapes footplate into the oval window or explosive rupture of the round window. Progressive hearing loss or persistent disequilibrium in these settings is strongly suggestive of a traumatic PLF. Complete examination of the ear is necessary in patients experiencing these types of injuries. The integrity of the tympanic membrane is established. A pneumatic fistula test is performed to look for nystagmus. In this setting, observing nystagmus with pneumatic compression is suggestive of a PLF. Positional testing (Hallpike's maneuver) is also useful in patients complaining of position-induced vertigo. Vestibular tests entail electronystagmography (ENG) and an ENG fistula test. The ENG fistula test is monitored by recording electrodes placed horizontally near the lateral canthus of the eyes. Eye movements are recorded while positive and negative pneumatic tympanic membrane massage is applied with a Siegle otoscope or tympanometry bridge. The tracing is examined for nystagmus that is timed to manipulation of ear canal pressure (Fig. 119-1). Movement of the eyes can also be assessed with infrared video goggles placed over the eyes. This eliminates visual fixation and allows direct observation of eye deviation.

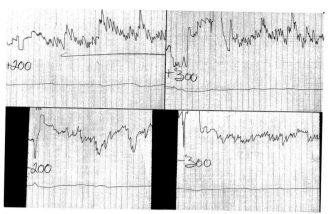

Figure 119-1. Electronystagmographic tracing of a positive fistula test. The *top row* shows that positive pneumatic pressure induces right-beating nystagmus at 200 and 300 mm H_2O. The *bottom row* demonstrates that negative pressure in the same ear reverses the direction of the nystagmus to left beating. Note the increase in beat frequency with greater pressure.

Unfortunately, the results of preoperative auditory and vestibular tests are variable and not specific to PLF. A positive pneumatic or ENG fistula test is certainly helpful in diagnosing a PLF, but negative explorations have been reported despite demonstrated affirmative preoperative findings. Conversely, PLFs have been identified in some patients despite normal preoperative test results.

Identification of the protein β_2-transferrin in perilymph has been offered as a diagnostic marker of PLF. Obtaining an adequate liquid sample of the middle ear fluid in question can be difficult. The volume may not be sufficient to aspirate and collect. Gelfoam has been used as an absorbent material from which the protein may be eluted. However, in a study of 20 samples of known perilymph collected at the time of cochlear implantation or labyrinthectomy, only 1 tested positive for β_2-transferrin. None of the control specimens demonstrated the protein.[6] This adds to the dilemma of confirming that a perilymph leak is truly present during middle ear exploration.

It was anticipated that communication between the scala tympani (perilymph) and cerebrospinal fluid (CSF) from the subarachnoid space through the cochlear aqueduct may provide a means to detect whether an active fistula is present. Fluorescein was injected by lumbar puncture in the CSF of 28 patients with suspected traumatic, idiopathic, iatrogenic, or inflammatory PLF. A few hours later the oval and round window niches were microscopically and endoscopically examined with white and blue light. Only two patients (7%) demonstrated fluorescence behind the round window membrane with blue light. Direct observation of perilymph in the setting of stapedectomy and semicircular canal fistulas revealed no staining. Despite the lack of reported neurologic complications from intrathecal fluorescein, this method for evaluating PLF was not recommended.[7]

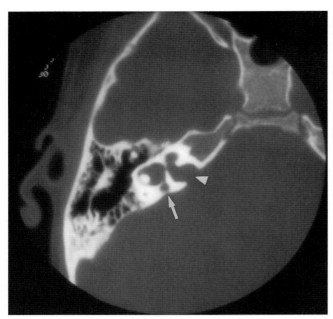

Figure 119-2. Bone-windowed computed tomography scan of a patient with progressive and fluctuating sensorineural hearing loss. Note the otic capsule abnormalities, including the bulbous vestibular aqueduct *(arrow)* and the dilated vestibule and internal auditory canal *(arrowhead).*

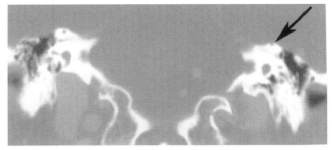

Figure 119-3. Coronal bone-windowed computed tomography scan showing dehiscence of the left superior semicircular canal *(arrow).*

There has been evidence that spontaneous PLFs may be associated with other congenital anomalies of the temporal bone.[2] Patients with abnormalities such as Mondini's dysplasia have a higher incidence of middle ear abnormalities and PLFs. Whether finding plus repairing a PLF halts the progressive nature of these anomalies or the PLF simply represents an epiphenomenon is unclear. In pediatric and young adult patients with progressive hearing loss and vestibular symptoms, radiographic imaging of the temporal bone is warranted. Demonstration of bilateral changes in hearing implies either metabolic, structural, or neural pathology. Although a demyelinating process is more effectively detected with magnetic resonance imaging, computed tomography (CT) better identifies anomalies of the otic capsule (Fig. 119-2). Because PLFs have been identified with congenital anomalies of the inner or middle ear, a patient with progressive hearing loss and an abnormal CT scan of the temporal bone may be a candidate for PLF exploration.

Physicians have varied opinions regarding the source of sudden, progressive, or fluctuating hearing loss in children. There is controversy as to whether PLF can be a possible cause. A retrospective study investigated hearing and vestibular outcomes in 160 ears of pediatric patients undergoing middle ear fistula surgery for sudden, progressive, or fluctuating hearing loss of great than 20 dB in three frequencies. Of the 103 ears with a fistula confirmed by visual inspection of leaking or reaccumulating fluid, 92% demonstrated stabilization or improvement of hearing after surgical repair of the leak. In the 57 ears in which a fistula was not identified but the oval and round windows were packed with muscle or connective tissue, 95% had stabilized or improved hearing. Based on observations from their parents, 70% of children with a positive fistula exploration for vertigo and disequilibrium had improvement in their symptoms after surgical repair.[8]

It is difficult to reach a meaningful conclusion about the potential role that a congenital PLF may have in causing sensorineural hearing loss in children. Why hearing levels may stabilize in ears in which a fistula is not identified yet still treated surgically is unclear. A plausible explanation is that at the time of exploration the leak is intermittent or not evident because the operative ear is facing up and thus perilymph is required to drain against gravity. It is reasonable to conclude that surgical repair (packing of tissue in the round and oval windows) does not result in a significant risk for postoperative hearing loss.

Our understanding of the etiology of hearing loss or vestibular problems, or both, has significantly expanded since the first edition of this textbook. Lloyd Minor is credited with characterizing the auditory and vestibular signs and symptoms associated with dehiscence of the superior semicircular canal (SCC).[9] Many of the symptoms, such as noise-induced dizziness, hearing loss, and disequilibrium precipitated by heavy lifting, belching, coughing, sneezing, or straining, are common to both PLF and dehiscence of the SCC. Similarly, a positive fistula test (nystagmus seen with pneumatic otoscopy) can occur in both clinical entities. An audiogram may show conductive hearing loss, but acoustic reflexes should still be present in SCC dehiscence. Vestibular evoked myogenic potentials are typically elicited at lower thresholds and can show enhanced amplitude responses. CT showing dehiscence of the SSC is critical in making the diagnosis. By using a multirow CT scanner, images of the temporal bone can be reconstructed parallel and perpendicular to the superior canal. We have shown that coronal images usually suffice in identifying the dehiscent canal (Fig. 119-3).[10]

PREOPERATIVE PLANNING

Patients in whom a PLF is suspected should undergo preoperative audiography to determine whether there has been a change from previous levels or to establish the baseline of hearing. Vestibular testing may be helpful if a unilateral paresis is identified or a positive PLF test (pneumatic otoscopy) is obtained. Imaging of the temporal bone may be informative after blunt or penetrating head trauma but provides limited additional information in cases of barotrauma or acoustic trauma. Imaging may be helpful after recent otologic surgery if a displaced prosthesis is of concern.

The choice of anesthesia is dependent on the age of the patient and the cause of the suspected PLF. Having the patient awake provides two benefits to the surgeon. First, the patient is able to follow commands, such as performing a Valsalva maneuver (breath holding with forceful straining against a closed glottis). It can be argued that similar results can be achieved with the patient under general anesthesia by having the anesthetist deliver sustained positive end-expiratory pressure (PEEP). Maintaining PEEP increases venous resistance, which causes increased intracranial pressure. Just as with a Valsalva maneuver, increased intracranial pressure may enhance transmission of fluid pressure to the inner ear perilymph fluid compartment and augment visualization of a latent PLF. However, iatrogenic injury to the inner ear cannot be readily ascertained under general anesthesia. The second benefit of having an awake patient is that it provides immediate feedback regarding the patient's subjective sensation of vertigo and dizziness. This is particularly beneficial in cases of recent otologic surgery or limited temporal bone trauma. Injudicious manipulation of a footplate that is subluxated or an oval window graft with fibrous adhesions to the saccule or utricle is detrimental to inner ear function. An awake, although sedated patient can directly communicate any feelings of disequilibrium to the surgeon.

Despite the cause of the suspected PLF, it is very difficult to perform exploratory ear surgery on children under local anesthesia. A young teenager or mature adolescent may tolerate this procedure with sedation. The surgeon, along with the parents, must decide which method of anesthesia is best for the patient and the surgeon. General anesthesia is generally necessary for exploratory tympanotomy performed on a child.

SURGICAL TECHNIQUES

The patient is positioned supine on the table with the involved ear up. A small area of postauricular hair may need to be shaved to provide access to suitable material for grafting or obliteration. Surgeons who routinely use a vein graft for stapedectomy would prepare and drape the dorsum of the hand if the integrity of the stapes footplate is in question. After adequate preoperative sedation or narcoleptic anesthesia is obtained, the operating microscope is positioned over the ear. Local anesthetic (2% lidocaine with 1:100,000 epinephrine) is infiltrated into the external meatus in four-quadrant fashion after inspection of the ear canal and tympanic membrane (Fig. 119-4). Local anesthesia with controlled vasoconstriction is necessary when exploring an ear for a PLF. Hemostasis is mandatory to minimize any

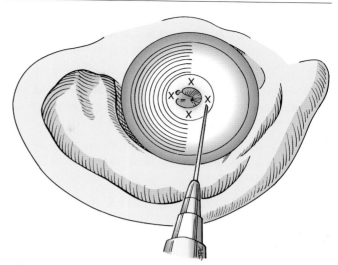

Figure 119-4. Local anesthetic solution is injected into the external auditory canal in four-quadrant fashion.

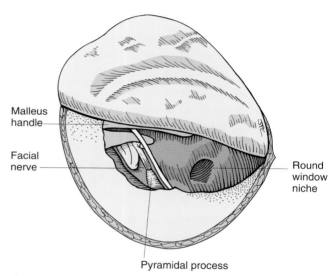

Figure 119-5. A tympanomeatal flap has been elevated. Bone from the posterosuperior canal wall has been removed by curette to maximize exposure of the oval and round window niches.

confusion that may occur as a result of serum leaking into the middle ear. It is recognized that some of the infiltrated local anesthetic may diffuse into the middle ear and appear as clear fluid welling up in the oval or round window niches.[11] The observer could falsely call this a PLF. Nonetheless, local injection is necessary to both anesthetize the ear canal and curtail bleeding. A tympanomeatal flap is elevated to enter the middle ear (Fig. 119-5). It is usually necessary to remove bone from the posterosuperior canal wall to achieve complete exposure of the oval window niche. Depending on the vascularity of the bone and middle ear, bleeding into the middle ear space may occur. Methods of controlling bleeding include placement of small Gelfoam pledgets impregnated with a topical vasoconstrictive solution from the local anesthetic, small pieces of Surgicel, or rarely, bipolar electrocautery. Once complete exposure is obtained, management, which is described later in this chapter, is dictated by the findings during surgery. The status of the middle ear mucosa and ossicular chain is examined.

Usually, the round window niche can be visualized by repositioning the microscope or the operating table without having to curette the posterior bony canal wall. The round and oval window niches are examined to look for reaccumulation of clear fluid despite repeated suctioning. A PLF may also be identified by recognizing a shifting light reflex from the operating microscope. Identifying a perilymph leak is facilitated by increasing intracranial pressure. If clear fluid is not noted, the patient is asked to perform a Valsalva maneuver. Other techniques used to enhance identification of a latent PLF include compression of the ipsilateral jugular vein, palpation of the ossicular chain to facilitate leakage, or placement of the patient in the Trendelenburg position.

At present, the diagnosis of a PLF is based on seeing reaccumulation of clear fluid or a change in the light reflex from the operating microscope. A more objective laboratory assay of the identified fluid would certainly help in understanding PLFs. There is ongoing investigation of the use of β_2-transferrin as a marker for perilymph fluid. Pieces of Gelfoam or Merocel are placed in each niche, and separately labeled samples are absorbed and collected. Electrophoresis with Western blot staining can identify isoforms of β-transferrin. Results of the assay are currently available in a minimum of 3 hours. Unfortunately, this information is not immediately available at the time of surgery to influence operative management. In addition, the true sensitivity and specificity of the assay have yet to be determined.[12]

Patients being explored for sudden or progressive hearing loss or vestibular symptoms after stapedectomy require specific management. Surgeons using tissue graft or vein graft for routine stapedectomy should be prepared to harvest a new graft before re-exploring an ear that has previously undergone otosclerosis surgery. The oval window niche is examined for a reparative granuloma in patients with rapidly progressive hearing loss and recent stapes surgery. If a granuloma is present, the prosthesis is removed and a new tissue seal is placed. If a granuloma is not present, the position of the prosthesis is inspected. If a tissue seal was used, its integrity and the covering of the vestibule are confirmed. Appropriate placement of the prosthesis is verified by palpation of the ossicular chain. Careful inspection to search for incomplete oval window coverage is undertaken (Fig. 119-6). The oval window niche is carefully examined for clear fluid. If concern exists regarding the integrity of the tissue seal, the prosthesis is removed and the tissue graft is replaced. Likewise, if a stapedotomy piston was used, displacement of the prosthesis from the fenestration site should be determined.

Patients subjected to blunt or penetrating trauma to the ear with ongoing dizziness and hearing loss

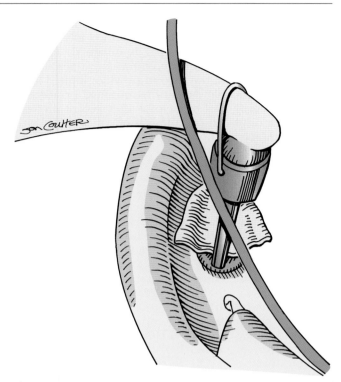

Figure 119-6. A cause of a perilymphatic fistula is a dehiscence in the tissue graft sealing the oval window after stapedectomy. The graft incompletely covers the posterior aspect of the oval window niche.

are managed similarly. The integrity of the ossicular chain is assessed. The incudostapedial joint may be compromised and the stapes footplate fractured, depressed, or subluxated into the vestibule. If this is determined, the incudostapedial joint is disarticulated. The dependent portion of the footplate is carefully elevated out of the vestibule. Should the patient complain of excessive vertigo or nausea, manipulation of the footplate is terminated. Potential tissue grafts that can be harvested include a vein from the hand, temporalis fascia, or tragal perichondrium. Our preference is areolar tissue or fascia overlying the temporalis muscle. After the mucosa is elevated from the margins of the oval window, the vestibule is sealed with the graft (Fig. 119-7).

Spontaneous PLFs are handled in a similar manner. The oval and round windows are inspected for clear fluid. If clear fluid is found, the mucosa near the stapes footplate is elevated (Fig. 119-8). The round window may have an overhang that should be removed with a curette or middle ear microdrill for better visualization. The mucosa is also elevated if a PLF is found in this area. The preferred material for sealing PLFs is fibrofascial tissue harvested from the postauricular area. Perichondrium from the tragus may also be used. Adipose tissue is purposely avoided because of its inherent properties of atrophy and resorption. Small pieces of fibrofascial tissue are placed in the oval or round windows and between the crura of the stapes (Fig. 119-9). Similarly, the round window niche is sealed after

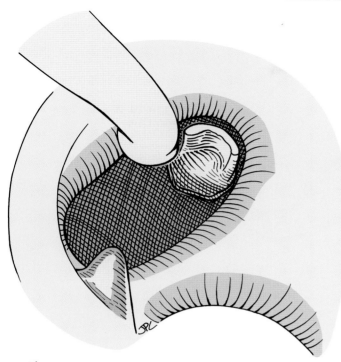

Figure 119-7. A portion of the anterior stapes footplate remains subluxated within the vestibule after trauma. A vein graft will be placed to completely cover the oval window niche.

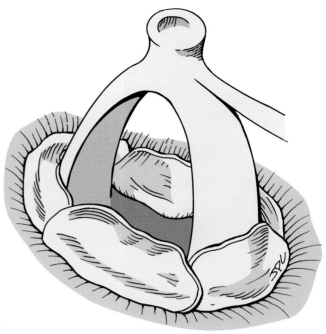

Figure 119-9. Small pieces of fibrofascial tissue are placed around the oval window niche to promote closure of a perilymphatic fistula.

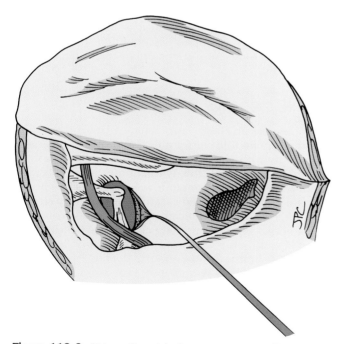

Figure 119-8. Using a fine pick, the mucosa surrounding the oval window niche is elevated to promote scarification with fibrous tissue grafts. *(From Bluestone CD, Stool SE: Atlas of Pediatric Otolaryngology. Philadelphia, WB Saunders, 1995, p 115.)*

the surrounding bone is denuded of mucosa. Methods to fix the tissue in place and promote scarring include the use of Avitene, Surgicel, or fibrin glue placed lateral to the tissue graft.

Another method of sealing the annular margin of the footplate is with a contoured graft. Fascia or perichondrium cut in the shape of a pair of pants or narrow U can be positioned around the anterior crux of the stapes with the limbs extending along the superior and inferior footplates. This provides a good seal of the anterior footplate and fistula ante fenestram (Fig. 119-10).

Along with the oval and round window niches, other areas should be inspected, including the area anterior to the footplate at the fistula ante fenestram and the area inferior to the round window niche, where microfissures have been reported.[13]

One of the more difficult decisions that one faces is what to do in the event that no PLF is identified. If clear fluid is not observed, it can certainly be argued that a PLF does not exist and that packing the niches is not warranted. There are anecdotal reports of hearing returning to normal in patients with negative explorations in which packing was not performed. Proponents of this philosophy argue that if routine packing is performed, one will never know whether the treatment was justified. On the other hand, one could argue that PLFs may be intermittent or difficult to identify when the involved ear is facing up at the time of surgery. The effects of gravity and minimal inner ear fluid pressure may hamper leakage of perilymph. In fact, authorities

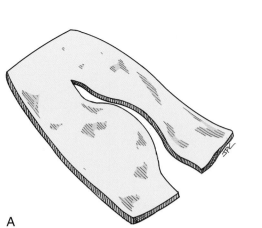

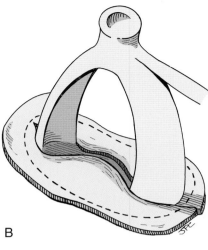

A

B

Figure 119-10. A, A fascia graft cut like a pair of pants has been prepared for the footplate area. **B,** The graft is placed around the stapes crura.

remain divided about what direction to take in the situation of negative exploration. Some surgeons pack routinely; others pack only if a PLF is identified. We recommend placing fascia (packing) at the time of exploration.

Management of a subluxated footplate can be difficult. Recent injuries, which limit the time for fibrous adhesions to develop, permit attempts at elevating the stapes from the vestibule. Should the patient complain of increasing vestibular symptoms during operative manipulation, further efforts are aborted. A similar approach is taken for an ear that is re-explored after stapes surgery. If a PLF is strongly suspected and none is obviously seen, the surgeon must decide whether the prosthesis should be replaced and the oval window regrafted or the symptoms should be ascribed to serous labyrinthitis. If surgery is being performed for unresolving vestibular problems in the presence of severe hearing loss, more aggressive intervention is warranted. Along with attempting to alleviate the vestibular symptoms, repairing communicating pathways from the middle ear to the perilymph and CSF may prevent potential otic meningitis. This approach is particularly applicable to younger patients with congenital otic capsule anomalies.

Recurrent symptoms after PLF repair are difficult to interpret and manage. Review of the patient's history and physical findings is necessary. A higher incidence of recurrent PLF has been reported when adipose tissue is used for grafting, presumably because of progressive atrophy of the adipose tissue graft. It is for this reason that we advocate fibrofascial tissue, muscle, or perichondrium for PLF repair.

Once the middle ear procedure is completed, the tympanomeatal flap is returned to its original position. The flap is secured with ointment, antibiotic-impregnated Gelfoam, or a silk sleeve compressed with small cotton balls and ointment. The tissue donor site is closed with 5-0 fast-absorbing suture and covered with a Steri-Strip.

POSTOPERATIVE MANAGEMENT

Patients can usually be discharged the same day unless severe nausea or vertigo is experienced. Oral narcotic analgesics are provided if needed. It is rarely necessary to provide wound care to the tissue donor site. A cotton ball in the external auditory meatus is changed as needed. Some serosanguineous drainage should be anticipated. Exposure of the ear to water, bending with heavy lifting, and sneezing with the nares occluded are to be avoided. The patient is seen 7 to 10 days postoperatively for removal of the Steri-Strips and packing. Restriction from water exposure is maintained for 3 more weeks. An audiogram is obtained 4 to 6 weeks after surgery to assess and document the status of auditory function.

COMPLICATIONS

The operative morbidity associated with surgical exploration of the middle ear for a PLF is minimal, especially in patients with significant preoperative hearing loss. Careful elevation of the tympanomeatal flap avoids potential tears in the tympanic membrane. The chorda tympani nerve is dissected carefully to minimize stretch and desiccation. Theoretically, packing of the round or oval windows should produce a conductive hearing loss. In reality, however, such packing does not lead to a significant clinical or audiometric deficit.

Packing of the round and oval windows should effectively prevent fluid from both exiting and entering the inner ear. As mentioned, symptoms, signs, and the diagnosis of PLF and Meniere's disease may overlap. Should intratympanic therapy with either an aminoglycoside (gentamicin) or steroid be necessary for subsequent intervention, access to the inner ear by injection into the middle ear may effectively be obstructed by the tissue graft. The subsequent treating physician should be aware of the patient's past medical history and details of the previous surgical procedures.

PEARLS

- Patients with sudden hearing loss or dizziness who have a history of recent barotrauma, physical ear injury, or otologic surgery should be suspected of having a PLF.
- Exploration of the middle ear should be carried out in patients in the pediatric age group who have sudden or fluctuating hearing loss and dizziness and middle or inner ear anomalies confirmed by CT.
- Identification of nystagmus elicited by pneumatic otoscopy may be enhanced by using infrared video goggles instead of directly observing the eyes for movement.
- Observation of a PLF is enhanced by having the patient perform a Valsalva maneuver if awake or having the anesthetist apply positive pressure ventilation if under general anesthesia.
- Because a fistula may be intermittent or difficult to elicit with the involved ear facing up at the time of middle ear exploration, both the oval and round windows should be packed with a tissue graft.

PITFALLS

- The symptoms and signs of pressure-induced vertigo and nystagmus are similar with acute endolymphatic hydrops, a stapes prosthesis located too deep in the vestibule, a PLF, and dehiscence of the superior semicircular canal.
- Complications of middle ear exploration should be rare, but great care should be taken to avoid a tear in the tympanic membrane or injury to the chorda tympani nerve.
- Excess fluid from injection of the local anesthetic and vasoconstrictor may permeate into the middle ear and be mistaken for perilymph.

- Adipose tissue should not be used for packing the PLF because it is more likely to atrophy and no longer occlude the area of PLF.
- Laboratory markers for identifying perilymph, such as β_2-transferrin or fluorescein, can be unreliable and their absence misleading.

References

1. Fee GA: Traumatic perilymphatic fistulas. Arch Otolaryngol 88:477-480, 1968.
2. Weber PC, Perez BA, Bluestone CD: Congenital perilymphatic fistula and associated middle ear abnormalities. Laryngoscope 103:160-164, 1993.
3. Gunesh RP, Huber AM: Traumatic perilymphatic fistula. Ann Otol Rhinol Laryngol 112:221-222, 2003.
4. Fitzgerald DC: Perilymphatic fistula and Meniere's disease. Clinical series and literature review. Ann Otol Rhinol Laryngol 110:430-436, 2001.
5. Sun GH, Simons JP, Mandell DL: Bilateral perilymphatic fistulas from a lightning strike: A case report. Laryngoscope 116:1039-1042, 2006.
6. Buchman CA, Luxford WM, Hirsch BE, et al: Beta-2 transferrin assay in the identification of perilymph. Am J Otol 20:174-178, 1999.
7. Gehrking E, Wisst F, Remmert S, et al: Intraoperative assessment of perilymphatic fistulas with intrathecal administration of fluorescein. Laryngoscope 112:1614-1618, 2002.
8. Weber PC, Bluestone CD, Perez B: Outcome of hearing and vertigo after surgery for congenital perilymphatic fistula in children. Am J Otolaryngol 24:138-142, 2003.
9. Minor LB: Clinical manifestations of superior semicircular canal dehiscence. Laryngoscope 115:1717-1727, 2005.
10. Branstetter BF, Harrigal C, Escott EJ, et al: Superior semicircular canal dehiscence: Oblique reformatted CT images for diagnosis. Radiology 238:938-942, 2006.
11. Wilson DF, Hodgson RS: Lidocaine in the middle ear. Laryngoscope 100:1059-1061, 1990.
12. Bassiouny M, Hirsch BE, Kelly RH, et al: Beta 2 transferrin application in otology. Am J Otol 13:552-555, 1992.
13. Kamerer DB, Sando I, Hirsch BE, et al: Perilymph fistula resulting from microfissures. Am J Otol 8:489-494, 1987.

Chapter 120

Intracranial Complications of Otitis Media

William A. Wood and Yael Raz

Complications from acute otitis media or chronic otitis media can be divided into extracranial complications (i.e., facial nerve paralysis, labyrinthitis, subperiosteal abscess) and intracranial complications. Intracranial complications of otitis media include meningitis, epidural abscess, subdural abscess (empyema), brain abscess, lateral sinus thrombophlebitis/sigmoid sinus thrombosis, otitic hydrocephalus, and Gradenigo's syndrome (Fig. 120-1). On occasion, an intracranial complication may be the initial symptom in a patient with a history of untreated otitis media. Multiple complications may coexist. Despite broad-spectrum antibiotics, complications of otitis media can result in high morbidity and even mortality, and surgical management is often necessary.

Spread of otitis media to intracranial structures may occur either directly or hematogenously. Direct extension can occur via multiple mechanisms:[1] preexisting congenital abnormalities such as a Mondini deformity, post-traumatic bony defects from temporal bone fracture, erosion of bony barriers as a result of cholesteatoma, normal communicating vein pathways from the mastoid to the intracranial space, and spontaneous or iatrogenic dehiscence of bone.[2] Meningitis, historically the most common intracranial complication of otitis media, frequently spreads in children via a hematogenous route or by extension from a local abscess.[3] With widespread *Haemophilus influenzae* type B and antipneumococcal vaccination of children, the incidence of meningitis as a complication of these two organisms has become very low.[1] Some recent series report a greater frequency of lateral sinus thrombophlebitis/sigmoid sinus thrombosis or brain abscess than meningitis. The frequency of various intracranial complications in a number of case series over the last decade is presented in Table 120-1.[4-17]

Patients may initially have the classic signs of otogenic infection, such as foul-smelling otorrhea, otalgia, headache, fever, vertigo, and sudden hearing loss. As the disease progresses, later signs include mental status changes such as confusion, obtundation or seizures, and cranial nerve palsies. Many patients with intracranial complications will have multiple complications, such as meningitis in addition to an abscess, and the otolaryngologist should seek to diagnose and treat all of these complications. Patients may have concurrent intratemporal complications such as subperiosteal abscess, labyrinthitis, and facial nerve paresis.

MENINGITIS

INDICATIONS AND PATIENT SELECTION

Patients with meningitis may have the classic signs and symptoms, such as headache, photophobia, spiking fevers, mental status changes, nausea, and vomiting. Physical signs that have been classically described for evaluating meningitis, such as Kernig's sign, Brudzinski's sign, and nuchal rigidity, were recently shown in a prospective study of patients suspected of having meningitis to have sensitivities of only 5% to 30%,[18] and hence clinical suspicion should remain high even when these signs are negative on examination. An early lumbar puncture is essential in suspected meningitis, followed immediately by empirical antibiotic treatment, pending culture results. In addition to opening pressure, cell counts, Gram stain, and culture, a cerebrospinal fluid (CSF)–serum glucose ratio of less than 0.5 is abnormal and greatly raises suspicion of meningitis.[19] Current practice guidelines for suspected bacterial meningitis recommend computed tomography (CT) before lumbar puncture for patients in the following categories: immunocompromised state, history of central nervous system disease (e.g., stroke), new-onset seizure, papilledema, abnormal level of consciousness, or focal neurologic deficit.[20]

Table 120-1	RECENT REPORTED SERIES OF INTRACRANIAL COMPLICATIONS OF OTITIS MEDIA IN CHILDREN, ADULTS, AND COMBINED GROUPS OF CHILDREN AND ADULTS								
Reference and Total Number of Patients	Patients with ICCOM	Meningitis	Epidural Abscess	Subdural Abscess/ Empyema	Brain Abscess	Lateral Sinus Thrombophlebitis or Sigmoid Sinus Thrombosis	Otitic Hydrocephalus	Other*
Pediatric Series								
Zanetti,[4] 2006, N = 45	13	6	3	0	1	7	0	2
Migirov,[5] 2005, N = 28 (11 children)	11	5	3	0	0	1	0	2
Leskinen,[6] 2004, N = 33	1	1	1	0	0	0	0	0
Luntz,[7] 2001, N = 223 (214 children)	19	7		1	1	6	0	5
Go,[8] 2000, N = 118	8	1	4	6	0	0	0	0
Kaftan,[9] 2000, N = 22 (3 of 22 <18 yr old)	3	3	0	0	0	0	0	0
Schwager,[10] 1997, N = 124	11 (4 patients had >1 ICCOM)	5	5	0	2	5	0	0

Adult Series

Study							
Leskinen,[11] 2005, N = 50	9	4 (1 death)	0	0	4	1	0
Migirov,[5] 2005, N = 28 (17 adults)	17	8	2	2	5	2 (1 transverse, 1 sigmoid)	0
Kaftan,[9] 2000, N = 22 (19 of 22 >18 yr old)	19	12	0	1	5	0	1 (Gradenigo's syndrome)
Barry,[12] 1999, N = 79 with otogenic meningitis	79	79	4	2	4	2	8

Series with Combined Children and Adults; Results Not Separated

Study							
Seven,[13] 2005, N = 32 with 59 ICCOMs	32	7	7	2	14	10	11
Penido,[14] 2005, N = 33	33	21	1	2	26 (3 deaths)	5	1
Matanda,[15] 2005, N = 343 (215 patients <20 yr old)	24	12	0	0	9	2	0
Goldstein,[16] 2000, N = 100 intratemporal complications of otitis media	16	2	7	1	1	5	2
Osma,[17] 2000, N = 93, 57 with ICCOMs (58% <20 yr old)	57	41	4	0	10	1	0

*Other includes cavernous sinus thrombosis, perisinus abscess, meningocele, petrous apex suppuration, internal jugular thrombosis, cerebritis, presuppurative encephalitis, and ventriculitis. Some patients had more than one intracranial complication.
ICCOM, intracranial complication of otitis media.

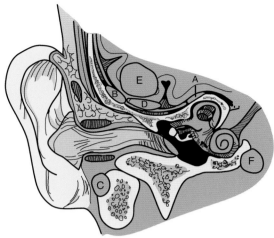

Figure 120-1. Intracranial complications of otitis media include meningitis (A), epidural abscess (B), lateral sinus thrombosis (C), subdural empyema (D), brain abscess (E), and petrous apicitis (F). *(Adapted from Vazquez E, Castellote A, Piqueras J, et al: Imaging of complications of acute mastoiditis in children. Radiographics 23:359-372, 2003.)*

Fine-cut CT of the temporal bone, with and without contrast enhancement, along with imaging of the brain allows evaluation of related intracranial complications such as a brain abscess, as well as detection of bone defects in the middle fossa or posterior fossa plate and other structural abnormalities. When otitis media is diagnosed or suspected, the otolaryngologist should perform a myringotomy and send the aspirate for immediate Gram stain, in addition to culture and sensitivity testing; a ventilation tube is placed. Antibiotics should then be adjusted to the results of culture of the middle ear aspirate and CSF. If the patient can tolerate magnetic resonance imaging (MRI), it should be performed because it has greater sensitivity for evaluating the extent and type of intracranial infection.[21]

SURGICAL TECHNIQUE

Aside from myringotomy and tube insertion, meningitis alone does not require additional surgical treatment. However, if the patient fails to respond adequately to systemic therapy, mastoidectomy should be considered when the patient is neurologically stable enough to tolerate the procedure, which may reveal a chronic underlying cause (Fig. 120-2). Hearing should be monitored closely. Possible sequelae include labyrinthitis ossificans with resultant sensorineural hearing loss, in which case early cochlear implantation should be considered.

EPIDURAL ABSCESS

INDICATIONS AND PATIENT SELECTION

Patients with coalescent mastoiditis or chronic suppurative otitis media with cholesteatoma are at risk for bony erosion into the intracranial epidural space and abscess formation. If the erosion occurs superiorly through the

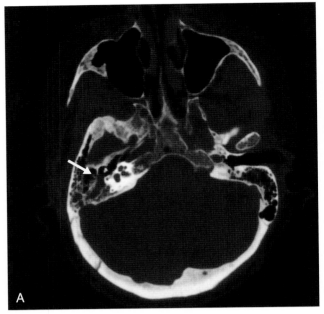

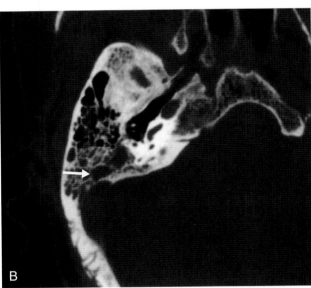

Figure 120-2. Chronic mastoiditis in a patient with meningitis. **A,** Antral block *(arrow),* chronic mastoiditis. **B,** Erosion of the posterior fossa plate overlying the sigmoid sinus *(arrow).* At the time of the scan, the patient was asymptomatic. She had severe cardiac risk and was observed without surgical intervention. However, 6 months later the patient was evaluated for otalgia, fever, and mental status changes. Workup revealed meningitis. A mastoidectomy was performed because of inadequate response to antibiotics. The antral block was found to be secondary to a cholesterol granuloma.

tegmen, the abscess will form in the middle fossa. Similarly, if the erosion occurs posteriorly, the abscess will form in the posterior fossa, often around the sigmoid sinus. Some authors refer to abscesses that are adjacent to the sigmoid sinus as perisinus abscesses or empyemas. One recent large series of patients with epidural abscesses found that 20% were secondary to otogenic infection, in contrast to almost two thirds that were secondary to infections of the paranasal sinuses.[22]

Patients with an otogenic epidural abscess classically have worsening temporoparietal headache in the region of the affected ear,[23] with or without mental status changes such as lethargy. However, "silent" abscesses may also be discovered on temporal bone CT performed to assess the condition of the mastoid and middle ear.[24] If an intracranial complication is suspected from the clinical or CT findings, MRI provides valuable additional information about the location and extent of such complications. When loculated purulent exudate, granulation tissue, or bony erosion is noted on mastoidectomy, evaluation of the integrity of the bony tegmen and surrounding bony confines of the intracranial space is necessary to rule out an epidural abscess. An epidural abscess may occur in association with other intracranial complications of otitis media, such as thrombophlebitis or thrombosis of the lateral or sigmoid sinus, and hence the otologist should have a high index of suspicion with regard to these other serious conditions.

SURGICAL TECHNIQUE

An isolated epidural abscess secondary to mastoiditis can usually be evacuated by a complete mastoidectomy, with careful unroofing of the affected bony plates to expose but not enter the dura (Fig. 120-3). Purulent material and granulation tissue should be sent for immediate Gram stain, culture, and sensitivity testing. The mastoid is then irrigated with antibiotic solution.

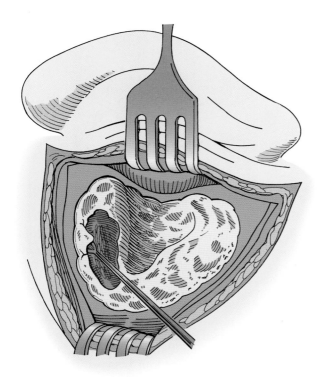

Figure 120-3. Exposure and drainage of an epidural abscess with wide exposure of the middle fossa dura.

If the abscess was not diagnosed preoperatively, follow-up imaging should be conducted to evaluate for the possible presence of other intracranial complications.

LATERAL SINUS THROMBOSIS

INDICATIONS AND PATIENT SELECTION

Inflammation of the dural sinuses secondary to otitis media can occur as a result of an adjacent epidural abscess or via direct extension from communicating venous channels between the mastoid and dural sinuses (Fig. 120-4) and may lead to thrombosis. Once the wall of a dural sinus is inflamed, a thrombus may form and can propagate in the lumen of the sinus. In severe cases it can lead to venous hemorrhage and cerebral infarction if collateral drainage is inadequate.

The lateral sinus is the combination of the transverse and sigmoid sinuses. Patients with lateral sinus thrombophlebitis and/or thrombosis (LST) secondary to otitis will typically complain of headache, fever, and photophobia, in addition to symptoms consistent with mastoiditis. Frequently, other intracranial complications such as an epidural or subdural abscess or otitic hydrocephalus coexist.[25] Intramural thrombi can often be diagnosed on contrast-enhanced CT, but MRI and MR venography are considered the "gold standards" for diagnosing and monitoring cerebral venous thrombosis (Fig. 120-5).[26]

A number of recent case series have demonstrated that the distribution of causes of LST is approximately equally divided between acute otitis media and chronic otitis media.[27,28] Other series report an exclusive association with chronic ear disease.[29] Most recent series have included fewer than 15 patients, thus indicating the relative rarity of this complication with effective early treatment of otitis media.

SURGICAL MANAGEMENT

Historically, the standard of care for LST has been, in addition to intravenous antibiotics, a complete mastoidectomy with exposure of the lateral sinus. Needle aspiration of the sinus may be used to determine whether purulent exudate is present (Fig. 120-6). If so, consideration should be given to incision and evacuation of the thrombus (Fig. 120-7). Bleeding from the lateral sinus can be controlled by extraluminal compression with Surgicel (Fig. 120-8). The medial wall of the sinus is maintained intact. Opening of the sinus plus removal of the clot are not necessary unless the sinus is grossly infected.[16] The role of postoperative anticoagulation is unclear.[31] In cases of noncoalescent mastoiditis, a conservative approach, including immediate myringotomy, tube placement, and topical and intravenous antibiotics, is reasonable.[32] The patient is monitored closely, and mastoidectomy and sinus exploration are performed if the patient fails to improve. A thrombosed sinus may recanalize spontaneously over a period of several weeks.[33]

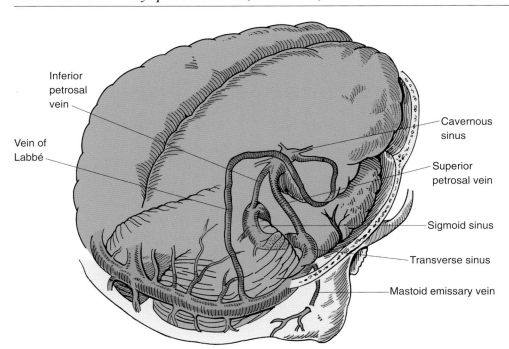

Inferior petrosal vein

Vein of Labbé

Cavernous sinus

Superior petrosal vein

Sigmoid sinus

Transverse sinus

Mastoid emissary vein

Figure 120-4. Anatomic relationship between the dural sinuses and the temporal bone.

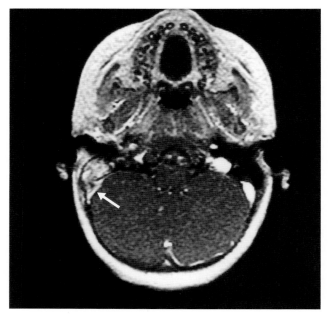

Figure 120-5. Magnetic resonance venogram showing a filling defect in the right sigmoid sinus indicative of thrombosis *(arrow)*; the patient also had an epidural abscess secondary to mastoiditis.

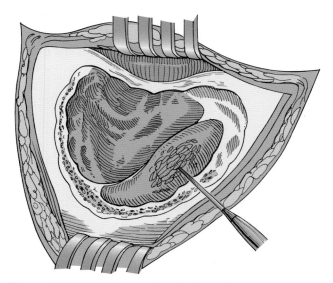

Figure 120-6. Palpation and aspiration of a thrombophlebitic dural sinus.

SUBDURAL ABSCESS (EMPYEMA)

INDICATIONS AND PATIENT SELECTION

Previously, otitis media was among the leading causes of subdural abscess[34]; however, over the last several decades it has become more infrequent. One retrospective review of 32 patients with subdural empyema since the 1970s found no cases secondary to otitis media[35]; another similar series noted that previous craniotomy was the most common risk factor for development of an abscess and had been performed in two thirds of cases. One very large series of 699 cases in a developing country found an otogenic source in about 9% of cases.[36]

Subdural empyema can develop via thrombophlebitis of small emissary veins traveling from an infected mastoid or middle ear centrally through the dura, where an abscess then develops between the dura and arachnoid. This complication may occur in conjunction with epidural abscess, meningitis, or brain abscess. Most patients have fever and meningismus. Even though

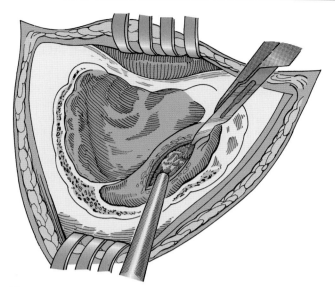

Figure 120-7. Incision and drainage of a thrombophlebitic dural sinus

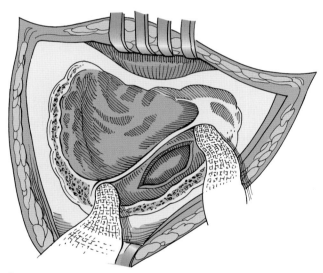

Figure 120-8. Extraluminal packing is used to control bleeding from the dural sinus.

focal signs such as hemiparesis will develop in many patients, almost 40% in the large series noted earlier had no focal signs. Empyema can progress rapidly to coma and death; when intracranial pressure rises acutely, papilledema may be absent.[37] Although imaging evaluation of a patient with suspected intracranial complications of otitis will usually include contrast-enhanced CT, one recent radiologic review recommends diffusion-weighted MRI to help distinguish subdural empyema from a reactive subdural effusion.[38]

SURGICAL TECHNIQUE

Subdural empyema needs to be evacuated on an emergency basis and the frequently accompanying increase

in intracranial pressure carefully monitored via lumbar puncture, along with the intravenous administration of antibiotics. Drainage can be achieved by craniotomy or CT-guided aspiration, in consultation with the neurosurgical service. If the otogenic source is chronic otitis media, mastoidectomy is indicated.

BRAIN ABSCESS

INDICATIONS AND PATIENT SELECTION

Brain abscess is an ominous complication that can still be fatal despite modern antibiotics and aggressive surgical treatment. The British writer Oscar Wilde died of an otogenic brain abscess near the turn of the last century; the postauricular Wilde incision is named for his father, Sir William Wilde, one of the founding fathers of otology.[39] Most recent case series are from developing countries because this complication is less frequently seen in wealthier societies with greater access to health care. A recent series of 41 patients from a university center in Turkey found approximately one case per year, with almost all patients having a history of cholesteatoma.[40] Another similar series of 36 patients from India reported that all patients had cholesteatoma at surgery, although one third had only granulation tissue on otoscopy.[41] A series of 20 patients with brain abscesses in an Italian center over a 16-year period, reported in the German literature, noted that 12 of them were of otogenic origin.[42]

Many patients with an otogenic brain abscess will have additional intracranial complications of otitis media, including meningitis and epidural abscess. The abscess usually forms by direct extension via osteitic bone. If there is a defect in the tegmen tympani, an abscess may form in the temporal lobe (Fig. 120-9); if there is a defect over the sigmoid sinus, an abscess may form in the cerebellum. The previously mentioned Indian series noted a larger prevalence of cerebellar abscess (17 versus 9), and the Turkish series reported 54% in the temporal lobe and 44% in the cerebellum. Patients will usually have a headache of several days' duration, along with foul-smelling otorrhea and often mental status changes. Temporal bone CT may miss a brain abscess, so imaging should also include brain CT with contrast enhancement.

SURGICAL TECHNIQUE

The abscess itself must be addressed on an emergency basis before rupture, which can lead to septicemia and death. Mastoidectomy is necessary to remove any precipitating cholesteatoma, and in some cases the abscess cavity itself may be drained through this approach. A multidisciplinary approach is coordinated with the neurosurgical service, and patients generally undergo craniotomy in conjunction with mastoidectomy. Sennaroglu and Sozeri[40] reported aspirating the abscess via mastoidectomy after preparing the dura with povidone-iodine, followed by irrigation and placement of drainage tubes, which are used for ongoing irrigation until

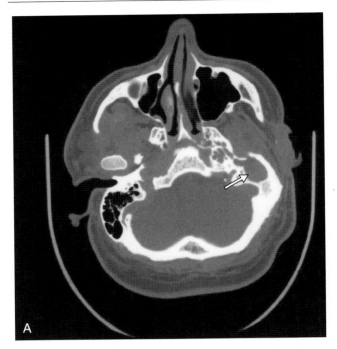

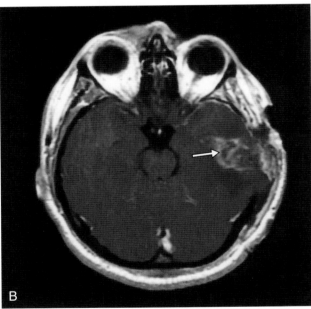

Figure 120-9. A, Computed tomography scan demonstrating a left-sided cholesteatoma *(arrow)* in a patient with canal atresia who had a brain abscess *(arrow)* as seen on magnetic resonance imaging (**B**).

the cavity shows collapse on follow-up CT. Antibiotics are adjusted to culture results of the aspirate. A similar approach was reported in a series of eight patients in rural India, where neurosurgical consultation was not available.[43] In a series of eight patients from Germany, two abscesses were drained by the neurotology team via a mastoid approach alone, and two other cases required a neurosurgical approach (all patients underwent mastoidectomy).[44] In the Italian series of 20 patients noted earlier, 17 underwent neurosurgical intervention.

OTITIC HYDROCEPHALUS

INDICATIONS AND PATIENT SELECTION

Otitic hydrocephalus is believed to occur as a result of lateral sinus thrombosis. It is a rare complication characterized by papilledema and ipsilateral abducens palsy in the majority of cases; the exact mechanism is not known and it can occur even if the contralateral lateral sinus is patent.[45] One series in India reported three cases of tubercular origin.[46] Previously it was believed that the pathophysiology must also involve the superior sagittal sinus, but this theory is debatable.[47]

Patients typically have signs of increased intracranial pressure, such as nausea, vomiting, and diplopia. Lumbar puncture may show opening pressures as high as 480 mm H_2O[48] with otherwise normal CSF findings and hence must be performed with great care (e.g., in the operating room with a compliant patient in the lateral decubitus position) if brain stem tonsillar herniation is a concern based on findings of papilledema. MRI and MR venography show transverse sinus thrombosis well.[49] Importantly, one series of five pediatric patients from Germany over a 4-year period found that all but one had already achieved resolution of acute otitis media with antibiotic treatment 1 to 4 weeks previously but were found to have diplopia.[50]

SURGICAL TECHNIQUE

In the recent German series,[50] all five patients improved only with surgical intervention; intravenous antibiotics alone were not sufficient treatment. Surgery included mastoidectomy, myringotomy, and in some cases a lumbar drain. If lateral sinus thrombosis is present, it may be aspirated by needle, with possible incision and drainage. Elevated intracranial pressure should be treated medically with mannitol, acetazolamide, or other diuretics.

PETROUS APICITIS/GRADENIGO'S SYNDROME

INDICATIONS AND PATIENT SELECTION

An aerated petrous apex may become infected as an extension of mastoiditis and otitis media and be disposed to associated intracranial complications, including epidural abscess, abducens palsy, and trigeminal irritation, among others. The classic triad described by Gradenigo in 1904 and 1907 included suppurative otitis media, abducens paralysis, and deep facial or retrobulbar pain secondary to trigeminal involvement, although only 42% (24 of 57) of the patients in his series had the complete triad (Fig. 120-10).[51] Petrositis can be associated with involvement of cranial nerves V and VI. As noted by Gradenigo, abducens palsy occurs in a minority of cases of petrous apicitis, but symptoms vary, and rarely this may be the only manifestation.[52] The syndrome may occur in conjunction with other

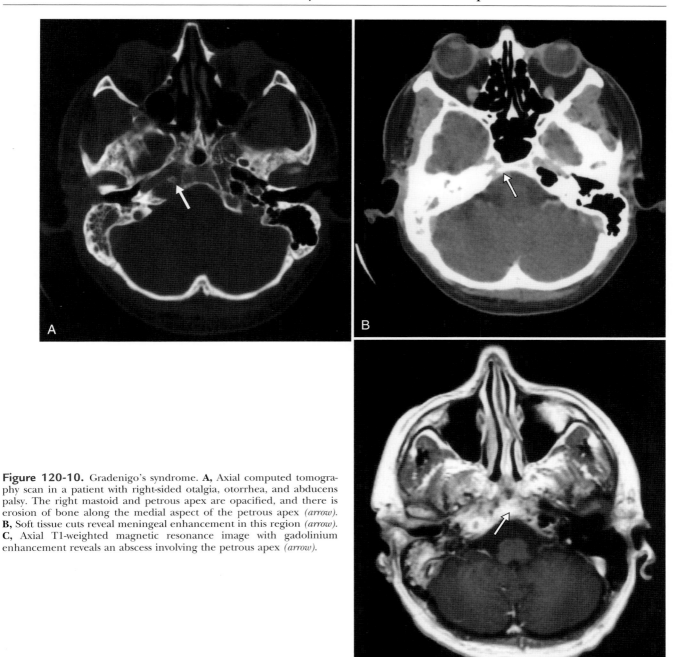

Figure 120-10. Gradenigo's syndrome. **A,** Axial computed tomography scan in a patient with right-sided otalgia, otorrhea, and abducens palsy. The right mastoid and petrous apex are opacified, and there is erosion of bone along the medial aspect of the petrous apex *(arrow).* **B,** Soft tissue cuts reveal meningeal enhancement in this region *(arrow).* **C,** Axial T1-weighted magnetic resonance image with gadolinium enhancement reveals an abscess involving the petrous apex *(arrow).*

intracranial complications, and hence possible additional pathologies such as meningitis and lateral sinus thrombophlebitis should be thoroughly evaluated concurrently.

Petrous apicitis can occur secondary to acute otitis media and as a complication of chronic ear disease. Pneumatized petrous apices generally communicate with mastoid air cells, thereby providing a route of spread for infection, and some authors report that even nonpneumatized or sclerotic petrous apices may become inflamed.[53] Anatomic studies have also demon-

strated venules forming conduits from the cavernous to the inferior petrosal sinus or jugular bulb.[54] Inflammation of the petrous apex can irritate the abducens, which travels under the petroclinoid ligament in Dorello's canal.[55] Similarly, the trigeminal (gasserian) ganglion or branches can become involved and result in pain throughout the affected distribution.

Both CT and MRI have important roles in diagnosing petrositis.[56] CT with contrast enhancement can show bony erosion, fluid-filled opacification, and possibly abscess formation, but the contralateral petrous apices cannot be assumed to be equivalently anatomically aerated for comparison. MRI can distinguish between marrow, CSF, and purulence.

SURGICAL TECHNIQUE

If a trial of intravenous antibiotics does not lead to the resolution of petrositis or if imaging shows areas of necrotic bone, surgical management is indicated. One recent case report detailed resolution of Gradenigo's syndrome without surgery in both a 6-year-old child in whom the condition developed after acute otitis media and a 70-year-old with a history of chronic ear disease.[57] Another report noted one case in three resolving with antibiotics, but the other two patients required surgery.[58]

The petrous apex has been described as the least surgically accessible portion of the temporal bone.[59] Mastoidectomy and tympanostomy tube placement may be sufficient to allow drainage of the petrous apex air cell tracts.[60] Surgical approaches to an inflamed petrous apex depend on the patient's hearing status and temporal bone anatomy and on the surgeon's training and include the infralabyrinthine, transcanal infracochlear, transsphenoidal, translabyrinthine or subtotal petrosectomy, and middle fossa approaches (discussed in Chapter 102).[61,62]

POSTOPERATIVE CARE/COMPLICATIONS

Complications of mastoidectomy and postoperative care are described in Chapter 115. Additional surveillance is necessary in a patient with intracranial complications, including monitoring for CSF otorrhea/rhinorrhea, cerebral edema, seizures, and pneumocephalus. Monitoring in an intensive care unit with imaging within 24 hours after surgical intervention is warranted. Prolonged bed rest and possible neurologic impairment leave patients predisposed to pulmonary emboli, and prophylaxis may be warranted. A multidisciplinary team that includes neurosurgery and infectious disease consultants is recommended. Long-term intravenous antibiotics may be indicated (with a peripherally inserted central catheter) for all intracranial complications of otitis media.

The otolaryngologist must be alert to the possible development of intracranial complications of otitis media and, when suspected, must remain aware that more than one such complication will often occur simultaneously. For any patient with otorrhea, temporal bone imaging should be considered. Early and effective treatment of acute otitis media with antibiotics has made the development of subsequent complications more subtle and less fulminant. Temporal bone imaging should be done on an urgent basis and should include brain imaging if otitis is accompanied by headache, fever, mental status changes, visual complaints, or other signs or symptoms that may indicate a disease process involving more than just the middle ear. Ambiguous or inconclusive findings on contrast-enhanced CT should be followed by MRI, and a low threshold for admission

and further workup should be maintained until the possibility of intracranial complications can be confidently excluded.

PEARLS

- Patients often have more than one intracranial complication.
- When evaluating for the possibility of intracranial complications of otitis media, MRI provides better detail of intracranial structures than CT.
- Hearing should be monitored closely after meningitis with consideration given to early cochlear implantation if hearing loss is accompanied by radiologic evidence of labyrinthitis ossificans.
- Some complications (i.e., empyema) may progress very rapidly, and emergency surgical intervention is warranted.

PITFALLS

- Classic signs of meningitis (Kernig's sign, Brudzinski's sign) are not very sensitive and may be absent in a patient with otitic meningitis.
- Temporal bone imaging may miss an intracranial abscess; suspicion should prompt dedicated brain CT or MRI with contrast enhancement.
- Intracranial complications may occur several weeks after treatment of an acute ear infection; thus, if there is a history of recent acute otitis media, the possibility of intracranial involvement should not be dismissed on the basis of a normal otoscopic examination.
- In patients with radiologic evidence of severely elevated intracranial pressure, lumbar puncture may result in cerebral herniation; particularly in patients with otitic hydrocephalus, this procedure should be performed with great care, preferably in the operating room.

References

1. Harker LA, Shelton C: Complications of temporal bone infections. In Cummings CW, Flint PW, Haughey BH, et al (eds): Cummings' Otolaryngology Head and Neck Surgery, 4th ed. St Louis, Elsevier Mosby, 2005, pp 3013-3039.
2. Migirov L, Eyal A, Kronenberg J: Intracranial complications following mastoidectomy. Pediatr Neurosurg 40:226-229, 2004.
3. Harris JP, Kim DW, Darrow DH: Complications of otitis media. In Nadol JB, McKenna MJ (eds): Surgery of the Ear and Temporal Bone, 2nd ed. Philadelphia, Lippincott Williams & Wilkins, 2005, pp 219-240.
4. Zanetti D, Nassif N: Indications for surgery in acute mastoiditis and their complications in children. Int J Pediatr Otorhinolaryngol 70:1175-1182, 2006.
5. Migirov L, Duvdevani S, Kronenberg J: Otogenic intracranial complications: A review of 28 cases. Acta Otolaryngol 125:819-822, 2005.

6. Leskinen K, Jero J: Complications of acute otitis media in children in southern Finland. Int J Pediatr Otorhinolaryngol 68:317-324, 2004.

7. Luntz M, Brodskky A, Nusem J, et al: Acute mastoiditis—the antibiotic era: A multicenter study. Int J Pediatr Otorhinolaryngol 57:1-9, 2001.

8. Go C, Bernstein JM, de Jong AL, et al: Intracranial complications of acute mastoiditis. Int J Pediatr Otorhinolaryngol 52:143-148, 2000.

9. Kaftan H, Draf W: Otogene endokranielle Komplikationen—trotz aller Fortschritte weiterhin ein ernst zu nehmendes Problem. Laryngorhinootologie 79:609-615, 2000.

10. Schwager K, Carducci F: Endokranielle Komplikationen der akuten und chronischen Otitis media bei Kindern und Jugenlichen. Laryngorhinootologie 76:335-340, 1997.

11. Leskinen K, Jero J: Acute complications of otitis media in adults. Clin Otolaryngol 30:511-516, 2005.

12. Barry B, Delattre J, Vie F, et al: Otogenic intracranial infections in adults. Laryngoscope 109:483-487, 1999.

13. Seven H, Coskun BU, Calis AB, et al: Intracranial abscesses associated with chronic suppurative otitis media. Eur Arch Otorhinolaryngol 262:847-851, 2005.

14. Penido NDO, Borin A, Iha LCN, et al: Intracranial complications of otitis media: 15 years of experience in 33 patients. Otolaryngol Head Neck Surg 132:37-42, 2005.

15. Matanda RN, Muyunga KC, Sabue MJ, et al: Chronic suppurative otitis media and related complications at the University Clinic of Kinshasa. B-ENT 2:57-62, 2005.

16. Goldstein NA, Casselbrant ML, Bluestone CD, Kurs-Lasky M: Intratemporal complications of acute otitis media in infants and children. Otolaryngol Head Neck Surg 119:444-454, 1998.

17. Osma U, Cureoglu S, Hosoglu S: The complications of chronic otitis media: Report of 93 cases. J Laryngol Otol 114:97-100, 2000.

18. Thomas KE, Hasbun R, Jekel J, et al: The diagnostic accuracy of Kernig's sign, Brudzinski's sign, and nuchal rigidity in adults with suspected meningitis. Clin Infect Dis 35:46-52, 2002.

19. Tunkel AR: Approach to the patient with central nervous system infection. In Mandell GL, Bennett JE, and Dolin R (eds): Mandell's Principles and Practice of Infectious Diseases, 6th ed. Philadelphia, Churchill Livingstone, 2005.

20. Tunkel AR, Hartman BJ, Kaplan SL, et al: Practice guidelines for the management of bacterial meningitis. Clin Infect Dis 39:1267-1284, 2004.

21. Falcone S, Post MJ: Encephalitis, cerebritis, and brain abscess: Pathophysiology and imaging findings. Neuroimaging Clin N Am 10:333-353, 2000.

22. Nathoo N, Nadvi SS, van Dellen JR: Cranial extradural empyema in the era of computed tomography: A review of 82 cases. Neurosurgery 44:748-753, 1999.

23. Dobben GD, Raofi B, Mafee MF, et al: Otogenic intracranial inflammations: Role of magnetic resonance imaging. Top Magn Reson Imaging 11:76-86, 2000.

24. Bizakis JG, Velegrakis A, Papadakis CE, et al: The silent epidural abscess as a complication of acute otitis media in children. Int J Pediatr Otorhinolaryngol 45:163-166, 1998.

25. Syms MJ, Tsai PD, Holtel MR: Management of lateral sinus thrombosis. Laryngoscope 109:1616-1620, 1999.

26. Wasay M, Azeemudin M: Neuroimaging of cerebral venous thrombosis. J Neuroimaging 15:118-128, 2005.

27. Kaplan DM, Kraus M, Puterman M, et al: Otogenic lateral sinus thrombosis in children. Int J Pediatr Otorhinolaryngol 49:177-183, 1999.

28. Manolidis S, Kutz JW Jr: Diagnosis and management of lateral sinus thrombosis. Otol Neurotol 26:1045-1051, 2005.

29. Seven H, Ozbal AE, Turgut S: Management of otogenic lateral sinus thrombosis. Am J Otolaryngol 25:329-333, 2004.

30. Neely JG: Facial nerve and intracranial complications of otitis media. In Jackler RK, Brackmann DE (eds): Neurotology, 2nd ed. Mosby, Philadelphia, 2005.

31. Bradley DT, Hashisaki GT, Mason JC: Otogenic sigmoid sinus thrombosis: What is the role of anticoagulation? Laryngoscope 112:1726-1729, 2002.

32. Wong I, Kozak FK, Poskitt K, et al: Pediatric lateral sinus thrombosis: Retrospective case series and literature review. J Otolaryngol 34:79-85, 2005.

33. Agarwal A, Lowry P, Isaacson G: Natural history of sigmoid sinus thrombosis. Ann Otol Rhinol Laryngol 112:191-194, 2003.

34. Hlavin ML, Kaminski HF, Fenstermaker RA, White RJ: Intracranial suppuration: A modern decade of postoperative subdural empyema and epidural abscess. Neurosurgery 34:974-980, 1994.

35. Dill SR, Cobbs CG, McDonald CK: Subdural empyema: Analysis of 32 cases and review. Clin Infect Dis 20:372-386, 1995.

36. Nathoo N, Nadvi SS, van Dellen JR, Gouws E: Intracranial subdural empyemas in the era of computed tomography: A review of 699 cases. Neurosurgery 44:529-535, 1999.

37. Greenlee JE: Subdural empyema. Curr Treat Options Neurol 5:13-22, 2003.

38. Wong AM, Zimmerman RA, Simon EM, et al: Diffusion-weighted MR imaging of subdural empyemas in children. AJNR Am J Neuroradiol 25:1016-1021, 2004.

39. Mai R, Rutka J: The irony of being Oscar: The legendary life and death of Oscar Wilde. J Otolaryngol 29:239-243, 2000.

40. Sennaroglu L, Sozeri B: Otogenic brain abscess: Review of 41 cases. Otolaryngol Head Neck Surg 123:751-755, 2000.

41. Kurien M, Job A, Mathew J, Chandy M: Otogenic intracranial abscess: Concurrent craniotomy and mastoidectomy—changing trends in a developing country. Arch Otolaryngol Head Neck Surg 124:1353-1356, 1998.

42. Marchiori C, Tonon E, Boscolo P, et al: [Brain abscesses after extracranial infections of the head and neck area.] HNO 51:813-822, 2003.

43. Hippargekar PM, Shinde AD: Trans-mastoid needle aspiration for otogenic brain abscesses. J Laryngol Otol 117:422-423, 2003.

44. Kempf HG, Wiel J, Issing PR, Lenarz T: [Otogenic brain abscess.] Laryngorhinootologie 77:462-466, 1998.

45. Kuczkowski J, Dubaniewicz-Wybieralska M, Przewozny T, Narozny W: Otitic hydrocephalus associated with lateral sinus thrombosis and acute mastoiditis in children. Int J Pediatr Otorhinolaryngol 70:1817-1823, 2006.

46. Grewal DS, Hathiram BT, Agarwal R, et al: Otitic hydrocephalus of tubercular origin: A rare cause. J Laryngol Otol 114:874-877, 2000.

47. Tomkinson A, Mills RGS, Cantrell PJ: The pathophysiology of otitic hydrocephalus. J Laryngol Otol 111:757-759, 1997.

48. Bari L, Choksi R, Roach ES: Otitic hydrocephalus revisited. Arch Neurol 62:824-825, 2005.

49. Unal FO, Sennaroglu L, Saatci I: Otitic hydrocephalus: Role of radiology for diagnosis. Int J Pediatr Otorhinolaryngol 69:897-901, 2005.

50. Koitschev A, Simon C, Lowenheim H, et al: Delayed otogenic hydrocephalus after acute otitis media in pediatric patients: The changing presentation of a serious otologic complication. Acta Otolaryngol 125:1230-1235, 2005.

51. Chole RA, Donald PJ: Petrous apicitis: Clinical considerations. Ann Otol Rhinol Laryngol 92:544-551, 1983.

52. Price T, Fayad G: Abducens nerve palsy as the sole presenting symptom of petrous apicitis. J Laryngol Otol 116:726-729, 2002.

53. Neely JG, Arts HA: Intratemporal and intracranial complications of otitis media. In Bailey BJ, Johnson JT (eds): Bailey's Otolaryngology Head and Neck Surgery, 4th ed. Lippincott Williams & Wilkins, Philadelphia, 2006, pp 2041-2056.

54. Gadre AK, Brodie HA, Fayad JN, O'Leary MJ: Venous channels of the petrous apex: Their presence and clinical importance. Otolaryngol Head Neck Surg 116:168-174, 1997.

55. Chole RA, Sudhoff HH: Chronic otitis media, mastoiditis, and petrositis. In Cummings' Otolaryngology Head and Neck Surgery, 4th ed. St Louis, Elsevier Mosby, 2005, pp 2988-3012.

56. Singh ML, Rejee R, Varghese AM: Gradenigo's syndrome: Findings on computed tomography and magnetic resonance imaging. J Postgrad Med 48:314-316, 2002.

57. Burston BJ, Pretorius PM, Ramsden JD: Gradenigo's syndrome: Successful conservative treatment in adult and paediatric patients. J Laryngol Otol 119:325-329, 2005.

57. Minotti AM, Kountakis SE: Management of abducens palsy in patients with petrositis. Ann Otol Rhinol Laryngol 108:897-902, 1999.

59. Chole RA: Petrous apicitis: Surgical anatomy. Ann Otol Rhinol Laryngol 94:251-257, 1985.

60. Goldstein NA, Casselbrant ML, Bluestone CD, Kurs-Lasky M: Intratemporal complications of acute otitis media in infants and children. Otolaryngol Head Neck Surg 119:444-454, 1998.

61. Brackmann DE, Giddings NA: Drainage procedures for petrous apex lesions, In Brackmann DE, Shelton C, Arriaga MA (eds): Otologic Surgery, 2nd ed. Saunders, Philadelphia, 2001, pp 466-477.

62. Brackmann DE, Toh EH: Surgical management of petrous apex cholesterol granulomas. Otol Neurotol 23:529-533, 2002.

Facial Nerve

Chapter 121

Tumors of the Facial Nerve

Barry E. Hirsch and Michele St. Martin

Primary tumors of the facial nerve are relatively rare. Bell's palsy is the most common disorder that primarily affects the facial nerve. Facial paralysis frequently results from other pathologic processes affecting the posterior fossa, temporal bone, parotid gland, and infratemporal fossa. Secondary involvement of the facial nerve can occur as a result of trauma or erosive tumor such as cholesteatoma, primary squamous cell carcinoma, glomus tumors, acoustic neuroma, meningioma, malignant neoplasms of the parotid gland, and tumors metastatic to the temporal bone.

The most common primary tumors of the facial nerve are neuromas and hemangiomas. Other less common primary tumors of the facial nerve include neurofibroma, granular cell tumor, meningioma, and primary glomus tumors. Malignant epithelioid cranial nerve sheath tumor involving the facial and trigeminal nerves has also been described,[1] but most malignant tumors of the facial nerve are the result of metastasis or perineural invasion. Cancer of the parotid gland, such as adenoid cystic carcinoma and mucoepidermoid carcinoma, is known to invade the facial nerve at the skull base.[2] Breast, lung, and renal cancers can also metastasize to the facial nerve, most often in the internal auditory canal (IAC).[3] Although primary tumors of the facial nerve are relatively rare, the admonition of Sir Terence Cawthorne, "All that palsies is not Bell's," must be considered when slowly progressive facial paresis develops.[4]

This chapter focuses on facial nerve neuroma and hemangioma.

The nomenclature for neurogenic tumors of the facial nerve includes the terms *neurinoma*, *schwannoma*, and *neurilemmoma*, although *neuroma* is used in this chapter to describe this tumor. Neuromas arise from Schwann cells, the myelin-producing cells peripheral to the axon, and are usually located eccentrically and compressing the nerve. The histopathology may follow one of two patterns. The first is that of a dense array of cells in a regular pattern (Antoni A), and the second demonstrates areas of loose stroma and vacuolation (Antoni B) (Fig. 121-1). Often there is a mixture of both patterns, although neither suggests any prognostic implications. This is in contrast to neurofibromas, which arise from endoneurial connective tissue. These tumors are more typically associated with neurofibromatosis 1, or von Recklinghausen's disease.

Neuroma of the facial nerve is considered to be a slowly growing tumor. It appears grossly as a diffuse bulge of the facial nerve but characteristically involves multiple segments along its course. A neuroma may arise anywhere along the course of the facial nerve from the root entry zone in the cerebellopontine angle (CPA) to the extratemporal trunk of the nerve within the parotid gland. Figure 121-2 combines the results of two publications reviewing 287 cases of facial nerve neuroma.[5,6] The tympanic segment is most commonly

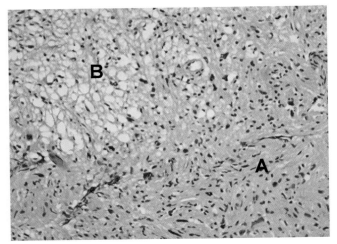

Figure 121-1. Histopathologic patterns of cellular distribution in facial neuroma. A, Antoni A (cellular, more organized); B, Antoni B (loose stroma, fewer cells, myxoid change).

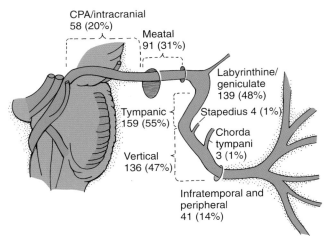

Figure 121-2. Segmental distribution and frequency of facial neuromas in 287 cases. These tumors characteristically involve multiple nerve segments. CPA, cerebellopontine angle.

involved, followed by the geniculate/labyrinthine and vertical segments.

It is reported that up to 50% of patients with primary neuroma do not present with signs or symptoms of facial nerve dysfunction.[7] The structures of the IAC, otic capsule, and middle ear are subject to encroachment and erosion by an expanding tumor of the facial nerve. Common initial symptoms, other than facial nerve paresis, include hearing loss, tinnitus, and vertigo or dysequilibrium.

The existence of neuroma of the facial nerve isolated to the porus of the IAC and CPA has been questioned. Published reports of such tumors have provided insight into radiologic findings that preoperatively may differentiate an acoustic neuroma from a facial nerve

neuroma. Acoustic neuromas are usually centered on the IAC. Demonstrating the bulk of tumor to be eccentric to the axis of the IAC raises suspicion of facial nerve neuroma.[7] Facial nerve neuroma limited to the IAC or fallopian canal may not demonstrate bony expansion on computed tomography (CT). Contrast-enhanced magnetic resonance imaging (MRI) is more sensitive in revealing tumors of the facial nerve isolated to the IAC.

Hemangioma is considered to be a vascular hamartoma composed of blood vessels. The blood supply to the facial nerve originates from three separate sources, thus creating a vascular arcade. The intracranial and intrameatal segments of the facial nerve are vascularized by the internal auditory artery, which originates from the anterior inferior cerebellar artery. The geniculate ganglion area is supplied by the petrosal artery, which follows the course of the greater superficial petrosal nerve. The petrosal artery is a branch of the middle meningeal artery. The third blood supply to the vertical and horizontal facial nerve segments is from the stylomastoid artery. This source has its origin from the posterior auricular or occipital arteries. These vessels create a prominent watershed vascular plexus over the geniculate ganglion area.

Depending on the size of the vessel involved, hemangiomas of the facial nerve are categorized as *capillary* or *cavernous* hemangioma. Similar to neuromas, this histologic subclassification does not have prognostic implications. Hemangiomas of the facial nerve predominantly occur at the geniculate ganglion and the IAC. They rarely originate more distally along the horizontal or vertical segments of the facial nerve. Hemangiomas usually arise eccentrically from the nerve and initiate remodeling of the surrounding trabeculated bone, on which they create spicules and centers of ossification. Because of their extrinsic origin, it was believed that hemangiomas could be dissected from the underlying nerve more easily than is the case with schwannomas. However, recent publications suggest that hemangiomas of the geniculate ganglion often infiltrate the facial nerve, thus requiring sacrifice of the nerve with cable graft repair for complete resection.[8]

The initial symptoms of hemangioma of the facial nerve are dependent on the location. In contrast to neuroma, hemangiomas of the facial nerve typically manifest signs of facial nerve paresis or paralysis unless they are isolated to the IAC. In this location, they frequently cause progressive sensorineural hearing loss with reduced word discrimination, similar to an acoustic neuroma. In contrast, hemangiomas of the geniculate ganglion predominantly produce slowly progressive facial paralysis occurring over a period of months to years. Facial nerve hemangioma is also an uncommon cause of atypical hemifacial spasm.[9,10] The degree of facial paresis seen with hemangioma is considered to be more severe than that occurring with a neuroma of the same size. The gross appearance of hemangioma of the facial nerve is similar to that of a red sponge. Small tumors may cause severe symptoms and, until recently, defied easy detection.

Radiographic imaging plays an important role in the differential diagnosis of these tumors. Similar to facial neuroma, identification of hemangioma of the facial nerve requires high-resolution bone-windowed CT and MRI focused along the course of the facial nerve. Recent reports suggest that gadolinium-enhanced MRI has greater sensitivity than CT in detecting and differentiating hemangiomas from other tumors of the geniculate ganglion area.[11] The CT findings may demonstrate irregular, indistinct bone margins containing bone spicules within the tumor. This honeycomb appearance has been termed *ossifying hemangioma*.[12] It must be emphasized that the patient's history and diagnostic imaging studies provide the critical information necessary to make a presumptive diagnosis of primary neoplasm of the facial nerve.

PATIENT SELECTION

Complete examination of the head and neck is necessary. Examination of the face must include all branches of the facial nerve, with attention directed to gross and fine motor function. Evidence of synkinesis, mass motion, and fasciculations is sought. These signs may be further elicited by asking the patient to squeeze the eyelids closed and perform a sustained exaggerated smile or grimace. These maneuvers evoke latent fasciculations or demonstrate subsequent weakness. Based on the degree of paresis and synkinesis, the level of facial function is defined by the House-Brackmann grading system (Table 121-1).[13] This system was devised to describe recovery of facial function after surgery, inflammation, or trauma. It has been adapted to describe

abnormalities ranging from mild weakness to complete paralysis at initial examination.

The parotid gland and neck are palpated for evidence of tumor or adenopathy, respectively. The fifth cranial nerve is tested for evidence of motor or sensory abnormalities. Findings on otoscopy are usually normal, although a mass in the middle ear aural polyp may be evident. The results of tuning fork testing would be reversed (bone greater than air or a negative Rinne test) when ossicular chain movement is impeded by the tumor. Significant asymmetrical sensorineural hearing loss may also be identified with tuning fork testing.

Radiologic imaging is critical in establishing a presumptive diagnosis. Both high-resolution CT and MRI can demonstrate a primary tumor of the facial nerve. Thorough and precise radiologic imaging is mandatory for tracing the entire course of the facial nerve from the brain stem to the parotid gland. CT is better able to show bone expansion or changes such as those seen with ossifying hemangioma. This honeycomb appearance with evidence of bone remodeling and ossification is highly suggestive of hemangioma (Fig. 121-3). In addition, the structures of the otic capsule and middle ear are more readily identified on CT, and their degree of involvement can be defined (Fig. 121-4). Radiologic diagnosis of facial nerve neuromas can be based on the location of nerve enlargement, surrounding bone changes, or evidence of enhancement. MRI is more sensitive for demonstrating such enhancement. Tumor expansion of the geniculate ganglion area will be evident on both MRI and CT, but diffuse facial nerve involvement is readily apparent on gadolinium-enhanced MRI (Fig. 121-5).

Intracranial or intrameatal (IAC) neuromas of the facial nerve are more frequently diagnosed as

Table 121-1	HOUSE-BRACKMANN FACIAL NERVE GRADING SYSTEM	
Grade	**Description**	**Characteristics**
I	Normal	Normal facial function in all areas
II	Mild dysfunction	*Gross:* Slight weakness noticeable on close inspection; may have very slight synkinesis *At rest:* Normal symmetry and tone *Motion:* Forehead—moderate to good function; eye—complete closure with minimal effort; mouth—slight asymmetry
III	Moderate dysfunction	*Gross:* Obvious but not disfiguring difference between the two sides; noticeable but not severe synkinesis, contracture, or hemifacial spasm *At rest:* Normal symmetry and tone *Motion:* Forehead—slight to moderate movement; eye—complete closure with effort; mouth—slightly weak with maximal effort
IV	Moderately severe dysfunction	*Gross:* Obvious weakness and/or disfiguring asymmetry *At rest:* Normal symmetry and tone *Motion:* Forehead—none; eye—incomplete closure; mouth—asymmetrical with maximal effort
V	Severe dysfunction	*Gross:* Only barely perceptible motion *At rest:* Asymmetry *Motion:* Forehead—none; eye—incomplete closure; mouth—slight movement
VI	Total paralysis	No movement

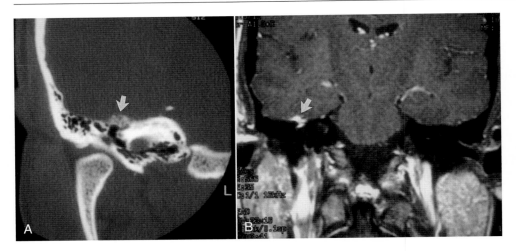

Figure 121-3. The patient is a 32-year-old woman with facial weakness and synkinesis. **A,** Bone-windowed computed tomography scan demonstrating a tumor of the geniculate ganglion with honeycomb trabeculation *(arrow).* B, T1-weighted contrast-enhanced magnetic resonance image showing enhancement of the geniculate ganglion region *(arrow).*

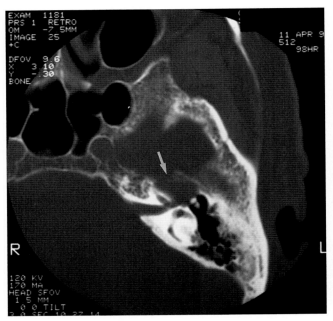

Figure 121-4. Bone-windowed computed tomography scan showing a facial nerve neuroma eroding the cochlea and impinging on the head of the malleus *(arrow).*

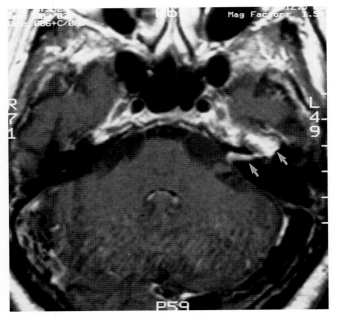

Figure 121-5. T1-weighted enhanced magnetic resonance image (same patient as in Fig. 121-4) demonstrating facial nerve neuroma of the geniculate ganglion and diffuse involvement of the facial nerve from the porus to the geniculate ganglion *(arrows).*

acoustic neuroma. However, lateral extension into the labyrinthine segment and geniculate ganglion areas should alert the radiologist and otolaryngologist to the likelihood of a primary tumor of the facial nerve. Certainly, enlargement of the tympanic (horizontal) and mastoid (vertical) segments of the facial nerve is suggestive of neuroma of the facial nerve. Secondary involvement from a primary tumor of the parotid gland or metastatic cancer must be ruled out. Primary neuroma of the facial nerve in the extratemporal (parotid) portion of the facial nerve has been reported.[14]

Options for management include surgical resection, decompression, stereotactic radiosurgery, or observation. Removal of the bony compartment encasing the facial nerve (fallopian canal) permits tumor expansion with less entrapment, thereby allowing facial weakness to progress more slowly over time. The detriment in waiting for complete paralysis to develop is that ongoing, irreversible degenerative changes are occurring in both the proximal and distal portions of the nerve along with atrophy of the denervated facial muscles. Optimal results with facial reanimation procedures occur when paresis/paralysis is of shorter duration. The longer the duration of paralysis, the worse the outcome. To formulate a treatment plan, one attempts to predict the natural history and progression of an untreated tumor whose presumptive histopathologic diagnosis is based on the interpretation of radiologic imaging.

The status of the patient's hearing must also be considered. It must be anticipated that a patient will probably lose residual hearing if the tumor erodes into the otic capsule or is causing retrocochlear hearing loss. In patients with poor contralateral hearing, removal of an ipsilateral tumor of the facial nerve should not be recommended if injury to the cochlear nerve or otic capsule is likely. In this situation, surgical decompression, stereotactic radiosurgery (SRS), or watchful waiting is suggested unless the tumor has imminent potential to create other significant neurologic sequelae. Similarly, if tumor growth results in severe ipsilateral sensorineural hearing loss, resection is undertaken and amplification or cochlear implantation is performed on the contralateral side.

The physician may be faced with various options that require careful deliberation regarding the optimal management of facial nerve tumors. The most straightforward situation occurs in a patient with symptoms of slowly progressive facial paralysis and evidence of synkinesis, hemifacial spasm, or a tic developing over a period of a few weeks to months. Similarly, a patient with complete facial paralysis in whom Bell's palsy is diagnosed and who fails to demonstrate any return of motor function within 6 months should be presumed to have a tumor.

Recurrent episodes of Bell's palsy should also arouse suspicion of a tumor of the facial nerve, especially when complete return of function does not occur and each episode results in subsequent worsening or permanent dysfunction. Patients often experience twitching, tics, or fasciculations with concomitant synkinesis and mass movement and may complain of eye symptoms because of an inability to blink or close the eye. The patient's facial nerve function grade is recorded.

The ideal surgical candidate is a patient who has slowly progressive facial paresis with House-Brackmann grade III or worse and normal hearing on the contralateral side. Assuming that the patient has no medical conditions posing unacceptable surgical risks or contraindications to a potentially lengthy general anesthetic, the patient is a candidate for surgical removal of the tumor. The radiographic size, location, and involvement of nearby structures will dictate the most advantageous surgical approach.

One of the more difficult decisions to be made is recommending treatment of a presumed tumor of the facial nerve when a patient has normal facial function or is presenting with subtle facial paresis, synkinesis, or fasciculations. This situation arises when a patient is scanned for other symptoms, such as sensorineural hearing loss, unrelenting pain, pulsatile tinnitus, or atypical vestibular complaints. If a tumor of the facial nerve is presumptively diagnosed because of its location and enhancement characteristics, a comprehensive discussion of treatment options, risks, and benefits should take place with the patient and family. When the tumor is small, there is a greater likelihood of complete removal with anatomic preservation of the facial nerve. This affords the patient the greatest chance of normal or nearly normal facial function. A small hemangioma located in the area of the labyrinthine segment, geniculate ganglion, or horizontal segment can frequently be removed with preservation of the underlying facial nerve. However, both the patient and the surgeon must be prepared for the possibility that the tumor has infiltrated the facial nerve and requires resection and nerve grafting. This would obviously result in complete paralysis, which is a marked change requiring psychological adjustment in view of the fact that minimal dysfunction was present preoperatively. Larger hemangiomas filling the IAC are more likely to require facial nerve sacrifice and repair.

Thus, patients with normal facial function and a presumed tumor of the facial nerve must decide whether they wish to proceed with surgical removal or wait until facial paresis/paralysis develops. It must be emphasized to such patients that the longer facial paralysis has been present, the poorer the outcome after primary nerve repair. The timing for intervention is influenced by the surgeon's technical skills and experience in managing tumors in this site. Special mention should be made of the rare cystic facial neuroma. Rapid growth of the cyst can make facial weakness worse or accentuate other symptoms. A recent publication advocates drainage and marsupialization of the cyst through a retrosigmoid approach to manage this subset of patients.[15]

The surgeon may incidentally discover a primary tumor of the facial nerve when surgery is being carried out for other indications. Otologic procedures during which the horizontal or vertical segments of the facial nerve may be visualized include exploratory tympanotomy, tympanomastoidectomy, and cochlear implantation. In this situation, the planned procedure should be completed if the anatomy permits. Rather than removing the tumor in a patient with normal preoperative facial function, the findings and subsequent evaluation should be discussed once the patient is fully awake. Although there are rare exceptions to this principle, the patient and family should understand the nature of the pathology and participate in the subsequent course of management given the potential for facial nerve paralysis.

Medium to large primary tumors of the facial nerve are frequently accompanied by facial weakness. Occasionally, in a patient with normal facial function preoperatively, a tumor of the facial nerve is identified intraoperatively during surgery for a posterior fossa tumor. In particular, during surgery for an enhancing IAC and CPA tumor presumed to be an acoustic neuroma, it may be discovered that the tumor is indeed a neuroma or, less likely, a hemangioma of the facial nerve. It is usually well into the tumor removal stage that the origin of the tissue is clearly identified. Decompression may buy additional time for paralysis to occur, but once the tumor is partially resected, facial paresis will probably result. Because facial paralysis is a known risk and complication of acoustic neuroma surgery, the surgeon should proceed with tumor removal. In this situation, the patient is informed after tumor resection and reconstruction have been completed. However, if it can be demonstrated early in the procedure that a small tumor originates from the facial nerve, decompression of the surrounding bone provides additional time for less restricted tumor growth. Retrospective review of the radiologic images may demonstrate findings that in the future would raise suspicion of a primary facial nerve tumor.

Dissatisfaction with the possibility of worsening facial weakness after microsurgical resection has led to a search for treatment alternatives for facial nerve neuroma. Recent reports in the literature have discussed the use of SRS for nonacoustic schwannomas, including facial nerve neuroma. SRS has been well established as a treatment modality for acoustic neuroma that affords excellent tumor control with a low rate of new cranial nerve deficits. Several publications have discussed the use of both gamma knife– and linear accelerator–based radiosurgery to treat nonacoustic neuromas. Pollock and colleagues reported on the treatment of 11 patients with either trigeminal or jugular foramen schwannomas.[16] Tumor growth was controlled in 100% of patients with trigeminal schwannomas and 75% of patients with jugular foramen schwannomas at mean follow-ups of 21 and 10 months, respectively. None of the patients experienced worsening of cranial nerve deficits after treatment. Mabanta and associates published a series of 18 patients with nonacoustic schwannomas who were treated with linear accelerator SRS.[17] Two of the 18 patients had a facial neuroma; the remaining patients had a trigeminal or jugular foramen tumor. The authors reported a 100% control rate. Three patients suffered complications, including progression of preexisting facial weakness, new hearing loss, and ataxia. However, five patients experienced improvement in neurologic symptoms. A French series of nine patients with facial neuroma treated with gamma knife radiosurgery was published in 2004.[18] Follow-up ranged from 2 to 7 years, during which time no patient experienced worsening of facial function. Additionally, two case reports from the Japanese literature discuss the use of SRS for facial neuroma.[19,20]

PREOPERATIVE PLANNING

Complete examination of the head and neck with attention directed to facial nerve function is performed. The House-Brackmann grading system is used to record the degree of facial nerve weakness or paralysis. The patient is instructed to attempt complete and forceful eye closure. If the patient demonstrates a poor Bell phenomenon and is unable to adequately protect the cornea, the benefit of insertion of a gold weight should be addressed. Various gold weights are temporarily taped to the upper eyelid to determine whether improved eye closure and comfort are achieved. If ectropion is present, a lower lid–tightening procedure should be planned. The ear is inspected with an operating microscope. The status of the external auditory canal, tympanic membrane, and middle ear is noted.

Audiometric analysis will determine the hearing status of both ears. Identification of ipsilateral conductive hearing loss suggests that ossicular chain involvement may require disarticulation and reconstruction and that the middle ear will require exploration. If poor hearing is identified in the contralateral ear and it is anticipated that hearing will be compromised on the side with the tumor, careful deliberation must be given to the options of tumor management. In this situation, observation, radiation therapy, or surgical decompression to provide more room for tumor growth are all reasonable management alternatives.

Stapes reflex testing may be helpful in determining the site of the lesion. An intact stapes reflex in the presence of facial paralysis would indicate facial nerve involvement in the distal vertical segment or its extratemporal course. Vestibular testing does not provide enough information to alter the treatment strategy.

Preoperative electrophysiologic facial nerve tests are occasionally helpful. When facial paresis is present, electroneuronography (ENoG) demonstrates decreased responses. The ENoG data obtained from patients with normal facial function or minimal paresis may occasionally be of benefit. Elicitation of 50% or greater reduction in the ENoG amplitude provides additional support demonstrating compromised neural integrity. Patients with normal facial function and surgeons may be more willing to entertain surgical excision when objective verification of facial nerve involvement is established. However, ENoG is rarely useful when complete facial paralysis has been present for more than a few weeks. In the setting of facial paresis or paralysis, facial electromyography of the peripheral facial muscles may provide evidence of fibrillation (denervation) and polyphasic voluntary motor unit (reinnervation) potentials. This provides confirmatory evidence that an ongoing destructive and reparative process is occurring.

Preoperative diagnosis of a presumed tumor of the facial nerve depends on radiologic imaging. The surgeon must carefully review the scans to ensure that complete data have been compiled. Both contrast-enhanced CT and MRI are often needed to determine the extent and size of the lesion, whether the otic capsule is eroded, and which segments of the facial nerve are affected. Facial nerve neuromas are prone to multiple areas of involvement. Imaging will identify whether the labyrinthine segment of the nerve enhances or is widened, whether the greater superficial petrosal nerve is involved, and whether middle ear growth has affected the ossicular chain. The MRI or CT scanning protocol should extend beneath the skull base to trace the course of the facial nerve through the parotid. This information is needed to determine which operative approach is most appropriate, who should be part of the surgical team, what surgical and ancillary equipment is necessary (such as facial nerve monitoring), and whether other autologous tissue is needed for nerve repair and wound closure. These latter areas include the neck for a greater auricular nerve graft, the lateral lower part of the leg for a sural nerve graft, or the abdomen for a free fat graft.

The appropriate surgical approach is dictated by the size and location of the tumor and the type and degree of hearing loss. Although unusual and difficult to diagnose, presumed tumors of the facial nerve isolated to the CPA are removed through a retrosigmoid craniotomy. The more common location for these tumors is between the lateral IAC and the vertical segment of the facial nerve. A middle fossa approach is necessary for tumors of the facial nerve in the IAC, labyrinthine segment, and geniculate ganglion areas if hearing is to be preserved. Tumors confined to the horizontal or vertical fallopian canal are managed by a transmastoid approach. A combined middle fossa–transmastoid approach is necessary for larger tumors centered around the geniculate ganglion because access to the proximal and distal nerve stumps for repair will be needed. When hearing in the ipsilateral ear is compromised (speech reception threshold >50 dB, discrimination <50%), a translabyrinthine or transcochlear approach permits direct access to the tumor and facilitates primary repair of the facial nerve.

Hemangiomas of the facial nerve are, by definition, vascular tumors. However, they rarely achieve sufficient size to warrant arteriography and embolization. Nevertheless, blood typing and screening are performed when an intracranial procedure is planned.

A comprehensive discussion of the natural course of the tumor and the risks and benefits of surgical resection must take place with the patient and significant family members. The patient should understand that temporary or permanent facial paralysis will probably occur and that subsequent care will be dictated by the intraoperative management of the tumor. Unilateral complete hearing loss may result despite undertaking a hearing preservation approach.

SURGICAL TECHNIQUES

All procedures are performed with the patient under general endotracheal anesthesia with inhalational and intravenous narcotic agents. In patients with preoperative facial function, muscle relaxants are avoided to permit facial nerve monitoring. The patient is placed in the supine position with the head turned toward the contralateral ear when undergoing transmastoid, translabyrinthine, middle fossa, or a combined procedure. The more medial access needed for the retrosigmoid approach often requires placement of support rolls beneath the patient's shoulder and hip to rotate the patient into a semidecubitus position. A Mayfield head holder and pins are secured to the patient and the table when a retrosigmoid approach is used (Fig. 121-6A and B). The upper part of the neck is included in the operative field to provide access to the greater auricular nerve. The ipsilateral leg is also prepared and draped if the tumor is known to be extensive and could require a longer nerve graft. The left lower quadrant of the abdomen is prepared for a fat graft when a translabyrinthine or middle fossa approach is planned. Perioperative antibiotics are given when opening the dura is anticipated.

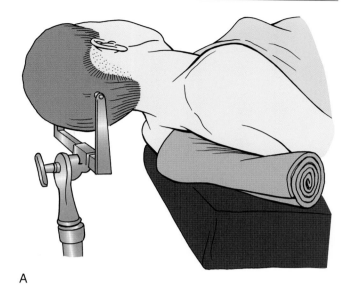

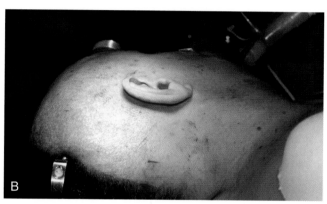

Figure 121-6. A, Positioning of a patient for a retrosigmoid approach to the posterior fossa. **B,** Photograph of a patient in a three-pin Mayfield head holder.

Transmastoid Approach

A curvilinear incision is made 1 cm posterior to the postauricular sulcus through the skin, subcutaneous tissue, and fibroperiosteal layer over the mastoid cortex. The periosteum is elevated posteriorly and anteriorly until the level of the bony external auditory canal is encountered. Self-retaining retractors are placed, and a transcortical mastoidectomy is performed. The antrum and horizontal semicircular canal serve as important initial surgical landmarks for this approach. The sinodural angle is delineated. Bone over the sigmoid sinus and posterior bony canal wall is thinned to provide the necessary exposure to the vertical portion of the facial nerve.

The short process of the incus is identified. It serves as a helpful landmark for the facial recess, which must be surgically defined. Regardless of whether the tumor is located in the horizontal or vertical portion of the facial nerve, the middle ear and mastoid portions are exposed to obtain access to the margins. The tumor should be evident at this time. Using continuous suction

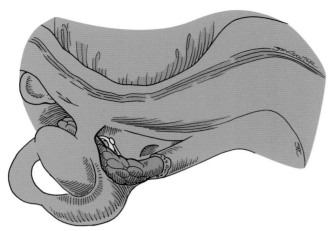

Figure 121-7. A complete mastoidectomy via a facial recess approach provides exposure of the epitympanum and the vertical segment of the facial nerve. The incus has been removed to reveal the tumor. The head of the malleus is intact.

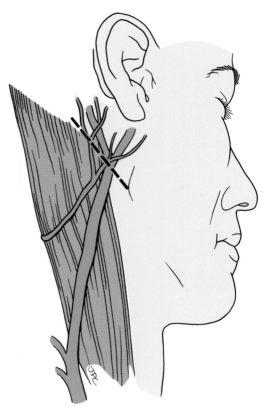

Figure 121-8. Methods for identifying the greater auricular nerve with pertinent anatomic landmarks. The greater auricular nerve exits posterior to the sternocleidomastoid muscle at the junction of its upper and middle thirds. The greater auricular nerve can also be found midway between the angle of the mandible and the mastoid tip.

irrigation and diamond burrs, the bone overlying the facial nerve and tumor is thinned. Access to the horizontal (tympanic) segment of the facial nerve often requires removal of the incus (Fig. 121-7), which is accomplished through the facial recess unless the tumor is so large that it obliterates this space. In this situation, the ear is returned to its anatomic position and a tympanomeatal flap is elevated through the ear canal. Bone from the posterosuperior canal wall is removed by curette to provide exposure of the incudostapedial joint. The joint is separated and the incus is removed (see Chapter 117) (see Video 121-1).

This approach provides access to the facial nerve from the geniculate ganglion to the stylomastoid foramen. If additional exposure is necessary at the proximal horizontal segment of the facial nerve, the head of the malleus is removed. The eggshell-thinned bone of the fallopian canal is removed. If the tumor extends toward the distal aspect of the vertical segment of the facial nerve, the chorda tympani nerve is sacrificed and dissection of the facial recess is extended. The tumor is removed with a 59S Beaver blade by sharply dividing the tumor from the nerve. Fine spring scissors facilitate this dissection. If the tumor cannot be separated from the nerve, sharp transection is performed to remove the nerve segment and tumor together (see Videos 121-2 and 121-3). Frozen section examination is used to examine the margins of resection and histologically confirm complete removal of the tumor. The nerve is repaired with an interposition graft from the greater auricular nerve (see the next section, "Greater Auricular Nerve Graft"). The graft is carefully positioned in the fallopian canal without tension, between the remaining segments of the facial nerve. It is difficult and unnecessary to suture the ends together. A small piece of fascia or fibrin glue may be placed over each anastomosis to minimize mobility. If the head of the malleus has not been removed, the incus can be returned to its anatomic position and supported by

Gelfoam. Absence of the head of the malleus requires ossicular chain reconstruction by means of an incus interposition. This procedure is detailed in Chapter 114. If the ear canal was entered for exposure or ossicular chain reconstruction, the tympanic membrane is returned to its anatomic position and supported with a silk sleeve or Gelfoam. The postauricular incision is closed in the usual fashion, and a sterile dressing is applied to the mastoid and neck.

Greater Auricular Nerve Graft

Various characteristics of the greater auricular nerve make it an ideal donor for facial nerve repair. The nerve is in close proximity to the surgical field. Although it supplies sensation to the pinna and preauricular area, sacrifice of this nerve leaves only a small area of anesthesia. The anatomy of the nerve is relatively constant, thus providing consistent localization.

Two methods are used for localizing the greater auricular nerve (Fig. 121-8). Dividing the sternocleidomastoid (SCM) muscle into thirds, the nerve is identified at the posterior border of the SCM, between the upper and the middle thirds. The other method locates the nerve midway along a line connecting the mastoid tip and the angle of the mandible. An incision in a skin crease over this area is taken through subcutaneous tissue. This may be incorporated with the mastoid incision or, preferably, through a separate incision. The greater auricular nerve is found lying lateral to the SCM, exiting from its posterior surface. Retrograde dissection along the nerve by retracting the SCM anteriorly permits more proximal harvesting of the nerve from its origin in the cervical plexus.

Translabyrinthine Approach

A postauricular curvilinear incision is positioned approximately 3 to 4 cm posterior to the postauricular crease. A transcortical mastoidectomy is performed as described previously. Similar to the approach for an acoustic neuroma, bone posterior to the sigmoid sinus is removed and the sigmoid sinus is skeletonized. This facilitates retraction of the posterior fossa dura and sigmoid sinus. A labyrinthectomy is performed to expose the IAC. The bone surrounding the IAC and porus is removed. Tumor extending distal to the labyrinthine segment is exposed (Fig. 121-9). Involvement of the horizontal segment may require removal of the head of the malleus and the incus to get to the distal tumor margin. The facial nerve is decompressed beyond the area of enlargement. All drilling should be completed before opening the dura of the IAC and posterior fossa.

The posterior fossa and IAC dura are opened. The labyrinthine segment of the facial nerve is a critical anatomic landmark in translabyrinthine surgery. However, it may not be evident when the nerve is encased by tumor. Its location in the anterosuperior

quadrant of the IAC and medial to the eighth nerve complex in the CPA is traced proximally and confirmed with a nerve stimulator if facial function was present preoperatively. The vestibular nerves are sharply divided and sacrificed. Tumor that is extrinsic to the nerve is sharply dissected from the underlying facial nerve. Hemangioma of the facial nerve is vascular with a gritty texture because of the bony trabeculations that are often present in the labyrinthine segment and geniculate ganglion areas. Sacrifice of the facial nerve is necessary if the tumor cannot be sharply dissected from the nerve. The tumor is removed and the margins checked by frozen section examination.

The method of nerve repair depends on the length of facial nerve graft resected. If a small section of nerve has been sacrificed, primary repair is accomplished by mobilizing the horizontal and vertical portions of the facial nerve from the fallopian canal. This posterior transposition provides 1 to 2 cm of additional length to perform the anastomosis (Fig. 121-10). The proximal nerve stump is supported with Gelfoam. Placement of 9-0 or 10-0 nylon suture may be difficult near the porus or CPA. Satisfactory reapproximation with one suture is sufficient. Because of the lack of epineurium covering the proximal facial nerve, a single suture passed through the diameter of the nerve stabilizes the anastomosis.[21] Resection of a larger segment of the facial nerve may require a cable graft. The greater auricular nerve usually provides both adequate length and similar diameter to that of the facial nerve. If there is a noticeable difference in diameter between the two ends of the nerve graft, with the proximal end being larger, the distal end of the nerve graft is sutured to the proximal end of the

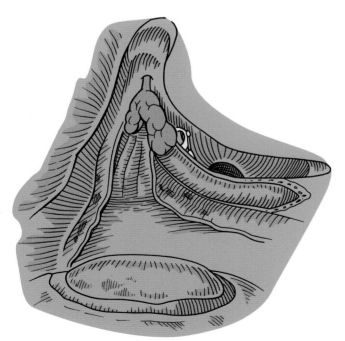

Figure 121-9. Translabyrinthine approach to a tumor of the facial nerve proximal to the geniculate ganglion. An island of bone remains over the sigmoid sinus. The dura of the internal auditory canal is intact. The tumor extends from the fundus to the second genu.

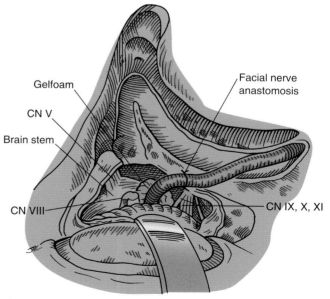

Figure 121-10. Horizontal and vertical segments of the facial nerve mobilized to permit primary repair of the facial nerve (cranial nerve [CN] VII). The brain stem, trigeminal nerve (CN V), cochleovestibular nerves (CN VIII), and lower cranial nerves (CN IX, X, XI) are demonstrated. Gelfoam supports the proximal nerve for suturing.

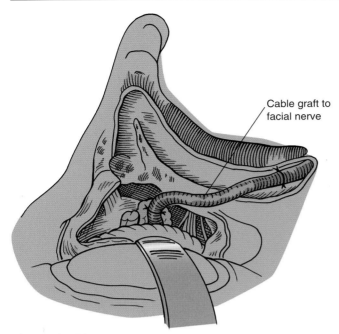

Figure 121-11. Greater auricular nerve interposition cable graft to the facial nerve from the porus to the distal vertical segment.

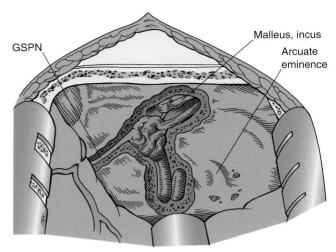

Figure 121-12. Middle fossa approach to a tumor of the facial nerve located at the geniculate ganglion. The labyrinthine and proximal horizontal segments are exposed. GSPN, greater superficial petrosal nerve.

facial nerve to ensure that all graft fascicles at this anastomosis are present in the distal nerve. The distal anastomosis is secured with 8-0 nylon suture and has the additional support of the fallopian canal (Fig. 121-11).

Fat is harvested from the left lower quadrant of the abdomen. The abdominal wound should be closed over a Penrose drain. The abdominal fat is soaked in bacitracin solution, and the wound is copiously irrigated with bacitracin solution. Strips of abdominal fat are placed around the nerve to support the anastomosis. The remainder of the cavity is filled with abdominal fat. The wound is closed in three-layer fashion, and a sterile mastoid pressure dressing is applied.

Middle Fossa Approach

Detailed surgical techniques involving the middle fossa approach are comprehensively described in Chapter 124. The patient is placed in a supine position on the operating table with the head fully turned toward the contralateral ear. A preauricular incision begins in a skin crease anterior and superior to the tragus. The incision is gently curved to the superior temporal line to expose the temporal fascia. The skin flaps are undermined posteriorly and anteriorly, and a self-retaining retractor is placed. A temporalis muscle flap pedicled on its inferior origin is elevated to the level of the zygomatic root. A middle fossa temporal craniotomy measuring 4×5 cm is created, and the bone flap is removed. The middle fossa dura is elevated from the temporal bone. It is typically necessary to remove additional bone inferiorly to a level flush with the floor of the middle fossa. When the floor of the middle fossa is reached, it is safer to elevate the dura in a posterior-to-anterior

direction to avoid injury to the greater superficial petrosal nerve. Hemangiomas of the facial nerve involving the geniculate ganglion should be evident at this time. Another important landmark is the arcuate eminence. Unfortunately, this structure is inconsistently present and may be confused with other ridges on the floor of the middle fossa. Drilling medially over the meatal plane toward the superior petrosal sinus is safe and avoids injury to the otic capsule. Drilling with suction irrigation is directed inferiorly until the roof of the IAC is encountered. The underlying periosteum and dura are left intact until all bone work is completed. The IAC is demarcated laterally to expose its roof until the labyrinthine segment of the facial nerve is identified. Tumor extending distal to the geniculate ganglion requires further bony dissection. The tegmen tympani is removed with caution because of the underlying ossicular chain. If additional access to the epitympanum and horizontal facial nerve is needed, a transmastoid approach should be performed as well. Preoperative imaging should have prepared the surgeon to anticipate the need for a combined approach.

Once adequate bone exposure is achieved, the IAC dura is opened to expose the tumor and proximal facial nerve (Fig. 121-12). The tumor is sharply dissected from the underlying facial nerve, if possible. Often during removal of a hemangioma, a plane can be developed between the facial nerve and the tumor. Sometimes a neuroma of the facial nerve, if located eccentrically, may be excised while continuity of the underlying nerve is maintained. If the nerve must be sacrificed because of tumor involvement, reconstruction will require a graft. For this short distance, the greater auricular nerve is readily accessible and of appropriate length and diameter.

If there is a minimal weakness of facial nerve function, decompression of the involved segment of the nerve is a treatment strategy. The overlying bone of the

IAC, labyrinthine segment, and geniculate ganglion is drilled to eggshell thickness and carefully removed. Despite bleeding that may occur from a hemangioma, the use of bipolar cautery should be avoided around the facial nerve.

Proximal anastomosis of the facial nerve is technically challenging through a middle fossa approach. Size 9-0 or 10-0 nylon suture is secured to the proximal end of the nerve graft. A single suture is then passed into the cut end of the proximal facial nerve. The distal end of the nerve graft is positioned without tension next to the distal facial nerve. If the tumor is located laterally in the fundus and geniculate ganglion areas, the greater auricular nerve graft is placed in a bone trough connecting the labyrinthine and proximal horizontal segments of the fallopian canal. Suturing in this area is usually unnecessary (Fig. 121-13). Either a free temporalis muscle graft or a small piece of abdominal fat is used to plug the IAC to prevent a cerebrospinal fluid (CSF) leak.

During closure, attention must be focused on the tegmen tympani. If it is absent, support is provided by sagittally splitting the craniotomy bone plate and positioning a bone segment over the epitympanum. The dura is tacked with 4-0 Nurolon to the edges of the craniotomy defect. The craniotomy bone plate is replaced and secured with 2-0 absorbable suture or miniplates. The temporalis muscle is returned to its anatomic position and secured with 2-0 and 3-0 absorbable suture. The skin is closed in two layers, and a compression dressing is applied.

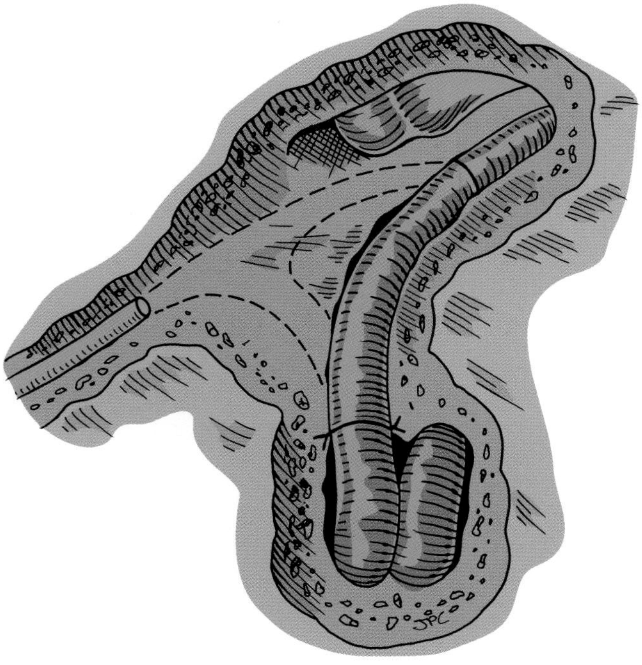

Combined Middle Fossa–Transmastoid Approach

This approach is used when a tumor of the facial nerve is proximal to the geniculate ganglion and distal to the head of the malleus in the horizontal segment of the nerve. This approach is also undertaken if hearing is to be preserved. Otherwise, a translabyrinthine approach is more direct and efficient. The incision for the combined approach is the standard postauricular one. The superior limb extends beyond the route of the helix to the preauricular area. The incision continues anteriorly and superiorly, parallel to the hairline toward the temporal area. The incision courses superiorly and curves posteriorly, parallel to the superior temporal line. It forms the shape of a question mark (Fig. 121-14). The posteriorly based temporal skin flap is retracted with either suture or large self-retaining retractors. This combined approach provides additional access to the horizontal and vertical portions of the facial nerve, as described in the section "Transmastoid Approach," earlier in this chapter.

The choice of donor nerve is dictated by the length of the resected facial nerve. Usually, the greater auricular nerve provides adequate length for repair. However, should a longer segment be needed, a sural nerve is harvested (see the next section, "Sural Nerve Graft"). The surrounding areolar and adventitial layers should be débrided from the end of the nerve graft and the thin epineurium left for suturing (see Video 121-4).

In this combined approach the tegmen tympani is removed to expose the tumor and the course of the facial nerve. As mentioned in the previous section, this area is repaired with bone taken from the middle fossa craniotomy plate. Care must be taken to not compress

Figure 121-13. Interposition cable graft repair from the facial nerve in the distal internal auditory canal to the horizontal segment.

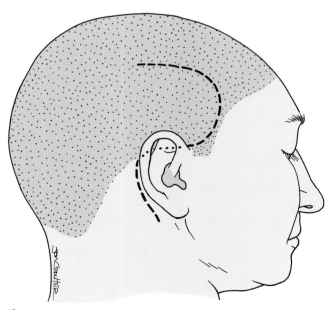

Figure 121-14. Incision for a combined middle fossa–transmastoid approach.

the facial nerve graft or to impede ossicular chain reconstruction. Again, the IAC must be diligently packed with fat or muscle to prevent leakage of CSF from the IAC into the middle ear space. Wound closure follows as described in the previous section.

Sural Nerve Graft

The sural nerve is a cutaneous sensory nerve that innervates the posterolateral aspect of the foot and back of the leg (Fig. 121-15). It is identified 2 cm posterior to the lateral malleolar process and deep to the lesser saphenous vein. The sural nerve is of greater diameter than the auricular nerve and has a higher neural population. There are two methods for harvesting the nerve. The first is by multiple stepped transverse incisions over the posterolateral aspect of the leg and blind dissection of the nerve with a vein stripper (Fig. 121-16A and B). The other technique dissects the nerve with a continuous vertical incision. This method creates more postoperative morbidity but provides better control of bleeding and minimizes trauma to the nerve.

Retrosigmoid Approach

It is unusual to preoperatively diagnose a neuroma of the facial nerve that is isolated to the posterior fossa and IAC. An enhancing tumor in this area would be most consistent with an acoustic neuroma. The operative approach and techniques are detailed in Chapter 124. Primary anastomosis is not feasible when surgical exposure is limited to the posterior fossa. A translabyrinthine approach would be required to mobilize the facial nerve in the temporal bone. Cable nerve grafting in this area is also technically difficult, especially when tumor extends out to the fundus, and may necessitate a combined transmastoid and retrosigmoid approach.

Stereotactic Radiosurgery

Fractionated external beam radiation therapy has been the conventional method for radiation treatment. Newer techniques using a frame-based linear accelerator, gamma radiation from cobalt delivered through a gamma knife, or electron beam from a mobile linear accelerator such as the CyberKnife are available for single or multiple focused treatments (fractions) and provide millimeter accuracy in delivery of treatment. We prefer the CyberKnife system for various reasons. It is a mobile linear accelerator that delivers photon beams measured in megavolts (Fig. 121-17). It is a frameless system that avoids the minor morbidity of placing a head frame on the patient, thus making it ideal for fractionated treatment. More important, the system allows treatment of tumors that extend below the skull

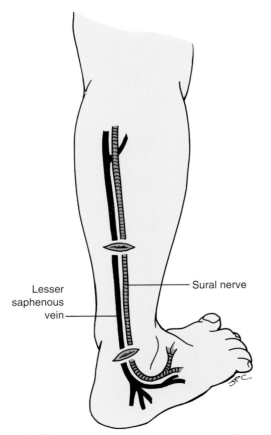

Figure 121-15. Landmarks and anatomy of the sural nerve. Note the relationship to the lesser saphenous vein and lateral malleolus.

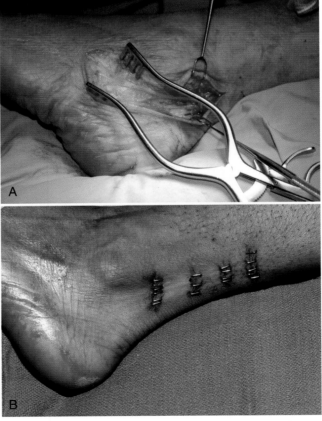

Figure 121-16. A, Surgical exposure for harvesting a sural nerve graft. **B,** Closure of incisions with a stair-step approach.

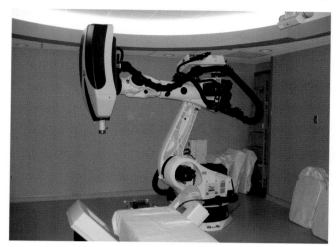

Figure 121-17. CyberKnife Robotic Radiosurgery system manufactured by Accuray, Sunnyvale, CA.

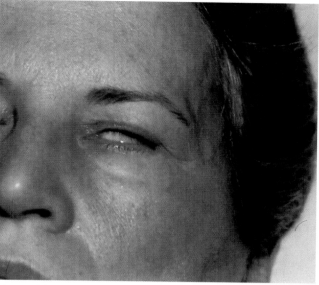

Figure 121-18. Left facial paralysis with incomplete eye closure. A good Bell phenomenon is present, with the lower cornea just visible.

base. The gamma knife system has its field of delivery limited to the head and skull base.

Both CT and MRI are performed, fused, and displayed by overlapping the images. The tumor map is contoured so that the field of interest is outlined by using information from both the CT and MRI scans, although treatment is based on CT confirmation. The soft tissue signal from MRI allows the tumor to be outlined. The bony anatomy of the temporal bone is also used to verify the location of the tumor and identify other important structures to be protected from the full dose of delivered radiation. These are termed critical structures. At our institution, this process of contouring the tumor is done jointly by both the surgeon and the radiation oncologist. The planned treatment is then reviewed with the radiation physicist. The tumor is irradiated with 18 to 21 Gy to the 80% isodose line in three fractions. For 18 Gy, each treatment fraction would be 6 Gy given during three sessions delivered every other day. The dose at the margin of the tumor is usually close to the prescription dose of 18 to 21 Gy, unless there is a critical structure immediately adjacent to the tumor. Minimizing treatment to a critical structure would lower the dose at the margin of the tumor. The maximum tumor dose is 22.5 to 26.25 Gy at the 100% dose. A mask made of Aquaplast is fit tightly to the patient's head, face, and neck to provide immobilization. Each treatment is given for approximately 30 minutes delivered every other day. No sedation, intravenous fluids, or hospitalization is necessary.

Conventional external beam radiation therapy may incur long-term complications such as osteonecrosis, chronic otitis externa, breakdown of skin, eustachian tube dysfunction, and the potential development of a malignant tumor. Acute cranial nerve dysfunction (hearing loss, imbalance or vertigo, facial paresis, vocal fold weakness, dysphagia) can occur and may be transient. The use of focused stereotactic radiation therapy should minimize these risks.

POSTOPERATIVE MANAGEMENT

Unless medical conditions indicate otherwise, patients undergoing transmastoid or extratemporal surgery do not require intensive care management in the postoperative period. In contrast, patients undergoing a translabyrinthine, suboccipital, or middle fossa approach should be observed in an intensive care setting. Neurologic symptoms and potential complications are monitored for 24 hours. The compression dressing is maintained for 3 days. If an abdominal drain was placed at the site of a fat graft, it is removed when drainage is minimal.

Patients are relatively immobilized when a sural nerve graft is taken. An elastic wrap is left in place for approximately 1 week. Active ambulation in the immediate postoperative period is uncomfortable and discouraged. Physical therapy consultation and the use of a walker are most helpful for early rehabilitation. Sutures or staples are removed 7 to 10 days after surgery.

Paresis or paralysis of the face is often present postoperatively. Critical attention is directed toward protection of the cornea during the recovery period. Lubrication with artificial tears during the day and ointment at night is prescribed. A moisture chamber is also beneficial to maintain humidity around the eye. If a nerve-grafting procedure was undertaken, facial recovery is not anticipated for at least 6 months, depending on the site of nerve sacrifice and repair. The patient is asked to attempt eye closure while noting the degree of scleral and corneal show (Fig. 121-18). If eye symptoms are bothersome and corneal protection is compromised, a gold weight is temporarily affixed to the upper lid to determine whether lid closure is facilitated and irritation is alleviated. A variety of gold weights (0.6 to

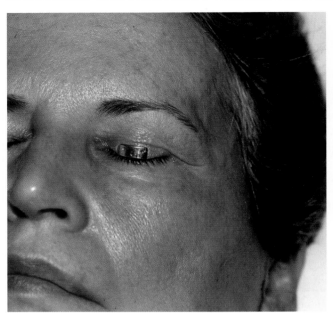

Figure 121-19. A gold weight (1.2 g) is taped to the upper eyelid to provide complete eye closure.

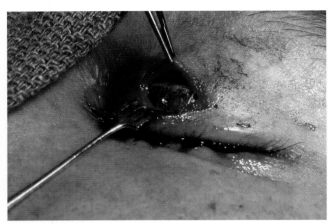

Figure 121-20. A pocket is created deep to the orbicularis oculi muscle and superficial to the tarsal plate for insertion of a gold weight.

1.6 g) are sampled to determine the optimal size (Fig. 121-19). Insertion of the gold weight is subsequently performed during the hospital stay. Topical tetracaine hydrochloride (Pontocaine) ophthalmic drops are placed in the eye. A scleral shield is placed over the cornea for protection. Intravenous sedation is given, and a local anesthetic is injected into the upper eyelid.

The incision in a supratarsal crease is taken through the skin and orbicularis oculi muscle. Westcott scissors are used to dissect a plane deep to the orbicularis oculi muscle and superficial to the tarsal plate. A pocket is created to insert the appropriate size of gold weight, as determined preoperatively (Fig. 121-20). A 1.2-g gold weight is well tolerated by most patients. The gold weight is sutured to the tarsal plate with 8-0 nylon. The orbicularis oculi muscle is reapproximated with 6-0 Dexon, and the skin is closed with running fast-absorbing catgut. A ⅛-inch Steri-Strip is applied over the incision.

Patients not complaining of or demonstrating preoperative vestibular symptoms may experience acute nausea and become vertiginous if the vestibular nerve has been sacrificed or the otic capsule is entered during the procedure. Supportive care is provided over the first few days, pending central compensation for the unilateral vestibular injury.

Patients who are stable and able to ambulate are discharged within 2 to 6 days postoperatively, depending on whether an intracranial approach was undertaken. Hearing is preliminarily assessed by gross measures such as whispering or using a telephone. Tuning forks are also useful. If the middle ear was not involved but surgery was in close proximity to the cochlear nerve or artery or the otic capsule, an audiogram is obtained while the patient

is in the hospital. If ossicular chain reconstruction was performed, a formal audiogram is obtained 4 to 6 weeks after surgery. Sutures are removed from the operative site 7 to 10 days after surgery.

There are several choices regarding the optimal radiologic method for monitoring the tumor postoperatively. If details regarding the bony anatomy need to be critically assessed, CT scanning is appropriate. Otherwise, MRI provides important information on soft tissue densities. Fat suppression techniques will reduce the signal of adipose tissue and more readily differentiate tumor from a fat graft. A baseline scan is obtained 3 months postoperatively and repeated 1 year later. Any postoperative changes should be less intense and contracted than on the baseline scan. The schedule for future scans is based on whether complete tumor removal was achieved and the findings on the 15-month postoperative scan.

Hearing status is assessed during the postoperative period. An audiogram is performed to determine whether a conductive, sensorineural, or mixed hearing loss remains. Significant conductive loss can be repaired electively if the middle ear space was not obliterated during wound closure. Hearing aid amplification may also be offered for conductive or sensorineural loss if word recognition is good.

Return of facial function is monitored over time. Evidence of reinnervation is initially manifested by an increase in facial tone and redefinition of the nasolabial fold. Recovery may occur within 6 weeks if tumor removal permitted preservation of the facial nerve. Facial recovery can take 12 to 15 months if nerve or cable grafting was performed in the IAC/CPA region. When return of function is delayed close to one year, needle electromyographic recordings may demonstrate polyphasic potentials indicating that reinnervation is taking place. This reassures both the surgeon and the patient that more time is needed to observe for ongoing recovery.

COMPLICATIONS

Vascular Injury

Intraoperative arterial or venous bleeding should be readily recognized and managed. The surgeon should be aware of the anatomic variability of the sigmoid sinus and jugular bulb. The sigmoid sinus may be located extremely laterally or anteriorly within the mastoid as the facial nerve is approached. This applies to any transmastoid procedure. Furthermore, approaches that require dissection medial to the plane of the vertical segment of the facial nerve may encounter the jugular bulb. Constant awareness of this structure will minimize inadvertent damage. Injury to the sigmoid sinus usually responds to local compression with Surgicel and neuroplasty. The carotid artery should not be subject to injury with any of the approaches described unless the cochlea has been extensively eroded by tumor. This would be evident on preoperative images, and appropriate meticulous surgical technique should be used. During a translabyrinthine or retrosigmoid approach, the anterior inferior cerebellar artery should be identified and protected. Injury to this vessel results in anacusis, vertigo, facial paralysis, hemiparesis, and possibly death.

Cerebrospinal Fluid Leak

The potential morbidity of CSF otorrhea, rhinorrhea, or a cutaneous fistula is the development of meningitis. Meningitis is a serious complication that if not recognized and treated early, may prove fatal. High clinical suspicion for a leak or meningitis is maintained throughout the postoperative period. The patient is instructed to avoid straining or sneezing with a closed mouth and to report any suspicious watery drainage. A leak through the wound is repaired by placing interrupted sutures across the dehiscent site. Topical collodion liquid is another adjunctive method for sealing the incision. A compression dressing is reapplied. If the wound is not ballotable and rhinorrhea is present, a subarachnoid lumbar drain is placed for 3 to 5 days. Drainage is maintained at 6 to 10 mL/hr (~150 to 240 mL/day). Almost all CSF leaks respond to this regimen. Failure to stop the leak will require re-exploration and possible obliteration of the eustachian tube.

Hearing Loss and Vertigo

Depending on the location of the tumor and the operative approach used, hearing loss may occur. Complete sensorineural loss (anacusis) is a known risk rather than a complication when a tumor is located in the IAC and CPA. Similarly, if the CT scan demonstrates otic capsule erosion, there is a greater likelihood of hearing compromise. Persistent conductive hearing loss would occur from unrecognized ossicular chain involvement, unsuccessful ossicular chain reconstruction, or persistent fluid in the middle ear space.

Unless there has been ongoing vestibular loss, sudden sacrifice of the vestibular nerves or injury to the labyrinth results in acute vestibular vertigo. Supportive measures are provided, and assuming that complete denervation has occurred, central compensation should provide return of balance function over the next 6 weeks. Patients experiencing difficulty in recovery of balance are referred to a physical therapist trained in vestibular rehabilitation.

Facial Nerve Repair

Certain principles must be adhered to when facial nerve repair is undertaken. The ends of the nerve or cable graft should be sharply freshened before anastomosis. The proximal end of the facial nerve in the CPA, bathed in CSF, is not likely to become desiccated. Immediately after tumor removal, if the facial nerve is resected, isolating plus wrapping the proximal stump in moistened Gelfoam protects the nerve and eliminates confusion regarding its true identity when the anastomosis is performed. There should be no tension on the anastomosis. If during a translabyrinthine approach a transposed nerve is reapproximated, it should be further supported with the fat used for obliteration and packing. Monofilament nylon suture (9-0 or 10-0) is used for the proximal neurorrhaphy when the dural extension or epineurium is absent. An epineurium-to-epineurium repair is performed more peripherally with 8-0 suture.

PEARLS

- Up to one half of all patients with primary tumors of the facial nerve will have normal facial nerve function.
- Both CT and MRI with gadolinium enhancement are essential in establishing the diagnosis of primary tumors of the facial nerve.
- Resection of the nerve and cable grafting are often required to achieve complete tumor resection, and the surgeon should always be prepared for this possibility.
- MRI with fat suppression should be used postoperatively to evaluate for tumor recurrence.
- Stereotactic radiosurgery appears to be an effective means of tumor control for facial nerve neuromas and should be considered in elderly patients, patients who are higher surgical risks, patients with good facial nerve function, and those with only one hearing ear.

PITFALLS

- Patients with a primary tumor of the facial nerve and good preoperative facial function present a difficult management problem, and consideration should be given to surgical decompression, stereotactic radiosurgery, or observation.
- Attempts to resect a tumor of the facial nerve in an only-hearing ear should be avoided if the tumor involves the IAC or cochlea.

- Resection of a hemangioma of the facial nerve may involve significant bleeding, but use of bipolar cautery should be avoided near the facial nerve.
- A primary tumor of the facial nerve may be identified intraoperatively after having been diagnosed preoperatively as an acoustic neuroma; in this case, the surgeon should notify the patient's family and proceed with tumor resection.
- Failure to plug the IAC with fat or muscle during a middle fossa approach may lead to CSF rhinorrhea or otorrhea.
- Tumor may involve a long length of the nerve not detected by MRI.

References

1. Fisher BJ, Dennis KE: Malignant epithelioid cranial nerve sheath tumor: Case report of a radiation response. J Neurooncol 78:173-177, 2006.
2. Selesnick SH, Burt BM: Regional spread of nonneurogenic tumors to the skull base via the facial nerve. Otol Neurotol 24:326-333, 2003.
3. Suryanarayanan R, Dezso A, Ramsden RT, et al: Metastatic carcinoma mimicking a facial nerve schwannoma: The role of computerized tomography in diagnosis. J Laryngol Otol 119:1010-1012, 2005.
4. Cawthorne T: Bell's palsies. Ann Otol Rhinol Laryngol 72:774-779, 1963.
5. Lipkin AF, Coker NJ, Jenkins HA, et al: Intracranial and intratemporal facial neuroma. Otolaryngol Head Neck Surg 96:71-79, 1987.
6. O'Donoghue GM, Brackmann DE, House JW, et al: Neuromas of the facial nerve. Am J Otol 10:49-54, 1989.
7. Fagan PA, Misra SN, Doust B: Facial neuroma of the cerebellopontine angle and the internal auditory canal. Laryngoscope 103:442-446, 1993.
8. Isaacson B, Telian SA, McKeever PE, et al: Hemangiomas of the geniculate ganglion. Otol Neurotol 26:796-802, 2005.
9. Asaoka K, Sawamura Y, Tada M, et al: Hemifacial spasm caused by a hemangioma at the geniculate ganglion: Case report. Neurosurgery 41:1195-1197, 1997.
10. Friedman O, Neff BA, Willcox TO, et al: Temporal bone hemangiomas involving the facial nerve. Otol Neurotol 23:760-766, 2002.
11. Martin N, Sterkers O, Nahum H: Haemangioma of the petrous bone: MRI. Neuroradiology 34:420-422, 1992.
12. Fisch U, Ruttner J: Pathology of intratemporal vascular tumors. Laryngoscope 91:867-876, 1981.
13. House JW, Brackmann DE: Facial nerve grading system. Otolaryngol Head Neck Surg 93:146-147, 1985.
14. Prasad S, Myers EN, Kamerer DB, et al: Neurilemmoma (schwannoma) of the facial nerve presenting as a parotid mass. Otolaryngol Head Neck Surg 108:76-79, 1993.
15. Rodrigues SJ, Fagan PA, Biggs ND: Management of cystic facial neuromas: An alternative approach. Otol Neurotol 25:183-185, 2004.
16. Pollock BE, Kondziolka D, Flickinger JC, et al: Preservation of cranial nerve function after radiosurgery for nonacoustic schwannomas. Neurosurgery 33:597-601, 1993.
17. Mabanta SR, Buatti JM, Friedman WA, et al: Linear accelerator radiosurgery for nonacoustic schwannomas. Int J Radiat Oncol Biol Phys 43:545-548, 1999.
18. Mdarhri D, Touzani A, Tamura M, et al: [Gamma knife surgery for VII nerve schwannomas.] Neurochirurgie 50:407-413, 2004.
19. Hasegawa T, Kobayashi T, Kida Y, et al: [Two cases of facial neurinoma successfully treated with gamma knife radiosurgery.] No Shinkei Geka 27:171-175, 1999.
20. Isono N, Tamura Y, Kuroiwa T, et al: [Combined therapy with surgery and stereotactic radiosurgery for facial schwannoma: Case report.] No Shinkei Geka 30:735-739, 2002.
21. Brackmann DE, Hitselberger WE, Robinson JV: Facial nerve repair in cerebellopontine angle surgery. Ann Otol Rhinol Laryngol 87:772-777, 1978.

Chapter **122**

Facial Nerve Decompression

Yu-Lan Mary Ying and Elizabeth H. Toh

Facial paralysis causes significant functional and aesthetic defects that often lead to great psychosocial distress. The potential causes of acute facial paralysis are numerous and listed in Table 122-1. This chapter focuses on management of the most common causes of facial paralysis that are amenable to surgical decompression, including Bell's palsy, facial paralysis associated with acute and chronic otitis media, and facial paralysis resulting from surgical trauma. Facial paralysis associated with temporal bone trauma is discussed in Chapter 128.

The goal of management in patients with facial paralysis of any etiology is to maximize functional recovery and minimize cosmetic deformity. In an effort to improve our understanding of neural injury and recovery, Sunderland introduced a histopathophysiologic classification system for nerve injuries that remains widely used today.[1] Injuries that induce only a conduction block within the nerve (neuropraxia, first-degree injury) do not disrupt axoplasmic continuity, and neural discharges can still be conducted if an electrically evoked stimulus is presented distal to the conduction block. The gross nerve structure remains intact. Second-degree injury involves axonal disruption (axonotmesis), without disruption of surrounding Schwann cell and neural connective tissue integrity. Full recovery usually occurs with the first two degrees of injury. Third- and fourth-degree injuries involve damage to the endoneurium and perineurium, respectively. The most severe forms of injury are characterized by complete neural tube disruption (neurotmesis, fifth-degree injury). In second- to fifth-degree injuries, the facial nerve undergoes distal wallerian degeneration. As a result, these nerves are not able to propagate electrically generated evoked potentials distal to the site of injury.

During recovery, if the axon regenerates through an intact neural tubule, complete return of motor function occurs without synkinesis. However, any violation of the neural support structures (endoneurium, peri-neurium, and epineurium) will result in misdirection of the regenerating neural fibers and cause synkinesis and incomplete motor recovery. When complete paralysis is due to either anatomic discontinuity or irreversible neural degeneration, the facial nerve requires repair or decompression for the most optimal functional and aesthetic results. Nonetheless, with completely severed nerves, some residual weakness and synkinesis are to be expected, even with the best surgical outcomes.

PATIENT SELECTION

Electrical Testing

Electrical testing constitutes the primary diagnostic modality for surgical decision making in patients with facial paralysis. Surgical management of a patient with facial paralysis is based on the premise that decompression or repair of the injured nerve will lead to better long-term functional outcomes than is the case with spontaneous recovery in a conservatively managed patient. Several electrical tests are available to evaluate the status of the facial nerve, estimate the severity of nerve injury, and prognosticate spontaneous recovery. Because most injuries to the facial nerve affect the intratemporal portion of the nerve, which is not usually readily accessible for evaluation, assessment of injury is based on measuring downfield potentials in the degenerating distal nerve. The extent and rate of progression of wallerian degeneration after injury are used as relative indicators of the severity of neural injury. Rapid wallerian degeneration is associated with neurotmesis, whereas nerves that degenerate more slowly are more likely to exhibit axonotmesis. The two most reliable and objective electrical tests for facial nerve assessment are electroneuronography (ENoG) and facial muscle electromyography (EMG). Because complete or nearly complete recovery is to be expected with incomplete

Table 122-1	DIFFERENTIAL DIAGNOSIS OF FACIAL PARALYSIS	

Birth
Traumatic vaginal delivery
Myotonic dystrophy
Möbius' syndrome (facial diplegia associated with other cranial nerve deficits)

Traumatic
Cortical injuries
Basilar skull fractures
Brain stem injuries
Penetrating injury to the middle ear
Facial injuries
Barotrauma

Neurologic
Opercular syndrome (cortical lesion in the facial motor area)
Millard-Gubler syndrome (abducens palsy with contralateral hemiplegia because of a lesion in the base of the pons involving the corticospinal tract)

Infectious
Malignant otitis externa
Acute or chronic otitis media
Cholesteatoma
Meningitis
Parotitis
Chickenpox
Herpes zoster oticus (Ramsay Hunt syndrome)
Encephalitis
Poliomyelitis (type I)
Mumps
Mononucleosis
Leprosy
Human immunodeficiency virus and acquired immunodeficiency syndrome
Influenza
Coxsackievirus
Malaria
Syphilis
Tuberculosis
Botulism
Mucormycosis
Lyme disease

Genetic and Metabolic
Diabetes mellitus
Hyperthyroidism
Pregnancy
Alcoholic neuropathy
Bulbopontine paralysis
Oculopharyngeal muscular dystrophy

Neoplastic
Facial nerve neuroma
Facial nerve hemangioma
Vestibular schwannoma
Glomus jugulare tumor
Meningioma
von Recklinghausen's disease
Cholesterol granuloma
Carcinoma (invasive or metastatic from the breast, kidney, lung, stomach, larynx, prostate, or thyroid)

Toxic
Thalidomide (Miehlke's syndrome: involvement of cranial nerves VI and VII with atretic external ears)
Tetanus
Diphtheria
Carbon monoxide
Lead intoxication

Iatrogenic
Mandibular block anesthesia
Antitetanus serum
Vaccine treatment of rabies
Otologic, skull base, and parotid surgery
Embolization

Idiopathic
Bell's palsy
Melkersson-Rosenthal syndrome (recurrent facial palsy, furrowed tongue, fasciolabial edema)
Hereditary hypertrophic neuropathy (Charcot-Marie-Tooth disease, Dejerine-Sottas disease)
Autoimmune syndromes of temporal arteritis, periarteritis nodosa, and other vasculitides
Guillain-Barré syndrome (ascending paralysis)
Multiple sclerosis
Myasthenia gravis
Sarcoidosis (Heerfordt's syndrome, uveoparotid fever)
Wegener's granulomatosis
Eosinophilic granuloma
Amyloidosis
Hyperostoses (e.g., Paget's disease, osteopetrosis)
Kawasaki disease (infantile acute febrile mucocutaneous lymph node syndrome)

Vascular
Benign intracranial hypertension
Intratemporal aneurysm of the internal carotid artery

Data modified from May M: Differential diagnosis by history, physical findings and laboratory results. In May M (ed): The Facial Nerve. New York, Thieme-Stratton, 1986.

facial paralysis, electrical testing is of value only in assessing a patient with complete facial paralysis.

ENoG measures facial motor activity in response to a suprathreshold electrical stimulus applied to the facial nerve distal to the site of injury. Compound muscle action potentials are measured with surface electrodes placed in the nasolabial fold. The amplitudes of compound muscle action potentials elicited on the normal and involved sides are compared. In the first 3 days after the onset of complete facial paralysis, the distal facial nerve will continue to stimulate normally until wallerian degeneration occurs. ENoG testing is therefore delayed until at least 3 days after the onset of acute facial paralysis and continued every second or third day until day 14. Reduction of the ENoG response relative to the unaffected side correlates with the degree of facial muscle denervation, which in turn reflects the extent of neural degeneration on the paralyzed side. Because severe neural degeneration is associated with poor functional recovery, surgical decompression is offered when ENoG testing indicates greater than a 90% decrease in function on the affected side versus the normal side.

EMG with needle electrodes placed within the facial musculature measures spontaneous and voluntary electrical activity in the facial muscles. It is useful for assessing the presence and extent of muscle denervation and reinnervation. EMG testing is a necessary adjunct to the interpretation of ENoG results if surgical decompression is being considered. Deblocking of the regenerating nerve fibers results in asynchronous firing of electrical potentials and therefore the absence of measurable compound action potentials on ENoG testing with skin surface electrodes. Because voluntary motor unit action potentials measured on needle EMG testing do not require synchronous electrical activity, they may be detected early in the recovery of facial nerve function and indicate a favorable prognosis. In addition, polyphasic action potentials on voluntary facial muscle contraction indicate muscle reinnervation and may precede clinical signs of recovery by 6 to 12 weeks. Spontaneous fibrillation potentials detected 2 to 3 weeks after injury indicate significant muscle denervation and poor recovery.

Bell's Palsy

Bell's palsy, by far the most common cause of acute facial paralysis, accounts for approximately 70% of cases.[2] There is enough evidence to support the concept that the facial paralysis associated with Bell's palsy is the result of an inflammatory response to herpes simplex virus type 1 that induces edema and vascular compromise, which results in functional impairment.[3,4] This entrapment neuropathy is believed to occur in the labyrinthine segment of the facial nerve, where the fallopian canal is narrowest in diameter.

Unilateral facial paralysis affecting all branches of the nerve begins suddenly over the course of 24 to 48 hours and may progress to complete paralysis within 3 to 7 days. Symptoms may be preceded by otalgia on the affected side. With the exception of facial dysfunction and, rarely, an erythematous chorda tympani nerve, no other abnormalities are typically detected on clinical examination of these patients. Hearing and balance are not affected. Progressive loss of facial function beyond 2 weeks, absence of recovery by 4 months, fluctuating function, ipsilateral recurrence, and the presence of facial twitching should alert the physician to the possible presence of an underlying tumor and prompt early imaging of the facial nerve. Bell's palsy may recur in up to 15% of patients, although it more commonly occurs on the contralateral side.

Sixty-five percent to 85% of these patients regain good facial function with medical treatment alone consisting of systemic steroids with or without antiviral therapy. The prognosis for satisfactory recovery of

women in whom Bell's palsy with complete facial paralysis develops during pregnancy is significantly worse.[5] Facial movement usually begins in these patients approximately 3 weeks after onset of the paralysis. Permanent residual weakness or secondary abnormalities, such as synkinesis or facial spasm, occur in 15% to 35% of patients. In patients with electrical tests indicating severe neural degeneration, surgical decompression may offer improved recovery of facial function. In a multicenter prospective clinical trial involving individuals with Bell's palsy who had 90% or greater degeneration on ENoG testing within the first 14 days of onset of complete paralysis and absence of motor unit potentials on voluntary EMG testing, surgical decompression of the facial nerve at the meatal foramen, labyrinthine segment, and geniculate ganglion resulted in a 91% chance of good outcome 7 months after paralysis as opposed to a 42% chance of good recovery in patients with the same ENoG and EMG parameters who were treated with steroids only.[6] The results of this study suggest that surgical decompression of the labyrinthine facial nerve may be beneficial for a select group of patients with Bell's palsy who meet electrical test criteria for unfavorable recovery. However, some controversy remains regarding the benefit of surgical decompression for these patients.[7]

All patients seen within the first 2 weeks after the onset of acute facial paralysis should be treated with systemic steroid therapy (prednisone, 1 mg/kg/day for 10 days with an additional 5-day taper). Additionally, a 10-day course of antiviral therapy may be prescribed (acyclovir, 800 mg five times a day, famciclovir, 500 mg three times a day, or valacyclovir, 1 g two times a day).[8,9] Antiviral therapy should preferably be commenced within 72 hours of the onset of symptoms.[10,11] With the exception of protective eye care, no additional treatment is necessary for patients with incomplete paralysis. Those who progress to complete paralysis should undergo electrical testing beginning 3 days after complete loss of clinical function. If ENoG testing indicates greater than 90% degeneration within the first 2 weeks after the onset of paralysis, the patient has a 50% chance of residual facial weakness and synkinesis. Surgical decompression may be offered to these patients if additional EMG testing fails to reveal any evidence of neural regeneration.

Herpes Zoster Oticus

Herpes zoster oticus (Ramsay Hunt syndrome) is a syndrome of acute peripheral facial paralysis associated with otalgia and varicelliform lesions of the auricle and external auditory canal. It is distinguished from Bell's palsy by the characteristic viral eruptions, a higher incidence of associated cochlear and vestibular dysfunction, and a poorer prognosis for recovery of facial function. Primary treatment of herpes zoster oticus is antiviral agents such as acyclovir or famciclovir and high-dose systemic corticosteroids. Unlike Bell's palsy, there is no literature to support surgical decompression of the facial nerve in these patients.

Acute Facial Paralysis Resulting from Surgical Trauma

Traumatic injuries to the facial nerve from temporal bone fractures, penetrating trauma, and iatrogenic injury represent the second most common cause of facial paralysis. The facial nerve is at risk for injury during surgery on the parotid gland, temporal bone, and cerebellopontine angle. Complications from parotid gland or temporomandibular joint surgery can result in injuries that affect the facial nerve from the stylomastoid foramen to the facial musculature. In the cerebellopontine angle, facial nerve disruption generally results during removal of an acoustic neuroma. The lack of a tough epineural sheath and anatomic distortion by the tumor make the nerve particularly prone to injury in this site.[12]

Within the temporal bone, iatrogenic injuries to the facial nerve occur most commonly during middle ear and mastoid surgery. The incidence of unexpected injury to the facial nerve as a result of an operative procedure is highest during surgery for chronic otitis media with or without cholesteatoma, and such injury occurs in up to 2% to 4% of cases. In surgery for chronic ear conditions, the facial nerve is most vulnerable to injury at three sites: the tympanic segment, the second genu, and the mastoid segment. The facial nerve is especially vulnerable in the tympanic segment because the fallopian canal is naturally dehiscent at this site in up to 30% of individuals.[13] Furthermore, this site is frequently involved with granulation tissue or cholesteatoma, which can cause erosion of the fallopian canal. If the fallopian canal is dehiscent or eroded, dissection of diseased mucosa or cholesteatoma from the nerve sheath can injure the nerve. The tympanic segment of the facial nerve is also at risk for injury caused by drilling, especially during removal of the posterior canal wall in a canal wall down mastoidectomy. The vertical portion of the facial nerve can be injured during drilling of the mastoid when the posterior canal wall is taken down, when the facial recess is opened, or when the retrofacial air cell tracts are opened. The key to avoiding iatrogenic injuries in temporal bone surgery is thorough knowledge of facial nerve anatomy within the temporal bone.[14]

Iatrogenic facial nerve trauma is best prevented by acquiring a thorough understanding of the course of the nerve through the temporal bone and by clearly identifying landmarks within the middle ear and mastoid that relate closely to the nerve. Injuries to the facial nerve detected at the time of surgery should be addressed immediately whenever possible. Surgical decompression of the fallopian canal 1 cm proximal and distal to the site of an injury is usually adequate if the nerve is intact but contused. The epineurium may be incised if the nerve is significantly edematous or contused. By contrast, if more than 50% of the nerve has been transected, repair by primary neurorrhaphy or interposition grafting is warranted. If facial nerve paralysis is unexpected and noted immediately in the recovery room, any packing in the ear should be removed, and the patient should be observed for 2 hours to allow any effect of the lidocaine used during the procedure to dissipate. Operative trauma to the facial nerve must be suspected if the facial paralysis persists. Neural integrity can also be confirmed by the presence of voluntary motor unit action potentials on needle EMG testing in the immediate postoperative period. Surgery to explore and repair the facial nerve should be arranged within 24 to 48 hours. Delayed facial paralysis may also occur after mastoid surgery and is generally a result of neural edema and secondary entrapment neuropathy after mild manipulation of the facial nerve in a dehiscent segment. Packing should be removed from the mastoid and ear canal, and serial ENoG testing should be performed to detect any significant neural degeneration. All patients with facial paralysis resulting from surgical trauma should be treated with high-dose systemic corticosteroids (prednisone, 1 mg/kg/day for 10 days with an additional 5-day taper).

Acute Facial Paralysis Associated with Acute and Chronic Otitis Media

Facial paralysis associated with acute suppurative otitis media is typical in children or young adults who have clinical signs and symptoms of a middle ear abscess. The facial paralysis usually progresses rapidly over a period of 2 to 3 days and is associated with the acute onset of otalgia and otorrhea. The pathophysiology appears to be related to the presence of natural bony dehiscences in the fallopian canal along the tympanic segment of the facial nerve that allow inflammatory products to produce inflammation and edema of the nerve.

Management of facial paralysis associated with acute otitis media should be aggressive. Myringotomy is performed immediately to drain the purulent exudate and to obtain material for culture and sensitivity testing. A ventilation tube is placed to maintain aeration of the middle ear. Intravenous broad-spectrum antibiotics are begun empirically and may be modified when the results of the culture and sensitivity testing are available. Topical antibiotic otic drops are started, and daily aspiration of the middle ear is performed. Corticosteroids (prednisone, 1 mg/kg/day) are prescribed for 10 days. If computed tomography (CT) of the temporal bone reveals coalescent mastoiditis or intracranial extension of the infection, a cortical mastoidectomy should be performed. Patients with intracranial complications should be managed in consultation with the neurosurgical service. The prognosis for recovery of function in those with facial paralysis secondary to acute otitis media is good without surgical decompression.[15]

In chronic otitis media, facial nerve paralysis is most commonly associated with cholesteatoma or chronic inflammatory granulation tissue involving the tympanic and vertical segments of the facial nerve.[16] As with acute otitis media, facial nerve dysfunction may be caused by inflammation, edema, and subsequent entrapment neuropathy. Alternatively, extraneural and intraneural compression may also result from an enlarging choles-teatoma or abscess. Chronic otitis media complicated by facial paralysis is usually managed surgically. Removal of cholesteatoma, with or without surgical decompres-sion of the affected facial nerve segment, intravenous antibiotics, and corticosteroid therapy usually result in favorable functional recovery. Patients with chronic suppurative otitis media without cholesteatoma appear to have a better functional outcome than do those with cholesteatoma.[17] The prognosis for recovery of facial function in these patients is related to the time of intervention.[18]

Acute Facial Paralysis Associated with Tumors

The most common neoplasms causing facial paralysis are malignant tumors of the parotid gland. Facial nerve neuroma, acoustic neuroma, and primary brain tumors are less common causes of facial paralysis. Surgical man-agement is dictated by tumor pathology and is described in detail in other chapters of this textbook.

PREOPERATIVE PLANNING

Electrical tests, including ENoG and EMG, are used to determine surgical candidacy when no clinical function is observed. General guidelines for offering surgical decompression include 10% or less muscle function on the affected side versus the normal side as determined by ENoG performed between days 3 and 14 after the onset of complete facial paralysis, along with the absence of motor unit action potentials on EMG testing.

High-resolution axial and coronal CT scanning of the temporal bone using a bone algorithm should be performed if surgery is planned. This is of particular value in patients with facial paralysis resulting from otitis media and trauma. CT enables the surgeon to localize the site of pathology preoperatively. Magnetic resonance imaging will demonstrate enhancement of the labyrinthine facial nerve in all cases of Bell's palsy but is not routinely performed before surgical decom-pression unless there is clinical suspicion of underlying neoplastic disease.

Audiometric testing should be performed in all cases of facial nerve paralysis to detect any associated hearing loss, which may aid in the diagnosis, especially of any injury to the cochlea, and help dictate the surgi-cal approach. It also provides a baseline for monitoring recovery in the postoperative period.

Determination of which regions of the facial nerve require exploration and the approach to be used is based primarily on the cause of the facial paralysis and the expected site of injury. In Bell's palsy, the labyrin-thine segment and perigeniculate region are decom-pressed via a middle fossa approach. In facial paralysis caused by acute or chronic otitis media, the mastoid and tympanic segments are explored, depending on the site and extent of disease. Canal wall down mastoid-ectomy may be required to properly exteriorize a cho-lesteatoma involving the facial nerve. Surgery for facial

paralysis secondary to intraoperative injury is directed at the site of surgical injury.

Lubrication and protection of the affected eye should be instituted at the time of initial diagnosis and continued until adequate eye closure is achieved. An ophthalmologic opinion should be obtained if expo-sure keratitis is present.

SURGICAL APPROACHES

Selection of the surgical approach is determined by the location of the facial nerve injury and hearing status in the affected ear (Fig. 122-1).

Transmastoid Approach

This approach is used when facial nerve injury is limited to the tympanic and mastoid segments of the intratem-poral facial nerve. The mastoid cortex is exposed through a standard postauricular incision and soft tissue dissection as described in Chapter 115. A com-plete mastoidectomy is performed until the mastoid antrum is entered medially. The lateral semicircular canal is identified and bone dissection is continued anterosuperiorly to expose the body of the incus in the epitympanum. Great care should be taken to avoid inadvertently drilling on the ossicular chain and violat-ing the tegmen when drilling in the epitympanum.

The mastoid segment of the facial nerve is identi-fied by two important surgical landmarks: the lateral semicircular canal superiorly and the digastric ridge inferiorly (Fig. 122-2). The lateral semicircular canal is the most important landmark for the facial nerve because it defines both the anteroposterior and the mediolateral location of the facial nerve at the second genu. As the digastric ridge is followed anteriorly, the underlying fascia spirals to form the sheath of the facial nerve at the stylomastoid foramen. Thus, the course of the mastoid segment of the facial nerve can be pre-dicted by visualizing a line connecting the lateral semi-circular canal and the anterior aspect of the digastric ridge.

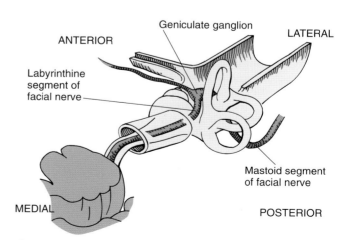

Figure 122-1. Anatomic course of the facial nerve.

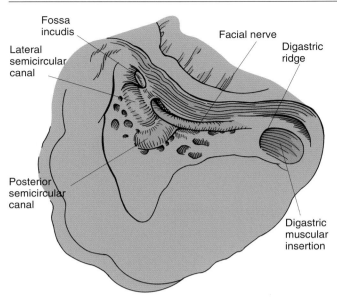

Figure 122-2. Surgical landmarks for the mastoid segment of the facial nerve.

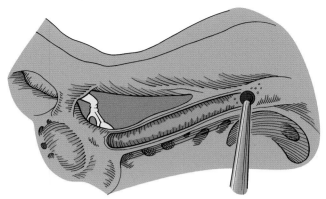

Figure 122-4. The mastoid segment of the facial nerve is decompressed.

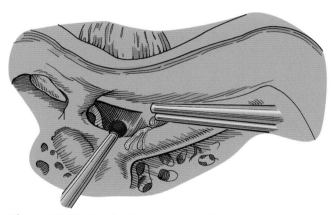

Figure 122-3. The facial recess is opened.

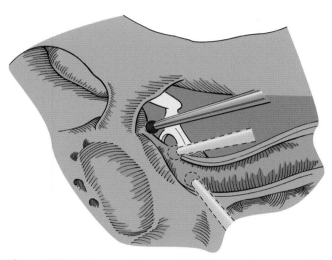

Figure 122-5. The second genu and distal tympanic segment of the facial nerve are decompressed.

Once the course of the mastoid segment of the facial nerve is identified, the facial recess is opened with 1- to 3-mm diamond burrs (Fig. 122-3). Drilling should be carried out parallel to the course of the nerve with the use of copious irrigation to minimize the risk of thermal injury to the nerve. A narrow bridge of bone is preserved along the inferior border of the fossa incudis to protect the incus. Bone is removed over the lateral surface of the facial nerve until a thin shell of bone remains. Inferior and lateral exposure of the facial recess is limited by the chorda tympani nerve. Anterior and slightly medial to the facial nerve, additional bone removal is often necessary to maximize exposure within the facial recess.

At this point, exposure of the facial nerve is sufficient to allow decompression of the mastoid segment, second genu, and distal tympanic segment. Decompression begins by exposing the thick periosteum of the stylomastoid foramen with a 2- to 2.5-mm diamond burr while leaving the thick fibrous sheath around the facial

nerve intact in this location. The circumference of the facial nerve should be exposed for 180 degrees along its posterior and superior surface, between the lateral semicircular canal and the stylomastoid foramen (Fig. 122-4).

A small diamond drill burr is then used to decompress the second genu and distal tympanic segment of the facial nerve by rotating the diamond burr from the posterior surface of the nerve to the lateral and antero-lateral surface of the nerve. This maneuver, called *barber poling*, prevents fenestration of the lateral semicircular canal (Fig. 122-5).

Depending on the position of the incus, the distal tympanic segment and second genu of the facial nerve may be decompressed with a microdrill and microcurette while leaving the incus intact in some individuals (Fig. 122-6). If the relative proximity of the incus to the fallopian canal does not allow safe dissection of the nerve, the incus should be removed for exposure and replaced at the completion of the procedure.

The ability to expose the perigeniculate region via the transmastoid approach depends on the position of

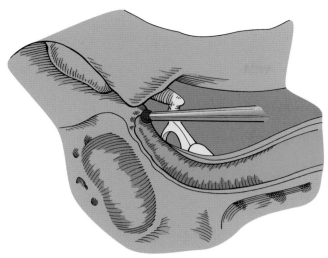

Figure 122-6. The proximal tympanic segment is decompressed with the incus in place if space permits.

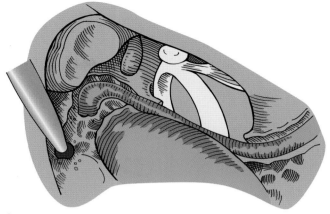

Figure 122-7. The perigeniculate and distal labyrinthine segments of the facial nerve are decompressed.

the middle fossa plate within the epitympanum and requires removal of the incus and occasionally the head of the malleus. The incudostapedial joint is separated through the facial recess, and the incus is rotated posteriorly out through the epitympanum by placing a 90-degree hook under the incus body. The tympanic facial nerve lies superior to the oval window and then courses between the cochleariform process inferiorly and the cog superiorly before diving medially toward the geniculate ganglion. The proximal tympanic segment is decompressed up to and beyond the cochleariform process with a microdrill and microcurette. The junction of the facial nerve and geniculate ganglion is reached with further anterior and medial dissection under the head of the malleus (Fig. 122-7).

The facial nerve turns abruptly posterior, medial, and inferior at the geniculate ganglion as it enters the labyrinthine segment. The ampulla of the superior canal blocks further exposure of the labyrinthine facial nerve through the transmastoid approach. Complete exposure of the labyrinthine segment of the facial nerve requires a middle fossa approach (if hearing is present) or a translabyrinthine approach (if hearing is absent).

Once the fallopian canal in the tympanic and mastoid segments has been exposed, any residual impinging bony spicule is removed. The nerve sheath is opened at the site of injury and for a short distance proximal and distal to the site of injury to assess the severity of injury to the fascicles. If the fascicles are intact, the decompression procedure is complete. If more than 50% of the nerve fascicles have been violated or the nerve is completely transected, primary neurorrhaphy or cable grafting is indicated.

The removed incus is replaced at the end of the procedure and supported in place with saline-soaked Gelfoam pledgets. If removal of the malleus head was necessary for surgical exposure, the incus may be sculpted and interposed between the stapes capitulum and malleus handle. The postauricular wound is closed

in layers with absorbable suture, and a mastoid dressing is applied to the operated ear for 24 hours. Postoperative hospitalization for transmastoid decompression alone is not necessary.

Translabyrinthine Approach

This approach is used to decompress the facial nerve proximal to the geniculate ganglion in a nonhearing ear. The surgical technique is identical to that used for translabyrinthine removal of acoustic neuromas and is detailed in Chapter 124.

Middle Fossa Approach

The primary advantage of the middle fossa approach is that it provides optimal exposure of the perigeniculate and labyrinthine facial nerve while preserving residual hearing in the operated ear. This is the approach used for surgical decompression of carefully selected patients with Bell's palsy and temporal bone fracture. It may also be used in combination with a transmastoid approach if complete intratemporal facial nerve decompression is necessary.

The patient is positioned supine with the head turned so that the operated ear is facing up. Intraoperative facial nerve monitoring is established at the beginning of the procedure. Paralytic agents are not used after induction of general anesthesia. Although the facial nerve is paretic, direct electrical stimulation of the intratemporal facial nerve during surgery may sometimes identify the site of conduction block. Brain stem auditory evoked responses are also monitored routinely because hearing preservation is desired. Perioperative medications administered include broad-spectrum antibiotics with good cerebrospinal fluid (CSF) penetration (ceftriaxone), furosemide (Lasix), 20 mg mannitol, 0.5 gm/kg, and dexamethasone, 10 mg. Bacitracin (50,000 units/L of saline solution) is used in the irrigation fluid.

An incision is made in the preauricular crease, starting at the level of the lower border of the zygoma and extending superiorly above and behind the auricle to form a reverse question mark (Fig. 122-8). Anterior

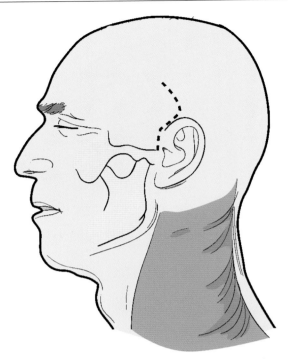

Figure 122-8. Skin incision for the middle fossa approach.

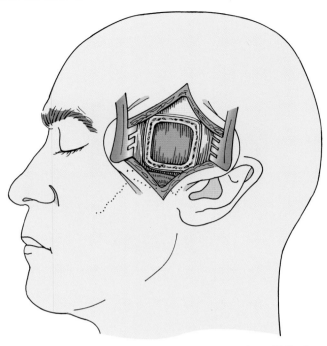

Figure 122-9. Temporal craniotomy used in the middle fossa approach.

and posterior skin flaps lateral to the temporalis fascia are elevated to expose the temporalis muscle. An anteroinferiorly based temporalis muscle flap is created by incising the muscle along linea temporalis with Bovie electrocautery. A 4- × 5-cm craniotomy centered two thirds anterior and one third posterior to the external auditory canal and inferiorly based at the root of the zygoma is created with a 4-mm cutting burr (Fig. 122-9). The bone flap is carefully elevated from underlying dura with a dural elevator, removed, and soaked in bacitracin solution until the end of the procedure. Any bleeding from the dura may be controlled with bipolar electrocautery. The inferior border of the craniotomy is then lowered to the level of the middle fossa floor. Dura is carefully elevated off the middle fossa floor in a posterior-to-anterior direction to expose the anatomy of the floor of the middle fossa (Fig. 122-10). The limits of exposure are the middle meningeal artery anteriorly, the sulcus of the superior petrosal sinus medially, and the arcuate eminence overlying the dome of the superior semicircular canal posteriorly. Dura over the greater superior petrosal nerve (GSPN) tends to be densely adherent to the nerve. Great care is needed in dissection at this point because of the possibility of injuring a dehiscent geniculate ganglion. The dura is elevated in a posterior-to-anterior direction to minimize injury to the GSPN and geniculate ganglion (Fig. 122-11). Once exposure of the floor of the middle fossa is complete, the tongue of the middle fossa self-retaining retractor is secured at the sulcus of the superior petrosal sinus to retract the temporal lobe (Fig. 122-12).

The GSPN is used as the primary anatomic landmark for locating the facial nerve along the middle

fossa floor. The arcuate eminence overlying the dome of the superior semicircular canal is located, and the positions of the cochlea, facial nerve, internal auditory canal (IAC), and middle ear ossicles are estimated. The location of the IAC is determined by bisecting the angle formed by the GSPN and arcuate eminence (Fig. 122-13). The roof of the middle ear is opened to identify the head of the malleus and the cochleariform process. The perigeniculate region is exposed by following the GSPN posteriorly and the tympanic segment of the facial nerve anteriorly into the geniculate ganglion with a 1-mm diamond burr (Fig. 122-14).

Bone over the labyrinthine facial nerve is then carefully removed by following the nerve from the geniculate ganglion posteriorly and medially into the IAC (Fig. 122-15). The labyrinthine facial nerve lies immediately lateral to the upper basal turn of the cochlea. The diameter of the fallopian canal in the labyrinthine segment is less than 1 mm, and it runs between the upper basal turn of the cochlea and the ampulla of the superior semicircular canal. The distance between the upper basal turn of the cochlea and the ampulla of the superior semicircular canal is 5.5 ± 1.0 mm (Fig. 122-16). A 1-mm diamond burr is used to uncover the superior surface of the labyrinthine segment. To prevent inadvertent fenestration of the cochlea, the area immediately anterior to the labyrinthine segment is closely observed for the blue line of the upper basal turn of the cochlea. Similarly, the area posterior to the labyrinthine segment is observed for the blue line of the ampulla of the superior semicircular canal. If the cochlea is inadvertently fenestrated, suctioning should be avoided in the area and the bone defect immediately plugged with bone wax. Bone over the tegmen tympani

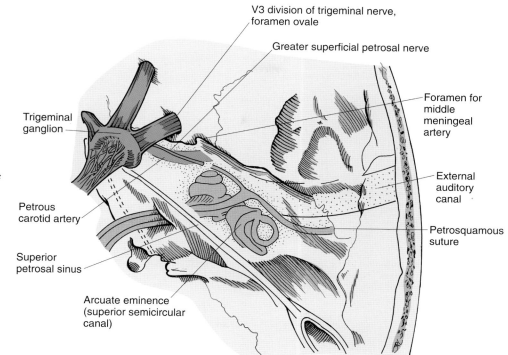

V3 division of trigeminal nerve, foramen ovale

Greater superficial petrosal nerve

Foramen for middle meningeal artery

Trigeminal ganglion

External auditory canal

Petrous carotid artery

Petrosquamous suture

Superior petrosal sinus

Arcuate eminence (superior semicircular canal)

Figure 122-10. Anatomy of the floor of the middle fossa.

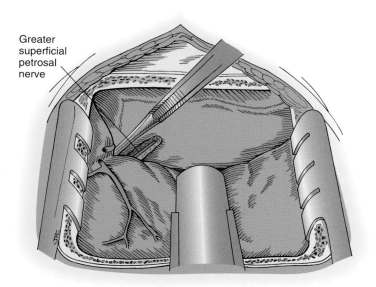

Greater superficial petrosal nerve

Figure 122-11. The greater superficial petrosal nerve is identified and preserved.

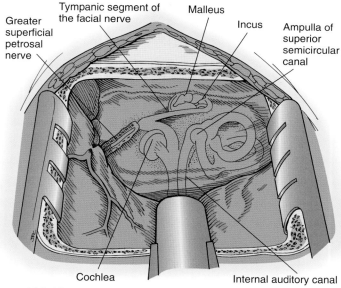

Greater superficial petrosal nerve

Tympanic segment of the facial nerve

Malleus

Incus

Ampulla of superior semicircular canal

Cochlea

Internal auditory canal

Figure 122-12. The floor of the middle fossa is exposed, and the self-retaining middle fossa retractor is secured.

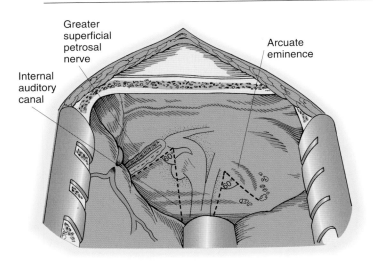

Figure 122-13. The position of the internal auditory canal is identified by using the anatomic relation of the greater superficial petrosal nerve and the arcuate eminence.

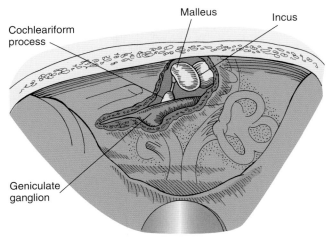

Figure 122-14. The tegmen tympani is unroofed to identify the malleus, incus, and cochleariform process. The geniculate ganglion is exposed. The perigeniculate and labyrinthine segments of the facial nerve are identified.

is removed to complete bony decompression of the perigeniculate facial nerve. Once bony exposure of the facial nerve has been achieved, the dura of the IAC and any dural thickening surrounding the meatal foramen are incised. The periosteum and perineurium of the facial nerve are split to a point just distal to the geniculate ganglion (Fig. 122-17).

Before closure, any open mastoid air cells are occluded with bone wax and the resultant epitympanic defect covered with temporalis fascia. The roof of the IAC is sealed with a small abdominal fat graft. A free bone graft is harvested from the temporal craniotomy flap for placement over the fascia to provide additional structural support and prevent herniation of dura/brain into the middle ear. The middle fossa retractor is released and removed to allow the temporal lobe to expand back over the middle fossa floor. The remainder of the craniotomy flap is replaced and secured by

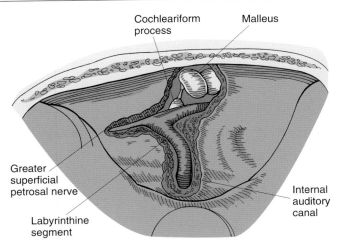

Figure 122-15. The labyrinthine segment of the facial nerve is exposed.

reapproximating the overlying temporalis muscle. The skin flap is then reapproximated in two layers without the use of any drain. A mastoid dressing is placed over the operated ear for 3 days postoperatively, and the patient is hospitalized for 4 to 5 days. The patient is monitored postoperatively in routine manner for intracranial surgery, with attention paid to CSF leakage from the wound or nose. Placement of a lumbar drain usually resolves this problem.

Facial Nerve Repair

Restoration of anatomic continuity of the facial nerve without tension is the primary goal of facial nerve repair. In general, the earlier that repair of the injured facial nerve takes place, the better the functional outcome. In patients with neural transection from surgery or trauma, immediate exploration and primary repair are advocated. If not possible, delayed exploration and repair should be performed as soon as medically feasible (within 30 days) for the best functional outcome.[9] The transected ends of the facial nerve should preferably be tagged to facilitate identification of the nerve endings at the time of secondary surgery.

Three anastomotic techniques have been reported in the literature. Epineural nerve repair is the most common anastomosis technique. It involves placing nonabsorbable suture through the epineurium on each side of the anastomosis and reapproximating the ends. The potential disadvantage is that it fails to approximate the individual nerve fascicles. Perineural repair consists of suturing the individual perineurium of each fascicle. The epineurium is sutured as a second layer. The advantage of this technique is that better contact of individual nerve fascicles may be achieved. Fascicular and interfascicular nerve repair involves individually approximating the fascicles. Natural fiber, fibrinogen adhesives, or fine sutures (10-0 or 11-0 nylon) are used to coapt the individual fascicles. To date, no definitive studies have documented the superiority of tubulization or enclosing the anastomosis to prevent tissue invasion and abnormal axon growth.[9] Accurate surgical approximation remains the primary goal. It is impor-

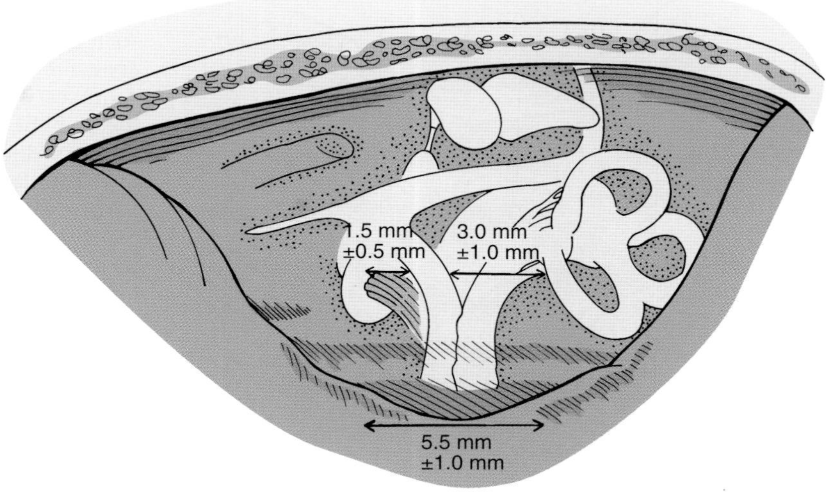

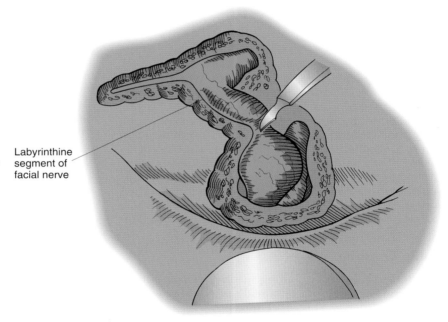

Figure 122-16. Average anatomic measurements between the labyrinthine segment of the facial nerve, the upper basal turn of the cochlea, and the ampulla of the superior semicircular canal.

Figure 122-17. The dura of the internal auditory canal and the periosteum and perineurium of the facial nerve are incised.

Labyrinthine segment of facial nerve

tant to remember that the working portion of the nerve is the endoneural surface and not the nerve ends. Therefore, epineurium needs to be trimmed back to uncover the endoneural surface for good axonal volume match at the anastomotic sites.

In general, partial or complete transection of the facial nerve should be repaired by primary neurorrhaphy or cable grafting when the proximal and distal ends of the facial nerve are accessible.

Primary Repair

Primary repair is the ideal surgical option whenever feasible because there will be only one anastomosis and minimal size incongruency of the reapproximated nerve endings. For this reason, some surgeons prefer

nerve mobilization and primary anastomosis over other techniques.

Intratemporal rerouting of the distal nerve segment involves a translabyrinthine exposure, sectioning of the GSPN and chorda tympani branches, and complete skeletonization of the facial nerve within the fallopian canal to gain another 1.5 cm in length for tension-free anastomosis. The disadvantage of this approach is that the blood supply to the distal nerve segment may be disrupted and lead to further neural injury. The cut endings of the nerve are freshened by sharply trimming the endings back to normal-appearing nerve tissue. Any excess surrounding soft tissue is trimmed to allow proper identification of the nerve sheath. In delayed repairs, fibrous scarring or traumatic neuromas at the

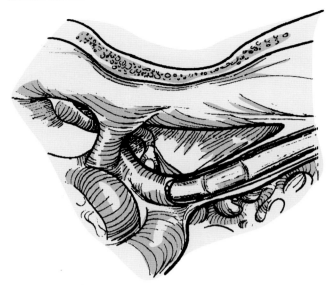

Figure 122-18. Interposition nerve graft laid in the mastoid segment of the fallopian canal.

proximal end of the cut nerve should be excised before repair. Suture anastomosis of the nerve is generally unnecessary within the temporal bone. When outside the fallopian canal, one to two 9-0 monofilament sutures are used to reapproximate the epineural layer. At the cerebellopontine angle, the lack of a resilient epineural layer may necessitate a single through-and-through suture to secure the cut ends of the nerve together. The suture is passed through the distal end first to avoid placing tension and traction on the proximal end, which may lead to tearing of the proximal end. After suture repair, the anastomosis may be further reinforced with fibrinogen. Use of nerve tubes and conduits is unnecessary.

Cable Grafting

Cable or interposition grafting involves placing a free nerve graft between the proximal and distal segments of the facial nerve. This procedure provides a conduit for growth of axons to the facial musculature. It is indicated when tension-free primary anastomosis cannot be performed. Disadvantages of this technique are the requirement for two anastomoses and decreased axon availability.

The great auricular nerve is the most widely used donor nerve in the head and neck for most short-segment facial nerve defects because of its close proximity to most surgical fields, excellent size match, and limited donor site morbidity. Its limitations are its relatively short length (up to 8 cm), restricted branching pattern, and potential for involvement by malignant disease. The great auricular nerve is located midway between the mastoid tip and clavicle along the posterior border of the sternocleidomastoid muscle.

The sural nerve is the second most popular donor nerve for facial nerve reconstruction. It provides excellent size match, is available in lengths of up to 40 cm

for grafting, and has an extensive arborization pattern. It is an ideal choice for near-total facial nerve reconstruction after oncologic procedures, as well as for cross-facial grafting. Harvesting of the sural nerve requires a second operative site. The sural nerve is located between the lateral malleolus and Achilles tendon, deep or posterior to the saphenous vein.

Details on the technique of harvesting great auricular and sural nerve grafts are provided in Chapter 121. Neural anastomosis is accomplished in a fashion similar to primary anastomosis. Cable grafts laid within the fallopian canal may be supported with Gelfoam alone without suture approximation (Fig. 122-18).

POSTOPERATIVE MANAGEMENT

Patients undergoing transmastoid exploration of the facial nerve are discharged home on the same day. If a craniotomy is performed, the patient will require hospitalization for several days for close observation. Perioperative antibiotics are routinely administered for all craniotomy cases. The patient is instructed about eye protection, and this is reinforced until good eye closure is restored. Static reanimation of the eye with an upper eyelid gold weight or palpebral spring is recommended at the time of facial nerve repair or grafting in patients requiring neurorrhaphy, because recovery of facial function is not anticipated for 6 to 12 months. Reanimation is also recommended for patients with facial paralysis who lack a normal Bell phenomenon and those with a decreased or absent corneal reflex in the affected eye.

COMPLICATIONS

Potential complications of transmastoid facial nerve decompression include further surgical trauma to the facial nerve, hearing loss (either conductive or sensorineural), vertigo, CSF leak, and wound infection. All drilling along the facial nerve should be performed with a diamond burr and copious irrigation to prevent thermal injury. The inner ear is most at risk at the lateral semicircular canal during decompression of the mastoid segment and second genu of the nerve. The ampullated ends of the superior and lateral canals are at risk during exposure of the perigeniculate region from the transmastoid approach. It is important to recognize inadvertent fenestration of the inner ear as soon as it occurs and to seal the fenestration with bone wax. Sensorineural hearing loss can also occur from inadvertently drilling on the ossicular chain. This injury is prevented by disarticulating and removing the incus if there is not enough room to safely decompress the tympanic segment without touching the incus. Care should be taken to avoid trauma to the middle fossa dura to prevent CSF leakage. To minimize trauma to the dura, it is important to use the properly sized burr, watch all edges of the burr while drilling, and switch to a diamond burr when in tight areas or when the dura has been exposed. If the dura is violated, repair with fascia, muscle, bone, or any combination of these tissues is necessary. Techniques for repair of dural and tegmen defects are described in Chapter 127.

Potential intraoperative and postoperative complications of the middle fossa approach include sensorineural hearing loss, vertigo, edema of the temporal lobe or contusion, subdural hematoma, CSF leak, and meningitis. Sensorineural hearing loss and vertigo result from inadvertent fenestration of the cochlea and vestibular labyrinth during exposure of the labyrinthine facial nerve and IAC. Should fenestration occur, the site should be immediately occluded with bone wax. Temporal lobe edema or contusion (or both) and subdural hematoma may occur as a result of direct injury during craniotomy or temporal lobe retraction. These complications are avoided by taking steps to reduce intracranial pressure at the start of surgery (e.g., reducing Pco_2; administering intravenous mannitol, furosemide, and dexamethasone). If the temporal lobe is tight, a small incision in the dura can be made to release CSF before retracting the temporal lobe. If injury to the temporal lobe is suspected, a CT scan of the head should be performed postoperatively to assess the degree of edema, and a neurosurgeon should be consulted.

Although functional outcome does not seem to be related to the length of the nerve graft, nerve grafts placed distal to the meatal foramen appear to do better. Timing of repair after injury is also a critical factor in determining recovery. The best functional recovery after nerve repair or grafting still results in mild to moderate facial weakness with synkinesis. Facial movement may not be clinically evident until at least 6 months after surgery and may continue to improve for 2 years or more after neurorrhaphy. Therefore, adjuvant facial reanimation procedures (see Chapter 88) may be indicated if poor oral and ocular sphincter control is bothersome.

PEARLS

- Incomplete facial paralysis portends a favorable prognosis and should be managed conservatively.
- ENoG and EMG testing should be used to identify patients who would potentially benefit from surgical decompression of the facial nerve.
- Thorough understanding of temporal bone anatomy and the intratemporal course of the facial nerve is critical in preventing iatrogenic trauma to the nerve.
- Tension-free anastomosis is critical for the best functional results after neurorrhaphy.
- Static facial reanimation procedures should be considered after facial nerve repair if significant oral or ocular sphincter deficiencies are encountered.

PITFALLS

- ENoG results alone may underestimate the extent of recovery in a regenerating nerve and should therefore never be used independently to determine candidacy for surgical decompression.

- Temporal lobe retraction is poorly tolerated in elderly individuals and results in an unacceptably high risk of intracranial complications.
- Inadvertent drilling on the incus or stapes during decompression of the distal tympanic facial nerve will result in postoperative sensorineural hearing loss.
- Thermal injury to the facial nerve may occur if inadequate irrigation is used while decompressing the fallopian canal with a diamond drill burr.
- Mobilization of the facial nerve from the fallopian canal to gain nerve length for primary anastomosis entails a moderate risk of further nerve devascularization and trauma.

References

1. Sunderland S: Nerves and nerve injuries. Baltimore, Williams & Wilkins, 1968.
2. Niparko JK: The acute facial palsies. In Jackler R, Brackman D (eds): Neurotology. St Louis, Mosby–Year Book, 1994.
3. Burgess RC, Michaels L, Bale JF Jr, et al: Polymerase chain reaction amplification of herpes simplex viral DNA from the geniculate ganglion of a patient with Bell's palsy. Ann Otol Rhinol Laryngol 103:775-779, 1994.
4. Murakami S, Mizobuchi M, Nakashiro Y, et al: Bell palsy and herpes simplex virus: Identification of viral DNA in endoneurial fluid and muscle. Ann Intern Med 124:27-30, 1996.
5. Gillman GS, Schaitkin BM, May M, et al: Bell's palsy in pregnancy: A study of recovery outcomes. Otolaryngol Head Neck Surg 126:26-30, 2002.
6. Gantz BJ, Rubinstein JT, Gidley P, et al: Surgical management of Bell's palsy. Laryngoscope 109:1177-1188, 1999.
7. Friedman RA: The surgical management of Bell's palsy: A review. Am J Otol 21:139-144, 2000.
8. Adour KK, Ruboyianes JM, Von Doersten PG, et al: Bell's palsy treatment with acyclovir and prednisone compared with prednisone alone: A double-blind, randomized, controlled trial. Ann Otol Rhinol Laryngol 105:371-378, 1996.
9. Axelsson S, Lindberg S, Stjernquist-Desatnik A: Outcome of treatment with valacyclovir and prednisone in patients with Bell's palsy. Ann Otol Rhinol Laryngol 112:197-201, 2003.
10. Alberton DL, Zed PJ: Bell's palsy: A review of treatment using antiviral agents. Ann Pharmacother 40:1838-1842, 2006.
11. Hato N, Matsumoto S, Kisaki H, et al: Efficacy of early treatment of Bell's palsy with oral acyclovir and prednisolone. Otol Neurotol 24:948-951, 2003.
12. Fucci MJ, Buchman CA, Slattery WH: Neurorrhaphy techniques for facial paralysis. Facial Plast Surg Clin North Am 5:223-240, 1997.
13. Di Martino E, Sellhaus B, Haensel J, et al: Fallopian canal dehiscences: A survey of clinical and anatomical findings. Eur Arch Otorhinolaryngol 262:120-126, 2005.
14. Weber PC: Iatrogenic complications from chronic ear surgery. Otolaryngol Clin North Am 38:711-722, 2005.
15. Redaelli de Zinis LO, Gamba P, Balzanelli C: Acute otitis media and facial nerve paralysis in adults. Otol Neurotol 24:113-117, 2003.
16. Harker LA, Pignatari SS: Facial nerve paralysis secondary to chronic otitis media without cholesteatoma. Am J Otol 13:372-374, 1992.
17. Makeham TP, Croxson GR, Coulson S: Infective causes of facial nerve paralysis. Otol Neurotol 28:100-103, 2007.
18. Quaranta N, Cassano M, Quaranta A: Facial paralysis associated with cholesteatoma: A review of 13 cases. Otol Neurotol 28:405-407, 2007.

TEMPORAL BONE

Chapter 123

Carcinoma of the Temporal Bone

Barry E. Hirsch, C. Y. Joseph Chang, and Stephanie Moody Antonio

Primary malignant tumors arising in the temporal bone are rarely seen in the typical community practice of otology. The external auditory canal (EAC) is the most common site of origin. Squamous cell carcinoma of the EAC has a reported incidence of about 1 per one million per year and is the major focus of this chapter. Primary malignancies of the temporal bone may also arise in the middle ear and mastoid and rarely in the jugular foramen and petrous apex. Secondary tumors of the temporal bone commonly develop as a result of spread from adjacent structures such as the concha, pinna, and parotid gland. Metastasis to the temporal bone from distant sites can also occur, often at the petrous apex. Each region of the temporal bone is affected by unique tumor types, clinical manifestations, and examination findings. Because it is common for a tumor to involve overlapping anatomic regions, no area can be considered in isolation, and broad understanding of the temporal bone and its surrounding structures is vital.

Basal cell carcinoma is the most common tumor of the pinna and concha and occurs four times as frequently as squamous cell carcinoma. Melanoma and Merkel cell cancer are less common. Melanoma of the pinna and EAC account for about 10% of head and neck melanomas.[1] Malignancies arising from the medial EAC and middle ear include squamous cell carcinoma, adenocarcinoma, adenoid cystic carcinoma, and rarely, Merkel cell carcinoma, lymphoma, and malignant melanoma. Rhabdomyosarcoma originates in the

middle ear and mastoid and is the most common malignancy of the temporal bone in children. Other tumor types occurring in the middle ear and mastoid include melanoma, squamous cell carcinoma, endolymphatic sac tumor (papillary adenocarcinoma), adenocarcinoma, and lymphoma. Malignant schwannomas and neuromas have been identified in the middle ear and jugular foramen. Unique tumor types in the petrous apex include chondrosarcoma, neuroendocrine carcinoma, meningioma, and hemangiopericytoma. Adenoid cystic carcinoma, mucoepidermoid carcinoma, sarcoma, plasmacytoma, fibrosarcoma, multiple myeloma, and osteosarcoma have also been reported in the temporal bone. Metastasis to the temporal bone from breast, colon, and renal cell carcinomas have all been reported.

A patient with long-standing otorrhea, otalgia, or a mass in the EAC should be presumed to have carcinoma until proved otherwise. Bleeding, hearing loss, facial paralysis, a periauricular swelling or mass, lymphadenopathy of the parotid or upper part of the neck, and lower cranial nerve palsies may indicate a cancer lesion in the temporal bone. It is important to be mindful of the possibility of malignant otitis externa because its clinical picture is very similar to cancer in this site.

Sun exposure contributes to the development of basal cell and squamous cell carcinomas of the pinna and lateral EAC. A genetic predisposition to skin cancer may also exist and is manifested by the development of skin cancer in sites not exposed to sunlight, as well as in sun-exposed areas. Chronic otitis media and cholesteatoma are common in patients with cancer of the temporal bone and have been implicated as etiologic factors. Squamous metaplasia resulting from chronic inflammation could result in dysplastic changes and lead to cancer.[2-4] Human papillomavirus has been implicated in squamous cell carcinoma of the middle ear.[5-7] Included in these series are cases of temporal bone cancer induced by radiation exposure. Patients with these cancers had a particularly poor outcome.

PERTINENT TEMPORAL BONE ANATOMY

The pinna and temporal bone have traditionally been divided into anatomic subunits that correspond to the depth of resection of the various procedures used for surgical correction. The EAC is divided into cartilaginous (lateral) and bony (medial) portions. The cartilaginous portion is a poor barrier against the spread of neoplasm. Tumors in this area can erode through skin, cartilage, and soft tissue to invade the parotid gland anteriorly or the concha and postauricular sulcus posteriorly (Fig. 123-1A and B [1 and 2]). The fissures of Santorini are vertical fissures in the cartilaginous EAC that allow direct access of cancer from the skin of the EAC to periparotid tissues (Fig. 123-2). In contrast, the bony canal provides a more resistant barrier to direct invasion. Cancer in this area tends to track medially through the tympanic membrane into the middle ear and mastoid spaces (see Fig. 123-1A and B [3]). The foramen of Huschke provides a potential pathway between the bony EAC and the soft tissues of the parotid area and temporomandibular joint (TMJ). This structure is a defect in the anterior inferior tympanic ring that usually closes by 5 years of age but persists in 7% of adults (Fig. 123-3).[8]

The middle ear and mastoid cavities provide minimal resistance to the spread of cancer. Anteriorly, cancer may invade through tissue surrounding the eustachian tube and involve the internal carotid artery (ICA), Meckel's cave, and the cavernous sinus (see Fig. 123-1A and B [5]). Superiorly, cancer can penetrate the tegmen tympani and tegmen mastoideum to involve the middle fossa dura and temporal lobe (see Fig. 123-1A and B [4]). Medially, the otic capsule provides a good barrier to the spread of cancer, but several areas are vulnerable. The round and oval windows can be penetrated and result in invasion through the vestibule into the internal auditory canal (IAC) and posterior fossa (see Fig. 123-1A and B [6]). In addition, the facial nerve can provide a pathway for the spread of cancer intracranially through the petrous apex, as well as into the infratemporal fossa (ITF) through the stylomastoid foramen (see Fig. 123-1A and B [7]). Posteriorly, cancer can invade the posterior fossa plate, dura, and sigmoid sinus (see Fig. 123-1A [8]). Finally, the air cell system of the temporal bone provides a multidirectional highway for the spread of cancer. Cancer within the middle ear and mastoid follows air cells as a pathway into the petrous apex and IAC and inferiorly into the jugular bulb and can penetrate the ITF and posterior fossa (see Fig. 123-1A and B [5, 6, and 9]).

Lymphatic drainage of the EAC extends anteriorly to the parotid and periparotid lymph nodes, inferiorly to the internal jugular lymph nodes, and posteriorly to the mastoid lymph nodes. The lymphatic drainage pathways from the middle ear and mastoid have not been well elucidated, but they are believed to be of only minor importance, because nodal metastasis from a malignancy limited to the middle ear and mastoid is rare.

STAGING OF TEMPORAL BONE MALIGNANCIES

A systematic and useful staging system for cancer of the temporal bone has not been universally accepted. A major obstacle to the development of a useful preoperative staging system in the past was the difficulty of cancer mapping because the medial portion of the cancer could not be visualized and spread to the skull base and intracranial cavity was difficult to evaluate. The development of multiaxial imaging modalities such as computed tomography (CT) and magnetic resonance imaging (MRI) has helped overcome this problem. A useful system proposed by the University of Pittsburgh uses imaging to determine the extent of tumor involvement and has become widely accepted for squamous cell carcinoma.[9-14]

The staging system for cancer of the temporal bone involves the same tumor-node-metastasis (TNM) model used for staging cancers in other anatomic sites. Tumor extent is defined as T1 through T4, depending on the degree of bone, cartilage, and soft tissue involvement of the ear canal and tympanic, mastoid, and petrous bones (Table 123-1). The N and M portions of the classification and the staging system follow the same format as for other sites according to the American Joint Committee on Cancer.[15] In our recent series of patients with squamous cell carcinoma of the temporal bone staged in this manner, the 2-year disease-free survival rate was 100% for T1, 100% for T2, 56% for T3, and 17% for T4, thus demonstrating that this staging system can be predictive of outcome.[9] We modified the Pittsburgh staging system after further review of patients from an extended series.[16] In the modified staging system, facial nerve weakness is considered an indicator of T4 cancer and has a worse prognosis than T3 cancer. We observed that facial nerve paresis did not occur in cancers classified as limited T1, T2, or T3 lesions. Involvement of the facial nerve would otherwise be classified as T4 based on the anatomic area of involvement, including the medial wall of the middle ear (horizontal segment), extensive bony erosion in the mastoid (vertical segment), or involvement of the stylomastoid foramen. In the T4 group, survival was similar in patients with and without facial paralysis. A few reports have used the modified staging system,[16,17] but further study on the importance of facial paralysis in cancer of the temporal bone is

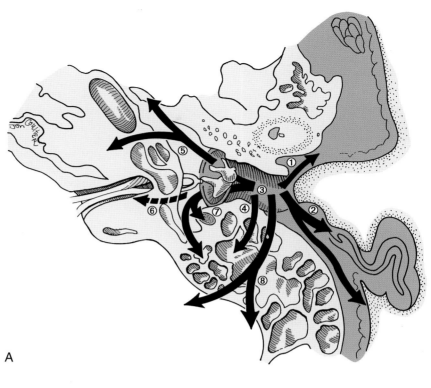

Figure 123-1. Axial **(A)** and coronal **(B)** temporal bone anatomy identifying pathways of the spread of cancer. Cancer can spread (1) anteriorly through the cartilaginous ear canal into the parotid gland; (2) through the concha into the postauricular sulcus; (3) through the tympanic membrane into the middle ear; (4) posteriorly into the mastoid; (5) into the anterior mesotympanum to the carotid artery and eustachian tube; (6) into the inner ear through the round window or otic capsule; (7) along the facial nerve into the infratemporal fossa; (8) through the mastoid, posterior fossa dura, and sigmoid sinus; and (9) beneath the skull base to the jugular fossa, carotid artery, and lower cranial nerves.

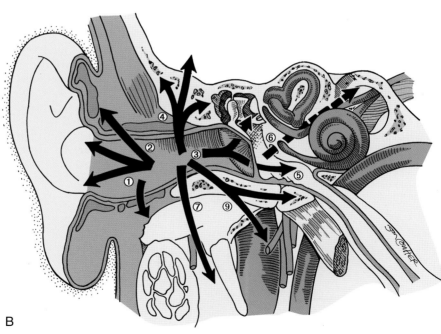

needed to support standardization of this staging system.

TREATMENT

The first systematic discussion of the management of cancer of the temporal bone was presented by Politzer in 1883.[18] Refinements in this approach have evolved over the past century. Radical mastoidectomy with radi-ation therapy was previously the recommended treatment, but cure rates were quite low. In 1954, Parsons and Lewis described the technique of en bloc subtotal temporal bone resection.[19] Lederman presented the first large series of patients treated by radiation therapy in 1965 and espoused the concept of combined therapy at a time when the role of radiation in treating cancer of the temporal bone was not yet well accepted.[20] In 1984, Graham and colleagues reported total en bloc resection of the temporal bone, including the ICA.[21]

Historically, overall 5-year survival with temporal bone cancer was low. In Conley and Novack's series of patients undergoing surgical resection, the cure rate

Table 123-1	CARCINOMA OF THE TEMPORAL BONE: TUMOR STAGING SYSTEM
T1	Tumor limited to the EAC; no bone erosion or soft tissue extension
T2	Tumor with limited bone erosion to the EAC or <0.5 cm of soft tissue involvement
T3	Tumor with full-thickness EAC bone erosion, <0.5-cm soft tissue involvement, or tumor in the middle ear or mastoid
T4	Tumor eroding the cochlea, petrous apex, medial wall of the middle ear, carotid canal, jugular foramen, or dura; or >0.5-cm soft tissue involvement; or facial nerve paresis
EAC, external auditory canal.	

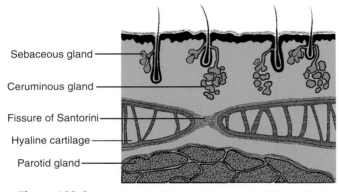

Figure 123-2. The fissures of Santorini are vertical fissures in the cartilaginous external auditory canal. Tumor spreads easily through these pathways into the periparotid soft tissues.

was 18%, but the operative mortality rate was 27%.[22] Lederman reported a cure rate of 33% at 5 years for combined surgical and radiation treatment versus 11% for radiation alone.[20] Despite advocating en bloc subtotal temporal bone resection and occasional adjuvant radiation therapy, Lewis and Page achieved a 28% cure rate.[23] The cure rate remains low despite the innovative work of surgeons and radiation oncologists and the use of aggressive therapy. Patients with cancer limited to the EAC have been reported to have an 85% to 100% disease-free survival rate with surgery with or without radiation therapy.[10,16,24,25] Cancer extending to the middle ear, mastoid, and soft tissues is associated with a poor outcome, and even with extensive surgery and radiation therapy, the survival rate is little more than 50%.

It has not been clearly established what treatment modalities provide the best outcome given the extent of disease. The relatively low incidence of cancer of the temporal bone makes randomized clinical trials impossible. As a consequence, every published study is essentially an analysis of a case series, with inconsistent treatment protocols often being used. This, along with the lack of a universal staging system and variability in surgical nomenclature, limit making use of published data in a meaningful analysis.

Surgical Therapy

Primary surgical therapy should be performed to remove the cancer in its entirety. The issue of whether piecemeal resection as opposed to en bloc resection compromises survival has not been resolved. It is clear that piecemeal resection of the temporal bone medial to the EAC is a more controlled operation than the en bloc technique is. Once the cancer has spread to the medial wall of the middle ear and invades the mastoid air cells, the prognosis becomes quite poor unless clear margins are achieved with radical therapy. A positive margin is associated with a very poor chance of cure.

The treatment program depends primarily on the extent of the cancer. The margins of resection for

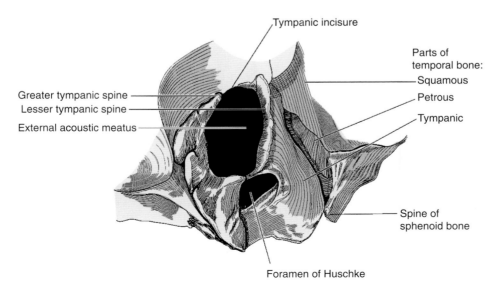

Figure 123-3. Foramen of Huschke. During development, two prominences (greater and lesser tympanic spines) extend from the tympanic ring and separate the space into the external auditory canal and the foramen of Huschke. These processes approach each other and fuse during the first year of life. With continued growth of bone from the inferior part of the tympanic bone, the foramen eventually fills with bone. Occasionally, the foramen remains patent. (*Adapted from Anson BJ, Donaldson JA: Surgical Anatomy of the Temporal Bone. The Middle Ear. Philadelphia, WB Saunders, 1967, p 122.*)

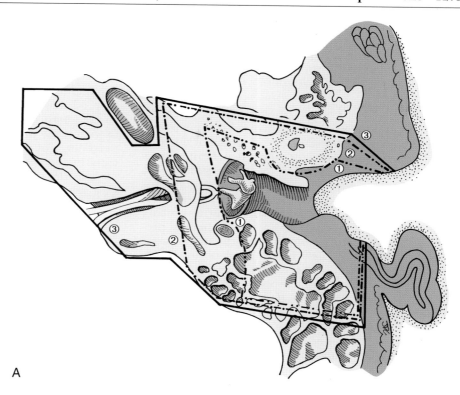

Figure 123-4. Axial **(A)** and coronal **(B)** illustrations demonstrating (1) lateral resection of the temporal bone, (2) subtotal resection of the temporal bone, and (3) total resection of the temporal bone. The carotid artery is preserved in this illustration.

A

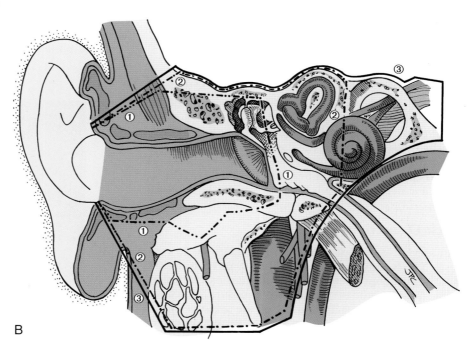

B

lateral, subtotal, and total temporal bone resection are illustrated in Figure 123-4. Cancer limited to the EAC (T1, T2) should be treated by lateral temporal bone resection with superficial parotidectomy and preservation of the facial nerve. Rarely, the cancer may be small, isolated in the lateral cartilaginous aspect of the EAC, and not eroding bone, thereby permitting sleeve resection of the external canal skin, lateral to the tympanic

membrane. In practice, sleeve resection is probably not oncologically adequate. Cancer that has invaded the middle ear and mastoid cavities (T3) should be addressed by subtotal temporal bone resection. Total temporal bone resection (sometimes called radical temporal bone resection) is performed when cancer extends to the petrous apex. Cancer extending to the TMJ, neck, dura, or ITF (T4) will require resection of these structures. Although involvement of dura and brain is considered by some to indicate unresectable disease, Moffat and coauthors reported on two patients with squamous cell cancer involving the brain who survived after resection and radiation therapy.[13]

Adjuvant Therapy

Radiotherapy as a single modality has not been very successful in curing any stage of carcinoma of the temporal bone. Although the additional benefit of postoperative radiation therapy has been questioned for limited tumors excised with adequate margins and for larger tumors with positive margins,[26] it is generally believed that combined therapy consisting of primary surgical resection followed by radiation therapy provides the best chance to control the cancer and improve survival.[10,13,16] We routinely recommend postoperative radiation therapy unless the cancer is well isolated in the EAC with very little bone erosion. Fifty to 60 Gy are delivered to the primary site, parotid region, ITF, and ipsilateral neck.

The role of chemotherapy is evolving. Traditionally, it has not been effective for primary treatment. A group of patients treated by preoperative chemoradiation therapy and temporal bone resection had better survival than did patients treated by surgery or radiation therapy alone.[27] In cases in which medical conditions preclude a safe procedure or the extent of disease prohibits a reasonable chance of adequate resection, palliative radiation therapy and chemotherapy may be offered.

Management of the Parotid Lymph Nodes

Parotidectomy is routinely performed in conjunction with temporal bone resection. In this way, the first echelon of lymphatic drainage for the anterior EAC may be reviewed. Ideally, the parotid is resected en bloc with the temporal bone. However, for T1 and T2 cancers, superficial parotidectomy is sufficient. For T3 and T4 cancers and if the facial nerve is to be resected, total parotidectomy is performed.

Neck Dissection

Supraomohyoid neck dissection is performed in most cases. The lymphatic drainage of pinna and EAC lesions is not entirely predictable but will often extend to the upper jugular nodal chain. Also, exposure of cervical structures provides safe control of the great vessels, if needed. In a clinically N0 neck, neck dissection can be done as a staging procedure to assist in the decision as whether to proceed with postoperative radiation therapy. The survival benefit provided by elective neck dissection is unclear. Metastasis to the lymph nodes is a significant indicator of a poor prognosis. In Moffat and associates' report of 39 patients with squamous cell carcinoma of the temporal bone, 9 (23%) had positive nodes in the neck. All these patients succumbed to the disease within 27 months.[13] In our experience, neck dissection and parotidectomy are commonly carried out at the time of temporal bone resection, which pro-

vides good local/regional control but does not seem to affect survival.[16]

PATIENT SELECTION

In general, less extensive cancers are more readily cured than advanced cancers that have invaded the middle ear and mastoid. A major difficulty in the management of cancer of the temporal bone has been the small percentage of patients in whom the diagnosis is made early in the course of their disease. Because chronic otitis media or otitis externa with purulent otorrhea is very common, otorrhea caused by cancer is often assumed to be secondary to inflammatory disease. Other symptoms of hearing loss and tinnitus are not specific to cancer of the temporal bone. All too frequently, biopsy is delayed until the disease is no longer limited to the EAC (Fig. 123-5).

The signs and symptoms of cancer arising in the temporal bone, especially early in its course, may be difficult to distinguish from those of chronic otitis externa and otitis media. However, the presence of persistent, deep-seated, unrelenting pain may be a differentiating symptom because appropriate treatment of routine chronic ear infections usually provides relatively rapid relief of discomfort. Chronic petrositis (Gradenigo's syndrome) is associated with deep chronic pain and otorrhea, although a mass lesion is absent. Spontaneous bleeding is also an unusual feature in purely infectious ear disease unless canal cholesteatoma has caused bone erosion with neovascularization. Malig-

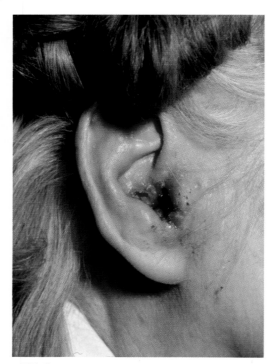

Figure 123-5. This patient with pathology of the right external auditory meatus failed to respond to medical therapy. Early biopsy in this case is warranted.

nant external otitis, which can closely mimic the signs and symptoms of malignancy, can be difficult to distinguish from cancer. Cases of malignant external otitis that were eventually diagnosed as cancer have been reported, thus underscoring the importance of early biopsy in suspicious cases.[28] In summary, any condition of the EAC that does not respond to topical and systemic antibiotic treatment should be suspected of harboring a malignancy, and biopsy should be performed early. Biopsy is performed by direct incision; a staging mastoidectomy is not appropriate because it reduces the reliability of staging radiography and may compromise the surgical margins of resection.

Depending on the stage of disease, surgical treatment of cancer arising in the temporal bone is potentially a major undertaking. The risk of morbidity and mortality increases with factors such as advanced age and medical conditions such as coronary artery disease, pulmonary disease, diabetes mellitus, and peripheral vascular disease. However, because combined-modality therapy that includes major surgery appears to be the only treatment that offers any reasonable chance of control of cancer, there is no absolute medical contraindication to surgical treatment. Aggressive preoperative, perioperative, and postoperative care must be given to minimize the chance of a major medical complication. Each patient and physician will need to decide whether the proposed treatment and its potential benefit are worth the risk. For example, a patient with cancer of the temporal bone who has a life expectancy of less than one year for other medical reasons will probably derive minimal benefit from aggressive treatment.

The second issue regarding the decision to proceed with treatment is the extent of the cancer. Extension into certain areas such as the cavernous sinus and brain parenchyma makes total tumor extirpation nearly impossible,[29] and the possibility of cure becomes unlikely, even with the addition of aggressive adjuvant radiation therapy and chemotherapy. In these cases there is little potential for improving the patient's prognosis. Involvement of the internal carotid canal is also problematic but it is not an absolute contraindication to total resection of cancer. Some patients will be able to tolerate resection of the ICA but will require preoperative studies to determine eligibility, as described in a later section.

PREOPERATIVE PLANNING

History, physical examination, and radiologic imaging remain the most important methods of determining the extent of the cancer. Evidence of the spread of cancer beyond the anatomic limits of the EAC is evaluated. The cancer and associated inflammation often obliterate the EAC, thereby restricting examination of the tympanic membrane and middle ear. However, the presence of severe conductive hearing loss, unilateral sensorineural hearing loss, otitis media, vertigo, taste dysfunction, or facial nerve paralysis may indicate invasion into the middle ear, eustachian tube, and otic

capsule. The presence of Horner's syndrome, transient ischemic attacks, or syncope may indicate involvement of the ICA. Trismus, TMJ dysfunction, and lower cranial nerve palsies suggest the spread of cancer into the jugular foramen ITF. The presence of seizures, dysphasia, and other cognitive deficits warrant investigation for intracranial spread of tumor. The patient should be examined carefully for physical evidence of a mass in the neck, parotid gland, soft palate, and postauricular region. An audiogram is obtained to establish the type and degree of hearing loss. The status of the hearing is important because preservation of hearing is possible only if lateral resection of the temporal bone is performed. However, the amount of resection is determined by the extent of the cancer and not by the degree of residual hearing function.

The full extent of the cancer should be mapped in accordance with physical findings and multiaxial imaging consisting of CT for delineation of the bony anatomy of the temporal bone and MRI for visualization of soft tissues and intracranial structures. The initial radiologic study for definition of the tumor is high-resolution CT with and without contrast enhancement. It can accurately map tumors in the temporal bone and predict invasion of cancer outside the EAC. CT is especially well suited for detecting bony abnormalities. Extension of tumor into the bone of the EAC, middle ear, mastoid, labyrinth, eustachian tube, carotid canal, sigmoid sinus, ITF, and intracranial cavity can be seen (Fig. 123-6). MRI with gadolinium enhancement is superior to CT in certain respects, especially in delineating soft tissue detail. MRI is more accurate in differentiating effusion in the middle ear and mastoid

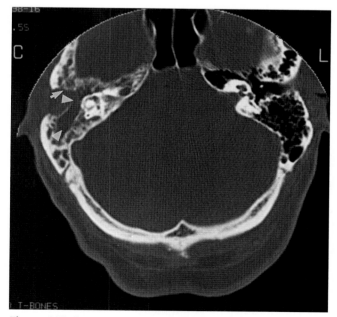

Figure 123-6. Computed tomography scan of extensive squamous cell carcinoma of the temporal bone with erosion through the bone of the right external auditory canal into the anterior soft tissue *(arrow)*, middle ear, and mastoid *(arrowheads)*. *(Courtesy of M. Arriaga, M.D.)*

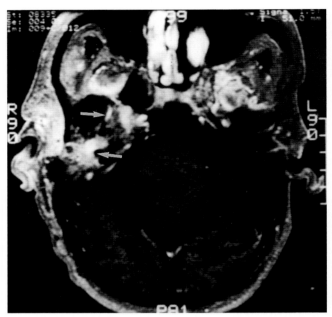

Figure 123-7. Magnetic resonance image of the same patient as in Figure 123-2 with carcinoma of the temporal bone. A T1-weighted contrast-enhanced image demonstrates enhancement of the middle ear and infratemporal fossa *(arrows)*. *(Courtesy of M. Arriaga, M.D.)*

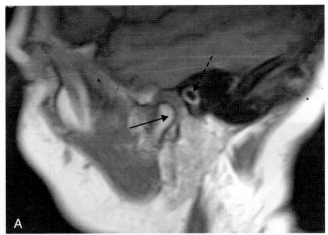

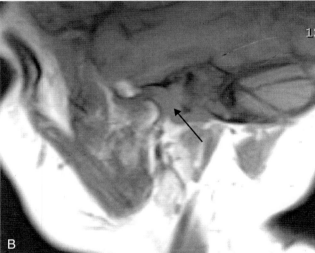

Figure 123-8. Sagittal T1-weighted magnetic resonance image of the temporomandibular joint (TMJ). **A,** There is a normal soft tissue interface between the external auditory canal *(dashed arrow)* and the condyle *(solid arrow)*. **B,** Tumor from the external canal extends through the bony canal into the glenoid fossa *(arrow)*.

from cancer, although such differentiation may be difficult with either modality. MRI is significantly better than CT in determining the interface between cancer and normal tissue. Therefore, MRI is quite sensitive in detecting invasion of cancer into the dura and soft tissues of the ITF (Fig. 123-7) and temporomandibular region (Fig. 123-8). Usually, both MRI and CT will be required to adequately stage the disease process.

Once a tumor map has been created, the need for further studies will become apparent. Encroachment of cancer in the region of the ICA should be investigated with angiography to help determine whether invasion into the vessel has occurred. Because there is a significant risk of injury to the carotid artery if tumor resection is performed near this vessel, the patient's tolerance of permanent occlusion of the ICA should be determined preoperatively by balloon test occlusion with xenon/CT.[30] The venous phase of the angiogram demonstrates the venous anatomy of the brain. Specifically, the location of the vein of Labbé and the dominance of the ipsilateral sigmoid and jugular drainage are noted. In a few patients, the ipsilateral venous drainage is so dominant that sacrifice of the jugular vein or sigmoid sinus on this side can lead to venous cerebral infarction. Thus, careful consideration of the patency of the contralateral side must be undertaken if it is anticipated that the sigmoid sinus or jugular vein may be sacrificed.

The presence of metastatic cancer, especially in the neck, should be detected before therapy. Metastasis to the neck is unusual in cancer of the temporal bone, but a thorough physical examination and CT or MRI with contrast enhancement should detect lymph node involvement. Spread of cancer to the lymph nodes in the superficial lobe of the parotid gland is more common, so the superficial lobe of the parotid gland is usually removed during surgery with preservation of the facial nerve. If the pathology is squamous cell carcinoma, a metastatic evaluation consisting of chest radiography and liver function testing is adequate. In malignant tumors with a high predilection for systemic spread such as melanoma, CT scanning of the chest, abdomen, and pelvis, as well as whole-body bone scanning, should be performed. The recent introduction of positron emission tomography (PET)/CT scanning has made identification of metastasis more accurate.

Preoperative staging determines the scope of the planned procedure and the necessity for a team approach. Neurosurgical participation is appropriate when surgery requires intracranial resection. Similarly, wound closure after tumor removal may necessitate transfer of regional or distant tissue, thus warranting consultation with a reconstructive surgeon.

Surgical treatment of cancer of the temporal bone usually requires a long duration of anesthesia and can entail major blood loss and fluid shifts, intracranial manipulation, and postoperative stress, including fluid and electrolyte abnormalities, pulmonary and cardiac stress, coagulation abnormalities, and the possibility of aspiration. The patient's medical status should be optimized before surgery. Significant conditions such as coronary artery disease, chronic obstructive pulmonary disease, diabetes mellitus, bleeding disorders, and malnutrition should be identified and treated preoperatively to minimize potential major medical complications.

SURGICAL TECHNIQUES

The surgical approach is dictated by the location and extent of cancer relative to the temporal bone. Lateral resection of the temporal bone is performed for cancer limited to the EAC (T1, T2). Subtotal resection of the temporal bone is performed for cancer that has penetrated into the middle ear and mastoid cavities (T3). The medial extent of resection incorporates the otic capsule. Extratemporal dissection is dictated by the areas of cancer infiltration and is specifically focused toward the ITF, jugular bulb, or dura, as indicated. Invasion into the petrous apex by cancer is managed by total resection of the temporal bone.

General oral endotracheal anesthesia is achieved with inhalational agents, intravenous narcotics, and hypnotics. Neuromuscular blocking agents are avoided during the procedure to permit monitoring of motor nerve activity. A short-acting agent, such as succinylcholine, is frequently used at the start of the procedure for safe induction and intubation. The patient is placed supine with the head turned toward the contralateral ear. Sequential compression stockings are worn to prevent deep venous thrombosis. Cranial nerves VII, IX, X, and XI are monitored if they need to be identified and preserved. Monitoring for cerebral and brain stem traction or injury during subtotal or total temporal bone resection is achieved with somatosensory evoked potentials and contralateral auditory brain stem response recordings, respectively. Regions to be prepared include not only the primary surgical site but also any areas needed to provide graft material, such as the abdomen for fat; neck or leg for nerve grafts; and chest, abdomen, or back for pedicled or free flaps. A third-generation cephalosporin with cerebrospinal fluid (CSF) penetration, such as ceftriaxone, is administered perioperatively. Furosemide (Lasix), 10 mg, and mannitol, 0.25 to 0.5 g/kg, are given intravenously 30 minutes before the intracranial portion of the procedure to decompress the subarachnoid space if retraction of the temporal lobe or cerebellum is anticipated.

Lateral Temporal Bone Resection

The anatomic unit removed with lateral resection of the temporal bone is the EAC. Boundaries of resection include the middle ear cavity medially, the TMJ capsule anteriorly, the zygomatic root superiorly, the mastoid cavity posteriorly, and the ITF inferiorly. Laterally, the resection can include the concha, as well as portions of the pinna, depending on the extent of the cancer. Occasionally, the entire pinna must be removed. Lateral resection of the temporal bone is appropriate for cancer limited to the EAC without penetration medially through the tympanic membrane. Spread of cancer anteriorly or inferiorly into the TMJ or ITF can be treated by extension of the surgical resection into these areas. Significant spread of cancer into the middle ear or mastoid cavity requires more extensive resection of the temporal bone.

The lateral margins of resection depend on the location of the cancer. In general, if the cancer is situated within the EAC, only the conchal bowl is included. The proposed incision sites are injected with 2% lidocaine with 1:100,000 epinephrine for hemostasis. A circumferential incision is made around the concha for cancer involving only the EAC, and the tragus is left with the skin flap if the cancer does not involve the lateral and anterior external auditory meatus. Otherwise, the tragus is included with the lateral circumferential skin margin (Fig. 123-9). If the subcutaneous layer of the concha, tragus, and antihelix is involved by cancer, more of the central portion of the pinna is resected (Fig. 123-10). If a substantial portion of the pinna is involved, the entire pinna is resected.

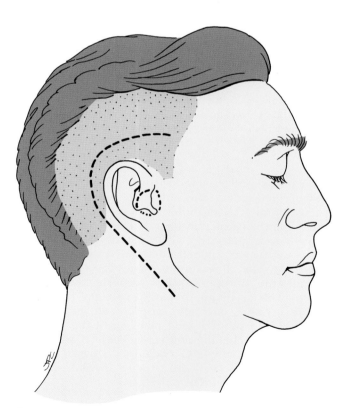

Figure 123-9. Postauricular and meatal incisions for resection of the temporal bone. This illustration demonstrates inclusion of the tragus with the specimen.

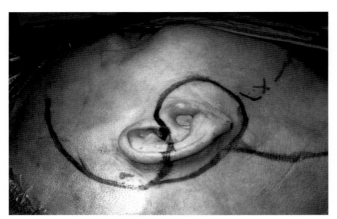

Figure 123-10. Skin incision when tumor infiltrates the tragus and conchal bowl.

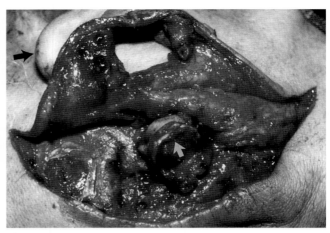

Figure 123-12. The anteriorly based skin flap containing the pinna *(black arrow)* is reflected anteriorly, with the external auditory canal *(white arrow)* and surrounding soft tissue left behind.

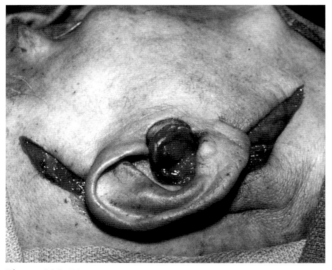

Figure 123-11. The anteriorly based skin flap containing the pinna is separated from the core of the external auditory meatus. The meatus has been oversewn to prevent tumor spillage.

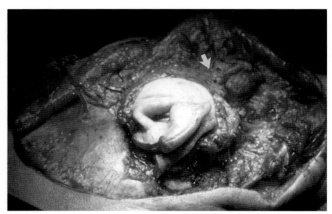

Figure 123-13. Most of the pinna remains with the specimen (see Fig. 123-10). The skin flap is secured anteriorly to expose the parotid gland *(arrow)*. The superior limb of the incision is extended toward the forehead in preparation for an infratemporal fossa approach.

A postauricular incision is made 3 cm behind the postauricular sulcus and extended superiorly toward the temporal area and inferiorly over the mastoid tip into a high cervical skin crease. The neck incision is brought more inferiorly if neck dissection is anticipated. The postauricular skin incision is raised a short distance anteriorly. The dissection is then directed medially through the fibroperiosteal layer over the mastoid cortex. This facilitates obtaining a tight three-layer closure if CSF is encountered. The soft tissue flap is dissected in a subperiosteal plane until the posterior part of the conchal incision is reached. To avoid inadvertent entry into the EAC, a hemostat is placed through the posterior aspect of the conchal incision into the postauricular wound. Once this plane of dissection has been established, the conchal incision is connected circumferentially with the postauricular wound, thus isolating the conchal bowl, EAC, and tumor from the skin flap containing the remainder of the pinna (Fig.

123-11). If there is any doubt about the adequacy of the lateral skin margin, a crescent-shaped segment of skin from the conchal bowl of the pinna is sent for frozen section analysis. The lateral part of the EAC is sutured closed to prevent tumor spillage. The skin flap is dissected anteriorly while staying superficial to the deep temporalis fascia superiorly, the sternocleidomastoid fascia inferiorly, and the parotid fascia anteriorly (Fig. 123-12) until the masseter muscle is identified. This develops an anterior-based skin flap that is retracted forward to expose the entire parotid gland (Fig. 123-13). The skin flap is secured with sutures and rubber bands.

Using a large cutting burr, a complete mastoidectomy is performed to expose the sinodural angle posteriorly, the tegmen mastoideum superiorly, the bony ear canal anteriorly, and the digastric ridge inferiorly. Care is taken to not thin the bony ear canal to the point of exposing the cancer. The horizontal semicircular canal is identified for orientation, and the bone of the zygo-

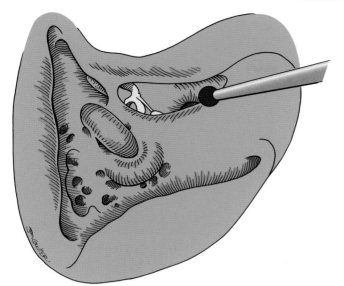

Figure 123-14. The facial recess is dissected to expose the chorda facial angle and the incudostapedial joint.

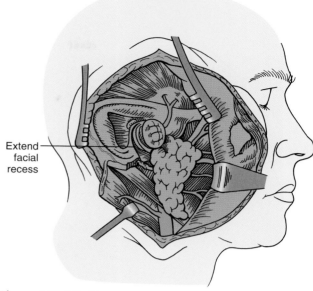

Extend facial recess

Figure 123-15. The operative field is demonstrated. The facial recess is extended inferiorly and then anteriorly by dissecting medial to the tympanic annulus. The stylomastoid foramen is exposed, but the nerve is not dissected free from its surrounding fascia and fibrous tissue.

matic root is drilled to expose the epitympanum and bony plate of the tegmen tympani. Drilling in this area is directed anteroinferiorly toward the posterior aspect of the glenoid fossa. Dissection directed anteriorly poses the risk of penetrating the dura of the middle fossa. The anterior limit of this dissection is the capsule of the TMJ.

A large diamond burr is used to identify the vertical portion of the facial nerve from the second genu to the stylomastoid foramen while maintaining the horizontal semicircular canal and digastric ridge as landmarks. Once the facial nerve has been identified, the facial recess is opened with a small cutting burr, followed by a diamond burr (Fig. 123-14). The middle ear is inspected through the facial recess to verify the absence of penetration of the cancer through the tympanic membrane. The incudostapedial joint is disarticulated and the incus is removed. The tensor tympani tendon is transected. The facial recess is then extended inferiorly by sacrificing the chorda tympani nerve to expose the posterior portion of the hypotympanum. Using a cutting burr, the inferior portion of the tympanic ring is drilled toward the anterior wall of the EAC (Fig. 123-15). Care is taken to not thin the bony EAC extensively to avoid exposure of the cancer. The more medial orientation of the anterior tympanic membrane requires infratympanic drilling directed anteromedially to avoid inadvertent entry into the anterior sulcus of the EAC. This is accomplished by continuing the dissection of the facial recess anteromedially while always keeping the hypotympanum in view. The anterior limit of this dissection is the periosteum between the temporal bone, the ITF, and the capsule of the TMJ. In this area, the surgeon must remain oriented to the location of the eustachian tube orifice to avoid injury to the carotid artery.

Once this bony dissection has been completed, the EAC is attached anteriorly by anteromedial section of

bone just lateral to the eustachian tube. A superficial parotidectomy is performed by identifying the facial nerve distal to its exit from the stylomastoid foramen. After retracting the tail and body of the parotid gland, the main trunk of the facial nerve is traced peripherally to isolate the lateral or superficial portion of the gland. Details of this technique can be found in Chapter 62. Dissection of the facial nerve in the stylomastoid foramen can be difficult because the nerve is surrounded by a thick cuff of fibrous tissue. Meticulous dissection in this area and isolation of the nerve often result in facial paresis or paralysis, which is usually temporary. It is preferable to maintain this cuff of tissue lateral to the facial nerve because less aggressive dissection can allow preservation of facial function. Once the superficial lobe of the parotid gland has been dissected, the EAC and parotid specimens are removed in continuity with the extratemporal portion of the facial nerve under direct vision.

An osteotome is inserted through the extended facial recess to the bone just lateral to the eustachian tube orifice. A few gentle taps on the osteotome will complete the osteotomy, and the EAC can be dissected from the TMJ capsule (Fig. 123-16). During this maneuver care must be taken to avoid injury to the ICA by the osteotome, which lies just medial to the eustachian tube. At this point the specimen is attached only to the parotid gland, the superficial lobe of which can be removed in continuity with the specimen and the facial nerve preserved.

If the operative resection creates a large and deep cavity, the posterior one half of the temporalis muscle is rotated into the surgical defect and secured with 2-0 absorbable suture (Fig. 123-17). The skin flap is

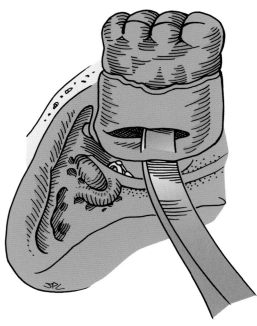

Figure 123-16. The remaining anterior bony attachment is freed with a small osteotome positioned medial to the anterior tympanic annulus.

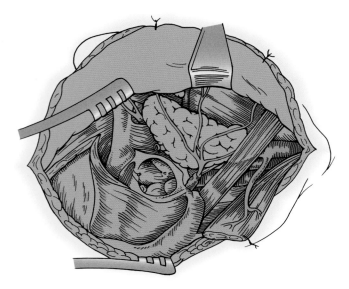

Figure 123-17. A superficial parotidectomy is performed to remove the parotid with the lateral temporal bone specimen. The posterior one half of the temporalis muscle is rotated into the mastoid cavity.

returned to its anatomic position. Hemovac drains are placed both superiorly and inferiorly while avoiding suction trauma to the facial nerve (Fig. 123-18). Small to medium defects are closed with a split-thickness skin graft that is secured with bolster packing consisting of silk ligatures tied over a Xeroform bolster. This technique is described under "Reconstruction" later in this chapter. Larger skin and cavity defects are closed with free or pedicled myocutaneous flaps. A compression

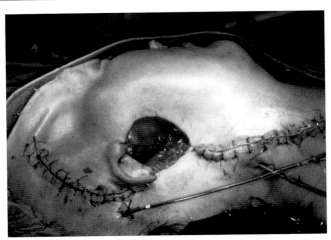

Figure 123-18. Skin closure with Hemovac drains in place. The central cavity defect will be closed with a skin graft.

dressing is applied unless microvascular anastomosis has been performed.

Subtotal Temporal Bone Resection

Cancer extending medial to the tympanic membrane and invading the middle ear, hypotympanum, otic capsule, facial nerve, or mastoid is managed by subtotal resection of the temporal bone. In the past, an en bloc technique of resection was advocated to encompass the tumor. It has been noted that en bloc resection of the EAC with surrounding soft tissue structures followed by piecemeal resection of tumor and structures medial to the middle ear provides better operative control and probably does not negatively influence the cure rate.[24] The strategy is to perform a largely extradural and subperiosteal resection of the temporal bone with margins at the middle fossa dura superiorly, the posterior fossa dura and sigmoid sinus posteriorly, the ICA anteriorly, the base of the skull and jugular bulb inferiorly, and the petrous apex medially. Extension of cancer beyond these boundaries signifies a grave prognosis, but the resection can be extended in certain cases, as discussed later.

The approach for lateral resection of the temporal bone is performed as described previously, with examination of the middle ear through the facial recess and mastoid cavity for cancer. If cancer is present, the more encompassing resection is warranted. If facial nerve function is normal preoperatively and it is visibly clear of tumor as noted during the procedure, a decision is made, based on the extent of cancer, whether the nerve should be sacrificed and included with the specimen. If the nerve is to be preserved, piecemeal resection of the cancer is planned. If the facial nerve is uninvolved, it will be mobilized and preserved as the dissection proceeds. Bone is removed over the sigmoid sinus and posterior fossa dura. The tegmen and posterior fossa plates of bone are first thinned with a cutting burr and then resected piecemeal after dural elevation. These segments of bone are sent for permanent section. Care is taken to not injure the superior petrosal sinus at this

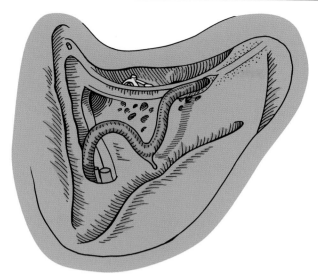

Figure 123-19. The facial nerve, if it is to be preserved, is mobilized by transecting the greater superficial petrosal nerve and transposing the facial nerve posteriorly. The vestibular nerves are divided to gain access to the facial nerve. The cochlear nerve remains intact.

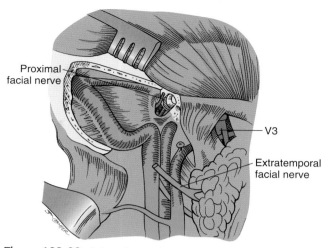

Figure 123-20. Subtotal resection of the temporal bone with the medial margin through the internal auditory canal and cochlea. The vertical portion and genu of the carotid artery are dissected. The vaginal process between the jugular bulb and the carotid artery has been drilled. The extratemporal facial nerve is intact.

stage. Translabyrinthine dissection exposes the IAC and jugular bulb. If cancer is not present at the jugular bulb, no further resection is performed in this area.

If the facial nerve is to be preserved, it is skeletonized along the labyrinthine, geniculate, horizontal, and vertical segments down to the stylomastoid foramen. The eggshell-thin pieces of bone on the anterior, lateral, and posterior aspects of the nerve are removed with a dissector. The dura of the IAC is opened to allow mobilization of the facial nerve at the porus acusticus. The greater superficial petrosal nerve is transected from the geniculate ganglion, and the facial nerve is gently dissected out of its bony canal and mobilized posteriorly (Fig. 123-19). If the facial nerve is to be sacrificed, the dissection and mobilization are omitted, but the IAC is still opened. Both the facial and the vestibulocochlear nerves are transected, and the proximal ends of these nerves are examined by frozen section analysis to ensure a tumor-free medial margin of resection. The remaining tympanic ring inferiorly is then drilled to the periosteum of the skull base. This periosteum protects vascular and neural structures in the ITF and is not resected unless cancer is identified in this area. Bone resection continues along the periosteum anterosuperiorly until the capsule of the TMJ is encountered. Medially, bone dissection is continued until the vertical portion of the ICA is encountered. Care is taken to keep the periosteal covering over this artery intact while drilling with a diamond burr.

If cancer has not infiltrated into the protympanum, the anterior limit of resection can be performed without resection of the mandibular condyle. Absence of cancer in this area can be confirmed intraoperatively by obtaining a frozen section of the mucosal edge near the eustachian tube orifice. The bone lateral and posterior to the vertical portion of the ICA above the jugular bulb

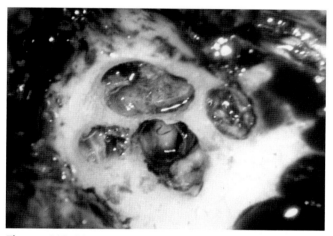

Figure 123-21. Intraoperative dissection through the internal auditory canal and cochlea modiolus for subtotal resection of the temporal bone.

is drilled with a diamond burr to isolate the artery from the otic capsule. Once this has been accomplished, the remainder of the otic capsule containing the cochlea is drilled (Figs. 123-20 and 123-21). The vaginal process between the jugular bulb and the ICA is also drilled out, with only the petrous apex remaining.

Dissection of the Jugular Foramen

If cancer has infiltrated into the jugular bulb, total removal of the cancer requires resection of the sigmoid sinus. If only the lateral aspect of the sigmoid sinus or jugular bulb is involved, resection can be achieved without much added morbidity. Resection of cancer involving the medial wall or pars nervosa of the jugular foramen results in injury to the lower cranial nerves and possibly a larger dural defect.

For cancer that involves only the lateral wall of the sigmoid sinus and jugular bulb, total resection of tumor can be achieved with an ITF approach similar to the Fisch type A. The subtotal temporal bone resection is completed after dissection and isolation of the internal jugular vein (IJV) and cranial nerves IX, X, XI, and XII in the neck. The facial nerve has been either transected or mobilized out of the way. The soft tissues between the posterior belly of the digastric muscle and the IJV are dissected in layers to expose the vein from the skull base to the jugular bulb. The IJV is doubly ligated in the neck with 2-0 silk and divided. The sigmoid sinus inferior to the takeoff of the superior petrosal sinus is tied with 2-0 silk by making stab incisions in the dura on either side of the sigmoid sinus, passing a curved aneurysm needle into and out of the dural opening, and passing the tie around the sigmoid sinus (see Chapter 125, Figs. 125-10 and 125-11). The dural incisions are repaired primarily or with plugs of muscle secured with 4-0 Nurolon. The sigmoid sinus can also be controlled proximally by extraluminal packing with oxidized cellulose.

The retrosigmoid dura is decompressed to the jugular foramen with a diamond drill. The vaginal process has already been resected during the subtotal temporal bone resection. The cancer in the region of the jugular bulb is debulked without entering the lumen. To resect the lateral wall of the sigmoid sinus and jugular bulb, the inferior petrosal sinus feeding into the lumen must be controlled. A large incision is made on the lateral aspect of the jugular bulb, and the medial wall is quickly packed with oxidized cellulose to control bleeding. Once adequate hemostasis has been achieved, the lateral wall of the sigmoid sinus from the superior ligation to the jugular foramen is removed along with the IJV. The medial wall of the lumen is inspected for residual cancer, and the packing in the jugular bulb is reinforced as needed (Fig. 123-22).

If cancer is present on the medial wall of the jugular bulb, the resection must be extended into the pars nervosa. If a decision is made to do this, the medial wall of the jugular bulb is removed, and the contents of the par nervosa are resected, including cranial nerves IX, X, and XI. The adequacy of margins of resection of these nerves proximally and distally is verified by frozen sections, and further resection is completed as necessary. A positive margin proximally will require nerve resection in the posterior fossa, which can be performed through a retrosigmoid approach or through the exposure created by resection of the jugular bulb. The residual bone anteromedial to the jugular foramen can be drilled to the ICA anteriorly and the hypoglossal canal anteromedially. The inferior petrosal sinus may need to be packed again during this maneuver. Any dural defects should be repaired with fascia or pericranium.

If the lower cranial nerves were functional preoperatively and required transection intraoperatively, a tracheotomy is performed for pulmonary toilet and care of aspiration, and a nasogastric feeding tube is placed. Medialization of the vocal cord via a type I thy-

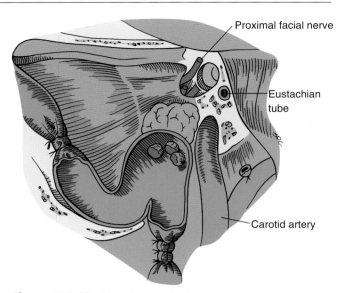

Figure 123-22. Dissection of the jugular foramen when cancer invades the hypotympanum and vaginal process. Resection of the inferior sigmoid sinus and lateral jugular bulb is demonstrated. Oxidized cellulose is packed in the openings in the inferior petrosal sinus. The facial nerve has been resected proximally to the labyrinthine segment. The cochlea has been partially removed. The eustachian tube can be seen.

roplasty or arytenoid adduction can also be performed intraoperatively (see Chapter 41).

Dural Resection

If inspection of the dura reveals residual cancer after subtotal resection of the temporal bone, resection of the dura is performed in collaboration with a neurosurgeon. For cancer in the subtemporal dura, an incision is made in the dura laterally while being careful to not injure the vein of Labbé. The temporal lobe is retracted superiorly to expose the involved dura inferiorly, which is excised with adequate margins. The defect is closed with a fascial or pericranial graft. The presence of invasion into brain parenchyma should have been detected preoperatively. Resection of involved brain tissue may be technically possible, but the probability of cure is exceedingly low.

Involvement of the posterior fossa dura by cancer is treated similarly. Adequate exposure can frequently be obtained through a presigmoid dural incision. The cerebellum is retracted, and the involved dura is excised with appropriate margins. If the medial wall of the sigmoid sinus is involved, the craniectomy is extended posteriorly with a drill to make a retrosigmoid opening in the dura. The lateral wall of the sigmoid has already been resected, and hemostasis at the inferior petrosal sinus has been achieved. The cerebellum is retracted, the involved dura is resected with margins, and the defect is repaired with a fascial or pericranial patch.

Infratemporal Fossa Resection

When cancer infiltrates into the protympanum, additional anterior exposure is needed to transpose the carotid artery and excise soft tissue around the eustachian tube. The superior portion of the incision is extended anterosuperiorly toward the frontotemporal hairline to expose the temporalis muscle. Elevation of the skin flap is performed superficial to the deep temporal fascia until the region of the frontal branch of the facial nerve is reached, at which point the dissection is carried deep to the fascia in the superficial temporal fat pad while avoiding injury to the frontal branch of the facial nerve. This dissection is carried to the lateral rim of the orbit anteriorly and the zygomatic arch inferiorly. Using electrocautery, the periosteum is incised along the lateral edge of the orbital rim and the superior edge of the zygomatic arch. The soft tissue lateral, medial, and inferior to the zygomatic arch is dissected in a subperiosteal plane to release it from the masseter muscle. A V-shaped osteotomy is made in the malar eminence, which consists of the anterior zygoma and lateral maxilla. The zygomatic arch is removed and saved after the osteotomy is completed in the posterior zygomatic root. The temporalis muscle is then dissected off the underlying bone and remains pedicled on the coronoid process of the mandible (Fig. 123-23).

Total parotidectomy is performed by dissecting out the branches of the facial nerve. If the nerve is to be sacrificed and included with the temporal bone dissection, the peripheral branches are identified, tagged, and transected. The superficial temporal artery is divided and the soft tissues overlying the condylar portion of the mandible are resected. Using an oscillating saw, the mandibular condyle is transected at the level of the coronoid notch. The frontal branch of the facial nerve may require transection to provide access to the mandible.

With the temporalis muscle reflected inferiorly, the contents of the ITF are separated from the skull base by dissection in a subperiosteal plane starting anteriorly. The lateral pterygoid plate is encountered first. The foramen ovale is located approximately 1 cm posterior and just medial to this structure, and the foramen spinosum is situated about 0.5 cm posterior to the foramen ovale (Fig. 123-24). The middle meningeal artery is coagulated with bipolar cautery and transected. Now, with the vertical portion of the ICA in view at the skull base, the periosteum of the skull base is elevated in a posterior-to-anterior direction to connect to the dissection at the foramen ovale.

If any tumor is seen within the ITF, it may be resected at this time because the important structures in the region have been identified. The lateral pterygoid muscle is transected in the region of the mandibular osteotomy. The dissection is performed in layers while taking care to not lacerate the internal maxillary artery inadvertently. Any vascular structures that are in the way can be divided and controlled with ties or clips. The venous plexus in the pterygoid region can be the source of significant bleeding, which must be controlled by bipolar cautery and packing with oxidized cellulose.

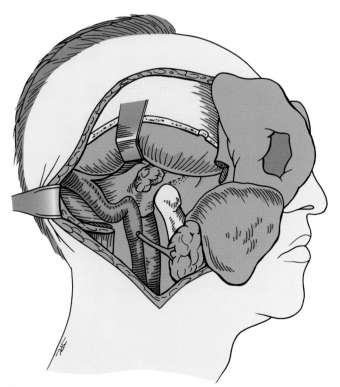

Figure 123-23. Infratemporal fossa approach for cancer invading the eustachian tube and petrous apex. The zygomatic arch has been removed, and the temporalis muscle has been mobilized inferiorly. The mandibular condyle and the parotid gland remain intact.

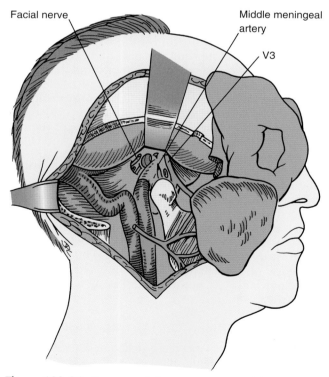

Figure 123-24. Exposure of the petrous apex and infratemporal fossa. A total parotidectomy has been completed. The middle meningeal artery is divided, and the trigeminal nerve (V3) is exposed.

A temporal craniotomy is performed to provide access to the floor of the middle fossa. The middle fossa dura is elevated to expose the IAC posteriorly, the superior petrosal sinus medially, and the foramen ovale and V3 anteriorly. The floor of the middle fossa is then resected posterior to V3 and medial to the eustachian tube with a cutting burr or rongeurs. If tumor invades the eustachian tube with extension into the petrous apex, total resection of the temporal bone is performed.

Total Temporal Bone Resection

Total en bloc resection of the temporal bone with clear margins is conceptually the procedure needed for oncologic control. The vital structures that surround the temporal bone demand that a meticulously controlled approach be performed to avoid catastrophic vascular and neurologic consequences. Even if the carotid artery is to be sacrificed with the specimen, proximal and distal control must be achieved. Similarly, the brain, dura, and cranial nerves must be dissected and isolated. Although a "no-touch" tumor approach remains the technique to which we aspire, it is often not accomplished to safely obtain access to the petrous portion of the temporal bone.

After completion of subtotal temporal bone dissection, proximal control of the ICA is obtained either at the skull base or in the neck. Distal control is achieved in the floor of the middle cranial fossa via middle fossa craniotomy. The carotid artery posterior to V3 is exposed so that a clip can be placed on it for distal control if necessary. The bone lateral to the ICA at the genu is removed, and the ICA is dissected free from its canal from the skull base to the foramen ovale. A thick, fibrous ring of tissue surrounds the ICA at the carotid foramen. When mobilizing this portion of the ICA, it is safer to first dissect circumferentially around the fibrous tissue rather than along the carotid itself because the risk of carotid laceration is high. The fibrous ring can be left intact while the ICA is mobilized. Once adequate exposure has been achieved, the remainder of the otic capsule containing the cochlea is drilled. Anteriorly, the petrous apex is drilled to complete total resection of the temporal bone (Fig. 123-25). The eustachian tube lies inferolateral to the carotid canal at the genu and travels anteromedially. The eustachian tube can be resected anteriorly to the level of the foramen ovale. If cancer is found anterior to this area, nasopharyngeal resection and possibly cavernous sinus dissection will be necessary to achieve total resection, which is beyond the scope of this chapter. The transected end of the eustachian tube is sutured closed to prevent CSF rhinorrhea.

Reconstruction

The goals of soft tissue reconstruction after temporal bone resection include alleviation of cosmetic deformity, prevention of CSF leak, and promotion of adequate healing. In most cases, these objectives are best accomplished with a vascularized flap. To prevent com-

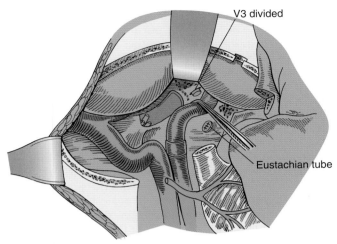

Figure 123-25. Total temporal bone resection. The mandibular condyle is resected. The carotid artery has been spared and is retracted to provide safe access to the petrous apex. Removal of the otic capsule has left a large dural defect. V3 has been divided and the eustachian tube has been suture-ligated. The infratemporal fossa is dissected down to the pharyngobasilar fascia.

munication between the nasopharynx and the middle ear space after lateral temporal bone resection, the eustachian tube is obliterated by scarifying the mucosa and filling the lumen with ossicles, bone dust, Surgicel, or a plug of muscle.

The resultant defect after lateral resection of the temporal bone is similar to that after radical mastoidectomy, and there is usually little risk of CSF leak, so adequate tissue coverage can be accomplished with a split-thickness skin graft to create a mastoid cavity. However, because most patients require radiation therapy after surgery or have previously undergone radiation therapy, we believe that a vascularized flap to promote adequate healing provides the optimal result. The posterior one half of the temporalis muscle is separated from the anterior portion, and while pedicled inferiorly, the posterior portion of the muscle is rotated into the mastoid cavity.

The surgical defect after subtotal temporal bone resection extends medially through the otic capsule and poses a greater likelihood of a CSF leak. If ITF dissection has not been performed, the resultant defect is not significantly larger than one resulting from lateral temporal bone resection. Usually, a pedicled posterior temporalis flap provides adequate coverage. Other options include a lower island trapezius or pectoralis major myocutaneous flap. If these flaps cannot be mobilized superiorly to cover the temporal bone defect adequately, a free flap with microvascular anastomosis to the superficial temporal or facial artery system can be used. The most commonly used free flap is the rectus abdominis, although a scapular or latissimus dorsi free flap can also be used. The TMJ is not reconstructed routinely.

If the facial nerve has been resected and there is an adequate proximal stump, it is reconstituted with a

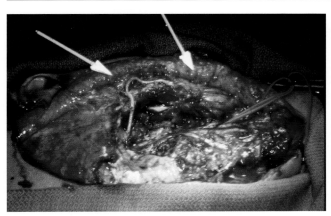

Figure 123-26. Right total temporal bone resection, including the condyle of the mandible. The facial nerve is repaired with a long sural nerve graft (*arrows* at the upper and lower divisions of the remaining nerve).

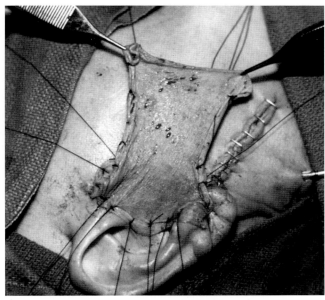

Figure 123-27. A split-thickness skin graft is sutured to the posterior skin margins with 3-0 silk.

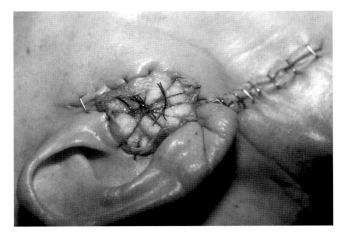

Figure 123-28. The skin graft is contoured to the cavity, immobilized with Xeroform gauze, and secured with 3-0 silk sutures tied over the packing.

cable nerve graft. Most frequently, we use the sural nerve (see Chapter 121). The greater auricular nerve can be used if the length required is less than 6 cm. Otherwise, a sural nerve graft is necessary to obtain a longer donor graft for anastomosis between the proximal and distal ends of the facial nerve (Fig. 123-26). If facial nerve resection has been performed distal to the pes anserinus, both the upper and lower branches are reconstructed. If the proximal stump of the facial nerve has been resected at the brain stem with an inadequate length left for anastomosis, a hypoglossal-to-facial (XII to VII) nerve anastomosis can be performed.

If a CSF leak is a potential problem, the wound should be closed in at least three layers with two layers of 2-0 Vicryl or Dexon for the deep tissues followed by a running and locking horizontal mattress suture consisting of 4-0 Surgilon for the skin. If a conchal defect is closed with a skin graft, this area must be isolated from the remainder of the wound before skin grafting by completely obliterating the space between the pinna flap and the underlying muscle flap with 2-0 and 3-0 absorbable suture.

A split-thickness skin graft (0.015 inch) is secured to 180 degrees of the pinna defect. Sutures of 3-0 silk are kept long to serve as bolster ties. A piecrust technique is used, similar to that for grafting oral cavity lesions. The central aspect of the skin graft is contoured within the cavity defect, and the remaining skin is trimmed to the appropriate size and further secured to the wound margins (Fig. 123-27). The graft is usually packed with Xeroform gauze and secured with a tie-over bolster dressing (Fig. 123-28).

After wound closure, a mastoid dressing is placed and the patient is extubated before transport to the recovery area. Unless a watertight CSF closure has been achieved, drains for the wound are placed to gravity drainage. Continuous suction is applied when the likelihood of CSF permeating the wound is negligible.

POSTOPERATIVE MANAGEMENT

Most patients who undergo lateral resection of the temporal bone require postoperative care comparable with that after routine mastoidectomy, except that the flap requires monitoring. The head should be elevated 30 degrees, and diet and ambulation are advanced as tolerated. The mastoid dressing is removed on the first postoperative day, and any skin graft bolsters are removed on the fifth day. The remaining pinna may have a tenuous blood supply, especially if a large, anteriorly based skin flap was raised. This is usually manifested by increased venous congestion, which can compromise the auricle and the remainder of the wound. If the pinna appears to be in jeopardy, we have used medical-

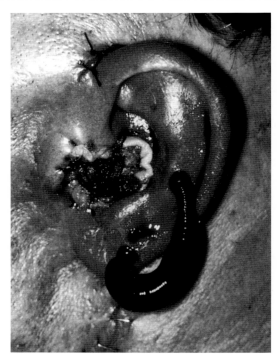

Figure 123-29. Severe venous congestion compromises the auricle. Options for management include stab incisions or leeches, as demonstrated.

grade leeches to assist venous decompression and mobilization of fluid (Fig. 123-29).

If a significant dural defect was created or a considerable amount of brain retraction was necessary during surgery, the patient is managed in a monitored care situation for the first 24 hours for frequent neurologic evaluation and monitoring of vital signs. The level of care needed, which is similar to that after translabyrinthine acoustic tumor surgery, can be given in an intensive care unit or a step-down unit. The patient's intake and output, as well as blood count and electrolytes, are monitored. The mastoid dressing is kept in place for 3 to 5 days, although on the second postoperative day the dressing is removed to check the wound and then replaced. The patient is monitored for CSF rhinorrhea or CSF leak through the wound, and any suspicious fluid is sent for β_2-transferrin testing. The patient is instructed to not strain or perform a Valsalva maneuver for 3 weeks. We do not routinely place a lumbar drain intraoperatively, although it has been done on occasion if a large dural defect is expected or if neck dissection has been performed and there is possible communication between the neck wound and the subarachnoid space. The patient can be transferred to surgical floor care if no significant intracranial complications have occurred.

If ITF dissection with resection of the mandibular condyle has been performed, the patient is encouraged to mobilize the mandible as soon as possible to promote maintenance of a proper occlusal relationship and to decrease the risk of fibrous ankylosis. Our colleagues in oral surgery are consulted to oversee this aspect of the patient's recovery.

If a free flap has been performed, the patient and wound are closely monitored by clinical findings and Doppler ultrasound examination of the vascular anastomosis. Care is taken to not place any ties around the patient's neck that could potentially constrict the vascular pedicle to the flap. Any evidence of significant flap ischemia should be detected early so that intervention to salvage the flap, which may include revising the anastomoses, can be performed immediately.

Patients who have facial nerve palsy or paralysis postoperatively are treated with eye drops during the day and ointment at night to avoid exposure keratitis and corneal ulceration. A plastic eye shield (moisture chamber) is useful in protecting the eye. If facial nerve function is expected to return within 4 to 6 weeks, as occurs after facial nerve transposition, the patient usually requires no further treatment. If recovery from facial nerve dysfunction is expected to take longer or if the dysfunction may be permanent, a gold weight is placed in the upper eyelid and a lateral tarsal strip is performed if ectropion becomes a problem. These procedures are performed in the early postoperative period (see Chapter 121). If facial nerve function fails to recover, a hypoglossal-to-facial (XII to VII) nerve anastomosis can subsequently be performed.

A patient with new iatrogenic lower cranial nerve palsy or paralysis is at significant risk for aspiration and resultant pulmonary infection. The patient should be placed in a step-down unit for frequent suctioning through the tracheostomy. Nutrition is provided through a feeding tube while the patient undergoes swallowing rehabilitation coordinated by a speech pathologist. This rehabilitation includes clinical assessment as well as evaluation by modified barium swallow and performance of various swallowing exercises customized for each patient. Once the patient is handling secretions adequately with competent glottic function, the tracheotomy tube is removed to enhance recovery of deglutition. The feeding tube is removed when the patient is able to ingest adequate nutrition by mouth. If adequate swallowing function cannot be attained, a gastrostomy tube is placed.

Immediate postoperative scans are not performed unless the patient is showing evidence of an intracranial complication such as hemorrhage, abscess, hydrocephalus, or pneumocephalus. Baseline postoperative scans consisting of MRI or CT, or both, are obtained within 3 months after surgery to help monitor for recurrent disease. These scans are repeated every 6 months for the next 2 years and yearly thereafter.

Reconstruction with a split-thickness skin graft over a vascularized muscle flap creates minimal cosmetic deformity (Fig. 123-30). If the entire pinna has been resected, reconstruction options are a prosthetic ear or multistaged procedures in a surgical bed that is compromised. Given the problems inherent in reconstruction of the pinna, our preference is for a prosthesis. Using either the preoperative ipsilateral ear or a reverse moulage of the contralateral ear, a synthetic prosthesis can be created that is both functionally and cosmetically acceptable (Fig. 123-31).

Radiation treatment is begun approximately 6 weeks after surgery, when adequate wound healing has occurred. The most common area of recurrence of cancer is locally, in the skull base, dura, or ITF, so these areas are treated specifically. The neck is also treated, especially zones II and III, although the risk of failure here is much less than the risk of failure locally.

COMPLICATIONS

The goal of surgical treatment of cancer of the temporal bone is to achieve total removal of the cancer with minimal morbidity. Avoidance of complications is critical to successful rapid rehabilitation of the patient post-operatively. Aggressive temporal bone resection may be associated with major intracranial complications. Extensive brain retraction can result in lower cranial nerve palsy with aspiration, cerebellar or temporal lobe edema

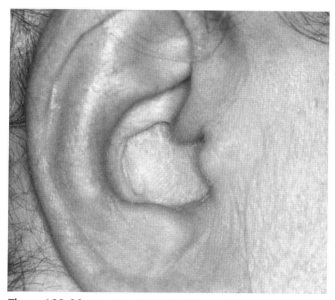

Figure 123-30. A well-healed split-thickness skin graft at the meatal opening. The size of the defect does contract to provide an acceptable cosmetic appearance.

and dysfunction, and cerebral infarction. The vein of Labbé is particularly vulnerable, and compression of this vein can lead to temporal lobe venous infarction. Dissection of the ICA can result in embolic stroke, injury with bleeding, and stroke. The dura must be carefully reconstructed because CSF leaks in this setting can be difficult to control and are a major risk for meningitis.

Vascular

Major arterial injuries can cause disastrous consequences, and all precautions should be taken to prevent these injuries. Most moderate-sized vessels such as branches of the internal maxillary artery can be controlled adequately, even in the event of inadvertent laceration. However, the ICA requires more complex management. The need for possible surgical dissection near the ICA should be ascertained preoperatively by CT and MRI and by angiography if necessary. If it is determined that carotid mobilization or dissection may be required, preoperative balloon test occlusion with xenon/CT is performed. The data obtained provide an estimate of ipsilateral regional cerebral blood flow while the carotid is temporarily occluded for 15 minutes. These results place patients in one of three risk groups for the development of major cerebral ischemia in the event of abrupt carotid interruption: high, intermediate, and low. Approximately 80% of patients will be in the low-risk group, and these patients are likely to tolerate permanent carotid occlusion. About 10% will be in the high-risk group. These patients will not tolerate any duration of carotid occlusion, so operative therapy involving carotid manipulation should be avoided unless bypass to the middle cerebral artery is performed initially. The remaining 10% of patients will be in the intermediate-risk group. These patients require carotid revascularization if the ICA is sacrificed and the use of adjuvant methods to minimize cerebral ischemia, such as induced hypertension, barbiturate coma, and hypothermia.[30]

Intraoperatively, before manipulation of the ICA, proximal control of the vessel in the neck or at the skull base and distal control in the horizontal portion of the intrapetrous carotid artery should be obtained. In this way, should an inadvertent injury to the ICA occur,

Figure 123-31. A, Total auricular resection with only the tragus remaining. **B,** A prosthetic pinna provides excellent cosmetic appearance and function.

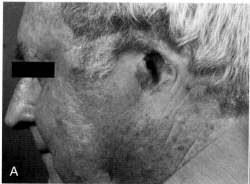
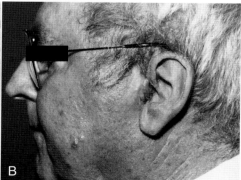

rapid control of the situation can be achieved so that the injury can be managed in an expeditious and controlled fashion. If a laceration of the ICA occurs, it is managed by either primary repair, repair with a patch, bypass grafting using the saphenous vein, or sacrifice of the ICA without reconstruction.

Venous complications are also possible after temporal bone resection, especially if manipulation or resection of the sigmoid sinus is performed. The vein of Labbé is an important route of venous outflow from the temporal lobe, and damage to this vein can lead to significant temporal lobe infarction with aphasia if on the dominant side and seizures. The best strategy for managing this complication is prevention. When packing or ligating the sigmoid or transverse sinus it is important to stay far anterior to the insertion of the vein of Labbé into the transverse sinus. Once an infarct occurs, therapy consists of speech and language rehabilitation, neurologic support, and administration of antiseizure medications such as phenytoin (Dilantin) and phenobarbital.

Cerebrospinal Fluid Leak

The main morbidity of a CSF leak is increased risk for the development of meningitis. Because meningitis can be a life-threatening condition, prevention plus control of CSF leaks is very important. CSF leaks occur when there is inadequate closure of the dura in conjunction with a path for egress of CSF through the soft tissues to the external environment. The usual sites of leakage are the eustachian tube, incision site, and remnant of the EAC.

Prevention is the most efficacious method of management. All dural closures should be made as watertight as possible. Any potential dead spaces should be obliterated by placement of muscular flaps or autologous fat grafts. The final barriers to CSF flow, skin closure and the eustachian tube, should be closed or obliterated in watertight fashion. A drain is not placed in the wound. Postoperatively, the patient's head is kept elevated and the patient is instructed to avoid straining or performing a Valsalva maneuver. A pressure dressing is maintained for 5 days.

Despite preventive treatment, CSF leaks can occur, and when they do, prompt management can prevent serious consequences. The critical factor is early diagnosis. The patient should be instructed to report any egress of clear fluid from the nose or any drip down the nasopharynx. Oftentimes, the diagnosis is obvious and no further testing is required. β_2-Transferrin testing of fluid will identify CSF.[31] However, if the physician is clinically suspicious that a CSF leak has occurred, action must be taken despite test results to the contrary.

If the leakage occurs through an incision, the area of dehiscence is reinforced with horizontal mattress sutures. Topical collodion liquid is also useful. Most CSF leaks that persist for more than 24 hours despite maintenance of a pressure dressing and head elevation can be controlled with the placement of a lumbar drain. The lumbar drain is allowed to drain approximately 150 mL/day, or 50 mL per 8-hour shift. Care must be taken to not overdrain CSF, because severe headaches may develop and there is the potential that the negative pressure may permit air and other nonsterile fluids to enter the subarachnoid space from the wound. The use of antibiotics prophylactically in the setting of a CSF leak is controversial. In the event of a CSF leak into a clean surgical wound, the authors think that antibiotic prophylaxis does not reduce the incidence of meningitis and may in fact increase the risk of having a resistant organism in patients in whom bacterial meningitis does develop.

If the CSF leak persists after 3 to 5 days of lumbar drainage, a surgical procedure to stop the leak is indicated. Usually, the uncontrolled CSF leak is through the eustachian tube. A transmastoid procedure through the previous incision is performed to access the eustachian tube and obliterate it in a more complete fashion. This can be accomplished by further scarification of the mucosa followed by insertion of bone dust, Surgicel, and muscle plugs. Occasionally, the source of a CSF leak in the dural repair will be visible. In such cases, the dural closure can be reinforced with patches of fascia or muscle sewn over the dural defect. The wound is closed in multiple layers, as described previously, in watertight fashion, and a mastoid dressing is placed for 5 days. Lumbar drainage is continued for the next 3 days and the drain removed if there is no further CSF leak.

A very difficult problem occurs if an extensive neck procedure is performed at the time of temporal bone resection with dural resection. Because the neck requires drainage temporarily after surgery, a CSF leak into the neck can occur quite readily. This becomes a potentially serious problem when a tracheostomy is in place. Great effort is necessary to ensure that the tracheostomy wound does not communicate with the neck dissection. Otherwise, CSF will readily pass subcutaneously through the neck into the trachea and exit out the tracheotomy wound. Similarly, tracheal secretions colonized with bacteria can infect the neck and CSF space by retrograde contamination and create a very serious infection.

Infection

Wound infections occur infrequently after resection of the temporal bone. Appropriate treatment is no different from treatment elsewhere in the head and neck. A more feared complication is meningitis or other intracranial infection such as a brain abscess. The risk of meningitis developing after resection of the temporal bone and requiring intracranial surgery is low in the absence of a CSF leak, so prompt and effective treatment of such leaks is critical. Symptoms of meningitis include fever, severe headache, backache, and altered sensorium. There may or may not be focal neurologic deficits. The diagnosis is made by lumbar puncture. A third-generation cephalosporin is administered intravenously after samples are obtained for culture. A CT scan with contrast enhancement is obtained to rule out an intracranial abscess. It is difficult to differentiate aseptic meningitis from bacterial meningitis based on clinical findings and laboratory values, so antibiotics are continued until culture results are available in 2 days. If the cultures are negative and clinical suspicion of bacterial meningitis is not high, the antibiotics are stopped and steroids (dexamethasone [Decadron], 4 mg intravenously every 6 hours) are given and tapered over a period of several weeks. If the cultures are positive or the patient's clinical status is suggestive of bacterial meningitis, the antibiotics are tailored to the culture results and continued for 10 to 14 days.

Aspiration pneumonia is a possible complication after temporal bone resection, especially if previously functional lower cranial nerves are sacrificed or injured during surgery. In these cases, a type I thyroplasty with or without vocal cord medialization and a tracheotomy are usually performed at the time of surgery. The patient is fed through a feeding tube until aspiration stops and the patient is able to swallow. Aggressive pulmonary toilet is provided while the patient undergoes rehabilitation for deglutition and airway protection. Aspiration pneumonia is treated with culture-specific antibiotic therapy and further aggressive pulmonary toilet.

Intracranial Hemorrhage and Hypertension

Although neurosurgical procedures have become relatively safe, there is still a risk of acute intracranial complications after temporal bone resection involving intradural manipulation. One of the most rapidly progressive and potentially fatal complications is acute intracranial hemorrhage, which if not treated promptly can lead to irreversible cerebral injury with uncontrolled cerebral edema or brain stem herniation and even death. Preventing this complication obviates the urgent management necessary for this event. All patients should be screened by history and physical examination for bleeding disorders. If detected, the disorder should be treated adequately before surgery. Intraoperatively, all bleeding sites must be well controlled before closure of the wound. Postoperatively, the patient should remain normotensive and refrain from vigorous activities.

The signs of acute intracranial hemorrhage are due to increased intracranial pressure, as manifested by altered sensorium or loss of consciousness. Focal neurologic deficits, including fixed and dilated pupils and systemic signs such as bradycardia and hypertension, can also occur, but lack of these changes does not rule out an intracranial hemorrhage. The location of hemorrhage can be extradural, subdural, or intraparenchymal. Most extradural hematomas are due to bleeding from dural vessels or dural sinuses. Subdural hemorrhage occurs as a result of dural bleeding, as well as uncontrolled bleeding from intracranial vessels. Intraparenchymal hemorrhage is rare after the resection of extra-axial lesions.

Once an intracranial hemorrhage is suspected, a CT scan without contrast enhancement is performed to confirm the diagnosis. The patient's condition is temporized by the administration of mannitol, 0.25 to 0.5 g/kg intravenously, and hyperventilation after intubation. If the patient's vital signs are unstable or there is evidence of brain stem herniation, the patient is brought directly to the operating room without scanning. A lumbar puncture should never be performed in this setting for fear of inducing brain stem herniation through the foramen magnum. A ventriculostomy can be performed to rapidly decompress the increased intracranial pressure. The craniectomy or craniotomy is reopened, and the blood clot is evacuated. The source of bleeding is sought and controlled.

Postoperatively, the patient is monitored in an intensive care unit setting with maintenance of ventriculostomy pressure under 15 mm Hg. A CT scan is obtained to rule out further hematoma, and the patient is allowed to recover.

Wound

Management of wound complications after temporal bone resection is similar to that in other areas of the head and neck, except that CSF leak is a potential problem, as discussed previously. The integrity of the flap used to obliterate the operative defect is vital to keep the subarachnoid space separated from the outside environment. Complications that can compromise this function are ischemia and separation of the flap from the wound.

It is unusual for ischemia to develop in pedicled flaps, but it occurs occasionally if the flap is stretched too far or if strangulation of the vascular pedicle occurs as a result of significant constriction placed inadvertently around the neck. Injury to the vascular pedicle intraoperatively can also occur but is rare. If the pedicled flap becomes nonviable, it should be replaced immediately with an alternative flap, whether it is another pedicled flap or a free flap. Free flaps are more susceptible to ischemic complications than pedicled flaps are, and careful monitoring in the postoperative period by clinical evaluation and Doppler ultrasound is performed to detect any impending vascular pedicle compromise. If vascular compromise does occur, the patient is taken back to the operating room to revise the vascular anastomosis.

Flap separation leading to wound dehiscence occurs most frequently at the distal edge of a pedicled flap. The cause is usually placement of the flap under too much tension or local necrosis of the distal portion of the flap. If an intact bed of granulation exists within the wound and there is no evidence of a CSF leak, conservative wound management with dressing changes to allow healing by secondary intention is adequate. In the presence of a CSF leak, the wound should be revised immediately. If the tip of the flap is necrotic but an adequate extra length of flap is available, the flap revision is performed by advancing the new distal end to cover the entire wound. If there is not enough length, a second pedicled or free flap should be used to either close the residual wound or replace the old flap entirely.

SUMMARY

Cancer of the temporal bone is a challenging disease to treat effectively. Modern management of this disease consists of combined-modality therapy, including surgery to remove all evident disease and radiation therapy to treat the margins of resection. The surgical procedure of choice depends on the extent of disease and consists of lateral resection of the temporal bone; subtotal resection of the temporal bone; subtotal resection of the temporal bone with extension to the ITF, jugular foramen, or dura; and total resection of the temporal bone, which also includes removal of the petrous apex. In the event of facial nerve sacrifice, primary reconstruction with a cable graft is performed. Postoperative radiation therapy should encompass the resection margins, residual parotid gland, ITF, and ipsilateral neck.

PEARLS

- Always consider the possibility of cancer in a patient with chronic otorrhea, especially if the patient has severe pain, a mass or ulcer, or facial paralysis or if the patient does not respond appropriately to medical management.
- Perform both CT and MRI to assess the bone and soft tissue anatomy and the extent of disease.
- Management of temporal bone cancer includes adequate resection, usually with lateral or subtotal temporal bone resection, and in most cases, postoperative radiation therapy.
- The cure rate is 80% to 100% for T1 and T2 cancers but remains limited for late-stage disease, with a mortality rate of 50% or higher.
- Compromise of facial nerve function requires diligent care of the eye.

PITFALLS

- Performance of a mastoidectomy for staging or biopsy is never appropriate.
- Failure to achieve adequate margins will probably ultimately result in treatment failure.
- Large defects should not be closed by local tissue advancement; free flaps are more appropriate in selected patients.
- Failure to obliterate the eustachian tube may result in nasopharyngeal reflux and infection or CSF rhinorrhea when the dura is incompletely closed.
- Insufficient venous drainage may compromise the vascular integrity of the remaining pinna.

References

1. Devaney KO, Boschman CR, Willard SC, et al: Tumours of the external ear and temporal bone. Lancet Oncol 6:411-420, 2005.
2. Kenyon GS, Marks PV, Scholtz CL, et al: Squamous cell carcinoma of the middle ear. A 25-year retrospective study. Ann Otol Rhinol Laryngol 94:273-277, 1985.
3. Lim V, Danner C, Colvin GB, et al: Primary basal cell carcinoma of the middle ear presenting as recurrent cholesteatoma. Am J Otol 20:657-659, 1999.
4. Takahashi K, Yamamoto Y, Sato K, et al: Middle ear carcinoma originating from a primary acquired cholesteatoma: A case report. Otol Neurotol 26:105-108, 2005.
5. Jin YT, Tsai ST, Li C, et al: Prevalence of human papillomavirus in middle ear carcinoma associated with chronic otitis media. Am J Pathol 150:1327-1333, 1997.
6. Lim LH, Goh YH, Chan YM, et al: Malignancy of the temporal bone and external auditory canal. Otolaryngol Head Neck Surg 122:882-886, 2000.
7. Lustig LR, Jackler RK, Lanser MJ: Radiation-induced tumors of the temporal bone. Am J Otol 18:230-235, 1997.
8. Donaldson JA: Surgical Anatomy of the Temporal Bone, 4th ed. Philadelphia, Lippincott Williams & Wilkins, 1992.
9. Arriaga M, Curtin H, Takahashi H, et al: Staging proposal for external auditory meatus carcinoma based on preoperative clinical examination and computed tomography findings. Ann Otol Rhinol Laryngol 99:714-721, 1990.
10. Austin JR, Stewart KL, Fawzi N: Squamous cell carcinoma of the external auditory canal. Therapeutic prognosis based on a proposed staging system. Arch Otolaryngol Head Neck Surg 120:1228-1232, 1994.
11. Gillespie MB, Francis HW, Chee N, et al: Squamous cell carcinoma of the temporal bone: A radiographic-pathologic correlation. Arch Otolaryngol Head Neck Surg 127:803-807, 2001.
12. Leonetti JP, Smith PG, Kletzker GR, et al: Invasion patterns of advanced temporal bone malignancies. Am J Otol 17:438-442, 1996.
13. Moffat DA, Wagstaff SA, Hardy DG: The outcome of radical surgery and postoperative radiotherapy for squamous carcinoma of the temporal bone. Laryngoscope 115:341-347, 2005.
14. Zhang B, Tu G, Xu G, et al: Squamous cell carcinoma of temporal bone: Reported on 33 patients. Head Neck 21:461-466, 1999.
15. American Joint Committee on Cancer Staging: Manual for Staging of Cancer, 3rd ed. Philadelphia, JB Lippincott, 1988.
16. Moody SA, Hirsch BE, Myers EN: Squamous cell carcinoma of the external auditory canal: An evaluation of a staging system. Am J Otol 21:582-588, 2000.
17. Nyrop M, Grontved A: Cancer of the external auditory canal. Arch Otolaryngol Head Neck Surg 128:834-837, 2002.
18. Politzer A: A Textbook of Diseases of the Ear. London, Baillier Tindadl & Cox, 1883.
19. Parsons H, Lewis JS: Subtotal resection of the temporal bone for cancer of the ear. Cancer 7:995-1001, 1954.
20. Lederman M: Malignant tumours of the ear. J Laryngol Otol 79:85-119, 1965.
21. Graham MD, Sataloff RT, Kemink JL, et al: Total en bloc resection of the temporal bone and carotid artery for malignant tumors of the ear and temporal bone. Laryngoscope 94:528-533, 1984.
22. Conley JJ, Novack AJ: The surgical treatment of malignant tumors of the ear and temporal bone. Part I. Arch Otolaryngol 71:635-652, 1960.
23. Lewis JS, Page R: Radical surgery for malignant tumors of the ear. Arch Otolaryngol 83:114-119, 1966.
24. Kinney SE: Squamous cell carcinoma of the external auditory canal. Am J Otol 10:111-116, 1989.
25. Spector JG: Management of temporal bone carcinomas: A therapeutic analysis of two groups of patients and long-term followup. Otolaryngol Head Neck Surg 104:58-66, 1991.
26. Prasad S, Janecka IP: Efficacy of surgical treatments for squamous cell carcinoma of the temporal bone: A literature review. Otolaryngol Head Neck Surg 110:270-280, 1994.
27. Nakagawa T, Kumamoto Y, Natori Y, et al: Squamous cell carcinoma of the external auditory canal and middle ear: An operation combined with preoperative chemoradiotherapy and a free surgical margin. Otol Neurotol 27:242-248, discussion 249, 2006.

28. Grandis JR, Hirsch BE, Yu VL: Simultaneous presentation of malignant external otitis and temporal bone cancer. Arch Otolaryngol Head Neck Surg 119:687-689, 1993.

29. de Vries EJ, Sekhar LN, Horton JA, et al: A new method to predict safe resection of the internal carotid artery. Laryngoscope 100:85-88, 1990.

30. Ariyan S, Sasaki CT, Spencer D: Radical en bloc resection of the temporal bone. Am J Surg 142:443-447, 1981.

31. Skedros DG, Cass SP, Hirsch BE, et al: Beta-2 transferrin assay in clinical management of cerebral spinal fluid and perilymphatic fluid leaks. J Otolaryngol 22:341-344, 1993.

Chapter 124

Acoustic Neuroma

Barry E. Hirsch, Michele St. Martin, and Amin B. Kassam

Acoustic neuroma (AN) is the most common benign tumor arising in the posterior cranial fossa. The term *acoustic neuroma* is a misnomer, in that the tumor typically arises from the vestibular rather than the auditory division of the eighth cranial nerve and is of Schwann's cell origin. Thus the proper nomenclature would be *vestibular schwannoma*. These tumors are thought to originate near Scarpa's ganglion where the density of Schwann's cells is greatest. The origin of the tumor is equally divided between the superior and the inferior divisions of the vestibular nerve. Typically, these tumors are benign and slow growing, increasing in size, on average, from 1 to 2 mm a year; however, more rapid or slower growth characteristics are also observed. The consistency can be soft, firm, or mixed, with cystic components as well.

HISTORY

Surgery of AN was first described in the late 19th century. Early successful surgical resection was accomplished through a suboccipital craniotomy, removing the tumor by finger dissection.[1] Surgical mortality was unacceptably high owing to the fact that many patients were moribund preoperatively. Two of the early pioneers in AN surgery were Harvey Cushing and his protégé, Walter Dandy. During the first 3 decades of the 20th century, Cushing refined his philosophy of management of AN to recommend a bilateral suboccipital craniectomy approach and advocated unhurried resection and meticulous hemostasis. He also employed partial cerebellar resection when necessary. His techniques for hemostasis included the use of bone wax, silver clips, and electrocautery.[2,3] Unfortunately, he gutted only the core of the tumor; thus many patients subsequently died of tumor regrowth.

The concept of total tumor removal was advanced by Dandy, who reintroduced a unilateral suboccipital approach with gentle but complete resection of the tumor capsule.[4] The first translabyrinthine craniotomy was performed by F. H. Quix in 1911.[5] This approach was condemned by the neurosurgical community until the early 1960s when the translabyrinthine approach was perfected by William House in conjunction with his neurosurgical colleague, William Hitselberger. Their use of an operating drill and microscope to directly access the tumor with preservation of the facial nerve set the stage for the new era of surgery for AN.[6]

Methods for diagnosing AN have significantly improved over the past century. Tomography has enabled the identification of enlargement of the internal auditory canal (IAC). Myelography required injection of contrast material into the subarachnoid space; the contrast was floated into the IAC by patient positioning. Contrast-enhanced computed tomography (CT) eliminated much of the morbidity associated with myelography, reduced the amount of radiation exposure, and increased the sensitivity of diagnostic radiographic tests. Since the mid-1980s, magnetic resonance imaging (MRI) has become the state-of-the-art in diagnosing ANs. Tumors as small as 1 to 2 mm may be readily identified on MRI.

Audiometric tests have undergone similar sophisticated improvements over time. A battery of special tests, including Bekesy's audiometry, alternating binaural loudness balance test, short-increment sensitivity index, and tone decay, are now of only historical importance for use in categorizing cochlear or retrocochlear hearing loss. Identifying decay of the acoustic reflex or reduced word discrimination at higher presentation levels (rollover) is suggestive of retrocochlear pathology. The auditory brain stem response (ABR) test is now the most specific and sensitive objective audiometric test for diagnosing AN. It had been reported that an abnormal ABR might be identified in 96% of tumors. Recent publications have shown that the ABR test may be normal (false-negative) in 31% of patients with tumors less than 1.0 cm.[7] The greater sensitivity of MRI testing now allows discovery of small tumors limited to the IAC.

PATIENT PRESENTATION

Patients with a small tumor isolated to the IAC typically complain of unilateral hearing loss, tinnitus, and occasionally vestibular dysfunction. A few patients experience sudden hearing loss. Recurrent acute attacks of vertigo are an unlikely presentation for AN. However, disequilibrium with motion intolerance may be present. Patients may describe unilateral difficulty in discerning speech. This becomes more apparent when the telephone is used in the involved ear. Patients complaining of this problem should be evaluated with MRI. Facial nerve dysfunction is a rare presenting sign. Slow progressive weakness may occur with larger tumors. Patients complaining of headaches prompt the request for MRI, which may demonstrate an otherwise asymptomatic acoustic neuroma.

Very large tumors not only compromise hearing and facial function (paresis, synkinesis) but also may affect other cranial nerves causing hypesthesia, analgesia, dysesthesia, dysphagia, aspiration, and hoarseness. Coarse-beating nystagmus on ipsilateral gaze, fine-beating nystagmus on contralateral gaze (Brun's nystagmus), and ataxia with a broad-based gait are manifestations of compression of the brain stem and cerebellum.

PATIENT SELECTION AND COUNSELING

Since the mid-1980s, MRI has evolved to be the state-of-the-art in identifying AN. Enhanced CT with thin cuts taken 0.6 mm apart through the IAC is also capable of identifying tumors as small as 3 to 5 mm, but this is less sensitive than MRI.

Management of posterior fossa tumors suspected of being an AN is dependent on numerous factors. Currently, there are three options for therapy: surgery, irradiation, and observation. In the first option (surgical resection), surgery can be performed through three main approaches along with their modifications—the middle fossa, translabyrinthine, and retrosigmoid approaches. It is assumed that complete resection will be accomplished, although on rare occasion, subtotal removal may be planned. In the second form of therapy (irradiation), methods for delivery include cobalt radiation by gamma knife surgery and photon beam radiation by a linear accelerator. Stereotactic radiation has traditionally been delivered by neurosurgeons; however, neurotologists are now actively participating in this treatment modality as well.[8] The third option for management is to perform no immediate intervention but to observe and monitor tumor growth with serial MRI.

Goals of treatment include either complete resection in the case of surgery, or prevention of growth in the case of radiation, while minimizing morbidity and mortality.[9] Preservation of facial nerve function and hearing function are secondary goals. Surgical mortality is typically less than 1% for acoustic neuroma resection, with an overall morbidity rate of 22%.[9] Recurrence following surgical resection is approximately 1.5%.[9] In their discussion, Kaylie and McMenomy conclude that microsurgery is the treatment of choice for acoustic neuroma due to higher growth rates following radiation versus surgery, comparable postoperative cranial nerve function, and the risk of radiation-induced malignancy.[9] However, the authors acknowledge that following radiation, the quality of life measures are better, and return to work occurs more quickly.

Many physicians agree that observation is often appropriate for older patients or those with small tumors. Patients opting for observation must be informed of the natural history of AN, particularly the risk of hearing deterioration or sudden hearing loss. A recent publication from Denmark found that 89% of tumors less than 1.5 centimeters that were observed for 3 to 4 years demonstrated tumor growth and/or further hearing loss.[10] However, a meta-analysis of 903 patients treated initially with observation found that only 20% ultimately required intervention.[11] It has also been reported that 50% of patients with class A or B hearing will lose useful hearing if observed.[12] Patients must be aware of potentially increased surgical risk if intervention becomes necessary at an older age.[13]

The best results of microsurgery are seen in centers with high patient volumes and experienced surgical teams.[13] Additionally, better results are seen in the later stages of a surgeon's career due to the learning curve.[14] The advantage of surgical resection is the ability to achieve complete tumor removal with very low rates of recurrence. However, recurrence rates of up to 20% can be seen in cases of subtotal resection.[11] Meta-analysis of 5005 patients undergoing microsurgery between 1972 and 1999 indicates a good facial nerve outcome (House-Brackmann Grade 1-2) in 87%, and a 36% rate of useful hearing preservation.[11] Potential complications include hearing loss, cerebrospinal fluid (CSF) leak, facial weakness, headaches, meningitis, cerebrovascular accident, and death. In the best case scenario, hearing may be preserved in approximately 50% of patients who have useful hearing preoperatively.[13,15] Hearing preservation rates vary by approach: 53% of patients had useful hearing preserved via the middle fossa approach, while this rate dropped to 30% with the retrosigmoid approach as reported by Harsha.[15] Therefore patients should be aware of the risk of hearing loss. Patients should be made aware of subsequent alternatives for aural rehabilitation including the CROS, BiCROS, and Baha hearing devices.

Facial nerve outcomes are affected by the size of the tumor, with tumors larger than 1.5 cm having an increased risk of facial weakness postoperatively. Facial

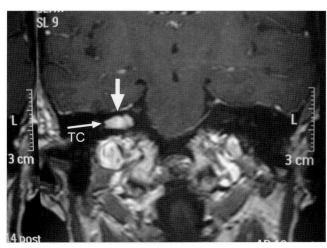

Figure 124-1. T1-weighted magnetic resonance image with contrast showing a right internal auditory canal acoustic neuroma located laterally in the fundus *(arrow)*, above and below the transverse crest (TC).

nerve outcomes are better when surgery is performed in a center doing a high volume of such surgery. Rates of good facial nerve function are 93% for middle fossa, 97% for retrosigmoid, and 78% for translabyrinthine approaches in series of at least 100 patients.[15] However, it should be noted that patients' self-reports of facial nerve function are often worse than the surgeon's assessment.[16]

The case of a patient with good preoperative hearing but tumor located laterally in the IAC deserves special mention. When the tumor extends laterally into the fundus, particularly if it is of inferior vestibular nerve origin, the transverse crest will likely preclude total tumor resection via the middle fossa approach (Fig. 124-1). Additionally, it is difficult to achieve full tumor resection while preserving hearing through a retrosigmoid approach in this case as well. Therefore such patients may opt for a translabyrinthine approach, knowing that hearing loss will be traded for more complete tumor resection and possibly a lower chance of facial weakness.[13]

Radiosurgery offers the advantage of outpatient treatment and minimal recovery time, and affords excellent tumor control with low rates of cranial nerve dysfunction.[17,18] Many reports indicate that improved hearing and facial nerve results are seen following stereotactic radiosurgery (SRS) compared with microsurgery.[19-21] In a series of patients treated at the University of Pittsburgh with gamma knife radiosurgery using a median dose of 13 Gy, a 97.1% rate of tumor control was achieved with 1.1% rate of facial weakness, 2.6% rate of trigeminal nerve dysfunction, and 71% rate of "hearing level preservation."[22] However, high-frequency hearing loss following SRS has been shown to correlate with maximal cochlear dose and transient evoked otoacoustic emissions (TEOAEs) worsened in 75% of patients who had measurable TEOAEs before treatment.[23] At the University of Florida, linear accelerator-based SRS results on 108 patients with AN treated after 1994 included a 93% rate of radiologic control, 5% rate

of facial neuropathy, and 2% trigeminal neuropathy.[24] A meta-analysis of 1475 patients treated with gamma knife radiosurgery between 1969 and 2000 documented an 8% rate of tumor growth and an 8% rate of trigeminal or facial neuropathy, and 4.6% of patients ultimately required microsurgery.[25] Hydrocephalus may also develop following radiosurgery, requiring placement of a ventriculoperitoneal shunt.[26] Patients must be informed of the eight cases of possible malignant transformation reported in the literature, as well as the possibility that future surgical resection may be more difficult.[13,24,27] Some centers also offer conventionally fractionated radiotherapy for AN.[28] The principles and details regarding our use of CyberKnife SRS are provided in Chapter 125.

Recent investigations have addressed quality of life following treatment for AN. Several studies suggest that SRS offers improved posttreatment quality of life compared with microsurgery.[20,29] Myrseth and colleagues reported better facial nerve function, as well as better Glasgow Benefit Inventory and SF-36 scores, in patients treated with gamma knife versus microsurgery. A prospective trial conducted at the Mayo Clinic showed that patients undergoing microsurgery experienced a decline in several subscales of the Health Status Questionnaire postoperatively; this decline was not seen in patients treated with gamma knife radiosurgery.[20] Additionally, the Dizziness Handicap Inventory scores were better for the gamma knife group.[20]

Understanding the typical growth characteristics of AN facilitates the physician's decision regarding what treatment should be offered to the patient. Overall, we consider surgical resection to be the preferred method in the management of AN in young (younger than 65 years of age), healthy patients. An estimation of the patient's longevity must be considered. Patients who are otherwise healthy and have a family history of survival into their late ninth decade can be considered for surgical intervention. Patients between 65 and 70 years of age are evaluated on the basis of factors that include their health, neurologic examination, tumor size, tumor location, rate of growth, hearing status in each ear, and family medical history. We acknowledge that gamma, electron, or proton beam radiation should also be considered effective alternative methods for stopping tumor growth. In the face of documented growth of the tumor, we recommend radiation for patients older than 70 years of age or for patients who have tumors beyond the IAC who are medically unstable. We offer the option of photon beam or gamma radiation to patients who have a recurrence of a previously resected tumor. We also recommend radiation to patients who have had subtotal removal of a large tumor where total resection might have the potential to produce adverse surgical morbidity. In the elderly or medically compromised patient, a small tumor without associated neurologic symptoms other than unilateral hearing loss can be followed over time, observing for evidence of tumor growth. Repeat MRI is obtained in 6 months to compare tumor size. If tumor growth becomes manifest, radiation treatment is suggested, and if no growth has occurred, the MRI scan will be repeated in 6 months. The interval increases to yearly and then every 3 years if there is no change in the size of the tumor.

A treatment program must be individually tailored for each patient with bilateral ANs (neurofibromatosis-2 [NF-2]). NF-2 patients may have other associated intracranial tumors or tumors of the spinal cord and must be diligently examined and imaged to determine the tumor status as well as their medical stability for intracranial surgery. The size of the tumors and the hearing status must be accurately determined. Management options include surgical resection, surgical decompression to allow for tumor growth, radiation, and observation. Until recently, we considered radiation therapy to be a reasonable alternative in the management of bilateral tumors. However, the poor hearing results following gamma radiation do not justify this method as the preferred, exclusive treatment alternative when hearing is intact. Furthermore, the long-term outcome of irradiating NF-2 tumors is unknown at this time. Given that these tumors often present in young people, it may be necessary to follow them for periods up to 50 years. If tumor growth occurs despite radiation therapy, complete surgical removal may be technically more difficult because of the radiation therapy, with greater likelihood of neurologic consequences. We have had experience using an auditory brain stem implant inserted at the time of tumor removal for patients with bilateral ANs. The device provides sound awareness to an anacoustic ear but has not provided the excellent speech recognition achieved with cochlear implants. In summary, one must judiciously decide which patient would be ideally suited for radiation therapy.

Other than the exceptions noted previously, most patients are considered to be surgical candidates for excision of the tumor. Various factors must be evaluated in order to formulate a treatment plan. The status of the patient's hearing is the predominant issue that dictates the surgical approach. There is great controversy as to what is considered useful hearing. Patients with hearing thresholds better than 50-dB speech reception threshold (SRT) and 50% speech discrimination (DISC) (word recognition) are considered candidates for a hearing preservation procedure. However, the size and location of the tumor must be taken into account when attempting to save hearing. It can be argued that any hearing should be preserved in order to provide sound localization. Thus hearing levels of 70 dB SRT and 30% DISC may be considered usable hearing suitable for a hearing aid. Hearing in the contralateral side must also be considered. If hearing function is normal in the uninvolved ear, then preservation of poor hearing will not be psychoacoustically useful to the patient. Patients with tumors that extend greater than 2 cm into the cerebellopontine angle (CPA) are unlikely to have preservation of hearing regardless of the preoperative hearing status. However, if preoperative hearing is good, it is reasonable to attempt hearing preservation through a retrosigmoid approach if the tumor does not extend laterally to the fundus of the IAC.

The translabyrinthine approach is used to remove tumors in most patients with hearing levels greater than 50-dB SRT and less than 50% DISC. This approach may also be used in patients with good hearing, if the tumor extends past the transverse crest in the IAC and the patient is willing to sacrifice hearing for more complete tumor resection. The translabyrinthine approach is reported to have a 9% rate of postoperative CSF leak, and depending on the size of the tumor, a 73% rate of House-Brackmann Grade I-II facial function. This rate increases to 78% in high-volume centers.[15] The translabyrinthine approach is also used for NF-2 patients with poor hearing in whom an auditory brain stem implant is anticipated.

The retrosigmoid approach is useful for patients with serviceable hearing and greater than 0.5-cm tumor extension into the CPA. We also favor the retrosigmoid approach for removing very large tumors when the brain stem is compressed and shifted to the contralateral side. The disadvantage of this approach is its limited access to the lateral IAC. The retrosigmoid approach has been reported to have a 30% rate of hearing preservation overall, a 92% rate of House-Brackmann Grade I-II facial function at all centers, and an 11% rate of postoperative CSF leak. Notably, there is a 21% rate of postoperative headache following this approach.[15]

The middle fossa approach is useful for excising tumors that are contained within the IAC or that extend less than 0.5 cm into the CPA at the porus. Furthermore, caution must be observed for patients older than 60 years of age. The dura in these patients is often thin and subject to lacerations. This may be accompanied by annoying venous bleeding, making the middle fossa dissection challenging and making obtaining a watertight dural closure difficult. This approach offers a 53% rate of hearing preservation overall and an 89% rate of House-Brackmann Grade I-II facial function.[15] Rates of hearing preservation correlate with tumor size and vary by center, and may be improved with near field whole eighth nerve monitoring in small tumors.[30] For tumors with more than 10-mm extension into the CPA, there is a higher postoperative rate of hearing loss and facial weakness when the middle fossa approach is used.[31] There is a 6% rate of postoperative CSF leak and 8% incidence of postoperative headaches.[15]

PREOPERATIVE PLANNING

A complete history is obtained regarding symptoms including hearing status and tinnitus. Patients are questioned regarding difficulty with ambulation, dysequilibrium, and vertigo. A history of headaches, facial twitching, hypesthesia, or difficulty with voice or swallowing is sought.

Physical examination is focused on cerebellar function and the cranial nerves of the posterior fossa. Extraocular movements are observed, looking for gaze-evoked nystagmus. Facial and corneal sensations are tested in order to evaluate the sensory distribution of the trigeminal nerve. Facial movements are observed, seeking evidence of weakness. The lower cranial nerves are assessed by testing oropharyngeal tactile sensation and vocal cord mobility. The patient's tandem gait is observed, and other evidence of cerebellar dysfunction, including dysmetria and dysdiadochokinesia, is sought.

A complete audiogram, consisting of air and bone pure-tone thresholds and speech audiometry, is obtained. Identifying rollover (worsening word recognition with increased presentation levels) further supports a retrocochlear lesion. Despite knowing that a patient has a posterior fossa tumor suggestive of an AN, ABR is frequently obtained, especially when hearing function is present. Evidence of interpeak latency shifts or change in waveform morphology is investigated. Furthermore, if good waveforms are readily identifiable, the ABR test provides a useful baseline for intraoperative auditory monitoring if a hearing preservation procedure is undertaken (Fig. 124-2).

Once a presumed diagnosis of AN is made, vestibular testing may be obtained. The findings on caloric stimulation provide information regarding the degree of vestibular loss owing to the tumor. A significantly reduced vestibular response informs the surgeon and patient that postoperative vertigo and dizziness should be at a minimum. The findings of reduced responses on caloric stimulation are considered to be indicative of superior vestibular nerve function. This information may be useful when planning a middle fossa approach. Normal residual caloric responses imply sparing of the superior vestibular nerve and the tumor originating from the inferior vestibular nerve. Unfortunately, the finding of a reduced vestibular response to caloric stimulation is not diagnostic of superior vestibular nerve tumor origin. It has been shown that a reduced caloric response can be demonstrated in 60% of tumors arising from the inferior division (Fig. 124-3).[32] In summary, we do not routinely obtain vestibular testing in diagnosing or planning treatment for patients suspected of having an AN.

Radiologic imaging is critical in diagnosing and managing a tumor in the posterior fossa. A presumptive diagnosis of an AN is determined by the location and shape of the tumor along with its signal characteristics without and with contrast. The tumor size has an inverse relation to the likelihood of preserving preoperative hearing. The larger the tumor, the less likely that the cochlear nerve and function can be maintained. As tumors get larger than 2 cm, hearing preservation is rarely successful. The same concern exists for the facial

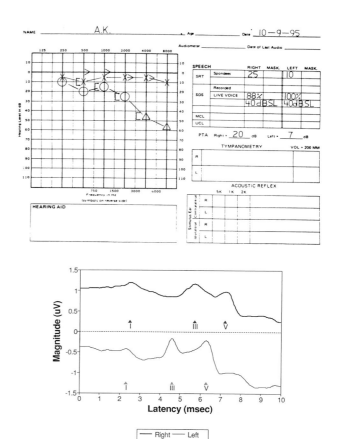

Figure 124-2. A, Audiogram of a 24-year-old patient complaining of right hearing loss. Note high-frequency sensorineural loss with reduced word recognition score. **B,** Auditory brain stem response of the same patient demonstrating a right interpeak latency shift of I-III and I-V intervals consistent with retrocochlear pathology.

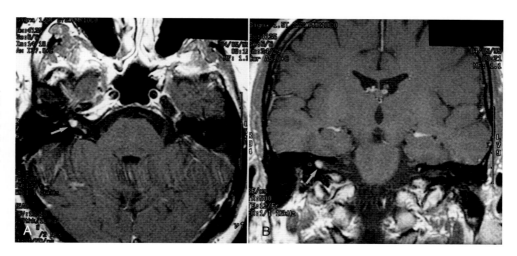

Figure 124-3. T1-weighted contrast-enhanced axial **(A)** and coronal **(B)** magnetic resonance imaging scans. Note the right inferior vestibular nerve schwannoma *(arrows)* located in the posteroinferior fundus of the internal auditory canal (IAC).

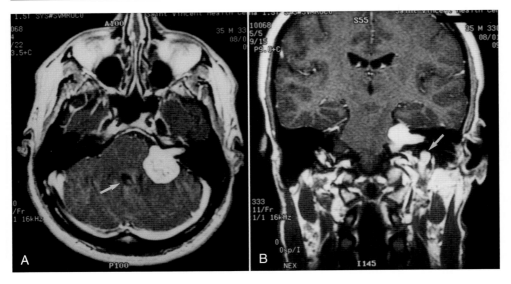

Figure 124-4. T1-weighted contrast-enhanced magnetic resonance imaging scan of a left acoustic neuroma. **A,** Axial image showing a 3-cm tumor with compression of the brain stem. The fourth ventricle is patent *(arrow)*. **B,** Coronal image demonstrating the inferior extent of the tumor. Note the relationship to the jugular fossa *(arrow)*.

nerve. The removal of large tumors is more likely to produce postoperative facial paresis or paralysis. Also, facial nerve outcomes in cystic tumors have been reported to be worse than in solid tumors.[33]

The MRI scan demonstrates the relationship of the tumor to the surrounding brain. Brain stem compression may obstruct the fourth ventricle with resultant hydrocephalus. The scan is also reviewed to determine whether the tumor impinges on the fifth or lower cranial nerves. Removal of large tumors may produce postoperative corneal and facial hypesthesia from manipulation of the trigeminal nerve. Similarly, tumor extending inferiorly low in the posterior fossa can affect cranial nerves IX, X, and XI (Fig. 124-4). The surgeon and patient must both be prepared for a possible postoperative swallowing and laryngeal dysfunction.

The MRI scan is also reviewed in order to determine the lateral extent of the tumor. Patients with good hearing and tumor limited to the IAC and extending to the fundus are candidates for a middle fossa approach (Fig. 124-5). Patients with good hearing and tumor 0.5 cm beyond the IAC into the CPA should undergo a retrosigmoid approach if hearing is to be preserved. However, tumor extending and filling the fundus cannot be removed under direct microscopic vision. Owing to limitations posed by the otic capsule, the posterior wall of the IAC cannot be completely drilled laterally, exposing the fundus. Identifying tumor within the fundus on MRI requires thorough evaluation of this area at the time of surgery.

The location of the jugular bulb can be determined from the MRI scan. Blood and flow signal can be seen on T1- and T2-weighted images. However, a more accurate assessment of the bony and vascular anatomy of the temporal bone is obtained with a CT scan. We frequently obtain a thin-cut bone-windowed CT scan when a hearing preservation procedure is planned or when the jugular bulb is suspected on MRI of creating an anatomic obstacle. The noncontrast bone-windowed

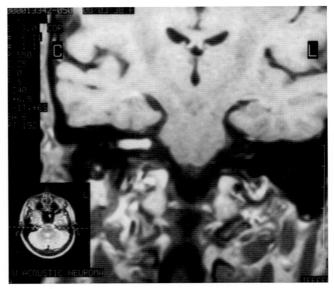

Figure 124-5. T1-weighted contrast-enhanced magnetic resonance imaging scan of a right acoustic neuroma extending toward the fundus, filling the internal auditory canal. The transverse crest is not well outlined.

study shows the pneumatization of the temporal bone relative to the IAC (Fig. 124-6). Knowing preoperatively that the petrous bone is well pneumatized provides additional landmarks when drilling around the IAC via a middle fossa or retrosigmoid approach.

Collating the data presented previously helps determine which surgical approach is most appropriate and provides information that may be predictive of successful preservation of hearing. Negative predictive factors include tumor size greater than 2.0 cm, evidence of widening of the IAC, tumor extension laterally to the fundus, and poor waveform morphology on ABR testing.[34,35]

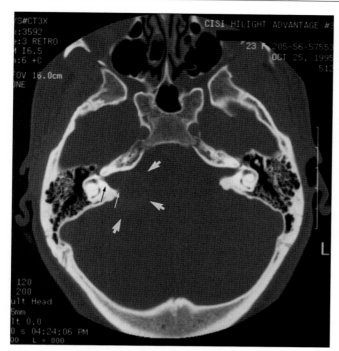

Figure 124-6. Bone algorithm computed tomography scan of a right acoustic neuroma. Note widening of the internal auditory canal. Approximately 7 mm of bone from the posterior lip of the porus acusticus can be drilled safely before the posterior semicircular canal is entered (*small arrows*). *Large arrows* outline the margin of the tumor.

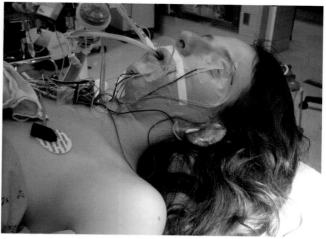

Figure 124-7. Before turning the patient into the appropriate position for the procedure, electrodes are inserted for monitoring the cranial nerves and somatosensory potentials.

Informed Consent

An excellent discussion of informed consent in acoustic neuroma treatment was published in 2005.[13] The author stressed the importance of a balanced and unbiased discussion of treatment options, which is most easily afforded by a multidisciplinary team having experience with both radiation and surgical modalities of treatment. The decision process must be individualized for each patient. There are numerous factors that must be considered when formulating a treatment plan, both in the mind of the physician and in what is proposed to the patient. These factors include the chronologic and physiologic age and health of the patient; characteristics of the tumor such as size, location, and rate of growth; a family history or presence of multiple intracranial tumors (NF-2); hearing status of the ipsilateral and contralateral ear, ABR waveform morphology, if obtained; and the functional status of their vestibular system. Surgeons should be aware that patients make their treatment choices using information given to them by physicians, patient education pamphlets, Internet searches, discussions with other patients, and published data.[36] The inclination of the patient regarding their preference for surgical or radiation treatment influences their thought process. Some patients wish to avoid surgery at any cost; other people are distressed with the realization that tumor is present within their head and prefer surgical excision. The importance of a comprehensive and understandable informed consent cannot be overemphasized. It is most important to discuss with the patient and family the location of the tumor and its relationship to the surrounding vascular, dural, and neural structures. The treatment options of observation, surgical removal, or radiation therapy are reviewed. The risks, benefits, and outcomes are explained. Although the physician may influence the patient's thinking, the final decision for treatment rests with the patient.

SURGICAL TECHNIQUE

Anesthesia

Removal of an AN is performed with the patient under general endotracheal anesthesia. Long-acting muscle relaxants are avoided in order to permit monitoring of the facial nerve. Short-acting muscle relaxants are employed at the start of the procedure during induction and intubation and following completion of tumor removal when final facial nerve thresholds are determined. Anesthesia is maintained with inhalation agents, narcotics, and barbiturates. Neurophysiologic monitoring is conducted for all procedures. This consists of electrode placed to monitor cranial nerves V, VI, VII, VIII, and X. Even if hearing is absent or to be sacrificed with a translabyrinthine approach, the contralateral ear is monitored because it provides feedback regarding the status of the contralateral brain stem. Somatosensory potentials are also evaluated during the case, reflecting the integrity of the lower brain stem and peripheral nervous system (Fig. 124-7). A urinary catheter is inserted, and antithrombotic stockings with sequential compression devices are placed. The infraumbilical area of the abdomen is shaved and prepared for potential removal of an adipose tissue graft.

Translabyrinthine Approach

A postauricular C-shaped incision begins 2 cm superior to the root of the auricle. The incision extends

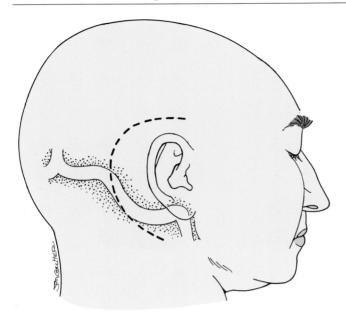

Figure 124-8. Incision for a translabyrinthine approach. The transverse and sigmoid sinuses are illustrated.

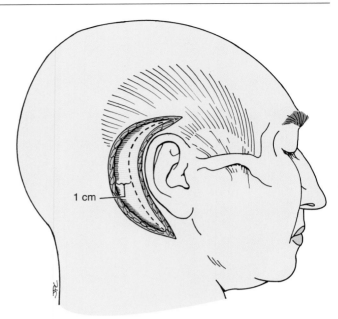

Figure 124-9. The deeper incision divides the temporalis muscle just superior to the linea temporalis and continues in a curvilinear direction through the fibroperiosteal layer over the mastoid cortex, 1 cm anterior to the posterior skin flap.

posteriorly and inferiorly 4 cm posterior to the postauricular sulcus. It continues inferior and anterior to the mastoid tip (Fig. 124-8). Superiorly, the skin incision extends to the depth of the temporalis fascia. An anterior-based skin flap is developed superficial to the temporal fascia and fibroperiosteum overlying the mastoid cortex. A second or more medial anterior-based flap is created, consisting of incised temporalis fascia and muscle and mastoid fibroperiosteum. This is developed just anterior to the posterior edge of the skin incision (Fig. 124-9). A small piece of temporalis muscle deep to the temporalis fascia is harvested from the superior limit of this flap.

Two self-retaining retractors are placed 90 degrees to one another. Using a large cutting burr and suction irrigation, a transcortical mastoidectomy is performed. Once the antrum has been identified, the bone dissection is enlarged to expose the lateral and inferior aspect of the middle fossa dura, sinodural angle, sigmoid sinus, and mastoid tip. The posterior bony canal wall is thinned to fully expose the antrum, fossa incudis, epitympanum, and air cells over the facial recess. The bone overlying the sigmoid sinus and retrosigmoid posterior fossa dura must be removed. This is initially accomplished with cutting and then using diamond burrs. Preservation of an island of bone (Bill's island) over the sigmoid sinus minimizes direct trauma to the wall of the sinus from retraction (Fig. 124-10).

In order to obtain a watertight closure and avoid CSF rhinorrhea, the eustachian tube is obliterated through an extended facial recess approach. The incus is separated from the stapes and removed. The posterior buttress is drilled to increase exposure of the middle ear. Pieces of Surgicel and muscle are placed through the enlarged facial recess directly into the

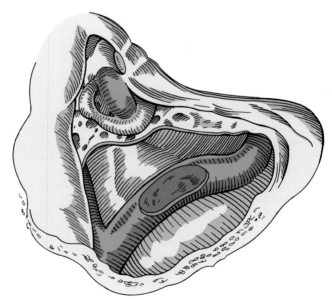

Figure 124-10. The transmastoid approach requires exposure of the middle and posterior fossa dura, leaving an island of bone over the sigmoid sinus. The antrum is opened, and the incus is identified. The posterior bony canal wall is thinned, with a bone remaining over the vertical facial nerve. The digastric ridge is outlined inferiorly.

eustachian tube (Fig. 124-11). If space permits, the short process and body of the incus are also placed into the eustachian tube after removing the incus long process. Additional small pieces of Surgicel and muscle are placed into the eustachian tube orifice.

A labyrinthectomy is then performed. The dissection continues through the horizontal semicircular

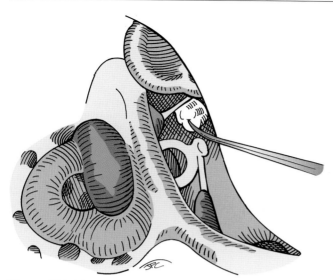

Figure 124-11. The incus is removed from the fossa incudis, and the facial recess is extended by drilling the posterior buttress. The eustachian tube is packed with Surgicel and muscle using a curved pick.

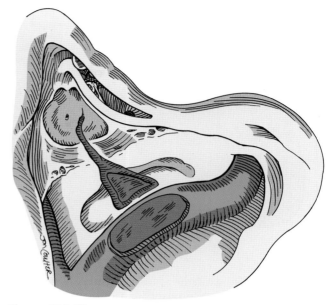

Figure 124-12. A labyrinthectomy has been completed, opening into the vestibule. The more medial bone of the middle fossa tegmen and posterior fossa is removed. The endolymphatic duct and sac are identified. The subarcuate artery may persist in the solid angle.

canal, which is used as the initial landmark for the horizontal segment and second genu of the facial nerve. A thin shell of bone is left over the distal horizontal, second genu, and vertical portions of the facial nerve. The pink color of the nerve can be seen through the bone. The labyrinthectomy is taken through the vestibule and the medial wall of the otic capsule. It is necessary to remove all bone from the middle and posterior fossa dura, sinodural angle, and jugular bulb. This is initially accomplished with cutting and then using diamond burrs. Once the bone is of appropriate thickness, it can be removed with a dissecting instrument such as a Lempert, Penfield, duckbill, Freer, or Cottle elevator (Fig. 124-12).

The IAC is skeletonized for at least 180 degrees of its posterior circumference. It is important to remove bone both superior and inferior to the IAC. During the exposure of the inferior aspect of the IAC and dome of the jugular bulb, the cochlear aqueduct is entered and CSF is typically encountered (Fig. 124-13). The trough superior to the IAC and inferior to the middle fossa dura is drilled cautiously. The lateral aspect of the IAC is further dissected with a small diamond burr. In addition to drilling the IAC laterally to the fundus, a trough superior to the IAC is developed to provide access to the superior and lateral aspect of the tumor (see Video 124-1). The final bony dissection is over the labyrinthine portion of the facial nerve. At this point, Bill's bar, separating the facial nerve and superior division of the vestibule nerve, is identified.

The dome of the jugular bulb may extend superiorly to the level of the IAC. This limits the working space for addressing both the IAC and CPA portions of the tumor. It is necessary to decompress this area of its overlying bone. The lining over the jugular bulb is thin so caution is needed when drilling over this area. Once the bone is removed, a neuropatty may be used to

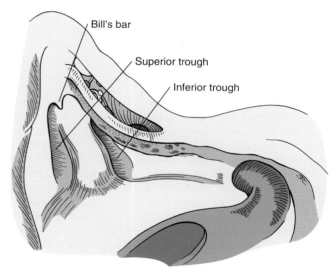

Figure 124-13. The IAC is skeletonized, creating a superior and an inferior trough. Bill's bar is identified. Bone from the posterior lip of the porus acusticus must be removed. The cochlear aqueduct is located superior to the jugular bulb.

further compress the bulb inferiorly. Placing Surgicel under the neuropatty provides compression and packing of this area. The inferior trough can then be completed with jugular bulb displaced inferiorly from the surgical field (see Video 124-2).

The presigmoid dura is coagulated with bipolar cautery to obtain surface hemostasis. The dura and periosteum of the IAC are cut in a lateral-to-medial direction to give access to the IAC. The posterior fossa dura is cut sharply beginning just anterior to the sigmoid

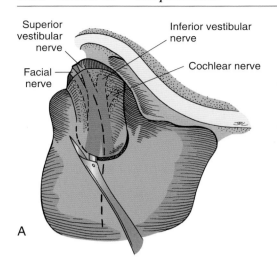

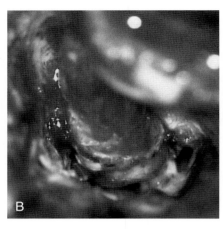

Figure 124-14. **A,** The incisions in the IAC and posterior fossa dura are demonstrated. **B,** The IAC is dissected circumferentially, creating a superior and an inferior trough. The posterior fossa dura is opened.

sinus. The incision of the dura continues toward the dural ring, defining the posterior rim of the porus. It then continues both superior and inferior to the IAC, providing wide access to the posterior fossa (Fig. 124-14; see also Video 124-3). The dural over the IAC is then opened. A McElveen knife permits dissection with a rounded tip and then cutting of the dural with the sharp portion of the instrument (see Video 124-4). The lateral insertion of the superior vestibular nerve is sharply dissected away from the facial nerve. Tumor present laterally in the fundus will be encountered at this time and is also sharply dissected away from the facial nerve.

Small tumors limited to the IAC and the area of the porus can be removed in a lateral-to-medial direction. Unless the cochlear nerve is involved, it is best to leave it undisturbed, so as to avoid any potential injury to the perineural vessels that may also supply the facial nerve. The facial nerve monitor and stimulator are invaluable for performing this procedure. The minimal current output of the nerve stimulator should be used in order to establish current thresholds.

When operating on large tumors, the specimen will need to be removed in a piecemeal fashion. The tumor is initially dissected in a subarachnoid plane. Prominent surface vessels are coagulated with bipolar cautery. When most of the tumor is in the CPA, the capsule of the tumor is entered with sharp dissection (Fig. 124-15). Tumors with a firm consistency may need to be softened with cup forceps. Sections of the tumor are then removed with scissors dissection or Takahashi's forceps. Bipolar cautery not only assists in control of hemostasis but also shrinks the tumor, facilitating removal. The location of the facial nerve must be verified before cautery is applied. More rapid debulking of the central part of the tumor is accomplished with ultrasonic aspiration. The facial nerve is usually stretched over the anterior and medial surface of the tumor but, in some cases, may be located either inferiorly or superiorly. Rarely, the facial nerve is in a posterosuperior location. Debulking of the central part of the tumor leaves the tumor capsule with the adherent facial nerve. Identifi-

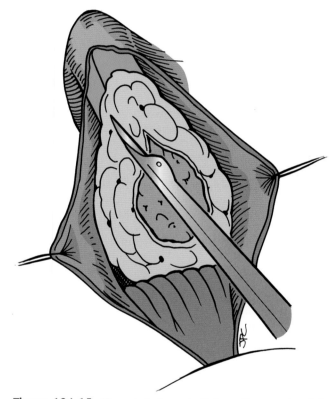

Figure 124-15. Hemostasis is controlled on the capsule of the tumor with bipolar cautery. The tumor surface is entered with sharp dissection. The core of the tumor is then removed. The facial nerve is frequently located on the anterosuperior pole of the tumor.

cation of the facial nerve and cochlear vestibular complex at the brain stem facilitates removal of residual tumor. Care is taken to identify and preserve the anterior inferior cerebellar artery (AICA), which often lies between the seventh and the eighth nerves. The tumor capsule is moved posteriorly and inferiorly. The facial nerve stimulator is used to locate the facial nerve or its root entry zone on the brain stem. Cutting the proximal stump of the eighth nerve facilitates removal of the

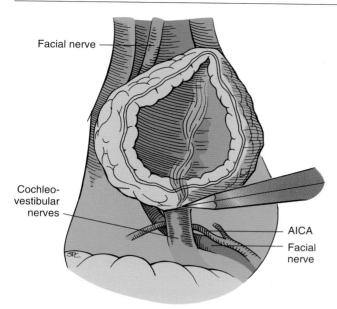

Figure 124-16. After the tumor is debulked, the capsule may be moved posteriorly and inferiorly to identify the proximal facial nerve and cochleovestibular bundle. A loop of the anterior inferior cerebellar artery (AICA) is frequently found between the nerves. The proximal end of the tumor is coagulated with the bipolar cautery and the cochleovestibular nerves are transected.

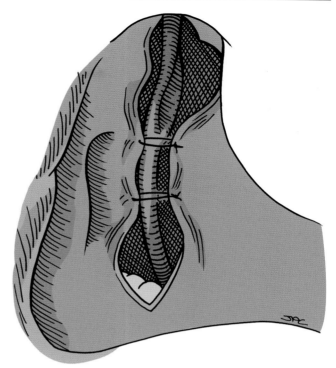

Figure 124-17. The remaining edges of the porus and posterior fossa dura are reapproximated to support the fat graft. Note the ribbon-like attenuation of the facial nerve at the porus.

tumor (Fig. 124-16; see also Video 124-5). Dissection is then continued from the medial to the lateral direction. The remaining tumor capsule is sharply dissected away from the facial nerve. The wound, dura, and posterior fossa are irrigated with saline solution. Hemostasis is ensured with bipolar coagulation.

Disrupting the facial nerve in order to completely remove an AN is a rare occurrence. However, when it does occur, effort should be made to repair the nerve primarily. With the nerve having been stretched by the enlarging tumor, primary reapproximation may be feasible. Owing to the lack of epineurium, it may be difficult to get more than one 8-0 nylon suture placed to reapproximate the disrupted ends of the facial nerve. A few drops of fibrin glue may be used to further secure the anastomosis. This is facilitated by placing small pledgets of Gelfoam around the reapproximated nerve ends. If there is inadequate length to perform a primary anastomosis, then a cable graft using the sural or greater auricular nerve is performed.

The edges of the posterior fossa dura are reapproximated using interrupted or running 4-0 dural sutures (silk or Nurolon). A convenient needle to use in this tight area is an Ethicon TF-4.[11] Complete closure is not possible owing to the dural defect at the IAC. Similar to a clothesline, the suture spans the dura defect, providing a lattice support for the next step of obliteration of the wound with adipose tissue (Fig. 124-17; see also Video 124-6). Abdominal fat, harvested from the infraumbilical area of the abdomen, is soaked in the bacitracin solution. Pieces of fat and temporalis muscle that were obtained earlier in the procedure are placed through the facial recess, filling the middle ear. The

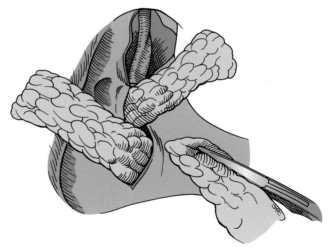

Figure 124-18. The ends of strips of fat are placed through the dural openings into the posterior fossa.

aditus is completely blocked with muscle. A small piece of Surgicel secures the muscle plug. The abdominal fat is then cut into strips and advanced through the dural defect (Fig. 124-18). The remainder of the mastoid cavity is also packed with abdominal fat. Fibrin glue is applied around the fat (see Video 124-7). The wound is closed in three layers. The mastoid cortical defect is covered with a titanium plate fixed to the temporal bone with self-tapping screws. The fibroperiosteal and temporalis muscle fascial flap is closed with interrupted sutures. The subcutaneous skin flap is also approximated with the same suture. A running interlocking 4-0 Nurolon suture closes the skin. Skin staples may also be used. Antibiotic ointment and a Telfa pad are placed over the incision, and a sterile pressure dressing is applied.

Middle Fossa Approach

The patient is positioned supine on the table and placed in a Mayfield head holder with the head turned with the involved ear facing the ceiling. The hair is shaved in the preauricular region from the tragus to the superior temporal line. Electrodes for facial nerve monitoring are placed. In order to monitor the ABR, a sound source is placed into the ear canal affixed with a foam rubber plug and bone wax to secure the ear phone. This is covered with an Op-Site dressing, and the area is prepared and draped. Extraction of fluid from the soft tissue of the brain permits easier retraction of the temporal lobe. Techniques used to shrink and soften the brain include removal of CSF via a spinal drain, mild dehydration using intravenous mannitol and furosemide, and lowering the patient's partial pressure of carbon dioxide (Pco_2) through hyperventilation. A lumbar drain, although not used routinely, is inserted after induction of general anesthesia by turning the patient in a lateral position. The patient is returned to the supine position once the catheter has been secured. Mannitol and furosemide are given at the time the skin incision is made.

The design of the skin incision depends in part on the surgeon's preference but also on the goal of the surgery. Figure 124-19 shows three common modifications of the preauricular skin incision used for the middle fossa approach to the IAC. We prefer an inci-

sion that extends vertically with a slight curve at the superior extent depicted by line B. The incision is outlined, and a solution of 1% lidocaine (Xylocaine) with 1 : 100,000 epinephrine is injected to help with hemostasis during the initial elevation of the skin flap. Once the skin and subcutaneous tissues have been incised and the skin flaps undermined, the area of the temporalis fascia and muscle above the root of the zygoma will be exposed. The temporalis muscle is incised in order to create an inferiorly based pedicled flap at its origin. The temporalis muscle is cut along the linea temporalis above the mastoid and continues vertically and superiorly to the superior temporal line. A cuff of fascia and periosteum is preserved superiorly for suture reapproximation at the conclusion of the procedure. Anteriorly, the descending temporalis muscle incision divides the muscle body as it extends toward the zygomatic arch. A periosteal elevator is used to mobilize the temporalis muscle inferiorly to the root of the zygoma. Hemostasis is obtained with bipolar coagulation or bone wax. The temporalis muscle is also retracted inferiorly with a 2-0 Dexon or silk suture. The external auditory canal, root of the zygoma, and glenoid fossa are important landmarks.

A temporal craniotomy is then performed over the squamous portion of the temporal bone. The craniotomy flap is positioned approximately one-third posterior to and two-thirds anterior to the external auditory canal. It measures approximately 5 cm in the vertical dimension and 4 cm in anteroposterior width. The inferior aspect of the craniotomy is based on the root of the zygoma and should be placed as low as possible. The flap is dissected with a medium cutting burr that defines the perimeter of the bone flap (Fig. 124-20). Another method of turning the bone flap is to place four burr holes at each corner of the bone dissection. A craniotome with a footed attachment on a high-speed drill is used to finely cut the two vertical and superior horizontal bone cuts, connecting the burr holes. Because of anatomic limitations, it is often difficult to use the footed attachment for the inferior horizontal cut. The inferior horizontal cut is made with a round cutting or matchstick burr. Using an elevator, the bone flap is lifted while the underlying dura is cautiously detached from the inner table. The dura underlying the craniotomy site is elevated. Hemostasis is secured with bipolar coagulation. Once the bone flap is removed, the inferior aspect of the craniotomy should be lowered to the level of the floor of the middle fossa using a rongeur or cutting burr (Fig. 124-21). Rough edges of the craniotomy site and bone flap are smoothed with a rongeur or drill. The dura is elevated from the floor of the middle fossa. Dissection requires patience and slow but progressive retraction of the temporal lobe. Adequate brain softening should have been achieved from the previously administered osmotic agents.

Familiarity with the surface anatomy of the floor of the middle fossa is essential to facilitate this operative approach. The most lateral adhesion of dura occurs at the petrosquamous suture. Anteriorly, the middle meningeal artery enters through the foramen spinosum.

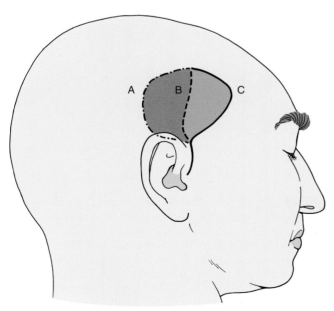

Figure 124-19. Skin incisions available for a middle fossa approach to an acoustic neuroma. Our preference is B.

The lesser and greater superficial nerves run parallel from the sphenopetrosal groove. The greater superficial petrosal nerve (GSPN) courses from posterior to anterior, leaving the geniculate ganglion through the facial hiatus. Deep to the GSPN lies the horizontal portion of the petrous carotid artery. Lateral to the carotid artery is the tensor tympani muscle above and the eustachian tube below. The internal carotid artery courses medially and inferiorly to the mandibular division of the trigeminal nerve (V3). The arcuate eminence lies posteriorly and medially on the floor of the middle fossa. This is the bony convexity of the superior semicircular canal. Posterior to the arcuate eminence is the tegmen of the mastoid. The superior petrosal sinus runs obliquely from posterolateral to anteromedial and forms the medial boundary separating the middle from the posterior fossa. This anatomy relative to the ossicles, geniculate ganglion, facial nerve, IAC, vestibular labyrinth, and cochlea is demonstrated in Figure 124-22.

Using an operating microscope, a Lempert elevator, and small suction, the dura is elevated from the floor of the middle fossa in a lateral-to-medial and posterior-to-anterior direction. Laterally, within the first 10 mm of dural elevation, the petrosquamous suture line is encountered. The dura may be firmly attached along this suture line, and occasionally, a few small perforating veins will be noted and can be coagulated or waxed. Further medially and anteriorly, the next landmark along the floor of the middle fossa is the middle meningeal artery. Commonly, venous bleeding from a periarterial venous plexus will be encountered and should be controlled with bipolar electrocautery or small pledgets of Surgicel. The middle meningeal artery is isolated by circumferential dissection around the artery. Although not routinely necessary, if extended exposure is needed, the artery is cauterized and then divided using microscissors. It is helpful to dissect the artery far enough to allow a small cuff of vessel to be retained on both the cranial and the dural sides. Unsuccessful hemostasis is controlled with a hemoclip.

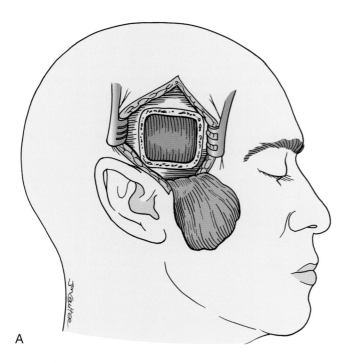

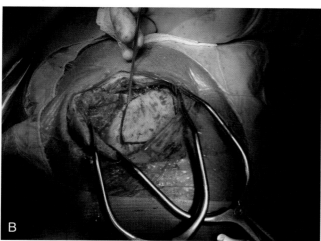

Figure 124-20. A, A craniotomy, 5 × 4 cm, is developed with a medium-sized cutting burr. It is positioned two-thirds anterior and one-third posterior to the external auditory canal. **B,** Photograph of right ear showing the outline of the bone flap before elevation. The temporalis muscle is transposed anteriorly and inferiorly.

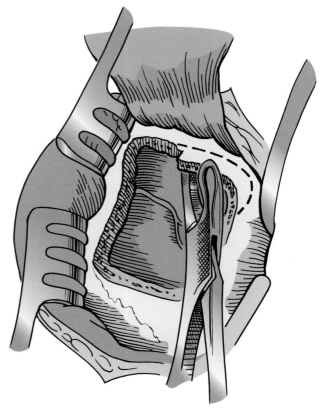

Figure 124-21. The inferior aspect of the craniotomy site is enlarged, removing sharp protruding edges. A rongeur or drill burr is used to smooth the edges.

Dissection of the dura from posterior to anterior avoids injury to the geniculate ganglion from retrograde elevation of the GSPN. The prominence in the floor of the middle fossa is the arcuate eminence, which is another key landmark. The middle fossa dura is elevated medially until the edge of the petrous bony ridge is palpated. Care is taken not to tear the superior petrosal sinus. The dura is dissected along the ridge of the petrous bone. Once the middle fossa dura has been dissected to the level of the sulcus of the superior petrosal vein, a retractor is repositioned and secured. Two methods of retracting the dura and temporal lobe have been used. The first method is with a Greenberg retractor secured to a Mayfield head holder. The second method is to use a House-Urban or Fisch middle fossa retractor. The rigid blade elevating the temporal lobe is then placed.

Important landmarks for identifying the IAC are the arcuate eminence and the GSPN leading posteriorly toward the geniculate ganglion (Fig. 124-23). The course of the GSPN and arcuate eminence form an angle of approximately 120 degrees. A line bisecting this angle forms a 60-degree angle with both the GSPN and the arcuate eminence. This line, parallel with the external auditory canal, overlies the course of the IAC. If the anatomy is uncertain, then the arcuate eminence is bluelined to define the superior semicircular canal. Another method for identifying the IAC is by retrograde dissection of the GSPN. This will identify the geniculate ganglion and, in turn, the labyrinthine segment of the facial nerve. Meticulous and careful dissection is necessary in the labyrinthine segment because the basal turn of the cochlea lies immediately anterior and lateral to this structure.

Once the important landmarks are determined, drilling is begun at the most medial aspect of the presumed location of the IAC. This area provides a wide margin of error, allowing the surgeon to work in a safe but rapid fashion. If the arcuate eminence is not obvious, drilling posteriorly will identify the mastoid tegmen and air cells. These can then be followed anteriorly until the dense otic capsule bone of the superior semicircular canal is identified. An additional method for identifying the anatomic structures is by drilling over the tegmen tympani to identify the ossicles, horizontal portion of the facial nerve, and geniculate ganglion. The nerve can then be traced proximally toward the IAC. It is necessary to expose at least 180 degrees of circumference of the IAC, especially medially. As the dissection

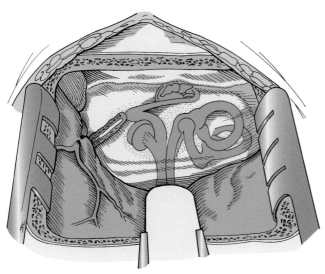

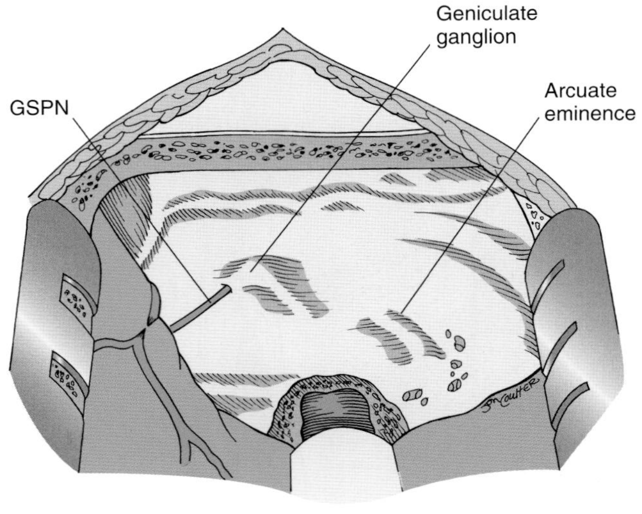

Figure 124-22. The anatomy deep to the floor of the middle fossa is illustrated. The middle meningeal artery has been divided. The greater superficial petrosal nerve can be traced posteriorly in the geniculate ganglion. The facial nerve courses between the basal turn of the cochlear and ampullated end of the superior semicircular canal. The ossicles are demonstrated.

Figure 124-23. The greater superficial petrosal nerve (GSPN) exiting the facial hiatus and the arcuate eminence are noted. Dissection begins medially where the proximal IAC and the superior lip of the porus acusticus are identified.

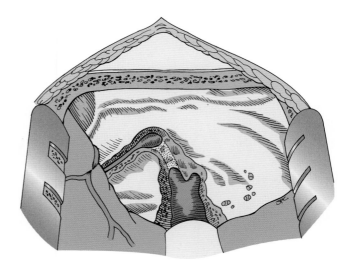

Figure 124-24. Drilling over the IAC is continued laterally, exposing the proximal fallopian canal containing the labyrinthine segment of the facial nerve. The IAC may also be identified by retrograde dissection of the greater superficial petrosal nerve to the geniculate ganglion.

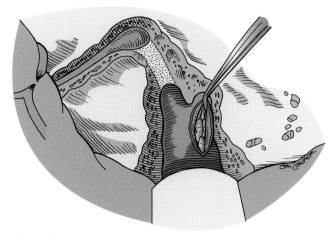

Figure 124-25. The dura overlying the superior vestibular nerve is incised along the posterior wall of the IAC. Tumor is evident through the dural opening.

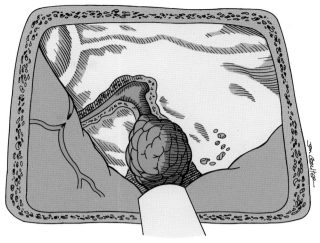

Figure 124-27. Fat is placed in the defect in the dura over the roof of the internal auditory canal. The middle fossa dura will be tacked laterally to the edges of the craniotomy defect when the retractor is removed.

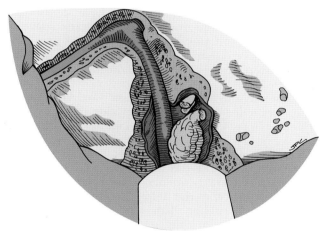

Figure 124-26. The tumor is separated sharply from the facial nerve. In this situation, the superior vestibular nerve is divided distally and the tumor is dissected from lateral to medial.

of the IAC progresses from medial to lateral, the extent of circumferential dissection of the IAC must be reduced so that the upper basal turn of the cochlea and ampullated portion of the superior semicircular canal are not inadvertently entered (Fig. 124-24).

Following completion of all bone drilling exposing the IAC, the IAC is entered. The dura is opened most safely on the posterior aspect of the IAC, away from the facial nerve, reflecting the dura anteriorly (Fig. 124-25). It is important to dissect the tumor away from the facial nerve carefully and sharply. If the tumor originates from the inferior vestibular nerve, the fascicles of the superior vestibular nerve are sharply divided and dissected. This also facilitates identification and isolation of the facial nerve. It is preferable to remove the tumor from a medial to a lateral direction, avoiding stretch and injury to the labyrinthine segment of the facial nerve and the cochlear nerve. The proximal end of the vestibular nerve is cut, and the tumor is carefully dis-

sected laterally. However, if the tumor obscures the CPA it may need to be debulked or removed from lateral to medial (Fig. 124-26). If hearing is to be preserved, care is taken not to cauterize vessels that are running along the course of the cochlear nerve.

Despite having a flap of dura and periosteum over the IAC, a watertight closure cannot be obtained. Fat is harvested from the abdomen and is soaked in bacitracin solution, and small pledgets are placed into the roof of the IAC. Hemostasis is ensured over the middle fossa dura. Any other tears or defects in the dura are primarily closed or repaired (Fig. 124-27). Two dura tacking sutures reapproximate the dura to the edges of the craniotomy through burr holes made previously. The bone flap is then replaced over the dura and secured with miniplates. The temporalis muscle flap is carefully reapproximated with absorbable sutures. A Jackson-Pratt drain is placed subcutaneously attached to a closed system and the wound is drained overnight. Skin is closed subcutaneously with 2-0 Dexon or Vicryl sutures. The skin closure is completed with a running 4-0 nylon suture or staples.

Retrosigmoid Approach

The patient is placed supine on the table and general oral endotracheal anesthesia is induced. Appropriate venous and arterial lines are secured. Electrodes for facial nerve and ABR testing are placed. A sound source and ear mold are secured within the external auditory meatus of both ears. The patient is repositioned by elevating the ipsilateral shoulder, back, and hip, which are supported with wedges of rolled blankets or pillows. This assists with access to the suboccipital region. Gel pads lining the operating room table avoids pressure necrosis to the dependent hip and lateral thorax. Additional exposure is accomplished with neck flexion and head rotation toward the contralateral ear. A Mayfield head holder with three-point skeletal fixation is secured. The postauricular hair is shaved and a curvilinear

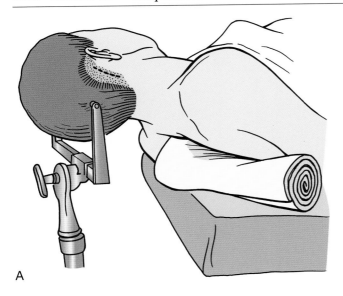

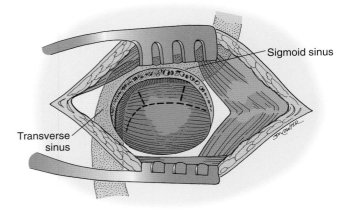

Figure 124-29. The retrosigmoid craniotomy is limited by the transverse sinus superiorly and the sigmoid sinus anteriorly. The curvilinear and stellate incision in the dura is illustrated.

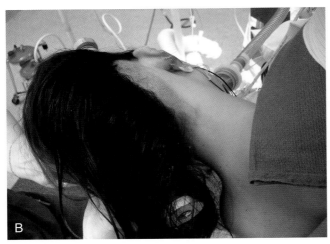

Figure 124-28. A, The patient is positioned supine on the operating table, using an ipsilateral shoulder roll for additional rotation. Mayfield pin fixation secures the head position. The incision is marked on the skin. **B,** Positioning of patient for right retrosigmoid procedure. (*A, Redrawn from Sekhar LN, Janecka IP [eds]: Surgery of Cranial Base Tumors. New York, Raven Press, 1993.*)

oblique skin incision is marked over the retrosigmoid suboccipital area 2 cm medial to the mastoid process or 1 cm medial to the hairline (Fig. 124-28). The patient is prepared and draped in the usual sterile fashion.

The incision is carried down to the suboccipital muscles. The occipital bone is exposed by subperiosteal muscle dissection and elevation in line with the incision. This exposes the lateral suboccipital bone medially and the mastoid process laterally. An emissary vein is typically encountered and requires bipolar coagulation, ligation, or compression with bone wax.

Using a high-speed drill, a suboccipital craniotomy is performed, exposing the dura of the cerebellar hemisphere. The limits of the exposure are the transverse sinus superiorly and the sigmoid sinus anteriorly. Hemostasis is obtained throughout the wound. Air cells that have been opened into the mastoid are obliterated with

bone wax. Opening of the posterior fossa dura is performed to maximize exposure and facilitate closure. This depends on the anatomy of the transverse and sigmoid sinus and the posterior fossa exposure. The incision may be either semilunar or cruciate. The dural incision frequently used is demonstrated in Figure 124-29.

Entrance into the posterior fossa should be inferior to permit medial and superior elevation of the cerebellar hemisphere. This technique facilitates entry into the subarachnoid space and opening of the cerebellopontine cistern, which permits further relaxation of the cerebellum once CSF has been drained. The dura of the posterior fossa is opened. The operating microscope is brought into the field. The cerebellum is protected with a rubber dam and neuropatties. The arachnoid membrane encasing the cisterna magna needs to be opened. This allows egress of CSF, which reduces the pressure in the posterior fossa avoiding potential herniation of the cerebellum out of the wound. The lower cranial nerves IX through XI are identified. Further dissection inferiorly and medially provides exposure to the hypoglossal nerve as demonstrated in Video 124-8. If exposure cannot be maintained easily, a self-retaining Greenberg retractor is placed into position. The cerebellar hemisphere and flocculus are identified and retracted in a superomedial direction. This technique further relaxes the cerebellum, thereby providing exposure of the tumor (Fig. 124-30). Similarly, the root entry zone of the seventh and eighth cranial nerves is identified. The position and integrity of the seventh nerve should be verified initially with electrical stimulation. The origin from the brain stem can be located at the root entry zone of the ninth cranial nerve. Once the location and integrity of the proximal facial nerve is confirmed, a Teflon felt pledget is placed over the nerve for protection and subsequent identification (see Video 124-9). If the cochlear division of the eighth cranial nerve is identified, a direct nerve monitoring electrode is placed at its root entry zone if a hearing preservation procedure is

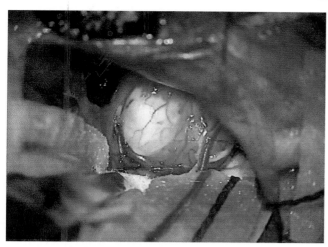

Figure 124-30. Right retrosigmoid approach to an acoustic neuroma. A Greenberg retractor blade over a cottonoid patty gently retracts the cerebellum, exposing the tumor.

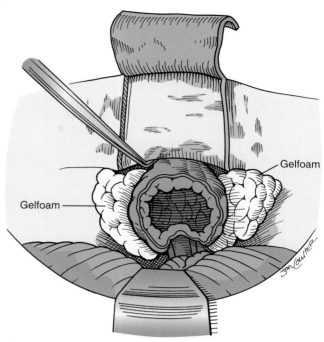

Figure 124-31. The tumor has been partially gutted and resected. A right-angled hook is used to palpate the posterior bony meatus of the porus acusticus. A medially (posteriorly) based dural flap is incised and elevated. Gelfoam is placed superior and inferior to the tumor in preparation for drilling.

undertaken. If the nerve is not identified, the wire electrode is placed in the vicinity of the lateral recess, superior to the ninth cranial nerve, which is in close proximity to the cochlear nucleus. If the tumor is too large to permit direct visualization of the brain stem, the tumor must be debulked.

Excision of the tumor is done in a systematic fashion incorporating identification of the facial nerve, control of surface and parenchymal bleeding, and tumor removal. The dissection is carried out in a subarachnoid plane. The location of the facial nerve should be determined before removing tumor. A stimulator is used to map the surface of the tumor, assuring the facial nerve is not displaced on the posterior surface of the tumor. Once this is verified, bipolar forceps are used to coagulate vessels located on the surface of the tumor. Sharp dissection provides an entry point to the parenchyma of the tumor. The capsule of the tumor is opened and a representative portion is taken with a cup forceps for frozen section confirmation of the pathology. This will also assure that a specimen has been received by the pathology laboratory. The core of the tumor is progressively removed ("gutted") using an ultrasonic aspiration device leaving the outer walls of the tumor intact. Much of the bulk of the tumor resection is executed in this manner. The contents within the suction portion of this instrument are not readily available for histologic analysis, emphasizing the need for sending a frozen section. Decompressing the central core of the tumor thins the capsular walls allowing for further dissection of the tumor capsule away from normal structures such as the brain stem, tentorium, and trigeminal nerve. The surface of the tumor is again stimulated, looking for the position of the facial nerve. When it is verified that the nerve is not over the area being dissected, the capsule is again bipolared, controlling any surface vessels or bleeding. The capsule is then resected, diminishing the size of the remaining tumor in the CPA. Video 124-10 demonstrates this sequence and techniques for excision of the tumor.

If changes in auditory brain stem evoked potentials should occur, this part of the procedure is curtailed and retraction loosened. If ABR changes occur despite elimination of retraction, pieces of Gelfoam soaked in papaverine may inhibit vasoconstriction.

The facial nerve typically travels over the anterosuperior aspect of the tumor. Tumor dissection is continued until the walls of the anterior and superior capsule remain. Care is taken to avoid trauma to the AICA or the posterior inferior cerebellar artery (PICA) during the dissection. Neuropatties or rolled Teflon felt pledgets are used between the tumor capsule and the surrounding cerebellum, brain stem, cranial nerves, vessels, or tentorium. It may be necessary to dissect tumor from the fifth cranial nerve, depending on the size and location. The petrosal vein (Dandy's vein) is located superiorly and laterally in the posterior fossa, just inferior to the tentorium. Excessive stretch on this vessel leads to tear, resulting in bleeding that may be difficult to control. It is prudent to identify the vein and divide it using bipolar coagulation and microscissors. The petrosal vein can be safely sacrificed if it obstructs access to the tumor or if bleeding occurs. Video 124-11 demonstrates sacrificing the petrosal vein.

The tumor is further mobilized from the inferior aspect of the capsule. The direction of the dissection is between the brain stem and the capsule, keeping in mind the location of the facial nerve. Once the dissection plane is defined, pledgets of Teflon are placed to maintain separation of tumor from the surrounding normal structures (see Video 124-12).

In most cases, tumor is present in the IAC. The lateral extent can be determined from the contrast-enhanced T1-weighted MRI or CT scan. When adequate debulking is achieved or if the tumor is of small size, the porus of the IAC is identified. This can be confirmed by palpating the posterior edge of the lip with a right-angled hook. Bipolar coagulation is performed over the posterior surface of the petrous bone outlining the rectangular flap. A number 15 blade is used to cut the posterior flap of dura, which can be based either laterally or medially (posteriorly) along the petrous bone to the level of the operculum (see Video 124-13). This can usually be palpated with a Rosen dissector (Fig. 124-31). Care is taken to preserve the endolymphatic sac when hearing preservation is attempted. Gelfoam is placed superior and inferior to the tumor to avoid excessive bone dust from settling in the operative field.

Using a cutting burr, the posterior aspect of the porus and IAC is drilled. This is continued in a semicircumferential fashion, outlining the superior and inferior aspects of the IAC (see Video 124-14). Dissection is continued approximately 7 mm laterally. However, the extent of dissection is determined by the lateral extent of the tumor. In addition, a bone-windowed CT scan defines the relationship of the lateral aspect of the tumor to the posterior semicircular canal and vestibule. Similarly, although bone detail is absent, MRI clearly identifies whether tumor extends to the fundus. Drilling is continued initially with a cutting burr and then with smaller diamond burrs to create a trough both superior and inferior to the IAC (see Video 124-15). The exposure necessary requires the posterior 180 to 270 degrees of the IAC to be drilled.

The edges of the remaining IAC should be palpated with a narrow elevator. The dura is initially elevated from the underlying bone both superiorly and inferiorly. It is at this point that the surgeon can determine whether the amount of bone that has been removed is sufficient (see Video 124-16). The dura covering the posterior aspect of the IAC is then opened inferiorly exposing the underling tumor (Fig. 124-32). The tumor is then dissected away from the dura lining the IAC superiorly and inferiorly (see Video 124-17).

If the tumor does not extend to the fundus, the lateral extent of the tumor is identified. A facial nerve monitor and stimulator are crucial to the success of this part of the procedure. Removal of tumor from the IAC can begin once the facial nerve has been identified. The facial nerve is routinely positioned in the anterior superior quadrant of the IAC. A facial nerve stimulator-dissector is used to initially confirm the location of the facial nerve (see Video 124-18). It is typically a distinct nerve at the distal fundus. Dissection can be accomplished with an excavator carefully separating the tumor from the facial nerve (see Video 124-19). The direction of dissection at this point is from lateral to medial. In a hearing preservation procedure, great care must be taken to avoid traction of the cochlear nerve as it is rolled medially. As the tumor is rolled out medially, it may remain attached to the lateral vestibular nerve. Sharp dissection is necessary to divide the vestibular nerve to release the tumor from the facial nerve (see Video 124-20). The facial nerve can be severely flattened along the anterior canal wall, especially at the anterior lip of the porus (see Video 124-21).

It is difficult to directly view the extreme lateral extent of the tumor occupying the fundus. The last 2 to 3 mm of the posterior bony wall of the IAC remains intact in hearing preservation procedures. Curved excavators are used to scoop out the remaining tumor (Fig. 124-33). Favorable dissection and excision occur when

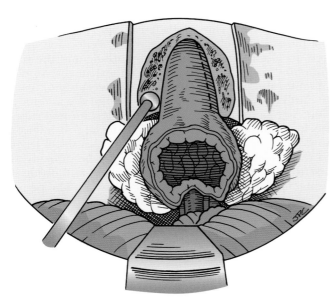

Figure 124-32. The internal auditory canal is outlined by drilling a trough superiorly and inferiorly. The dura of the IAC is incised inferiorly *(dotted line),* away from the facial nerve.

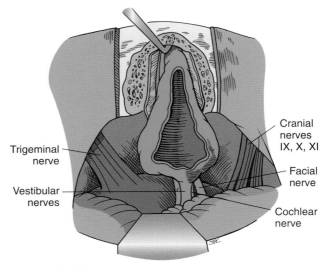

Trigeminal nerve

Vestibular nerves

Cranial nerves IX, X, XI

Facial nerve

Cochlear nerve

Figure 124-33. The tumor is debulked centrally but extends into the fundus. The fundus is attenuated in the proximal internal auditory canal. A curved excavator rolls the most lateral extent of the tumor medially.

the lateral tumor is blunted and rolls out intact. Care is taken when dissecting the fibers of the vestibular nerve laterally in order to avoid injury to the underlying facial nerve entering the labyrinthine segment. Angled rigid telescopes occasionally help view this area to determine whether complete resection has been achieved.

The central aspect of the tumor is removed from the IAC. Kartush stimulating dissectors are frequently used in this part of the procedure. The facial nerve is identified anterosuperiorly using a nerve stimulator. The facial nerve is frequently flattened, and meticulous dissection is performed, removing tumor from the nerve. Similar techniques are employed for the cochlear nerve, which is located anterior and inferior within the IAC. The focus of attention in the IAC dissection shifts between the facial nerve and the cochlear nerve, if hearing is to be preserved. Alteration in the ABR fifth-wave latency or amplitude warrants cessation of dissection in that area and relaxing the retractors if in place. Similarly, it is best to cease dissection around the facial nerve if the monitoring device indicates spontaneous neural firing, suggesting irritation or injury. Attention is turned to other areas of dissection.

Once the facial nerve is identified, the bulk of tumor in the CPA must be further debulked and removed. The ultrasonic aspirator can quickly vaporize the tumor. The facial nerve requires ongoing protection as the dissection proceeds. As the dissection proceeds, pledgets of Teflon felt are positioned over the critical structures (brain stem, cranial nerves, and significant vessels) for protection. Various instruments are available to sharply remove the tumor including scissors, a round knife, and sharp facial nerve stimulator/dissectors (see Video 124-22).

The residual tumor lies at the anterior face of the petrous bone. Meticulous dissection is undertaken from both a medial and lateral direction. The protective felt pledgets are removed from the nerve proximally to keep the nerve in view as the tumor is sharply dissected (see Video 124-23). The most difficult region is at the anterior wall of the petrous bone, central to the lip of the anterior porus, where the facial nerve is most often flattened and attenuated. Tumor must be meticulously dissected, often in a small piecemeal fashion (see Video 124-24). We accept leaving microscopic foci of tumor on the facial nerve if total removal would significantly compromise the integrity of the nerve. Resection of any residual tumor from the porus acusticus and CPA is completed. The vestibular nerves are divided proximally near the brain stem. Hearing preservation is attempted if a plane of dissection is obtained between the vestibular nerve and the cochlear nerve. Care is taken to avoid injury to the internal auditory artery (Fig. 124-34).

Once tumor excision is completed, hemostasis is secured. The anesthesiologist is notified that monitoring is no longer necessary, permitting the use of paralytic agents. This facilitates a smoother emergence from general anesthesia. The wound is then irrigated with bacitracin solution. To prevent CSF rhinorrhea postoperatively, the bony edges of the IAC are checked for

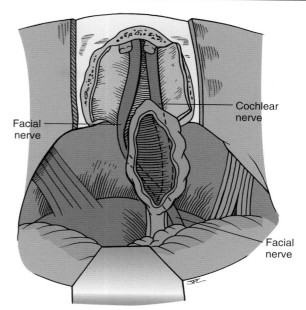

Figure 124-34. The tumor remains pedicled on the vestibular nerves. The facial nerve runs medial and superior to the tumor. The cochlear nerve is intact inferiorly. Hearing preservation requires meticulous dissection of the tumor away from the proximal cochlear nerve.

opened air cells. Bone wax on a cottonoid patty is compressed into open cells. If the temporal bone is well pneumatized, a muscle plug is gently placed within the IAC and supported with a piece of Surgicel. All neuropatties and rubber dams are removed.

The edges of the posterior fossa dura are reapproximated with 4-0 Nurolon. If desiccation has occurred, it may be necessary to supplement the dural closure with homograft dura, pericardium, or fascia. Isolation of the dura from the suboccipital muscles likely minimizes long-term headaches. A wafer of Gelfoam or Duragen is compressed and placed over the dura. A cranioplasty over the occipital and mastoid bony defect is performed using a titanium mesh plate. The wound is closed in multiple layers using uninterrupted sutures of Dexon. Skin is closed using staples or 4-0 Nurolon. A sterile pressure dressing is applied, and the procedure is terminated. The anesthetic is reversed, and depending on its depth and concern for the patient's neurologic status, extubation may be done in the operating room or subsequently in the recovery room.

PATHOLOGY

The histopathology of acoustic neuroma can vary. There may be gross and microscopic cystic areas. There are two predominant patterns of cellular architecture. The first is called *Antoni A*, which is characterized by sheets of dense, organized, palisading nerve cells. The other pattern is *Antoni B*, demonstrating a looser array with a cystic stroma (Fig. 124-35). It is unclear whether the morphology of these patterns has direct implication toward the biologic activity of these tumors.

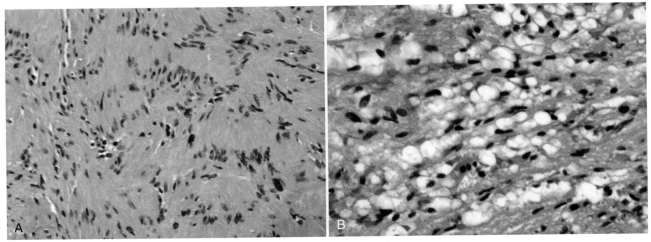

Figure 124-35. Histologic patterns of cellular architecture in acoustic neuroma. **A,** Antoni A. **B,** Antoni B.

POSTOPERATIVE MANAGEMENT

Regardless of the approach, a sterile pressure dressing is applied and remains in place for 2 days. Patients are monitored in an intensive care unit in the immediate postoperative period. Hourly vital signs and neurologic checks are recorded while the patient is in the intensive care unit. Blood pressure and urine output are carefully monitored for evidence of increased intracranial pressure, diabetes insipidus, or the inappropriate secretion of antidiuretic hormone. The risk of pulmonary emboli is minimized postoperatively with continued use of sequential compression devices until the patient is ambulating. Depending on the patient's degree of alertness, oral intake is advanced from clear liquids to solids as tolerated.

Immediate-onset or delayed facial paresis may occur. Patients with a poor Bell's phenomenon are at greater risk for corneal exposure. If inadequate eye closure is noted, comprehensive care of the cornea is provided to avoid desiccation and ulceration. Topical artificial tears are instilled every 2 hours or as needed. Ophthalmic ointment is placed in the lower conjunctival fornix at night. A clear eye shield or moisture chamber is used during the day for further protection.

Patients are encouraged to ambulate as soon as possible. Depending on the degree of residual vestibular function existing before surgery, patients may experience mild to severe vertigo and dysequilibrium following surgery. Patients with tumors that eliminated vestibular function preoperatively will experience less dysequilibrium. Nystagmus toward the contralateral side is often evident during the first few postoperative days. The long-term use of vestibular suppressants, such as meclizine, is avoided. Supportive care with antinauseants is provided as needed.

Patients are carefully observed for CSF leakage. This may occur directly through the incision or via the eustachian tube and out the nose. Clear watery rhinor-

rhea is evidence of a CSF leak. If the fluid content is in question, the specimen is sent for β_2-transferrin analysis. Management of this problem is reviewed under Complications later in this chapter. The dressing is removed on the second postoperative day. Bulging and pulsation of the wound following a translabyrinthine approach warrant replacement of a pressure dressing for a few more days. This finding has been minimized with the use of a miniplate over the transmastoid craniotomy and fat graft. Wound care consisting of twice-daily cleansing with peroxide and the application of an antibiotic ointment is provided. The abdominal wound used for a fat graft is inspected daily. The Penrose or Jackson-Pratt drain is removed when minimal drainage appears on the bandage, usually between the first and the third day postoperatively. Patients are discharged 4 to 6 days following the surgery, depending on the integrity of dural closure, nutrition, and ability to ambulate. MRI scanning is routinely obtained postoperatively. Patients manifesting a change in mental status or focal neurologic deficits also warrant urgent imaging to determine whether there is evidence of a bleed, hematoma, or vascular compromise. Sutures or staples are removed 10 to 14 days postoperatively. An MRI scan is obtained 6 months following surgery. This provides a baseline scan from which to compare subsequent images. The next scan is obtained 1 year later or 18 months following surgery. Dural enhancement often seen on the first scan is stabilized or less intense on subsequent scans. A third scan is obtained in 3 years. If this is also normal, a final scan is obtained in 5 years (Table 124-1).

COMPLICATIONS

Regardless of the surgical approach, patients undergoing excision of AN may experience complications. These may occur both intraoperatively or postoperatively. Problems that may occur during the surgical procedure are similar to those of any other intracranial

Table 124-1	POSTOPERATIVE MAGNETIC RESONANCE IMAGING SCHEDULE	
Time Following Surgery		**Interval**
3 mo		3 mo
15 mo		1 yr
51 mo		3 yr
111 mo		5 yr

operation. The skin flaps and dura should be handled in an atraumatic fashion. Undue retraction and desiccation must be avoided. In particular, during the middle fossa approach, tears in the dura may be created during elevation of the temporal lobe. Once recognized, the tear should be repaired primarily at that time.

Bleeding may be arterial or venous. The most common sources of venous bleeding are from the sigmoid or transverse sinuses during translabyrinthine or retrosigmoid approaches. A superior petrosal sinus may also be lacerated during the middle fossa or translabyrinthine approach. Small defects may be closed with bipolar forceps. Larger defects should be covered with Surgicel and compression applied. The superior petrosal sinus may need to be ligated or clipped and divided in order to secure hemostasis. Arterial bleeding in the posterior fossa is a serious complication. This must be controlled. Bleeding from small vessels may be stopped with bipolar coagulation. Serious neurologic sequelae may result from injury to the AICA or PICA. These vessels are carefully dissected away from the tumor and, if necessary, isolated with neuropatties. Other methods that may be used to control bleeding include topical microfibular collagen hemostat (Avitene), bipolar coagulation, and hemoclips.

Compression or retraction on the brain stem may be manifested by changes in the ABRs and somatosensory potentials. More significant consequences result in hemodynamic instability manifested by hypertension or hypotension with bradycardia.

Large tumors approached through the posterior fossa may be in proximity to cranial nerves V, IX, X, and XI. Meticulous surgical technique must be exercised in order to avoid trauma to these nerves. Although sequelae may not be evident intraoperatively, a vocal cord paresis at the time of extubation may compromise laryngeal function and protection.

Another rare but serious intraoperative complication is air embolus. This occurs secondary to the opening of a large venous sinus, permitting air to be sucked into the vessel. A change in the auditory output of the precordial Doppler stethoscope is one of the earlier indicators of this event. The patient's hemodynamic status is subsequently compromised. Management consists of occluding the open vessel and turning the patient to the left side, head down. If a Swan-Ganz catheter is in place, air can be aspirated from the right atrium. A large piece of Surgicel is packed into the sinus, and compression with a neuropatty is applied.

POSTOPERATIVE COMPLICATIONS

Facial Paresis/Paralysis

Facial paralysis is not actually a complication of the procedure but rather an accepted risk. In the immediate postoperative period, this is more likely to occur with a middle fossa approach but is also dependent on the size and adherence of the tumor. If a mild paresis exists (less than House-Brackmann grade III), then comprehensive eye care may not be needed. However, with incomplete eye closure, poor Bell's phenomenon, and slow blinking, artificial tears, ophthalmic ointment, and a clear moisture chamber are provided. An anatomically intact facial nerve with low stimulation thresholds at the conclusion of the procedure implies a good prognosis for facial recovery. However, if large stimulation intensities were necessary to evoke a response, then return of function may not be evident for many months. In this event, we suggest that a gold weight be inserted. Ectropion may develop in older patients with increased skin laxity. Tightening of the lower lid with a lateral tarsal strip may be warranted. Rarely, the facial nerve must be divided in order to accomplish complete tumor removal. In this case, immediate end-to-end anastomosis or cable grafting provides the best functional outcome. Approximately 46% of patients who undergo cable grafting will recover to a House-Brackmann grade III, and an additional 25% will recover to grade IV.[37]

Hearing Loss

Similar to facial nerve injury, hearing loss is another risk that frequently occurs following tumor resection, despite attempts at hearing preservation. Despite having good ABR waveforms at the conclusion of the procedure, complete hearing loss may still occur. The risk of hearing loss increases with tumor size, particularly for those tumors with greater than 15 mm in the CPA.[38] Worse preoperative hearing, increasing wave V latency, and inferior vestibular nerve origin have also been reported to increase the risk of hearing loss.[39] Postoperative hearing loss is more common in patients with significant adhesion between the tumor and cochlear nerve.[40] Additionally, patients who initially have preserved hearing following the retrosigmoid approach may go on to lose hearing in the operated ear at a rate exceeding that in the contralateral ear.[41] This result is contradicted by a report from the House Ear Institute, which found that surgery did not affect the postoperative progression of hearing loss in the operated ear.[24]

Cerebrospinal Fluid Leak

When CSF leak occurs, it is usually evident through the incision or manifested as clear, watery rhinorrhea. It is unusual to observe CSF otorrhea in that the tympanic membrane and external auditory canal should not have been violated. A ballotable collection of CSF underneath the skin flaps is treated with a pressure dressing. The head of the bed should remain elevated. If clear fluid leaks through the incision, then the skin closure is augmented with single interrupted sutures. Liquid collodion is an effective skin sealant and can be painted over the wound if a slow leak persists. If this is not adequate for controlling the leak, then a lumbar drain is placed. The catheter is connected to a Buretrol device, which provides accurate monitoring of CSF drainage. By adjusting the height of the Buretrol device, a drainage rate of 6 to 10 mL/hr is maintained. The lumbar drain remains in place for 3 to 4 days. If the CSF leak or rhinorrhea persists but is subsiding, an additional 2 days may be needed. However, if an active leak remains despite 5 days of lumbar drainage, then reexploring the wound is necessary. Careful obliteration of any exposed air cells with bone wax, muscle, or fat will minimize the risk of CSF leak; some surgeons employ endoscopes to inspect the temporal bone for unseen exposed air cells.[42] For patients in whom petrous apex air cells open directly into the eustachian tube, obliteration of the entire length of the tube can be accomplished using a combined transaural/transnasal approach.[43]

Meningitis

Patients developing new-onset headache with fever, vomiting, and a change in mental status should be immediately evaluated for meningitis. Bacterial meningitis occurs in approximately 2.5% of patients, although aseptic meningitis may be seen in up to 20% of patients.[13] A spinal tap identifies increased white blood cell counts with a shift to the left, elevated protein, and reduced glucose levels. A Gram stain may identify an organism that will direct one's choice for antibiotic coverage. Vancomycin and an aminoglycoside or a third-generation cephalosporin, such as ceftazidime or ceftriaxone, are used. If the Gram stain is negative and the culture shows no growth, antibiotics may be discontinued, and a presumed diagnosis of aseptic meningitis given. However, if the culture is positive, antibiotics are continued for 7 to 10 days.

Intracranial Bleeding

Delayed postoperative bleeding usually occurs during the first 3 to 5 days. This may be intracerebral or cerebellar bleeding or a subdural collection or hematoma. Patients may manifest symptoms of altered mental status, lethargy, somnolence, limb weakness, or aphasia. An emergency CT scan is obtained to identify the nature of intracranial pathology. A noncontrast study is adequate to demonstrate a bleed or hematoma. In addition, hydrocephalus may be evident on the scan. Management is dictated based on the findings of the scan.

Seizures

Seizures following translabyrinthine or retrosigmoid resection of ANs are rare. These are more likely to occur with a supratentorial injury following middle fossa retraction. Problems with receptive or expressive aphasia may occur from excessive retraction and injury to the left temporal lobe. The surgeon must be aware of the degree of temporal lobe retraction exerted

through a middle fossa approach. Emergent treatment consists of intravenous diazepam and a loading dose of phenytoin. Oral phenytoin is continued postoperatively for 4 to 6 months.

Trigeminal Nerve Dysfunction

Large ANs can extend superiorly through the tentorium and anteriorly to the petrous apex. Injury to the trigeminal nerve more typically affects V1 and V2 (sensory divisions) as opposed to V3 (the motor division). Facial hypesthesia and analgesia may result. This deficit, in conjunction with a facial nerve paralysis, is a potentially devastating combination injury. The hypesthesia of the cornea along with lagophthalmos intensifies the likelihood of corneal injury. Despite comprehensive prophylactic eye care, it may be necessary to perform medial and lateral tarsorrhaphies to minimize the dystrophic and erosive changes that may occur in the cornea. Similarly, the lateral ala of the nose is subject to ischemic necrosis. Patients can manually traumatize the involved insensate nares, initiating destruction of the alar rim.

Lower Cranial Nerve Injury

Tumors that extend inferiorly are in close approximation to cranial nerves IX, X, and XI. The multiple fine fascicles of these cranial nerves may be injured during dissection. Despite anatomic integrity of these cranial nerves, pharyngeal and laryngeal dysfunction may result. Patients may develop dysphagia, dysphasia, aspiration, and breathy voice. Nasogastric tube feeding may be necessary if aspiration persists. Temporary resolution may be augmented with Gelfoam injection of the involved vocal cord. If the surgeon believes that substantial intraoperative injury has occurred, then a type I thyroplasty, which is reversible, can provide longer-lasting relief (see Chapter 38).

Headache

Postoperative pain in the incision is common with any procedure. Patients undergoing a middle fossa approach may experience pain on mastication owing to temporary temporalis muscle dysfunction. Similarly, pain in the posterior aspect of the neck frequently occurs following a suboccipital approach. Symptoms are usually relieved with application of heat, parenteral or oral narcotics, and eventually, nonsteroidal anti-inflammatory medication. Regardless of the approach, headache and stiffness of the neck may develop 5 to 7 days postoperatively. Lumbar puncture and fluid analysis are warranted to rule out bacterial or aseptic meningitis. Xanthochromic CSF with few white cells, secondary to red blood cell breakdown, is the likely cause of meningeal irritation. Steroids are usually prescribed if routine analgesics are ineffective. Long-term postoperative headache is associated with the retrosigmoid approach. Symptoms may present for upward of 1 year. Treatment consists of nonsteroidal anti-inflammatory medications, nerve block, and rarely wound revision or rhizotomy.

PEARLS

- Given the current accepted alternatives of management, patients must receive a comprehensive discussion addressing surgical removal, stereotactic radiation treatment, and monitoring the tumor for further growth over time.
- Consideration should be given to observing the tumor with serial MRI scans in people older than age 70 years with small tumors.
- CT imaging can be helpful to identify a high jugular bulb providing useful information in anticipation of a translabyrinthine approach.
- Every effort should be given to complete all bone drilling and dissection before the dura is opened.
- Temporary placement of Teflon pledgets, which are less adherent than neuropatties, protect critical structures that are isolated as the dissection proceeds.

PITFALLS

- Inadequate exposure will significantly impede safe and complete access to the tumor for total removal.
- Proceeding with tumor dissection in the presence of the facial nerve monitor device indicating neurotonic discharge (irritation) may result in preventable irreversible injury. Attention should be directed to another area.
- Excessive manipulation and retraction of the temporal lobe during middle fossa surgery may result in brain injury, seizures, and dysphasia, especially on the left side.
- The use of the bipolar electrocautery adjacent to the facial nerve may cause permanent injury.
- Aggressive retraction and dissection of the tumor from the fundus can avulse the delicate cochlear and facial nerve fibers, resulting in hearing loss and facial weakness.

References

1. Ballance C: Some points in surgery of the brain and its membranes. London, Macmillan, 1907, p. 276.
2. Cushing H: Further concerning acoustic neuromas. Laryngoscope 31:209-228, 1921.
3. Cushing H, Bovie WT: Electrosurgery as an aid to the removal of intracranial tumors. Surg Gynecol Obstet 47:751-784, 1928.
4. Dandy WE: An operation for the total extirpation of tumors in the cerebellopontine angle: A preliminary report. Johns Hopkins Medical Bulletin 33:344-345, 1922.
5. Quix FH: Ein fall von translabyrinthine operiertem tumor acusticus. Verh Dtsch Otol Ges 21:245-252, 1912.
6. House WF: History of the development of the translabyrinthine approach. In Silverstein H, Norell H (eds): Neurological Surgery of the Ear. Birmingham, Aesculapius, 1977, pp 235-238.
7. Gordon ML, Cohen NL: Efficacy of auditory brainstem response as a screening test for small acoustic neuromas. Am J Otol 16:136-139, 1995.
8. Wackym PA, Runge-Samuelson CL, Poetker DM, et al: Gamma knife radiosurgery for acoustic neuromas performed by a neurotologist: Early experiences and outcomes. Otol Neurotol 25:752-761, 2004.
9. Wootten CT, Kaylie DM, Warren FM, et al: Management of brain herniation and cerebrospinal fluid leak in revision chronic ear surgery. Laryngoscope 115:1256-1261, 2005.
10. Charabi S, Balle V, Charabi B, et al: Surgical outcome in malignant parotid tumours. Acta Otolaryngol Suppl 543:251-253, 2000.
11. Yamakami I, Uchino Y, Kobayashi E, et al: Conservative management, gamma-knife radiosurgery, and microsurgery for acoustic neurinomas: A systematic review of outcome and risk of three therapeutic options. Neurol Res 25:682-690, 2003.
12. Massick DD, Welling DB, Dodson EE, et al: Tumor growth and audiometric change in vestibular schwannomas managed conservatively. Laryngoscope 110:1843-1849, 2000.
13. Wackym PA: Stereotactic radiosurgery, microsurgery, and expectant management of acoustic neuroma: Basis for informed consent. Otolaryngol Clin North Am 38:653-670, 2005.
14. Wiet RJ, Mamikoglu B, Odom L, et al: Long-term results of the first 500 cases of acoustic neuroma surgery. Otolaryngol Head Neck Surg 124:645-651, 2001.
15. Harsha WJ, Backous DD: Counseling patients on surgical options for treating acoustic neuroma. Otolaryngol Clin North Am 38:643-652, 2005.
16. Martin HC, Sethi J, Lang D, et al: Patient-assessed outcomes after excision of acoustic neuroma: Postoperative symptoms and quality of life. J Neurosurg 94:211-216, 2001.
17. Chung WY, Liu KD, Shiau CY, et al: Gamma knife surgery for vestibular schwannoma: 10-year experience of 195 cases. J Neurosurg 102(Suppl):87-96, 2005.
18. Lunsford LD, Niranjan A, Flickinger JC, et al: Radiosurgery of vestibular schwannomas: Summary of experience in 829 cases. J Neurosurg 102(Suppl):195-199, 2005.
19. Karpinos M, Teh BS, Zeck O, et al: Treatment of acoustic neuroma: stereotactic radiosurgery vs. microsurgery. Int J Radiat Oncol Biol Phys 54:1410-1421, 2002.
20. Pollock BE, Driscoll CL, Foote RL, et al: Patient outcomes after vestibular schwannoma management: A prospective comparison of microsurgical resection and stereotactic radiosurgery. Neurosurgery 59:77-85; discussion 77-85, 2006.
21. Regis J, Pellet W, Delsanti C, et al: Functional outcome after gamma knife surgery or microsurgery for vestibular schwannomas. J Neurosurg 97:1091-1100, 2002.
22. Flickinger JC, Kondziolka D, Niranjan A, et al: Results of acoustic neuroma radiosurgery: An analysis of 5 years' experience using current methods. J Neurosurg 94:1-6, 2001.
23. Ottaviani F, Neglia CB, Ventrella L, et al: Hearing loss and changes in transient evoked otoacoustic emissions after gamma knife radiosurgery for acoustic neurinomas. Arch Otolaryngol Head Neck Surg 128:1308-1312, 2002.
24. Friedman RA: The surgical management of Bell's palsy: A review. Am J Otol 21:139-144, 2000.
25. Yamakawa K, Shitara N, Genka S, et al: Clinical course and surgical prognosis of 33 cases of intracranial epidermoid tumors. Neurosurgery 24:568-573, 1989.
26. Hayhurst C, Dhir J, Dias PS: Stereotactic radiosurgery and vestibular schwannoma: Hydrocephalus associated with the development of a secondary arachnoid cyst: A report of two cases and review of the literature. Br J Neurosurg 19:178-181, 2005.
27. Battista RA, Wiet RJ: Stereotactic radiosurgery for acoustic neuromas: A survey of the American Neurotology Society. Am J Otol 21:371-381, 2000.
28. Andrews DW, Suarez O, Goldman HW, et al: Stereotactic radiosurgery and fractionated stereotactic radiotherapy for the treatment of acoustic schwannomas: Comparative observations of 125 patients treated at one institution. Int J Radiat Oncol Biol Phys 50:1265-1278, 2001.
29. Myrseth E, Moller P, Pedersen PH, et al: Vestibular schwannomas: Clinical results and quality of life after microsurgery or gamma knife radiosurgery. Neurosurgery 56:927-935; discussion 927-935, 2005.

30. Meyer TA, Canty PA, Wilkinson EP, et al: Small acoustic neuromas: Surgical outcomes versus observation or radiation. Otol Neurotol 27:380-392, 2006.

31. Satar B, Jackler RK, Oghalai J, et al: Risk-benefit analysis of using the middle fossa approach for acoustic neuromas with >10 mm cerebellopontine angle component. Laryngoscope 112(8 Pt 1): 1500-1506, 2002.

32. Linthicum FHJ: Electronystagmography findings in patients with acoustic tumors. Semin Hearing 4:47-53, 1983.

33. Fundova P, Charabi S, Tos M, et al: Cystic vestibular schwannoma: Surgical outcome. J Laryngol Otol 114:935-939, 2000.

34. Cohen NL, Lewis WS, Ransohoff J: Hearing preservation in cerebellopontine angle tumor surgery: The NYU experience 1974-1991. Am J Otol 14:423-433, 1993.

35. MacDonald CB, Hirsch BE, Kamerer DB, et al: Acoustic neuroma surgery: Predictive criteria for hearing preservation. Otolaryngol Head Neck Surg 104:128, 1991.

36. Kondziolka D, Lunsford LD, Flickinger JC: Comparison of management options for patients with acoustic neuromas. Neurosurg Focus 14:e1, 2003.

37. Falcioni M, Taibah A, Russo A, et al: Facial nerve grafting. Otol Neurotol 24:486-489, 2003.

38. Yates PD, Jackler RK, Satar B, et al: Is it worthwhile to attempt hearing preservation in larger acoustic neuromas? Otol Neurotol 24:460-464, 2003.

39. Brackmann DE, Owens RM, Friedman RA, et al: Prognostic factors for hearing preservation in vestibular schwannoma surgery. Am J Otol 21:417-424, 2000.

40. Moriyama T, Fukushima T, Asaoka K, et al: Hearing preservation in acoustic neuroma surgery: Importance of adhesion between the cochlear nerve and the tumor. J Neurosurg 97:337-340, 2002.

41. Chee GH, Nedzelski JM, Rowed D: Acoustic neuroma surgery: The results of long-term hearing preservation. Otol Neurotol 24:672-676, 2003.

42. Sanna M, Taibah A, Russo A, et al: Perioperative complications in acoustic neuroma (vestibular schwannoma) surgery. Otol Neurotol 25:379-386, 2004.

43. Selesnick SH, Liu JC, Jen A, et al: Management options for cerebrospinal fluid leak after vestibular schwannoma surgery and introduction of an innovative treatment. Otol Neurotol 25:580-586, 2004.

Chapter 125

Glomus Tumors

Barry E. Hirsch

Paraganglioma or glomus tumor is a tumor of the neuroendocrine system derived from neural crest cells and chemoreceptor cells. The tumor was termed a *chemodectoma* by Mulligan in 1950.[1] The ability to pick up chromium salts led to the designation of the histologic staining characteristic as chromaffin or nonchromaffin positive. The largest concentration of paraganglionic cells is with the adrenal medulla. The other predominant locations of paraganglionic tissue are found in the branchiomeric chemoreceptor system of the aortic arch, carotid bifurcation, and temporal bone. Guild described the location of other glomus bodies within the temporal bone, identifying an average of 2.82 foci, half of which were in the jugular bulb and one fourth on the promontory of the cochlea.[2] The term commonly accepted to describe neoplastic tumors of the paraganglionic receptors is *glomus tumor.* Glomus tumors of the temporal bone are neoplasms arising from normally occurring paraganglionic bodies or formations that are located on the dome of the jugular bulb and along the course of Jacobson's nerve (ninth cranial nerve) onto the cochlear promontory. On rare occasions, these tumors take origin from the facial nerve.[3] The tumors of the temporal bone may be grouped into two categories: those arising from the middle ear (promontory) and those arising from the jugular bulb. These are termed *glomus tympanicum tumors* and *glomus jugulare tumors.* As tumor expansion occurs, it may be difficult to distinguish the precise origin of the lesion. Thus larger tumors involving both the middle ear and the jugular bulb are termed *jugulotympanic glomus tumors.*

Although most tumors are sporadic, familial glomus tumors may occur in 20% of patients with glomus tumors. Many of the tumors are multicentric and bilateral at the time of presentation, which typically occur at an earlier age in successive generations in families harboring genetic mutations. Investigation into the hereditary patterns of familial paraganglioma has resulted in the identification of four loci termed *PGL1, PGL2, PGL3,* and *PGL4.* The first two loci were found on chromosome 11 at bands 11q23.1 and 11q13.1. Both regions are associated with an autosomal dominant pattern and maternal imprinting. Inheriting the gene from the mother portends a lower incidence of transmission compared with passing the gene onto offspring from the father. Mutation in genes responsible for production of proteins that are critical components of a cellular oxygen-sensing system may permit proliferation of chief cells in paraganglionic cells. The loci for PGL3 and PGL4 are on chromosome 1. Heth wrote an excellent review of the basic science of glomus jugulare tumors.[4]

Glomus tumors are slow-growing, invasive, highly vascular neoplasms that are in critical proximity to the lower cranial nerves. Although locally destructive, glomus tumors are rarely considered to be malignant. It may be difficult to determine whether a glomus tumor is malignant. Some of the histologic features suggestive of malignancy include increase in mitotic activity, necrosis in the center of the cell nests, and vascular invasion. The hallmark of aggressive malignant behavior is the presence of tumor in the regional lymph nodes or distant organs confirmed with histologic examination.

Metastatic tumors have been found in the vertebrae, ribs, spleen, and lungs. In a series of 175 temporal bone glomus tumors, 5.1% were classified as malignant. Conventional external beam radiation therapy (XRT) is not advocated as the primary modality of treatment because viable tumor cells can remain following radiation treatment. Five-year survival for malignant glomus tumors of the temporal bone is 71.2%.[5]

Table 125-1	GLOMUS TUMOR CLASSIFICATION: FISCH
Type	**Description**
A	Tumor limited to middle ear cleft (promontory)
B	Tumor confined to middle ear, hypotympanum, and mastoid
C_1	Tumor eroding jugular bulb and carotid foramen; not invading carotid artery
C_2	Tumor involving infralabyrinthine and apical temporal bone; erosion of vertical carotid artery
C_3	Tumor involving infralabyrinthine and apical temporal bone; erosion of horizontal carotid artery
C_4	Tumor involving infralabyrinthine and apical temporal bone; tumor grows to foramen lacerum and cavernous sinus
D_1	Intracranial tumor <2 cm
D_2	Intracranial tumor >2 cm; *e*, extradural; *i*, intradural
Di_3	Unresectable intracranial extension

Data from Fisch U: Infratemporal fossa approach for glomus tumors of the temporal bone. Ann Otol Rhinol Laryngol 91:474-479, 1982; and Fisch U, Mattox D: Classification of glomus temporal tumors. In Fisch U, Mattox D (eds): Microsurgery of the Skull Base. Stuttgart and New York, Georg Thieme, 1988, pp 149-153.

Table 125-2	GLOMUS TUMOR CLASSIFICATION: GLASSCOCK-JACKSON
Type	**Description**
	Glomus Tympanicum
I	Small mass limited to promontory
II	Tumor completely filling middle ear space
III	Tumor filling middle ear and extending into mastoid
IV	Tumor filling middle ear, extending into mastoid or through tympanic membrane to fill external auditory canal; may extend anterior to carotid
	Glomus Jugulare
I	Small tumor involving jugular bulb, middle ear, and mastoid
II	Tumor extending under internal auditory canal; may have intracranial extension
III	Tumor extending into petrous apex; may have intracranial extension
IV	Tumor extending beyond petrous apex into clivus or infratemporal fossa; may have intracranial extension

Data from Jackson CG, Glasscock ME, Harris PF: Glomus tumors: Diagnosis, classification, and management of large lesions. Arch Otolaryngol 108:401-410, 1982.

Two classification systems have been offered for nomenclature and staging. Fisch described and modified a classification system based on the size and extent of the tumor (Table 125-1).[6,7] There are four categories (A, B, C, and D) of staging tumors, from limited to the middle ear cleft (type A) to large lesions demonstrating intracranial extension (type D). The Glasscock and Jackson classification system divides the tumors into tympanic or jugulare tumors (Table 125-2).[8] Each group is further subdivided into four types of progressively larger tumors, from small lesions limited to the site of origin to more extensive tumors involving regional areas of the temporal bone. Although the latter system attempts to define the anatomic origin of the tumor, both classifications address the pertinent issues of tumor size, petrous apex or carotid artery involvement, and intracranial extension. This provides critical information necessary to design an operative approach and plan.

PATIENT SELECTION

Patients with glomus tumors frequently report a history of symptoms of pulsatile tinnitus, hearing loss, aural fullness, and not uncommonly, cranial nerve dysfunction such as facial paresis, dysphasia, or hoarseness. Patients should be questioned regarding symptoms including tachycardia, palpitations, headaches, pallor, excessive perspiration, nausea, and problems of control of blood pressure, all of which are related to excess catecholamine secretion by the tumor. A complete otologic and head and neck examination is required. The tympanic membrane and middle ear space are inspected for tumor. When tumor is in the middle ear, a red mass is noted behind the tympanic membrane, and pulsation can be observed under high magnification (Fig. 125-1). The patient should be evaluated for evidence of weakness or dysfunction of cranial nerves VII, VIII, IX, X, XI, and XII. Both sides of the neck are palpated for mass lesions in the jugulodigastric and carotid bifurcation areas. Audiometry should be performed to determine the presence of a conductive, mixed, or sensorineural hearing loss.

Once a glomus tumor has been presumptively diagnosed by the history and physical examination, the diagnosis and evaluation of the type and extent of the tumor are required. Along with a history of pulsatile tinnitus or the presence of a vascular mass in the middle ear, radiologic imaging can demonstrate characteristic features strongly suggestive of glomus tumor. On computed tomography (CT) scanning, these features include the location of the lesion, bone erosion around the jugular bulb and carotid artery, and enhancement following administration of contrast. Large glomus tympanicum tumors can extend inferiorly into the hypotympanum and erode trabeculated bone toward the jugular bulb. Similarly, glomus jugulare tumors expand superiorly toward the hypotympanum and middle ear. It can occasionally be difficult to definitively characterize the site of origin. The differential diagnosis of an

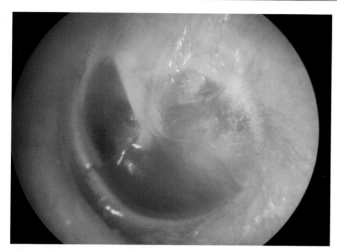

Figure 125-1. Left tympanic membrane with a pulsatile circumscribed vascular tumor filling the inferior portion of the middle ear.

expanding, bone-eroding enhancing tumor in the jugular fossa region include neurofibroma, schwannoma, lymphoma, meningioma, and metastatic disease. Biopsy is to be avoided owing to the vascular nature of the tumor. Only after the extent of tumor is defined (middle ear, jugular bulb, carotid artery, clivus, intracranial, or intradural extension) can decisions regarding optimal management be made. Glomus tumors are rarely malignant. However, because of their propensity for progressive and invasive growth and involvement of major vessels and lower cranial nerves, treatment is routinely required. It is only the occasional asymptomatic small tumor in an older person that can be followed up radiographically for evidence of growth.

Paragangliomas can also occur with other endocrine tumors associated with familial syndromes. Such tumors include carcinoma of the thyroid gland, medullary carcinoma of the thyroid, and those found with multiple endocrine neoplasia (MEN) type I, consisting of pituitary adenoma, parathyroid adenoma, and pancreatic islet cell adenoma.

Treatment options for glomus tumors of the temporal bone include observation with serial scanning to monitor for growth, microsurgical excision, and radiation therapy. Complete surgical resection minimizes the chance for recurrence but may entail significant morbidity. Radiation therapy does not eliminate the tumor but is intended to halt tumor progression. Proponents for surgery suggest radiation is indicated for palliation, following incomplete tumor excision or for patients who are medically infirm or elderly. However, there is strong evidence indicating that radiotherapy could also be considered the definitive treatment strategy for skull base glomus tumors. Glomus jugulare tumors have traditionally been treated by fractionated XRT. Hinerman and colleagues summarized their experience of 53 patients with 55 temporal bone tumors (46 were glomus jugulare and 9 were glomus tympanicum tumors). Patients received megavoltage radiation over a continuous course. With almost half of the patients followed up for 15 years, local tumor control was achieved in 93% of the previously untreated tumors and 92% of those previously treated.[9] The long-term results using stereotactic radiosurgery remain to be seen, but some early experience suggests there may be insufficient control of tumor if the planning treatment volume is kept too tight.[10] In a series of 42 patients treated with gamma knife surgery, 19 received radiation as their primary therapy and 23 patients for recurrent glomus jugulare tumor. The mean follow-up was 44 months (range 6 to 149 months). Although this is considered a relatively short period of time, tumor control was accomplished, in that 31% decreased in size, 67% were unchanged, and the only one that grew was in a patient who failed previous radiation therapy.[11]

We propose that healthy, young (younger than 65 years of age) patients should consider surgical resection. Large glomus tumors usually encroach on the ninth and tenth cranial nerves, putting them at risk during resection. Asymptomatic patients must be assessed as to whether they could tolerate the consequences of pharyngeal and laryngeal dysfunction. If sacrifice of the ninth and tenth cranial nerves is anticipated, patients with limited pulmonary reserve would be unlikely surgical candidates. In contrast, patients with a history of dysphagia or hoarseness who demonstrate vocal cord dysfunction can better tolerate sacrifice of the ninth and tenth cranial nerves. These people have typically developed compensatory mechanisms to minimize problems with swallowing and aspiration.

Large glomus jugulare tumors in relatively asymptomatic patients pose a significant dilemma in their optimal management. Specifically, patients having large tumors where surgical resection will likely incur new postoperative lower cranial nerve deficits often results in significant morbidity. The possible need for a tracheotomy, nasogastric tube placement, or percutaneous gastrostomy feeding tube, along with complications of aspiration, pneumonia, inanition, and weakness of the shoulder and tongue, must be considered by the patient and their family as well as the physicians and surgeons involved with the patient's care. Although radiation treatment in a relatively young person is not without short- or long-term risk, the aforementioned complications may have immense impact on the patient's future quality of life. Long-term results following total resection of class C and D tumors revealed that full rehabilitation may take 1 to 2 years. In a series by Briner and colleagues, 97% of patients finally resumed improved function, deeming their postoperative dysphasia tolerable and allowing a more normal social life.[12]

The optimal management program for patients 65 years of age and older should be individualized. Older patients with compromised pulmonary function or other chronic unstable medical conditions are not good surgical candidates. Radiation therapy has been shown to be an effective method for tumor palliation and thus is a reasonable alternative treatment.

PREOPERATIVE PLANNING

The granules contained within the chief cells of these tumors contain the precursors for catecholamine synthesis. Patients with intermittent or labile hypertension or those with signs and symptoms of a hypermetabolic state should be evaluated for a secreting tumor. Unlike the adrenal gland, glomus tumors lack the enzyme phenylethanolanine N-methyltransferase, which converts norepinephrine to epinephrine. This is why norepinephrine is the mostly commonly secreted chemotransmitter. Urine collected for 24 hours is screened for metanephrine, vanillylmandelic acid, epinephrine, and norepinephrine. Because the incidence of secreting glomus tumors is low (1% to 3%), elevated levels of these vasoactive peptides should also prompt investigation for pheochromocytoma. A CT scan of the abdomen is used to rule out a retroperitoneal adrenal or extra-adrenal tumor. Magnetic resonance imaging (MRI) can also be used, but it may be plagued by movement artifact. Further diagnostic evaluation is necessary when elevated levels of serum or urine catecholamine precursors and metabolites are identified. The workup for potential metastatic disease may also demand other radiographic techniques to locate sites of distant spread. Imaging with ^{123}I MIBG (metaiodobenzylguanidine) scintigraphy is picked up by active endocrine tissue such as paraganglioma, pheochromocytoma, and neuroblastoma. Anesthesia consultation for coordinating pharmacologic blockade is warranted for patients with elevated catecholamine levels. Both α- and β-adrenergic blockers such as phentolamine and propranolol, respectively, may be necessary.

Patients considered to be surgical candidates must have the extent of tumor involvement delineated. This entails imaging techniques that define the relationship of the tumor to critical anatomic structures. Currently, the diagnosis is usually made with contrast-enhanced CT or MRI scans. Bone-windowed, thin-cut (1.5-mm) CT images define the relationship of the tumor to the carotid artery, sigmoid sinus, jugular bulb, pars nervosa, middle ear, facial nerve, otic capsule, and posterior fossa (Fig. 125-2). MRI enhances the evaluation of glomus tumors of the temporal bone and skull base. Contrast-enhanced MRI identifies the tumor often with a speculated pattern described as "salt and pepper" vascularity with greater sensitivity in demonstrating tumors of the skull base. In addition to delineating the tumor, MRI demonstrates the relationship of the surrounding soft tissues and major vessels.

The soft tissue resolution and information obtained from MRI scans help differentiate tumor from surrounding soft tissue, brain parenchyma, and mucosal changes within the temporal bone (Fig. 125-3). The relatively new technique of magnetic resonance angiography (MRA) also shows the relationship of the tumor to carotid artery, sigmoid sinus, and jugular bulb (Fig. 125-4). MRA shows the proximity of the tumor or displacement of the major vessels along with the predominant blood supply. MR venography highlights the anatomy of the transverse, sigmoid, and petrosal sinuses;

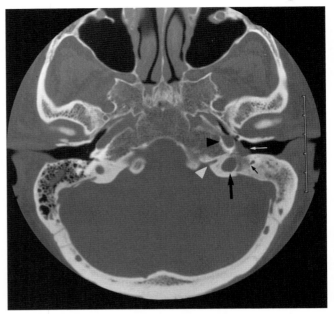

Figure 125-2. Bone-windowed computed tomography (CT) scan demonstrating the left middle ear and a hypotympanic mass *(white arrow)* infiltrating and eroding bone between the carotid artery *(black arrowhead)*, the jugular vein *(large black arrow)*, and the medial aspect of the facial nerve *(small black arrow)*. The pars nervosa is not affected *(white arrowhead)*.

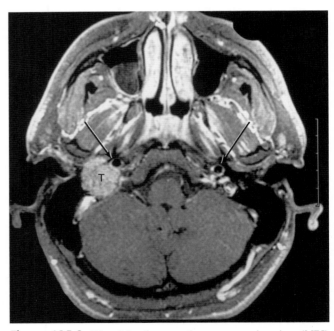

Figure 125-3. T1-weighted magnetic resonance imaging (MRI) scan with contrast showing a glomus tumor (T) occupying the right jugular fossa extending to the skull base. Note the internal carotid arteries *(arrows)*.

the jugular bulb; and the descending jugular vein. It is most helpful if the patency of these venous structures can be verified or if thrombosis is present. Although occasionally fraught with difficulty in interpretation, information regarding flow characteristics in these vessels may be helpful in determining the degree of tumor involvement and obstruction to flow.

Until the techniques and interpretation of MRA become consistently reliable and comprehensively informative, four-vessel cerebral angiography remains necessary. Angiography should be obtained when CT imaging identifies a large tumor or when carotid artery involvement is suspected or identified. The data gained from this study provide critical information needed to institute a management plan. The location and extent of tumor are identified by the vascular blush. The four-vessel study also identifies other paragangliomas that may be present in the head and neck area (Fig. 125-5). Patients with multiple paragangliomas have a higher incidence of similar tumors being identified in other family members.

An effective method of screening these individuals is with a contrast-enhanced CT scan of the temporal bone (skull base) and neck, down to the level of the carotid bifurcation. It is imperative to know whether multiple paragangliomas or carotid body tumors are present on the ipsilateral or contralateral side in order to avoid the potential devastating complications related to bilateral lower cranial nerve compromise. Arteriography demonstrates the blood supply to the lesion. The major blood supply of glomus jugulare tumors is from the ascending pharyngeal artery. When a significant feeding vessel is identified, selective angiography and embolization using polyvinyl alcohol or Gelfoam is performed. Large lesions (glomus jugulare) are routinely embolized 1 to 2 days before surgical resection (Fig. 125-6).

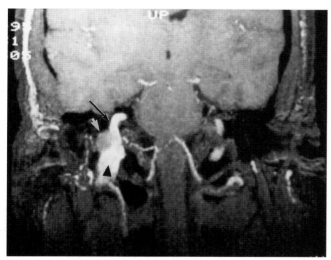

Figure 125-4. Magnetic resonance angiography (MRA) scan showing a tumor *(white arrow)* in the right skull base compressing the vertical portion of the carotid artery *(black arrow)*. The carotid artery and jugular vein are superimposed *(black arrowhead)*.

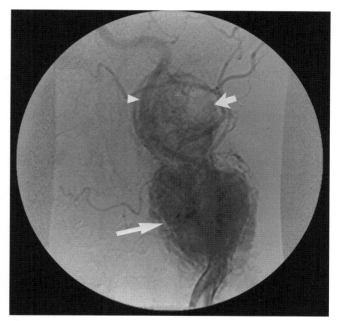

Figure 125-5. Left common carotid arteriogram of a patient with contralateral glomus jugulare demonstrating carotid body *(large arrow)* and glomus vagale *(small arrow)* tumors. The internal carotid artery is anteromedially displaced *(arrowhead)*.

Figure 125-6. A, Preembolization arteriogram revealing right glomus jugulare tumor with characteristic blush *(arrowhead)*. **B,** Postembolization study confirms effective occlusion of major feeding vessels. Tumor blush is significantly diminished.

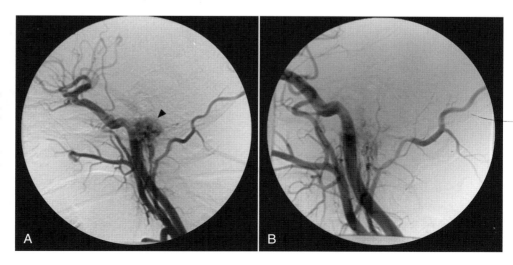

Based on CT scan findings demonstrating extensive involvement, intraoperative carotid artery injury, repair, or resection may be anticipated. In this situation, at the time of the arteriogram, a balloon catheter is also used to functionally test the competency of the contralateral cerebral blood supply and circle of Willis. Balloon test occlusion (BTO) of the ipsilateral internal carotid artery (ICA) helps determine whether the patient can tolerate carotid artery occlusion or sacrifice. Xenon blood flow studies during BTO provide an objective and quantitative measure of cerebral blood flow. This information helps the surgical team determine whether carotid artery sacrifice will be tolerated. Failure to successfully tolerate BTO or if inadequate blood flow is demonstrated indicates that carotid artery repair or bypass will be necessary if injury or sacrifice occurs. Other members of the skull base team (neurosurgeons, vascular surgeons) are alerted if intracranial tumor is present or vascular repair is likely.

Finally, the venous phase of the arteriogram also reveals whether the sigmoid sinus is patent or occluded, demonstrates other venous outflow pathways, and indicates the status of the contralateral sigmoid sinus and jugular vein (Fig. 125-7). If no venous obstruction is shown, then the venous drainage of the dominant side is also demonstrated. The relationship of the ipsilateral vein of Labbé to the transverse sinus should be defined. Although tumor does not usually extend this far proximal in the venous drainage system, this information should be confirmed.

Large glomus jugulare tumors are more likely to encroach on the ICA and the lower cranial nerves. The option of subtotal resection of a large tumor could be considered if cranial nerve function is normal preoperatively and compromise or sacrifice is anticipated to achieve complete resection. Determination is made

based on imaging, assessing whether the pars nervosa (medial aspect of the jugular bulb) is involved. Intradural extension of tumor in this area would define the need for resection of the entire jugular bulb and pars nervosa. This approach is planned preoperatively based on the patient's preference for maintaining normal physiologic function of phonation, respiration, and swallowing. Similar strategy for planned subtotal resection can be given if the carotid artery is involved.

Perioperative systemic antibiotics are not given for glomus tumors isolated to the middle ear or mastoid space. Prophylaxis is provided if cerebrospinal fluid (CSF) exposure is anticipated. Patients with large lesions (glomus jugulare) should have blood held for type and screen. Autologous donation for potential transfusion can be planned in advance.

The importance of a comprehensive and understandable informed consent cannot be overemphasized. It is most important to discuss with the patient and family the location of the tumor and its relationship to the surrounding vascular, dural, and neural structures. The treatment options of observation, surgical removal, or radiation therapy are reviewed. The risks, benefits, and outcomes are explained. The discussion must be delivered to assure that the patient understands the significance of potential loss of lower cranial nerve function. The potential need for additional surgical procedures to manage complications following tumor removal should be discussed. These include eye protection with a gold weight and possible lower lid tightening, tracheotomy, vocal cord medialization procedures, gastrostomy tube, or CSF lumbar drainage. Delivery of a comprehensive informed consent should be documented in the patient's medical record.

STEREOTACTIC RADIOSURGERY

Fractionated XRT has been the conventional method for radiation treatment. Newer techniques using a frame-based linear accelerator, gamma radiation from cobalt delivered through the gamma knife, or photon beam from a robot-mounted mini-linear accelerator such as the CyberKnife are available for single or multiple focused treatments (fractions) providing submillimeter accuracy in treatment delivery. This author prefers the CyberKnife system for various reasons. It is a robotic-assisted mini-linear accelerator delivering 6 megavolts of photon beams with 6 additional degrees of freedom compared with conventional gantry-mounted accelerator (Fig. 125-8A). It is a frameless localization and delivery system that avoids the minor morbidity of placing a head frame on the patient, making it ideal for fractionated treatment. More important, the system allows for treatment of tumors that extend below the skull base, such as glomus jugulare tumors that grow inferiorly within the jugular vein or glomus vagale tumors located high in the neck. The gamma knife system has its field of delivery limited at the skull base.

A variety of imaging modalities such CT, positron emission tomography, and MRI can be fused and

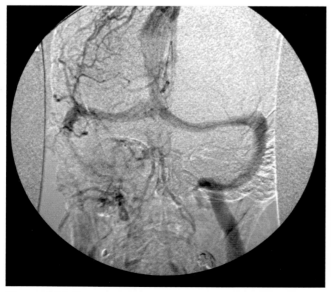

Figure 125-7. Venous phase of a carotid arteriogram showing marked attenuation of right sigmoid sinus and jugular vein flow with patency of the contralateral side.

anatomy of the temporal bone is also used to verify the location of the tumor and identifies other important structures to be protected from the full dose of delivered radiation. These are called *critical structures* and serve as avoidance structures that can be preferentially protected during treatment. At our institution, contouring the tumor is done both by the surgeon and radiation oncologist. The planned treatment is then created and reviewed with the radiation physicist and ultimately approved by the radiation oncologist. The tumor is radiated with 18 or 21 Gy to the 80% isodose line in three fractions. The dose at the margin of the tumor is usually close to the prescription dose of 18 or 21 Gy, unless there is a critical structure immediately adjacent to the tumor. Minimizing treatment to a critical structure would lower the dose at the margin of the tumor. The maximum tumor dose is 22.5 or 26.25 Gy at the 100% dose (see Fig. 125-8B). A thermoplastic mask (Aquaplast) is created at the time of simulation and tightly immobilizes the patient's head and neck, and offers similar degrees of accuracy to the more invasive gamma knife frame. Each of three treatments is given for approximately 30 minutes delivered every other day. No sedation, intravenous fluids, or hospitalization are necessary (see Fig. 125-8C).

Radiation therapy may incur long-term complications such as osteonecrosis, chronic otitis externa, breakdown of skin, eustachian tube dysfunction, and the potential development of malignant tumor. Acute cranial nerve dysfunction (hearing loss, imbalance or vertigo, facial paresis, vocal fold weakness, dysphagia) can occur and may be transient.

SURGICAL TECHNIQUES

Unless the lesion is small and clearly limited to the middle ear promontory, all procedures are performed with the patient under general endotracheal anesthesia using inhalation and intravenous techniques. Muscle relaxants are avoided, so that intraoperative monitoring of cranial nerves VII, IX, X, XI, or XII can be performed.

Glomus Tympanicum Tumors

The surgical approach for glomus tympanicum tumors is dictated by the size of the lesion. Small tumors limited to the mesotympanum and hypotympanum without involvement of the jugular bulb are removed through a transcanal approach. Larger lesions usually require a postauricular approach to provide greater exposure. A postauricular approach is also necessary when the inferior annulus is not adequately visualized through the external auditory meatus. This is often due to a prominent bulge from the anterior wall or a high floor of the ear canal.

Under the operating microscope, local anesthesia is injected as a four-quadrant block into the skin of the external auditory meatus. The same local solution is infiltrated into the skin of the postauricular sulcus. Lateral canal incisions at 12 o'clock and 6 o'clock are made and connected with a vertical incision

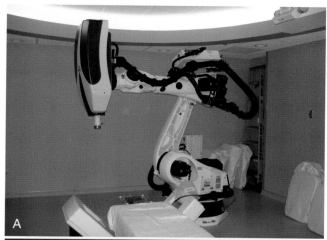

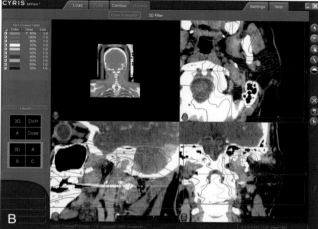

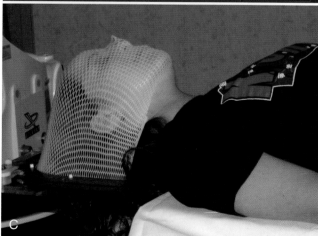

Figure 125-8. A, CyberKnife robotic radiosurgery system manufactured by Accuray, Sunnyvale, California. **B,** Contour and isodose treatment plan for a left jugular paraganglioma extending into the upper neck. **C,** Patient positioned on the CyberKnife treatment table secured by Aquaplast mask.

displayed by overlapping the images. The tumor map is contoured, outlining the field of interest using information from the fused scan, although treatment is based on CT confirmation. The soft tissue signal from the MRI scan allows the tumor to be outlined. The bony

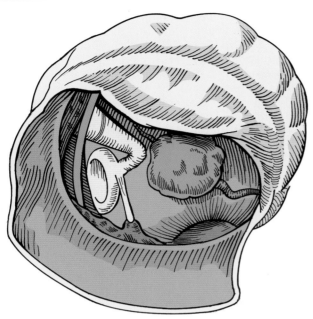

Figure 125-9. Transtympanic approach to a glomus tumor isolated within the middle ear.

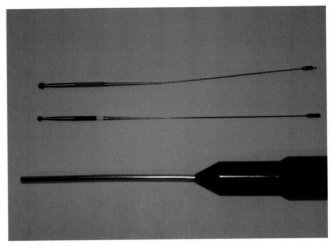

Figure 125-10. A microear drill is used to access narrow or small areas. Drill bits are available as cutting and diamond burrs.

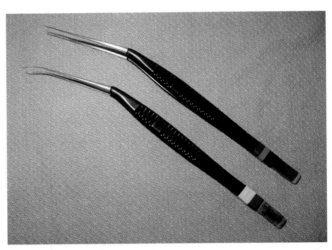

Figure 125-11. Microbipolar forceps facilitate cautery in the middle ear and can be used through an ear speculum.

approximately 5 mm from the annulus. The posterior canal skin flap that is based laterally is back-elevated within the canal. The flap is also known as the *vascular strip.* A postauricular incision is made and carried down to cortical mastoid bone. The spine of Henle is a good landmark for the slope of the posterior bony ear canal. The postauricular and canal flap incisions are connected and the ear is retracted anteriorly with a self-retaining retractor.

A tympanomeatal flap based on the anterior third of the medial ear canal is created. This incision extends from the 12-o'clock to the 4-o'clock position in a right ear or from the 12-o'clock to the 8-o'clock position in a left ear. The incision should preserve 5 mm of skin lateral to the annulus. The tympanomeatal flap is elevated, preserving the chorda tympani nerve. The margins of the tumor are dissected and elevated to isolate the vascular supply to the lesion (Fig. 125-9). Excision of a tumor that involves the hypotympanum requires greater exposure by removal of the inferior tympanic ring with a microear drill (Fig. 125-10). When the inferior margin of the tumor cannot be visualized, the tympanic bone can be taken down to the floor of the hypotympanum. If tumor infiltrates the trabeculated air cells of the hypotympanum, these cells and tumor are removed using a diamond burr. The use of microbipolar forceps facilitates hemostasis during removal of the tumor (Fig. 125-11). Often a pedicled vessel feeding the tumor can be found and should be electrocoagulated (see Video 125-1).

The vascular supply from the tympanic plexus is isolated and cauterized. If this is not possible, then the tumor is coagulated with the bipolar cautery and removed, and subsequent hemostasis is obtained. Small cotton balls soaked with 1 : 1000 epinephrine are useful to temporarily compress sites of bleeding during tumor removal from the middle ear. Oxidized cellulose compressed over the tumor is another effective method for obtaining temporary hemostasis. After the tumor is removed and hemostasis is obtained, the tympanomeatal flap is returned to its anatomic position. Depending on the extent of hypotympanic exposure, it may be necessary to support the inferior aspect of the flap with a medially placed temporalis fascia graft or Gelfoam placed in the hypotympanum. A silk sleeve supported with cotton balls or Gelfoam is used for a canal dressing.

Jugulotympanic Glomus Tumors

Jugulotympanic tumors that involve the middle ear, jugular bulb, and hypotympanic air cells are usually too large to remove through a transcanal approach. The tumor may erode bone near the carotid artery (Fisch type C$_1$, Glasscock-Jackson tympanicum type IV, or jugulare type I). It is usually not necessary to develop the exposure of the infratemporal fossa (ITF) and upper neck required for large glomus jugulare tumors. The initial transcortical mastoid approach is similar to that described for mastoidectomy (see Chapter 115). An incision is made 1 cm posterior to the postauricular crease. The skin, subcutaneous tissue, and fibroperiosteal layer over the mastoid cortex are incised and elevated from a posterior and anterior direction. Dissection is taken to the spine of Henle and the posterior aspect of the external auditory meatus. A transcortical mastoidectomy is performed with cutting burrs and suction irrigation. Landmarks to be identified are the antrum, mastoid tegmen, horizontal semicircular canal, fossa incudus, and short process of the incus. The sigmoid sinus is skeletonized to provide maximal exposure between the sigmoid sinus and the vertical portion of the facial nerve. The tumor may be encountered in the infralabyrinthine retrofacial air cells. Following an imaginary line drawn along the body of the incus and short process, the facial recess (posterior tympanotomy) is developed with cutting and then diamond burrs. Extending the facial recess toward the tympanic ring greatly improves exposure to the posterior mesotympanum and hypotympanum. It is necessary to sacrifice the chorda tympani nerve with an extended facial recess approach.

Attention is then turned to the external auditory canal (EAC). A tympanomeatal flap is developed from the 12-o'clock to the 5-o'clock position (for a right ear). Elevation of the tympanic membrane exposes the middle ear portion of the tumor. At this point, the surgeon must determine whether tumor can be removed with the given exposure. If extensive tumor involves the tympanic bone and hypotympanum, the infratympanic facial recess approach is extended (Fig. 125-12).[13] It may be necessary to create a "fallopian bridge" by skeletonizing the distal vertical portion of the facial nerve in order to remove all tumor. The margins of the tumor are dissected and defined. Hemostasis and tumor shrinkage are obtained with bipolar or microbipolar forceps. Tumor is removed with cup forceps (see Video 125-2). A cotton ball with epinephrine is used to temporarily control bleeding (see Video 125-3). If the exposure is still inadequate, the posterior canal wall may need to be taken down. If the tumor is more extensive than anticipated, management follows the description for glomus jugulare tumors (see Glomus Jugulare Tumors [Fisch types C_1 and C_2] later in this chapter).

Whether the canal wall is left up or taken down, tympanic membrane and ossicular chain reconstruction are undertaken as needed. When the incus is removed in order to facilitate tumor removal from the area around the stapes, an incus interpositioning is performed. If the malleus is absent, then stapes augmentation is achieved with either a partial ossicular replacement prosthesis or an ossicular remnant of the incus body or malleus head (see Chapter 114).

If the posterior canal wall is intact, the posterior canal skin flap (vascular strip or Koerner's flap) is

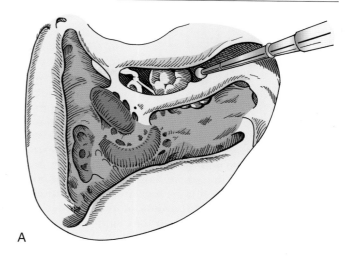

A

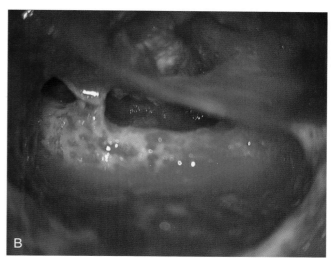

B

Figure 125-12. Access to the glomus tumor in the middle ear and hypotympanic space is achieved by extending the facial recess approach. Opening the retrofacial infralabyrinthine air cells provides exposure of the posterior margins of the tumor.

replaced along the posterior bony wall and the ear is returned to its anatomic position. A pack is placed in the external ear canal. Options for this include a silk sleeve, rosebud packing, Gelfoam, continuous gauze, or ointment. The author's group's preference is to use a silk sleeve bolstered with antibiotic-impregnated cotton balls.

If the posterior canal wall is taken down, a medial rosebud packing is placed (see Chapter 113). (Gelfoam may also be used to secure the tympanic membrane or graft.) The pinna is then returned to its anatomic position, placing the posterior canal wall skin flap into the mastoid cavity. A packing of antibiotic-impregnated continuous gauze is placed through the external auditory meatus and into the mastoid cavity. For both approaches, the postauricular incision is closed using 4-0 Nurolon suture. A sterile mastoid dressing is applied.

Glomus Jugulare Tumors
(Fisch Types C_1 and C_2)

Skin Incision

Preoperative determination of tumor extension provides information for the operative approach. Jugulare tumors with limited carotid involvement (Fisch types C_1 and C_2) may permit preservation of the posterior bony canal wall. A postauricular mastoidectomy incision located 3 cm posterior to the pinna extends over the lower border of the mastoid tip, through an upper neck skin crease, toward the greater cornu of the hyoid bone (Fig. 125-13). A second, deeper incision positioned 1 cm anteriorly through the musculoperiosteum layer over the mastoid cortex creates a "stepped" flap that facilitates closure at the end of the procedure. The musculoperiosteum layer cortex is elevated anteriorly toward the EAC. The neck incision goes through the subcutaneous tissue and platysma muscle, with preservation of the greater auricular nerve, which is harvested to its maximal length.

Neck Dissection

Dissection in the upper neck provides identification and isolation of cranial nerves X, XI, and XII and the great vessels. The neck dissection isolates the tail of the parotid from the sternocleidomastoid muscle (SCM). The spinal accessory nerve (CN XI) is identified at the anterior border of the SCM. Using cutting cautery, the SCM is released from its mastoid attachment and retracted posteriorly. The 11th cranial nerve is followed superiorly toward the jugular vein, identifying the 10th and 12th cranial nerves and the common, internal, and external carotid arteries. The tail of the parotid is elevated superiorly and anteriorly in order to identify the

posterior belly of the digastric muscle. The posterior belly of the digastric muscle is dissected from the digastric groove and retracted superiorly in order to expose the inferior contents of the jugular fossa and stylomastoid foramen (Fig. 125-14). The jugular vein, common carotid artery, ICA, and cranial nerves are isolated and tagged with appropriately colored vascular loops. The ascending pharyngeal and occipital arteries are usually encountered and need to be ligated. The lower cranial nerves, jugular vein, and carotid artery are further dissected superiorly to the inferior aspect of the tumor.

Transtemporal Dissection

A transcortical mastoidectomy is performed. The pertinent landmarks to be identified are the horizontal semicircular canal, incus, mastoid tegmen, sinodural angle, and sigmoid sinus. Management of the posterior bony canal wall depends on the extent of the tumor. Tumors with extensive involvement of the carotid artery (Fisch types C_3 and C_4), extension into the clivus, invasion into the cochlea (anacousis), or destruction of lateral perifacial air cells often require a canal wall down procedure, along with transposition of the facial nerve. Tumors that are less extensive may be removed through an extended facial recess approach. Similar to the approach for a small jugulotympanic glomus tumor, the extended facial recess approach begins superiorly at the chorda facial recess. Using the vertical portion of the facial nerve as the medial dissection limit, the tympanic bone is drilled from a superior-to-inferior-to-anterior direction. The chorda tympanic nerve is sacrificed. The lateral limit of the extended facial recess is the tympanic ring. Retrofacial and infralabyrinthine air cells and bone are removed to the stylomastoid foramen. The facial nerve is skeletonized, leaving eggshell-thin coverage surrounding a "fallopian bridge" (see Fig. 125-12).

The digastric ridge is delineated within the mastoid cavity. Dissection is continued anteriorly toward the stylomastoid foramen. Thinning the bone to eggshell thickness along the lateral inferior aspect of the digastric ridge facilitates removal of the mastoid tip using a rongeur. It is necessary to expose the posterior fossa dura both posterior and anterior to the sigmoid sinus. Some bone is left over the proximal sigmoid sinus near

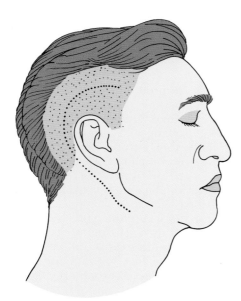

Figure 125-13. Skin incision for large glomus tumor when the carotid artery, jugular vein, and lower cranial nerves must be identified.

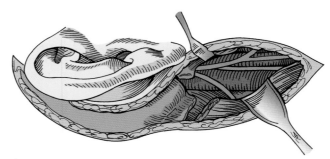

Figure 125-14. The postauricular incision is carried into the neck. The carotid artery, jugular vein, and lower cranial nerves are isolated. The sternocleidomastoid and digastric muscles are retracted.

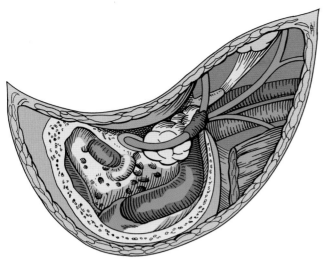

Figure 125-15. Transmastoid tumor dissection isolating the sigmoid sinus, vertical facial nerve along the extended facial recess, digastric ridge, neck vessels, and lower cranial nerves.

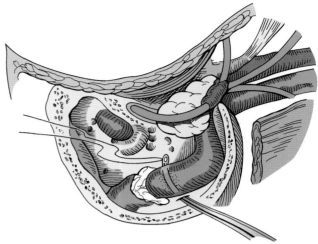

Figure 125-16. The extended facial recess approach exposes the tumor in the hypotympanum. The vertical portion of the facial nerve remains in place. The proximal sigmoid sinus can be isolated by extraluminal packing or suture ligation.

the sinodural angle (above Donaldson's line). The sigmoid sinus is carefully dissected free from the overlying roof of bone. This exposure provides access to extraluminal packing or suture ligation of the sinus. Dissection with the drill is continued along the sigmoid sinus toward the jugular bulb. All bone must be removed from this area. The tumor is now removed.

This approach provides exposure of, but limited controlled access to, the infratemporal carotid artery (Fig. 125-15). Preoperative imaging determines whether distal and proximal control of the petrous carotid artery is necessary to safely remove all tumor. If the tumor does not erode the bone surrounding the carotid artery, this canal wall-up, extended facial recess approach provides appropriate exposure.

Tumor Isolation and Removal

Venous bleeding may occur from the sigmoid sinus, jugular vein, condylar vein, or inferior petrosal sinus. The first two are controlled at the onset of tumor removal. The sigmoid sinus may be occluded by either extraluminal packing or ligation. Extraluminal occlusion is performed with oxidized cellulose that is packed under a retained shelf of bone covering the proximal sigmoid sinus. If this is not successful or feasible, ligation of the sinus is performed by making small openings in the dura anterior and posterior to the sigmoid sinus. An aneurysm needle is passed from posterior to anterior deep to the sigmoid sinus. The needle is blindly passed medial to, but hugging, the sigmoid sinus, avoiding injury to the intracranial contents (cerebellum). A long 2-0 silk ligature is passed through the aneurysm, needle up to its mid length, and the aneurysm needle is withdrawn. The suture is then cut in half, so as to leave two separate ligatures (Fig. 125-16). A small piece of muscle is harvested and placed over the sigmoid sinus, and the first suture is tied and secured. The

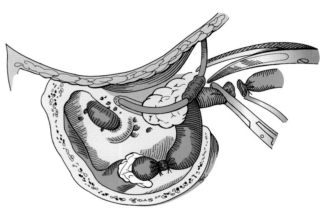

Figure 125-17. Proximal control of the sigmoid sinus is achieved. Surgicel packing can also be used to occlude the proximal sigmoid sinus. The jugular vein is divided, and the proximal segment is dissected into the jugular fossa. The anterior plane of dissection is along the carotid artery, which is not shown (see Fig. 125-16).

second suture is similarly tied, thus providing double ligation and occlusion of the sigmoid sinus.

The jugular vein in the neck is doubly ligated at this time. The proximal stump of the jugular vein in the neck is dissected superiorly toward the jugular bulb and fossa (Fig. 125-17). Care is taken to preserve the spinal accessory nerve. It is usually necessary to pass the proximal stump of the jugular vein medial to the spinal accessory nerve in order to facilitate the superior dissection. The distal extratemporal ICA should be in direct view as the jugular vein is dissected toward the jugular bulb. The styloid process and its muscular attachments may need to be removed in order to gain access to the skull base.

The sigmoid sinus is opened distal to the ligatures in order to inspect the intraluminal contents. Usually, the medial wall of the sigmoid sinus is not invaded by tumor unless there is intracranial extension. The inferior aspect of the sigmoid sinus is incised in a longitudinal direction toward the jugular bulb. The tumor is sequentially isolated from a posterior-to-anterior direction, dissecting the superior, lateral, and inferior walls of the sigmoid sinus from the medial wall. Bipolar coagulation is usually needed to obtain hemostasis and shrink the tumor. The lateral and superior aspect of the jugular bulb are dissected toward the superior extent of the tumor. Tumor often occludes the jugular bulb. However, once the tumor is removed from this area, brisk bleeding may be encountered from the multiple orifices of the inferior petrosal sinus and condylar vein. The medial jugular fossa is packed with oxidized cellulose. This dissection is performed medial (deep) to the vertical portion of facial nerve and stylomastoid area. Care must be taken to avoid trauma or pressure to the medial (deep) surface of the facial nerve. Tumor often remains in the hypotympanum and middle ear. This is removed by working both medial and lateral to the facial nerve.

Certain intraoperative findings may necessitate a canal-wall-down procedure. The first is the need for increased exposure of tumor invading the carotid artery. Also, limited space in the retrofacial and infralabyrinthine areas may require transposition of the facial nerve in order to provide adequate exposure of the tumor. Reconstruction of the tympanic membrane and ossicular chain can still be performed as needed.

Unless the medial wall of the jugular bulb or sigmoid sinus is removed, CSF is not encountered. However, the dead space created by the removal of bone and tumor requires partial obliteration with abdominal fat. Packing of the ear canal is identical to that described previously. A Hemovac drain is placed deep to the neck skin flaps. The postauricular wound is closed in three layers, reapproximating the musculoperiosteum, subcutaneous tissue, and skin.

Large Glomus Jugulare Tumors (Fisch Type C$_2$ or Greater)

A large postauricular C-shaped incision begins 3 cm superior to the pinna. If it is known that an ITF dissection is necessary to gain access to the distal ICA, then the incision begins anterior and superior to the pterion. The incision extends posteriorly and inferiorly 3 to 4 cm posterior to the helical rim, continues inferiorly across the lower border of the mastoid tip, and through upper neck skin crease toward the greater cornu of the hyoid bone in anticipation of isolation of the great vessels and lower cranial nerves. This creates an anteriorly based flap, which will include the pinna. The superior incision and dissection are taken down to the level of the temporalis fascia.

The EAC is transected medial to the cartilaginous bony junction. The skin of the proximal canal is dissected away from the underlying cartilaginous canal, and the cartilage is removed. This leaves a cuff of external auditory meatus skin that will be everted by placing superior and inferior sutures in the canal skin. The

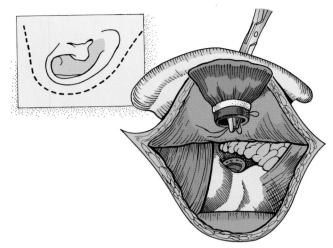

Figure 125-18. The ear canal is transected. A fibroperiosteal flap based on the posterior canal has been created. The ear canal skin is everted with a horizontal suture passed through the distal cuff of canal skin. (*Redrawn from Gantz BJ, Fisch U: Modified transotic approach to the cerebellopontine angle. Arch Otolaryngol 109:253, 1983. Copyright 1983, American Medical Association.*)

ends of these sutures are passed retrograde through the EAC. This facilitates eversion of the cuff of the external auditory meatus skin, which is reapproximated in a linear fashion with interrupted sutures of 4-0 Dexon (Fig. 125-18). A deep flap of fibroperiosteum is developed in order to create a second layer for closure of the external meatus. This 2.5- × 2.5-cm flap is based on the posterior aspect of the subcutaneous tissue of the EAC. It is sutured anteriorly to the subcutaneous tissue of the skin just deep to the tragus.

Neck Dissection

The approach and dissection in the neck are identical to that previously described for smaller glomus jugulare tumors. The great vessels and cranial nerves are isolated and tagged with vessel loops. A moistened lap sponge is left in the wound during the infratemporal fossa dissection.

Infratemporal Fossa Dissection

Preoperative evaluation will determine the degree of involvement of the carotid artery or clivus. Extensive tumors involving the horizontal portion of the carotid artery and petrous apex require dissection of the ITF. This approach provides necessary exposure for control of the distal ICA. The upper limb of the skin incision must be extended toward the forehead, just superior to the pterion. The superior skin flap is elevated superficial to the temporalis fascia down to the level of the zygomatic arch. Care is taken to go medial to the deep cervical fascia in order to avoid injury to the temporal branches of the facial nerve. Dissection with electrocautery facilitates removal of the attachments of temporalis fascia to the arch and body of the zygoma. Similarly, the fascial attachment of the masseter muscle is removed from the inferior surface of the zygomatic arch, which

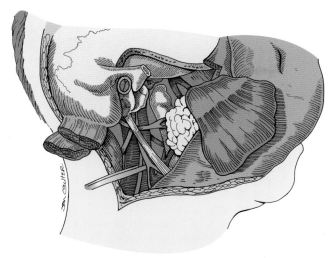

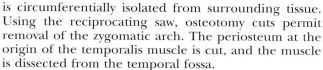

Figure 125-19. Removing the zygomatic arch permits mobilization of the temporalis muscle, exposing the infratemporal fossa. Soft tissue dissection isolating the extratemporal facial nerve, great vessels, and lower cranial nerves is demonstrated. The tumor has not been exposed in the temporal bone.

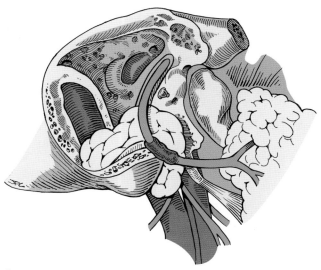

Figure 125-20. Radical mastoidectomy has been performed by removing the posterior canal wall medially to the skeletonized facial nerve. The digastric ridge is dissected in preparation for removing the mastoid tip and mobilizing the facial nerve. The tumor in the middle ear and mastoid is evident.

is circumferentially isolated from surrounding tissue. Using the reciprocating saw, osteotomy cuts permit removal of the zygomatic arch. The periosteum at the origin of the temporalis muscle is cut, and the muscle is dissected from the temporal fossa.

The dissection is continued in a subperiosteal plane into the ITF (Fig. 125-19). Venous bleeding is often encountered and controlled with bipolar coagulation and oxidized cellulose. Inferior and anterior retraction of the mandibular condyle widens the exposure. However, should complete exposure and control of the carotid artery be necessary, then resection of the mandibular condyle improves surgical access to the vertical segment of the carotid. The attachment of the pterygoid muscle to the neck of the condyle is divided with electrocoagulation. The condyle may be removed with a reciprocating saw. Dissection in the ITF is directed toward the foramen ovale (trigeminal nerve V3) and foramen spinosum (middle meningeal artery). Control of the carotid artery is obtained by performing an inferior frontotemporal craniotomy. A craniotomy is performed by placing burr holes through which the underlying dura is elevated and bone flap removed. Additional exposure of the petrous apex and carotid artery at the infratemporal skull base is accomplished with a dissecting drill and rongeurs. The horizontal segment of the petrous ICA is identified and isolated by this extradural middle fossa dissection. This approach facilitates the subtemporal ITF exposure of pertinent petrous artery landmarks: V3, greater superficial petrosal nerve, and middle meningeal artery.

Transtemporal Dissection

Complete mastoidectomy is performed. The approach and dissection are identical to that previously described for smaller glomus jugulare tumors (Fisch type C_2 or

greater). Exposure of the dura of the posterior fossa anterior and posterior to the sigmoid sinus must be performed in anticipation of opening the dura, possible resection of the dura, and removal of the tumor. Most tumors require complete exposure of the middle ear and necessitate removing the posterior canal wall along with the epithelium of the medial EAC and tympanic membrane. Reconstruction of the middle ear is usually not feasible owing to the extent of the lesion and the need to obliterate the eustachian tube to avoid CSF rhinorrhea. If function of the cochlea is to be preserved, the incudostapedial joint is separated through the facial recess approach. The ossicles lateral to the stapes and the tympanic membrane may be removed. The posterior bony canal wall is taken down to the level of the horizontal and vertical portion of the facial nerve. Similarly, the anterior canal wall must be removed to the level of the parotid gland and periosteum of the glenoid fossa. Tumor extending into the middle ear is encountered at this time. The vertical segment of the facial nerve interferes with access to large tumors filling the jugular fossa and invading the carotid artery. Facial nerve transposition is usually necessary to achieve optimal exposure. The facial nerve is decompressed from the geniculate ganglion to the stylomastoid foramen with cutting and then diamond burrs. Favorable anatomy may permit more limited mobilization of the facial nerve from its second genu (Fig. 125-20).

Precise dissection and isolation of the facial nerve in the stylomastoid foramen is difficult. The transposition is facilitated by cutting the remaining tendon and fibers of the digastric muscle within the mastoid proximal to the stylomastoid foramen. The muscle, along with the contents of the stylomastoid foramen, is elevated from the underlying bone in a posterior-to-anterior direction. The facial nerve is then dissected

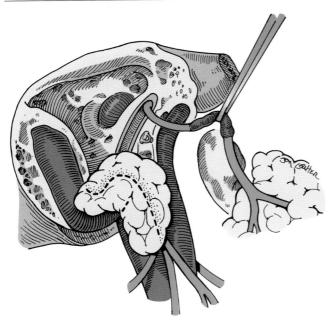

Figure 125-21. The facial nerve has been mobilized anteriorly, exposing the tumor in the mastoid, middle ear, and jugular bulb areas. The tendons attached to the styloid process have been divided. Retraction of the mandible permits isolation of the carotid artery.

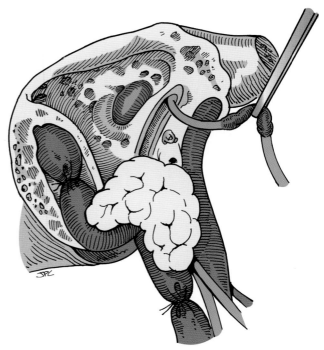

Figure 125-22. The proximal sigmoid sinus and jugular vein are suture ligated. The tumor is carefully dissected off the carotid artery. The lateral sigmoid sinus is opened.

away from the fallopian canal. The cuff of fibrous tissue surrounding the facial nerve is sutured anteriorly to the periparotid fascia, providing retraction of the vertical and horizontal facial nerve. Complete removal of the tympanic ring and remaining mastoid tip can then be accomplished. The styloid process is identified and removed by releasing the stylohyoid and styloglossal tendons from the tip of the styloid (Fig. 125-21).

Tumor Isolation and Removal

The tumor is removed. The sigmoid sinus is isolated proximally, and the jugular vein is ligated in the upper neck (Fig. 125-22). Resection of the tumor follows the same sequence as that previously described for less extensive glomus jugulare tumors. Tumor found superior to the jugular bulb and into the middle ear is dissected away from the otic capsule. If erosion into the inner ear occurs, further drilling of the otic capsule facilitates removal of the tumor.

Remaining tumor is carefully dissected off the carotid artery in a subadventitial plane, which completes the extradural dissection and removal of the tumor. The fibrocartilaginous ring surrounding the carotid artery at the skull base must be divided to achieve this plane (Fig. 125-23).

If intracranial tumor is found, the dura of the posterior fossa is opened. The medial wall of the sigmoid sinus and jugular bulb typically require resection. Care is taken to preserve the neural contents of the pars nervosa. Significant intracranial extension of tumor and jugular bulb involvement obviate successful nerve preservation. Tumor is removed from the cerebellopontine angle (Fig. 125-24). Often the intracranial

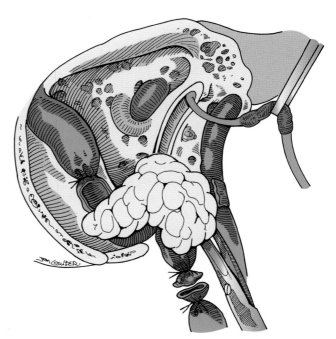

Figure 125-23. The sigmoid sinus and jugular vein have been divided. The inferior aspect of the tumor is dissected off the carotid artery in a subadventitial plane.

portion of the tumor has been devascularized by the skull base dissection. Should a large amount of intracranial tumor remain with limited exposure, then a retrosigmoid craniotomy is performed. This additional exposure would be anticipated based on preoperative

Chapter 125   **Glomus Tumors**   **1333**

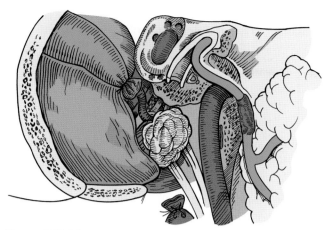

Figure 125-24. The dura is resected when tumor invades the posterior fossa and additional exposure is needed. Tumor in this area often requires sacrifice of lower cranial nerves. Dural grafting is necessary. (*Redrawn from Sekhar LN, Janecka IP [eds]: Surgery of Cranial Base Tumors. New York, Raven Press, 1993.*)

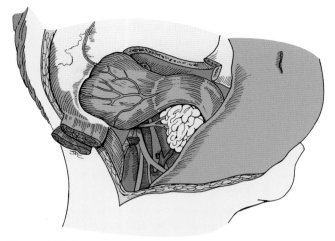

Figure 125-25. The temporalis muscle is rotated posteriorly and inferiorly to provide a vascularized graft, facilitating wound closure.

imaging and planning. A second-stage procedure may be required if a large amount of residual tumor is present. When all tumor has been removed and hemostasis achieved, the wound is then closed. Care is taken to ensure obliteration of the eustachian tube to avoid postoperative CSF rhinorrhea. The body of the incus, a small piece of muscle, and oxidized cellulose are packed into the eustachian tube. Large defects in the dura are repaired primarily with grafts of temporalis fascia, although watertight closure in this area can be difficult. Other fascial tissue available include galea, pericranium, and fascia lata. It also may be necessary to close the small openings in the dura where the sigmoid sinus was ligated. Small pieces of muscle are bolstered over these defects with figure-of-eight sutures in the dura. Fat is harvested from the abdominal wall. The wound is copiously irrigated with a bacitracin solution, and the fat is placed into the temporal bone defect area.

Patients with large lesions requiring removal of posterior fossa dura and grafting are at greater risk for CSF leaks. Additional tissue may be necessary to provide watertight closure of the wound. The temporalis muscle can be elevated and transposed posteriorly and inferiorly in order to facilitate this closure. It is usually necessary to remove the root of the zygoma in order to pedicle and rotate the entire temporalis muscle. The edges of the temporalis muscles are approximated to the SCM and semispinalis and splenius capitis muscles (Fig. 125-25). Extensive tumors that require a transotic capsule approach with large areas of temporal bone resection create considerable dead space that may not be adequately obliterated with abdominal fat. In some cases, it may be necessary to fill the defect with a free flap of rectus abdominis muscle. The SCM and proximal posterior belly of the digastric muscles are also reapproximated to the fibroperiosteal tissue on the skin flap that covered the mastoid cortex. A small Hemovac drain is tunneled through a stab incision in the posterior neck and placed in the inferior aspect of the neck

dissection and left to gravity drainage overnight. The skin flap is returned to its anatomic position and closed in a three-layer fashion. A running locking suture reapproximates the skin. Staples may also be used. A sterile compression mastoid and neck dressing are applied.

POSTOPERATIVE CARE

The level and intensity of postoperative monitoring and management are dictated by the extent of the surgical procedure and the neurovascular structures encountered. Small lesions that were approached through an endaural incision receive basic postoperative care. Vital signs are monitored on a routine basis. The ear packing is changed as needed. The patient should be ready for discharge the following morning.

Tumors excised by a combined transmeatal postauricular approach are managed in a similar fashion. A mastoid dressing that was placed postoperatively is removed the following morning. Patients are instructed to change the external canal cotton ball as needed. The postauricular incision is cleaned with peroxide or alcohol, and a topical antibiotic ointment is applied twice a day. Patients are seen 7 to 10 days postoperatively. Those patients with an endaural approach have the packing removed and the tympanic membrane inspected for integrity. Those with a combined approach have their sutures and outer ear canal packing removed. The patient is instructed to use topical ear drops twice a day, and the inner packing is removed 1 week later.

Patients with more extensive tumors requiring resection of dura frequently have the external ear canal closed as a blind sac. If a Hemovac neck drain is placed, it is removed the day following surgery. A pressure dressing remains for 3 days. Patients are carefully assessed for function of the lower cranial nerves. Oral intake is commenced if dysphagia and aspiration do not occur. Corneal protection with a moisture chamber, artificial tears, and ointment at night are provided if facial paresis is present. Patients are encouraged to be out of bed the following day. Management of complications or cranial nerve injury is detailed in the following section. Sutures are removed 7 to 10 days postoperatively. In order to assess the status of the excised tumor, a baseline scan is obtained postoperatively at 3 months. MRI with fat suppression technique helps differentiate the varied tissue densities within the operative site. Any suspicious areas identified on the scan prompt a repeat scan in 6 months. Otherwise, imaging is obtained in 1 year. If this is negative for tumor, a scan is obtained 1 year later.

COMPLICATIONS

The potential complications following glomus tumor surgery are numerous and depend on the location and extent of the tumor. The postoperative complications following glomus tumor surgery can be divided into those that pertain to problems with the wound, bleeding, CSF leak, neurologic, and cranial nerve deficits.

A seroma or hematoma may compromise wound healing. Glomus jugulare tumors require a large skin flap and dissection into the neck. Obtaining a watertight closure may be difficult with regard to the integrity of the dura. For this reason, a Hemovac drain remains only until the following day. It is kept to gravity drainage as opposed to negative pressure. A pressure dressing is also applied to the wound to minimize the possibility of seroma or hematoma. A collection of CSF (pseudomeningocele) is managed by maintaining a pressure dressing and elevating the head. If the CSF collection continues to expand, then lumbar drainage is instituted for 3 to 5 days.

Injury to cranial nerves results in functional deficits that must be addressed. Transposition of the facial nerve usually results in temporary facial paresis or paralysis. It is difficult to predict when the return of facial function will occur. Corneal protection is necessary if the patient has inadequate eye closure. Topical artificial tears are used throughout the day. Ophthalmic ointment is placed in the lower conjunctival sulcus at night. Additional daytime protection with a clear plastic moisture chamber provides comfort and minimizes corneal desiccation. Long-term eye protection is effectively provided with placement of a gold weight in the sub orbicularis oculi muscle/pretarsal space (see Chapter 121). A lower lid–tightening procedure is recommended for patients with laxity of the lower lid or those demonstrating ectropion.

Complications related to the tympanic membrane and ossicular chain can occur when excising tympanic or jugulotympanic glomus tumors. During an endaural approach with the tympanomeatal flap elevated, inadvertent contact with a microbipolar forceps to the tympanic membrane may result in ischemia and necrosis. A tympanic membrane perforation may result, requiring a patch or formal myringoplasty (see Chapter 113). Persistent conductive hearing loss as a result of ossicular chain reconstruction can be subsequently revised or treated with a hearing aid. The maximal conductive hearing loss that results from obliteration of the middle ear space and closure of the ear canal is more difficult to manage. Unless a deep cuff of tissue is constructed to create an external auditory meatus that would fit an ear mold, the use of a hearing aid will not be successful.

Injury or sacrifice to the ninth and tenth cranial nerves in patients who previously were asymptomatic results in problems of dysphagia, aspiration, and hoarseness. Despite the patient being under general anesthesia, it is reasonable to perform an intraoperative vocal cord medialization procedure (thyroplasty type I) while the neck is open (see Chapter 41). If the 10th cranial nerve is anatomically intact, then postoperative assessment is determined when the patient is awake.

Injury to the spinal accessory nerve results in shoulder drop and dysfunction. Postoperative physical rehabilitation therapy should be requested once the patient is ambulatory.

Tumors that extend inferiorly into the neck may put the hypoglossal nerve at risk. This would be unusual unless there is an associated large glomus vagale or carotid body tumor. Dysmotility of the tongue may result in mild dysarthria and problems with deglutition. Functionally, this injury alone is usually well tolerated. However, in combination with injury to the ninth and tenth cranial nerves, hypoglossal injury puts the patient at greater risk for dysphagia and aspiration. Thus patients who are clinically symptomatic postoperatively should be evaluated for a vocal cord medialization procedure. An arytenoid adduction procedure augments the closure of the posterior glottic chink, which further minimizes the potential for aspiration. Tracheotomy may still be necessary for uncontrolled aspiration and pulmonary toilet. Cricopharyngeal myotomy further relaxes the upper esophageal sphincter, which facilitates swallowing.

Watertight closure may be difficult when the dura is resected and repaired. Avoidance of a CSF leak is accomplished by meticulous obliteration of the eustachian tube, packing of the mastoid cavity with fat, and three-layer closure to the muscle and fibroperiosteum, subcutaneous tissue, and skin. Due to the critical structures adjacent to glomus tumors including the lower cranial nerves, carotid artery, jugular vein and venous sinuses, the dura, brain and spinal fluid serious complications of lateral skull base surgery do occur. The mortality from management of the carotid artery has resulted from cerebrovascular complications. In a large series of glomus tumors of the temporal bone treated surgically, the rate of CSF leak was 11.6% and incidence of aspiration pneumonia was 5.3%.[5] The incidence of postoperative CSF leak dropped to 4.5% when dural closure or reconstruction involved a vascularized local, regional, or free flap.[14]

If CSF leak occurs through the skin or nose despite a pressure dressing, lumbar drainage is instituted. This is maintained at 6 to 10 mL/hr over 3 to 5 days. Although rarely necessary, persistent CSF leak may warrant wound reexploration.

Ongoing problems with aspiration may prevent resumption of oral intake. In the immediate postoperative period, nutritional support is provided by nasogastric feeding. Despite efforts to provide glottic competence with swallowing therapy, a gastrostomy or jejunostomy feeding tube may be necessary.

Management of intraoperative injury to the ICA is dictated by results of BTO and xenon blood flow studies. Demonstration of inadequate contralateral perfusion requires preservation of the ipsilateral carotid. Laceration or tear is either primarily repaired or replaced with a saphenous vein graft. Despite data providing assurance of adequate contralateral flow, ligation of the carotid artery may result in progressive thrombus formation and possible emboli. Patients in whom a carotid artery was repaired or grafted should have postoperative studies, such as Doppler ultrasound, MRA, or trans-femoral arteriography, to determine the status of the ICA. Patients exhibiting ischemic neurologic compromise should be considered for embolectomy or heparinization.

- Intraoperative severe and difficult to control hypertension may occur in patients with unrecognized preoperative symptoms and signs of a vasoactive-secreting tumor.
- Incomplete assessment of patients with a family history of paraganglioma may proceed toward subsequent growth of multicentric tumors resulting in more difficult management decisions affecting the cranial nerves and great vessels of the head and neck.
- Following resection of a glomus jugulare tumor, sacrifice of a patent sigmoid sinus and jugular vein when the contralateral central venous outflow is insufficient may result in intracranial hypertension.
- Unexpected facial nerve injury can result if involvement of the vertical portion of the facial nerve from posterior tumor extension in the middle ear and hypotympanum is not recognized.

PEARLS

- Arteriography and venous outflow studies are helpful for large tumors by identifying the blood supply of the tumor, the proximity of the major vessels, occlusion of the ipsilateral jugular vein, patency of the contralateral venous drainage system, and the opportunity for tumor embolization before surgical resection.
- Stereotactic radiotherapy may provide effective control of tumor when given as the primary modality of treatment, following recurrence of tumor, or as part of the planned strategy for subtotal resection.
- Small cotton balls soaked with 1 : 1000 epinephrine are useful to temporarily compress sites of bleeding during tumor removal from the middle ear.
- Rotation of a vascularized temporoparietal fascia/muscle flap is an effective reconstructive technique for closure of a cranial and dural defect, minimizing the risk of CSF leak.
- The potential morbidity of newly acquired cranial nerve dysfunction (CN VII-XII) following resection of large glomus jugulare tumors demands a comprehensive discussion with the patient and family and documentation of the informed consent containing the options, risks, and benefits of the treatment.

PITFALLS

- Failure to recognize potential compromise of the lower cranial nerves following resection of large glomus jugulare tumors may incur significant postoperative morbidity and changes in the quality of life.

References

1. Mulligan RM: Chemodectomy in the dog. Am J Pathol 26:680-681, 1950.
2. Guild SR: The glomus jugulare, a nonchromaffin paraganglion, in man. Ann Otol Rhinol Laryngol 62:1045-1071, 1953.
3. Bartels LJ, Pennington J, Kamerer DB, et al: Primary fallopian canal glomus tumors. Otolaryngol Head Neck Surg 102:101-105, 1990.
4. Heth J: The basic science of glomus jugulare tumors. Neurosurg Focus 17:E2, 2004.
5. Manolidis S, Shohet JA, Jackson CG, et al: Malignant glomus tumors. Laryngoscope 109:30-34, 1999.
6. Fisch U: Infratemporal fossa approach for glomus tumors of the temporal bone. Ann Otol Rhinol Laryngol 91(5 Pt 1):474-479, 1982.
7. Fisch U, Rouleau M: Facial nerve reconstruction. J Otolaryngol 9:487-492, 1980.
8. Jackson CG, Glasscock ME 3rd, Harris PF: Glomus tumors. Diagnosis, classification, and management of large lesions. Arch Otolaryngol 108:401-410, 1982.
9. Hinerman RW, Mendenhall WM, Amdur RJ, et al: Definitive radiotherapy in the management of chemodectomas arising in the temporal bone, carotid body, and glomus vagale. Head Neck 23:363-371, 2001.
10. Feigenberg SJ, Mendenhall WM, Hinerman RW, et al: Radiosurgery for paraganglioma of the temporal bone. Head Neck 24:384-389, 2002.
11. Pollock BE: Stereotactic radiosurgery in patients with glomus jugulare tumors. Neurosurg Focus 17:E10, 2004.
12. Briner HR, Linder TE, Pauw B, et al: Long-term results of surgery for temporal bone paragangliomas. Laryngoscope 109:577-583, 1999.
13. Jackson CG: The infratympanic extended facial recess approach for anteriorly extensive middle ear disease: A conservation technique. Laryngoscope 103(4 Pt 1):451-454, 1993.
14. Jackson CG, McGrew BM, Forest JA, et al: Lateral skull base surgery for glomus tumors: Long-term control. Otol Neurotol 22:377-382, 2001.

Chapter **126**

Cholesterol Granuloma and Congenital Epidermoid Tumors of the Temporal Bone

Barry E. Hirsch and Alec Vaezi

Expansile destruction of the petrous apex may be due to congenital epidermoid tumor or cholesterol granuloma. The etiology, incidence, and management of cholesterol granuloma and congenital epidermoid tumor within the temporal bone are different. Distinguishing between these two processes was difficult before the advent of computed tomography (CT) and magnetic resonance imaging (MRI), especially when the lesion or tumor originated medially and anteriorly within the petrous apex.

Pathology extending in this area challenges the neurotologic team to comprehensively evaluate and effectively manage these lesions. Abnormalities in the petrous apex may be silent for many years because of the depth and isolation of this area. Once the pathology encroaches on surrounding vital structures such as the dura and brain, carotid artery, orbit, 4th through 11th cranial nerves, and otic capsule, symptoms and signs will become apparent. Pathology in the petrous apex is often identified incidentally or when diagnostic imaging is performed for vaguely described symptoms such as lightheadedness; retro-orbital, ear, vertex, or occipital head pain; tinnitus; visual blurriness; or diplopia. Just as the causes and radiologic findings differ, so do the management strategies and surgical approaches.

PERTINENT ANATOMY

The petrous apex is a wedge-shaped structure that occupies the medial and anterior aspect of the temporal bone. The petrous apex is inferior, medial, anterior, and superior to the otic capsule. The superior surface forms the floor of the middle cranial fossa. Along this surface pass the greater and lesser superficial petrosal nerves and is the exit point for the middle meningeal

artery through the foramen spinosum. At the tip of the petrous apex lies a depression containing the gasserian ganglion of the trigeminal nerve. The petroclinoid ligament forms the attachment of the tip of the petrous apex to the sphenoid bone. This area is termed *Meckel's cave,* through which passes the fifth cranial nerve. The sixth cranial nerve is located just medially and passes through Dorello's canal. The horizontal portion of the carotid artery lies posteromedial to V3, and its bony covering is often dehiscent. The anterolateral surface of the petrous bone contains the genu of the carotid artery and its horizontal segment. The bony opening of the eustachian tube passes in an anterior, inferior, and medial direction toward the nasopharynx. The jugular bulb and vein exit the inferior surface of the petrous bone through the jugular foramen. The 9th, 10th, and 11th cranial nerves also leave the skull base through the pars nervosa of the jugular fossa. The carotid foramen lies anterior to the jugular bulb on the inferior surface of the petrous bone. The posteromedial surface of the temporal bone faces the posterior fossa. Openings into this surface include the internal auditory canal (IAC), which contains the cochlear, vestibular, facial, and intermedius nerves; the operculum, which contains the endolymphatic duct and sac; and the aperture for the subarcuate artery. The posterior aspect of the temporal bone contains the mastoid cavity and faces the sigmoid sinus and posterior fossa (Fig. 126-1).

The petrous bone can be conceptually and functionally divided into anterior and posterior compartments.[1] This division is in a coronal direction passing through the IAC. Pathology in the posterior compartment is readily accessed through a transmastoid or translabyrinthine approach. Congenital cholesteatomas of the middle ear are frequently

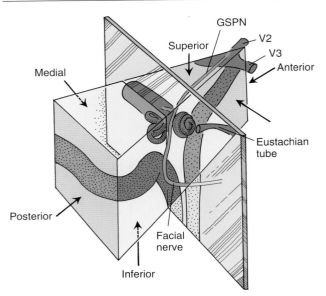

Figure 126-1. Petrous portion of the temporal bone. A coronal plane through the internal auditory canal separates the posterior and anterior petrous apex. The greater superficial petrosal nerve (GSPN) runs along the superior surface of the petrous bone. The gasserian ganglion and the mandibular division of the trigeminal nerve are located in the apex.

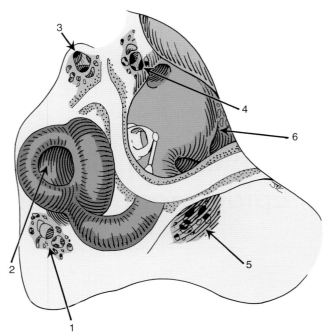

Figure 126-2. Drainage approaches to the petrous apex. 1, Supralabyrinthine tract inferior to the middle fossa dura; 2, subarcuate tract beneath the superior semicircular canal; 3, air cells of the zygomatic root; 4, small triangular region of bone between the genu of the carotid artery and the cochlea; 5, retrofacial infralabyrinthine tract; 6, infracochlear air cell tract.

accessed via the external auditory meatus. Abnormalities in the anterior compartment, including the petrous apex, require more complex approaches.

Access to the Petrous Apex

Approaches to the petrous apex require an understanding of the anatomy of the temporal bone and surrounding vital structures of the skull base and posterior, middle, anterior, and infratemporal fossae. Access to the petrous apex is limited because of its anatomic location. The position of the otic capsule, facial nerve, and carotid artery obviates direct and complete exposure to this centrally located area.

Before the availability of antibiotics, suppurative disease of the petrous apex was a common sequela of otitis media and was associated with high morbidity and mortality. Historically, various transtemporal approaches have been described to gain access to the relatively isolated area of the petrous apex via the air cell tracts surrounding the otic capsule. These approaches were predominantly used for the management of infectious complications of otitis media causing petrous apicitis (Fig. 126-2). The various routes through the temporal bone include

1. The supralabyrinthine tract inferior to the middle fossa dura
2. The subarcuate tract beneath the superior semicircular canal
3. The air cells of the zygomatic root
4. The small triangular region of bone between the genu of the carotid artery and the cochlea
5. The retrofacial infralabyrinthine tract
6. The infracochlear air cell tract

The first four routes are effective for draining an abscess or suppurative inflammation in the petrous apex but may not adequately provide permanent aeration to this remote area. The latter two routes do provide a more reliable and wider opening to the petrous apex. The infracochlear approach was described by Farrior and then modified by Brackmann and coworkers to adapt the approach for drainage of petrous apex cholesterol granuloma.[2,3]

The development of advanced endoscopic techniques and instrumentation has provided access to the petrous apex though the nose, nasopharynx, sphenoid sinus, and base of the skull. The transnasal approach enters the petrous bone anteriorly and is medial to the carotid artery. The conventional lateral approaches passing superior or inferior to the temporal bone require careful consideration of the carotid artery and otic capsule. Specific indications and limitations must be recognized when planning surgical treatment of pathology in the petrous apex.

Lesions of the Petrous Apex

With more extensive use of high-definition CT and MRI, lesions of the petrous apex are now often identified before they become large and destructive. Most lesions of the petrous apex remain quiescent and grow slowly until they affect neighboring neurovascular structures, including the cranial nerves, brain, orbit, or carotid artery, or extend into the middle ear. Patients suffering from lesions of the petrous apex most often complain of hearing loss, dizziness, tinnitus, and headache (40% to 60%). Abnormalities of the cranial nerves causing symptoms and signs such as facial twitching or weakness or diplopia are less common (5% to 15%) but raise greater suspicion for pathology in the petrous apex. Extension of disease into the middle ear may result in conductive hearing loss, but perforation of the tympanic membrane with subsequent otorrhea is rare (5%).[4,5] Facial numbness, amaurosis fugax, vertigo, transient ischemic attacks, ataxia, dysmetria, and incoordination can also occur.

Lesions of the petrous apex can be classified into three categories: cystic, solid, and radiographic anomalies. A retrospective study analyzing lesions of the petrous apex determined cystic lesions to be the most common source of pathology.[4] Such lesions include cholesterol granuloma (60%), cholesteatoma (10%), and mucocele (3%). Second in frequency are solid tumors, a heterogeneous group that includes chondrosarcoma (6%), chondroma (3%), cavernous hemangioma (3%), and metastatic carcinoma (2%). The least common category is radiographic anomalies such as retained secretions (6%) and asymmetrical pneumatization (3%). That said, lesions of the petrous apex are quite rare and represent only about 0.5% of pathology found on MRI performed for sudden hearing loss, vestibular symptoms, or tinnitus.[6]

Cholesterol Granuloma

Cholesterol granuloma is a comprehensive term describing a loculated cystic or solid foreign body reactive process directed against cholesterol crystals resulting from the by-products of degraded blood. Terms synonymous with cholesterol granuloma include *cholesterol, chocolate, dark brown,* or *blue dome cysts.* Cholesterol granuloma was originally described by Politzer in 1869 as idiopathic hemotympanum.[7] In 1929, Shambaugh introduced this term to the English literature.[8] Cholesterol granuloma was not reported in the petrous apex until House and Brackmann described the finding in 1982, which was subsequently recognized as a distinct clinical entity in 1985.[9,10] Although these cysts represent the most common lesion of the petrous apex, they remain quite rare, with an incidence of less than 0.6 case per million per year.[11]

Cholesterol granuloma may develop in diverse locations, including the peritoneal cavity, pleura, and paranasal sinus. Cholesterol granuloma originating in the temporal bone can be divided into two categories: cholesterol granuloma of the tympanomastoid compartment and cholesterol granuloma of the petrous apex. Each type has distinctive clinical behavior and pathogenesis. Cholesterol granuloma of the tympanomastoid compartment is typically painless and preceded by chronic otitis, is associated with limited pneumatization in the temporal bones, and rarely erodes bone. Cholesterol granuloma also frequently forms outside the middle ear in patients with well-pneumatized temporal bones who have acute and chronic mastoid inflammation associated with obstruction of the aditus ad antrum. This process is often isolated to one or a few mastoid air cells located toward the mastoid tip or cortex. In contrast, cholesterol granuloma of the petrous apex is often found in patients with dry ears and highly pneumatized temporal bones and is associated with chronic deep otic or retro-orbital pain, as well as neuropathy of cranial nerves V, VI, and occasionally VII. These lesions extensively erode or expand bone.

The pathogenesis of cholesterol granuloma is unknown and somewhat controversial. The inciting event is presumed to be inflammation and hemorrhage in an area of compromised aeration and drainage. Anaerobic breakdown of blood leads to the formation of cholesterol crystals and a subsequent sterile foreign body reaction. The granuloma blocks ventilation, and as a consequence the reaction propagates and results in growth of the cyst. Thus, maintaining good aeration of the cyst is imperative to prevent recurrence after drainage. Curiously, petrous apex cholesterol granuloma develops preferentially in hyperpneumatized temporal bones. Extensive pneumatization is possibly associated with a defect in bone marrow–air cell separation observed on CT. Highly vascular bone marrow may provide a continuous source of bleeding to the growing cyst.[12] The supply of blood may also result from newly described venules located preferentially in the well-pneumatized petrous apex.[13]

The contents of cholesterol granuloma demonstrate a characteristic appearance by both gross observation and histologic examination. The contents of the cyst typically include a yellow-brown, viscous glue-like fluid with glittering crystals detectable by the unaided eye. The brown discoloration is thought to be derived from metabolized hemosiderin. A green-yellow color is a manifestation of its lipid contents, and the glistening refractive properties are attributed to the cholesterol crystals. Histologically, the cyst is characterized by cholesterol crystals surrounded by foreign body reactive giant cells and fibrous connective tissue containing round cells, macrophages, and evidence of neovascularization (Fig. 126-3). Cholesterol granuloma does not contain squamous epithelium or keratin debris. Similar to congenital epidermoid tumor, cholesterol granuloma of the petrous apex is an indolent, slowly growing cystic tumor eroding bone that eventually becomes symptomatic once the lesion has extended to involve the dura and brain, cavernous sinus, carotid artery, orbit, cranial nerves, or otic capsule.

Congenital Epidermoid Tumors

Congenital epidermoid tumors of the temporal bone can have their origin in the middle ear, geniculate ganglion area, mastoid process, squamous epithelium, petrous apex, jugular foramen, or posterior fossa. Congenital epidermoid tumors are also termed *congenital cholesteatoma, keratosis, primary keratoma, inclusion cyst,* and *pseudomucocele,* especially when they are located within the middle ear.[14] The histopathology of congenital cholesteatoma or epidermoid tumor demonstrates a squamous epithelium–lined cyst filled with keratin debris. There are no additional dermal elements other than a surrounding outer layer of connective tissue that

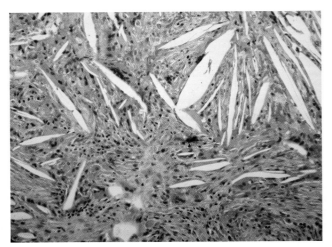

Figure 126-3. Histopathology of cholesterol granuloma. Note the large cholesterol crystal surrounded by a foreign body reaction with giant cells, macrophages, and fibrous connective tissue.

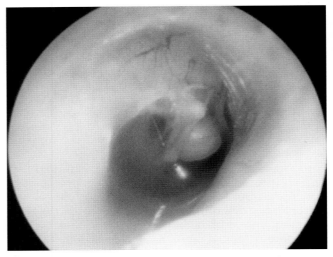

Figure 126-4. Congenital cholesteatoma located in the antero-superior quadrant of the right ear behind an intact tympanic membrane.

may be moderately vascular. The theory that these tumors may originally develop from congenital epithelial cell rests was proposed by Von Remak in 1854.[15]

According to Schuknecht, congenital epidermoid tumors occur in five sites in the temporal bone: (1) the petrous apex, (2) the middle ear, (3) the mastoid, (4) the cerebellopontine angle (CPA), and (5) the external auditory canal (EAC).[14]

Congenital epidermoid tumors of the petrous apex are believed to originate in the foramen lacerum during cephalic flexure of the head in early embryonic development with trapping of epithelial components. The cyst grows slowly. Similar to cholesterol granuloma, the symptoms relate to the space-occupying nature of the mass. These lesions become symptomatic by progressively compressing the eustachian tube, the trigeminal nerve, or the IAC and its contents or by stretching the dura. Congenital epidermoid tumors of the petrous apex may extend into the middle ear space. These tumors remain quiescent until they affect the cranial nerves, brain, orbit, or carotid artery or extend into the middle ear and cause further hearing loss or otorrhea. Hearing loss is the most common initial symptom.[16] Signs and symptoms of facial nerve involvement characterized by paresis, synkinesis, twitching, and paralysis are the second most common manifestation of congenital epidermoid tumors of the petrous apex.[17]

Establishing that a cholesteatoma of the middle ear is of congenital origin can be controversial. It is argued that eustachian tube dysfunction, retraction of the tympanic membrane, middle ear infections, and epithelial migration from insertion of a myringotomy tube are the forces that trap epithelium in the middle ear space. However, Michaels clearly demonstrated an epidermoid formation in the anterior superior middle ear mucosa in 54% of embryos examined at 10 weeks of gestation.[18] With normal development of the temporal bone, the epidermoid formation should undergo regression by 33 weeks of gestational age. The cause of congenital cho-

lesteatoma is considered to be lack of regression and continued growth of the epidermoid formation.

The differential diagnosis of a white mass within or medial to the tympanic membrane also includes congenital cholesteatoma of the petrous apex extending to the middle ear, osteoma of the tympanic ring or scutum, tympanosclerosis, or an inclusion cyst originating within the tympanic membrane. It is presumed that congenital epidermoid tumors are present from birth and continue to grow. Congenital cholesteatoma of the middle ear is most commonly identified at 4 years of age, but the age at diagnosis may range from infancy to the second decade of life.[19] Congenital cholesteatoma of the middle ear is often diagnosed on routine physical examination or during evaluation of a child with unilateral or bilateral hearing loss or otorrhea. When detected early, the epithelial pearl is typically located in the anterosuperior quadrant of the middle ear space (Fig. 126-4). Progression of disease with breakdown of the cyst laterally through the tympanic membrane results in bacterial colonization and otorrhea. Breakdown within the middle ear permits extension of disease throughout the middle ear, mastoid, and temporal bone and results in chronic otitis media and mastoiditis. Once recurrent otorrhea and middle ear involvement are established, it is almost impossible to distinguish congenital cholesteatoma of the middle ear from acquired cholesteatoma. Congenital middle ear epidermoid or cholesteatoma may extend into the petrous apex, but they are not usually as extensive as primary lesions originating in this area. Furthermore, growth of a congenital middle ear epidermoid generally results in early identification because of signs and symptoms of conductive hearing loss and otorrhea.

Congenital epidermoid tumors of the mastoid are also proposed to be of embryologic origin. They develop in patients lacking a history of recurrent otitis media, eustachian tube dysfunction, and attic retraction. Frequently, epidermoid tumor of the mastoid is manifested as hearing loss associated with destruction of the ossicular chain or perforation of the tympanic membrane. As it progressively expands into the middle ear, epidermoid tumors of the mastoid may be difficult to differentiate from middle ear cholesteatoma.

Intracranial epidermoid cysts are most commonly located in the CPA. Congenital epidermoid tumors account for 6% to 7% of all tumors found in the CPA. It has been proposed that epidermoid tumors in the CPA arise from either multipotential embryonic cells or displaced cells of the otic capsule. They usually become manifested during the third and fourth decades of life, with a slight increased predilection in males.[20] Because of the close proximity of the cranial nerves, congenital epidermoid tumors of the CPA are often accompanied by symptoms of hearing loss, tinnitus, or vertigo. Facial nerve signs of twitching and progressive weakness also occur. Infiltration of the dura by the tumor triggers the trigeminal nerve and causes headaches. As the tumor expands, cerebellar compression becomes manifested by postural instability, ataxia, and dysarthria. Extension anterosuperiorly and inferiorly will affect the 5th through 12th cranial nerves and create increased intracranial pressure, thereby causing headaches, nausea, vomiting, and potential loss of consciousness.[21] Because of their propensity for causing central neurologic symptoms and signs, congenital (primary) epidermoid tumors of the posterior fossa are seen more frequently by neurosurgeons.

Radiologic Imaging

Contemporary radiologic imaging modalities have introduced a new era into the diagnosis and management of temporal bone pathology. MRI can accurately define the soft tissue characteristics of these lesions and detect intracranial extension and involvement of the carotid artery and sigmoid sinus. CT demonstrates not only the specific pattern of rearrangement and destruction induced by the lesion but also the anatomic relationships of the tumor to the otic capsule, middle ear, carotid artery, and posterior and middle fossae. Despite the concern for cost containment in contemporary

medicine, this is one area in which obtaining both imaging formats greatly assists the surgeon in formulating the diagnosis and planning the operative approach. Differentiation of lesions of the petrous apex is achieved by observing characteristic findings on both MRI and CT (Table 127-1).

Data obtained from the variable stimulating and capture techniques used with MRI (T1 versus T2 weighting) help determine the nature of the temporal bone pathology. A bright or hyperintense signal is observed on unenhanced (non–contrast-enhanced) T1-weighted images as a result of the presence of proteinaceous fluid, blood, or fat. A bright or hyperintense signal on conventional spin-echo T2-weighted sequences is indicative of fluid. Because cholesterol granuloma is composed of both methemoglobin breakdown products with paramagnetic properties and serous fluid, it is characteristically bright on both T1- and T2-weighted images (Fig. 126-5). The use of intravenous contrast agents such as gadolinium does not provide significant additional information for this purpose. Although the capsule of the cyst may demonstrate slight enhancement with gadolinium because of localized neovascularization, it is not usually evident because of the bright signal already present on the non–contrast-enhanced T1-weighted image. In addition to establishing the diagnosis, MRI is useful to track recurrence of cholesterol granuloma after surgical drainage. When faced with the presence of an opacified surgical bed, MRI effectively differentiates fluid retention from accumulation of cystic contents because only recurrence appears bright on T1-weighted images. Similarly, epidermoid cysts also have a characteristic appearance on MRI. An epidermoid tumor is usually isodense relative to brain and appears hypointense on T1-weighted imaging. However, similar to cholesterol granuloma, epidermoid tumors are bright on T2-weighted images. Also similar to cholesterol granuloma, epidermoid cysts do not significantly enhance with gadolinium, but slight peripheral enhancement corresponding to the capsule may be seen.[22] However, if the cyst is infected or infiltrated with granulation tissue, it will demonstrate frank contrast

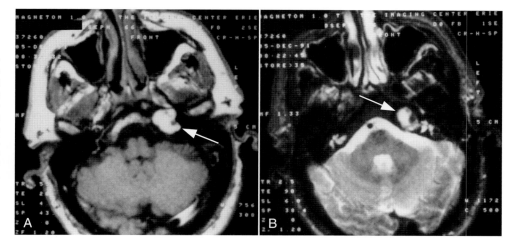

Figure 126-5. Petrous apex cholesterol granuloma, preoperative views. **A,** T1-weighted magnetic resonance image (MRI), without contrast enhancement, demonstrating a bright left petrous apex lesion (arrow) that is isointense with fat. **B,** T2-weighted MRI showing a bright left petrous apex lesion (arrow) that is isointense with cerebrospinal fluid and perilymph.

Table 126-1	CHARACTERISTIC RADIOLOGIC FINDINGS OF CHOLESTEROL GRANULOMA AND CONGENITAL EPIDERMOID TUMOR				
	MRI			*CT*	
Lesion	T1-Weighted	Contrast Enhancement	T2-Weighted	Bone-Eroded Margin	Contrast Enhancement
Cholesterol granuloma	Hyperintense	No	Hyperintense	Smooth	Occasional rim enhancement
Congenital epidermoid tumor	Hypointense	No	Hyperintense	Smooth	No
CT, computed tomography; MRI, magnetic resonance imaging.					

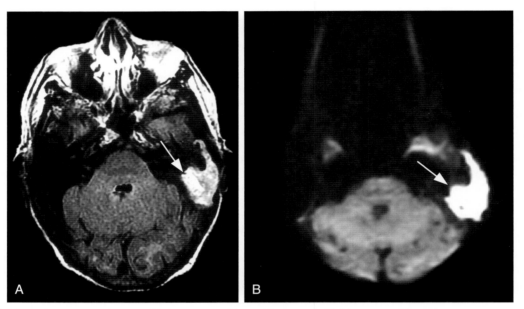

Figure 126-6. Magnetic resonance images of left petrous epidermoid tumor. **A,** Fluid-attenuated inversion recovery sequence showing a bright signal in the petrous and lateral temporal bone *(arrow)*. This excludes arachnoid cyst from the differential diagnosis. **B,** Diffusion-weighted image showing a bright signal in the same location, which strongly suggests it to be consistent with an epidermoid tumor *(arrow)*.

enhancement. Arachnoid cysts may be difficult to differentiate from epidermoid; both are filled with fluid and demonstrate low T1 and high T2 signal. In this case, fluid-attenuated inversion recovery (FLAIR) sequence will help differentiate these two pathologies because epidermoid cysts are bright on FLAIR sequences and arachnoid cysts are not. Chondrosarcoma; metastasis from breast, kidney, and prostate cancer; and mucocele are other pathologies of the petrous apex that are bright on T2-weighted images but can be distinguished from epidermoid by differential examination of CT and MRI (see Table 126-1).

Newer MRI pulse sequences have been developed that further help differentiate pathology in petrous bone. FLAIR sequences appear similar to T2-weighted sequences except that free fluid such as cerebrospinal fluid (CSF) is suppressed. Proteinaceous fluid, as seen in most air cell pathology, remains bright. Most tumors, including epidermoid tumors, will be bright on FLAIR sequences, just as they are on T2-weighted sequences. Diffusion-weighted imaging is a method of evaluating

the brownian motion of water molecules. Restricted water diffusion, thought to be due to the waxy consistency of epidermoid tumors, results in high signal intensity (Fig. 126-6).

CT scanning provides significant additional information regarding the characteristics of petrous apex lesions. Cholesterol granuloma and cholesteatoma both appear as a smoothly marginated expanding mass. They appear isointense or mildly hypointense relative to nearby brain on soft tissue windowing. MRI with intravenous contrast does not show significant enhancement or provide additional information unless the cyst is infected or infiltrated by granulation tissue. However, data obtained from a bone window algorithm are most useful. The presence of temporal bone pneumatization suggests that the lesion is probably a cholesterol granuloma. Congenital cholesteatoma is thought to inhibit normal temporal bone aeration, development, and thus pneumatization. The edges of cholesteatoma are sclerosed, eroded, and scalloped. Capsular calcification is occasionally seen. The size and location of the expan-

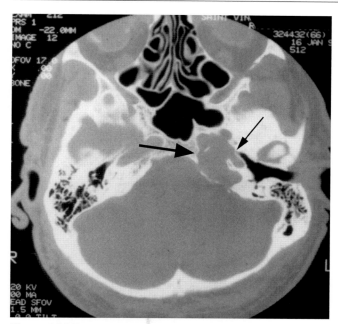

Figure 126-7. Bone-windowed computed tomography scan revealing an expansile left petrous apex lesion with smooth margins and isointense with brain *(large arrow)*, consistent with cholesterol granuloma. Note the relationship to the carotid artery *(small arrow)*.

sile lesion are clearly demonstrated. The relationship of the lesion or tumor to the otic capsule, ossicles, facial nerve, IAC, internal carotid artery (ICA), jugular bulb, and posterior fossa can be defined (Fig. 126-7). A bone-windowed CT scan in combination with MRI and MR angiography provides a road map for planning the operative approach.

PREOPERATIVE EVALUATION

Patients with congenital cholesteatoma or cholesterol granuloma will have had a presumptive diagnosis made that was based on initial signs, symptoms, and radiologic findings. Patients are questioned regarding their otologic history and previous surgical procedures. It should be determined whether they have had otorrhea, hearing loss, tinnitus, vestibular symptoms, facial paresis or twitching, diplopia, amaurosis fugax, or transient ischemic attacks. They are also asked about the location and severity of pain.

A complete neuro-otologic and head and neck physical examination is performed. The status of the tympanic membrane and middle ear space is evaluated. Facial and corneal sensations are tested for evidence of trigeminal nerve involvement. The full range of extra-ocular motion should be confirmed. Facial nerve function is carefully examined to look for evidence of fasciculation, weakness, or synkinesis.

A complete assessment of hearing consisting of air and bone conduction and speech audiometry is obtained. It is important to evaluate auditory function in both the involved and uninvolved ears. Operative management may necessitate closing the ear canal, which results in maximal conductive hearing loss. On

rare occasion, cochlear function may have to be sacrificed to completely remove an invasive cholesteatoma or congenital epidermoid tumor. Therefore, the contralateral ear should have normal hearing or be suitable for aural rehabilitation with amplification.

Radiologic imaging is critical in diagnosing and planning treatment of cholesterol granuloma and congenital epidermoid tumors. These two pathologic processes affecting the temporal bone are similar in that both CT and MRI are necessary to formulate the diagnosis and treatment plan. MRI defines the differential diagnosis based on the characteristic signals generated by the soft tissue and fluid content of the tumor or cyst. The tumor or cyst and the pneumatization tracts of the temporal bone are identified by bone-windowed CT. A well-developed pneumatized temporal bone is more amenable to exteriorization of epidermoid tumor and to drainage and aeration of cholesterol granuloma than a sclerotic temporal bone is. The location of the pathology in the petrous apex in relation to the sphenoid sinus should be examined. Expansion anteriorly toward a large sphenoid sinus allows the surgeon to consider a transnasal-transsphenoidal approach for management of the lesion. The relationship of the jugular bulb to the facial nerve and otic capsule is critical when a drainage procedure inferior to the otic capsule is likely. A high and lateral jugular bulb obstructs retrofacial infralabyrinthine access to the petrous apex. In this situation, axial and coronal images are carefully reviewed to determine whether the aeration and anatomy will permit a transcanal infracochlear approach.

The surgeon may also obtain a CT scan with fiducial markers in anticipation of performing surgery with image guidance technology. Intraoperative localization from an anterior approach is fairly accurate because the skull base contains numerous bony landmarks that allow registration of known anatomic sites. However, despite proposed intraoperative accuracy to less than 2 mm,[23] image guidance is not widely used in lateral skull base approaches because of technical problems with accurate registration and the fact that a 2-mm error may be catastrophic in the small operative window afforded by the infracochlear or infralabyrinthine approaches.

Large tumors within the petrous apex that approximate or encase the carotid artery warrant further evaluation. MR angiography is useful in preoperative planning to evaluate the anatomic relationship with the vessel. It must be determined whether blood flow from the contralateral side through the circle of Willis is adequate if it is expected that the ipsilateral carotid artery may be retracted, temporarily occluded, or resected during the procedure. Balloon test occlusion of the ipsilateral ICA provides reliable data for predicting the patient's tolerance to ICA manipulation or sacrifice; however, 15% of patients with normal collateral supply may still experience a stroke if the artery is sacrificed.[24]

It is important to reach a presumptive preoperative diagnosis based on physical examination and radiologic imaging findings to provide the surgeon with the ability to plan both the surgical approach and optimal management of the lesion. The specific surgical approach depends on the presumed pathology; the location of the tumor or cyst; the status of hearing, balance, and facial nerve function; the likelihood of encountering CSF; and the integrity of the carotid artery and the middle and posterior fossa dura. Depending on the nature, location, and extent of the pathology, the likelihood of encountering CSF, the patient's hearing status, and facial nerve involvement, the surgeon can anticipate whether total resection or exteriorization is advisable. Meticulous preoperative planning allows more aggressive and complete resection of recurrent tumors, thereby decreasing the need for salvage surgery.

The need for intraoperative facial nerve monitoring is dictated by the proximity of the pathology to the facial nerve and the likelihood that dissection, drainage, or resection of the tumor or cyst may place the facial nerve in jeopardy. As with most otologic procedures performed with the patient under general anesthesia, paralytic agents are avoided. General anesthesia is maintained with inhalation agents, narcotics, and hypnotics. Blood is typed and cross-matched for transfusion or collected for autotransfusion if the carotid artery is to be manipulated. The goals and risks of the procedure along with the limited alternatives are reviewed with the patient and family.

SURGICAL MANAGEMENT

Cholesterol Granuloma

Management of cholesterol granuloma and epidermoid tumor is different. In contrast to a true cyst, the walls of a cholesterol granuloma lack an epithelial lining. It is therefore unnecessary to remove the capsule entirely to successfully prevent recurrence or expansion of the granuloma. As long as adequate drainage and ventilation are maintained, the cyst should not recur. That said, surgery is not always warranted. Because of the indolent clinical course of cholesterol granuloma, small, asymptomatic, or inaccessible cysts with tolerable symptoms can be managed expectantly with frequent clinical follow-up and serial radiologic imaging. Several published series include long-term follow-up of patients managed expectantly, and quite often the clinical symptoms and cyst dimensions remain stable.[11,25]

The specific surgical treatment of cholesterol granuloma of the petrous apex depends on both the patient's hearing status at the time of surgery and the anatomic relationship of the tumor with surrounding neurovascular structures. For patients with nonserviceable hearing, good surgical exposure becomes more important than preservation of residual cochleovestibular function (Table 126-2). Thus, when sensorineural hearing loss is greater than 70 dB and word discrimination is less than 30%, cholesterol granuloma is drained via a translabyrinthine or combined translabyrinthine-transcochlear approach. The translabyrinthine approach provides greater exposure and drainage than the retrofacial infralabyrinthine approach alone does. Dissection through the temporal bone superior and inferior to the IAC increases ventilation to the petrous apex. If additional exposure is needed, the cochlea is sacrificed.

There are two management philosophies for treatment of patients with serviceable hearing. Some surgeons argue that total excision of the cyst wall best prevents reaccumulation of the cyst's contents. The approach can involve a combination of middle, posterior, or infratemporal fossa techniques for access. Recurrence rates are low, and stenting is not necessary when the entire cyst is removed.[25] The drawback is the

Table 126-2	DECISION MAKING FOR MANAGEMENT OF CHOLESTEROL GRANULOMA AND EPIDERMOID TUMOR		
Cholesterol Granuloma			
Good Hearing		Poor Hearing	Asymptomatic/Tolerable Symptoms with Difficult Access
Complete Excision	*Drainage*		
No Stent	With Stent	With or without Stent	
Middle + posterior fossa Middle fossa + transpetrosal	Infracochlear Infralabyrinthine Middle fossa Transsphenoidal	Translabyrinthine Transcochlear	Observe Serial magnetic resonance imaging or computed tomography
Epidermoid Tumor			
Preservation of Hearing		Sacrifice of Hearing	
Canal wall down mastoidectomy Preauricular subtemporal + infratemporal Middle fossa + occipital		Translabyrinthine Transcochlear Transotic	

possibility of entry through the dura with subsequent potential complications, including CSF leak and chemical meningitis. However, most authors, including ourselves, favor continuous drainage of the cyst into the pneumatized mastoid or middle ear cavities with placement of a permanent stent. Such drainage can be accomplished through the nose into the sphenoid sinus and nasopharynx. The transtemporal approaches of choice are the transmastoid infralabyrinthine and the transcanal infracochlear. Since 1990 the transcanal infracochlear approach has been supplanting the infralabyrinthine approach because the infracochlear approach for drainage of the cyst is achievable even in the presence of a high jugular bulb.[26] The success and complication rates of the two surgeries are similar. Overall, one can expect symptomatic relief in 80% of patients with minimal complications.[27] The drawback of long-term drainage with permanent stenting is a high recurrence rate of 15% to 60%, usually associated with obstruction of the stent.[28] The older literature described the highest recurrence rate of 60% in patients drained via a transethmoid, transsphenoid approach.[28] A recent retrospective series by Brackmann and Toh is very encouraging for transtemporal drainage procedures; a recurrence rate of only 3% was reported for cases in which a stent was placed.[27]

A middle fossa or keyhole middle fossa approach may produce adequate exposure but is not recommended because it is technically difficult to maintain cyst ventilation/drainage into the mastoid cavity or eustachian tube via stenting.[29] However, if establishment of drainage is successful, recurrence rates are similar to those of the infralabyrinthine approach.[27] A middle fossa approach with stenting is a valid option.

Transsphenoid drainage is an alternative to consider in cases in which the cholesterol granuloma abuts the posterior wall of the sphenoid sinus. This technique, originally described by Montgomery in 1977, was performed through a contralateral external ethmoidectomy approach.[30] Knowledge of the surgical anatomy plus the use of contemporary instrumentation such as endoscopic sinus telescopes permits endonasal access to the petrous apex tip directly through the sphenoid sinus. However, inability to maintain a patent fistula through this approach may result in recurrence of the cystic lesion. It is possible to enhance drainage of the cyst when intraoperative navigation is used in conjunction with endoscopy; more aggressive drainage may be achieved while avoiding damage to vital structures lying behind the sinus wall.[31]

The development of minimally invasive endoscopic neurosurgery may provide a valid option in the near future for resection of petroclival tumors. The expanded endonasal approach provides excellent access to petrous apex tumors and has been applied to drainage procedures for cholesterol granuloma and other tumors of the anterior petrous bone. At this juncture the lack of sufficient follow-up makes it difficult to predict the appropriateness of this type of approach for tumors of the petrous apex. The procedure includes bilateral

sphenoidotomy and posterior maxillary antrostomy with drilling of the petrous bone encasing the ICA. Lateral mobilization of the carotid artery can be performed to gain greater access to the petrous apex. Marsupialization of the granuloma into the sphenoid is performed. Kassam and colleagues, experienced in resection and debulking of petroclival tumors via the expended endonasal approach, propose to use this method for resection of cholesteatoma in addition to cholesterol granuloma.[32] It remains to be seen whether the newer techniques of endoscopic nasal surgery will provide more permanent drainage and lower the incidence of recurrence.

Epidermoid of the Petrous Apex

In contrast to cholesterol granulomas, epidermoid tumors must be excised completely; if tumor is left behind, the cyst will recur. However, the tumor is often tightly adherent to surrounding neurovascular structures and dura. It is believed that microrupture of the capsule may occur and induce an inflammatory reaction that binds the tumor to surrounding structures. Complete resection bears considerable risk because epidermoid tumors frequently encase vital structures. At the time of initial examination by an otolaryngologist, cranial nerves are involved in the majority of patients (85%). Hearing loss, vestibular deficits, and facial weakness are the most common, followed by deficits in function of cranial nerves V and VI. In addition to affecting nerves, tumors often involve major vessels (80%), including the carotid artery in 50% of cases.[33]

It is important to completely excise the tumor despite its intimate involvement with neurovascular structures. Recurrence is likely when the surgeon tries to preserve cranial nerve function and leaves epidermoid lining in these areas. Ultimately, cranial nerve deficits are not spared because salvage procedures will probably result in additional morbidity and sacrifice. In summary, the goal of resection of epidermoid tumors is safe but complete removal of tumor, which is facilitated by thorough preoperative planning and excellent surgical exposure.

For wide exposure of the petrous apex, we recommend the translabyrinthine approach. If the surgeon needs good exposure of the carotid artery, conversion to a transcochlear approach is possible. In the transotic procedure described by Fisch, the EAC is closed, the tympanic membrane and ossicles are removed, and the facial nerve is transposed anteriorly.[34] In the transcochlear approach originally described by House and colleagues, the facial nerve is displaced posteriorly.[35] The drawbacks of these approaches are sacrifice of cochlear and vestibular function, risk of CSF leak, and facial nerve palsy secondary to mobilization of the facial nerve to improve access, which may result in facial weakness in up to 75% of cases.[36] To avoid such complications, some surgeons advocate a middle fossa approach.

In the presence of intact cochlear function, we prefer to manage congenital epidermoid tumors with a canal wall down procedure if adequate exposure and exteriorization of disease can be achieved. This requires a well-pneumatized temporal bone with a high tegmen tympani. Unfortunately, congenital epidermoid tumors often originate in poorly pneumatized, contracted temporal bones, thus making it difficult to adequately exteriorize the tumor with the cochlea intact. Exposure is enhanced by sacrificing the cochlea and therefore hearing.

Occasionally, wide marsupialization of an epidermoid tumor is inadequate or unsafe. Total resection becomes necessary when exteriorization results in a CSF leak, when the dura or the carotid artery is exposed and at risk for desiccation in an open cavity, or when the opening of the marsupialized epidermoid cavity results in a very narrow, circuitous tract that makes postoperative examination and débridement difficult. In this situation, the entire tumor and its epithelial lining are removed and the wound is obliterated.

Surgical Techniques

Tympanomeatal Approach for Congenital Middle Ear Cholesteatoma

This approach is directed at isolated congenital middle ear cholesteatoma characteristically located in the anterosuperior quadrant of the middle ear. The patient is positioned supine on the operating room table with the head turned toward the contralateral ear. Using the operating microscope, the ear canal is injected in four-quadrant fashion with 2% lidocaine (Xylocaine) with 1:100,000 epinephrine. In young children, the anesthetic solution is diluted by half. After adequate local anesthesia and vasoconstriction have been achieved, a tympanomeatal flap based inferiorly is elevated. An incision is made lateral to the annulus from the 3- to the 9-o'clock positions. The tympanomeatal flap is elevated to enter the middle ear in the posterosuperior quadrant. The tympanic membrane, including the pars flaccida, is carefully dissected off the scutum and over the short process of the malleus. A sharp sickle knife or curved pick is used to incise the thin layer of mucoperiosteum along the posterior aspect of the malleus handle. The tympanic membrane is retracted inferiorly toward the umbo to expose the epithelial tumor (Fig. 126-8). The extent of inferior dissection of the tympanic membrane is dictated by the size and location of the mass. Using suction, right-angled picks, and curved excavators, the tumor is carefully freed from its attachments to bone and ossicles and removed (Fig. 126-9). Great care is taken to remove the epithelial pearl intact and avoid spillage of keratin in the middle ear and mastoid. Once the pearl is removed, the ossicular chain is examined for integrity and mobility, and the tympanic membrane is carefully inspected for a tear or perforation. If a defect is identified, it is repaired with a small piece of wet Gelfoam or an underlay connective tissue graft placed medial to the area. The tympanic membrane is returned to its anatomic position. A silk sleeve is placed over the tympanic membrane and supported by cotton balls with ointment. The ear canal may also be packed with Gelfoam moistened with antibiotic ear drops.

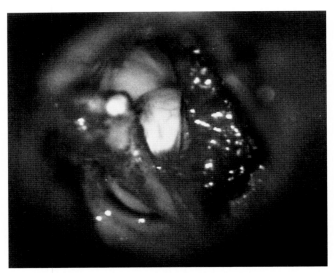

Figure 126-8. An inferiorly based tympanomeatal flap attached to the umbo exposes the encapsulated keratin pearl.

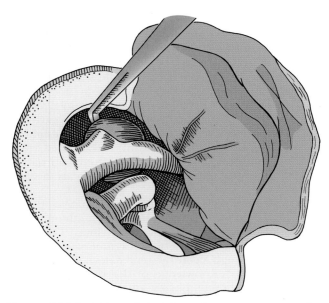

Figure 126-9. Right-angled picks and excavators are used to remove the keratin pearl intact.

More extensive primary cholesteatoma occupying the epitympanum may require additional exposure via a cortical mastoidectomy. Drilling is continued anteriorly through the root of the zygoma to expose the body of the incus and head of the malleus. Tumor located in this area frequently creates a conductive hearing loss. Removal of the incus and possibly the head of the malleus may be necessary to obtain access to the anterior epitympanum. The canal wall may have to be taken down to exteriorize any epitympanic disease that cannot be completely removed. Reconstruction of the ossicular chain is reviewed in Chapter 114. When the epithelial lining of the cyst ruptures into either the middle ear or the EAC, primary cholesteatoma of the middle ear becomes difficult to distinguish from acquired chronic otitis media with cholesteatoma. Surgical management is dictated by the extent and location of the cholesteatoma matrix within the middle ear and mastoid. This subject is reviewed in Chapter 115.

Transcanal Infracochlear Approach

Because of the limited opening into the petrous apex, this drainage procedure is better suited for treatment of cholesterol granuloma than epidermoid tumor. This approach is preferred when a high jugular bulb inhibits adequate exposure via the retrofacial infralabyrinthine approach. It has the advantage that problems arising from blockage of a Silastic shunt tube can be addressed through an inferior myringotomy.[3]

After induction of general anesthesia, the head is turned toward the contralateral ear. The facial nerve is electrically monitored throughout the procedure. Under the operating microscope, 2% lidocaine with 1:100,000 epinephrine is injected into the four quadrants of the EAC, as well as the postauricular skin. After adequate hemostasis is obtained, 12- and 6-o'clock incision are made from the mid–bony canal medially toward the external meatus laterally. The inferior incision stops at the conchal cartilage. These two incisions are connected vertically to create a long conchal flap. A postauricular incision is made, the posterior canal skin is elevated to the level of the endaural incisions, tracheostomy tape is placed through the meatus, and the auricle is reflected anteriorly.

Tympanomeatal incisions are made at the 10-o'clock position (right ear) and brought laterally and obliquely from the annulus. The lateral and inferior aspect of the tympanomeatal flap is incised at the prominence of the bulge in the canal wall (Fig. 126-10). Elevation of the meatal skin flap is taken down to the level of the annulus. The middle ear is entered posteriorly, and the annulus is elevated to create a flap that is based superiorly and pedicled on the umbo of the malleus. The anterior, posterior, and inferior bony canal walls are enlarged toward the hypotympanum. When the posterior canal wall is drilled, care must be taken to avoid

injury to the vertical portion of the facial nerve. If the chorda tympani nerve is used as the posterior limit of dissection, injury from the drill can be avoided (Fig. 126-11). The inferior tympanic ring is drilled to expose the hypotympanic air cells. Drilling is continued inferiorly to expose the genu of the carotid artery and jugular bulb. The posterosuperior limit of dissection is the round window. A triangle consisting of the carotid artery anteriorly, the jugular bulb posteriorly, and the basal turn of the cochlea superiorly forms the area for continued dissection. From measurements in cadavers, the size of the operating window averages 9.4 × 7.3 mm. Sometimes the space between the great vessels is small, less than 5 mm, thus restricting the usefulness of this approach for biopsy and drainage only rather than resection of cholesteatoma.[26] Cutting and then diamond burrs are used to continue the dissection in a medial and slightly superior direction (Fig. 126-12). This brings

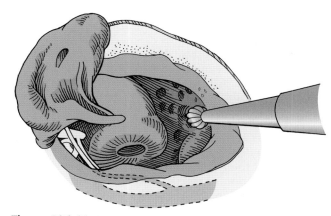

Figure 126-11. The superiorly based tympanomeatal flap is elevated to expose the mesotympanum and hypotympanum. A cutting burr is used to remove the prominence of the lateral canal wall and the inferior tympanic ring for further exposure of the hypotympanum. Care is taken posteriorly to avoid the vertical portion of the facial nerve.

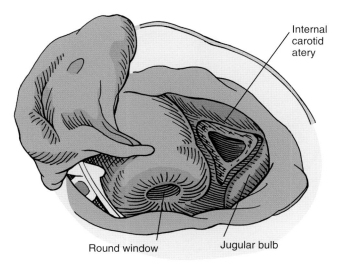

Internal carotid atery

Round window   Jugular bulb

Figure 126-12. A diamond burr is used to remove the hypotympanic air cells. The limits of dissection are the internal carotid artery anteriorly, the jugular vein posteroinferiorly, and the basal turn of the cochlea superiorly.

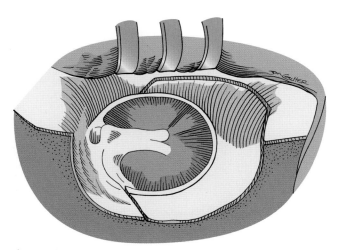

Figure 126-10. The superiorly based tympanomeatal flap is incised. The prominent anteroinferior bony canal wall will be removed.

the dissection inferior to the cochlea and anteroinferior to the IAC.

The air cells lateral to the cholesterol granuloma often appear dark. Once the cyst is entered, the characteristic thick, yellow-brown fluid and cholesterol crystals are encountered. The fistula opening into the cyst is enlarged while keeping the carotid artery and jugular vein in view. Cup forceps are used to remove some of the lateral inferior lining of the cyst wall. The cavity is evacuated of its fluid contents. The size of the opening is maximized by drilling to the limits of the carotid artery, jugular bulb, and basal turn of the cochlea. The cavity is irrigated with bacitracin-saline solution. If the cyst is multiloculated and the surgical approach gives limited exposure, endoscopy may be helpful. A sinus (2.7 mm) or otologic (1.9 mm) endoscope may facilitate visualization of hidden parts of the cystic lesion. In combination with suction and irrigation, endoscopy facilitates débridement and efficient drainage of septated cholesterol granuloma or eradication of cholesteatoma limited to the inferior petrous apex.[37]

The area is stented and drained with silicone or Silastic tubing. If not available, Silastic sheeting (0.02 inch) is cut in a rectangular shape and rolled to make a cylinder (Fig. 126-13). The inferior and lateral aspect of the Silastic tubing is trimmed so that it is contained completely within the middle ear and hypotympanic spaces. Gelfoam impregnated with an antibiotic suspension is placed in the newly created hypotympanum and along the medial floor of the new bony EAC. The inferior aspect of the tympanomeatal flap is returned to its anatomic position. A small graft of fascia positioned medial to the tympanomeatal skin flap and extended laterally toward the ear canal may be needed to cover a residual defect. Gelfoam with antibiotic suspension is placed lateral to the tympanic membrane and along the flap of the meatal skin. The auricle is returned to its anatomic position while ensuring that the posterior conchal skin flap is laid flat against the posterior bony canal wall. The lateral cartilaginous canal is packed with lateral rosebud packing, Gelfoam, or a Merocel sponge. The postauricular incision is closed with 4-0 resorbable suture braided subcutaneously and 5-0 fast-absorbing suture in the skin and covered with Steri-Strips, and a sterile mastoid dressing is applied.

The transcanal infracochlear approach requires exposure of the sigmoid sinus and drilling under the cochlea, which can potentially lead to complications. A modification was proposed in which only exposure of the ICA is required and a surgical window is drilled anterior to the cochlea, thereby presumably reducing the risk of injury to the jugular bulb and round window. The tradeoff for increased safety is a smaller working space averaging 4.7 × 3.2 mm instead of 7.3 × 9.4 mm with a traditional infracochlear approach.[38]

Retrofacial Infralabyrinthine Approach

The patient is positioned supine on the table with the head turned toward the contralateral ear. One centimeter of postauricular hair is shaved, and the ear is prepared in usual fashion. Two percent lidocaine with 1:100,000 epinephrine is infiltrated into the skin 2 cm posterior to the postauricular sulcus. A curvilinear incision is made through the skin. Fibroperiosteal tissue is elevated from the mastoid cortex, and self-retaining retractors are placed.

A complete transcortical mastoidectomy is performed. The sigmoid sinus is decompressed, and 1 cm of bone posterior to the edge of the sinus is removed. The horizontal semicircular canal is delineated. The aditus ad antrum is opened as widely as possible to maximize ventilation into the epitympanic and middle ear spaces. Further ventilation through the middle ear is accomplished by opening the facial recess if communication between the aditus ad antrum of the mastoid and the epitympanum of the middle ear is insufficient.

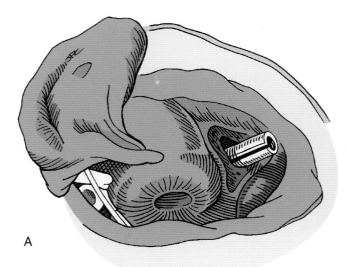
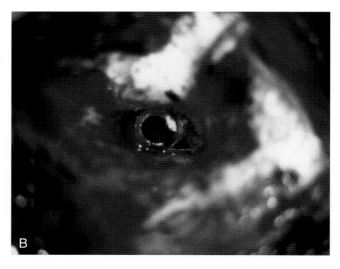

Figure 126-13. **A,** A rolled Silastic sheet is placed in the opening of the fistula from the cystic cavity to the hypotympanum. **B,** The Silastic sheeting in place.

The posterior semicircular canal is outlined with a diamond drill. The vertical portion of the facial nerve is defined, and a thin covering of bone is left for protection. Additional bone is removed to expose the mastoid tip and digastric ridge.

Using a cutting burr, drilling is continued through the air cells posterior to the vertical portion of the facial nerve. Dissection is carried in an anteromedial direction. The continuation of the sigmoid sinus into the jugular bulb must be defined. To obtain adequate access through this route, a high jugular bulb must not be present. This anatomic variation would have been identified on preoperative bone-windowed CT scanning. In patients with a high jugular bulb, the procedure can be converted into an infracochlear approach.[26] Posterior compression of the sigmoid sinus enhances the exposure and angle necessary to gain access to the petrous apex cyst. Once it is opened, the contents of the cyst are evacuated. Cup forceps are used to completely remove the lining of the posterolateral cyst wall. This opening is maximized through the confines of the area limited by the facial nerve anteriorly, the ampullated end of the posterior semicircular canal superiorly, the posterior fossa dura posteriorly, and the jugular bulb inferiorly.

The cavity is irrigated with bacitracin solution. A Silastic tube or sheeting rolled into a cylinder is placed in the cavity and trimmed to an appropriate length so that it lies within the inferior aspect of the mastoidectomy (Fig. 126-14). The postauricular incision is closed with 4-0 resorbable braided suture, and a sterile mastoid dressing is applied.

Translabyrinthine Approach

The translabyrinthine approach for drainage of the petrous apex is identical to that for resection of an acoustic neuroma (Chapter 124). This approach is undertaken if hearing is significantly compromised or absent. Bone is removed 1 cm posterior to the sigmoid sinus, and the middle fossa tegmen is thinned. A complete labyrinthectomy is performed. The IAC is carefully outlined while taking care to not enter the dura of the IAC, the posterior fossa, or the middle fossa.

The incus is removed, and the fossa incudis is drilled to maximize communication between the mastoid and the epitympanic space. A trough is created superior to the IAC if the bony anatomy permits. Entrance into the petrous apex can be achieved through suprameatal air cells, if present. Care must be taken to avoid injury to the facial nerve in its labyrinthine segment.

The bone inferior to the IAC is removed with a diamond burr (Fig. 126-15). The location of the jugular bulb is noted. Caution should be exercised when working in the area superior to the jugular bulb and inferior to the IAC. The cochlear aqueduct enters the vestibule in this area, and entry into the cochlear aqueduct results in leakage of CSF into the wound. This is difficult to suture and may need to be plugged with fat or muscle. If it cannot be occluded in watertight fashion and sealed from potential communication with the cyst, the cholesterol granuloma drainage procedure must be terminated. Abdominal fat is packed into the cavity, and muscle is plugged into the epitympanum.

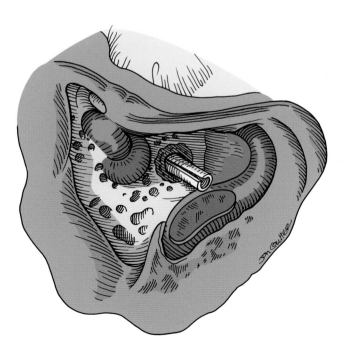

Figure 126-14. Retrofacial infralabyrinthine approach. A transcortical mastoidectomy is performed to identify the antrum, posterior semicircular canal, facial nerve, digastric ridge, and jugular bulb. A Silastic tube from the mastoid into the cyst provides drainage and aeration.

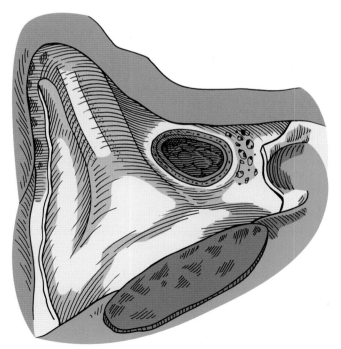

Figure 126-15. Translabyrinthine approach to the petrous apex. The IAC is skeletonized to create an inferior and superior trough around the porus acusticus. Care is taken to avoid the cochlear aqueduct and jugular bulb. The labyrinthine segment of the facial nerve is noted.

The inframeatal exposure of the petrous apex should drain and ventilate the cyst adequately. More aggressive removal of cyst lining is possible with wider exposure. Drainage with a catheter or Silastic sheeting is unnecessary if a large opening in the fistula is created. The wound is copiously irrigated with bacitracin solution. The skin is closed in two layers, and a sterile mastoid dressing is applied.

Transcochlear Approach

The transcochlear approach is reserved for patients who have a large tumor of the petroclival region with preexisting hearing loss. It is a modification of the translabyrinthine approach in which the cartilaginous EAC is closed in a cul-de-sac. A canal wall down mastoidectomy is then performed with unroofing of the sigmoid sinus and exposure of the dura of the posterior and middle fossae. The IAC is identified and the facial nerve is decompressed from the stylomastoid foramen to the IAC. The facial nerve is dissected free from the fallopian canal and transposed posteriorly. This requires identification and sacrifice of the greater superficial petrosal nerve (GSPN). After liberation of the geniculate ganglion, the labyrinthine, tympanic, and vertical portions of the facial nerve are successively released and transposed posteriorly toward the dura of the posterior fossa. The nerve is immobilized with fibrin glue. The cochlea and fallopian canal are then drilled to expose the vertical portion of the ICA. Additional anterior exposure requires drilling the anterior wall of the EAC and displacing the mandibular condyle anteriorly. The horizontal portion of the IAC is then exposed. At the end of the procedure, the eustachian tube is plugged with muscle, Surgicel, and fat harvested from the abdomen, which is then covered with a temporalis myofascial flap.

Although this approach is fairly safe and allows good exposure, it is frequently complicated by cranial nerve palsy. For instance, in a review of 66 cases, every patient in whom the facial nerve was transposed had facial nerve weakness, with only 5% of patients recovering normal facial nerve function 1 year after the procedure. Most of the patients (60%) recovered to House-Brackmann grade III function. Other postoperative deficits included weakness of cranial nerves IV (6%) and VI (9%).[39]

Tympanomastoid Exteriorization

A petrous apex epidermoid tumor or cholesterol granuloma can be marsupialized or drained directly into the tympanic space. This approach almost always entails a canal wall down mastoidectomy. Whether the ossicular chain can be reconstructed depends on the location of the disease, the status of the hearing preoperatively, and the procedure that was performed.

The patient is positioned supine on the operating table with the head turned toward the contralateral ear. The supra-auricular and postauricular hair is shaved, and the ear is prepared and draped in the usual sterile fashion. A longer Koerner flap is made in the EAC in anticipation of a canal wall down mastoidectomy. A postauricular incision is made, and dissection is continued into the EAC. The posterior canal skin flap is elevated and retracted into the ear canal with tracheotomy tape. The auricle is retracted anteriorly. A transcortical mastoidectomy is performed. Because the approach is directed toward the anterior epitympanic area, creation of a large mastoid cavity is to be avoided. Therefore, bone from the mastoid tip and sinodural angle does not have to be extensively removed unless the temporal bone is pneumatized and mucosal disease is present.

The aditus ad antrum, horizontal semicircular canal, and incus are identified. Attention is then turned to the EAC. A tympanomeatal flap is elevated to identify and disarticulate the incudostapedial joint. The incus is removed and saved if it is not involved with cholesteatoma. The posterior bony canal wall is taken down, the anterior and posterior buttress is removed, and the facial ridge is lowered to the level of the EAC. Using a malleus nipper through the neck of the malleus, the head of the malleus is removed. Drilling and dissection are continued anteriorly through the zygomatic route. The geniculate ganglion is noted, and dissection is continued along the GSPN. If greater exposure is necessary inferiorly, the malleus and tensor tympani tendon are removed as well. Although it may permit drainage of a cholesterol cyst, the tympanomastoid approach is predominantly used to marsupialize cholesteatoma located in this area (Fig. 126-16).

The invasive and expansive nature of petrous apex epidermoid tumors is likely to cause sensorineural

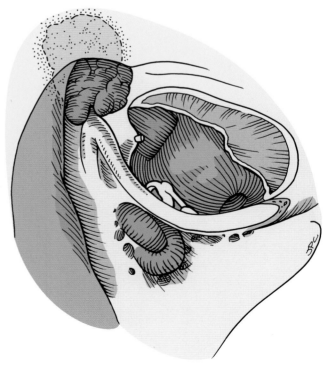

Figure 126-16. Tympanomastoid exteriorization. A canal wall down mastoidectomy is used to expose the anterior epitympanum and the cholesteatoma in the petrous apex. Dissection along the greater superficial petrosal nerve opens the petrous apex through the air cells of the zygomatic route.

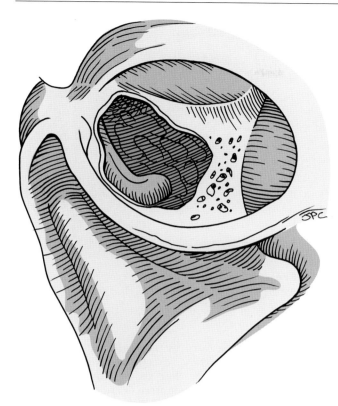

Figure 126-17. Transcochlear approach to the petrous apex. The contents of the epidermoid tumor are removed while leaving the matrix lining intact.

hearing loss. If cochlear function has been compromised preoperatively (speech reception threshold >70 dB, discrimination <30%), greater exposure is achieved by continuing the dissection through the cochlea. The inferior limits of this opening are the eustachian tube and genu of the carotid artery. Drilling is continued through and parallel to the plane of the cochlea. The proximal modiolus and lateral fundus of the IAC should be avoided to prevent a CSF leak. The contents of the petrous apex cholesteatoma are evacuated with blunt instruments such as suction, cup forceps, curettes, and smooth elevators. The epithelial matrix is usually left intact (Fig. 126-17). The cavity is copiously irrigated with bacitracin solution.

Despite the use of meticulous surgical technique while removing or exteriorizing an epidermoid tumor or cholesterol granuloma, CSF leakage may occur as a result of attenuation of the dura. Another situation in which a transepitympanic petrous apex exteriorization approach may need to be converted to obliteration is when the carotid artery becomes significantly exposed. Concern for desiccation of the adventitia of the carotid artery in a marsupialized cavity demands soft tissue protection and coverage. This routinely entails obliteration of the cavity with a temporalis muscle flap or abdominal fat. If the cavity must be obliterated because of a CSF leak, wide exposure of the carotid artery, or excessive exposure of the dura, great effort is taken to completely remove the wall of the granuloma or the epidermal

matrix lining. The external auditory meatus is closed in a two-layer technique (see Chapter 125). An abdominal fat graft is most effective in sealing the CSF leak and obliterating the cavity. The posterior portion of the temporalis muscle is divided, rotated inferiorly, and sutured to the sternocleidomastoid muscle and subcutaneous tissue of the posterior skin.

If cochlear function was not sacrificed, reconstruction of the ossicular chain is undertaken. These techniques are reviewed in Chapter 114. When performing an exteriorization procedure, the epidermoid cavity is packed with continuous gauze impregnated with antibiotic ointment. The packing is placed through the external auditory meatus and positioned in the depth of the epidermoid cavity. The packing is continued through the epitympanic space and mastoid cavity to secure the Koerner flap posteriorly. The postauricular wound is closed with 4-0 resorbable braided suture subcutaneously and 5-0 fast-absorbing suture in the skin supported by Steri-Strips, and an external mastoid dressing is applied.

Preauricular Subtemporal Infratemporal Approach

This approach is used when complete excision of cholesterol granuloma or epidermoid tumor of the petrous apex is necessary. If normal cochlear function is present preoperatively, a hearing conservation procedure is warranted. The patient is positioned supine on the table with the head turned toward the contralateral ear. Should lateral neck rotation be limited, an ipsilateral shoulder roll is placed to provide additional rotation. A strip of hair is shaved from the lateral side of the scalp. The head is placed in three-point fixation with pins using a Mayfield head holder. The preauricular incision is outlined in curvilinear fashion toward the hairline of the forehead (Fig. 126-18). A solution of 1% lidocaine with 1 : 100,000 epinephrine is injected into the planned incision. The skin is incised, and the dissection is taken down to the level of the temporal fascia. Anterior and posterior skin flaps are elevated. Anteriorly, the frontal or temporal branch of the facial nerve must be preserved by incising the deep temporalis fascia in the area just superior to the temporal fat pad. Dissection is continued anteroinferiorly beneath the level of the deep temporalis fascia to protect the frontalis branch within the anterior skin flap from transection, although it is still subject to being stretched (Fig. 126-19). The root and arch of the zygoma are palpated and isolated by incising the periosteal attachments superior and inferior to the arch. Using a Freer or Adson elevator, the medial surface of the zygomatic arch is freed of its muscular attachments.

The attachment of the temporalis muscle is incised along its borders of insertion. A margin of the fibrous attachment along the superior temporal line is preserved to facilitate subsequent reapproximation and wound closure. The temporalis muscle is incised posteriorly, superiorly, and anteriorly and elevated from the temporal fossa. The inferiorly based temporalis muscle flap is dissected well into the infratemporal fascia.

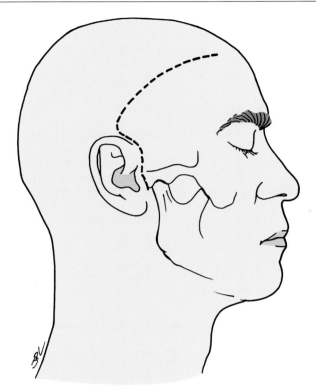

Figure 126-18. Incision for a preauricular subtemporal infratemporal fossa approach.

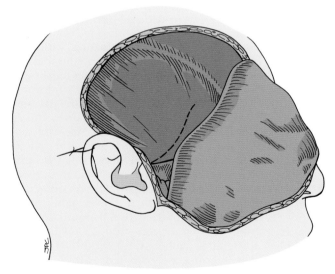

Figure 126-19. The anterior flap is elevated. The frontal branch of the facial nerve is preserved by incising the superficial and deep layers of the temporalis fascia superior to the level of the temporal fat pad.

The zygomatic arch containing the lateral glenoid fossa and part of the body of the zygoma are removed as one unit. This permits further retraction of the inferiorly pedicled temporalis muscle flap and provides greater exposure of the infratemporal fossa (Fig. 126-20).

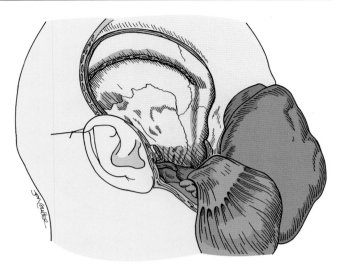

Figure 126-20. The zygomatic arch and glenoid fossa are removed. The temporalis muscle, pedicled on its origin, is retracted inferiorly.

If access to the vertical portion and genu of the carotid artery is necessary, resection of the mandibular condyle is undertaken. Soft tissue surrounding the mandibular condyle is elevated. Venous bleeding is often encountered but is controlled with bipolar coagulation. The neck of the condyle is freed of its periosteum, and the bone is cut with a reciprocating or sagittal saw. If proximal exposure of the carotid artery is not necessary, the capsule and meniscus of the temporomandibular joint are dissected from the glenoid fossa, and the condyle is retracted inferiorly.

The subtemporal approach is continued by performing a temporal craniotomy centered over the infratemporal fossa. The inferior aspect of the craniotomy should be made as low as possible (Fig. 126-21). The base of the skull consisting of the inferior squamous portion, part of the petrous portion, and the posterior extent of the sphenoid bone is further removed with a cutting burr. The middle fossa dura is elevated medially in a posterior-to-anterior direction to the level of the superior petrosal sinus. The temporal lobe is gently elevated and retracted superiorly with a Greenberg retractor. The middle meningeal artery is identified and divided via bipolar coagulation. The third or mandibular division of the trigeminal nerve is identified. Along the floor of the middle cranial fossa, the GSPN is identified and provides a landmark for the geniculate ganglion. The geniculate ganglion also serves as a superior landmark for the cochlea. The GSPN is then transected to avoid traction injury to the facial nerve. Further drilling in this area with cutting and then diamond burrs provides initial exposure of the carotid artery.

The horizontal portion of the carotid artery must be dissected for identification, retraction, or possibly temporary clipping. Bone between the facial hiatus and the foramen spinosum is removed with a drill and rongeurs to unroof the carotid artery. Dissection lateral to

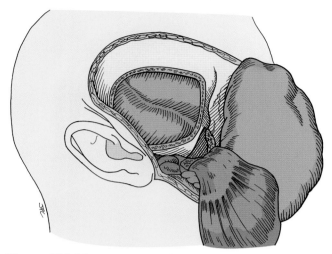

Figure 126-21. A frontotemporal craniotomy is performed to provide access to the middle (subtemporal) and infratemporal fossae.

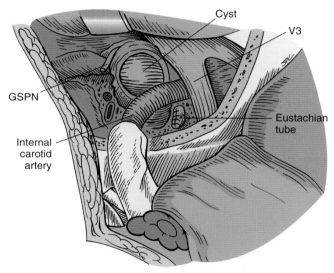

Figure 126-22. Bone separating the subtemporal dura from the infratemporal fossa is removed to expose V3. The greater superficial petrosal nerve (GSPN) has been divided to permit decompression of the internal carotid artery. This exposure allows excision of a petrous apex cholesterol granuloma if a drainage procedure is unsuccessful or resection of an isolated epidermoid tumor if hearing is intact.

the artery exposes the tensor tympani muscle and the eustachian tube. The eustachian tube is transected, and its cartilaginous portion is suture-ligated if the carotid artery is mobilized anterolaterally.

Drilling is continued in the central aspect of the petrous apex. An expansile tumor or cyst should be readily apparent at this time (Fig. 126-22). The area is entered, and its contents are evacuated. Once a cavity has been created, meticulous dissection of the epidermal matrix or cyst wall is performed. Care must be taken when the cyst lining is removed from the carotid artery because of possible attenuation of the adventitia and wall of the carotid artery. Attention is also given to

the dura from which the cyst wall lining was removed. The integrity of the dura must be verified to prevent postoperative CSF leakage. When the entire cyst wall has been removed, the cavity is copiously irrigated with bacitracin solution. The residual cavity defect warrants soft tissue obliteration with abdominal fat. The lateral craniotomy bone flap is returned to its anatomic position and secured with miniplates or 2-0 Vicryl sutures, the temporalis muscle is reattached to its insertion with multiple 2-0 Vicryl sutures, and the zygomatic arch is secured in its original position with miniplates or sutures. The skin is closed in three-layer fashion, and a sterile pressure dressing is applied.

Expanded Endoscopic Transnasal Approach

Since writing of the first edition of this textbook, surgeons at the University of Pittsburgh Medical Center have developed and mastered transnasal endoscopic procedures directed to the pituitary gland, anterior skull base, anterior cranial fossa, infratemporal fossa, and posterior fossa. These surgical techniques have been adapted to gain access to the petrous bone from an anterior approach despite development of the sphenoid sinus.[32] The dissection through the sphenoid bone is medial to the carotid artery. The petrous apex is the point of entry for access and drainage of cholesterol granuloma.

POSTOPERATIVE MANAGEMENT

The intensity of immediate postoperative care is determined by the extent of the operative procedure undertaken and whether the cranial nerves, the carotid artery, the dura, or the otic capsule were affected or compromised by the procedure. Patients undergoing a drainage procedure for cholesterol granuloma via the infracochlear or infralabyrinthine route can be discharged from the hospital on the same or the following day, depending on their tolerance for the procedure and reaction to general anesthesia. Patients are seen 7 to 10 days postoperatively for ear canal packing and removal of the postauricular Steri-Strips. If the medial external canal covering the tympanomeatal flap was filled with Gelfoam, antibiotic suspension drops are prescribed twice daily. The patient is seen every 2 to 3 weeks to suction out the remaining Gelfoam and ensure that healing of the inferior canal wall is taking place. After a few weeks, the middle ear can be assessed. It takes 4 to 6 weeks for the inferior canal and hypotympanum to heal. The patient's middle ear is observed in the interim to monitor for resolution of postoperative serous effusion. Concern for compromised middle ear aeration via the eustachian tube is managed by placement of a myringotomy tube in the anterosuperior quadrant. An audiogram is obtained after complete healing to assess the status of postoperative hearing.

A pressure dressing is maintained over wounds that were obliterated with fat or a transposed temporalis muscle. Drains are not placed within the operative site routinely. However, if an abdominal fat graft was obtained and a Penrose drain was placed in the abdominal wound, the drain is removed once drainage diminishes. In patients with congenital epidermoid tumor who are able to have the disease exteriorized by marsupialization, the mastoid dressing is removed the day after surgery. A cotton ball placed in the external auditory meatus is subject to serosanguineous drainage and is changed frequently. When the patient is seen 7 to 10 days postoperatively, the postauricular Steri-Strips and part of the continuous-strip gauze packing are removed. The packing is withdrawn until there is significant resistance to removal or mild bleeding is encountered. Topical antibiotic ear drops are prescribed, and the remainder of the packing is removed the following week. Oral antibiotics are not prescribed, although oral narcotic analgesics are provided for pain relief.

Patients requiring extensive dissection or resection are at risk for CSF leak and injury to the cranial nerves, otic capsule, carotid artery, dura, and brain. Patients are closely monitored for symptoms or signs related to these neurovascular structures. The patient's neurologic status is monitored frequently when a CSF leak is encountered or a subtemporal approach was performed. Patients are evaluated for signs of mental status change or evidence of meningitis. Those requiring a transpetrous or subtemporal infratemporal fossa approach for total resection of cholesterol granuloma or epidermoid tumor are usually hospitalized for a few days. The wound and patient are observed for infection, subdural hematoma, and CSF accumulation, otorrhea, or rhinorrhea. Further details regarding skull base approaches are reviewed in Chapter 102.

The presence or development of facial nerve dysfunction requires supportive care. Particular attention is devoted to protection of the cornea. Weakness of the orbicularis oculi with symptomatic lagophthalmos is managed by artificial tears during the day and ointment at night. A clear moisture chamber is provided if topical drops alone do not adequately relieve the dryness and irritation. Placement of a gold weight within the upper eyelid is recommended for assisted lid closure and corneal protection if it is anticipated that facial paralysis will be present for more than a brief time (see Chapter 121). Persistent erythema with eye irritation warrants ophthalmic consultation.

Inadvertent or intentional entry into the otic capsule usually results in vertigo if vestibular function was present preoperatively. Supportive measures consisting of antiemetic medications such as phenothiazine or droperidol should be taken. Assisted ambulation will enhance central vestibular recovery. The physical therapy department is consulted to initiate a rehabilitation treatment plan. Physiologically young patients will adapt centrally to the unilateral vestibular loss. At our institution, patients who continue to exhibit uncompensated disequilibrium are subsequently referred to the vestibular rehabilitation physical therapist for ongoing outpatient care. Coping strategies and vestibular retraining exercises are the focus of their program.

If a hearing preservation procedure was performed, a postoperative audiogram is obtained at approximately

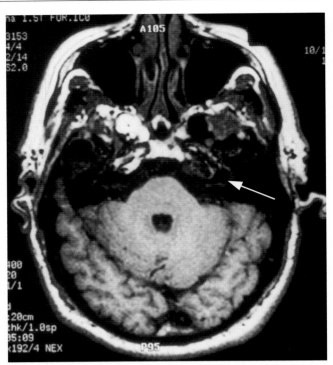

Figure 126-23. Postoperative magnetic resonance image of the cholesterol granuloma shown in Figure 121-5. This non–contrast-enhanced T1-weighted image demonstrates lack of signal in the petrous apex *(arrow)*, indicative of excellent aeration and resolution of the cyst.

1 month. Unless the procedure consisted of marsupialization into a large mastoid cavity, it is necessary to monitor for recurrence with radiologic imaging. Given that the tumor or cystic lesion demonstrated bone expansion with smooth remodeling, a CT scan can be used to effectively evaluate changes in the cavity. Regardless of whether the procedure entailed drainage and ventilation or resection with obliteration, a CT scan obtained 3 months postoperatively will provide the baseline for future comparisons. MRI does have a role in postoperative monitoring (Fig. 126-23). If there is concern for recurrence of pathology despite a stable CT scan, MRI readily differentiates changes in tissue density. If the cavity was obliterated with fat, fat suppression MRI techniques can be used to critically assess the contents of the bony cavity. A subsequent scan is obtained 1 year after the baseline scan. If the petrous apex is found to contain air, adequate ventilation has been achieved. If the cavity was obliterated and the patient shows no new clinical signs or symptoms, a CT scan is obtained 3 years later.

COMPLICATIONS

The problems and complications that arise after management of cholesterol granuloma and large epidermoid tumors depend on the surgical approach and completeness of the procedure. In addition to the problem of persistent or recurrent disease, complications can be grouped by cranial nerve deficits, central nervous system sequelae, vascular injury and bleeding, and problems related to the wound.

A preexisting conductive hearing loss may remain or increase in magnitude, depending on the operative management of the ossicular chain and tympanic membrane. The first goal of the procedure is to effectively eradicate or exteriorize the pathologic process for which the procedure was performed. This may require radical mastoidectomy, which by definition may maximize a conductive hearing loss. Under this circumstance, the conductive hearing loss is an accepted outcome from the procedure rather than a risk or complication. However, if the ossicular chain was reconstructed and a conductive hearing loss persists, subsequent aural rehabilitation can be provided by revision surgery or hearing aid amplification.

Despite normal cochlear function, the procedure may occasionally require sacrifice of the otic capsule to eliminate the cyst or tumor. Again, this would be not a complication but rather a planned outcome. However, if it was unplanned, sensorineural hearing loss may result from inadvertent injury to the otic capsule or ossicular chain. Planned or unintended entry into the inner ear typically results in vestibular signs of nystagmus, vomiting, and postural instability and symptoms of nausea, vertigo, and disequilibrium.

Middle ear effusion develops when the eustachian tube is sacrificed during the subtemporal infratemporal fossa approach. The resultant conductive hearing loss is treated with a ventilation tube. It is best to wait approximately 4 to 6 weeks before tube insertion to allow complete healing of any potential dural defects.

Resection of large tumors of the petrous apex extending toward the cavernous sinus may also put the third, fourth, fifth, and sixth cranial nerves at risk. Patients with petrous apex involvement occasionally have preoperative symptoms of facial hypoesthesia. Care should be taken to minimize further trauma to the trigeminal nerve. Similarly, the immediate proximity of the sixth nerve to Meckel's cave requires that it be identified during intradural procedures to avoid excessive manipulation. Injury to this nerve results in paresis of the lateral rectus muscle. If the nerve was stretched during the procedure, return of function can be expected within a few months. Sacrifice of the sixth cranial nerve or paralysis that does not resolve warrants consultation with an ophthalmologist for corrective muscle surgery.

Injury to the seventh cranial nerve may result in paresis or paralysis of the facial musculature. If it is known that dissection around the facial nerve left the nerve anatomically intact, supportive care is provided as described previously under "Postoperative Management." Sacrifice of the seventh nerve is corrected by reconstruction with a hypoglossal-to-facial nerve anastomosis if primary or cable graft repair could not be performed at the time of the procedure.

The lower cranial nerves may also be affected by large epidermoid cysts or cholesterol granuloma of the petrous apex. However, direct invasion is relatively rare. Intraoperative injury to these nerves results in dysphagia, aspiration, hoarseness, and inanition. Temporary dysfunction is managed by injection of Gelfoam into the vocal cord and enteral supplementation via nasogastric feeding. Permanent injury to the vagus nerve resulting in hoarseness, dysphagia, and aspiration is managed by a type I thyroplasty and cricopharyngeal myotomy.

Infralabyrinthine or infracochlear drainage procedures require intimate dissection around the jugular bulb. Intraoperative extradural venous bleeding can be quite bothersome, but it is usually controlled with Surgicel, bone wax, or bipolar cautery. Dissection of the petrous apex requires careful attention to the carotid artery. Preoperative testing with balloon occlusion provides an indication of how the patient will tolerate temporary intraoperative occlusion to repair injury to the ICA. It is best to avoid a potential injury to the carotid artery by meticulous dissection and protection of the vessel. If the dura into the posterior fossa is opened, similar respect is given to the intracranial vessels. Repair of these small vessels is technically most difficult, and clipping or bipolar coagulation may be necessary. This may result in serious central nervous system deficits in the cerebellum, midbrain, and brain stem.

Procedures in which resection or drainage is attempted in an extradural fashion may still be complicated by CSF otorrhea and rhinorrhea. Leakage around the otic capsule into a closed middle ear space will be manifested as CSF rhinorrhea. Canal wall down procedures (radical mastoid cavity) in which tympanic membrane reconstruction was not undertaken will have CSF leaking directly through the aural wound. The risk for meningitis demands repair of the fistula. Lumbar drainage of CSF is rarely effective in controlling the leak once a fistula has developed in an open cavity. Operative intervention requiring soft tissue obliteration with wound compression is usually necessary for effective control.

Wound infection is a rare complication of otologic surgery. Soft tissue infection and cellulitis are treated with systemic antibiotics. Formation of an abscess such as in the epidural space requires drainage, culture for an organism, and appropriate parenteral antibiotics. Drainage procedures for cholesterol granuloma provide a potential pathway for retrograde infection into the cystic cavity. If the expansion process had thinned the wall of the cavity and exposed the carotid artery, carotid hemorrhage may result. A bacterial or fungal infection may become established in the cancellous bone, with the subsequent development of temporal bone osteomyelitis.[18]

Excessive retraction of or direct injury to the temporal lobe may occur from procedures directed at the petrous apex via the subtemporal infratemporal fossa or direct transtemporal approaches. Injury to the left temporal lobe may result in expressive or receptive aphasia. Though rare, ischemia and infarction may produce temporary or permanent hemiparesis and hypoesthesia.

PEARLS

- Both CT and MRI are necessary for determining the type of pathology affecting the petrous apex.
- Transnasal/transpetrous approaches to pathology of the petrous apex should be considered when reviewing images showing the anatomy of related structures.
- Sacrifice of the eustachian tube results in middle ear effusion when the tympanic membrane remains intact or is reconstructed. Delayed ventilation of the middle ear should be planned after extensive procedures to avoid the risk of CSF otorrhea.
- Temporary or permanent injury to the facial nerve requires early aggressive eye care to protect the cornea from desiccation or further injury.
- Placement of a ventilation tube in the tympanic membrane may obviate early occlusion of a Silastic drainage tube positioned between the petrous apex and the hypotympanum after an infracochlear approach.

PITFALLS

- Underestimating the exposure necessary for complete removal or creating suboptimal drainage of pathologic processes of the petrous apex will result in persistence or recurrence of disease.
- CSF otorrhea or rhinorrhea after approaches to the petrous apex may not respond to lumbar drainage; operative intervention will probably be necessary.
- Subtotal removal of the epithelial matrix of an epidermoid cyst may be temporizing and represents the first stage of subsequent procedures.
- Performing a procedure that drains the petrous apex and creation of a radical mastoid cavity without coverage of an exposed carotid artery may result in desiccation and rupture.
- A middle fossa approach to cholesterol granuloma of the petrous apex may not afford adequate drainage into the middle ear. The entire cyst and its lining will need to be removed.

References

1. Chole RA: Petrous apicitis: Surgical anatomy. Ann Otol Rhinol Laryngol 94:251-257, 1985.
2. Farrior JB: Anterior hypotympanic approach for glomus tumor of the infratemporal fossa. Laryngoscope 94:1016-1021, 1984.
3. Giddings NA, Brackmann DE, Kwartler JA: Transcanal infracochlear approach to the petrous apex. Otolaryngol Head Neck Surg 104:29-36, 1991.
4. Muckle RP, De la Cruz A, Lo WM: Petrous apex lesions. Am J Otol 19:219-225, 1998.
5. Terao T, Onoue H, Hashimoto T, et al: Cholesterol granuloma in the petrous apex: Case report and review. Acta Neurochir (Wien) 143:947-952, 2001.
6. Schick B, Brors D, Koch O, et al: Magnetic resonance imaging in patients with sudden hearing loss, tinnitus and vertigo. Otol Neurotol 22:808-812, 2001.
7. Politzer A: Uber bewegliche Exudate in der Trommelfellhohle [The membrane in health and disease]. Vienna, Wien Med Presse (Wm Wood), 1869.
8. Shambaugh GE: The blue drum membrane. Arch Otolaryngol 10:238-240, 1929.
9. House JL, Brackmann DE: Cholesterol granuloma of the cerebellopontine angle. Arch Otolaryngol 108:504-506, 1982.
10. Graham MD, Kemink JL, Latack JT, Kartush JM: The giant cholesterol cyst of the petrous apex: A distinct clinical entity. Laryngoscope 95:1401-1406, 1985.
11. Mosnier I, Cyna-Gorse F, Grayeli AB, et al: Management of cholesterol granulomas of the petrous apex based on clinical and radiologic evaluation. Otol Neurotol 23:522-528, 2002.
12. Jackler RK, Cho M: A new theory to explain the genesis of petrous apex cholesterol granuloma. Otol Neurotol 24:96-106, discussion 106, 2003.
13. Gadre AK, Brodie HA, Fayad JN, O'Leary MJ: Venous channels of the petrous apex: Their presence and clinical importance. Otolaryngol Head Neck Surg 116:168-174, 1997.
14. Schuknecht H: Pathology of the Ear. Philadelphia, Lea & Febiger, 1993.
15. Von Remak R: Beitrag zur Entwicklungsgeschichte der krebshaften Geschwulste. Dtsch Klin 6(170B):174, 1854.
16. Pyle GM, Wiet RJ: Petrous apex cholesteatoma: Exteriorization vs. subtotal petrosectomy with obliteration. Skull Base Surg 1:97-105, 1991.
17. Glasscock ME 3rd, Woods CI 3rd, Poe DS, et al: Petrous apex cholesteatoma. Otolaryngol Clin North Am 22:981-1002, 1989.
18. Michaels L: An epidermoid formation in the developing middle ear: Possible source of cholesteatoma. J Otolaryngol 15:169-174, 1986.
19. McGill TJ, Merchant S, Healy GB, Friedman EM: Congenital cholesteatoma of the middle ear in children: A clinical and histopathological report. Laryngoscope 101:606-613, 1991.
20. Nager G: Epidermoids (Congenital Cholesteatomas). Baltimore, Williams & Wilkins, 1992.
21. Yamakawa K, Shitara N, Genka S, et al: Clinical course and surgical prognosis of 33 cases of intracranial epidermoid tumors. Neurosurgery 24:568-573, 1989.
22. Pisaneschi MJ, Langer B: Congenital cholesteatoma and cholesterol granuloma of the temporal bone: Role of magnetic resonance imaging. Top Magn Reson Imaging 11:87-97, 2000.
23. Van Havenbergh T, Koekelkoren E, De Ridder D, et al: Image guided surgery for petrous apex lesions. Acta Neurochir (Wien) 145:737-742, discussion 742, 2003.
24. de Vries EJ, Sekhar LN, Horton JA et al: A new method to predict safe resection of the internal carotid artery. Laryngoscope 100:85-88, 1990.
25. Eisenberg MB, Haddad G, Al-Mefty O: Petrous apex cholesterol granulomas: Evolution and management. J Neurosurg 86:822-829, 1997.
26. Haberkamp TJ: Surgical anatomy of the transtemporal approaches to the petrous apex. Am J Otol 18:501-506, 1997.
27. Brackmann DE, Toh EH: Surgical management of petrous apex cholesterol granulomas. Otol Neurotol 23:529-533, 2002.
28. Thedinger BA, Nadol JB Jr, Montgomery WW, et al: Radiographic diagnosis, surgical treatment, and long-term follow-up of cholesterol granulomas of the petrous apex. Laryngoscope 99:896-907, 1989.
29. Cristante L, Puchner MA: A keyhole middle fossa approach to large cholesterol granulomas of the petrous apex. Surg Neurol 53:64-70, discussion 70-71, 2000.
30. Montgomery WW: Cystic lesions of the petrous apex: Transsphenoid approach. Ann Otol Rhinol Laryngol 86:429-435, 1977.
31. DiNardo LJ, Pippin GW, Sismanis A: Image-guided endoscopic transsphenoidal drainage of select petrous apex cholesterol granulomas. Otol Neurotol 24:939-941, 2003.
32. Kassam AB, Gardner P, Snyderman C, et al: Expanded endonasal approach: Fully endoscopic, completely transnasal approach to the middle third of the clivus, petrous bone, middle cranial fossa, and infratemporal fossa. Neurosurg Focus 19(1):E6, 2005.

33. Kaylie DM, Warren FM 3rd, Haynes DS, Jackson CG: Neurotologic management of intracranial epidermoid tumors. Laryngoscope 115:1082-1086, 2005.

34. Fisch U: Infratemporal fossa approach to tumours of the temporal bone and base of the skull. J Laryngol Otol 92:949-967, 1978.

35. House WF, De La Cruz A, Hitselberger WE: Surgery of the skull base: Transcochlear approach to the petrous apex and clivus. Otolaryngology 86:770-779, 1978.

36. Selesnick SH, Abraham MT, Carew JF: Rerouting of the intratemporal facial nerve: An analysis of the literature. Am J Otol 17:793-805, discussion 806-809, 1996.

37. Mattox DE: Endoscopy-assisted surgery of the petrous apex. Otolaryngol Head Neck Surg 130:229-241, 2004.

38. Gerek M, Satar B, Yazar F, et al: Transcanal anterior approach for cystic lesions of the petrous apex. Otol Neurotol 25:973-976, 2004.

39. Sanna M, Zazzoni A, Saleh E, et al: The system of the modified transcochlear approach: A lateral avenue to the central skull base. Am J Otol 19:88-98, 1998.

Chapter 127

Cerebrospinal Fluid Otorrhea and Encephalocele

Elizabeth H. Toh

Temporal bone cerebrospinal fluid (CSF) otorrhea may occur from a variety of congenital or acquired etiologies (Table 127-1). Leakage of CSF through the temporal bone represents a fistula from the fluid-filled subarachnoid space into the pneumatized temporal bone. Subsequent egress of CSF through a defect in the mastoid cavity, tympanic membrane, or external auditory canal presents as otorrhea. Rhinorrhea represents drainage of CSF through the eustachian tube and may occur with or without otorrhea. An encephalocele is a protrusion of the brain, with or without overlying dura, beyond the confines of the cranial cavity into the mastoid or middle ear. A true encephalocele contains prolapsed brain tissue, whereas a meningoencephalocele contains brain and meninges. The terms *CSF otorrhea* and *encephalocele* both imply an anatomic pathway between the subdural space and the exterior. For this reason, both have equal potential for central nervous system complications and infections.

Gacek demonstrated that aberrant arachnoid granulations may occur in the vicinity of the temporal bone as well as in other areas of the skull base.[1] Unlike classic arachnoid granulations, these aberrant structures do not have an absorptive role associated with CSF. Although arachnoid granulations of the middle or posterior cranial fossa are not routinely encountered during mastoid surgery, the incidence of these structures in temporal bone histopathologic studies of the surface of the middle fossa is as high as 22%. The most common locations of these aberrant arachnoid granulations are lateral to the cribriform plate in the anterior cranial fossa, and on the floor of the middle fossa. Occasionally they may occur in the posterior fossa plate between the sigmoid sinus and the bony labyrinth. Intermittent increases in spinal fluid pressure are hypothesized to cause gradual increase in size of these

aberrant arachnoid granulations and erosive changes in the underlying bone, with eventual protrusion through the tegmen or posterior fossa plate. It is thought that these granulations are the largest single cause of spontaneous CSF leaks in adults. The typical presentation of spontaneous CSF leaks in adults is unilateral serous otitis media with no preceding upper respiratory infection, which is refractory to decongestant and antibiotic therapy. Myringotomy and ventilation tube placement usually results in persistent clear watery drainage that does not respond to conventional ototopical therapy. A high index of clinical suspicion is necessary to diagnose this entity.

Perilymphatic fistulas are another potential source of communication between the middle ear and the subarachnoid space. These defects rarely result in any clinically significant accumulation of fluid within the middle ear and therefore typically do not present like other causes of CSF otorrhea or rhinorrhea. Leakage typically occurs from the otic capsule through a dehiscence in the stapes footplate. The diagnosis is usually made in childhood, and typically presents as recurrent meningitis with hearing loss in the affected ear. Perilymphatic fistulas are discussed in detail in Chapter 119.

Spontaneous meningoencephaloceles of the skull base have been reported since early in this century. The most common location for encephaloceles of the temporal bone is along the floor of the middle cranial fossa. The posterior fossa of the temporal bone may also be affected, although rarely. Defects are frequently identified in multiple locations at the time of presentation. Congenital defects in the bone of the skull base predispose to progressive formation of dural and arachnoid herniations. Prolapse into the epitympanum and middle ear may cause conductive hearing loss or present with a mass in the middle ear (Fig. 127-1). Retrograde bacte-

Table 127-1	CAUSES OF CEREBROSPINAL FLUID OTORRHEA	
Congenital	**Acquired**	**Spontaneous**
Meningoencephalocele, secondary to congenital skull base defects	Posttraumatic (temporal bone fractures, surgery)	Arachnoid granulations
Perilymphatic fistulas	Chronic otitis media Neoplasia Postirradiation	

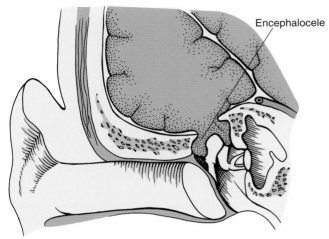

Encephalocele

Figure 127-1. Herniation of brain tissue from the middle cranial fossa into the epitympanum.

rial contamination from the nasopharynx, paranasal sinuses, or middle ear may result in the development of meningitis. Therefore this disorder occurs most frequently in childhood.

Trauma to the temporal bone may occur as a result of blunt head trauma or surgery of the temporal bone. CSF otorrhea secondary to temporal bone fractures is discussed in Chapter 128. Diagnosis is straightforward in these cases, and the majority of these patients respond to conservative management. Bed rest and head elevation results in spontaneous resolution in up to 90% of patients with temporal bone fractures. Most of the remaining cases can be controlled by intermittent or continuous lumbar drainage, leaving only a few patients who require surgical intervention.[2] Iatrogenic trauma to the dura during surgery of the temporal bone can eventually lead to weakening of the dura with resultant meningoencephalocele, encephalocele, and CSF otorrhea. Dural exposure alone, without violation, does not usually result in herniation of brain tissue or CSF leak. If CSF leak is noted at the time of iatrogenic trauma, surgical repair should be performed immediately.

CSF otorrhea and encephaloceles related to chronic otitis media may occur with or without cholesteatoma, usually in patients with an antecedent history of oto-

logic surgery. Cholesteatomas may erode into the otic capsule as well as through the middle or posterior fossa plates. However, chronic otitis media and mastoiditis with granulation tissue alone may also lead to this defect over a long period. The erosive process from cholesteatoma and chronic inflammation most commonly affects the horizontal semicircular canal, but may extend superiorly to involve the mastoid and middle ear tegmen.

Primary tumors or tumors metastatic to the temporal bone or areas adjacent to it may also cause bone erosion, which may be associated with secondary CSF otorrhea. The most common tumor in children is rhabdomyosarcoma. The most common tumors in adults are epithelial tumors and paragangliomas.

PATIENT SELECTION

CSF leak of otogenic origin may present in several ways. If the tympanic membrane is violated, clear otorrhea is noted. With an intact tympanic membrane, the patient may complain of clear watery drainage from the nose, which usually occurs when bending over or straining. If leakage is minimal or intermittent, CSF may drain directly into the pharynx and esophagus without being noticed by the patient. The second clinical presentation occurring in individuals with an intact tympanic membrane, is hearing impairment and aural fullness as a result of middle ear effusion. Even in the absence of an antecedent upper respiratory infection, the diagnosis is presumed to be serous otitis media, and a myringotomy is often performed to drain the fluid. Following this procedure, the patient has continuous clear otorrhea, which persists despite antibiotic, antihistamine, and decongestant therapy. The latter presentation is typical of spontaneous otogenic CSF leaks in adults and a high index of suspicion is critical in making a timely diagnosis. The incidence of bilaterality in spontaneous otogenic CSF leaks may be up to 22%.[3]

Meningitis (single or repeated episodes) may be the initial presentation of a CSF leak. This is more common in children when they have been unaware of any hearing loss or aural fullness in the affected ear. Meningitis often leads to a profound sensorineural hearing impairment, which may often be the presenting problem in children. Any patient presenting with meningitis must be carefully evaluated for a potential otogenic source.

Patients complaining of hearing impairment occasionally will have a mass discovered within the middle ear, with or without hearing loss (Fig. 127-2). High-resolution computed tomography (CT) of the temporal bone usually identifies the origin of the soft tissue mass and points to any defects in the bony plates of the middle or posterior fossa. Anyone with previous tympanomastoid surgery presenting with otorrhea, a middle ear effusion, or rhinorrhea should be suspected of having a defect in the dura as a result of the original procedure. A history of prior trauma to the temporal bone should alert the examiner to the potential diagnosis of encephalocele or meningoencephalocele.

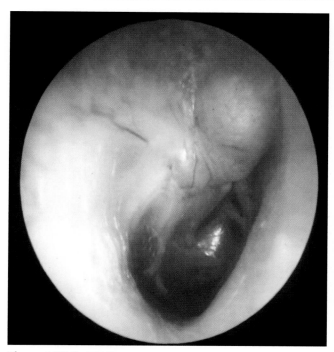

Figure 127-2. Middle ear mass visualized on otoscopy.

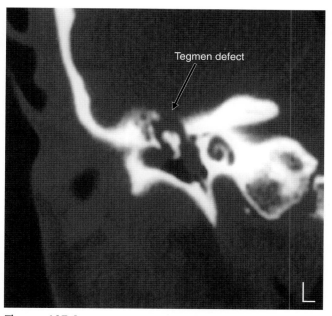

Tegmen defect

Figure 127-3. High-resolution coronal computed tomography scan of temporal bone showing the defect in the bone in the tegmen tympani and soft tissue in the epitympanum and middle ear *(arrow)*.

PREOPERATIVE PLANNING

Once CSF otorrhea, rhinorrhea, or encephalocele is suspected, efforts must proceed quickly to confirm the presence of a dural defect and furthermore to locate the defect precisely. The surgeon should attempt to elicit the symptoms of rhinorrhea. This can often be accomplished by having the patient bend forward and place the head between the knees for several minutes. It may also be accomplished by having the patient lie in a head-down position and then turn to the prone position to encourage active drainage. When CSF is observed clinically, there is usually no question about its origin. It appears as clear as water and is not cloudy or sanguinous. Difficulty in identification may be encountered only in trauma cases in which there is concomitant bleeding. In these cases, a telltale ring of CSF may be seen outside the stain left by blood and serum on a dressing or bed linens (halo sign), which may alert the physician to this problem.

Testing fluid for the presence of glucose, usually with a test strip, is notoriously unreliable and usually requires large amounts of fluid to produce consistent results. It is therefore no longer used as a primary diagnostic modality for confirmation of CSF. When the origin or nature of the drainage is in question, we prefer the technique of identifying β_2-transferrin within the fluid using immunoelectrophoresis. This testing requires remarkably scant quantities of CSF and may be submitted to the laboratory as free fluid or on a carrier material such as Gelfoam or Merocel. β_2-transferrin is present only in CSF and perilymph, and is not found in blood or serum. The sensitivity and specificity of this test is approximately 100% and 95%, respectively, and is not influenced by contamination with blood or other body fluids.[4]

High-resolution CT imaging of the temporal bone using a bone algorithm is the cornerstone of diagnosing and localizing CSF leaks in the temporal bone. Coronal cuts usually enable the examiner to identify the location and number of bony defects in the petrous temporal bone. CT imaging also helps in identifying soft tissue within the middle ear and mastoid, erosion of the bone of the otic capsule, or structural anomalies of the inner ear (Fig. 127-3). Magnetic resonance imaging of the brain plays a complementary role in determining the nature and origin of soft tissue in the middle ear and mastoid when a large defect in the tegmen is identified on CT imaging (Fig. 127-4). Neither radionuclide cisternography or CT cisternography provides any additional diagnostic information in the evaluation of CSF leaks.[5]

An audiogram should be obtained to evaluate the presence and extent of hearing impairment in the affected ear before surgical management. A hearing preservation approach is preferred in the presence of any aidable residual hearing in the operated ear.

SURGICAL APPROACHES

The surgical approach is dictated by the size, number, and location of bony defects, as well as the status of the hearing in the affected ear. Dehiscence of the posterior fossa plate, as well as of the posterior and lateral portions of the middle fossa plate, can almost always be repaired through a transmastoid approach (Fig. 127-5). Medial and anterior defects involving the tegmen tympani and petrous apex, respectively, require a

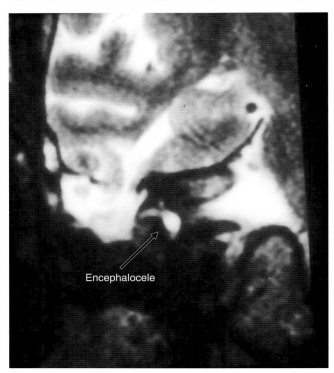

Figure 127-4. T2-weighted magnetic resonance imaging (MRI) of brain in coronal plane confirming soft tissue seen in Figure 127-3 as encephalocele *(arrow)*.

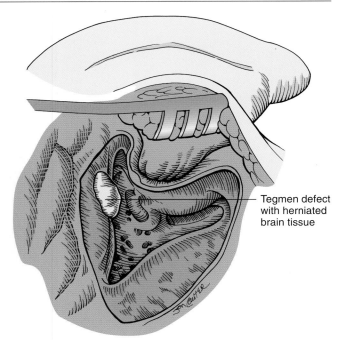

Figure 127-5. The transmastoid approach for repair of an encephalocele (right ear).

middle cranial fossa approach for repair. Large or multiple tegmen defects usually require a combined transmastoid and middle cranial fossa approach. Patients with chronic otitis media and defects eroding the otic capsule may require a canal wall-down mastoidectomy in order to obtain adequate exposure for surgical repair and exteriorization of disease if extensive cholesteatoma is identified.

Details of the techniques for each of these approaches are described in Chapters 115 and 124. The transmastoid approach provides the distinct advantage of extracranial visualization of the defect without temporal lobe retraction. However, bony defects exceeding 2 cm in diameter are more reliably repaired from above using a supplemental middle fossa approach. In these cases, the postauricular incision is extended superiorly and anteriorly, and a limited craniotomy is performed, centered around the location of the defect identified from below. Similarly, in a patient with previous canal wall-down mastoid cavity with residual hearing, the defect in the tegmen and the encephalocele should be repaired from above using the middle fossa approach.[6]

When CSF otorrhea is copious, a lumbar drain is placed at the time of surgery. During surgery, the drain can be clamped to aid localization of the site of the leak. The Valsalva maneuver, performed by the anesthetist, may also be helpful, when necessary.

When brain herniation is encountered, there is uniform agreement that this tissue is nonfunctional and may be removed. This lack of function is assumed to be the result of tissue strangulation, ischemia, and resultant edema of this tissue. In general, broad-based encephaloceles herniating through large bony defects are considered viable and may be reduced back into the cranial vault. Bipolar electrocautery is used to remove nonviable tissue until the margins of the bony defect through which it has extruded is well defined.

Many methods of repair of these defects have been advocated over the years. A multilayer closure using a combination of free grafts has remained the most reliable technique to repair the defects. A large variety of materials including both biologic tissues and synthetic materials have been used to repair the dura. Autologous temporalis fascia, pericranium, and fascia lata are preferred when available because they are easy to handle, nontoxic, inexpensive, and have favorable biologic behavior. Fascia lata may be obtained if temporalis fascia is lacking due to previous surgery, but obtaining fascia lata requires additional surgery, operating time, and donor site morbidity. The use of synthetic materials is no longer widely used because of local tissue reactions, excessive scar formation, meningitis, and hemorrhage. Solvent-preserved, gamma-sterilized Tutoplast bovine pericardium has also been widely used for dural substitution with favorable clinical outcomes.[7,8] The use of fibrin glue with primary closure alone does not appear to have any additional benefit.[2] Hydroxyapatite cement cranioplasty has been used in conjunction with autologous fat for prevention of CSF leak following vestibular schwannoma surgery and for primary repair of small defects in the tegmen in spontaneous CSF leaks.[9]

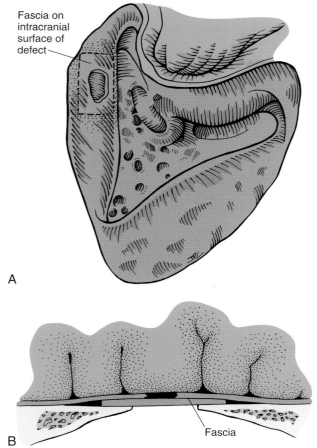

Figure 127-6. Use of fascia intracranially to form the first layer of repair of a dural defect.

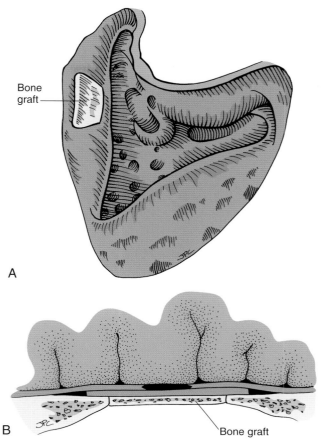

Figure 127-7. A shaped bone graft placed into the tegmen defect.

Two layers of temporalis fascia are used with a transmastoid approach, one on either side of the bony defect. Following removal of all soft tissue around the bony defect in the posterior or middle fossa, the intracranial dura is dissected with a duckbill or hockey-stick elevator until 1 cm of elevation is obtained circumferentially around the bony defect. At this point, dried temporalis fascia is placed within the bony defect and spread out over the intracranial surface between the dura and the tegmen (Fig. 127-6). Reexpansion of the brain contents ensures the retention of the fascial graft. The bony defect is then closed using a cancellous bone graft taken from the mastoid process, retrosigmoid area, or squamous portion of the bone, or using a conchal cartilage graft. This provides additional support for the primary graft material. When small bone defects are present, the bone graft or cartilage graft can be contoured to fit tightly into the exact shape of the space it is filling (Fig. 127-7). A tightly fitting graft in a small defect requires nothing further to keep it in place. A second layer of temporalis fascia is then placed over the bony defect on the mastoid side (Fig. 127-8), buttressed in place by means of temporalis muscle or abdominal fat.

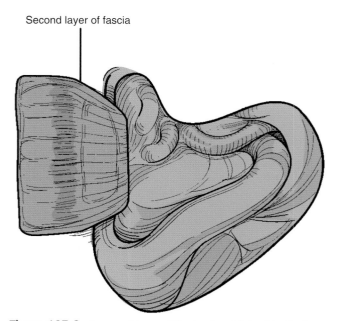

Figure 127-8. A second layer of fascia placed lateral to the bone graft.

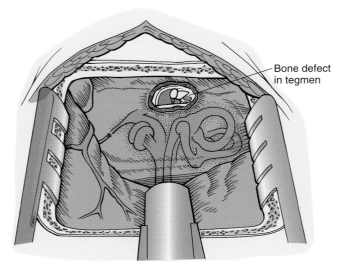

Figure 127-9. The middle fossa approach to repair showing the defect in the bone after removal of herniated tissue.

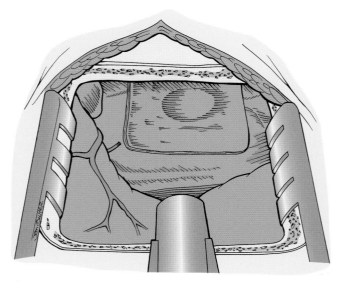

Figure 127-10. A large piece of dried temporalis fascia is used to cover the defect in the bone.

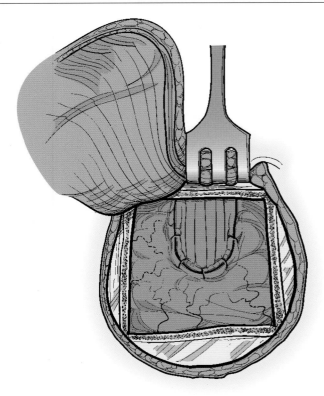

Figure 127-11. The temporalis muscle oversewn on the dura to repair the dural defect.

A middle cranial fossa approach may be used as the primary approach for repair when anterior, medial, or multiple defects are present. Following extradural elevation of the temporal lobe, soft tissue is once again carefully removed from the bony defect (Fig. 127-9). A large piece of dried temporalis fascia is next placed across the floor of the middle cranial fossa (Fig. 127-10), and the temporal lobe is allowed to reexpand and hold this tissue in place. Larger defects should be supported using an additional bone or cartilage graft placed over the fascial graft. In addition, an attempt is made to close the dural defect responsible for the leak. When this defect is small, it can be closed primarily by suturing. When the defect is larger, a small piece of temporalis muscle is oversewn with 6-0 Nurolon sutures (Fig. 127-11). Alternatively, the entire repair can be

done by an intradural technique.[10] Opening the dura on the lateral surface of the temporal lobe permits elevation of the brain from the underlying dura. This allows for close inspection of the herniated contents as well as the adjacent brain. Larger broad-based encephaloceles in uninfected fields may potentially be recranialized using this technique. The graft is placed on the dura, and the expanded brain then secures its fixation. In the rare case of a large defect with high-volume CSF drainage, vascularized tissue such as a pedicled temporalis muscle flap or pericranial flap should be rotated intracranially and secured to dura medial to the defect.

Defects in the otic capsule or tegmen plate associated with chronic middle ear disease are approached in the standard tympanomastoid fashion. In the absence of any useful hearing in the affected ear, the eustachian tube, mastoid, and middle ear may be obliterated and the ear canal closed. The malleus, incus, tympanic membrane, and skin of the medial external auditory canal are removed. It is also necessary to carefully seal the eustachian tube using bone and temporalis muscle (Fig. 127-12). The external auditory meatus is oversewn and closed in a layered fashion by means of absorbable Dexon sutures medially and nylon sutures laterally (Fig. 127-13). Temporalis muscle and abdominal fat are used to fill the bony defects (Fig. 127-14).

Following completion of repair and before wound closure, the head is elevated 45 degrees; this is continued in the recovery room and throughout the

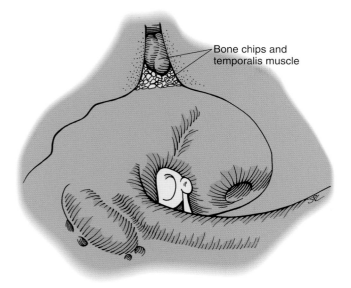

Figure 127-12. Obliteration of the eustachian tube with bone chips and temporalis muscle.

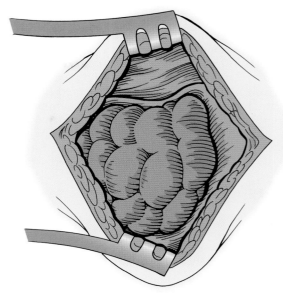

Figure 127-14. Obliteration of the mastoid with a fat graft taken from the abdominal wall.

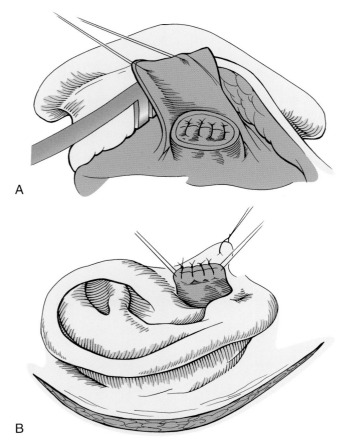

Figure 127-13. A, Sealing of the external meatus by sewing a fibro-fascial flap to its medial surface. **B,** Completion of the meatal closure with everting sutures placed.

hospitalization. Because of the potential for intracranial infection, a bolus of intravenous antibiotic is always given perioperatively. We use third-generation cephalosporins with broad-spectrum coverage. When purulent exudate is encountered at the time of surgery, cultures help determine the choice of antibiotic.

POSTOPERATIVE MANAGEMENT

Postoperatively, the head is elevated 45 degrees during the hospital stay and patients are encouraged to continue this for 7 to 10 days at home. Patients who have undergone craniotomy for repair of CSF leaks should be observed in the hospital for at least 3 to 4 days. Those who have undergone transmastoid surgery may generally be discharged home in 1 to 2 days. Antibiotic coverage is also continued intravenously until the patient is discharged, and then a similar agent is given orally for 7 days. When lumbar drainage has been placed preoperatively, it is continued for 24 to 72 hours postoperatively, depending on the extent of CSF leakage and size of defect repaired. The subarachnoid drain is then clamped for an additional 24 hours to confirm the absence of any further CSF leak, and then removed.

Persistent CSF leak is the most common complication following surgery. Because of the blood within the middle ear postoperatively, visualization of the tympanic membrane is not a good guide to successful cessation of CSF leakage in the immediate postoperative period. However, within 3 to 4 weeks, the middle ear should be pneumatized and clearly visualized. The patient is also questioned repeatedly and asked to report any incidence of nasal or posterior pharyngeal drainage, which might indicate continued CSF otorrhea. Restraints against lifting, straining, and exercise are encouraged for 2 weeks following surgery.

Although temporary aphasia and seizures are potential postoperative complications from temporal lobe resection or retraction, our patients have had no problems related to the excision of nonviable brain tissue. Neurologic deficits are not expected postoperatively, and headache has not been a significant problem. Meningitis and brain abscess are potential complications, but these have usually been seen preoperatively rather than postoperatively.

PEARLS

- The vast majority of traumatic CSF leaks resolve with conservative management alone.
- Dural exposure alone without violation at the time of otologic surgery does not lead to CSF leak.
- Due to a significant incidence of multiple tegmen defects in spontaneous CSF leaks, the middle fossa approach allows for thorough inspection of the middle fossa floor before surgical repair.
- The best results are obtained with multilayer closure techniques using autologous tissue.
- In a nonhearing ear, obliteration of the middle ear and mastoid with blind sac closure of the external auditory canal offers the most effective and reliable repair for CSF leaks and large encephaloceles.

PITFALLS

- Failure to recognize multiple defects on preoperative CT imaging may lead to incomplete repair and persistent postoperative CSF leak.
- Failure to circumferentially elevate dura around the bony defect will not allow for reliable graft placement and repair.

- Primary dural closure alone is usually not adequate for repair of CSF leaks.
- The use of fixatives, such as fibrin glue, does not improve surgical success rates.
- With large tegmen defects, the weight of the temporal lobe alone, without the use of a supporting bone or cartilage graft, is not adequate for supporting a soft tissue graft over the defect.

References

1. Gacek RR: Arachnoid granulation cerebrospinal fluid otorrhea. Ann Otol Rhinol Laryngol 99:854-862, 1990.
2. Savva A, Taylor MJ, Beatty CW: Management of cerebrospinal fluid leaks involving the temporal bone: Report on 92 patients. Laryngoscope 113:50-56, 2003.
3. Lundy LB, Graham MD, Kartush JM, et al: Temporal bone encephalocele and cerebrospinal fluid leaks. Am J Otol 17:461-469, 1996.
4. Skedros DG, Cass SP, Hirsch BE, et al: Beta-2 transferrin assay in clinical management of cerebral spinal fluid and perilymphatic fluid leaks. J Otolaryngol 22:341-344, 1993.
5. Stone JA, Castillo M, Neelon B, et al: Evaluation of CSF leaks: High-resolution CT compared with contrast-enhanced CT and radionuclide cisternography. AJNR Am J Neuroradiol 20:706-712, 1999.
6. McMurphy AB, Oghalai JS: Repair of iatrogenic temporal lobe encephalocele after canal wall down mastoidectomy in the presence of active cholesteatoma. Otol Neurotol 26:587-594, 2005.
7. Caroli E, Rocchi G, Salvati M, et al: Duraplasty: Our current experience. Surg Neurol 61:55-59; discussion 59, 2004.
8. Filippi R, Schwarz M, Voth D, et al: Bovine pericardium for duraplasty: Clinical results in 32 patients. Neurosurg Rev 24(2-3):103-107, 2001.
9. Kveton JF, Goravalingappa R: Elimination of temporal bone cerebrospinal fluid otorrhea using hydroxyapatite cement. Laryngoscope 110(10 Pt 1):1655-1659, 2000.
10. Jackson CG, Pappas DG Jr, Manolidis S, et al: Brain herniation into the middle ear and mastoid: Concepts in diagnosis and surgical management. Am J Otol 18(2):198-205; discussion 205-196, 1997.

Chapter **128**

Temporal Bone Trauma

Elizabeth H. Toh

Injuries resulting from trauma to the temporal bone range from temporary and minor disorders to severe and permanent ones. Identifiable fractures are usually associated with more severe neurologic deficits, but even in the absence of a fracture, the auditory and vestibular systems may have sustained concussive damage resulting in clinically significant functional sequelae. Dysfunction of the facial nerve occasionally occurs even in the absence of radiographically demonstrable fracture. Blows to the side of the head or penetrating trauma from foreign bodies introduced through the external auditory canal may result in trauma to the tympanic membrane, ossicular chain, inner ear, and, rarely, the facial nerve. Injuries to the middle ear generally can be dealt with using the same techniques outlined in Chapter 114. The scope of this chapter is restricted to management of the sequelae of temporal bone fractures.

PATIENT SELECTION

Fractures of the temporal bone have traditionally been classified anatomically into longitudinal, transverse, and mixed, based on their relationship relative to the long axis of the petrous pyramid (Figs. 128-1 and 128-2). This traditional scheme of classification has been shown to be of limited value in reliably predicting clinical complications resulting from injury to the temporal bone. With the advent of high-resolution computed tomography (HRCT) imaging, several authors have proposed the use of "otic capsule sparing" and "otic capsule violating" terminology to better define and prognosticate the clinical impact of these injuries.[1,2] The most serious injuries, and those most often requiring surgery, are the result of transverse or otic capsule–violating fractures. Table 128-1 lists the most common sequelae of temporal bone fractures. Facial nerve palsy

and the rare persistent cerebrospinal fluid (CSF) leak are the primary clinical conditions that require the determination of suitability for surgical intervention in the early postinjury setting. Hearing loss and dizziness do not generally require early intervention; in many cases, these conditions resolve spontaneously. Less common symptoms, such as facial hypesthesia and paresis of the abducens nerve, are also frequently self-limited. Any associated lacerations of the external auditory canal and violation of the tympanic membrane may initially be managed conservatively with dry ear precautions and ototopical antibiotics. Elective surgical repair of persistent perforations of the tympanic membrane may be offered for a safe dry ear or hearing improvement following a 6- to 8-week trial of conservative management. The risk of delayed meningitis and secondary cholesteatoma formation should be kept in mind in patients with temporal bone fractures.

Facial Paralysis

Weakness of the facial nerve may be immediate or delayed in onset, partial or complete. Although there is universal agreement that delayed-onset facial paralysis usually portends favorable clinical recovery and should be managed conservatively, much controversy surrounds the role and timing of surgery in the patient with immediate-onset weakness.[3-5] Most traumatic facial palsies resolve without surgical intervention and the decision to operate is usually based on predictors of poor functional outcome. We agree with the otologic consensus that surgical exploration is of benefit in patients with immediate-onset complete facial paralysis because of the greater likelihood that the nerve has been anatomically disrupted or is compressed by a bone spicule. Surgery in these patients appears to facilitate early recovery with minimal faulty regeneration.

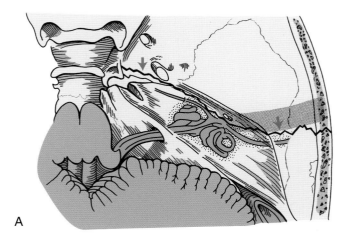

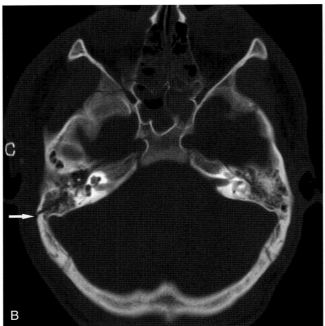

Figure 128-1. A, Longitudinal temporal bone fracture *(arrows)* sparing the otic capsule and internal auditory canal. **B,** Computed tomography scan showing a longitudinal fracture *(arrow)*.

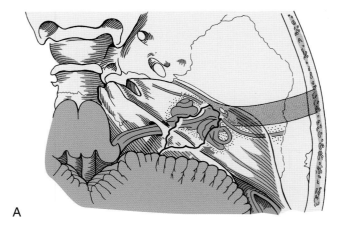

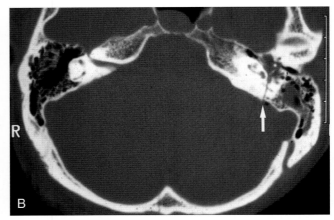

Figure 128-2. A, Transverse temporal bone fracture *(arrows)* with involvement of the otic capsule and the contents of the internal auditory canal. **B,** Computed tomography scan showing transverse fracture *(arrow)*.

Table 128-1	SYMPTOMS AND SIGNS FOLLOWING TEMPORAL BONE FRACTURE
Symptom/Sign	**Treatment**
Hearing loss	No immediate treatment necessary.
Dizziness	Vestibular suppression followed by rehabilitation.
Facial weakness	Early determination of status is necessary. Surgical exploration for immediate onset paralysis with poor prognostic indicators.
Cerebrospinal fluid otorrhea	Usually resolves spontaneously; not a surgical consideration for at least 7 days.

The following criteria form the basis for surgical selection with respect to facial paralysis in temporal bone trauma:

1. Immediate onset paralysis with progressive decline of electrical responses on electroneuronography (ENoG) to less than 10% of responses on the normal side within the first 14 days.
2. Immediate-onset paralysis with significant disruption of the fallopian canal demonstrated on HRCT.

The decision to intervene surgically is more challenging in patients with incomplete immediate-onset facial paralysis. Conservative management is the general rule when partial function remains. Aggressive eye care is critical while awaiting functional recovery in all patients. In the absence of any medical contraindications, the administration of a tapering course of systemic steroids (prednisone 1 mg/kg body weight or equivalent, tapered over 1 week) is generally thought to be helpful in reducing any traumatic neural edema and promoting early recovery. Care must be taken to rule out extratemporal nerve injuries in patients in whom only one or several branches are involved.

Cerebrospinal Fluid Leak

CSF leak associated with temporal bone fractures may manifest as otorrhea, rhinorrhea, or otorhinorrhea. A high percentage of CSF leaks associated with skull base fractures resolve with conservative management within a week. Strict bed rest, head elevation, and the administration of stool softeners usually suffice to control these leaks. Lumbar drainage is used with an indwelling catheter for approximately 3 to 4 days when spontaneous resolution does not occur within the first 3 days of bed rest and head elevation. When drainage persists despite these measures or when HRCT identifies obvious severe bone disruption, surgery is indicated. The overall incidence of meningitis following temporal bone trauma with an associated CSF leak is less than 10%.[3] The use of prophylactic antibiotics is recommended in select patients with increased risk of meningitis, including those with persistent CSF leaks beyond 7 days, those with concomitant infections elsewhere, and those who have a lumbar drain in place. Indiscriminate use of systemic antibiotics may mask the early signs and symptoms of meningitis. White blood cell counts help in early detection of meningitis, and diagnostic lumbar puncture should be performed when any clinical suspicion of infection arises.

PREOPERATIVE EVALUATION

Dedicated HRCT of the temporal bones at 1- to 1.5-mm thickness intervals using bone algorithm is the best imaging modality for evaluating temporal bone injury. Axial and true or high-resolution reconstructed coronal images should be requested. A routine CT scan of the head obtained for the purpose of ruling out intracranial trauma is inadequate for evaluating the intratemporal facial nerve and ossicular chain. When evaluating the fallopian canal, one should look for multiple fracture sites because this is more common than is usually recognized.[6] The status of the otic capsule and the ossicular chain can be ascertained as well. Longitudinal or otic capsule sparing fractures will most often compromise the facial nerve at or distal to the geniculate ganglion. Conversely, transverse or otic capsule involving fractures usually injure the facial nerve medial to the geniculate ganglion (Fig. 128-3). The degree of pneumatization of the mastoid and level of the middle fossa dural plate are of interest if surgical intervention is contemplated. The significance of these factors is discussed later in the chapter. Magnetic resonance imaging plays a complementary role in the evaluation of associated intracranial trauma.

Topographic testing of facial nerve function, including the Schirmer test, has been found to be unreliable in localizing the site of lesion and has limited clinical utility in this setting. Audiometric testing is a necessary component of a full clinical evaluation and should be obtained at the earliest feasible time. It is helpful not only to determine the type of hearing loss but in the case of sensorineural impairment, to decide whether residual function is useful. Hearing results do not

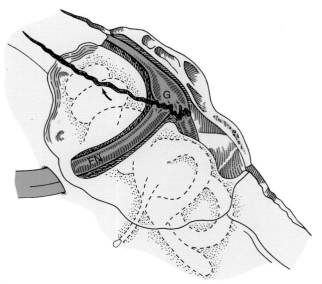

Figure 128-3. Superior view of a transverse fracture line *(arrow)* involving the facial nerve (FN) medial to the geniculate ganglion (G).

dictate the necessity for surgery in the early posttrauma period, but they do influence the selection of surgical approach, when it becomes necessary. Conductive hearing loss will often resolve spontaneously; hearing losses that remain can be surgically corrected later. Sensorineural hearing impairment is usually permanent, although it sometimes improves slightly over time. Vestibular testing plays no role in the early evaluation of fractures of the temporal bone. The vast majority of vestibular symptoms are expected to resolve and may, in any case, be delineated later.

When the decision has been made to surgically explore the facial nerve, empiricism dictates that undue delay is counterproductive. Once the patient is neurologically stable and the site of lesion identified on HRCT, surgery should proceed. The organization of blood clot and the development of scar and fibrous tissue can only affect results negatively. This active approach to these injuries is obviously not always possible because some patients are seen for the first time after many weeks or months have elapsed. These patients will nevertheless benefit from exploration, as long as they meet the criteria elaborated earlier.[7] When persistent CSF leak is the only indication for surgical intervention, closure should proceed after 7 to 10 days of conservative management because the risk of meningitis increases significantly thereafter.[3]

SURGICAL TECHNIQUES

Selection of surgical approach is dependent on both site of injury and hearing status in the involved ear. Injuries of the facial nerve at or distal to the geniculate ganglion can be approached via a standard transmastoid exposure. Injuries medial to the geniculate ganglion may be approached in several ways, depending on residual hearing in the affected ear and the degree of

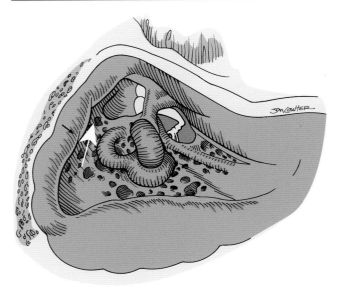

Figure 128-4. Transmastoid exposure of temporal bone that is suitable for transepitympanic exploration (*large arrow*) of the facial nerve because of a high middle fossa tegmen. (*Arrow,* level of middle fossa dura.)

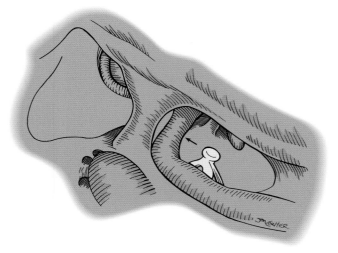

Figure 128-5. Exposure and decompression of the horizontal portion of the facial nerve (*arrow*). (Incus removed.)

pneumatization of the temporal bone. Severe sensorineural hearing loss allows for translabyrinthine exposure of the facial nerve. Conversely, when hearing conservation is indicated, the middle cranial fossa approach may be elected. In the case of a well pneumatized epitympanum in which the middle fossa dural plate is relatively high, the labyrinthine portion of the facial nerve may be exposed via a transmastoid transepitympanic approach (Fig. 128-4). This approach, however, does not provide adequate exposure for the meatal segment of the facial nerve.

Although repair of a disrupted tympanic membrane and defects of the ossicles may be accomplished simultaneously, it is often necessary to delay these reconstructive efforts due to edema of the mucosa, bleeding, and the friability of traumatized tissue within the middle ear. In cases of severe bony tegmen disruption with herniation of brain tissue, associated repair of the encephalocele is indicated.

Transmastoid Approach for Facial Nerve Injuries at or Distal to the Geniculate Ganglion

A complete mastoidectomy (see Chapter 115) is performed to access the mastoid antrum and locate the lateral semicircular canal. Bony dissection is then continued anterosuperiorly toward the epitympanum until the body of the incus is identified. The parasagittal plane of the incus is extrapolated posteriorly to identify the level of the facial recess, which is then opened and saucerized to delineate the vertical facial nerve within the mastoid. The mastoid segment of the nerve may also be identified at its point of exit from the stylomastoid foramen by following the digastric ridge anteriorly in the mastoid tip. Skeletonization of the fallopian canal should be performed with care using 2- to 3-mm

diamond burrs and copious irrigation. In most cases, the fracture line is often observed on the surface of the mastoid cortex and can be followed medially to the site of injury. Working alternately between the facial recess and the epitympanum, the surgeon can remove thin bone from the tympanic portion of the fallopian canal if bony decompression of this segment is indicated (Fig. 128-5). If necessary, the incus can be removed in order to improve exposure of the tympanic facial nerve. In this case, the incudostapedial joint is separated through the facial recess using a small sharp hook and the incus retrieved through the epitympanum, taking care not to sublux the stapes. Preserving a small bony bridge in the fossa incudis for support of the short process of the incus allows for easy replacement of the incus with little or no hearing deficit.

Injuries to the facial nerve produced by stretching or compression are managed with decompression of the fallopian canal proximal and distal to the injury until normal nerve is identified. The need for additional incision of the epineural sheath is controversial. Any bone chips impinging on the nerve should be removed. The integrity of the axonal bundles within the nerve sheath must also be determined. Transection of nerve fibers by trauma may be total or partial. It is generally considered advantageous to preserve the facial nerve when 50% or more of the diameter of the nerve appears intact. Complete transection may be repaired with primary end-to-end apposition. If tension-free reapproximation or reanastomosis cannot be accomplished or maintained, facial nerve rerouting for primary reanastomosis or interposition grafting should be considered. Eliminating the second genu of the facial nerve, for example, is an effective technique for shortening the distance of proximal and distal nerve segments lateral to the geniculate (Fig. 128-6A). Anastomosis might also proceed directly from the internal auditory canal (IAC) to the vertical segment of the facial nerve by dividing the greater superficial petrosal

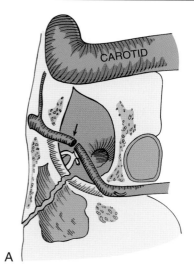

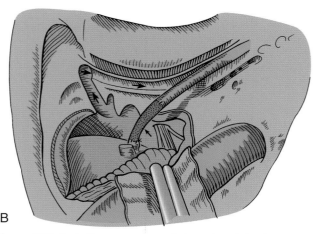

Figure 128-6. **A,** Reconstructive technique for gaining length and avoiding an interposition graft by eliminating the second genu of the facial nerve. (*Arrow,* transpositioned facial nerve.) **B,** Anastomotic technique using an interposition graft and "short-circuiting." (*Large arrows,* normal course of the facial nerve; *small arrow,* shortened course of the facial nerve.)

nerve at the geniculate ganglion, rerouting the intact distal segment, and interposing a cable graft (see Fig. 128-6B). For interposition nerve grafting (Fig. 128-7), the great auricular nerve is the preferred donor site because of the nerve's proximity and size compatibility. Epineurium must be carefully trimmed back and nerve fascicles sharply sectioned for optimal end-to-end contact. For both primary repair and interposition grafting of the labyrinthine, tympanic, and mastoid segments, the fallopian canal provides an excellent bed for anastomosis and usually the nerve does not require any suturing. With repair of the nerve within or medial to the IAC, one or two 8-0 monofilament sutures may be placed in the epineurium. Standard layered mastoidectomy wound closure and ear dressings are used.

Transmastoid Translabyrinthine Approach for Facial Nerve Injuries Medial to the Geniculate Ganglion without Useful Hearing

The procedure described in the preceding section is carried out and followed by a complete labyrinthectomy and skeletonization of the IAC from the porus acusticus to the fundus (see Chapter 124). When drilling through the semicircular canals, care should be exercised when following the posterior semicircular canal anteriorly under the second genu of the facial nerve to its ampulla. The superior limit of the lateral IAC is defined by the location of the superior vestibular nerve, which lies immediately anterior to the ampulla of the superior semicircular canal. The IAC is skeletonized laterally to permit identification of Bill's bar (vertical crest), which separates the facial nerve anteriorly from the superior vestibular nerve posteriorly. Skeletonization of the facial nerve is then continued anteriorly to the geniculate ganglion using a small diamond burr. The entire intratemporal course of the facial nerve can then be exposed (Fig. 128-8). If facial nerve rerouting is necessary to achieve tension-free repair, the greater superficial petrosal nerve is divided at the geniculate ganglion and the facial nerve gently elevated out of the fallopian canal. Grafting techniques are similar to those described earlier, except the repair of a transected nerve is considerably more difficult in the IAC because of gravity and the presence of CSF pulsations. Collagen or Silastic sleeves can add support to the anastomosis following suturing and add greater strength to the graft sites. Closure is similar to that described for translabyrinthine removal of acoustic neuromas and requires the obliteration of the eustachian tube and middle ear with temporalis muscle, packing of the mastoid cavity with abdominal fat, and layered wound closure. A pressure dressing should be maintained over the operated ear for 3 to 4 days to minimize the risk of postoperative CSF leakage.

Transmastoid Transepitympanic Approach for Facial Nerve Injuries Medial to the Geniculate Ganglion with Useful Hearing

Following a complete mastoidectomy, the incus is removed as described earlier under Transmastoid Approach for Facial Nerve Injuries at or Distal to the Geniculate Ganglion. The geniculate ganglion is identified and followed posteromedially, staying anterior to the ampullated end of the superior semicircular canal (Fig. 128-9). The superior semicircular canal is skeletonized, allowing for exposure of the labyrinthine portion of the facial nerve. This portion of the nerve can then be decompressed; in fact, CSF is routinely encountered. Preoperative review of the HRCT scans must ensure that injury is lateral to the meatal portion of the nerve in order to achieve adequate exposure using this approach. When adequate exposure is in doubt, or if grafting of the meatal or proximal facial nerve is anticipated, the middle fossa approach should be used.

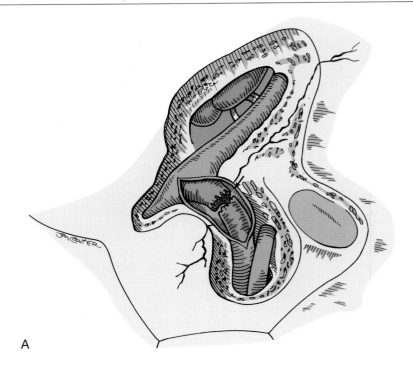

A

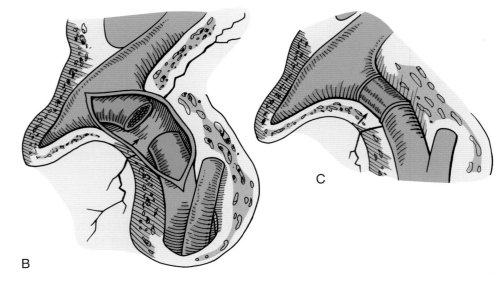

B   C

Figure 128-7. Use of an interposition graft for repair of a facial nerve defect in the internal auditory canal by the middle fossa approach. (*Arrows,* site of nerve transection, freshening, and repair.)

Middle Cranial Fossa Approach for Facial Nerve Injuries Medial to the Geniculate Ganglion with Intact Hearing

The superior surface of the temporal bone is exposed extradurally as described in Chapter 124. The extent of surgical exposure for decompression or repair of the facial nerve in this context is identification of the greater superficial petrosal nerve at its take off from the geniculate ganglion anteriorly. The nerve can then be followed proximally into the labyrinthine and IAC segments, recognizing the proximity of the labyrinthine facial nerve to the basal cochlear turn. Bone of the tegmen tympani may be removed to expose the tym-

panic segment of the nerve, taking care to avoid drilling directly on the head of the malleus and body of the incus. The middle fossa approach may be combined with a transmastoid exploration of the more distal nerve segment when indicated (Fig. 128-10). In that case, the transmastoid procedure should be completed first in order to fenestrate the middle fossa tegmen superior to the geniculate ganglion, thereby simplifying identification of the facial nerve and internal auditory canal through the middle fossa craniotomy. This combined exposure allows for surgical access to the entire intratemporal facial nerve from the cisternal segment to the stylomastoid foramen, while preserving hearing in the operated ear. Closure of the middle fossa craniotomy is

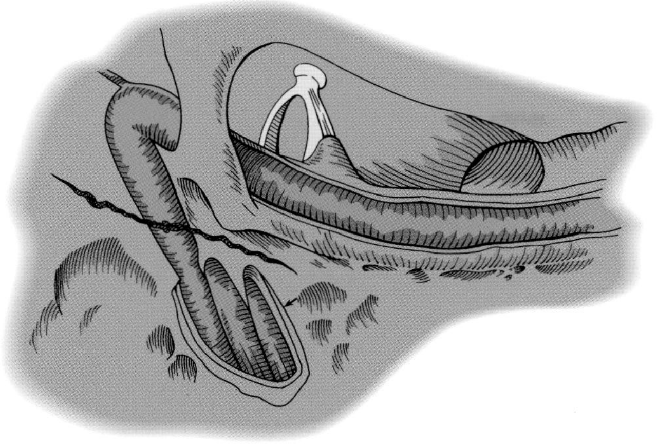

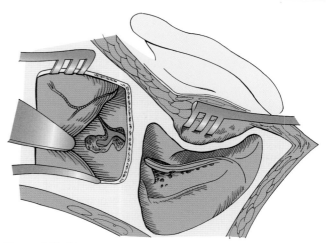

Figure 128-8. Transmastoid translabyrinthine exposure of the entire facial nerve. (*Arrow,* internal auditory canal.)

Figure 128-10. Combined middle fossa transmastoid approach to the facial nerve for hearing preservation.

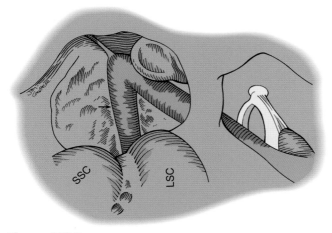

Figure 128-9. Transmastoid transepitympanic exposure of the labyrinthine portion of the facial nerve *(arrow)*. SCC, superior semicircular canal; LSC, lateral semicircular canal.

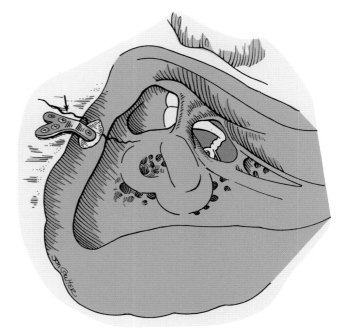

Figure 128-11. Bone grafting for repair of a middle fossa defect using a microplate *(arrow)*.

identical to that described for removal of tumor via the middle fossa (see Chapter 124). The mastoidectomy wound is closed in a standard layered fashion.

Repair of Cerebrospinal Fluid Leaks

Surgical techniques for the sole purpose of repairing CSF leaks resulting from temporal bone trauma are influenced by (1) site of leak, (2) hearing status of the affected ear, and (3) presence of brain herniation through the tegmen. For fractures through the tegmen mastoideum with persistent CSF leak, "sandwich" grafts consisting of fascia or freeze-dried dura are placed intracranially and extracranially using a combined transmastoid mini-middle fossa approach (see Chapter 127), and bone paté is placed along the fracture line. Large dehiscences of bone may require bony autografts, fashioned bone plugs, or microplating for temporal lobe support (Fig. 128-11).

When there is significant herniation of the temporal lobe through the fracture site, the devitalized brain tissue is débrided through a transmastoid exposure,

and the viable brain and dura elevated back through am extradural mini-middle fossa approach. The resultant dural defect may be repaired using temporalis fascia or freeze-dried dura. The bony defect is reinforced using autologous bone harvested from the craniotomy flap to prevent further prolapse of brain tissue into the mastoid or middle ear cavities.

In patients with anacusis following trauma, obliteration of the middle ear and mastoid with blind sac closure of the external auditory meatus may be performed using a standard two-layered technique. A complete mastoidectomy is performed. The skin of the external auditory canal, tympanic membrane, malleus, and incus are removed, leaving the stapes intact. The eustachian tube is obliterated with muscle, and the middle ear and mastoid cavities are packed with abdominal fat.

POSTOPERATIVE MANAGEMENT

Postoperative management in these patients is similar to that of chronic middle ear and mastoid surgery. With the exception of translabyrinthine craniotomies, mastoid dressings for all other cases are removed in 24 hours to check for hematoma, cutaneous CSF leaks, or wound infection. The dressing is reapplied as necessary. If the dura has been opened, perioperative antibiotic coverage is used for 48 hours and consists of either broad-spectrum cephalosporins or vancomycin in penicillin-allergic patients. In addition to achieving a watertight wound closure, elevation of the head by 30 degrees and use of stool softeners helps minimize postoperative CSF leakage. Steroids are given in moderate doses and tapered over 5 to 7 days unless medically contraindicated. The use of steroids in these cases, as in acoustic tumor surgery, has significantly decreased postoperative complaints of headache and neck pain. This is probably due to suppression of inflammation from the breakdown of red blood cells in the CSF. Supportive eye care is continued and varies greatly depending on age, skin laxity, and anticipated time for return of facial function. Young patients with good corneal coverage may require nothing but lubricants and moisture chambers. Others may require lateral tarsorrhaphy, gold weights, or even oculoplastic procedures if severe ectropion develops.

Early ambulation is encouraged for all the usual reasons, in addition to the benefits obtained in early vestibular compensation. Early enrollment in a formal vestibular rehabilitative and physical therapy program is helpful in older and multiply injured individuals. The early convalescent period is an appropriate time for more in-depth investigation of auditory and vestibular function in those who manifest persistent symptoms.

When the nerve has been determined to be intact or following adequate grafting, some return of function is to be expected. The repaired or grafted nerve will generally recover limited function with variable synkinesis. This is usually demonstrable within 6 months for lesions distal to the geniculate ganglion but may take up to 1 year for more proximal lesions. Failure of expected return of function within 1 year should motivate the surgeon to review the initial CT scan and perhaps even to repeat the study. Facial paralysis may persist in "old" temporal bone injuries long after spontaneous resolution should have occurred. Scarring and degeneration of the proximal nerve segment in these cases usually precludes successful primary repair. Anastomosis of the facial and hypoglossal nerves or nerve muscle pedicle reconstruction is advised in this instance.

Pseudoaneurysms of the internal carotid artery are very rarely seen following head trauma. These consist of disruption of the intima of the artery with consequent dissection of blood between the vessel wall and

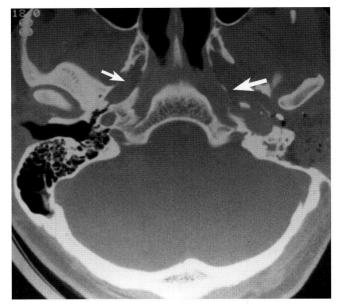

Figure 128-12. High-resolution computed tomography scan showing a posttraumatic pseudoaneurysm *(large arrow)* of the internal carotid artery. (*Small arrow,* normal carotid.)

the adventitial layer (Fig. 128-12). Stabilization may be spontaneous, but continued dissection of the aneurysm may require treatment. Following balloon occlusion and xenon flow studies to determine contralateral flow, balloons can be angiographically inserted proximal and distal to the site by an interventional radiologist. Failure of the contralateral flow testing would necessitate bypass grafting of the carotid artery.

PEARLS

- The primary indications for surgical intervention in temporal bone fractures are immediate complete facial paralysis with poor prognostic indicators, and persistent CSF leaks.
- Newer spiral CT scanners offer the ability to reconstruct high-resolution coronal images of the temporal bone, thus obviating the need for extreme neck extension needed to obtain true coronal images in these patients.
- Surgical approach is determined by hearing status in the affected ear and site of injury.
- When ENoG demonstrates less than 10% activity on the affected side, the adjunctive use of facial muscle electromyography to confirm the absence of electrical activity or appearance of fibrillation potentials is helpful in identifying surgical candidates for facial nerve decompression.[8]
- Facial nerve injuries distal to the geniculate ganglion are best accessed using the transmastoid approach, whereas facial nerve injuries medial to the geniculate ganglion may typically be accessed using the middle fossa approach in the hearing ear and using the translabyrinthine approach in the nonhearing ear.

PITFALLS

- Nerve repair under tension compromises microvascular circulation at the site of repair, resulting in scar formation, impaired axonal penetration, and uniformly poor functional outcome.
- Failure to recognize the presence of multiple sites of injury along the facial nerve will result in persistent facial paralysis following surgical decompression.
- Additional sensorineural hearing loss may result from drilling on the ossicular chain or violating the ampullated ends of the lateral and posterior semicircular canals when exposing the perigeniculate facial nerve through transmastoid approaches.
- Undue delay in surgical repair of persistent CSF leaks beyond 7 days may increase the risk of meningitis.
- When the external auditory canal is severely traumatized, cicatricial canal stenosis may develop with cholesteatoma formation medial to the stenotic segment.

References

1. Ishman SL, Friedland DL: Temporal bone fractures: Traditional classification and clinical relevance. Laryngoscope 114:1173-1741, 2004.
2. Dahiya R, Keller JD, Litofsky SN, et al: Temporal bone fractures: Otic capsule sparing versus otic capsule violating clinical and radiographic considerations. J Trauma 47:1079-1083, 1999.
3. Brodie HA, Thompson TC: Management of complications from 820 temporal bone fractures. Am J Otol 18:188-197, 1997.
4. Nosan DK, Benecke JE, Murr AH: Current perspective on temporal bone trauma. Otolaryngol Head Neck Surg 117:67-71, 1997.
5. McKennan KY, Chole RA: Facial paralysis in temporal bone trauma. Am J Otol 13:167-172, 1992.
6. Lambert PR, Brackmann DE: Facial paralysis in longitudinal temporal bone fractures: A review of 26 cases. Laryngoscope 94:1022-1026, 1984.
7. Quaranta A, Campobasso G, Piazza F, et al: Facial nerve paralysis in temporal bone fractures: Outcomes after late decompression surgery. Acta Otolaryngol 121:652-655, 2001.
8. Darrouzet V, Duclos JY, Liguoro D, et al: Management of facial paralysis resulting from temporal bone fractures: Our experience in 115 cases. Otolaryngol head Neck Surg 125:77-84, 2001.

Chapter **129**

Cochlear Implantation

Yu-Lan Mary Ying and Elizabeth H. Toh

Cochlear implants are implantable electronic prostheses designed to convert mechanical sound energy into electrical signals that directly stimulate the auditory nerve in severely to profoundly deaf individuals. They have become the standard of care for rehabilitating deafened individuals who no longer benefit from the use of conventional hearing aids. The Food and Drug Administration (FDA) approved the use of cochlear implant devices in the United States for adults in 1985 and for children in 1990. Since then, more than 80,000 devices have been implanted in this country.

The functional anatomy of the inner ear as it applies to cochlear implantation is briefly reviewed here. The cochlea consists of a central bony skeleton, the modiolus, and the surrounding bony otic capsule. Within the modiolus lies the auditory nerve with bipolar primary afferent neurons, their cell bodies (spiral ganglia), and efferent nerve fibers. The presence of at least 10,000 surviving cochlear neurons is vital for successful hearing outcomes using a cochlear implant device. The spiral ganglion neurons follow the spiral arrangement of the cochlear duct with maximal ganglion cell density located between the upper basal turn and lower middle turn of the cochlear duct. This has clinical significance in cochlear implantation for placing the electrode array close to the greatest density of cochlear neurons.

All cochlear implant systems have an externally worn device and an implanted internal component. The external hardware consists of an ear-level microphone, an ear-level or body-worn speech processor, and a transmitter placed behind the ear. The internal component consists of a receiver/stimulator, linked to an intracochlear electrode array via a lead wire. Sound received by the microphone is transduced into electrical signals, which are filtered, analyzed, and digitized by the speech processor, and forwarded to the transmit-

ting coil. The encoded signals are then delivered to the implanted receiver/stimulator by radio-frequency electromagnetic induction. This signal is reconverted to an electrical signal, which is then delivered to the implanted electrode within the scala tympani. Current applied to the electrodes radiates into the fluid of the scala tympani, spreads through the habenula perforata of the osseous cochlear modiolus, and stimulates the auditory nerve.

Three implant systems (Nucleus Freedom system, Harmony HiResolution Bionic Ear system, and Med-El Sonata$_{TI}^{100}$ and PulsarCI^{100} systems) are currently FDA approved for use in adults and children in the United States. All are multichannel systems with 16 to 24 electrodes designed to take advantage of the tonotopic organization of the cochlea. Incoming speech signals are filtered into a number of frequency bands, each corresponding to a given electrode in the array. The Nucleus Freedom and HiResolution Bionic Ear systems use precurved modiolar-hugging electrode arrays. The relative proximity of these precurved electrode arrays to spiral ganglion cells offers theoretical advantages of improved sound quality, speech recognition, and power efficiency. By contrast, the longer tapered straight electrode of the Med-El PulsarCI^{100} and Sonata$_{TI}^{100}$ systems are designed for deep intracochlear insertion and electrical stimulation of the full sound frequency range. Overall hearing outcomes as reflected by standard audiologic test scores have been comparable using devices from all three manufacturers. The selection of device to be implanted is, in most practices, left to the patient.

PATIENT SELECTION

Candidacy criteria for cochlear implantation in adults and children continue to evolve with advances in

Table 129-1	CANDIDACY CRITERIA FOR COCHLEAR IMPLANTATION IN ADULTS OLDER THAN 18 YEARS

- Bilateral severe to profound hearing loss: a three-frequency pure-tone average (500, 1000, 2000 Hz) unaided threshold in the better ear of greater than 70 dB
- Less than 20% word recognition score with consonant nucleus consonant (CNC) words bilaterally
- Minimal benefit from conventional hearing aids, as defined by hearing in noise sentence testing (HINT) recognition scores of less than 50% correct in the best aided condition
- No medical contraindications

Table 129-2	CANDIDACY CRITERIA FOR COCHLEAR IMPLANTATION IN CHILDREN

Children age 12 to 24 months:

- Bilateral profound hearing loss
- Lack of auditory skills development and minimal hearing aid benefit
- No medical contraindications
- Enrollment in an education program emphasizing auditory development

Children age 25 months to 18 years:

- Bilateral severe to profound hearing loss
- Lack of auditory skills development and minimal hearing aid benefit (open set word recognition scores of less than 30% correct)
- No medical contraindications
- Enrollment in an education program emphasizing auditory development

electrode design, surgical techniques for atraumatic electrode insertion, and speech processing strategies. Current devices use either precurved perimodiolar electrode arrays or slim-profile tapered arrays to minimize trauma to surviving neural elements within the cochlea. With the possibility of preserving residual hearing in the implanted ear, candidacy criteria have expanded to include individuals with more residual hearing.

Adults

Current candidacy criteria for cochlear implantation in adults are listed in Table 129-1. It is well established that individuals who lose hearing after acquiring speech and language skills (postlingually deafened) and those with a shorter duration of deafness before implantation perform better with cochlear implants. In fact, duration of deafness has been found to be the only reliable predictor of auditory performance.[1] Other variables, including age at implantation, age at onset of hearing loss, age of deafness, hearing aid use, side implanted, and preoperative audiologic test scores, have not consistently correlated with postimplantation performance. Prelingually deafened adults who have been habilitated using aural and oral education may receive some benefit from a cochlear implant.[2] There is no upper age limit for implantation in adults with good health.

Children

The selection procedure for children is more complex than for adults. In contrast to adults, both prelingually and postlingually deafened children are candidates for cochlear implantation. Research has shown that early auditory experience is critical for the development of central and peripheral auditory neural pathways. There exists an early period of language development in humans between ages 2 and 5, during which auditory input is paramount. Therefore, early hearing habilitation using a cochlear implant in children with congenital deafness and early profound acquired hearing loss is critical. Early implantation significantly improves the chance for development of normal speech and language in children.

Since the legislation of universal newborn hearing screening across the United States, many more infants with congenital hearing loss are being identified within the first few months of life. Current FDA guidelines permit implantation of children as young as 12 months of age. Exceptions to this lower age limit may be made in children with deafness resulting from meningitis. Earlier implantation in these children may allow for successful electrode insertion before the development of intracochlear ossification. Criteria for the pediatric age group are listed in Table 129-2. Appropriate family motivation, expectations, and support are also important factors in determining suitability of the child for implantation.

PREOPERATIVE EVALUATION

A complete history and physical examination are necessary to detect problems that may contraindicate surgery, or interfere with the patient's ability to complete postimplantation rehabilitation. Etiology of hearing loss is rarely a contraindication to implantation. Profound hearing loss associated with cochlear nerve aplasia is a rare congenital anomaly, in which the lack of auditory innervation obviates the option for cochlear implantation. Prior meningitis with cochlear ossification or fibrosis does not exclude a patient from implantation, but may necessitate modification of the surgical technique itself. The ear selected for implantation must be free of infection and ideally have an intact tympanic membrane.

An audiologic evaluation that characterizes hearing loss in both unaided conditions and in best binaurally aided conditions is performed. This includes measurement of pure tone thresholds, word, and sentence recognition testing. Aided speech recognition scores are the primary audiologic determinants of cochlear implant candidacy. Audiologic screening in children requires auditory brain stem evoked response testing, and otoacoustic emissions testing, in addition to conventional behavioral audiometry. A 6-month trial period using appropriate amplification, and intensive auditory and speech training is an integral component of candidacy assessment in children. The global evaluation of cochlear implant candidacy in children is considerably more challenging than in adults and is best approached by a dedicated team comprising speech and hearing professionals. The ultimate candidacy of a child is determined not only by a demonstrated physiologic need but also by the strength of the child's social and educational background.

Preoperative imaging necessarily includes a high-resolution, thin-cut computed tomography (CT) scan of the temporal bone in both the axial and coronal planes. This is used to determine the presence and patency of the cochlea, identify any congenital inner ear malformations, assess the caliber of the internal auditory canal, and assess the anatomy of the mastoid, middle ear, and facial nerve. Congenital malformations of the inner ear and cochlear ossification per se are not contraindications to cochlear implantation, although modifications in surgical technique or the use of nonstandard implant electrodes may be necessary and should be anticipated preoperatively. More recently, some implant teams have advocated the routine use of magnetic resonance imaging (MRI) of the internal auditory canals as the preoperative imaging modality of choice. In a retrospective review by Parry and colleagues, MRI was found to be more sensitive and specific in diagnosing soft tissue abnormalities in the inner ear than high-resolution computed tomography in cochlear implant candidates.[3] Using high-resolution T2-weighted sequences, MRI offers the capability for visualizing intracochlear fluid and is therefore more sensitive for detecting both bony and soft tissue obliteration of the cochlea. MRI can also be used to identify neural components within the internal auditory canal on sagittal reconstructions of the internal auditory canal to confirm the presence of a cochlear nerve.

In children, a comprehensive psychosocial evaluation is performed to identify factors that may affect subsequent adjustment to or benefit from the implant. Reasonable implant expectations and acceptance of the child or adult recipient by family members are addressed.

Several factors influence the selection of ear to be implanted. Generally, the ear with the shortest duration of deafness, the more consistent use of a hearing aid, and the most radiographically favorable anatomy (well-pneumatized mastoid, normal facial nerve anatomy, normal inner ear development, and patent cochlea) is selected for implantation. More recently, Friedland and colleagues have suggested that cochlear implantation of the poorer hearing ear does not compromise postoperative performance as measured using standard audiologic tests.[1] While duration of deafness was still the most consistent and significant determinant of postoperative speech recognition, the authors concluded that the overall auditory experience of the individual, rather than ear-specific criteria, was the best predictor of postoperative cochlear implant performance in the postlingually deafened adult. When both ears are

Table 129-3	GUIDELINES FOR MENINGITIS PROPHYLAXIS IN COCHLEAR IMPLANT CANDIDATES

- Children who have completed the pneumococcal conjugate vaccine (Prevnar) series should receive one dose of the pneumococcal polysaccharide vaccine (Pneumovax 23). If they have just received the pneumococcal conjugate vaccine, they should wait at least 2 months before receiving the pneumococcal polysaccharide vaccine.
- Children between 24 and 59 months of age who have never received either the pneumococcal conjugate vaccine or pneumococcal polysaccharide vaccine should receive two doses of pneumococcal conjugate vaccine 2 or more months apart and then receive one dose of pneumococcal polysaccharide vaccine at least 2 months later.
- Individuals age 5 years and older with cochlear implants should receive one dose of pneumococcal polysaccharide vaccine.

Source: http://www.cdc.gov/vaccines/vpd-vac/mening/cochlear/dis-cochlear-hcp.htm

equally suitable for implantation, the ear on the side of dominant hand is selected to facilitate usage of the device.

Of the more than 80,000 patients worldwide who have received cochlear implants, approximately 3500 have received bilateral cochlear implants.[4] Given the advantages of conventional binaural amplification for bilateral sensorineural hearing loss over monaural amplification, we should expect similar auditory performance with bilateral cochlear implantation. The reported benefits of bilateral implantation include significant decrease in head-shadow effect, improved speech understanding in noise, binaural summation, and sound localization. Implants may be placed sequentially at separate surgeries or simultaneously.

Children with cochlear implants have an increased risk for *Streptococcus pneumoniae* meningitis compared with children without cochlear implants. Routine preoperative pneumococcal vaccination is now recommended for all patients.[5] Guidelines for vaccination vary by patient age and are listed in Table 129-3.

SURGICAL APPROACHES

Surgery is performed under general anesthesia with the patient in the supine position. Continuous intraoperative facial nerve monitoring is routinely employed. The use of long-acting muscle relaxants is avoided for this reason. A single dose of a broad-spectrum antibiotic such as cefazolin (Ancef), 2 g, is administered at the time of anesthesia induction.

Device templates provided by the manufacturer are used to outline the position of the behind-the-ear (BTE) processor, internal receiver, and surgical incision. The internal receiver is placed above and behind the BTE processor, avoiding any overlap between the two components. The position of the internal receiver may be

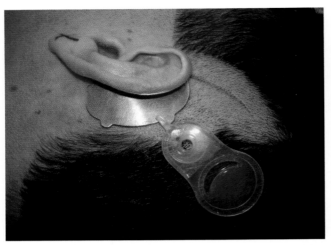

Figure 129-1. Implant template placement and surgical incision marking (Nucleus Freedom device).

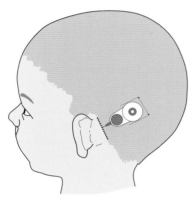

Figure 129-2. Minimal access incision for cochlear implantation. *(From O'Donoghue GM, Nikolopoulos TP: Minimal access surgery for pediatric cochlear implantation. Oto Neurotol 23:891-894, 2002. Reprinted with permission from Lippincott Williams & Wilkins, Optometry and Vision Science.)*

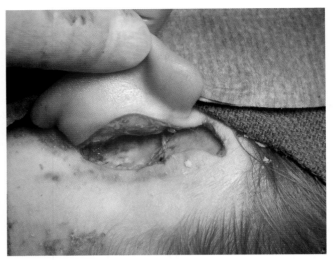

Figure 129-3. Skin incision and flap elevation.

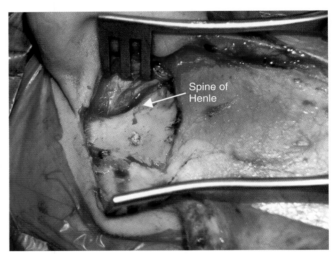

Figure 129-4. Musculoperiosteal flap elevated.

marked at this point using methylene blue and an 18-gauge needle if desired. A variety of skin flaps have been described, most of which are some variation of the standard postauricular incision used for routine mastoid surgery with a posterosuperior extension to provide surgical exposure for seating the internal receiver (Fig. 129-1). Minimal access approaches have been described for cochlear implant insertion if cosmesis is of concern to the patient. In this case, an oblique incision no greater than 3 cm in length, approximately 0.5 cm behind the postauricular crease, is made above and behind the pinna (Fig. 129-2).[6] After infiltration of the planned incision with 1% lidocaine with 1:100,000 epinephrine solution, the skin and subcutaneous tissue are incised down to the level of the temporalis fascia superiorly and mastoid periosteum inferiorly (Fig. 129-3). Skin flaps are then developed anteriorly to the ear canal and posteriorly to allow for placement of the internal receiver. An anteroinferiorly based musculoperiosteal flap is then created by incising the temporalis fascia, muscle, and periosteum. Posterosuperiorly, this flap

should be long enough to completely cover the electrodes as they emerge from the internal receiver. The mastoid cortex and retromastoid cranium are exposed by elevating this musculoperiosteal flap anteriorly until the spine of Henle is visualized (Fig. 129-4).

A complete mastoidectomy is performed using a combination of cutting and diamond drill burrs and continuous suction irrigation, without saucerization of the mastoid cavity. A bony overhang along the superior and posterior margins of the mastoid cavity is preserved for securing the electrode array within the cavity. Once the mastoid antrum is entered, the lateral semicircular canal is identified and drilling continues anterosuperiorly until the body of the incus is identified. The latter is used to define the level of the facial recess. Using 1- to 3-mm diamond burrs, the facial recess, bound by the chorda tympani nerve, facial nerve, and incus buttress, is carefully saucerized with copious irrigation to avoid thermal injury to the facial nerve (Fig. 129-5). Removal of bone anteromedial to the facial nerve in the facial

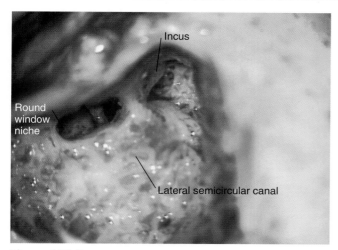

Figure 129-5. Facial recess opened for surgical access to round window.

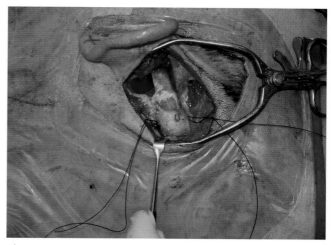

Figure 129-6. Bony recess and tunnel drilled for internal receiver and electrodes. Silk ties in place to secure internal receiver within recess.

recess is sometimes necessary to visualize the round window niche. When the facial recess is narrow, the chorda tympani nerve may need to be sacrificed to gain adequate exposure to the cochlea. In this situation, extreme caution should be exercised when removing bone lateral to the chorda tympani nerve to avoid violating the external auditory canal. Where a prominent round window lip is evident and obscures visualization of the round window membrane, the bony lip may be carefully drilled down using a 1- to 1.5-mm diamond burr. The mastoid cavity is then thoroughly irrigated with bacitracin solution (50,000 units bacitracin powder dissolved in 1000 mL normal saline solution) to remove any bone dust. The epitympanum and facial recess are plugged with Gelfoam or cotton prior to irrigation to avoid dispersing bone dust into the middle ear.

The position of the internal receiver is then confirmed at this point using the BTE and device templates. A dummy internal receiver is used to mark out the dimensions of the bony recess necessary to seat the internal receiver. Cutting and diamond drill burrs are used to develop this recess and the tunnel connecting this recess to the posterosuperior limit of the mastoid cavity. In pediatric patients, the limited thickness of the skull may necessitate removal of bone down to dura, leaving a central island of bone, to allow for adequate recessing of the device. Several techniques are available to secure the device within the bony recess, including the use of nonabsorbable sutures with or without screws, Gore-Tex strips, and microplates. We use four 4-0 silk sutures placed through suture tunnels created alongside the bony recess (Fig. 129-6).

Next, the cochleostomy is performed. Using a 1-mm diamond burr, a small cochleostomy is made immediately anterior and inferior to the round window membrane (Fig. 129-7). This allows surgical access directly into the scala tympani of the cochlear basal turn. Placement of the electrode array into this location is also possible directly through the round window membrane.

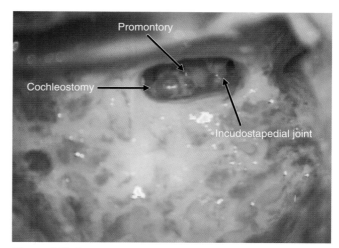

Figure 129-7. Placement of cochleostomy anterior and inferior to round window membrane.

The internal receiver is then placed in the bony recess previously created. The magnet of the internal device may be placed medial or lateral to the temporalis muscle (Fig. 129-8). Once the receiver has been secured in place, the electrode array is inserted into the scala tympani of the cochlea (Fig. 129-9). A variety of tools are provided by the implant manufacturers to facilitate electrode insertion. Undue force should not be used during electrode insertion to avoid electrode kinking within the cochlea and minimize insertional trauma to surviving neural elements within the cochlea. The cochleostomy is then plugged with small pieces of temporalis muscle or fascia. The ground electrode is then buried under the temporalis muscle anterosuperiorly. Once the implant is in place, only bipolar electrocautery should be used in order to minimize the risk of electrical current conduction through the device or into the cochlea. Intraoperative measurements (neural-response telemetry and impedance

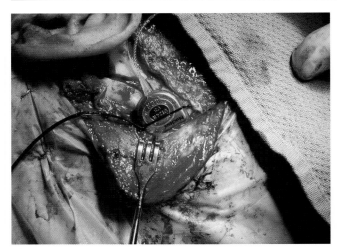

Figure 129-8. Device secured within bony recess and under temporalis muscle.

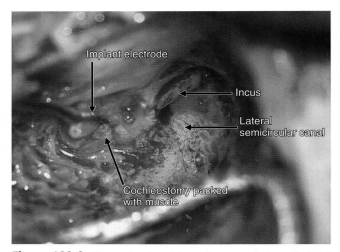

Figure 129-9. Electrode placed in scala tympani through facial recess.

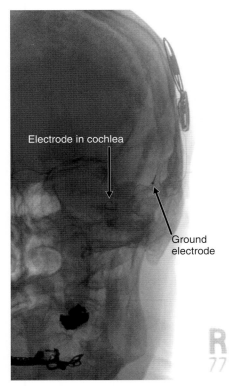

Figure 129-10. Anteroposterior radiograph of the skull showing good electrode placement within the cochlea.

testing) are obtained to confirm proper functioning of the device before or during wound closure. A plain anteroposterior view radiograph of the skull may be routinely or selectively obtained intraoperatively to confirm correct placement of the electrode array within the cochlea (Fig. 129-10). The wound is closed in layers without drainage. Care should be taken to ensure that the musculoperiosteal flap completely covers the mastoid cavity containing the electrode array. A mastoid dressing is applied to the operated ear for 24 hours.

POSTOPERATIVE MANAGEMENT

The patient is discharged home on the day of surgery with a 7-day course of oral antibiotics with antistreptococcal coverage. The patient is instructed to remove the mastoid dressing on postoperative day 1. The initial follow-up visit is in 1 week. The patient is fitted with a signal processor 4 weeks after surgery, and individual programming/rehabilitation begins. Regular follow-up visits with the implant physician and audiologist for the first several years with objective assessment of performance are planned.

COMPLICATIONS

Potential risks of the implant procedure are similar for chronic ear surgery: infection, facial nerve paralysis, dysgeusia, dizziness, cerebrospinal fluid (CSF) drainage, meningitis, risks of general anesthesia, and bleeding.

Wound infection that leads to failure of healing at the incision site is the most common problem associated with implant surgery. Breakdown of the skin flap with potential extrusion of the device can be prevented by keeping the skin incision at least 1 cm away from the edge of the internal receiver and maintaining a 6- to 7-mm thick skin flap overlying the internal receiver and magnet.[7] Any sign of cellulitis warrants aggressive treatment with broad-spectrum intravenous antibiotics. If implant exposure results from necrosis of the overlying skin flap, local rotational flaps may be necessary to cover the device (Fig. 129-11).

Facial nerve injury can occur as a result of surgery. Although intraoperative facial nerve monitoring may reduce this risk, a thorough knowledge of temporal

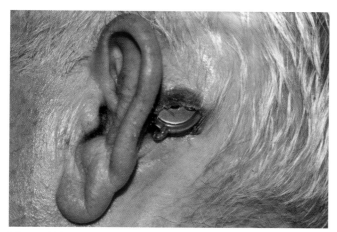

Figure 129-11. Wound breakdown over internal receiver with early extrusion of the device.

bone anatomy and meticulous surgical technique, along with copious irrigation while drilling in and through the facial recess, remain critical.

CSF leak has occurred when drilling the bony well for the internal receiver in patients with thin temporal squama. A small dural tear can be covered with temporalis fascia or repaired primarily. Firm packing of the cochleostomy site with connective tissue prevents perilymphatic fistulae following electrode array insertion. In patients with congenitally malformed inner ears, a postoperative CSF leak is anticipated based on the preoperative imaging findings. The eustachian tube should be temporarily obliterated before the cochleostomy. The elective placement of a lumbar drain in these cases is optional. If a significant postoperative CSF leak develops despite these measures, the eustachian tube and middle ear may be obliterated.

Worldwide meningitis cases in children and adult cochlear implant recipients reported in 2002 led the FDA and Centers for Disease Control and Prevention to develop recommendations for preoperative vaccination for all implant recipients. Studies have reemphasized the importance of packing the cochleostomy site with soft tissue to prevent bacteria from entering the inner ear and intracranial space.[8,9]

Intracochlear ossification can be anticipated preoperatively on CT imaging of the temporal bone. Surgical management options include drilling through the basal turn of the cochlea with partial electrode insertion,[10] insertion of a split electrode array through two separate cochleostomies in the basal and apical cochlear turns, respectively, to maximize the number of electrodes implanted.[11] The first cochleostomy is created at the standard site, just anterior to the round window membrane. The second cochleostomy is created approximately 2 mm anterior to the oval window.[12] An extensive drillout procedure to gain access to the upper basal turn has also been described by Gantz and colleagues for the ossified cochlea.[13]

PEARLS

- A limited cortical mastoidectomy with inferior exposure down to the level of the inferior external auditory canal is usually adequate for cochlear implantation.
- A combined transmastoid/transcanal approach, leaving the ear canal skin intact, may be helpful for added surgical exposure of the cochlea when a contracted mastoid is encountered.
- Removal of bone medial and anterior to the facial nerve within the facial recess may be necessary for exposure of the round window niche.
- Attention should be directed to inserting the cochlear implant electrode into the scala tympani with the electrode plates directed toward the modiolus.
- The musculoperiosteal flap should be reapproximated such that it completely covers the mastoid cavity with the carrier and ground electrodes within it.

PITFALLS

- Drilling lateral to the chorda tympani nerve when opening the facial recess may result in violation of the tympanic membrane or external auditory canal.
- Thermal injury to the facial nerve may occur while drilling in the facial recess if continuous irrigation is not applied.
- Inadequate surgical exposure and visualization of the round window may result in erroneous placement of the implant electrode within hypotympanic air cells.
- Suctioning at or within the cochleostomy may result in trauma to the surviving intracochlear neural elements, thus limiting postoperative auditory function.
- The presence of congenital inner ear malformations may increase the risk of postoperative CSF leak and meningitis.

References

1. Friedland DR, Venick HS, Niparko JK: Choice of ear for cochlear implantation: The effect of history and residual hearing on predicted postoperative performance. Oto Neurotol 24:582-589, 2003.
2. Waltzman SB, Cohen NL: Implantation of patients with prelingual long-term deafness. Ann Otol Rhino Laryngol 108:84-87, 1999.
3. Parry DA, Booth T, Roland PS: Advantages of magnetic resonance imaging over computed tomography in preoperative evaluation of pediatric cochlear implant candidates. Oto Neurotol 26:976-982, 2005.
4. Lustig LR, Wackym PA: Bilateral cochlear implantation. Oper Tech Otolaryngol 16:125-130, 2005.
5. Reefhuis J, Honein MA, Whitney CG, et al: Risk of bacterial meningitis in children with cochlear implants. N Engl J Med 349:435-445, 2003.

6. O'Donoghue GM, Nikolopoulos TP: Minimal access surgery for pediatric cochlear implantation. Oto Neurotol 23:891-894, 2002.

7. Luxford WM, Mills D: Cochlear implantation in adults. In Jackler RK, Brackmann DE (eds): Neurotology, 2nd ed. New York, Mosby, 2004, pp 1309-1314.

8. Cohen NL, Roland JT Jr, Marrinan M: Meningitis in cochlear implant recipients: The North American experience. Otol Neurotol 25:275-281, 2004.

9. O'Donoghue G, Balkany T, Cohen N, et al: Meningitis and cochlear implantation. Oto Neurotol 23:823-824, 2002.

10. Miyamoto RT, Kirk KI: Cochlear implantation. In Bailey BJ, Johnson JT (eds): Head & Neck Surgery—Otolaryngology, 4th ed. Philadelphia, Lippincott Williams & Wilkins, 2006, pp 2265-2277.

11. Millar DA, Hillman TA, Shelton C: Implantation of the ossified cochlea: Management with the split electrode array. Laryngoscope 115:2155-2160, 2005.

12. Lenarz T, Lesinski-Schiedat A, Weber BP, et al: The nucleus double array cochlear implant: A new concept for the obliterated cochlea. Oto Neurotol 22:24-32, 2001.

13. Gantz BJ, McCabe BF, Tyler RS: Use of multichannel cochlear implants in obstructed and obliterated cochleas. Otolaryngol Head Neck Surg 98:72-81, 1988.

Chapter 130

Microvascular Decompression of the Seventh Cranial Nerve

Johnathan A. Engh, Amin B. Kassam,
Michael Horowitz, Jeffrey Balzer, and John Y. K. Lee

Hemifacial spasm (HFS) is a relatively uncommon affliction with an estimated yearly incidence of approximately 1 per 10,000.[1] The disorder is characterized by involuntary unilateral contractions and twitching of the eye and face. The spasms are painless, yet they often cause significant social distress. In addition, many patients with HFS have difficulty reading, driving, or working. Medications generally offer no relief of symptoms. Botulinus toxin (Botox, Allergan, Inc.) injections have become increasingly popular as a temporizing measure for HFS, but do not have long-lasting efficacy. As a result of the lack of response of HFS to these conservative therapies, surgical interventions for HFS have emerged over the past half century.

The hypothesis that vascular compression of the seventh cranial nerve (CN VII) causes HFS opened the door for these surgical therapies. The theory was first proposed by Campbell and Keedy in 1947 as well as Laine and Nayrac in 1948.[2,3] Their proposal was based on Dandy's hypothesis that vascular compression of the dorsal root of the trigeminal nerve causes trigeminal neuralgia.[4] Subsequently, Gardner and Sava published their initial experience with decompression of the seventh nerve for HFS in 1962.[5,6] However, despite these early reports, decades would pass before Jannetta popularized microvascular decompression (MVD) of CN VII as the definitive treatment for hemifacial spasm.[7,8] Today, microvascular decompression of the seventh nerve stands alone as the single most effective and long-lasting treatment for HFS.

PATIENT SELECTION

HFS is a purely clinical diagnosis and therefore a careful history and physical examination must be obtained before consideration of craniotomy and MVD. Typically, HFS manifests as unilateral intermittent twitching of the facial muscles, usually beginning with orbicularis oculi. Subsequently, spasms spread contiguously to the other facial muscles. In atypical HFS, twitching begins in the lower facial muscles and subsequently spreads upward. The disease generally takes a relentless course and over a variable period of time progresses to all of the major muscles of one side of the face, including the frontalis, platysma, and stapedius muscles. The latter creates an odd clicking sound in the ipsilateral ear. Severe spasms may lead to tonic facial contractures (i.e., "tonus" phenomenon), which can be associated with facial muscle paresis. The cosmetic deformity of HFS is the most obvious concern for most patients, prohibiting normal social interactions. Moreover, HFS usually becomes a functional disability. Repetitive closure of the eyelids, especially when associated with tonus phenomenon, can impair vision and prohibit the pursuit of both occupational and leisure activities, including driving and reading.

HFS is slightly more common in women, and the left side of the face is more often affected than the right.[8] Symptoms may be exacerbated by fatigue and stressful activities. Although the spasms are involuntary, voluntary movements such as talking and smiling can

Table 130-1	DISTINGUISHING FEATURES OF HEMIFACIAL SPASM AND SIMILAR CONDITIONS			
Condition	**Spasm Location**	**Spasm Pattern**	**Spasm Laterality**	**Pain**
Hemifacial spasm	Orbicularis, with spread to other facial muscles	Arrhythmic and intermittent, may persist during sleep	Unilateral	Usually none
Blepharospasm	Orbicularis, may spread to the rest of the face	Symmetrical and forceful	Bilateral	Usually none, but may have photophobia and/or ocular dysesthesias
Post-paralytic synkinesis	Anywhere in facial nerve distribution	Associated with movement	Usually unilateral	Varies
Facial myokymia	All facial muscles	Movements exacerbated by fatigue; fine and continuous	Varies	Usually none
Tics and habit spasms	Usually outside the facial nerve distribution	Stereotyped and simple	Often bilateral	Usually none
Focal seizure activity	Anywhere in facial nerve distribution	Clonic, gross movements	Unilateral unless seizure generalizes	None

trigger contractions. Spasms continue during sleep, and no known medical conditions are associated with increased incidence of HFS. There is no apparent genetic transmission of HFS, although rare familial cases have been reported. No known toxin exposures appear to increase the incidence of this condition.

The differential diagnosis of hemifacial spasm includes postparalytic synkinesis, which occurs after facial nerve trauma or Bell's palsy. This phenomenon is usually brought on by facial movement and rarely occurs at rest. Other conditions that can be confused with hemifacial spasm include blepharospasm, tics or habit spasms, facial myokymia, Meige syndrome (combination of oromandibular dystonia and blepharospasm), and focal cortical seizures. Blepharospasm and myokymia typically occur bilaterally, whereas bilateral HFS is exceedingly rare. The distinguishing features of HFS and similar conditions are outlined in Table 130-1.

PREOPERATIVE EVALUATION

Although preoperative imaging cannot make or support the diagnosis of HFS, mass lesions such as neoplasms of the cerebellopontine angle, posterior circulation aneurysms, or arteriovenous malformations may be associated with HFS in 1% to 2% of cases. Therefore an essential part of the patient's preoperative evaluation is magnetic resonance imaging (MRI) scan with and without contrast to rule out the existence of such a mass lesion. If a mass lesion is discovered, both the mass lesion and the vascular compression source must be treated in order to achieve a cure. However, MRI and computed tomography (CT) scans should not be relied upon to identify vessels responsible for compression. A vessel (arterial or venous) of any size can be responsible

for the compression syndrome. If the MRI scan does demonstrate a large vessel near the CN VII root exit zone, the finding does not necessarily mean that this vessel is the primary source of compression or the only source of the compression. Thus, the role of preoperative imaging is to rule out other sources of vascular compression rather than guide the operative approach in most cases.

Once a patient is diagnosed with HFS and obtains adequate imaging, it is reasonable to refer the patient to a neurologist or neurophysiologist for electroneurophysiologic testing. The routine battery of tests that are performed includes baseline brain stem auditory evoked responses (BAERs), facial electromyography (EMG), and baseline lateral spread (LS) testing (see later text). Abnormalities are noted before any operations. Such testing is most critical in patients who have received Botox injections before seeking surgical treatment, because their baseline responses are often abnormal.

Patients with HFS have a characteristic electrophysiologic anomaly termed the *lateral spread response*. An understanding of the importance of this abnormal muscle response is critical, both to the diagnosis of HFS as well as the operation to cure it.[9] The LS can be evoked via percutaneous stimulation of one branch of the facial nerve while recording stimulus-evoked EMG from the various muscles of the face innervated by the facial nerve. In patients with HFS, when one branch of the facial nerve is electrically stimulated (e.g., zygomatic branch), not only do the muscles innervated by that branch (e.g., orbicularis oculi) display an evoked EMG response, but other facial muscles (e.g., mentalis) not innervated by that branch also demonstrate evoked EMG activity. This paradoxical EMG response can be evoked in the operating room and consists of a triphasic EMG potential followed by a series of after-discharge

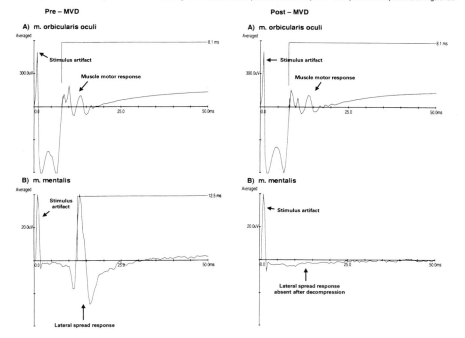

An intra-operative motor evoked potential (MEP) was obtained with supra-threshold stimulation of the zygomatic branch of cranial nerve VII on the operative side. The direct MEP was recorded in m. orbicularis oculi (**A**) with a peak latency of 8.1 msec and amplitude of 795 uV. Prior to microvascular decompression (**Pre - MVD**) the indirect "Lateral Spread" of evoked motor activity was recorded in m. mentalis (**B**) with a peak latency of 12.5 ms and amplitude of 67 uV. Following microvascular decompression of CN VII (**Post – MVD**) the lateral spread is extinguished.

Figure 130-1. Demonstration of the "lateral spread" phenomenon as visualized intraoperatively during an MVD for HFS.

potentials most typically recorded at a latency of 10 to 12 milliseconds. This response is obliterated following an adequate decompression of the seventh nerve (Fig. 130-1).

Most patients with hemifacial spasm are between the fourth and sixth decades of life, and are reasonable candidates for general anesthesia. Nonetheless, all of these patients require a formal perioperative risk assessment before any operation. Preoperative laboratory evaluations including electrolytes, complete blood counts, and coagulation profiles should be assessed. Electrocardiography and chest roentgenography help rule out occult cardiovascular disease. It is not necessary to keep blood products on hold in most cases. Any patient with a significant cardiac or other medical risk should have it addressed before craniotomy for MVD.

SURGICAL APPROACH

Patient Positioning and Preparation

The retrosigmoid or retromastoid approach is the standard surgical approach for MVD of the seventh nerve. Once anesthetized, the patient is placed in three-point head fixation with pins in the ipsilateral frontotemporal region and the contralateral mastoid. This approach maximizes access to the mastoid region on the treated side. When placing the pin fixation, it is important to keep the operative side pins anterior to a line running superiorly from the earlobe. If the pin is placed too far posteriorly, it will be difficult to insert the self-retaining retractor, because the handles will contact the head

holder. In addition, the squamosal portion of the temporal bone is to be avoided with the fixation pins, because this area of the skull is particularly thin and pinning in this area can lead to an epidural hematoma. Sixty pounds of pressure is usually adequate for rigid head fixation.

After pinning, the patient is rotated with the treated side up into the lateral decubitus position. All pressure points are padded, and an axillary roll is placed. The patient is taped to the table securely at the hip and underneath the axilla. In addition, the ipsilateral shoulder is pulled caudally with care not to stretch the brachial plexus. The neck is gently flexed and elevated from the lateral position such that two fingerbreadths are maintained between the chin and the sternum. This maneuver is designed to minimize the risk of jugular venous thrombosis. Proper patient positioning is demonstrated in Figure 130-2.

A Doppler monitor should be secured to the anterior chest wall in order to detect the occurrence of air embolism during venous sinus exposure. While lumbar cerebrospinal fluid (CSF) drainage is not routinely used, we do consider the use of CSF drainage if the patient is especially young (in which case the posterior fossa is fuller) or if the operation is a revision procedure (in which case the cerebellum may be adherent to the overlying dura). Furthermore, a lumbar drain is of additional value if the surgeon is less experienced at the procedure: lumbar drainage creates early cerebellar relaxation and minimizes the CSF pulsations that can make microsurgical dissection in this region more difficult.

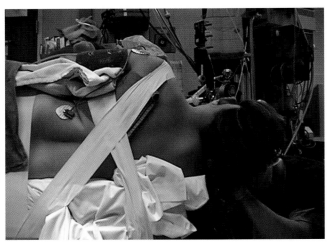

Figure 130-2. Proper lateral decubitus positioning for a seventh nerve decompression. This photograph and all subsequent operative photographs depict a left-sided operation.

Intraoperative Monitoring

Intraoperative BAERs are monitored, as are stimulus-evoked EMG responses from the orbicularis and mentalis muscle groups in response to stimulation of the zygomatic branch of the facial nerve. In addition, spontaneous EMG from cranial nerves IX and X is recorded to detect any injury potentials. The anesthesiologist should use only short-acting muscle relaxation for induction, thereby allowing for EMG monitoring and assessment of the presence of a lateral spread response before incision. The surgeon must ensure that an adequate recording of the lateral spread response is present before skin incision.

Surgical Exposure

A 3- × 5-cm area behind the ear is shaved. The mastoid eminence, digastric groove, and inion should be identified externally. The line between the inion and the external auditory meatus approximates the position of the transverse sinus. The digastric groove overlies the sigmoid sinus, and the junction of these two lines defines the transverse-sigmoid junction. A vertical incision is drawn 3 to 5 cm long, approximately 0.5 cm medial to the shaved hairline and parallel to it. A standard preoperative sterile skin preparation is applied. During draping of the operative field, the patient is administered 12.5 to 25 g of intravenous mannitol to facilitate cerebellar relaxation. Skin is opened with a scalpel. Deeper dissection uses monopolar electrocautery and bipolar sacrifice of the occipital artery. The initial periosteal dissection should always proceed medially before completing the lateral dissection, because the lateral periosteum is more loosely attached to the skull than is the medial periosteum, and the muscle thickness is greater medially than laterally. If the surgeon performs the muscle and periosteal dissection laterally (toward the ear) first, there is usually not enough tissue resistance to allow the Weitlaner retrac-

tor to force the medial tissue out of the surgical field. This situation makes visualization of the intracranial contents more difficult. If one should make the mistake of dissecting laterally first, the problem can be overcome in two ways: (1) by extending the incision superiorly and inferiorly to allow for more tissue mobilization or (2) by substituting skin hook and spring retractors for the Weitlaner self-retaining retractor.

Once the muscle and periosteum are mobilized and retracted, the underlying bony anatomy should be clearly identified. The mastoid emissary vein, which often marks the transverse-sigmoid sinus junction, will almost always be encountered and will need to be filled with wax for adequate hemostasis. The digastric groove must also be visualized; drilling along its medial border creates the dural exposure necessary for an adequate brain stem view.

Following periosteal dissection, the overlying bone may be removed via a craniectomy or craniotomy. Even though bone removal can be minimized to only a few centimeters, the authors prefer bone removal sufficient to expose the inferior edge of the transverse-sigmoid junction and the medial edge of the sigmoid sinus down to the level of the lower digastric groove. This 4- × 3-cm ovoid opening provides adequate inferolateral exposure to access the lateral cerebellomedullary cistern without significant cerebellar retraction. It is necessary to remove a portion of the posterior mastoid air cells in order to expose the edge of the sigmoid sinus. All the air cells are thoroughly waxed in order to avoid a postoperative CSF leak.[10]

Before dural opening, the Greenberg brain retractor system is attached to the three-point head holder in case fixed spatulas are required to control unforeseen intracranial bleeding. The system is not used in the vast majority of cases. The dura mater is then opened in a curvilinear fashion and reflected laterally with 4-0 monofilament suture. The dural reflection must lie immediately parallel to the descending sigmoid sinus so as to avoid a shelf of dura reducing subsequent lateral visualization. The medial dural cuff is maintained to allow for a watertight closure. A 3- × 0.5-cm rubber dam cottonoid sponge is placed along the lateral aspect of the cerebellar lobe to begin navigating around the cerebellum (Fig. 130-3).

Nerve Exposure

At this point, the operating microscope with a 325-mm objective lens is brought into the field. Dissection proceeds laterally around the edge of the cerebellum toward the lateral cerebellomedullary cistern, which contains the 11th cranial nerve. The brain is gently retracted with a cottonoid sponge. All cottonoids are moistened with saline and placed over an appropriately sized (0.5 × 3.0 cm) piece of latex (rubber dam) cut from a sterile surgical glove. The latex prevents trauma to the cerebellum and allows for easier advancement of the cottonoids. A rubber dam cottonoid and Teflon pledgets are pictured in Figure 130-4. Whereas we favor not using a retractor during the case, but rather retract-

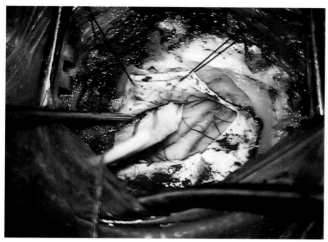

Figure 130-3. Rubber dam cottonoid placed on the lateral cerebellum in preparation for navigation around the cerebellar hemisphere.

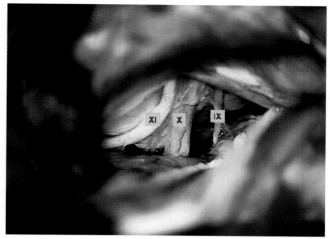

Figure 130-5. Visualization of the ninth (IX), tenth (X), and eleventh (XI) cranial nerves following arachnoidal dissection.

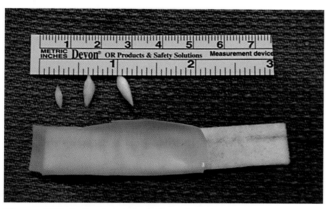

Figure 130-4. Patties and pledgets for microvascular decompression. Teflon pledgets are visualized superiorly, and a rubber dam cottonoid inferiorly.

ing with a controlled sucker (no. 3-4F), a 60-degree tapered retractor can be placed over the rubber dam cottonoid against the inferolateral aspect of the cerebellum. Following gentle navigation around the inferolateral cerebellar edge, the petrous dura overlying the 11th cranial nerve is visualized. Safe exposure of this landmark requires a dynamic dissection process with intermittent adjustments of both the patient's position and the operating microscope. Dissection around the lateral border of the cerebellum without adequate adjustment of the patient's position and/or the microscope's position may lead to cerebellar injury. This injury can be profound enough to cause lateral cerebellar infarction and brain herniation.

Beneath the petrous dura, the 11th nerve is visualized. If necessary, a portion of the overlying bone can be drilled off to facilitate cisternal visualization. The arachnoid between the nerve and the cerebellar flocculus is opened with an arachnoid knife. At this point the operator holds still, patiently allowing CSF egress

and cerebellar relaxation. The working zone of the posterior fossa is markedly increased by this maneuver. In addition, this maneuver allows for initial inspection of the lower cranial nerves (CN IX through XI). An overly superior approach to this cistern exposes the seventh and eighth nerves prematurely without adequate CSF drainage. An overly inferior approach to this cistern leads to the cerebellar tonsils near their termination at the foramen magnum.

Once CSF is drained and the cerebellum relaxes, the arachnoid over the lower cranial nerves is opened sharply with an arachnoid knife and microscissors (Fig. 130-5). The flocculus of the cerebellum and the choroid plexus protruding through the foramen of Luschka are exposed and gently retracted. Retraction at this point may result in changes in the BAER. If significant BAER changes occur (i.e., greater than 50% amplitude reduction or greater than 1 millisecond latency), retraction should be relaxed and the surgeon should pause until all responses return to their baseline configuration. Additional arachnoid around CN VIII may need to be cut to reduce transmitted retraction forces from the cerebellum as it is mobilized medially. It is important to watch the retractor (if used) or cottonoid frequently throughout the operative period because it is common for one of them to move against the lower cranial nerves and cause potential irreversible damage. Thorough, sharp arachnoidal dissection helps prevent cranial nerve injury during this portion of the procedure. In particular, removal of arachnoidal adhesions around the eighth nerve minimizes retraction injury to the cochlear nerve and cochlear nucleus. Any injury potentials are immediately reported to the surgeon during this critical portion of the dissection.

The facial nerve must be exposed along its entire course, especially at the brain stem root exit zone, the most common site of vascular compression. To visualize the root exit zone, it is important to completely dissect the flocculus and choroid plexus from the base of cranial nerves VIII, IX, and X. Looking toward the

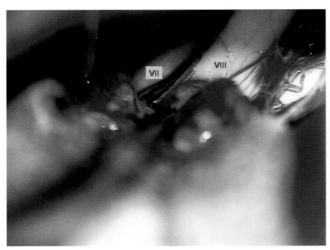

Figure 130-6. Visualization of the seventh nerve (VII) exiting the brain stem anterior and deep to the superficial eighth nerve (VIII). A small artery is compressing the nerve at its root exit zone.

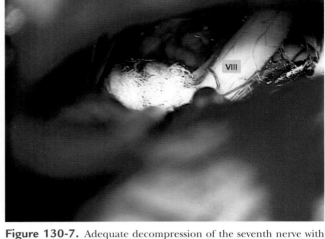

Figure 130-7. Adequate decompression of the seventh nerve with Teflon pledgets.

brain stem (achieved by angling the microscope inward and rotating the patient toward the surgeon), the surgeon should focus just medial to the ninth and tenth nerves. It is from this area that the facial nerve arises as it runs rostrally to follow the course of CN VIII, deep to it (Fig. 130-6). It is often necessary to work between CN IX and X and between CN VIII and IX to get the best view of the brain stem origin of the seventh nerve.

Microvascular Decompression

The most common vessels compressing the facial nerve are the posterior inferior cerebellar artery (PICA) and anterior inferior cerebellar artery (AICA).[8,11,12] Because of the proximity of the PICA origin from the vertebral artery (VA) to the compression site, the authors often first decompress the VA from the brain stem before decompression of PICA from the seventh nerve root exit zone. The VA is reliably located just medial to CN XI. The VA is elevated from the brain stem and large pieces of Teflon felt are placed between the vessel and the medulla so as to move the entire vascular complex laterally. This maneuver shifts the PICA and other VA perforators away from the brain stem as well as the CN VII exit zone. Early mobilization shifts PICA distally, reducing the need for neural tissue retraction during subsequent decompression. Once the VA is mobilized laterally, attention is turned to the CN VII root exit zone. Any arteries compressing this site are mobilized away from the brain stem and decompressed using Teflon pledgets (Fig. 130-7). At this point, the lateral spreads often begin to change morphology and amplitude or may even suddenly disappear. If they do not fully disappear, additional arterial sources of compression are sought. Some may be quite small and may be considered inconsequential to the spasm; however, by decompressing them the lateral spreads often completely resolve. If the spreads remain, a search for veins

contacting the CN VII exit zone is carried out. Often these veins can also be decompressed from the brain stem using sharp dissection and small pieces of Teflon. In other instances they need to be divided using a microknife, scissors, or hook. At no time should bipolar cautery be used in the region of CN VII or the brain stem; even small energy surges can lead to permanent CN VII and VIII dysfunction. Hemostasis from divided veins is readily achieved using gentle Teflon tamponade. When veins are found and eliminated, it often takes several minutes for the lateral spreads to completely disappear or fall to negligible levels. The reason for this delayed change is not clear; however, it is a reliable enough finding that the authors will wait several minutes for the lateral spreads to abate before searching for additional pathology. Such patience eliminates unnecessary dissection, which puts the cranial nerves and the brain stem at risk for iatrogenic injury.

Throughout the operation, close communication is maintained with the neurophysiology team. Any change in the BAER morphology mandates immediate action, because the eighth cranial nerve is especially sensitive to manipulation. If the amplitude drops by more than 50% or if the latency is increased by more than 1 millisecond, surgical manipulation ceases, and the BAER should be allowed to return to baseline. In less favorable circumstances, the surgeon should always wait until the latency drops below a 0.5-millisecond delay and the wave amplitude increases to at least 50% of baseline before resuming manipulation. Occasionally, the BAER will change after placement of a Teflon felt, necessitating removal. Sudden loss of BAER usually denotes a vascular injury to CN VIII either from vasospasm or vessel loss. Small perforator injury can lead to such changes, especially branches of AICA or the labyrinthine artery. Inadvertent spread of bipolar current can also lead to irreversible injury. The authors have frequently witnessed improvement of BAER recordings following irrigation of the eighth nerve with papaverine, implying that improvement of local micro-circulation can improve nerve function.

The neurophysiology team is essential for successful performance of a microvascular decompression of the seventh nerve. Accurate intraoperative monitoring prevents iatrogenic injury. In addition, tracking the lateral spread of impulses along the seventh nerve can lead the surgeon to the critical pathology, and lateral spread obliteration increases the surgeon's confidence that the patient will be cured. In certain cases, decompression of large vessels that appear to be clear culprits may in fact have no effect on lateral spreads. Furthermore, final decompression of small venules or arterioles can lead to ultimate resolution of abnormal electrical crosstalk and irritation. Therefore, neurophysiology input is critical to both novice and experienced microsurgeons.

Closure

At the conclusion of the decompression procedure, several Valsalva maneuvers to 40 mm Hg for 10 seconds are performed to ensure hemostasis. It is important to be sure the patient is pharmacologically paralyzed before Valsalva maneuvers are requested. The region is gently irrigated with warm saline bulb irrigation, and the dura is closed. Dural closure must be watertight. If the dura cannot be easily reapproximated, a small piece of muscle is sewn over the opening to seal off the leak. Larger defects are closed with a dural graft. Valsalva maneuvers are again performed to ensure the adequacy of the dural closure. If there is an inadvertent injury to a dural venous sinus during closure, then the area of the injury should be packed with hemostatic agents, such as Avitene, and allowed to stop spontaneously. Under no circumstances should such an injury be directly repaired with suture or vascular clips, which may worsen such an injury.

After dural closure, the bone edges of the mastoid air cells are thoroughly waxed once again. A pad of Gelfoam is placed over the dura to fill in any dead space. Sometimes, fibrin sealant glue can be applied to the dura as an additional barrier to CSF leakage. A wire mesh with titanium screws (KLS Martin, Jacksonville, FL) is fastened to the bony edges to reapproximate the shape of the skull. Care must be taken to avoid plunging into the subdural space with a slipped screw while attaching the cranioplasty plate. The authors have found that this technique prevents the adhesion of nuchal muscles to the dura, which may cause chronic postoperative headaches. The muscles are approximated with interrupted 2-0 absorbable sutures, and the fascia is closed in a similar fashion. The subcutaneous tissue and skin are closed with 3-0 absorbable sutures and a running 4-0 nylon suture. A sterile bandage is affixed with paper tape.

POSTOPERATIVE MANAGEMENT

As with any other patient status postcraniotomy with intradural manipulation, postoperative cardiac telemetry and respiratory monitoring is essential. Following a postoperative neurologic examination and a few hours of surveillance in the postanesthesia care unit, patients are transferred to the neurologic stepdown unit for overnight observation. Postoperative hypertension is to be avoided, because it entails an increased risk of late hemorrhage. The authors use intravenous short-acting antihypertensive agents (e.g., labetalol or hydralazine) to prevent elevation of the systolic blood pressure above 160 mm Hg for 24 hours. Postoperative nausea is treated with intravenous ondansetron, and other agents are added if necessary. Any patient with a severe headache undergoes an immediate non–contrast-enhanced head CT scan to rule out any postoperative hematoma. Patients with persistent headache not alleviated by medication and a negative scan undergo high-volume lumbar puncture. Approximately 15% to 20% of patients benefit from this method of treatment for mild postoperative intracranial hypertension. The cause of the intracranial hypertension is unclear, but it may be related to blood products and bone dust within the subarachnoid space, impairing CSF reabsorption.

Most patients are transferred from the stepdown unit to a regular floor on postoperative day 1. Diet is advanced, as well as activity. Most patients are ready to leave the hospital within an average of 3 days. Following discharge home, all patients are brought back to clinic within 10 to 14 days of the procedure for a wound check, neurologic examination, and audiogram. There is no role for routine postoperative imaging. The majority of patients are spasm-free at the time of discharge; in addition, patients with residual postoperative spasm tend to achieve delayed symptom resolution if the intraoperative decompression was adequate.[13-15] Cure rates generally range from 80% to 90% in experienced hands.

Complications include CSF leaks, wound infections, and cranial nerve injuries. Postoperative CSF leaks can present with rhinorrhea, otorrhea, or leakage directly through the incision. A lumbar drain with aggressive CSF drainage can eliminate an early postoperative leak, but if this therapy fails, then the wound needs to be revised in the operating room. Wound infections are uncommon, but they also necessitate operative washout and wound revision, along with appropriate antibiotics. Cranial nerve injuries are usually managed expectantly with two major exceptions: (1) patients with significant orbicularis weakness may require a gold weight for corneal protection, and (2) patients with significant vocal cord dysfunction may require a vocal cord injection.

MVD of the seventh nerve remains the gold standard therapy for hemifacial spasm. No other treatment has comparable long-term results. However, the procedure should not be taken lightly, because the complications of the operation can be serious. Results are best in experienced hands. Careful patient selection, meticulous operative technique, and reliable neurophysiologic monitoring are the three keys to successful treatment.

PEARLS

- The preoperative decision to perform an MVD for HFS is guided by clinical presentation, not by MRI.
- Correct preoperative patient positioning is critical to adequate exposure of the CN VII-VIII complex and minimization of brain retraction.
- The copious application of bone wax to the mastoid air cells both before dural opening and after dural closure prevents postoperative CSF leaks.
- Following dural opening, navigation around the cerebellar lobe toward the seventh nerve exit zone is a dynamic process with multiple adjustments of both microscope and patient position. Patience and sharp arachnoidal dissection facilitate safe CSF egress to minimize retraction injury.
- Entry into the cerebellomedullary cistern (i.e., the cistern of the 11th nerve) from below with subsequent dissection upward is the safest way to identify the eighth nerve (which runs quite superficially) and thus prevent injury to it. Cerebellar relaxation afforded by this maneuver facilitates subsequent dissection.

PITFALLS

- Tearing of a venous sinus during dural opening or closure can lead to significant blood loss, and hemostasis is difficult to obtain in this situation.
- Aggressive retraction of the lateral cerebellar lobe can lead to a cerebellar infarction postoperatively and, in rare cases, mass effect upon the brain stem.
- The eighth cranial nerve is extraordinarily sensitive to manipulation; attempts to adequately decompress the seventh nerve at the expense of eighth nerve manipulation rather than extensive arachnoidal dissection can lead to deafness.
- Attempts to directly coagulate small arterioles or venules at the root exit zone of the seventh nerve from the brain stem are prone to causing irreversible neural injury.

- Failure to keep the hand steady while affixing the cranioplasty plate can cause the screw to plunge into the subdural space, causing significant bleeding and necessitating redo wound closure.

References

1. Auger RG, Whisnant JP: Hemifacial spasm in Rochester and Olmsted County, Minnesota, 1960 to 1984. Arch Neurol 47:1233-1234, 1990.
2. Campbell E, Keedy C: Hemifacial spasm: A note on the etiology in two cases. J Neurosurg 4:342-247, 1947.
3. Laine E, Nayrac P: Hemispasme facial gueri par intervention sur la fossa posterieure. Rev Neurol 80:38-40, 1948.
4. Dandy WE: Concerning the cause of trigeminal neuralgia. Am J Surg 24:447-455, 1934.
5. Gardner WJ: Concerning the mechanism of trigeminal neuralgia and hemifacial spasm. J Neurosurg 19:947-958, 1962.
6. Gardner WJ, Sava GA: Hemifacial spasm—a reversible pathophysiologic state. J Neurosurg 19:240-247, 1962.
7. Jannetta PJ, Abbasy M, Maroon JC, et al: Etiology and definitive microsurgical treatment of hemifacial spasm: Operative techniques and results in 47 patients. J Neurosurg 47:321-328, 1977.
8. Barker FG, Jannetta PJ, Bissonette DJ, et al: Microvascular decompression for hemifacial spasm. J Neurosurg 82:201-210, 1995.
9. Moller AR, Jannetta PJ: Monitoring facial EMG responses during microvascular decompression operations for hemifacial spasm. J Neurosurg 66:681-685, 1987.
10. McLaughlin MR, Jannetta PJ, Clyde BL, et al: Microvascular decompression of cranial nerves: Lessons learned after 4400 operations. J Neurosurg 90:1-8, 1999.
11. Fukushima T: Microvascular decompression for hemifacial spasm: Results in 2870 cases. In Carter LP, Spetzler RF (eds): Neurovascular Surgery. New York, McGraw-Hill, 1995, pp 1133-1145.
12. Huang CI, Chen IH, Lee LS: Microvascular decompression for hemifacial spasm: Analyses of operative findings and results in 310 patients. Neurosurgery 30:53-56, 1991.
13. Ishikawa M, Nakanishi T, Takamiya Y, Namiki J: Delayed resolution of residual hemifacial spasm after microvascular decompression operations. Neurosurgery 49: 847-854, 2001.
14. Gotu Y, Matsushima T, Natori Y, et al: Delayed effects of the microvascular decompression on hemifacial spasm: A retrospective study of 131 consecutive operated cases. Neurologic Res 24:296-300, 2002.
15. Shin JC, Chung UH, Kim YC, Park CI: Prospective study of microvascular decompression in hemifacial spasm. Neurosurgery 40:730-735, 1997.

Chapter **131**

Surgery for Vertigo

William A. Wood and Elizabeth H. Toh

Vertigo may result from disorders of both the central and peripheral vestibular systems. The majority of patients may be managed conservatively with medical therapy and vestibular rehabilitation therapy. Critical to the management of patients with vertigo is the correct diagnosis of the underlying pathology. Those with peripheral vestibular disease who have symptoms refractory to medical management may benefit from surgery. Surgical options include those that address the specific pathology of the disease and those that ablate the peripheral vestibular organ. This chapter describes operative techniques for posterior semicircular canal occlusion (PSCO), endolymphatic sac decompression with or without shunting, labyrinthectomy, vestibular nerve section, and repair of superior semicircular canal dehiscence. Repair of perilymph fistulas is described in Chapter 119.

PATIENT SELECTION

Several criteria should be met before considering surgery for vestibular disease. First, a definitive diagnosis of a unilateral peripheral vestibulopathy should be made. This can usually be established following a comprehensive history, physical examination, and vestibular testing. The latter aids in localizing the site of pathology and excluding any underlying central vestibular problems that will impair vestibular compensation following ablative surgery. Bilateral and central vestibular dysfunctions are contraindications for ablative surgery such as labyrinthectomy and vestibular nerve section.

Next, graduated and comprehensive medical management of the vertigo should be instituted. This should include a trial of pharmacotherapy and for uncompensated peripheral vestibulopathy, a course of vestibular rehabilitation therapy. If symptoms persist despite non-surgical treatment and are disabling, surgical options may be considered.

Last, the age, comorbidities, and overall physical condition of the patient should be considered. In general, central vestibular compensation following ablative surgery is poorer in older individuals. Persistent disequilibrium may render that individual more disabled compared with their preoperative condition.

The most common peripheral vestibular disorders amenable to surgical intervention include benign paroxysmal positional vertigo (BPPV), Meniere's disease, uncompensated peripheral vestibulopathy, perilymph fistula, and superior semicircular canal dehiscence (SCDS) syndrome.

Benign Paroxysmal Positional Vertigo

The current canalolithiasis theory holds that the pathophysiology of BPPV likely results from free-floating otoconia within the posterior semicircular canal (PSC). Intraoperative observations of particulate matter in the PSC in some patients with BPPV support this hypothesis.[1] Positional changes cause movement of the otoconia within the canal, which in turn produces endolymph currents that deform the cupula and cause vertigo. BPPV is usually idiopathic, but may also begin after head trauma or vestibular neuritis. Patients often complain of sudden, short-lived severe vertigo related to changes in head position, particularly when going to, rolling over in, or arising out of bed.

A variant of the theory of pathogenesis of BPPV holds that these detached crystals adhere to either the gelatinous cupula of the crista ampullaris ("cupulolithiasis"). A competing theory is that there is loss of inhibitory input from the damaged otoliths.[2] Also, magnetic resonance imaging (MRI) of patients with permanent or "atypical" BPPV has shown fractures or filling defects in the semicircular canals that are not seen in control subjects.[3,4]

Particle repositioning is the mainstay of treatment for BPPV. A recent meta-analysis of nine randomized controlled trials with a total of 505 patients found that canalith repositioning is very effective, while noting that approximately one third of patients experience spontaneous resolution within 3 weeks.[5] The most recent published case series notes that in a practice with more than 3000 patients evaluated and treated for BPPV over a 7-year period, less than 1% of patients required surgical intervention.[6]

For the small subset of patients with intractable and multiply recurrent BPPV, occlusion of the PSC is offered (PSCO). Success rates for PSCO, as defined by significant relief of symptoms, are greater than 90% in most, if not all, series. Postoperative sequelae commonly include unsteadiness that may persist for only a few weeks to more than a year, and occasionally sensorineural hearing loss (SNHL), which some authors attribute to comorbidities (e.g., coexisting Meniere's disease and previous otologic surgery). Division of the singular nerve (singular neurectomy) that innervates the PSC is no longer performed for BPPV. Preoperatively, the patient should undergo an enhanced MRI scan of the internal auditory canals to evaluate for the rare presence of a retrocochlear lesion that may present with BPPV symptoms.[7]

Meniere's Disease

Meniere's disease is the traditional term for idiopathic symptomatic endolymphatic hydrops. Some authorities describe the classic constellation of symptoms—fluctuating hearing loss, vertigo, a sensation of aural fullness and/or tinnitus—as *Meniere's syndrome* and reserve the term *Meniere's disease* for the idiopathic form, because the symptom complex may also result from, for example, an infectious etiology such as syphilis.[8] The aural symptoms typically make localization self evident for the patient and physician, but the physician must elicit a directed and detailed history to narrow the differential diagnosis. The natural history of the disease varies greatly. A number of studies report long-term follow-up that seems to indicate some cases of Meniere's progressively worsen, whereas others stabilize. A number of longitudinal studies have noted progression to bilateral disease in one third or more of patients, increasing as the disease progresses.

The majority of patients with Meniere's disease experience control of vestibular symptoms with medical treatment alone, although hearing loss generally progresses with time. This includes a combination of dietary salt and caffeine restriction, and diuretic therapy (Dyazide). Other medications used with some success in Meniere's disease include vasodilators, histamines, and steroids. When a 6-month trial of medical therapy fails to adequately control vertigo attacks, treatment options include surgery, intratympanic steroid or gentamicin therapy, and use of the Meniett device. The indications and techniques for intratympanic therapy

are discussed in Chapter 107. All of these invasive treatment options aim to control the vertigo attacks only. Relief of tinnitus and aural fullness, and hearing stabilization or recovery is not consistently achieved. Surgical options for Meniere's disease include endolymphatic sac surgery, labyrinthectomy, and vestibular nerve section.

Endolymphatic sac surgery for Meniere's disease remains controversial. Surgery theoretically modulates endolymphatic sac function enough to control vertigo in approximately 60% of patients. The risk of additional hearing loss with sac surgery is minimal. Decompression alone is indicated for Meniere's disease in an only hearing ear because the theoretical risk of hearing loss is less compared with decompression with opening of the endolymphatic sac for shunt placement. One well-known randomized controlled trial comparing endolymphatic shunt placement with cortical mastoidectomy failed to show any therapeutic benefit of shunt surgery over mastoidectomy alone.[9] Subsequent statistical analyses of the same data set argue that the results support the efficacy of the shunt and do not support the placebo effect claimed by the original authors.[10] A subsequent randomized controlled study performed by Thomsen and colleagues compared shunt surgery with insertion of a tympanostomy tube and again failed to demonstrate any advantage to shunt surgery.[11]

Vestibular nerve section denervates the vestibular end organ with a small risk of additional hearing loss. Vertigo control for Meniere's disease alone using this procedure is greater than 90%. There are three surgical approaches for this procedure: retrolabyrinthine, middle fossa, and translabyrinthine. The retrolabyrinthine approach is the preferred approach for a hearing ear. The middle fossa approach is reserved for hearing patients with persistent vertigo following a retrolabyrinthine nerve section due to the presence of persistent vestibular nerve fibers in the distal internal auditory canal.

Labyrinthectomy involves surgical removal of the sensory epithelium of all five vestibular end organs and results in the loss of input to the central nervous system. The absence of this input facilitates better central compensation, as compared to aberrant input from an improperly functioning organ.[12] The procedure is offered only to patients with unilateral Meniere's disease and no useful residual hearing in the affected ear. Vertigo control is greater than 90%, although all residual hearing in the operated ear is sacrificed. For rare residual symptoms after labyrinthectomy, translabyrinthine vestibular neurectomy can be performed.

Surgery for Uncompensated Peripheral Vestibulopathy

Uncompensated unilateral peripheral vestibulopathy causes long-term persistence of disequilibrium and dizziness following a unilateral peripheral vestibular insult. Most cases result from trauma, Meniere's disease, and vestibular neuritis. Despite vestibular rehabilitation therapy, these patients continue to experience disabling symptoms. Some patients develop concurrent or subsequent BPPV, which can usually be treated successfully with repositioning.[13] For patients with ongoing symptoms beyond the inciting episode who do not respond adequately to medical management and vestibular rehabilitation, vestibular ablation of the affected ear should be considered. Treatment options include chemical ablation with intratympanic gentamicin therapy, vestibular neurectomy, and labyrinthectomy, as described for Meniere's disease.

Surgery for Superior Canal Dehiscence Syndrome

In 1998, Minor described a new syndrome with vertigo induced by sound (Tullio's phenomenon) or aural pressure (Hennebert's sign), and computed tomography (CT) evidence of dehiscent bone over the superior semicircular canal (SSC).[14] Valsalva maneuvers, sneezing, and other activities that increase intracranial pressure may produce vertigo. Office pneumatic otoscopy should elicit upward eye movement in the plane of the SSC. If elicited, this provides sufficient clinical suspicion to proceed with a high-resolution CT scan of the temporal bone. Additional testing may include vestibular evoked myogenic potentials (VEMPs), measured via contractions of the tonically active sternocleidomastoid muscle to loud click noises presented in the ipsilateral ear. Audiometric testing in these patients may show a conductive hearing loss with intact stapedial reflexes resulting from an inner ear conductive loss created by the dehiscent SSC segment behaving as a "third window."

Diagnosis of SCDS is confirmed on high-resolution CT imaging of the temporal bone in the coronal plane using a bone algorithm (Fig. 131-1). There is no advantage to additional Stenver and Pöschl views on CT imaging, which are digitally reformatted in planes perpendicular and parallel to the SSC, respectively.[15] One recent retrospective review evaluating radiologic findings alone in more than 400 temporal bone CT scans found evidence of a dehiscent-appearing SSC in 9% of studies, indicating a high sensitivity but low specificity for imaging in SCDS, given the apparent rarity of the clinical syndrome.[16]

Repair of the bony defect over the SSC may be offered for relief of severe and disabling noise- and pressure-induced vertigo. The SSC is surgically accessed through a middle fossa approach. The SSC is either plugged using a technique analogous to that used for posterior canal occlusion in BPPV, or the dehiscent canal is covered with a combination of fascia, bone, and fibrinogen glue. Minor reported a case series of 20 surgical repairs and found resolution of symptoms in 8 of 9 patients treated with plugging and 9 of 11 patients treated with capping without plugging.[17]

PREOPERATIVE PLANNING

Following a complete medical evaluation, the patient's vestibular complaints can usually be localized to the

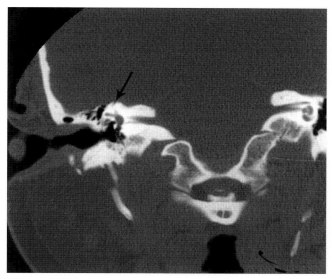

Figure 131-1. Coronal computed tomography of temporal bone showing dehiscence of superior semicircular canal *(arrow).*

central or peripheral vestibular organs. In the case of peripheral vestibular disease, when a reasonable trial of medical therapy fails to control vertigo and the patient is significantly disabled as a result of ongoing vestibular symptoms, the options for surgery and chemical ablation of the vestibular labyrinth should be discussed. The risks, complications, alternatives, and expected results of each procedure appropriate for the clinical situation are discussed with the patient.

A gadolinium-enhanced MRI scan of the brain and internal auditory canals is obtained as part of the initial diagnostic evaluation to exclude the presence of a retrocochlear or intracranial tumor. Additional CT imaging of the temporal bone as described earlier is obtained if there is clinical suspicion of SCDS. Vestibular function testing is used to localize the side of vestibular impairment and diagnose significant bilateral peripheral vestibular hypofunction or central vestibular dysfunction. The presence of bilateral or central vestibular dysfunction may significantly impair postoperative vestibular compensation and should therefore be taken into consideration when determining candidacy for vestibular ablation. The mobility and quality of life in older individuals with preexisting disequilibrium are severely impacted following any ablative procedure.

Preoperative hearing assessment is critical in selecting the appropriate surgical procedure and approach for each individual. Functional hearing is typically defined as a pure tone average of 50 dB or better and a word recognition score of 50% or better. These scores are used as general guidelines rather than absolute criteria for hearing preservation in vestibular surgery. The inability to perceive benefit from conventional amplification in the affected ear serves as an indicator of poor functional hearing in that ear. The hearing status of the contralateral ear is also assessed preoperatively. If treatment is being offered for an only-hearing ear, conservatism is the preferred approach.

SURGICAL APPROACHES

Posterior Semicircular Canal Occlusion

The patient is positioned and prepped as for standard mastoid surgery. Facial nerve monitoring is not routinely used. Broad-spectrum antibiotics may be administered intravenously at induction of general anesthesia. Through a standard postauricular approach, the surgeon performs a limited cortical mastoidectomy to expose the mastoid antrum and lateral semicircular canal (LSC) in the usual fashion. A saline-soaked Gelfoam pledget is placed into the aditus ad antrum to reduce the amount of blood and bone dust that enter the middle ear space. The PSC lies posterior and perpendicular to the LSC. The surgeon uses a small diamond burr to skeletonize and blue-line the PSC. A 1- × 3-mm oval window of bone over the mid portion of the PSC is then carefully thinned using a small diamond burr without violating the membranous labyrinth. The lumen of the PSC may be occluded using bone wax,[18] bone paste (bone dust mixed with fibrinogen glue),[19] or soft tissue (Fig. 131-2). The selected material should be prepared and ready for application before exposure of the membranous labyrinth. Bone dust and bone wax are applied to the PSC on the back of a duckbill elevator (see Video 131-1). Suction should not be applied to the opened canal because this may disrupt the membranous labyrinth and cause SNHL. After occlusion of the canal, the PSC defect may be covered with fascia, additional bone paste, and/or autologous blood. The surgical site is then closed in a layered fashion as described in Chapter 115.

Most published reports describe mechanical plugging as the mainstay of PSCO. The CO_2 laser may also be used for ablation of the membranous labyrinth as an adjunct to mechanical plugging of the PSC.[20] Either technique should prevent circulation of endolymph within the occluded membranous PSC and relieve the disabling symptoms of BPPV.

Endolymphatic Sac Decompression or Shunt

The patient is positioned and prepped as for standard mastoid surgery. Facial nerve monitoring is routinely used. Perioperative antibiotics are not routinely administered. A postauricular incision is made approximately 1 to 2 cm posterior to a standard postauricular incision for mastoid surgery because such an incision may be used in the future to perform a retrolabyrinthine nerve section for patients with persistent vertigo following endolymphatic sac surgery. A complete mastoidectomy is then performed. The mastoid antrum is entered and the LSC is identified. The sigmoid sinus is then skeletonized down to the proximal jugular bulb (Fig. 131-3). A saline-soaked Gelfoam pledget is placed into the aditus ad antrum to reduce the amount of blood and bone dust that enter the middle ear space.

The endolymphatic sac lies deep to the posterior fossa bone plate, between the PSC and the sigmoid sinus. It is consistently inferior to "Donaldson's line," an imaginary line extending posteriorly from the plane of the LSC. The vertical facial nerve is identified, using the LSC as a landmark, and skeletonized, as is the PSC, before opening the retrofacial air cells between the facial nerve laterally and the posterior fossa plate medially. The retrolabyrinthine air cell tract over the posterior fossa plate leads to the junction of the PSC and the posterior fossa dura, and removal of these air cells expose the operculum of the vestibular aqueduct (Fig. 131-4). Opening the retrofacial air cell tract exposes the junction of the ampullated limb of the posterior semicircular canal and posterior fossa plate overlying the endolymphatic sac.

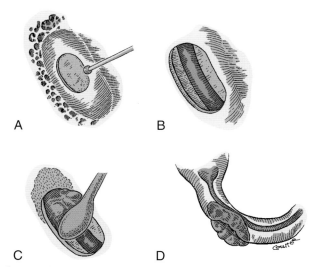

Figure 131-2. Technique for posterior semicircular canal (PSC). **A,** Skeletonization of midportion of PSC using small diamond burr. **B,** PSC fenestrated without violating membranous labyrinth. **C,** Bone wax, bone paste, or soft tissue is applied to the fenestrated portion of the PSC using a duckbill elevator. **D,** The membranous labyrinth within the PSC is compressed and occluded.

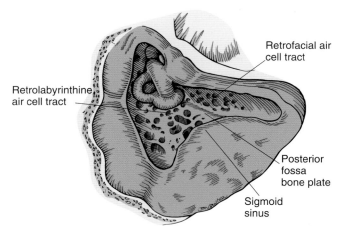

Figure 131-3. Complete mastoidectomy with skeletonization of the posterior semicircular canal, retrolabyrinthine and retrofacial air cells, sigmoid sinus, jugular bulb, and posterior fossa bone plate.

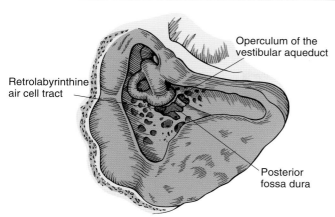

Figure 131-4. The retrolabyrinthine air cell tract is opened, leading to the junction of the posterior semicircular canal and the posterior fossa dura near the operculum of the vestibular aqueduct.

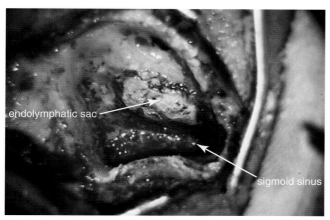

Figure 131-5. The dura of the posterior fossa is widely exposed. The endolymphatic sac is visible as a thickening of the dura fanning out from the posterior semicircular canal to the sigmoid sinus.

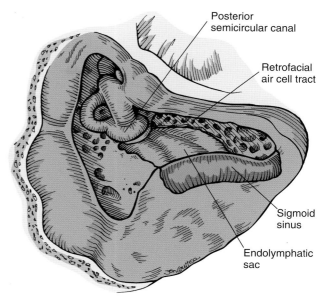

Figure 131-6. Location of the endolymphatic sac between the posterior semicircular canal and sigmoid sinus.

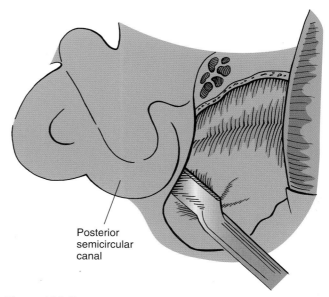

Figure 131-7. The dura medial to the posterior semicircular canal is palpated to define the operculum and endolymphatic duct.

Once the posterior fossa plate has been thinned to an eggshell thickness from the anterior border of the sigmoid sinus to the PSC, the thin remaining bone over the dura is removed using a Freer elevator or a large diamond burr to widely expose the endolymphatic sac (Fig. 131-5). The sac appears as a fan-shaped thickening of the dura spreading out from just deep to the PSC, posterolaterally toward the sigmoid sinus (Fig. 131-6). The dura medial to the PSC can be palpated to define the operculum and endolymphatic duct (Fig. 131-7).

At this point, decompression of the sac is complete and if shunting is not planned, the surgical wound is closed in a standard layered fashion. To open the endolymphatic sac, the surgeon carefully incises the lateral wall of the sac in a radial direction using a Beaver no. 5940 blade from the sigmoid sinus toward the operculum (Fig. 131-8). The medial and lateral walls of the sac are bluntly separated using an annulus elevator (Fig. 131-9). To place a shunt, the surgeon inserts a small piece of 0.005-inch thick silastic sheeting into the lumen of the sac (Fig. 131-10). The wound is then closed in

the standard layered fashion for mastoid surgery and a mastoid dressing is applied for 24 hours.

Surgical Labyrinthectomy

For the patient with disabling vertigo or disequilibrium resulting from a unilateral peripheral vestibulopathy and with no useful hearing in the affected ear, vestibular ablation is the treatment of choice. This may be done chemically using intratympanic gentamicin or surgically through a standard transmastoid approach. The neurosensory epithelium of the vestibular labyrinth is systematically and completely removed. This reliably

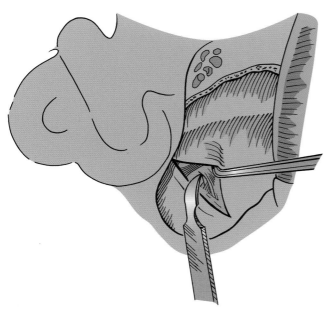

Figure 131-8. The lateral wall of the endolymphatic sac is incised.

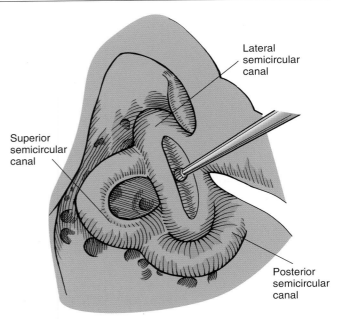

Figure 131-11. The superior wall of the lateral semicircular canal is removed. The inferior wall is left intact to protect the facial nerve.

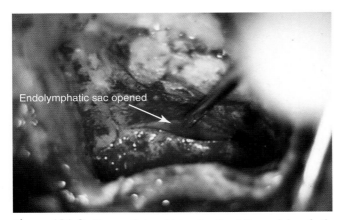

Figure 131-9. The medial and lateral walls of the endolymphatic sac are bluntly separated.

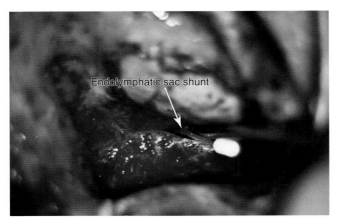

Figure 131-10. A silastic shunt is inserted in the lumen of the endolymphatic sac.

controls vertigo in most patients, but moderate to severe postoperative disequilibrium may necessitate a course of vestibular rehabilitation therapy to facilitate central vestibular compensation.

A transmastoid labyrinthectomy begins with a complete mastoidectomy through a standard postauricular incision, with intraoperative facial nerve monitoring. Perioperative antibiotics are not routinely administered for this procedure. Once the mastoid antrum is entered medially, the LSC is identified and drilling is continued anteriorly into the epitympanum until the body of the incus is identified. The perilabyrinthine air cells are carefully removed to expose all three semicircular canals. The surgeon should identify the course of the tympanic and mastoid segments of the facial nerve, but need not skeletonize it.

The semicircular canals are then opened sequentially to maintain surgical orientation of the canals during the labyrinthectomy. Using a 3-mm cutting burr and copious suction irrigation, the LSC is fenestrated superiorly along its entire length, beginning at the ampullated end and progressing posteriorly toward the PSC (Fig. 131-11). The inferior wall of the LSC protects the second genu of the facial nerve and should be left intact. The PSC is then fenestrated using the same size drill burr. Dissection is continued inferiorly and anteriorly under the facial nerve to expose the ampulla of the PSC. The inferior wall of the PSC should be left intact because it protects a high-riding jugular bulb. The PSC is then followed superiorly to the common crus, which will lead to the SSC. The SSC lies perpendicular to both the LSC and the PSC, on a deeper plane, and is carefully dissected in a posterior to anterior direction toward the ampulla (Fig. 131-12). Care is taken not to violate

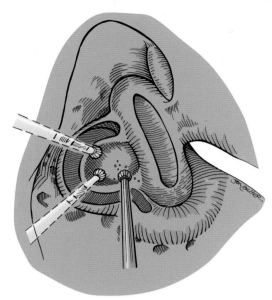

Figure 131-12. The common crus and superior semicircular canal are fenestrated from a posterior to anterior direction toward the superior semicircular canal ampulla.

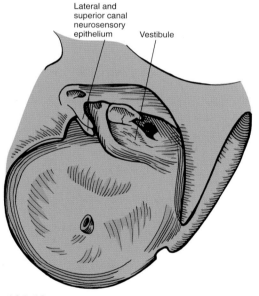

Figure 131-13. The neurosensory epithelium of the superior and lateral semicircular canal ampullae is exposed, the vestibule is opened, and the posterior semicircular canal is followed inferiorly to expose its ampulla.

the tegmen mastoideum and middle fossa dura during this portion of the bony dissection.

Anteriorly, the neurosensory epithelium of the superior and lateral ampullae is exposed and the vestibule is opened (Fig. 131-13). The medial wall of the superior and lateral ampullae should be left intact to prevent exposure of the internal auditory canal and facial nerve, cerebrospinal leak, and facial paralysis.

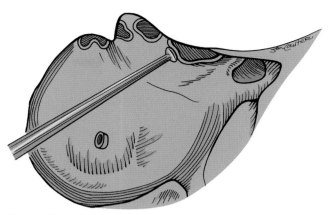

Figure 131-14. The five areas of neurosensory epithelium are exposed and removed systematically using a round knife or microcurette.

Once all five portions of neurosensory epithelium are exposed (the ampullae of the three semicircular canals, the utricle, and the saccule), each is removed systematically with a round knife or microcurette, taking care not to rupture the underlying bony cribrosa (Fig. 131-14). The area is inspected for cerebrospinal fluid leak. If there is no cerebrospinal fluid leak, closure of the surgical site proceeds in a layered fashion as for standard mastoid surgery. If a cerebrospinal fluid leak is detected, a free abdominal fat graft is used to obliterate the mastoid cavity. A mastoid dressing is applied over the ear for 24 hours.

Translabyrinthine Approach for Vestibular Nerve Section

This procedure is reserved for the rare patient who continues to experience disabling vestibular symptoms following a surgical labyrinthectomy. The goal is to remove Scarpa's ganglion with additional exposure of the internal auditory canal after the labyrinthectomy has been completed. This procedure carries an increased risk of facial nerve injury and cerebrospinal fluid leak compared with labyrinthectomy alone.

The preparation and surgical exposure for this procedure are as described for a transmastoid labyrinthectomy. Intraoperative facial nerve monitoring is routinely employed. Broad-spectrum antibiotics are administered intravenously at the time of induction of general anesthesia. A labyrinthectomy is completed as described above. The lateral one half of the internal auditory canal is then skeletonized using medium-sized diamond burrs and copious suction irrigation. The superior limit of the internal auditory canal is marked by the ampulla of the SSC, which is innervated by the superior vestibular nerve. The dura of the lateral internal auditory canal is exposed and the facial nerve is identified and electrically stimulated anterosuperiorly as it exits the internal auditory canal into the labyrinthine segment. At the fundus of the internal auditory canal, a vertical crest of bone (Bill's bar) separates the facial nerve anteriorly from the superior vestibular nerve posteriorly, and a

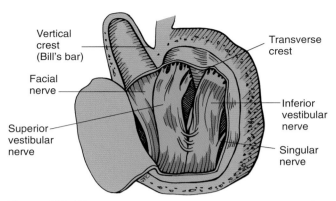

Figure 131-15. The transverse crest and Bill's bar are exposed at the fundus of the internal auditory canal. The dura of the internal auditory canal is opened. The facial, superior vestibular, inferior vestibular, and singular nerves are identified.

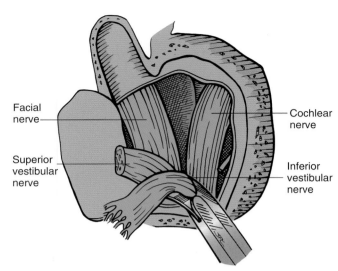

Figure 131-16. A segment of the vestibular nerve is resected.

transverse crest separates the superior vestibular nerve from the inferior vestibular nerve.

Dura along the posterior aspect of the internal auditory canal is incised, and superior and inferior dural flaps are developed to expose the contents of the internal auditory canal (Fig. 131-15). The superior vestibular nerve is then separated from the facial nerve from a lateral to medial direction using a blunt dissector. A 3- to 5-mm length of the superior vestibular nerve is resected. Similarly, the inferior vestibular nerve is separated from the cochlear nerve anteriorly by gentle blunt dissection from a medial to lateral direction to minimize traction on the cochlear nerve. A short segment of the inferior vestibular nerve is also resected (Fig. 131-16). The singular nerve is specifically identified and divided.

Once the nerve section is complete, the dura of the internal auditory canal is reopposed. In a well-aerated temporal bone with a large aditus ad antrum, the incus should be removed so that the eustachian tube and middle ear can be packed with temporalis muscle. The mastoid cavity is obliterated with free abdominal fat grafts. A watertight multilayer closure is then completed using a combination of absorbable and nonabsorbable sutures. A compressive mastoid dressing is applied for 3 days. The patient is discharged home on postoperative day 4 if no cerebrospinal fluid leak is apparent.

Posterior Fossa Approaches for Vestibular Nerve Section

The vestibular nerve may be exposed within the posterior fossa with an approach through the mastoid (retrolabyrinthine/presigmoid) or through a retromastoid/retrosigmoid craniotomy (retrosigmoid approach). Both approaches preserve hearing in the operated ear.

The posterior fossa approaches for vestibular nerve section are popular because they provide consistent and direct exposure of the cerebellopontine angle and expose the cochleovestibular and facial nerves between the porus of the internal auditory canal and the brain stem. Using these approaches, the facial nerve is easily identified anterior to the cochleovestibular nerve, and inadvertent injury to the facial nerve is uncommon.

The primary disadvantage of these approaches is that the vestibular nerve is exposed where the vestibular portion of the cochleovestibular nerve is not anatomically separate from the cochlear portion. Thus, location and division of the vestibular nerve must be based on the surgeon's knowledge of the anatomy of the cochleovestibular nerve. The presence of small blood vessels, which tend to demarcate the cochlear and vestibular nerve fibers, and subtle color differences between the two types of nerve fibers aid the surgeon in determining the plane between the vestibular versus cochlear nerve. Although there is a possibility of leaving some vestibular fibers uncut, the high rates reported for the control of vertigo suggest that leaving a few vestibular fibers uncut may be of limited clinical significance.

Retrolabyrinthine Approach for Vestibular Nerve Section

The patient is positioned supine with the head turned away from the surgeon. The ear is prepped and draped as for standard neuro-otologic surgery. Intraoperative facial nerve and evoked auditory brain stem responses are monitored routinely. A single dose of antibiotic is administered at the time of induction of general anesthesia. A wide C-shaped incision is made approximately 3 cm posterior to the postauricular crease and extended down to the temporalis fascia superiorly and mastoid periosteum inferiorly. Skin and subcutaneous tissue are then elevated in the subcutaneous plane anteriorly. The temporalis muscle and fascia and the periosteum are incised with an offset incision to allow for a good layered wound closure at the end of the proce-

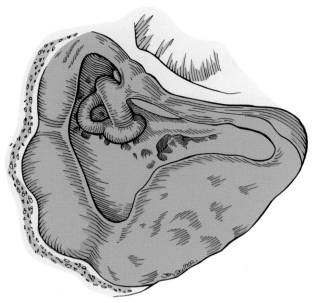

Figure 131-17. The mastoidectomy is completed by skeletonizing the semicircular canals and the bony plate overlying the posterior fossa dura.

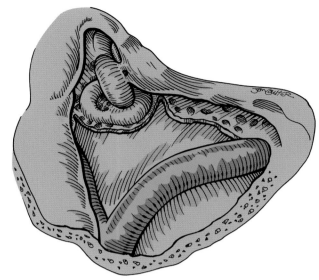

Figure 131-18. Dura overlying the posterior fossa and sigmoid sinus is exposed.

dure to prevent or contain cerebrospinal fluid leaks through the incision. An anteriorly based musculoperiosteal flap is then elevated to expose the mastoid cortex and secured in place with a large self-retaining retractor.

A complete mastoidectomy is performed and exposure down to the mastoid antrum allows for identification of the LSC. Bone overlying the middle fossa dura, sigmoid sinus, and posterior fossa dura is carefully removed using a large diamond burr. The vestibular labyrinth is exposed; particular attention is directed to fully skeletonizing the posterior semicircular canal (Fig. 131-17). Gelfoam is used to block the aditus ad antrum. The remaining bone over the posterior fossa dura between the sigmoid sinus and PSC is then removed with a Freer elevator or similar blunt dissector (Fig. 131-18). The endolymphatic sac and duct are preserved. The mastoid cavity is thoroughly irrigated with Bacitracin solution (Bacitracin 50,000 units/L of saline) once all bone dissection has been completed.

The dura anterior to the sigmoid is incised, creating an anteriorly based C- or U-shaped dural flap (Fig. 131-19). A $\frac{1}{2}$- × 3-cm neurosurgical cottonoid patty is placed over the cerebellum (Fig. 131-20). Cerebrospinal fluid is drained from the cerebellopontine cistern by opening the arachnoid in this location. The cerebellum falls away, allowing visualization of cranial nerves (CN) VII and VIII, centered within the field, with CN V anteromedially and CN IX, X, and XI laterally and inferiorly (Fig. 131-21).

Under high magnification, the courses of CN VII and CN VIII are examined and confirmed using electrical stimulation of CN VII (Fig. 131-22). Any small vessels intimately associated with CN VIII are gently dissected

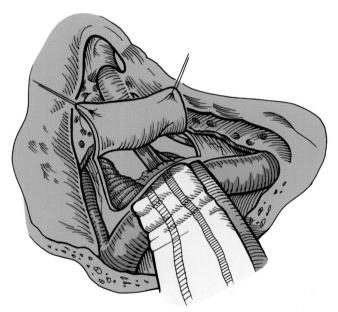

Figure 131-19. An anteriorly based U-shaped dural flap is developed, and the contents of the posterior fossa are exposed.

off the nerve. A surgical plane is then developed between the cochlear and vestibular portions of CN VIII. A recent cadaver study found that in an average of 75% of cases, the surgeon could visually identify a cleavage plane within the vestibulocochlear nerve near the porus acusticus, or develop it near that point with a ball-tipped dissector.[21] The vestibular division of CN VIII typically appears grayer than the cochlear division, which appears whiter. Often a minute blood vessel lies along this cleavage plane (Fig. 131-23). The vestibulocochlear nerve also rotates approximately 90 degrees as it passes from

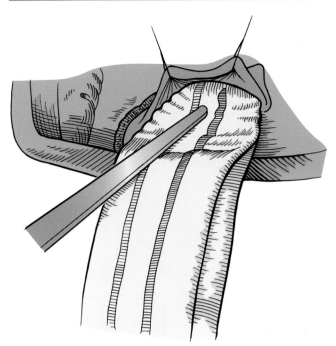

Figure 131-20. A ¹/₂- × 3-cm neurosurgical cottonoid patty is advanced between the anterior edge of the dura and the surface of the cerebellum.

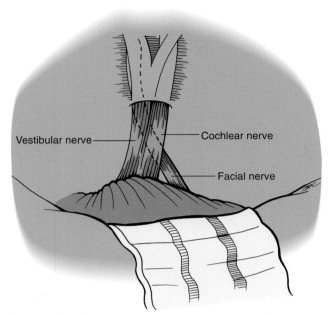

Figure 131-22. Anatomic relationships of the vestibular nerve, cochlear nerve, and facial nerve.

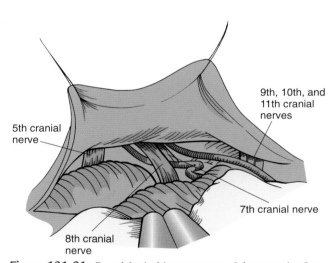

Figure 131-21. Retrolabyrinthine exposure of the posterior fossa.

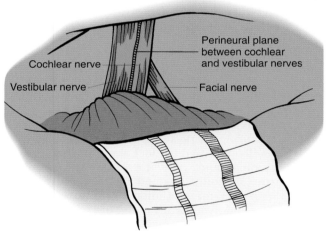

Figure 131-23. A perineural plane between the cochlear and vestibular nerves is frequently demonstrated by a small vessel or a slight depression in the nerve running longitudinally on the dorsal surface of the nerve.

the lateral internal auditory canal back toward the porus and brain stem, in a counterclockwise direction on the right side as viewed from the medial porus, and correspondingly clockwise on the left side.[22] Near the brain stem, the vestibular portion of CN VIII is usually more superior (closer to the tentorium); near the porus, it is usually superior or dorsal.

If a clear plane of demarcation can be identified, a no. 1 Roton dissector is used to separate the cochlear and vestibular divisions along this plane (Fig. 131-24). A bayoneted curved microscissors is then used to cut

the vestibular division of the eighth nerve starting from the superior-dorsal surface of the nerve (Fig. 131-25). The nervus intermedius commonly adheres to the ventral surface of the eighth nerve near the junction of the vestibular and cochlear divisions. The nervus intermedius is identified by its whiter appearance and can be traced back to the brain stem coursing between the seventh and eighth cranial nerves. Electrical stimulation of the nervus intermedius will excite the facial nerve but at a higher threshold than will direct stimula-

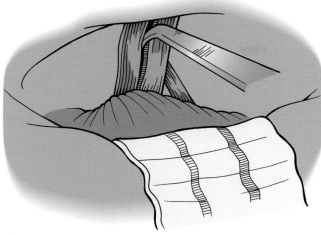

Figure 131-24. Separation of the cochlear and vestibular nerves.

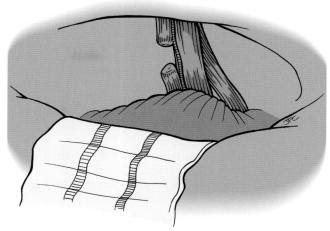

Figure 131-26. The completed vestibular nerve section.

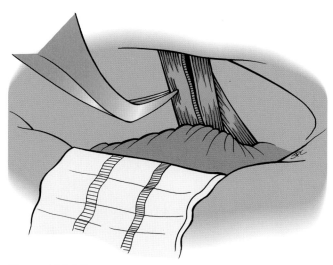

Figure 131-25. The vestibular nerve is divided starting from the superior-dorsal surface of the eighth cranial nerve.

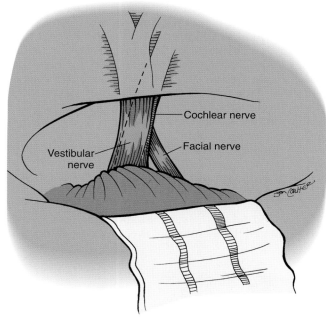

Figure 131-27. If a clear plane is not observed between the vestibular and cochlear nerves, the vestibular nerve is usually dorsal to the cochlear nerve.

tion of the facial nerve. To complete sectioning of the vestibular division, the eighth nerve is sectioned to the level of the nervus intermedius. The surgeon completes the neurectomy with removal of a 5- to 10-mm segment of nerve (Fig. 131-26).

If the plane of demarcation is not clear, the vestibular division probably has rotated from a superior to a more dorsal relationship to the cochlear division (Fig. 131-27). In this situation, a bayoneted, curved microscissors is used to begin the nerve section starting from the superior-dorsal margin of the nerve. A no. 3 Roton dissector is then used to dissect the cut fibers toward the brain stem. Additional fibers are then divided with microscissors and dissected medially. This technique is continued until the cochlear division and nervus intermedius are identified by color changes and perineural tissue planes appear.

After completion of the neurectomy, the neurosurgical patty is removed and hemostasis is secured. Dura is reapproximated with interrupted 4-0 Surgilon. Postoperative cerebrospinal fluid leak is prevented by packing the aditus ad antrum with a temporalis muscle graft and the mastoid cavity with free abdominal fat grafts. Layered wound closure is accomplished in the standard fashion, with additional skin closure using 4-0 nylon. A compressive mastoid dressing is then applied for 72 hours.

Retrosigmoid Approach for Vestibular Nerve Section

For a retrosigmoid vestibular nerve section, the patient is placed in a supine position, and a Mayfield head holder and pins are used to secure the head. A soft roll is placed under the ipsilateral shoulder, and the head is positioned in a 45-degree contralateral rotation and slight downward inclination. The bed is further rotated away to the contralateral side to optimize the angle of exposure of the posterior fossa (Fig. 131-28).

Intraoperative facial nerve and evoked brain stem audiometry monitoring is always used. Perioperative antibiotics are used for 24 hours, and dexamethasone (Decadron 10 mg) is given at the time of surgery. The anesthetist is instructed to keep the patient's PCO_2 below 30 mm Hg and to infuse 0.3 to 0.5 g/kg of mannitol at the beginning of the case to lower intracranial pressure.

An oblique linear skin incision is made approximately 4 cm behind the mastoid tip and angled anteriorly and superiorly for 5 cm (Fig. 131-29). Typically, the epidermis is incised with a knife, and cutting cautery is used to divide the dermis and subcutaneous tissues. The subcutaneous dissection is carried first posteriorly then medially down to the bony cranium. The subcutaneous tissues and deep musculature overlying the retromastoid cranium are elevated forward via a combination of blunt dissection and electrocautery. The mastoid emissary vein is isolated and divided, and the bony foramen of the vein is occluded with bone wax. The dissection is carried inferiorly until the cranium curves medially near the margin of the foramen magnum. Anteriorly, the posterior insertions of the digastric muscle are released, and superiorly the inferior margin of the temporalis muscle is exposed. Self-retaining retractors are positioned and hemostasis secured.

The courses of the sigmoid and transverse sinuses are estimated by examining the surface anatomy of the mastoid and retromastoid cranium (Fig. 131-30). A high-speed cutting burr is used to outline the posterior margin of the sigmoid sinus and inferior margin of the transverse sinus under magnification. A retrosigmoid craniotomy measuring approximately 2.5×2.5 cm (Fig. 131-31) is performed using a combination of high-speed drills and rongeurs. Before opening the dura, hemostasis is secured and all exposed mastoid air cells are occluded with bone wax. The dura is incised in a manner creating an anteriorly based U-shaped dural flap (Fig. 131-32). Bipolar electrocautery is used for hemostasis. Surgilon 4-0 sutures are placed through the dural flap and used to retract the flap anteriorly.

Exposure of the posterior fossa contents, and identification of and section of the vestibular nerve are then completed in the manner described for the retrolabyrinthine approach. The dura is then closed with 4-0 Surgilon sutures. Small pieces of free abdominal fat graft are placed over the dura in the craniotomy site. The craniotomy is reconstructed by securing the

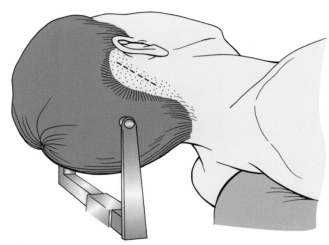

Figure 131-29. The skin incision for a retrosigmoid vestibular nerve section.

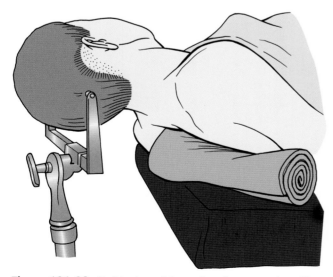

Figure 131-28. Positioning of the patient for a retrosigmoid vestibular nerve section.

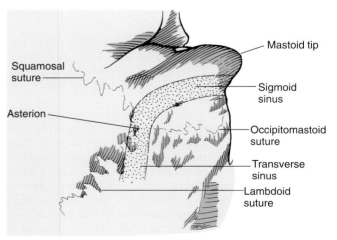

Figure 131-30. The surface anatomy of the mastoid and retrosigmoid cranium, and the estimated course of the transverse and sigmoid sinuses.

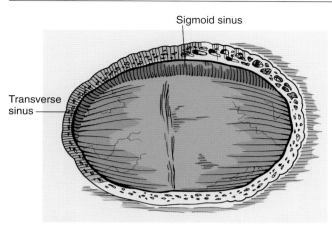

Figure 131-31. The retrosigmoid craniotomy bordered by the sigmoid and transverse sinuses.

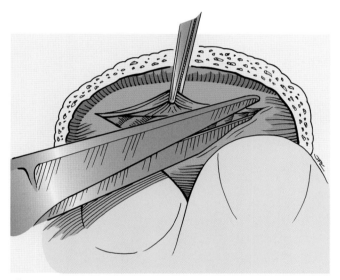

Figure 131-32. Creation of an anteriorly based dural flap with gentle pressure applied on the lateral surface of the cerebellum.

craniotomy flap in place using surgical plates or mesh. The incision is then closed in three layers with a deep layer of 2-0 Vicryl reapproximating the musculoperiosteal tissue over the cranium. The deep cutaneous tissues are closed with 2-0 Vicryl. The skin incision is closed with a running 4-0 nylon stitch, and a light dressing is applied for 24 hours.

Middle Fossa Approach for Vestibular Nerve Section

When hearing is present and the patient suffers from persistent vertigo after a retrolabyrinthine vestibular neurectomy, a middle fossa nerve section may be indicated to divide the vestibular components of CN VIII more distally and maintain hearing in the operated ear. This procedure is rarely used as the primary approach for vestibular nerve section. The advantage of this approach is that it enables visualization of the vestibular nerve where the superior, inferior, and singular nerves

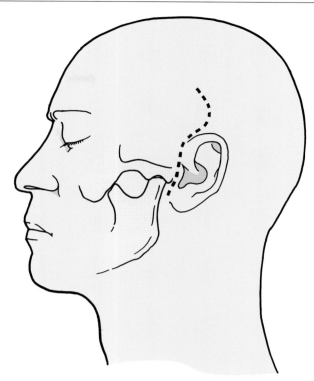

Figure 131-33. Skin incision for a middle fossa craniotomy.

have separated from the cochleovestibular trunk, thus increasing the likelihood of a complete nerve section. This approach is more technically demanding and of necessity involves some retraction of the temporal lobe for an extended period. The risk of facial nerve injury and SNHL is greater than that incurred using the posterior fossa approaches.

The patient is positioned supine with the head turned to the contralateral side so that the operated ear faces up. Intraoperative facial nerve and brain stem evoked audiometry responses are monitored routinely. Broad-spectrum antibiotics are administered intravenously at induction of general anesthesia. Diuretics and steroids are also used to reduce cerebrospinal fluid pressure. An incision is made in the preauricular crease, starting at the level of the lower border of the zygoma and extending superiorly above, behind the auricle to form a reverse-question mark (Fig. 131-33). Anterior and posterior skin flaps lateral to the temporalis fascia are elevated to expose the temporalis muscle. An anteroinferiorly based temporalis muscle flap is created by incising the muscle along the linea temporalis using Bovie electrocautery. A 5- × 5-cm craniotomy, centered two-thirds anterior and one-third posterior to the external auditory canal, and inferiorly based at the root of the zygoma is created using a 4-mm cutting burr (Fig. 131-34). The bone flap is carefully elevated from underlying dura using a dural elevator and soaked in Bacitracin solution until the end of the case. Any bleeding from the dura may be controlled with bipolar electrocautery. The inferior border of the craniotomy is then lowered to the level of the middle fossa floor. Dura is

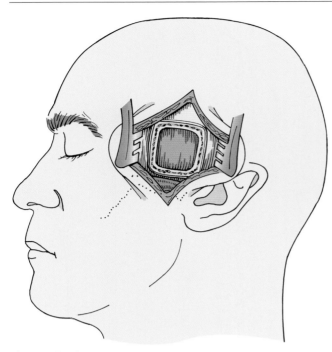

Figure 131-34. Middle fossa craniotomy.

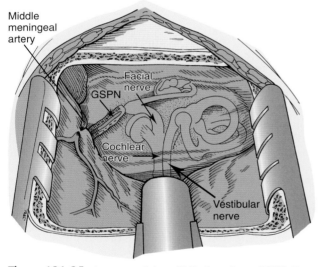

Figure 131-35. Anatomy of the middle fossa floor. GSPN, Greater superficial petrosal nerve.

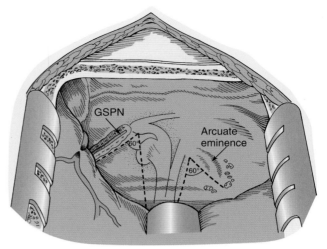

Figure 131-36. Locating the internal auditory canal. GSPN, Greater superficial petrosal nerve.

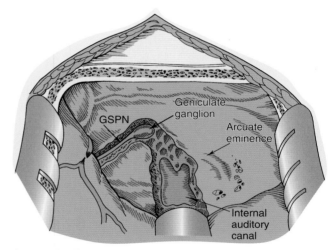

Figure 131-37. Exposure of the internal auditory canal. GSPN, Greater superficial petrosal nerve.

carefully elevated off the middle fossa floor in a posterior to anterior direction to expose the anatomy of the floor of the middle fossa (Fig. 131-35). The limits of exposure are the middle meningeal artery anteriorly, the sulcus of the superior petrosal sinus medially, and the arcuate eminence overlying the dome of the superior semicircular canal posteriorly. Dura over the greater superior petrosal nerve (GSPN) tends to be densely adherent to the nerve. Therefore, great care is needed in dissection at this point due to the possibility of a dehiscent geniculate ganglion. The dura is elevated in a posterior to anterior direction to minimize injury to the GSPN and geniculate ganglion. Once exposure of the middle fossa floor is complete, the tongue of the middle fossa self-retaining retractor is secured at the sulcus of the superior petrosal sinus to retract the temporal lobe.

The floor of the middle fossa is then inspected. Anatomic landmarks to be identified include the GSPN, the geniculate ganglion, and the arcuate eminence overlying the dome of the superior semicircular canal. The location of the internal auditory canal is determined by bisecting the angle formed by the GSPN and arcuate eminence (Fig. 131-36). The roof of the internal auditory canal is first skeletonized over the medial half of the canal. Once the canal has been definitively identified, it may be followed out laterally to the fundus using progressively smaller diamond burrs. At the fundus of the internal auditory canal, the proximity of the basal turn of the cochlea and the ampulla of the SSC limit bony exposure to a 90-degree circumference over the roof of the canal (Fig. 131-37). Bill's bar at the

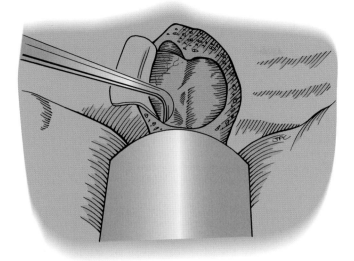

Figure 131-38. The dura of the internal auditory canal is incised.

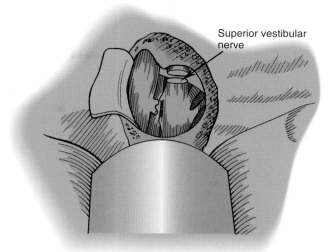

Figure 131-40. The superior vestibular nerve is divided distally.

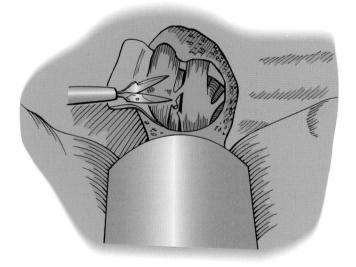

Figure 131-39. Vestibulofacial anastomotic fibers are divided.

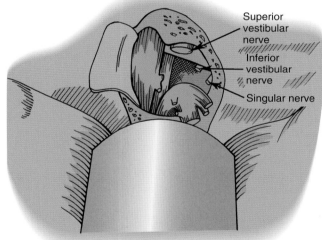

Figure 131-41. The inferior vestibular nerve and the singular nerve are divided distally.

lateral end of the internal auditory canal separates the facial nerve anteriorly from the superior vestibular nerve posteriorly.

Once the dura of the internal auditory canal is exposed, it is incised along the posterior one half of the internal auditory canal (Fig. 131-38). The contents of the canal are identified and the facial nerve course is confirmed using electrical stimulation. Vestibulofacial anastomotic fibers are divided (Fig. 131-39). The superior vestibular nerve is divided laterally and retracted medially to expose the inferior vestibular nerve (Fig. 131-40). The inferior vestibular nerve and the singular nerve are divided (Fig. 131-41). Finally, a segment of nerve containing Scarpa's ganglion is removed with microscissors. Care must be taken not to disrupt any blood vessels in the distal internal auditory canal, or else profound SNHL and facial paralysis can occur.

Once the nerve section is complete, the dural flaps are reopposed and the roof of the internal auditory canal is plugged with a free fat or muscle graft. The temporal lobe is allowed to reexpand over the middle fossa floor. The craniotomy bone plate is replaced. The surgical site is closed in layers to achieve a watertight seal. A light mastoid dressing is placed over the operated ear and kept in place for 24 to 72 hours. The patient is observed in the hospital for 3 to 4 days. Perioperative antibiotics are administered for 24 hours.

Repair of Superior Semicircular Canal Dehiscence Syndrome

Surgical repair of a symptomatic dehiscent SSC is performed using a middle fossa approach, as described above for middle fossa vestibular nerve section. Once the middle fossa floor is exposed and the self-retaining middle fossa retractor placed under the bony petrous ridge, the arcuate eminence is identified. The arcuate eminence corresponds to the SSC in most cases. The dehiscent segment of the SSC is identified and inspected.

We have adopted the practice of both plugging and capping the SSC in each case. A bone paste is made from bone dust from the craniotomy and bone wax, and compressed into the defect to occlude the membranous labyrinth. A split-thickness calvarial bone graft is then fashioned from the middle fossa craniotomy bone flap and placed over the bony defect in the floor of the middle fossa. Any defects laterally along the tegmen should also be either occluded with bone wax or covered with fascia. The temporal lobe is allowed to reexpand over the middle fossa floor after removal of the self-retaining retractor. The craniotomy flap is replaced, and temporalis muscle and skin incision are closed in multiple layers to achieve a watertight seal. A light mastoid dressing is placed over the operated ear and kept in place for 24 to 72 hours. The patient is observed in the hospital for 3 to 4 days. Perioperative antibiotics are administered for 24 hours.

POSTOPERATIVE MANAGEMENT

Most surgical procedures for vertigo will result in varying degrees of postoperative disequilibrium. Vestibular rehabilitation and physical therapy should be instituted early if symptoms are moderate to severe. Additional supportive care during this time includes antiemetic medications, pain control, and intravenous fluids. Nonablative procedures such as endolymphatic sac surgery and PSCO may also result in mild postoperative disequilibrium necessitating overnight observation in the hospital.

All patients undergoing intracranial surgery should receive broad-spectrum antibiotics intravenously for 24 hours. These patients are closely monitored in the postoperative period for potential complications including cerebrospinal fluid leak, meningitis, and intracranial bleeding.

COMPLICATIONS

Complications specific to surgery for vertigo include cerebrospinal fluid leak, meningitis, facial nerve injury, and further hearing loss. Management of postoperative cerebrospinal fluid leaks and iatrogenic facial nerve injuries are discussed elsewhere in this text. Potential risks and complications of each surgical procedure should be discussed with patients during the process of obtaining informed consent for surgery.

Posterior Semicircular Canal Occlusion

SNHL may occur if the vestibule is violated during skeletonization of the PSC. This usually occurs if the PSC is fenestrated too close to its ampulla, rather than midway between the ampulla and the common crus.

Suctioning should be avoided in and around the fenestrated PSC because this may disrupt the membranous labyrinth. Temporary SNHL may result from a serous labyrinthitis. Postoperative SNHL, dizziness, and vertigo may be reduced by minimizing the size of the PSC fenestration and administering perioperative steroids.

Endolymphatic Sac Surgery

Risks specific to this procedure include hearing loss, facial nerve injury, inadvertent fenestration of the PSC, bleeding resulting from trauma to the sigmoid sinus, and cerebrospinal fluid leak resulting from a dural tear. If the PSC is inadvertently fenestrated, the surgeon should avoid suctioning near the membranous labyrinth and immediately plug the defect with bone wax. The facial nerve is at risk for injury in the mastoid segment when skeletonizing the PSC and opening retrofacial air cells. Hearing loss resulting from endolymphatic sac surgery may be conductive or sensorineural in nature. Conductive hearing loss usually occurs as a result of blood in the middle ear after surgery. Delayed conductive hearing loss may occur if trapped bone dust in the middle ear causes bony ankylosis of the ossicular chain. This is prevented by plugging the aditus ad antrum with Gelfoam during the procedure. The posterior fossa dura may be violated when thinning the overlying bone at the time of initial exposure. Additionally, if the endolymphatic sac is not clearly identified, the posterior fossa dura may be mistakenly incised, resulting in cerebrospinal fluid leak. If the dural defect is small, it may be plugged with a small piece of muscle sutured in place with 4-0 Surgilon. A larger dural defect should be repaired with autologous tissue, and the middle ear and mastoid should be obliterated with muscle and fat, respectively, to prevent postoperative cerebrospinal fluid leak. Antibiotics are administered if a leak is detected at the time of surgery.

Labyrinthectomy

Facial nerve injury and cerebrospinal fluid leak may occur during a labyrinthectomy. Knowledge of the normal intratemporal course of the facial nerve is critical in avoiding iatrogenic trauma to the nerve. When the LSC is fenestrated, the inferior wall of the canal should be preserved to protect the second genu of the facial nerve. The ampulla of the PSC is found deep to and under the facial nerve. Drilling should proceed cautiously in this area to expose the neuroepithelial contents of the ampulla without violating the facial nerve. The labyrinthine facial nerve is protected by preserving the medial wall of the SSC and LSC ampullae.

Cerebrospinal fluid leak may occur if the lateral portion of the internal auditory canal is inadvertently opened at the level of the vestibule or if the dura of the posterior or middle fossa are violated. Cerebrospinal fluid leak can be avoided by preserving the medial wall of the vestibule. In addition, the neurosensory epithelium of the inner ear must be removed carefully, or the underlying bony cribrosa that transmits the vestibular nerve axons can be disrupted, causing a cerebrospinal fluid leak. If a cerebrospinal fluid leak occurs, the remaining labyrinthine capsule and mastoid should be obliterated with a free abdominal fat graft. Intravenous antibiotics are started intraoperatively and continued for 24 hours if a leak occurs.

Translabyrinthine Vestibular Nerve Section

Complications of translabyrinthine vestibular nerve section include facial nerve injury and cerebrospinal fluid leak. The risk of facial nerve injury is greater for translabyrinthine vestibular neurectomy than for labyrinthectomy because of the additional risk of facial nerve injury in the internal auditory canal and proximal labyrinthine segment. The facial nerve may be injured during bony exposure of the proximal fallopian canal and dissection of the nerve within the internal auditory canal.

The anterior inferior cerebellar artery may loop deep into the internal auditory canal and can be injured during dissection of the contents of the canal. If bleeding is encountered within the internal auditory canal, the source of bleeding should be clearly identified. Electrocautery should not be generally used within the internal auditory canal because spread of current may injure the facial nerve or anterior inferior cerebellar artery. In this situation, bleeding may be controlled with Surgicel.

Retrolabyrinthine and Retrosigmoid Vestibular Nerve Sections

Potential complications of both approaches include bleeding from a dural sinus, cerebellar edema, facial nerve injury, cochlear nerve injury, intracranial vascular injury, postoperative headache, and cerebrospinal fluid leak.

Trauma to the dural sinuses is best avoided by use of a gentle and patient technique when drilling near the sinuses. Rongeurs are used only after the dura has been freed from the overlying bone with dural elevators. The tip of the rongeur can easily tear a dural sinus if the tip is extended past the area of dura that has been elevated. A tear in the sigmoid sinus or mastoid emissary vein is usually managed by covering the area with Surgicel and applying light pressure. Larger tears may need to be repaired with 4-0 silk, with or without the addition of a small muscle plug.

Injury to the facial nerve is a rare but potential complication because of its proximity to the eighth nerve complex. Injury to the facial nerve is best avoided by clear identification of the nerve before the vestibular nerve section is performed. Electrical stimulation of the facial nerve is recommended to confirm the location and course of the nerve. Occasionally, the facial nerve is adherent to the ventral surface of the eighth nerve and will need to be separated from it before sectioning of the vestibular nerve. The facial nerve should be electrically stimulated at the end of the procedure to confirm its functional integrity. If the nerve does not respond to electrical stimulation, anatomic continuity should be confirmed by direct visualization of the course of the nerve. A transected nerve should be repaired primarily.

Trauma to the cochlear nerve is best avoided by using meticulous surgical technique. The arterial blood supply to the nerve must be maintained. Bipolar cautery near the eighth nerve should be used judiciously.

Headache in the immediate postoperative period may occur from sterile arachnoiditis, elevated intracranial pressure, or meningitis. To reduce the occurrence of sterile arachnoiditis and elevated intracranial pressure, one should use meticulous hemostasis. Dexamethasone is used perioperatively to reduce the severity of early postoperative headache. Retrosigmoid craniotomies should be reconstructed by replacing and securing the bone flap to avoid the development of chronic headaches. If headaches occur and persist, secondary reconstruction of the craniotomy defect, sensory nerve anesthetic block, or sensory nerve section may be required.

Middle Fossa Vestibular Nerve Section

Additional complications encountered with the middle fossa approach include SNHL, vertigo, facial paralysis, intracranial bleeding, and cerebrospinal fluid leak. A thorough knowledge of temporal bone anatomy as visualized from the middle fossa floor is helpful in avoiding iatrogenic trauma to the facial nerve, cochlea, and vestibular labyrinth.

Facial paralysis occurs more frequently with the middle cranial approach than with any other approach for vestibular nerve section. The facial nerve is primarily at risk while one is exposing and working within the internal auditory canal. The dura of the internal auditory should be opened posteriorly, over the superior vestibular nerve. The vestibulofacial anastomoses must be sharply divided to avoid traction injury to the facial nerve.

Temporal lobe edema, contusion, or subdural hematoma may occur from direct injury during the craniotomy or from retraction injury during elevation of the dura overlying the middle cranial fossa. These complications are avoided by taking steps to reduce intracranial pressure at the start of surgery (i.e., reducing Pco_2, intravenous mannitol, and dexamethasone). If the temporal lobe is tight, a small incision in the dura can be made to release cerebrospinal fluid before retraction of the temporal lobe. If temporal lobe injury is suspected, a head CT scan should be performed postoperatively to assess the degree of edema of the temporal lobe, and a neurosurgical colleague should be consulted.

Superior Semicircular Canal Dehiscence Repair

This procedure poses risks similar to those incurred with middle fossa vestibular nerve section. Because the surgeon is intentionally occluding the SSC, there is a risk of SNHL as well, just as in the PSC occlusion procedure.[23]

PEARLS

- Surgery is indicated only for control of disabling vestibular symptoms in patients with peripheral vestibulopathy who have failed medical treatment and vestibular rehabilitation.
- Vestibular ablation is contraindicated in those with bilateral peripheral or central vestibulopathy.
- Chemical vestibular ablation using intratympanic gentamicin has become the preferred primary treatment modality for disabling unilateral peripheral vestibulopathy because the risks of treatment are significantly lower than those incurred with surgical ablation.
- The retrosigmoid and retromastoid approaches are the preferred approaches for vestibular nerve section in patients with aidable hearing in the affected ear.
- The posterior semicircular canal should be fenestrated midway between its ampulla and the common crus for PSCO to minimize the risk of violating the vestibule and causing sensorineural hearing loss.

PITFALLS

- Vestibular ablation in the presence of bilateral peripheral vestibulopathy will result in disabling oscillopsia.
- Suctioning in the vicinity of a fenestrated or dehiscent semicircular canal may result in disruption of the membranous labyrinth and postoperative sensorineural hearing loss.
- Incomplete removal of the sensory neuroepithelium within the posterior semicircular canal ampulla is the most common cause of persistent vertigo following a labyrinthectomy.
- The absence of consistent clear demarcation between the cochlear and vestibular nerves in the cerebellopontine cistern increases the risk of inadvertent injury to the cochlear nerve in posterior fossa approaches for vestibular nerve section.
- Middle fossa approaches necessitate temporal lobe retraction for exposure of the middle fossa floor, which is poorly tolerated in older individuals.

References

1. Welling DB, Parnes LS, O'Brien B, et al: Particulate matter in the posterior semicircular canal. Laryngoscope 107:90-94, 1997.
2. Gacek RR: Pathology of benign paroxysmal positional vertigo revisited. Ann Otol Rhinol Laryngol 112:574-582, 2003.
3. Schratzenstaller B, Wagner-Manslau C, Alexiou C, et al: High-resolution three-dimensional magnetic resonance imaging of the vestibular labyrinth in patients with atypical and intractable benign positional vertigo. ORL J Otorhinolaryngol Relat Spec 63:165-177, 2001.
4. Schratzenstaller B, Wagner-Manslau C, Strasser G, et al: Intractable and atypical benign paroxysmal vertigo. Pathological results of high-resolution three-dimensional MR-tomography of the vestibular organ. HNO 53:1063-1066, 1068-1070, 1072-1063, 2005.
5. White J, Savvides P, Cherian N, et al: Canalith repositioning for benign paroxysmal positional vertigo. Otol Neurotol 26:704-710, 2005.
6. Shaia WT, Zappia JJ, Bojrab DI, et al: Success of posterior semicircular canal occlusion and application of the dizziness handicap inventory. Otolaryngol Head Neck Surg 134:424-430, 2006.
7. Dunniway HM, Welling DB: Intracranial tumors mimicking benign paroxysmal positional vertigo. Otolaryngol Head Neck Surg 118:429-436, 1998.
8. Minor LB, Schessel DA, Carey JP: Ménière's disease. Curr Opin Neurol 17:8-16, 2004.
9. Thomsen J, Bretlau P, Tos M, et al: Placebo effect in surgery for Ménière's disease. A double-blind, placebo-controlled study on endolymphatic sac shunt surgery. Arch Otolaryngol 107:271-277, 1981.
10. Welling DB, Nagaraja HN: Endolymphatic mastoid shunt: A reevaluation of efficacy. Otolaryngol Head Neck Surg 122:340-345, 2000.
11. Thomsen J, Bonding P, Becker B, et al: The non-specific effect of endolymphatic sac surgery in treatment of Ménière's disease: A prospective, randomized controlled study comparing "classic" endolymphatic sac surgery with the insertion of a ventilating tube in the tympanic membrane. Acta Otolaryngol 118:769-773, 1998.
12. Stockwell CM, Graham MD: Vestibular compensation following labyrinthectomy and vestibular neurectomy. Second International Symposium on Ménière's Disease. Kugler & Ghedini Publications, 1989.
13. Goebel JA, Gianoli G: Vestibular neuritis. In Jackler RK, Brackman DE (eds): Neurotology, 2nd ed. Philadelphia, Mosby, 2005, pp 484-488.
14. Minor LB, Solomon D, Zinreich JS, et al: Sound- and/or pressure-induced vertigo due to bone dehiscence of the superior semicircular canal. Arch Otolaryngol Head Neck Surg 124:249-258, 1998.
15. Branstetter BF 4th, Harrigal C, Escott EJ, et al: Superior semicircular canal dehiscence: Oblique reformatted CT images for diagnosis. Radiology 238:938-942, 2006.
16. Williamson RA, Vrabec JT, Coker NJ, et al: Coronal computed tomography prevalence of superior semicircular canal dehiscence. Otolaryngol Head Neck Surg 129:481-489, 2003.
17. Minor LB: Clinical manifestations of superior semicircular canal dehiscence. Laryngoscope 115:1717-1727, 2005.
18. Hirsch BE: Surgical treatment of vestibular disorders. Neurol Clin 23:875-891, viii, 2005.
19. Parnes LS: Posterior semicircular canal occlusion for benign paroxysmal positional vertigo. In Brackmann D, Shelton C, Arriaga M (eds): Otologic Surgery. Philadelphia: WB Saunders, 2001, pp 448-454.
20. Kartush JM, Sargent EW: Posterior semicircular canal occlusion for benign paroxysmal positional vertigo—CO_2 laser-assisted technique: Preliminary results. Laryngoscope 105(3 Pt 1):268-274, 1995.
21. Megerian CA, Hanekamp JS, Cosenza MJ, et al: Selective retrosigmoid vestibular neurectomy without internal auditory canal drill-out: an anatomic study. Otol Neurotol 23:218-223, 2002.
22. Ozdogmus O, Sezen O, Kubilay U, et al: Connections between the facial, vestibular and cochlear nerve bundles within the internal auditory canal. J Anat 205:65-75, 2004.
23. Hillman TA, Kertesz TR, Hadley K, et al: Reversible peripheral vestibulopathy: The treatment of superior canal dehiscence. Otolaryngol Head Neck Surg 134:431-436, 2006.

INDEX

Note: Page numbers followed by f or t indicate figures and tables, respectively.

Auricular reconstruction (*Continued*)
for protuberant ear, 791-797, 792f-795f. *See also* Otoplasty.
for skin cancer, 729, 730f
Auriculotemporal syndrome. *See* Frey's syndrome.
Autoimmune disease
laryngeal stenosis in, 359, 360f
tracheal stenosis in, 604
Autologous material, for vocal fold augmentation/injection, 319, 319t
Avulsion, in facial soft tissue injuries, 874, 876f

B

Baha system, 1209-1217, 1210f. *See also* Hearing aid, bone-anchored.
Baillarger's syndrome. *See* Frey's syndrome.
Ballenger swivel knife, in septoplasty, 21, 22f
Balloon catheter, in endonasal skull base reconstruction, 994
Balloon occlusion test, of internal carotid artery, 1324
Barium esophagography
in cervical esophageal cancer, 475-476, 476f
in Zenker's diverticulum, 461, 461f
Barotrauma, tympanostomy tube placement after, 1126
Basal cell carcinoma
of head and neck, 724, 724f
of lip, 185
Basal cell nevus syndrome, skin cancer in, 721
"Bath plug" graft, for skull defect repair, 134, 134f
Beckwith-Wiedemann syndrome, macroglossia in, 161-162
Belenky-Medina classification of first branchial cleft remnants, 646
Bell's palsy
in facial nerve tumor, 1245
facial paralysis in, 1259
Belmont-Grundfast model of first branchial cleft remnants, 646-647
Benign paroxysmal positional vertigo (BPPV), 1393-1394
Berry's suspensory ligament, transection of, in thyroid lobectomy, 548f, 550
Beta-trace protein (beta₂ transferrin)
in cerebrospinal fluid otorrhea, 1361
in cerebrospinal fluid rhinorrhea, 131, 132, 1054
in perilymphatic fistula, 1221, 1224
Bick procedures, in eye reanimation, 975-976, 976f-977f
Biliary cirrhosis, primary, 491-492
Bill's bar, in acoustic neuroma surgery, 1303, 1303f
Bilobed flap
for nasal reconstruction, 731, 732f
Zitelli's, for nasal skin coverage, 832, 834, 835f
Biofilm
chronic bacterial sinusitis with, 4-5
in otitis media with effusion, 1124
Bioform injection needle, 296
Bioimplantable material, for vocal fold augmentation/injection, 319, 319t

Biopsy
of external auditory canal mass, 1082-1084, 1083f, 1083t
fine-needle. *See* Fine-needle aspiration biopsy (FNAB).
of floor of mouth cancer, 244
of hard palate cancer, 207-208
of infratemporal fossa tumor, 999-1001
of juvenile angiofibroma, 41, 42f
laryngeal, office-based, 300, 300f
of lip cancer, 184
of maxillary sinus tumor, 78
of minor salivary glands of lip, 491-493, 492f-493f
of parotid gland tumor, 513
of sentinel lymph node, 686-687
of skin cancer, 723
of tumor involving nasal cavity and paranasal sinuses, 68
Bipedicled interposition flap, for nasal lining, 826f, 827, 827f-828f
Bite wounds, facial, 874, 875f, 876t, 882f
Blair incision, for superficial lobe parotidectomy, 513, 514f
Bleeding. *See* Hemorrhage.
Blepharoplasty, 857-870
anesthesia for, 858
complications of, 868-869
lower, 861-867
markings for, 864, 864f
pearls and pitfalls in, 869-870
postoperative management of, 867
transconjunctival approach to, 861-864, 862f-864f
transcutaneous approach to, 864-867, 864f-868f
patient selection for, 857
preoperative planning for, 857-858
upper, 858-861
markings for, 858-859, 859f
postoperative management of, 861
surgical technique for, 859-861, 859f-860f
Blepharospasm, 1386, 1386t
Blindness
after blepharoplasty, 869
from orbital emphysema, 141, 142f
Bondy-modified radical mastoidectomy, 1163, 1173, 1173f
Bone graft
for craniofacial skeleton reconstruction, 1064, 1065f
maxillary and alveolar cleft, 787-788, 787f
for middle fossa defect repair, 1373, 1373f
for midline nasal support, 829, 832f
for tegmen defect, 1363, 1363f
Bone invasion, survival and, 256, 258f
Bone-anchored hearing aid. *See* Hearing aid, bone-anchored.
Botulinum toxin injection, 292-295
approaches to, 292-293, 292f
with electromyographic guidance, 294, 295f
for essential voice tremor, 293
for Frey's syndrome, 495, 497-498, 497f
indications for, 291
with laryngoscopic guidance (two-person), 295
pearls and pitfalls in, 300-301

Botulinum toxin injection (*Continued*)
of posterior cricoarytenoid muscle, 294, 295f
postprocedure care/complications of, 299
preoperative planning for, 292, 292f
reconstitution and dilution procedure in, 292
serotypes for, 292
for spasmodic dysphonia, 293
of thyroarytenoid-lateral cricoarytenoid muscle complex, 294, 295f
for upper esophageal sphincter dysfunction, 460
for vocal fold granuloma, 293-294, 294f
Brachial plexus
anatomy of, 683f, 684-685
in radical neck dissection, 694, 694f
Brain abscess, in otitis media, 1235-1236, 1236f
Brainstem auditory evoked responses
in acoustic neuroma, 1299, 1299f
monitoring of, during facial nerve decompression, 1388, 1390
Branchial arch cyst infection, third, 648
Branchial cleft carcinoma, 648-649
Branchial cleft remnants, 645-656
developmental anatomy of, 645
differential diagnosis of, 645
first
description of, 645-647, 647f
excision of, 650-652, 650f, 651f
preauricular
description of, 646, 646f
excision of, 650, 651f
second and third
description of, 647-648, 647f-648f
excision of, 652-653, 652f-655f
surgical excision of
complications of, 653, 655
patient selection for, 648-649, 648f, 649f
pearls and pitfalls in, 655-656
postoperative management after, 653
preoperative planning for, 649-650, 649f
techniques for, 650-653
Bronchoscope(s)
flexible fiberoptic and "chip-tip," 566-567, 568f
rigid, 567-568, 568f
Bronchoscopy, 565-575
anatomic considerations in, 565, 566f
development of, 565-566
equipment for, 566-568, 567f-568f
flexible
equipment for, 566-567, 568f
technique for, 569-570
for foreign body removal, 573-574, 573f, 573t, 574f
in laryngeal carcinoma, 422
patient selection for, 568-569, 569t
rigid
equipment for, 567-568, 568f
technique for, 570-573, 570f-573f
techniques for, 569-574
Brow defect repair, 729
Brow incision, for superior orbital rim fracture repair, 918
Brow ptosis, blepharoplasty and, 857
Brow-lift, in eye reanimation, 974
Bubbles, on computed tomography of maxillary sinus accessory ostia, 52, 52f

Buccal space tumor, 533-538
  anatomic considerations in, 533, 534f
  differential diagnosis of, 534, 534t
  excision of
    complications of, 538
    pearls and pitfalls in, 538
    postoperative management after, 538
    preoperative planning for, 536
    techniques for, 536-538, 537f-538f
  preoperative evaluation of, 533-536,
    535f-536f
Buccogingival incision, 269, 270f. See also
  Gingivobuccal sulcus incision.
Burns
  caustic, laryngeal stenosis after, 358
  facial, 873

C

Cable graft, for facial nerve repair, 521, 521f
Calcification
  of cervical spine, 710, 712f
  in thyroglossal duct cyst, 636, 636f
Calcitonin, in medullary carcinoma, 542
Calcitriol, for hypoparathyroidism, 555
Calcium, administration of, for
  hypocalcemia, 555
Caldwell-Luc procedure. See Antrostomy,
  anterior (Caldwell-Luc procedure).
Canal cholesteatoma. See Cholesteatoma,
  canal.
Canal wall down mastoidectomy, 1163,
  1171-1173, 1172f-1173f
Canal wall up mastoidectomy, 1163,
  1167-1170, 1168f-1170f, 1175-1176
Cancer. See also specific anatomic site and
  neoplasm.
  of cervical esophagus, 473-483
  extracapsular spread of, 679, 680f
  of floor of mouth, 241-252
  of hard palate, 205-215
  of larynx, 379-391
  of lip, 183-193
  of nose, 728
  of oropharynx, 283-289
  periorbital, 727-728
  of skin, 719-736
  of soft palate, 199-202, 200f-202f
  staging of. See Staging.
  of supraglottic larynx, 393-409
  of temporal bone, 1271-1292
  of thyroid gland. See Thyroid cancer.
  of tongue, 217-227
Canine fossa
  anatomy of, 58, 59f
  exposure of, in anterior antrostomy,
    60-61, 61f
Canthal ligament, medial, repositioning of,
  in medial maxillectomy and lateral
  rhinotomy, 71
Canthopexy, lateral transorbital, in eye
  reanimation, 976
Canthotomy, lateral, with inferior
  cantholysis
  for orbital abscess, 140-141, 141f
  in orbital floor fracture repair, 918,
    919f-920f
  for retrobulbar hemorrhage, 139-140, 140f
Carbon dioxide laser, 383. See also Laser
  surgery.

Carcinoma. See also Adenocarcinoma;
  Cancer.
  adenoid cystic, of soft palate, 199
  basal cell
    of head and neck, 724, 724f
    of lip, 185
  branchial cleft, 648-649
  medullary, of thyroid gland, 542
  Merkel cell, of head and neck, 725-726
  papillary, arising in thyroglossal duct cyst,
    636-637, 636f
  sebaceous, of head and neck, 725
  squamous cell. See Squamous cell
    carcinoma.
  verrucous
    of cervical esophagus, 474
    of larynx, 381-382
Cardiopulmonary reserve, supraglottic
  laryngectomy and, 397-398
Carhart's notch, 1190, 1190f
Carotid artery
  aberrant, 1185-1186, 1186f
  anatomy of, 685
  identification of, in thyroid lobectomy,
    548f, 549
  infection of, 677
  internal
    ABOX-CT of, 999, 1000f, 1001t
    anatomy of, 144, 144f, 145f
    balloon occlusion test of, 1324
    encasement of, as contraindication to
      neck dissection, 688-689, 690f
    injury to
      during endonasal surgery, 1051
      during glomus tumor surgery, 1335
      during infratemporal fossa surgery,
        1019-1020
      during neck dissection, 704
      during temporal bone resection,
        1289-1290
    pseudoaneurysm of
      computed tomography angiography
        in, 145, 145f
      post-traumatic, 1374, 1374f
    segments of, 1046, 1046f
    surgical repair of
      postoperative management of, 149,
        149f
      preoperative planning for, 145-146,
        145f
  petrous
    exposure of, 148, 148f
    localization of, 1050, 1050f
    middle fossa approach to, 1024-1025,
      1027-1032, 1027f-1031f
Carotid body tumor
  diagnosis of, 664, 665f
  excision of, 667-668, 667f, 668f
  Shamblin classification of, 664, 666,
    666f
Carotid canal, 1046, 1047f
Carotid sheath
  in cervical spine surgery, 709, 710f
  in radical neck dissection, 695, 695f
Carotid-vertebral space, 710, 711f
Cartilage graft
  for microtia reconstruction, 798-799,
    798f-800f
  for nasal alar reconstruction, 829-830,
    833f

Cartilage graft (Continued)
  for nasal reconstruction, 830
  for posterior cricoid area, 370, 372f
Cartilage repair, in laryngeal trauma, 354,
  354f, 355f
Cartilage-contouring horizontal sutures, for
  otoplasty, 793-794, 794f
Cauliflower ear, 1079
Caustic burns, laryngeal stenosis after, 358
Cautery
  for anterior epistaxis, 3
  suction, for adenoidectomy, 36, 36f
  for tonsillectomy, 173, 176
Cellulitis, after foreign body removal from
  ear, 1097
Cephalic trim, in nasal tip surgery, 813, 813f
Cerebellar artery
  anterior inferior, injury to, during
    vestibular nerve section, 1409
  posterior inferior, decompression of, in
    hemifacial spasm, 1390
Cerebellopontine angle, congenital
  epidermoid tumor of, 1341
Cerebral blood flow, ABOX-CT of, 999,
  1000f, 1001t
Cerebral edema, after petrosal approach to
  cranial base tumor, 1042
Cerebral ischemia, after infratemporal fossa
  surgery, 1020
Cerebrospinal fluid analysis, in anterior
  cranial base tumor, 982
Cerebrospinal fluid leak
  after acoustic neuroma surgery,
    1315-1316
  after anterior cranial base surgery, 995
  classification of, 1053
  after cochlear implant surgery, 1383
  after endonasal surgery, 1051
  after facial nerve decompression, 1391
  after facial nerve tumor surgery, 1255
  after glomus tumor surgery, 1334
  after infratemporal fossa surgery,
    1020-1021
  after labyrinthectomy, 1408-1409
  after petrosal approach to cranial base
    tumor, 1041
  signs and symptoms of, 1360
  after temporal bone fracture, 1368,
    1373-1374, 1373f
  after temporal bone resection, 1290
  through ear. See Cerebrospinal fluid
    otorrhea.
  through nose. See Cerebrospinal fluid
    rhinorrhea.
Cerebrospinal fluid otorrhea, 1359-1366
  causes of, 1359-1360, 1360f, 1360t
  persistent, 1365-1366
  surgery for
    defect repair methods in, 1362-1364,
      1362f-1365f
    middle fossa approach in, 1361-1362,
      1364, 1364f
    patient selection in, 1360
    pearls and pitfalls in, 1366
    postoperative care in, 1365-1366
    preoperative planning of, 1361, 1361f,
      1362f
    techniques in, 1361-1365, 1362f-1365f
    transmastoid approach in, 1361, 1362,
      1362f, 1363, 1363f

Condyle, mandibular
  fracture involving, 897-898, 897f, 899f
  osteotomy of, in preauricular
    (subtemporal) infratemporal fossa
    surgery, 1004, 1005f
Congenital anomalies
  choanal atresia and, 27
  of middle ear, 1177-1187
Conjunctival incision, for lower lid
    blepharoplasty, 862
Continuous positive airway pressure, for
    obstructive sleep apnea, 151, 152f
Contrast material, for esophagography, 445
Contusion, facial, 872
Cordotomy, transverse, in glottic
    enlargement surgery, 312-313, 313f
Corneal injury, during lower lid
    blepharoplasty, 868
Coronal incision
  for Le Fort III fracture repair, 913-914,
    913f, 914f
  for orbital rim fracture repair, 914f, 918
Corticosteroids
  for Bell's palsy, 1259
  after ethmoid sinus endoscopic surgery,
    97
  for facial fracture, 931
  for facial paralysis, 1260, 1368
  injection of
    into frontal sinus, 4
    into inferior turbinate, 4
  intratympanic, 1084-1087, 1086f
  for laryngeal stenosis, 362
  for nasal polyps, 3-4
  after tonsillectomy, 178
  in tracheal stenosis surgery, 606
Cosmetic deformity, after infratemporal
    fossa surgery, 1020f, 1021
Costal cartilage
  for microtia reconstruction, 798-799,
    798f-800f
  for nasal reconstruction, 830
Cottle maneuver, 17, 20-21, 20f
Cranial base anatomy
  infratemporal, 1005, 1007, 1007f
  lateral, 1029f
Cranial base surgery
  anterior, 979-996
    complications of, 994-996
      central nervous system/skull base,
        995-996, 995f
      metabolic, 994-995
      vascular, 995
    craniotomy in, 987, 988f
    en bloc specimen removal in, 989, 990f
    endoscopic techniques in, 991-994,
      993f-994f
    extracranial approaches in, 984, 984f
    frontal lobe dura elevation in, 988-989,
      988f
    open, 985-991, 985f-991f
    orbital wall resection in, 989, 989f
    osteotomies in, 989, 989f, 993
    patient selection for, 981-984, 981f-984f
    pearls and pitfalls in, 996
    postoperative management of, 994
    preoperative planning for, 984-985
    reconstruction after
      endoscopic, 993-994, 993f-994f
      open, 989-991, 990f-991f

Cranial base surgery (Continued)
    scalp elevation in, 986-987, 986f, 987f
    scalp incisions for, 985-986, 985f, 986f
  endonasal, 1025, 1039-1040
  evolution of, 1045
  for infratemporal fossa tumor, 997-1021.
    See also Infratemporal fossa surgery.
  for middle and posterior fossae tumor,
    1023-1043. See also Petrosal approach
    to cranial base tumor.
  reconstruction after, 1061-1068
    complications of, 1065-1067
    free flap in, 749, 749f
    goals of, 1061, 1062t
    materials for, 1062t
    patient selection for, 1061
    pearls and pitfalls in, 1068
    postoperative care in, 1065
    preoperative planning for, 1061
    surgical techniques for, 1061-1065,
      1062f-1067f
Cranial base tumor
  anterior
    choice of therapy for, 982, 982t
    intracranial extension of, 979, 980f,
      983-984, 983f, 984f
    intranasal examination of, 981, 981f
    preoperative evaluation of, 981-984,
      981f-984f
    signs and symptoms of, 979, 981f
    types of, 979, 980t
  lateral, zoning classification for, 1024,
    1024f
  petrosal approach to, 1023-1043. See also
    Petrosal approach to cranial base
    tumor.
Cranial nerve injury
  after acoustic neuroma surgery, 1316
  after facial nerve decompression, 1391
  after glomus tumor surgery, 1334
  in laryngeal trauma, 351
  after petrosal approach to cranial base
    tumor, 1041-1042
Cranialization, of frontal sinus fracture,
    929-930, 931f
Craniofacial abnormalities, tympanostomy
    tube placement in patient with,
    1125-1126
Craniofacial complete dysjunction (Le Fort
    III fracture)
  preoperative evaluation of, 906, 906f
  treatment of, 913-914, 913f-915f
Craniofacial skeleton, reconstruction of,
    1064, 1065f, 1066f
Cribriform plate, 100
  cerebrospinal fluid rhinorrhea arising
    from, 133-134, 133f-135f, 1056
Cricoarytenoid joint, palpation of
  in glottic enlargement surgery, 312
  in posterior glottic stenosis, 314
Cricoarytenoid muscle, posterior
  in arytenoid adduction, 331, 332f
  localization and Botox injection of, 294,
    295f
Cricohyoidoepiglottopexy, laryngectomy
    with. See Laryngectomy, supracricoid
    partial, with cricohyoidoepiglottopexy.
Cricoid cartilage
  cancer involving, 411
  trauma to, 352, 354

Cricoid split, anterior, for subglottic stenosis
    in children, 371, 375, 375f
Cricopharyngeal achalasia, 461, 461f
Cricopharyngeal myotomy
  indications for, 459
  pearls and pitfalls in, 465
  postoperative management of, 465
  preoperative planning for, 462
  after supraglottic laryngectomy, 400
  technique of, 460, 462-463, 462f-463f
Cricopharyngeus muscle, dysfunction of,
    459-465, 460f-464f. See also Zenker's
    diverticulum.
Cricothyroid joint, disarticulation of, 403,
    404f
Cricothyroidotomy, laryngeal stenosis after,
    358
Cricothyrotomy, in laryngeal trauma,
    353
Cricotracheal resection, for tracheal stenosis,
    613
Crista galli, removal of, in endoscopic
    anterior cranial base surgery, 993
Cryosurgery, for skin cancer, 720
CT. See Computed tomography (CT).
Curettage with electrodesiccation, for skin
    cancer, 720
Curette, for adenoidectomy, 35-36, 36f
Cutting and diamond burrs, in canal wall
    reconstruction, 1109, 1110f
Cyanoacrylate tissue adhesives, for facial
    repair and reconstruction, 877
CyberKnife system
  for facial nerve tumor surgery, 1252-1253,
    1253f
  for glomus tumor surgery, 1324, 1325f
Cyst
  branchial cleft. See Branchial cleft
    remnants.
  epidermal, of tongue, 163f
  saccular, of larynx, 341-346. See also
    Laryngocele.
  thyroglossal duct. See Thyroglossal duct
    cyst.
  vocal fold, 303
Cystic neck mass, differential diagnosis of,
    633
Cytometry, flow, 630

D

Dacryocystitis, 967
Dacryocystorhinostomy, 967-972
  in medial maxillectomy, 70, 72f
  patient selection for, 967-968
  pearls and pitfalls in, 972
  postoperative management of, 971-972,
    972t
  preoperative evaluation for, 969
  surgical approaches for, 969-971,
    969f-971f
  in total maxillectomy, 80, 83f
Dacryoliths, 968
Dandy's vein, 1311
Danger space, 709
Deafness. See Hearing loss.
Débridement. See also Microdébrider.
  in facial soft tissue injuries, 872
Decannulation, in tracheostomy, 582-583
  accidental, 592

Hard palate, cancer of (Continued)
  surgery for
    anatomy in, 205
    complications of, 215
    neck dissection in, 211
    patient selection in, 205-207, 206f
    pearls and pitfalls in, 215
    postoperative management of, 214-215
    preoperative planning in, 207-209, 208f
    speech rehabilitation after, 211-214,
      213f-214f
    techniques in, 209-214, 209f-214f
  types of, 205, 206f
Hardy self-retaining speculum, in sphenoid
  sinus surgery, 110, 110f
Harmonic scalpel
  for cervical incision, 547
  for tonsillectomy, 172-173
Head and neck. See also Neck.
  cancer of
    extracapsular spread of, 679, 680f
    staging of, 679, 680f, 688, 689f
    mass in, fine-needle aspiration biopsy of,
      629-633
  skin cancer of, 719-736. See also Skin
    cancer.
Head holder, Mayfield horseshoe, 986, 1247,
  1247f
Headache
  after acoustic neuroma surgery, 1316
  after facial nerve decompression, 1391
  after vestibular nerve section, 1409
Hearing aid, bone-anchored, 1209-1217,
  1210f
  for aural atresia, 1115, 1116
  in children, 1215-1216
  drilling of fixture site for, 1211-1213,
    1212f
  insertion of, 1214-1215, 1214f, 1215f
  patient selection for, 1210
  pearls and pitfalls in, 1216-1217
  planning of skin flap for, 1210-1211, 1211f
  postoperative management of, 1216
  preoperative evaluation for, 1210
  soft tissue removal for, 1213-1214, 1213f
  surgical approach for, 1210-1216
Hearing assessment. See Audiologic testing;
  Audiometry.
Hearing loss
  in acoustic neuroma, 1299, 1299f
  after acoustic neuroma surgery, 1315
  in cerebrospinal fluid leak, 1360
  in children, progressive versus stable, 1179
  conductive
    assessment of, 1148, 1149f, 1178, 1179
    in middle ear malformations, 1177
  after endolymphatic sac surgery, 1408
  after facial nerve tumor surgery, 1255
  after glomus tumor surgery, 1334
  in infratemporal fossa tumor, 998
  after intratympanic gentamicin, 1084
  ossicular chain reconstruction for,
    1147-1162. See also Ossicular chain
    reconstruction.
  in otosclerosis, 1189-1190, 1190f
  after posterior semicircular canal
    occlusion, 1408
  sensorineural
    after mastoidectomy, 1175
    in perilymphatic fistula, 1222

Hearing loss (Continued)
    sudden, intratympanic dexamethasone
      for, 1084, 1085, 1086
    in tympanic membrane perforation, 1134
Hemangioma
  of facial nerve, 1242-1243, 1244f. See also
    Facial nerve, tumor of.
  macroglossia and, 162, 164f
Hematoma
  auricular, 1079-1081, 1080f
  after glomus tumor surgery, 1334
  after neck dissection, 705
  orbital, 950
  after orbital exenteration, 965
  after otoplasty, 795
  after prestyloid parapharyngeal space
    tumor excision, 530
  retrobulbar, after blepharoplasty, 869
  after rhytidectomy, 855
  septal, after septoplasty, 24
  after skin cancer surgery, 734
  after superficial lobe parotidectomy, 516
  after thyroid surgery, 553
Hemicoronal scalp incision
  for preauricular (subtemporal)
    infratemporal fossa surgery, 1002,
    1002f
  with Weber-Fergusson incision, in anterior
    transfacial approach, 1009, 1014,
    1014f
Hemifacial spasm
  differential diagnosis of, 1386, 1386t
  facial nerve decompression for, 1385-1392
    closure methods after, 1391
    monitoring during, 1388
    nerve exposure in, 1388-1390,
      1389f-1390f
    patient positioning and preparation in,
      1387, 1388f
    patient selection in, 1385-1386, 1386t
    pearls and pitfalls in, 1392
    postoperative management of, 1391
    preoperative evaluation in, 1386-1387,
      1387f
    surgical exposure in, 1388, 1389f
    technique of, 1390-1391, 1390f
Hemiglossectomy, 222. See also Glossectomy,
  partial.
Hemilaryngectomy. See Laryngectomy,
  vertical partial.
Hemochromatosis, neonatal, lip biopsy in,
  491
Hemorrhage
  during acoustic neuroma surgery, 1315
  during endoscopic sinus surgery, 143-150
  intracranial, after temporal bone
    resection, 1291
  after juvenile angiofibroma surgery, 48
  after laryngeal carcinoma endoscopic
    surgery, 390
  in midfacial and upper facial fracture, 905
  from nose. See Epistaxis.
  after percutaneous dilatational
    tracheostomy, 592
  retrobulbar, after endoscopic sinus
    surgery, 139-140, 140f
  after septoplasty, 24
  after tonsillectomy, 178-179
  after tracheostomy, 584
  during tracheostomy, 583

Hemostasis
  for facial soft tissue injuries, 871-872
  using electrocautery, for tonsillectomy,
    173, 176
Herpes zoster oticus, facial paralysis in, 1259
Hiatus semilunaris, 92
Histiocytoma, malignant fibrous, of head
  and neck, 726
HIV/AIDS, skin cancer in, 723
Hoarseness
  in laryngeal carcinoma, 382, 383
    after laryngeal carcinoma endoscopic
      surgery, 390
  in patients with cleft palate, 780, 780t
"Hockey stick" incision, for neck dissection,
  691, 692f
Hook, right-angled, for foreign body
  removal from ear, 1095, 1096f
Hot water irrigation, for epistaxis, 9
House-Brackmann grading system, for facial
  nerve tumor, 1243, 1243t
Human immunodeficiency virus (HIV)
  infection, skin cancer in, 723
Human papillomavirus infection
  chronic, skin cancer in, 723
  recurrent respiratory papillomatosis from,
    323
  vaccine for, 327
Hurd retractors, in styloid process surgery,
  196, 196f
Huschke, foramen of, 1272, 1274f
Hyaluronic acid, for vocal fold
  augmentation/injection, 319
Hydrocephalus
  high-pressure
    after facial nerve decompression,
      1391
    risk of, in patient with cerebrospinal
      fluid rhinorrhea, 1057-1058,
      1058f
    after temporal bone resection, 1291
  otitic, 1236
Hydroxyapatite
  for ossicular chain prosthesis, 1151, 1152f,
    1155, 1156f
  for vocal fold augmentation/injection,
    319
Hyoepiglottic ligament, in total
  laryngectomy, 426, 427f
Hypercalcemia, in hyperparathyroidism, 559
Hyperglycemia, after anterior cranial base
  surgery, 995
Hyperhidrosis
  assessment tools for, 496, 496t
  gustatory, 495-498, 496f, 497f
Hypernasality, in patients with cleft palate,
  780, 780t
Hyperparathyroidism, parathyroidectomy
  for, 559-564. See also Parathyroidectomy.
Hyperplastic polyp, of cervical esophagus,
  474
Hypersomnolence, in obstructive sleep
  apnea, 151, 152f
Hypertension, intracranial
  after facial nerve decompression, 1391
  risk of, in patient with cerebrospinal fluid
    rhinorrhea, 1057-1058, 1058f
  after temporal bone resection, 1291
Hyphema, as contraindication to orbital
  fracture repair, 939

Infection (*Continued*)
  after temporal bone resection, 1290-1291
  third branchial arch cyst, 648
  after tracheostomy, 584-585
Infectious diseases
  laryngeal stenosis in, 358-359, 359f
  tracheal stenosis in, 604
Inferior turbinate, steroid injection of, 4
Informed consent, for acoustic neuroma surgery, 1301
Infraorbital nerve, in anterior antrostomy, 61, 61f
Infraorbital neurovascular bundle, 58
Infratemporal fossa
  anatomic boundaries of, 997, 998t
  dissection of, in glomus tumor surgery, 1330-1331, 1331f
  resection of, in temporal bone resection, 1284-1286, 1285f
  tumor in
    biopsy of, 999-1001
    clinical evaluation of, 997-999, 999f-1000f, 1001t
    metastatic workup for, 1001
    reconstructive/rehabilitation considerations for, 1001
Infratemporal fossa surgery
  anterior transfacial (facial translocation) approach in, 1009, 1014-1015, 1014f-1016f
  complications of, 1019-1021, 1019f-1021f
  endoscopic, 1017-1018
  historical background on, 997, 998t
  patient selection for, 997-1001
  pearls and pitfalls in, 1021
  postauricular (transtemporal) approach in, 1008-1009, 1011f-1013f
  postoperative management of, 1018-1019
  preauricular (subtemporal) approach in, 1002-1008, 1002f-1011f
  preoperative planning for, 1001-1002, 1001t
  reconstruction after, 1001, 1007-1008, 1010f-1011f
  transorbital approach in, 1015, 1017, 1017f-1018f
Infratemporal skull base structures, identification of, 1005, 1007, 1007f
Injection, vocal fold. *See* Vocal fold augmentation/injection.
Injection needles, for transoral vocal fold augmentation, 296
Inlay graft, for skull defect repair
  epidural, 133, 133f
  subdural, 133-134, 134f
Inner ear
  anatomy of, 1377
  medication delivery to, 1084-1087, 1086f
Innominate artery rupture, after tracheostomy, 585, 586f
Insect, in external auditory canal, 1093, 1094-1095
Insufflation test, for tracheoesophageal puncture, 433
Intensive care unit, percutaneous dilatational tracheostomy in, 585-593, 588f-591f
Interarytenoid synechia, in posterior glottic stenosis, 314, 315f
Intercartilaginous incision, for medial maxillectomy, 74f

Interdomal suture, in nasal tip surgery, 813, 813f, 814, 814f, 815f, 817
Interferon, for recurrent respiratory papillomatosis, 326
Internal auditory canal
  exposure of, 1308-1309, 1308f
    in middle fossa vestibular nerve section, 1406, 1406f
  facial nerve repair in, 1371
  localization of, 1032, 1032f, 1308, 1308f
Intracranial bleeding, after acoustic neuroma surgery, 1316
Intracranial complications
  of otitis media, 1229-1238, 1230t-1231t, 1232f
  after temporal bone resection, 1291
Intracranial extension of anterior cranial base tumor, 979, 980f
Intracranial hypertension
  after facial nerve decompression, 1391
  risk of, in patient with cerebrospinal fluid rhinorrhea, 1057-1058, 1058f
  after temporal bone resection, 1291
Intracranial pressure, minimization of, in anterior cranial base surgery, 985
Intratympanic injections, 1084-1087, 1086f
Intubation
  endotracheal
    in anterior cranial base surgery, 986
    in infratemporal fossa tumor surgery, 1002
    in tracheal stenosis, 605
      tracheal stenosis after, 603-604
  laryngeal stenosis after, 358
  nasogastric, laryngeal stenosis after, 358
  in rigid bronchoscopy, 570, 570f
Iodine-131, after thyroid surgery, 555
Irrigation
  of ear canal, for foreign body removal, 1095, 1095f
  after ethmoid sinus endoscopic surgery, 97
  of facial soft tissue injuries, 871
  hot water, for epistaxis, 9
Isadora Duncan syndrome, 350
Ischemia
  cerebral, after infratemporal fossa surgery, 1020
  flap, after temporal bone resection, 1291
Island pedicle flap, for upper lip reconstruction, 730, 731f

J

Jackson-Pratt drain, in anterior cranial base reconstruction, 991
Jahn hydroxyapatite tube, 1129
Jejunal autograft, for esophageal reconstruction, 481
Jejunal free flap, 745
  disadvantages of, 745
  monitor loop of, 750, 750f
  for pharyngectomy defect, 748
  after total laryngopharyngectomy, 470, 471f
Jennings mouth gag, in partial glossectomy, 221, 221f
Jet ventilation
  high-frequency, during rigid bronchoscopy, 572-573, 573f
  in tracheal stenosis, 606

Jugular bulb
  glomus tumor arising from, 1319
    surgical management of, 1328-1333, 1328f-1333f
  high-riding, 1185, 1185f
Jugular foramen, dissection of, in temporal bone resection, 1283-1284, 1284f
Jugular vein, internal
  anatomy of, 685
  bilateral sacrifice of, 706
  in modified radical neck dissection, 697-698
  in radical neck dissection, 695-696, 696, 696f, 697f
  in selective neck dissection, 701, 703f
  septic thrombophlebitis of, 674, 674f, 676-677
Juvenile angiofibroma, 39-50
  biopsy of, 41, 42f
  history and physical examination in, 39, 40f
  imaging of, 39, 40f, 41, 41f
  staging of, 41, 42t
  surgical management of, 43-50
    approaches to, overview of, 43
    complications of, 48-49
    endoscopic techniques for, 43-44, 43f
    Le Fort I osteotomies for, 45-46, 47f-49f
    pearls and pitfalls in, 49
    postoperative care in, 47-48
    preoperative planning in, 41-42
    transpharyngeal or transpalatal approaches to, 44-45, 44f-46f
  therapeutic modalities for, 42-43

K

Karapandzic flap, for excision of large tumors of the lip, 188-189, 192f
Keel, in laryngeal trauma repair, 353-354, 354f
Keratin "pearl," in canal cholesteatoma, 1107, 1108f
Keratin plug, in keratosis obturans, 1107, 1108f
Keratoacanthoma, 724
Keratosis obturans, 1107-1111, 1108f
  complications of, 1110
  pearls and pitfalls in, 1110-1111
  postoperative management of, 1110
  preoperative evaluation of, 1109
  surgical management of
    patient selection for, 1109
    techniques for, 1109-1110, 1109f-1110f
Kerrison punch, in sphenoid sinus surgery, 111, 111f
Kerrison rongeur
  in anterior antrostomy, 61, 61f
  in juvenile angiofibroma surgery, 45, 45f
  in postoperative bleeding, 147, 147f
  in styloid process surgery, 196, 197f
Keyhole tongue reduction, 163, 164f
Kiesselbach's plexus, 7, 8f
Killian's triangle, 459, 460f
Kirschner wires, on free cartilage graft for posterior cricoid area, 370-371, 373f
Körner's septum, removal of, in mastoidectomy, 1169
Kuhn frontal sinus rescue procedure, 123, 124f

L

Labiomandibuloglossotomy, midline, 280, 281f

Labyrinthectomy. *See also* Translabyrinthine approach.
  for acoustic neuroma surgery, 1302-1303, 1303f
  for Ménière's disease, 1394
  partial, for cranial base tumor, 1025, 1037, 1037f
  surgical
    complications of, 1408-1409
    for vertigo, 1398-1399, 1398f-1399f

Laceration
  facial, 872, 873f
  trapdoor and circular/pedicled, 873

Lacrimal duct, transection of, in medial maxillectomy and lateral rhinotomy, 69, 70f

Lacrimal surgery, for tearing correction, 967-972. *See also* Dacryocystorhinostomy.

Lacrimal system
  anatomy of, 968f
  injury to, 878-879, 922

Lagophthalmos, after blepharoplasty, 868

LAHSHAL classification of clefts, 766, 766t

Lamina papyracea, 99

Laryngeal augmentation, for subglottic stenosis in children, 375

Laryngeal cancer, 379-391
  chemoradiation therapy for, 421-422
  early, 382-383, 383t
  endoscopic laser excision of
    complications of, 390
    contraindications to, 383t
    general procedure for, 384f, 385
    patient selection for, 379-380
    pearls and pitfalls in, 390-391
    positioning for, 385-386
    postoperative management in, 389-390
    preoperative planning for, 380-383, 381f, 382f
    technique for, 383-389, 384f, 386f-389f
  imaging of, 383, 383t
  laryngectomy for. *See also* Laryngectomy.
    horizontal partial, 393-409
    total, 421-430
    vertical partial, 411-419
  laryngocele and, 342-343, 343f
  neck dissection for, 422
  radiation therapy for, 380, 422
  staging of, 379-380, 380t
  with subglottic extension, 422
  supraglottic. *See* Supraglottic cancer.
  verrucous, 381-382

Laryngeal diversion technique, for aspiration, 595, 596

Laryngeal nerve
  recurrent
    identification of, in thyroid lobectomy, 548f, 549-550
    injury to
      in cervical spine surgery, 717
      during thyroid surgery, 554
    intraoperative monitoring of, 554
  superior
    injury to, during thyroid surgery, 554
    in lateral pharyngotomy, 237, 238f

Laryngeal office-based procedures, 291-301
  patient selection for, 291
  pearls and pitfalls in, 300-301
  postprocedure care/complications of, 299-300
  preoperative planning for, 292, 292f
  surgical techniques in, 292-299

Laryngeal papillomatosis
  recurrent, 325, 326
  tracheostomy in, 578, 578f

Laryngeal stenosis, 357-377. *See also* Tracheal stenosis.
  anatomic considerations in, 357
  antibiotics in, 362
  clinical assessment of, 360
  complications of, 376-377
  corticosteroids for, 362
  dilatation for, 361
  endoscopic microsurgery for, 361
  etiology of, 357-360, 359f-360f
  glottic, 314, 315f
    after recurrent respiratory papillomatosis surgery, 327
    surgical treatment of, 363-367, 365f-370f
  imaging of, 360-361, 361f
  mitomycin C for, 362
  pearls and pitfalls in, 377
  postoperative care in, 375-376
  post-traumatic, 355, 357-358
  preoperative planning in, 363
  stenting for, 361-362, 362f, 376
  subglottic
    in children, 371, 375, 375f
    surgical treatment of, 367, 370-375, 371f-375f
    with tracheal stenosis. *See* Tracheal stenosis.
  supraglottic, surgical treatment of, 363, 363f, 364f
  transcervical approaches to, 361
  "wait and see" approach to, 361

Laryngeal surgery, conservation. *See* Laryngectomy, horizontal partial; Laryngectomy, vertical partial.

Laryngeal trauma, 349-356
  airway management in, 350-351, 353
  blunt, 349-350, 350f
  in children, 349
  cranial nerve injury in, 351
  pearls and pitfalls in, 356
  penetrating, 350, 351f
  postoperative management of, 354-355
  preoperative assessment of, 351-352, 352f
  stenosis after, 355, 357-358
  strangulation as, 350, 352, 352f
  surgical management of, 353f-355f, 354-355
  vascular injury in, 351

Laryngectomy
  horizontal partial, 393-409
    anatomic considerations in, 394-395, 394f, 395f
    contraindications to, 398
    patient selection for, 395-396
    pearls and pitfalls in, 409
    preoperative evaluation in, 396-398, 396f, 397f
    techniques of, 398-409
    types of, 393, 394t

Laryngectomy (*Continued*)
  supracricoid partial, with cricohyoidoepiglottopexy, 403-408
    overview of, 393-394
    pearls and pitfalls in, 406, 408
    postoperative care in, 406
    preoperative evaluation in, 403
    technique of, 403-406, 404f-407f, 404t
  supraglottic
    extended, 401-402, 409
    overview of, 393
    pearls and pitfalls in, 402-403
    postoperative management of, 402
    technique of, 398-402, 399f-402f, 399t
    transcervical, 363, 363f, 364f
  total, 421-430
    neck dissection in, 422
    and partial pharyngectomy, 470
    patient selection for, 421-422
    pearls and pitfalls in, 430
    preoperative planning for, 422-423
    technique of, 423-430, 423t, 424f-429f
    tracheostomal stenosis after, 623-627, 625f-627f
    voice restoration after, 431-437, 432f-437f
  vertical partial, 411-419
    epiglottopexy with, 415, 417, 418f-419f
    frontolateral, 411, 412f
    patient selection for, 411-412, 412f, 413t
    pearls and pitfalls in, 419
    postoperative care in, 413t, 417
    preoperative planning for, 412, 412f
    technique of, 412-417, 413t, 414f-417f

Laryngocele, 341-346
  combined form of, 341, 342f
  complications of, 346
  excision of
    patient selection for, 343-344, 343f
    pearls and pitfalls in, 346
    postoperative management of, 346
    technique of, 344-346, 344f, 345f
  infected, 342, 343
  squamous cell carcinoma and, 342-343, 343f
  symptoms of, 342, 343

Laryngocutaneous fistula, after laryngofissure, 338

Laryngoesophagectomy, total, 468, 468f, 470, 470f

Laryngofissure, 335-339
  for anterior glottic stenosis, 365, 366f
  complications of, 338-339
  for laryngeal trauma surgery, 353, 353f
  patient selection for, 335
  for posterior glottic stenosis, 367
  preoperative evaluation in, 335-336
  technique of, 336-338, 336f-338f

Laryngopharyngectomy
  partial, 408-409, 409f, 468, 469-470
  total, 468, 470, 470f, 471f

Laryngopharyngoesophagectomy
  with colonic transposition, 481
  with free flaps, 481
  with gastric transposition and pharyngogastric anastomosis, 480, 480f
  postoperative management and complications of, 482

Lymphoma
  of hard palate, 205, 206f
  of soft palate, 199, 200f
  of thyroid gland, 542-543
  of tonsil, 283, 284f
Lynch's frontoethmoidectomy, 117-118, 118f

M

Macroglossia
  conditions causing, 161
  reduction procedures for, 161-167
    complications of, 166-167
    patient selection for, 161-162, 162f
    pearls and pitfalls in, 167
    postoperative management of, 166
    preoperative planning for, 162-163, 162f-164f
    types of, 163-166, 164f-166f
Magnetic resonance angiography (MRA)
  in glomus tumor, 1322-1323, 1323f
  in infratemporal fossa tumor, 999
  in temporal bone cholesterol granuloma and epidermoid tumor, 1343
Magnetic resonance imaging (MRI)
  in acoustic neuroma, 1299f, 1300, 1300f, 1314, 1315t
  in anterior cranial base tumor, 980f, 981-982, 982f, 983f
  in buccal space tumor, 535, 535f
  in cerebrospinal fluid otorrhea, 1361, 1362f
  in cerebrospinal fluid rhinorrhea, 132, 133, 1054, 1055f
  in cervical esophageal cancer, 477
  of cervical spine, 710f, 712
  in cochlear implant candidate, 1379
  in facial nerve tumor, 1243, 1244f, 1246
  in glomus tumor, 1322, 1322f
  in hemifacial spasm, 1386
  in hypopharyngeal tumor, 235-236
  in infratemporal fossa tumor, 999, 999f
  in juvenile angiofibroma, 39, 40f
  in laryngeal stenosis, 360-361
  in laryngocele, 343
  in laryngotracheal stenosis, 605
  in lip cancer, 185
  in maxillary sinus tumor, 78, 79f
  in maxillary sinusitis, 59-60
  in optic nerve decompression, 956f, 957
  in otosclerosis, 1192
  in plunging ranula, 500, 501f
  in prestyloid parapharyngeal space tumor, 525, 526f
  in temporal bone carcinoma, 1277-1278, 1278f
  in temporal bone cholesterol granuloma and epidermoid tumor, 1341-1342, 1341f, 1342f, 1342t, 1343, 1354, 1354f
  in thyroglossal duct cyst, 638
  in tongue base tumor, 230, 235-236
  in tongue cancer, 220, 220f, 223, 223f
  of tumor invasion into bone, 265, 265f
  of tumor involving nasal cavity and paranasal sinuses, 68, 69f
Malar eminence osteotomy, in preauricular (subtemporal) infratemporal fossa surgery, 1005, 1006f

Malleus, abnormalities of
  congenital, surgical correction of, 1183-1185, 1184f-1185f
  ossicular chain reconstruction for, 1159-1160, 1160f
Malocclusion
  after facial fracture repair, 932
  after infratemporal fossa surgery, 1019, 1019f
Malunion, after laryngofissure, 339
Mandible
  floor of mouth cancer involving, 243, 244f, 249-252, 250f-251f
  fracture of. See Mandibular fracture.
  reconstruction of
    distraction osteogenesis for, 267
    free flap for, 224, 250, 251f, 252, 273, 274f, 740f, 744f, 746-747
    methods of, 266-267, 266t
    plates for, 741f, 747
Mandibular advancement surgery. See also Maxillomandibular advancement surgery.
  for obstructive sleep apnea, 156-157, 156f, 157f
Mandibular alveolus, tumor arising on
  marginal mandibulectomy for, 263, 264f
  osteotomies for, 249, 251f
  radiography in, 264-265, 265f
  visor flap for, 249, 250f
Mandibular condyle osteotomy, in preauricular (subtemporal) infratemporal fossa surgery, 1004, 1005f
Mandibular fracture, 885-902
  classification of, 885, 886f
  involving angle, 894-896, 895f-896f
  involving body, 892-894, 893f-894f
  involving condyle, 897-898, 897f, 899f
  involving coronoid, 896
  involving ramus, 897
  involving symphysis and parasymphysis, 891-892, 891f
  involving teeth, 889-890
  after mandibulectomy, 260
  multiple, 898, 900f-902f
  open versus closed, 885
  pathologic, 265f
  treatment of, 888-898
    arch bar and maxillomandibular fixation in, 888-889, 889f-891f
    in children, 898, 899f
    open versus closed, 888
    patient selection for, 887
    pearls and pitfalls in, 902
    postoperative management after, 898
    preoperative planning for, 887-888
Mandibular osteoradionecrosis, segmental mandibulectomy for, 263
Mandibulectomy
  marginal, 255-260
    complications of, 260
    definition of, 264t
    indications for, 255-256, 256f, 257f
    for mandibular alveolar tumor, 263, 264f
    in mouth floor cancer surgery, 245, 246-247, 248f
    patient selection for, 257
    pearls and pitfalls in, 260
    postoperative management of, 260

Mandibulectomy (Continued)
    preoperative planning for, 257-258
    technique of, 258-260, 259f-260f
  segmental, 263-275
    definition of, 264t
    indications for, 263
    neck dissection before, 268
    patient selection for, 263-266, 264f-265f
    pearls and pitfalls in, 275
    postoperative management of, 273-274
    preoperative planning for, 267-268, 268f
    prosthetic rehabilitation after, 268
    reconstruction after, 272-273, 273f, 274f
    technique of, 268-273, 269f-273f
  in tongue base tumor, 229
  for total glossectomy, 224, 224f, 226
Mandibulotomy, 277-280
  definition of, 264t
  in excision of cancer of floor of mouth, 249, 249f-250f
  with midline tongue-splitting approach, 280, 281f
  patient selection for, 277
  pearls and pitfalls in, 282
  postoperative management of, 279-280
  preoperative evaluation for, 277-278
  prestyloid parapharyngeal space tumor excision with, 529-530
  technique of, 278-279, 278f, 279f
  in tongue base tumor excision, 229
  in total glossectomy, 226
  total parotidectomy with, 519, 519f
Mannitol
  for intracranial hypertension, 1291
  during temporal bone resection, 1279
Manometry, of upper esophageal sphincter, 462
Marginal incision, for rhinoplasty, 808, 808f, 809f
Marginal mandibular nerve
  injury to, in neck dissection, 704
  in neck dissection, 692, 692f
  in transcervical submandibular gland excision, 506-507, 507f, 508
Margins, positive, survival and, 256, 258f
Masseteric fascia, separation of, in preauricular (subtemporal) infratemporal fossa surgery, 1003, 1003f
Mastication, facial sweating and flushing during. See Frey's syndrome.
Mastoid, congenital epidermoid tumor of, 1340-1341
Mastoid dressing, in microtia reconstruction, 798
Mastoidectomy, 1163-1176. See also Transmastoid approach.
  anesthesia for, 1166
  Bondy-modified radical, 1163, 1173, 1173f
  canal wall down, 1163, 1171-1173, 1172f-1173f
  complications of, 1175-1176
  incisions for, 1166-1167, 1166f-1168f
  intact canal wall, 1163, 1167-1170, 1168f-1170f, 1175-1176
  meatoplasty with, 1173-1174, 1174f-1175f
  patient selection for, 1164, 1164f, 1165f
  pearls and pitfalls in, 1176
  posterior tympanotomy with, 1170-1171, 1170f, 1171f
  postoperative management of, 1174-1175

Nasal fracture
  patterns of, 910f
  preoperative evaluation of, 909-910, 910f
  surgical repair of, 920, 922, 923f
Nasal injuries, 882, 882f
Nasal lining, 822, 827-828
  bipedicled flap interposition for, 826f,
    827, 827f-828f
  free flap for, 828, 831f, 832f
  Menick's technique for, 827-828, 829f-830f
  septal mucoperichondrial flap for, 826f,
    827
  turnover/turn-in flap for, 822, 826f, 827
Nasal midline support, bone graft for, 829,
    832f
Nasal obstruction
  etiology of, 17, 18, 18t
  static facial reanimation for, 841
  surgical correction of, 17-25. See also
    Septoplasty; Turbinate reduction.
    complications of, 24-25
    patient selection for, 17-18
    pearls and pitfalls in, 25
    postoperative management in, 24
    preoperative planning for, 18-19, 19t
    techniques for, 19-24, 20f-24f
Nasal packing
  in endonasal skull base reconstruction,
    993-994
  for epistaxis, 9
  in septoplasty, 23
Nasal polypectomy, 100-101, 100f
Nasal polyps. See also Antrochoanal polyp.
  alligator forceps removal of, 4
  endoscopic sinus surgery for, 97
  with eosinophilic mucin, 3
  in-office microdébridement of, 4
  steroid injection for, 3-4
Nasal profile reduction/alignment, 810-812,
    811f-812f
Nasal prosthesis, 821, 822f
Nasal reconstruction, 821-837
  in bilateral cleft lip repair, 776
  nasal lining options in, 822, 826f-832f,
    827-828. See also Nasal lining.
  nasal skin coverage in, 830, 832, 833f-836f,
    834-836. See also Nasal skin coverage.
  in nasal-orbital-ethmoid (NOE) complex
    fracture, 923, 925f-926f
  patient selection for, 821
  pearls and pitfalls in, 836-837
  postoperative management of, 836
  preoperative planning for, 821-822,
    823f-825f
  skeletal support in, 828-830, 832f, 833f
  after tumor resection, 731-732, 732f-734f
  in unilateral cleft lip repair, 771, 772f, 773
Nasal septal button, placement of, 5
Nasal septum
  blood supply to, 7-9, 8f-10f
  caudal shortening of, in nasal tip surgery,
    814
  deviation of, 17
    etiology of, 18
    severe caudal, repair of, 21-22, 22f
    surgical correction of. See Septoplasty.
  evaluation of, after maxillary fracture
    repair, 915
  fracture of, 920
  hematoma of, after septoplasty, 24

Nasal septum (Continued)
  perforation of
    atrophic rhinitis with, 3
    biopsy of, 3
    after septoplasty, 24
Nasal skin coverage, 830, 832, 834-836
  composite chondrocutaneous graft for,
    832, 833f, 834f
  forehead flap for, 835-836
  full-thickness skin graft for, 830, 832
  nasolabial flap for, 834-835, 837f
  Zitelli's bilobed flap for, 832, 834, 835f
Nasal skin types, 822, 825f
Nasal subunits, 822, 825f
Nasal tip surgery, 812-817
  caudal septum shortening in, 814
  cephalic trim in, 813, 813f
  complications of, 818
  dorsal reduction in, 814, 818
  goals of, 812
  lateral crural overlay in, 815, 816, 816f
  medial crural overlay in, 817
  tip definition in, 812-814, 813f-815f
  tip graft in, 817
  tip projection in, 815-817, 816f-817f
  tip rotation in, 814-815, 815f-816f
  tip suturing in, 813, 813f, 814, 814f, 815f,
    817
  vertical dome division in, 813-814,
    814f-815f, 815, 817, 817f
Nasal valve, collapse of, with inspiration,
    2-3
Nasality, in patients with cleft palate, 780,
    780t
Nasal-orbital-ethmoid (NOE) complex
    fracture, 936
  preoperative evaluation of, 910, 910f
  surgical repair of, 922-923, 924f-926f
Nasoalveolar molding, for facial cleft,
    768-769, 769f
Nasoantral window
  for anterior antrostomy, 61, 61f
  for juvenile angiofibroma surgery, 43-44,
    43f
Nasogastric intubation, laryngeal stenosis
    after, 358
Nasolabial flap
  for nasal lining, 827, 827f-828f
  for nasal reconstruction, 731, 733f
  for nasal skin coverage, 834-835, 837f
Nasolacrimal duct obstruction, 967
Nasomaxillary complex (Le Fort II) fracture
  preoperative evaluation of, 906, 906f
  treatment of, 913
Nasopharyngeal airway, as stent, in choanal
    atresia repair, 30, 31f
Nasopharyngeal anesthesia, 295
Nasopharyngoscopy, in velopharyngeal
    incompetence, 782
Nasopharynx
  juvenile angiofibroma of. See Juvenile
    angiofibroma.
  stenosis of, after
    uvulopalatopharyngoplasty, 155,
    155f
Nasoseptal flap
  for endonasal skull base reconstruction,
    994
  harvesting of, 992
  for skull defect repair, 134, 134f-135f

Neck. See also Cervical entries; Head and
    neck.
  anatomy of, 681-686, 681f-686f
  skin cancer on, 728, 733
  trauma to
    deep neck abscess after, 674
    penetrating, 452, 452f
Neck abscess
  deep, 671-677
    bacteriology of, 674
    description of, 671-674, 672f-674f
    etiology of, 674, 674f
    incision and drainage of, 675-677, 676f
    pearls and pitfalls in, 677
    postoperative management of, 677
    preoperative evaluation of, 675, 675f
    in parapharyngeal space, 671-672,
      672f-673f, 675f, 676, 676f
    in prevertebral space, 673-674, 674f
    in retropharyngeal space, 672-673, 673f,
      676
    in submental-submandibular space, 671,
      672f
    in third branchial arch cyst infection, 648
Neck dissection, 679-707
  anatomic structures in, 681-686, 681f-686f
  in cervical esophageal cancer surgery, 478
  classification of, 687, 688f-689f
  complications of, 703-706
    intraoperative, 704
    postoperative, 704-706
    preoperative, 704
  extended, 687
  in floor of mouth cancer, 242, 247
  functional, 681
  in glomus tumor surgery, 1328, 1328f,
    1330
  in hard palate cancer, 211
  "hockey stick" incision for, 691, 692f
  in oropharyngeal cancer, 283, 287
  in partial laryngopharyngectomy, 408
  patient selection for, 688-689, 690f
  pearls and pitfalls in, 706-707
  posterolateral, 702-703
  postoperative management of, 703
  preoperative planning for, 689-690
  preoperative radiologic staging in, 688,
    689f
  versus radiation therapy, 690
  radical, 687, 688f
    description of, 680-681
    modified, 687, 688f-689f, 697-698,
      697f-698f
    steps in, 691t
    technique of, 690-697, 692f-697f
  in segmental mandibulectomy, 268
  selective
    advantages of, 689
    steps in, 691t
    techniques of, 698-702, 699f-703f, 707f
  in supraglottic carcinoma, 397
  techniques of, 690-703, 691t
  with temporal bone resection, 1276
  in thyroid surgery, 552-553, 553f
  in total laryngectomy, 422
Neck mass. See also Branchial cleft remnants.
  cystic, differential diagnosis of, 633
  midline. See also Thyroglossal duct cyst.
    differential diagnosis of, 635
    evaluation of, 637-638, 638f

Palate (Continued)
  local flaps for, 213
  prosthesis in, 212-213, 213f
  regional flaps for, 213, 214f
  tissue, 86
  dysfunction of, after transoral/transpalatal
    procedures, 1073
  hard. See Hard palate.
  soft. See Soft palate.
Palatine tonsils, 169-170, 170f
  removal of. See Tonsillectomy.
Palatomaxillary defects, classification of, 213,
  213t
Palatoplasty
  Furlow, 778-780, 779f
  revision, for velopharyngeal
    incompetence, 785
  two-flap, with intravelar veloplasty,
    776-778, 777f
  velopharyngeal incompetence after,
    781-782, 781f
Panendoscopy
  in floor of mouth cancer, 244
  in tongue base and hypopharyngeal
    tumor, 236
Pannus
  resection of, in transnasal procedures,
    1071
  rheumatoid, 1070, 1070f
Pansinusitis, 113
Papillary carcinoma, arising in thyroglossal
  duct cyst, 636-637, 636f
Papilloma, inverted
  endoscopic biopsy of, 4
  of sinonasal tract, medial maxillectomy
    and lateral rhinotomy for, 67, 68, 69f
Papillomatosis
  laryngeal, tracheostomy in, 578, 578f
  recurrent respiratory, 323-327, 324f-326f
Paraganglioma. See Glomus tumor.
Paraglottic space, cancer involving, 396,
  396f, 397f
Paralysis
  facial. See Facial paralysis.
  vocal fold. See Vocal fold, immobility/
    paralysis of.
Paranasal sinuses. See also specific sinus, e.g.,
  Ethmoid sinus.
  blood supply to, 143-144, 144f-145f
  tumor of, medial maxillectomy for, 68, 68f
Parapharyngeal space abscess, 671-672,
  672f-673f, 675f, 676, 676f
Parapharyngeal space tumor, 657-669
  anatomic considerations in, 657-660, 658f,
    659f
  complications of, 668-669
  histologic diagnosis of, 659t
  metastatic, 657, 660
  pearls and pitfalls in, 669
  poststyloid, 525, 527f, 664-668
    anatomic considerations in, 657
    excision of
      complications of, 669
      indications for, 666-667
      techniques for, 667-668, 667f, 668f
    types of, 664-666, 665f
  preoperative evaluation of, 660-661, 661t
  prestyloid
    anatomic considerations in, 525, 526f,
      657, 658f, 659f

Parapharyngeal space tumor (Continued)
  excision of, 525-531, 661-664
    complications of, 530-531, 668-669
    mandibulotomy for, 663-664
    parotid-submandibular incision for,
      662-663, 663f-664f
    patient selection for, 525, 527f
    postoperative management after, 530
    techniques for, 528-530, 528f-530f
    transcervical submandibular
      approach in, 661, 662f
    transoral, 530-531, 561
  fine-needle aspiration biopsy of, 528
  preoperative evaluation of, 525,
    527f-528f, 528
  signs and symptoms of, 660, 660f, 660t
  surgical approaches to, 661, 661t
Parascapular fasciocutaneous flap, 741
Parascapular free flap, 741
Parathyroid glands, identification of, in
  thyroid lobectomy, 548f, 549
Parathyroidectomy, 559-564
  approach to "localizing gland" in, 560-561,
    560f-561f
  approach to "nonlocalizing gland" in,
    561
  ectopic and nonectopic parathyroid tissue
    locations in, 561-563, 562f-563f
  endoscopic subtotal, 552
  patient selection for, 559
  pearls and pitfalls in, 564
  postoperative management of, 563
  preoperative planning for, 559-560
Parotid gland
  accessory lobe of
    anatomy of, 533
    tumor of, 533, 535f
  enlarged, in systemic disease, 513, 513f
  injury to
    Frey's syndrome after, 496
    traumatic, 879, 881
  tumor of
    benign, 511
    in buccal space, 535
    computed tomography of, 512, 512f,
      517, 518f
    fine-needle aspiration biopsy of, 512,
      633
    malignant, 511-512, 512f
    open biopsy of, 513
    in parapharyngeal space, 525, 527f,
      528f
Parotidectomy, 511-522
  facial nerve repair after, 521-522,
    521f-522f
  in first branchial cleft remnant excision,
    650-651
  Frey's syndrome after, 496, 516
  patient selection for, 511-512, 512f
  pearls and pitfalls in, 522
  preoperative evaluation for, 512-513,
    512f-513f
  radical, 519-521, 520f-521f
  for sialoadenitis, 487
  superficial lobe
    approaches to, 513-515, 514f
    postoperative management and
      complications of, 515-517, 517f
    prestyloid parapharyngeal space tumor
      excision with, 529, 530f

Parotidectomy (Continued)
  temporal bone resection in combination
    with, 1276
  total, with facial nerve dissection, 517-519,
    518f-519f
Parotid-submandibular incision, extended,
  for buccal space tumor excision,
  536-537, 537f-538f
Parotitis, chronic, 518
Particle repositioning, for benign
  paroxysmal positional vertigo, 1394
Passavant's ridge, 33
Passey-Muir valve, 582
Patient education, after skin cancer surgery,
  735-736
Pectoralis major myocutaneous flap
  complications of, 756
  for glossectomy defects, 744f, 747
  after lateral pharyngotomy, 239
  overview of, 753-756, 754f-755f
  after segmental mandibulectomy, 273
  skin island for, 755
  after total glossectomy, 223-224, 223f
Pectoralis myofascial graft, after lateral
  pharyngotomy, 239
Pedicle flap, 753-763
  cervicopectoral, 762, 762f
  deltopectoral, 761, 761f
  latissimus dorsi, 756-757, 756f
  pearls and pitfalls in, 762-763
  pectoralis major, 753-756, 754f-755f. See
    also Pectoralis major myocutaneous
    flap.
  sternocleidomastoid, 757
  temporalis, 759-761, 760f
  temporoparietal fascial, 758-759, 760f
  trapezius, 757-758, 758f
Percutaneous dilatational tracheostomy,
  585-593, 588f-591f
Pericranial flap, in anterior cranial base
  reconstruction, 990-991, 990f-991f,
  1061-1062, 1062f-1063f
Perilymphatic fistula, 1219-1227
  causes of, 1219-1220
  cerebrospinal fluid leak in, 1359
  post-traumatic, 1219, 1220
  revision stapes surgery for, 1201
  spontaneous, 1219
  after stapedectomy, 1207, 1224, 1224f
  surgical management of
    complications of, 1226
    patient selection for, 1220-1222,
      1221f-1222f
    pearls and pitfalls in, 1226
    postoperative care after, 1226
    preoperative planning for, 1222-1223
    techniques in, 1223-1226, 1223f-1226f
Perilymphatic gusher
  management of, 1182, 1186
  in middle ear reconstruction, 1178
  in stapes surgery, 1204
Periorbita
  cancer of, 727-728
  elevation of
    in anterior cranial base surgery, 986-987
    in preauricular (subtemporal)
      infratemporal fossa surgery, 1005,
      1006f
  injury to, 878-879, 879f, 880f
  repair of, 729

Thyroid nodule, solitary, 541, 542f, 544-545, 545f
Thyroid surgery, 541-555
  anesthesia for, 546
  cervical incision in, 546-547, 547f
  complications of, 553-555
  neck dissection in, 543, 552-553, 553f
  patient selection for, 541-544, 542f-543f
  pearls and pitfalls in, 555
  postoperative management of, 553
  preoperative evaluation for, 544-546, 545f-546f
  for substernal goiter, 551-552
  thyroid lobectomy in, 547-550, 548f-549f
  thyroidectomy in
    endoscopic, 552
    total, 550-551
Thyroiditis, chronic, 551
Thyroplasty, type I. See Laryngoplasty, medialization.
Thyrotomy
  lateral, for laryngocele excision, 344-346, 345f
  median. See Laryngofissure.
Tics, 1386t
Tinnitus, pulsatile, in otosclerosis, 1189
Tip, nasal. See Nasal tip surgery.
Tissue adhesives, cyanoacrylate, for facial repair and reconstruction, 877
Titanium
  for ossicular chain prosthesis, 1151, 1151f
  for stapes prosthesis, 1193
Titanium burr hole covers, in anterior cranial base reconstruction, 991, 991f
Titanium mesh
  for craniofacial skeleton reconstruction, 1064, 1066f
  for orbital reconstruction, 943, 1064-1065, 1067f
Titanium microplates
  in anterior cranial base reconstruction, 991
  in craniofacial skeleton reconstruction, 1064, 1065f
Tongue
  enlarged. See Macroglossia.
  epidermal cyst of, 163f
  neurofibroma of, 162, 162f, 165, 165f
  palpation of, 219, 220f
Tongue base
  suturing of, after supraglottic laryngectomy, 401, 401f
  tumor of, excision of
    lateral pharyngotomy for, 235-240. See also Pharyngotomy, lateral.
    mandibulectomy for, 229
    mandibulotomy for, 229
    suprahyoid pharyngotomy for, 229-233. See also Suprahyoid pharyngotomy.
Tongue cancer, 217-227
  deviation of tongue in, 219, 219f
  endophytic versus exophytic, 219, 219f
  metastasis of, 217, 218, 219-220, 220f
  neck dissection in, 218, 226
  partial glossectomy for, 218-223, 219f-222f
  postoperative management of, 226-227
  total glossectomy for, 223-226, 223f-225f
  treatment principles for, 217-218
  tumor thickness in, 219, 219f

Tongue flap, for palatal repair, 213, 787
Tongue-in-groove technique, in rhinoplasty, 817
Tongue-splitting approach, midline, mandibulotomy with, 280, 281f
Tonsil
  lymphoma of, 283, 284f
  metastasis to, 283, 284f
  pharyngeal. See Adenoid(s).
Tonsillectomy, 169-180
  adenoidectomy with, 33-34, 35, 170, 174
  complications of, 178-179
  hemostasis using electrocautery for, 173, 176
  indications for, 170, 171, 171t
  for obstructive sleep apnea, 177
  overview of, 169-170, 170f
  patient positioning for, 173, 174f
  patient selection for, 171, 171t
  in patients with cleft palate, 782-783
  pearls and pitfalls in, 180
  for peritonsillar abscess, 177-178
  postoperative care in, 178
  procedure for, 173-176, 175f-176f
  quality of life after, 176-177
  quinsy, 178
  types of procedures for, 172-173, 172t
  uvulopalatopharyngoplasty and, 153, 153f
Tooth (teeth)
  extraction of
    in marginal mandibulectomy, 259, 259f
    oral-antral fistula after, 63, 64-65, 64f, 65f-66f
  fracture of, 889-890
  injury to, in phonomicrosurgery, 309
  numbering system and descriptions of, 885, 886f
  rehabilitation of, after marginal mandibulectomy, 256, 257f, 258f
TORP (total ossicular replacement prosthesis), 1147, 1148, 1148f, 1158, 1159f, 1160, 1160f
Toxic shock syndrome, after septoplasty, 24
Trachea
  identification of, in thyroid lobectomy, 548f, 549
  penetrating injury to, management of, 455, 455f
  resection of
    in cervical esophageal cancer surgery, 478
    and end-to-end anastomosis, for tracheal stenosis, 611-613, 611f, 612f
Tracheal stenosis, 603-614, 605, 605f. See also Laryngeal stenosis.
  clinical evaluation of, 604-605, 604f
  complications of, 613
  definition of, 623
  dilatation for, 606
  endoscopic microsurgery for, 607, 607f
  imaging of, 605, 605f
  laryngotracheal reconstruction with cartilage autografts for, 608, 608f, 609f
  pathogenesis of, 603-604
  pearls and pitfalls in, 614
  postoperative management of, 613
  resection and end-to-end anastomosis for, 611-613, 611f, 612f

Tracheal stenosis (Continued)
  stenting for, 606-607
  sternocleidomastoid myoperiosteal flap for, 608, 610-611, 610f-611f
  surgical techniques for, 605-613
  after tracheostomy, 585
  transcervical procedures for, 607-608, 607f
Tracheal suctioning
  after mouth floor cancer excision, 247
  technique of, 582
Tracheobronchial anatomy, 565, 566f
Tracheobronchial foreign body, removal of, bronchoscopy for, 573-574, 573f, 573t, 574f
Tracheobronchitis, after tracheostomy, 585
Tracheocutaneous fistula, after tracheostomy, 617-621, 618f-620f
Tracheoesophageal fistula, tracheostomy and, 583, 585
Tracheoesophageal puncture
  contraindications to, 433
  after laryngotracheal separation, 596
  one-way valve used in, 432, 432f
  patient selection for, 432-433
  pearls and pitfalls in, 437
  postoperative care after, 437, 437f
  preoperative evaluation for, 433-434
  primary, 434, 434f
  role of speech-language pathologist in, 432
  secondary, 434-437, 435f-436f
  surgical closure of, 439-441, 440f
  in total laryngectomy, 427
Tracheolaryngeal separation. See Laryngotracheal separation.
Tracheomalacia, after tracheostomy, 585
Tracheoscopy, 565-575, 569t. See also Bronchoscopy.
  in cervical esophageal cancer, 477
Tracheostoma. See Stoma.
Tracheostomy, 577-593
  accidental extubation in, 592
  complications of, 583-585
    immediate postoperative, 584-585
    intraoperative, 583-584, 583f
    late postoperative, 585, 586f
  decannulation in, 582-583
    accidental, 592
  in glottic enlargement surgery, 312
  historical background on, 577
  before oropharyngeal cancer excision, 285
  in partial glossectomy, 221
  patient selection for, 578, 578f
  pearls and pitfalls in, 593
  percutaneous dilatational, 585-593, 588f-591f
    anesthesia for, 587
    complications of, 591-592
    instruments for, 587, 588f
    patient selection for, 586-587
    personnel for, 587
    postoperative considerations in, 590-591
    technique of, 587-590, 588f-590f
  postoperative care in, 582-583
  preoperative planning for, 578
  after supraglottic laryngectomy, 401, 402f
  surgical technique for, 579-581, 580f-581f
  in total laryngectomy, 428
  tracheocutaneous fistula and depressed scar after, 617-621, 618f-620f